Applied
Biopharmaceutics &
Pharmacokinetics

Applied Biopharmaceutics & Pharmacokinetics

Seventh Edition

EDITORS

Leon Shargel, PhD, RPh

Applied Biopharmaceutics, LLC
Raleigh, North Carolina
Affiliate Professor, School of Pharmacy
Virginia Commonwealth University, Richmond, Virginia
Adjunct Associate Professor, School of Pharmacy
University of Maryland, Baltimore, Maryland

Andrew B.C. Yu, PhD, RPh

Registered Pharmacist
Gaithersburg, Maryland
Formerly Associate Professor of Pharmaceutics
Albany College of Pharmacy
Albany, New York
Formerly CDER, FDA
Silver Spring, Maryland

New York   Chicago   San Francisco   Athens   London   Madrid   Mexico City
Milan   New Delhi   Singapore   Sydney   Toronto

Applied Biopharmaceutics & Pharmacokinetics, Seventh Edition

1 2 3 4 5 6 7 8 9 0   DOC/DOC   20 19 18 17 16 15

ISBN 978-0-07-183093-5
MHID 0-07-183093-6

This book was set in Times LT Std by Cenveo® Publisher Services.
The editor was Regina Y. Brown
The production supervisor was Rick Ruzycka.
The production manager was Tanya Punj, Cenveo Publisher Services.
The design was by Elise Lansdon; the cover design was by Barsoom Design, with cover art © Gregor Schuster/Corbis.
RR Donnelley was printer and binder.

This book is printed on acid-free paper.

Library of Congress Cataloguing-in-Publication Data

Shargel, Leon, 1941- , author.
    Applied biopharmaceutics & pharmacokinetics / Leon Shargel, Andrew B.C. Yu.—Seventh edition.
        p. ; cm.
    Applied biopharmaceutics and pharmacokinetics
    Includes bibliographical references and index.
    ISBN 978-0-07-183093-5 (hardcover : alk. paper)—ISBN 0-07-183093-6 (hardcover : alk. paper)
    I. Yu, Andrew B. C., 1945- , author.   II. Title.   III. Title: Applied biopharmaceutics and pharmacokinetics.
[DNLM: 1. Biopharmaceutics. 2. Pharmacokinetics. 3. Drug Administration Routes. 4. Models, Chemical.   QV 38]
RM301.4
615.7—dc23

                                                                                                    2015014810

McGraw-Hill books are available at special quantity discounts to use as premiums and sales promotions, or for use in corporate training programs. To contact a representative please e-mail us at bulksales@mcgraw-hill.com.

Contents

23. Application of Pharmacokinetics to Specific Populations: Geriatric, Obese, and Pediatric Patients   735

24. Dose Adjustment in Renal and Hepatic Disease   775

25. Empirical Models, Mechanistic Models, Statistical Moments, and Noncompartmental Analysis   817

Appendix A   Applications of Software Packages in Pharmacokinetics   851

Appendix B   Glossary   875

Contributors

S. Thomas Abraham, PhD
Associate Professor
Department of Pharmaceutical Sciences
College of Pharmacy & Health Sciences
Campbell University
Buies Creek, North Carolina

Michael L. Adams, PharmD, PhD
Associate Professor
Department of Pharmaceutical Sciences
College of Pharmacy & Health Sciences
Campbell University
Buies Creek, North Carolina

Antoine Al-Achi, PhD
Associate Professor
Campbell University
College of Pharmacy & Health Sciences
Buies Creek, North Carolina

Lily K. Cheung, PharmD
Assistant Professor
Department of Pharmacy Practice
College of Pharmacy & Health Sciences
Texas Southern University
Houston, Texas

Diana Shu-Lian Chow, PhD
Professor of Pharmaceutics
Director
Institute for Drug Education and Research (IDER)
College of Pharmacy
University of Houston
Houston, Texas

Philippe Colucci, PhD
Principal Scientist
Learn and Confirm Inc.
Sr. Laurent, QC, Canada

Dale P. Conner, Pharm.D.
Director
Office of Bioequivalence
Office of Generic Drugs
CDER, FDA
Silver Spring, Maryland

Barbara M. Davit, PhD, JD
Executive Director
Biopharmaceutics
Merck & Co.
Kenilworth, New Jersey

Hong Ding, PhD
Assistant Professor
Department of Immunology
Herbert Wertheim College of Medicine
Florida International University
Miami, Florida

John Z. Duan, PhD
Master Reviewer
Office of New Drug Products
Office of Pharmaceutical Quality
FDA/CDER
Silver Spring, Maryland

Murray P. Ducharme, PharmD, FCCP, FCP
President and CEO
Learn and Confirm Inc.
Sr. Laurent, QC, Canada
Professeur Associé
Faculté de Pharmacie
University of Montreal, Canada
Visiting Professor
Faculty of Pharmacy
Rhodes University, South Africa

Mathangi Gopalakrishnan, MS, PhD
Research Assistant Professor
Center for Translational Medicine
School of Pharmacy
University of Maryland
Baltimore, Maryland

Phillip M. Gerk, PharmD, PhD
Associate Professor
Department of Pharmaceutics
Virginia Commonwealth University
MCV Campus
School of Pharmacy
Richmond, Virginia

Charles Herring, BSPharm, PharmD, BCPS, CPP
Associate Professor
Department of Pharmacy Practice
College of Pharmacy & Health Sciences
Campbell University
Clinical Pharmacist Practitioner
Adult Medicine Team
Downtown Health Plaza of Wake Forest Baptist
Health
Winston-Salem, North Carolina

Christine Yuen-Yi Hon, PharmD, BCOP
Clinical Pharmacology Reviewer
Division of Clinical Pharmacology III
Office of Clinical Pharmacology
Office of Translational Sciences
Center for Drug Evaluation and Research
Food and Drug Administration
Silver Spring, Maryland

Minerva A. Hughes, PhD, RAC (US)
Senior Pharmacologist
Food and Drug Administration
Center for Drug Evaluation and Research
Silver Spring, Maryland

Manish Issar, PhD
Assistant Professor of Pharmacology
College of Osteopathic Medicine of the Pacific
Western University of Health Sciences
Pomona, California

Vipul Kumar, PhD
Senior Scientist I
Nonclinical Development Department
Cubist Pharmaceuticals Inc.
Lexington, Massachusetts

S.W. Johnny Lau, RPh, PhD
Senior Clinical Pharmacologist
Food and Drug Administration
Office of Clinical Pharmacology
Silver Spring, Maryland

David S.H. Lee, PharmD, PhD
Assistant Professor
Department of Pharmacy Practice
Oregon State University/Oregon Health and Science
University College of Pharmacy
Portland, Oregon

Patrick J Marroum, PhD
Director
Clinical Pharmacology and Pharmacometrics
AbbVie
North Chicago, Illinois

Shabnam N. Sani, PharmD, PhD
Assistant Professor
Department of Pharmaceutical and Administrative
Sciences
College of Pharmacy
Western New England University
Springfield, Massachusetts

Leon Shargel, PhD, RPh
Manager and Founder
Applied Biopharmaceutics, LLC
Raleigh, North Carolina
Affiliate Professsor
School of Pharmacy
Virginia Commonwealth University
Richmond, Virginia

Sandra Suarez Sharp, PhD
Master Biopharmaceutics Reviewer/Biopharmaceutics
Lead
Office of New Drug Products/Division of
Biopharmaceutics
Office of Pharmaceutical Quality
Food and Drug Administration
Silver Spring, Maryland

Rodney Siwale, PhD, MS
Assistant Professor
Department of Pharmaceutical and Administrative
Sciences
College of Pharmacy
Western New England University
Springfield, Massachusetts

Changquan Calvin Sun, PhD
Associate Professor of Pharmaceutics
University of Minnesota
Department of Pharmaceutics
College of Pharmacy
Minneapolis, Minnesota

He Sun, PhD
President and CEO
Tasly Pharmaceuticals Inc.
Rockville, Maryland
Professor and Chairman
Department of Pharmaceutical Economics and Policy
School of Pharmaceutical Science and Technology
Tianjin University
Tianjin, P. R. China

Vincent H. Tam, PharmD, BCPS (Infectious Diseases)
Professor Department of Clinical Sciences and
Administration
University of Houston College of Pharmacy
Texas Medical Center Campus
Houston, Texas

Dr. Susanna Wu-Pong, PhD
Associate Professor
Director
Pharmaceutical Sciences Graduate Program
VCU School of Pharmacy
Richmond, Virginia

Andrew B.C. Yu, PhD, RPh
Registered Pharmacist
Formerly senior reviewer, CDER, FDA
Associate Pharmaceutics Professor
Albany College of Pharmacy
Albany, New York

Corinne Seng Yue, BPharm, MSc, PhD
Principal Scientist
Learn and Confirm Inc.
Sr. Laurent, QC, Canada

Hong Zhao, PhD
Clinical Pharmacology Master Reviewer
Clinical Pharmacology Team Leader
Office of Clinical Pharmacology (OCP)
Office of Translational Sciences (OTS)
Center for Drug Evaluation and Research (CDER)
U.S. Food and Drug Administration (FDA)
Silver Spring, Maryland

HaiAn Zheng, PhD
Associate Professor
Department of Pharmaceutical Sciences
Albany College of Pharmacy and Health Sciences
Albany, New York

Preface

The publication of this seventh edition of *Applied Biopharmaceutics and Pharmacokinetics* represents over three decades in print. Since the introduction of classic pharmacokinetics in the first edition, the discipline has expanded and evolved greatly. The basic pharmacokinetic principles and biopharmaceutics now include pharmacogenetics, drug receptor theories, advances in membrane transports, and functional physiology. These advances are applied to the design of new active drug moieties, manufacture of novel drug products, and drug delivery systems. Biopharmaceutics and pharmacokinetics play a key role in the development of safer drug therapy in patients, allowing individualizing dosage regimens and improving therapeutic outcomes.

In planning for the seventh edition, we realized that we needed expertise for these areas. This seventh edition is our first edited textbook in which an expert with intimate knowledge and experience in the topic was selected as a contributor. We would like to acknowledge these experts for their precious time and effort. We are also grateful to our readers and colleagues for their helpful feedback and support throughout the years.

As editors of this edition, we kept the original objectives, starting with fundamentals followed by a holistic integrated approach that can be applied to practice (see scope and objectives in Preface to the first edition). This textbook provides the reader with a basic and practical understanding of the principles of biopharmaceutics and pharmacokinetics that can be applied to drug product development and drug therapy. Practice problems, clinical examples, frequently asked questions and learning questions are included in each chapter to demonstrate how these concepts relate to practical situations. This textbook remains unique in teaching basic concepts that may be applied to understanding complex issues associated with *in vivo* drug delivery that are essential for safe and efficacious drug therapy.

The primary audience is pharmacy students enrolled in pharmaceutical science courses in pharmacokinetics and biopharmaceutics. This text fulfills course work offered in separate or combined courses in these subjects. Secondary audiences for this textbook are research, technological and development scientists in pharmaceutics, biopharmaceutics, and pharmacokinetics.

This edition represents many significant changes from previous editions.

- The book is an edited textbook with the collaboration of many experts well known in biopharmaceutics, drug disposition, drug delivery systems, manufacturing, clinical pharmacology, clinical trials, and regulatory science.
- Many chapters have been expanded and updated to reflect current knowledge and application of biopharmaceutics and pharmacokinetics. Many new topics and updates are listed in Chapter 1.
- Practical examples and questions are included to encourage students to apply the principles in patient care and drug consultation situations.
- Learning questions and answers appear at the end of each chapter.
- Three new chapters have been added to this edition including, *Biostatistics* which provides introduction for popular topics such as risk concept, non-inferiority, and superiority concept in new drug evaluation, and *Application of Pharmacokinetics in Specific Populations* which discusses issues such as drug and patient related pharmacy

topics in during therapy in various patient populations, and *Biopharmaceutic Aspects of the Active Pharmaceutical Ingredient and Pharmaceutical Equivalence* which explains the synthesis, quality and physical/chemical properties of the active pharmaceutical ingredients affect the bioavailability of the drug from the drug product and clinical efficacy.

Leon Shargel
Andrew B.C. Yu

Preface to First Edition

The publication of the twelfth edition of this book is a testament to the vision and ideals of the original authors, Alfred Gilman and Louis Goodman, who, in 1941 set forth the principles that have guided the book through eleven editions: to correlate pharmacology with related medical sciences, to reinterpret the actions and uses of drugs in light of advances in medicine and the basic biomedical sciences, to emphasize the applications of pharmacodynamics to therapeutics, and to create a book that will be useful to students of pharmacology and to physicians. These precepts continue to guide the current edition.

As with editions since the second, expert scholars have contributed individual chapters. A multiauthored book of this sort grows by accretion, posing challenges editors but also offering memorable pearls to the reader. Thus, portions of prior editions persist in the current edition, and I hasten to acknowledge the contributions of previous editors and authors, many of whom will see text that looks familiar. However, this edition differs noticeably from its immediate predecessors. Fifty new scientists, including a number from out-side. the U.S., have joined as contributors, and all chapters have been extensively updated. The focus on basic principles continues, with new chapters on drug invention, molecular mechanisms of drug action, drug toxicity and poisoning, principles of antimicrobial therapy and pharmacotherapy of obstetrical and gynecological disorders. Figures are in full color. The editors have continued to standardize the organization of chapters: thus, students should easily find the basic physiology, biochemistry, and pharmacology set forth in regular type; bullet points highlight important lists within the text; the clinician and expert will find details in extract type under clear headings.

Online features now supplement the printed edition. The entire text, updates, reviews of newly approved drugs, animations of drug action, and hyper links to relevant text in the prior edition are available on the Goodman & Gilman section of McGraw-Hill's websites, *AccessMedicine.com* and *AccessPharmacy.com*. An Image Bank CD accompanies the book and makes all tables and figures available for use in presentations.

The process of editing brings into view many remarkable facts, theories, and realizations. Three stand out: the invention of new classes of drugs has slowed to a trickle; therapeutics has barely begun to capitalize on the information from the human genome project; and, the development of resistance to antimicrobial agents, mainly through their overuse in medicine and agriculture, threatens to return us to the pre-antibiotic era. We have the capacity and ingenuity to correct these shortcomings.

Many, in addition to the contributors, deserve thanks for their work on this edition; they are acknowledged on an accompanying page. In addition, I am grateful to Professors Bruce Chabner (Harvard Medical School/Massachusetts General Hospital) and Björn Knollmann (Vanderbilt University Medical School) for agreeing to be associate editors of this edition at a late date, necessitated by the death of my colleague and friend Keith Parker in late 2008. Keith and I worked together on the eleventh edition and on planning this edition. In anticipation of the editorial work ahead, Keith submitted his chapters before anyone else and just a few weeks before his death; thus, he is well represented in this volume, which we dedicate to his memory.

Laurence L. Brunton

About the Authors

Dr. Leon Shargel is a consultant for the pharmaceutical industry in biopharmaceutics and pharmacokinetics. Dr. Shargel has over 35 years experience in both academia and the pharmaceutical industry. He has been a member or chair of numerous national committees involved in state formulary issues, biopharmaceutics and bioequivalence issues, institutional review boards, and a member of the USP Biopharmaceutics Expert Committee. Dr. Shargel received a BS in pharmacy from the University of Maryland and a PhD in pharmacology from the George Washington University Medical Center. He is a registered pharmacist and has over 150 publications including several leading textbooks in pharmacy. He is a member of various professional societies, including the American Association Pharmaceutical Scientists (AAPS), American Pharmacists Association (APhA), and the American Society for Pharmacology and Experimental Therapeutics (ASPET).

Dr. Andrew Yu has over 30 years of experience in academia, government, and the pharmaceutical industry. Dr. Yu received a BS in pharmacy from Albany College of Pharmacy and a PhD in pharmacokinetics from the University of Connecticut. He is a registered pharmacist and has over 30 publications and a patent in novel drug delivery. He had lectured internationally on pharmaceutics, drug disposition, and drug delivery.

1 Introduction to Biopharmaceutics and Pharmacokinetics

Leon Shargel and Andrew B.C. Yu

Chapter Objectives

▶ Define drug product performance and biopharmaceutics.

▶ Describe how biopharmaceutics affects drug product performance.

▶ Define pharmacokinetics and describe how pharmacokinetics is related to pharmacodynamics and drug toxicity.

▶ Define the term clinical pharmacokinetics and explain how clinical pharmacokinetics may be used to develop dosage regimens for drugs in patients.

▶ Define pharmacokinetic model and list the assumptions that are used in developing a pharmacokinetic model.

▶ Explain how the prescribing information or approved labeling for a drug helps the practitioner to recommend an appropriate dosage regimen for a patient.

DRUG PRODUCT PERFORMANCE

Drugs are substances intended for use in the diagnosis, cure, mitigation, treatment, or prevention of disease. Drugs are given in a variety of dosage forms or *drug products* such as solids (tablets, capsules), semisolids (ointments, creams), liquids, suspensions, emulsions, etc, for systemic or local therapeutic activity. Drug products can be considered to be drug delivery systems that release and deliver drug to the site of action such that they produce the desired therapeutic effect. In addition, drug products are designed specifically to meet the patient's needs including palatability, convenience, and safety.

Drug product performance is defined as the release of the drug substance from the drug product either for local drug action or for drug absorption into the plasma for systemic therapeutic activity. Advances in pharmaceutical technology and manufacturing have focused on developing quality drug products that are safer, more effective, and more convenient for the patient.

BIOPHARMACEUTICS

Biopharmaceutics examines the interrelationship of the physical/chemical properties of the drug, the dosage form (drug product) in which the drug is given, and the route of administration on the rate and extent of systemic drug absorption. The importance of the drug substance and the drug formulation on absorption, and *in vivo* distribution of the drug to the site of action, is described as a sequence of events that precede elicitation of a drug's therapeutic effect. A general scheme describing this dynamic relationship is illustrated in Fig. 1-1.

First, the drug in its dosage form is taken by the patient by an oral, intravenous, subcutaneous, transdermal, etc, route of administration. Next, the drug is released from the dosage form in a predictable and characterizable manner. Then, some fraction of the drug is absorbed from the site of administration into either the surrounding tissue for local action or into the body (as with oral dosage forms), or both. Finally, the drug reaches the site of action. A pharmacodynamic response results when the drug concentration at the site of

1

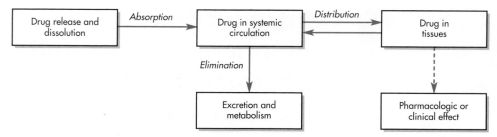

FIGURE 1-1   Scheme demonstrating the dynamic relationship between the drug, the drug product, and the pharmacologic effect.

action reaches or exceeds the *minimum effective concentration* (MEC). The suggested dosing regimen, including starting dose, maintenance dose, dosage form, and dosing interval, is determined in clinical trials to provide the drug concentrations that are therapeutically effective in most patients. This sequence of events is profoundly affected—in fact, sometimes orchestrated—by the design of the dosage form and the physicochemical properties of the drug.

Historically, pharmaceutical scientists have evaluated the relative drug availability to the body *in vivo* after giving a drug product by different routes to an animal or human, and then comparing specific pharmacologic, clinical, or possible toxic responses. For example, a drug such as isoproterenol causes an increase in heart rate when given intravenously but has no observable effect on the heart when given orally at the same dose level. In addition, the *bioavailability* (a measure of systemic availability of a drug) may differ from one drug product to another containing the same drug, even for the same route of administration. This difference in drug bioavailability may be manifested by observing the difference in the therapeutic effectiveness of the drug products. Thus, the nature of the drug molecule, the route of delivery, and the formulation of the dosage form can determine whether an administered drug is therapeutically effective, is toxic, or has no apparent effect at all.

The US Food and Drug Administration (FDA) approves all drug products to be marketed in the United States. The pharmaceutical manufacturers must perform extensive research and development prior to approval. The manufacturer of a new drug product must submit a *New Drug Application* (NDA) to the FDA, whereas a generic drug pharmaceutical manufacturer must submit an *Abbreviated New Drug Application* (ANDA). Both the new and generic drug

product manufacturers must characterize their drug and drug product and demonstrate that the drug product performs appropriately before the products can become available to consumers in the United States.

Biopharmaceutics provides the scientific basis for drug product design and drug product development. Each step in the manufacturing process of a finished dosage form may potentially affect the release of the drug from the drug product and the availability of the drug at the site of action. The most important steps in the manufacturing process are termed *critical manufacturing variables*. Examples of biopharmaceutic considerations in drug product design are listed in Table 1-1. A detailed discussion of drug product design is found in Chapter 15. Knowledge of physiologic factors necessary for designing oral products is discussed in Chapter 14. Finally, drug product quality of drug substance (Chapter 17) and drug product testing is discussed in later chapters (18, 19, 20, and 21). It is important for a pharmacist to know that drug product selection from multisources could be confusing and needs a deep understanding of the testing procedures and manufacturing technology which is included in the chemistry, manufacturing, and control (CMC) of the product involved. The starting material (SM) used to make the API (active pharmaceutical ingredient), the processing method used during chemical synthesis, extraction, and the purification method can result in differences in the API that can then affect drug product performance (Chapter 17). Sometimes a by-product of the synthetic process, residual solvents, or impurities that remain may be harmful or may affect the product's physical or chemical stability. Increasingly, many drug sources are imported and the manufacturing of these products is regulated by codes or pharmacopeia in other countries. For example, drugs in Europe may be meeting EP (European Pharmacopeia) and since 2006,

TABLE 1-1   Biopharmaceutic Considerations in Drug Product Design

Items	Considerations
Therapeutic objective	Drug may be intended for rapid relief of symptoms, slow extended action given once per day, or longer for chronic use; some drug may be intended for local action or systemic action
Drug (active pharmaceutical ingredient, API)	Physical and chemical properties of API, including solubility, polymorphic form, particle size; impurities
Route of administration	Oral, topical, parenteral, transdermal, inhalation, etc
Drug dosage and dosage regimen	Large or small drug dose, frequency of doses, patient acceptance of drug product, patient compliance
Type of drug product	Orally disintegrating tablets, immediate release tablets, extended release tablets, transdermal, topical, parenteral, implant, etc
Excipients	Although very little pharmacodynamic activity, excipients may affect drug product performance including release of drug from drug product
Method of manufacture	Variables in manufacturing processes, including weighing accuracy, blending uniformity, release tests, and product sterility for parenterals

agreed uniform standards are harmonized in ICH guidances for Europe, Japan, and the United States. In the US, the USP-NF is the official compendia for drug quality standards.

Finally, the equipment used during manufacturing, processing, and packaging may alter important product attribute. Despite compliance with testing and regulatory guidance involved, the issues involving

pharmaceutical equivalence, bioavailability, bioequivalence, and therapeutic equivalence often evolved by necessity. The implications are important regarding availability of quality drug product, avoidance of shortages, and maintaining an affordable high-quality drug products. The principles and issues with regard to multisource drug products are discussed in subsequent chapters:

Chapter 14	Physiologic Factors Related to Drug Absorption	How stomach emptying, GI residence time, and gastric window affect drug absorption
Chapter 15	Biopharmaceutic Considerations in Drug Product Design	How particle size, crystal form, solubility, dissolution, and ionization affect *in vivo* dissolution and absorption. Modifications of a product with excipient with regard to immediate or delayed action are discussed. Dissolution test methods and relation to *in vivo* performance
Chapter 16	Drug Product Performance, *In Vivo*: Bioavailability and Bioequivalence	Bioavailability and bioequivalence terms and regulations, test methods, and analysis examples. Protocol design and statistical analysis. Reasons for poor bioavailability. Bioavailability reference, generic substitution. PE, PA, BA/BE, API, RLD, TE
		SUPAC (Scale-up postapproval changes) regarding drug products. What type of changes will result in changes in BA, TE, or performances of drug products from a scientific and regulatory viewpoint
Chapter 17	Biopharmaceutic Aspects of the Active Pharmaceutical Ingredient and Pharmaceutical Equivalence	Physicochemical differences of the drug, API due to manufacturing and synthetic pathway. How to select API from multiple sources while meeting PE (pharmaceutical equivalence) and TE (therapeutic equivalence) requirement as defined in CFR. Examples of some drug failing TE while apparently meeting API requirements. Formulation factors and manufacturing method affecting PE and TE. How particle size and crystal form affect solubility and dissolution. How pharmaceutical equivalence affects therapeutic equivalence. Pharmaceutical alternatives. How physicochemical characteristics of API lead to pharmaceutical inequivalency
Chapter 18	Impact of Drug Product Quality and Biopharmaceutics on Clinical Efficacy	Drug product quality and drug product performance
		Pharmaceutical development. Excipient effect on drug product performance. Quality control and quality assurance. Risk management
		Scale-up and postapproval changes (SUPAC)
		Product quality problems. Postmarketing surveillance

Thus, biopharmaceutics involves factors that influence (1) the design of the drug product, (2) stability of the drug within the drug product, (3) the manufacture of the drug product, (4) the release of the drug from the drug product, (5) the rate of dissolution/release of the drug at the absorption site, and (6) delivery of drug to the site of action, which may involve targeting the drug to a localized area (eg, colon for Crohn disease) for action or for systemic absorption of the drug.

Both the pharmacist and the pharmaceutical scientist must understand these complex relationships to objectively choose the most appropriate drug product for therapeutic success.

The study of biopharmaceutics is based on fundamental scientific principles and experimental methodology. Studies in biopharmaceutics use both *in vitro* and *in vivo* methods. *In vitro* methods are procedures employing test apparatus and equipment without involving laboratory animals or humans. *In vivo* methods are more complex studies involving human subjects or laboratory animals. Some of these methods will be discussed in Chapter 15. These methods must be able to assess the impact of the physical and chemical properties of the drug, drug stability, and large-scale production of the drug and drug product on the biologic performance of the drug.

PHARMACOKINETICS

After a drug is released from its dosage form, the drug is absorbed into the surrounding tissue, the body, or both. The distribution through and elimination of the drug in the body varies for each patient but can be characterized using mathematical models and statistics. *Pharmacokinetics* is the science of the kinetics of drug absorption, distribution, and elimination (ie, metabolism and excretion). The description of drug distribution and elimination is often termed *drug disposition*. Characterization of drug disposition is an important prerequisite for determination or modification of dosing regimens for individuals and groups of patients.

The study of pharmacokinetics involves both experimental and theoretical approaches. The experimental aspect of pharmacokinetics involves the development of biologic sampling techniques,

analytical methods for the measurement of drugs and metabolites, and procedures that facilitate data collection and manipulation. The theoretical aspect of pharmacokinetics involves the development of pharmacokinetic models that predict drug disposition after drug administration. The application of statistics is an integral part of pharmacokinetic studies. Statistical methods are used for pharmacokinetic parameter estimation and data interpretation ultimately for the purpose of designing and predicting optimal dosing regimens for individuals or groups of patients. Statistical methods are applied to pharmacokinetic models to determine data error and structural model deviations. Mathematics and computer techniques form the theoretical basis of many pharmacokinetic methods. Classical pharmacokinetics is a study of theoretical models focusing mostly on model development and parameterization.

PHARMACODYNAMICS

Pharmacodynamics is the study of the biochemical and physiological effects of drugs on the body; this includes the mechanisms of drug action and the relationship between drug concentration and effect. A typical example of pharmacodynamics is how a drug interacts quantitatively with a drug receptor to produce a response (effect). Receptors are the molecules that interact with specific drugs to produce a pharmacological effect in the body.

The pharmacodynamic effect, sometimes referred to as the pharmacologic effect, can be therapeutic and/or cause toxicity. Often drugs have multiple effects including the desired therapeutic response as well as unwanted side effects. For many drugs, the pharmacodynamic effect is dose/drug concentration related; the higher the dose, the higher drug concentrations in the body and the more intense the pharmacodynamic effect up to a maximum effect. It is desirable that side effects and/or toxicity of drugs occurs at higher drug concentrations than the drug concentrations needed for the therapeutic effect. Unfortunately, unwanted side effects often occur concurrently with the therapeutic doses. The relationship between pharmacodynamics and pharmacokinetics is discussed in Chapter 21.

CLINICAL PHARMACOKINETICS

During the drug development process, large numbers of patients are enrolled in clinical trials to determine efficacy and optimum dosing regimens. Along with safety and efficacy data and other patient information, the FDA approves a label that becomes the package insert discussed in more detail later in this chapter. The approved labeling recommends the proper starting dosage regimens for the general patient population and may have additional recommendations for special populations of patients that need an adjusted dosage regimen (see Chapter 23). These recommended dosage regimens produce the desired pharmacologic response in the majority of the anticipated patient population. However, intra- and interindividual variations will frequently result in either a subtherapeutic (drug concentration below the MEC) or a toxic response (drug concentrations above the *minimum toxic concentration*, MTC), which may then require adjustment to the dosing regimen. *Clinical pharmacokinetics* is the application of pharmacokinetic methods to drug therapy in patient care. Clinical pharmacokinetics involves a multidisciplinary approach to individually optimized dosing strategies based on the patient's disease state and patient-specific considerations.

The study of clinical pharmacokinetics of drugs in disease states requires input from medical and pharmaceutical research. Table 1-2 is a list of 10 age adjusted rates of death from 10 leading causes of death in the United States in 2003. The influence of many diseases on drug disposition is not adequately studied. Age, gender, genetic, and ethnic differences can also result in pharmacokinetic differences that may affect the outcome of drug therapy (see Chapter 23). The study of pharmacokinetic differences of drugs in various population groups is termed *population pharmacokinetics* (Sheiner and Ludden, 1992; see Chapter 22). Application of Pharmacokinetics to Specific Populations, Chapter 23, will discuss many of the important pharmacokinetic considerations for dosing subjects due to age, weight, gender, renal, and hepatic disease differences. Despite advances in modeling and genetics, sometimes it is necessary to monitor the plasma drug concentration precisely in a patient for safety and multidrug dosing consideration. Clinical pharmacokinetics is also applied to

TABLE 1-2 Ratio of Age-Adjusted Death Rates, by Male/Female Ratio from the 10 Leading Causes of Death* in the US, 2003

Disease	Rank	Male:Female
Disease of heart	1	1.5
Malignant neoplasms	2	1.5
Cerebrovascular diseases	3	4.0
Chronic lower respiration diseases	4	1.4
Accidents and others*	5	2.2
Diabetes mellitus	6	1.2
Pneumonia and influenza	7	1.4
Alzheimers	8	0.8
Nephrotis, nephrotic syndrome, and nephrosis	9	1.5
Septicemia	10	1.2

*Death due to adverse effects suffered as defined by CDC.

Source: National Vital Statistics Report Vol. 52, No. 3, 2003.

therapeutic drug monitoring (TDM) for very potent drugs, such as those with a narrow therapeutic range, in order to optimize efficacy and to prevent any adverse toxicity. For these drugs, it is necessary to monitor the patient, either by monitoring plasma drug concentrations (eg, theophylline) or by monitoring a specific pharmacodynamic endpoint such as prothrombin clotting time (eg, warfarin). Pharmacokinetic and drug analysis services necessary for safe drug monitoring are generally provided by the *clinical pharmacokinetic service* (CPKS). Some drugs frequently monitored are the aminoglycosides and anticonvulsants. Other drugs closely monitored are those used in cancer chemotherapy, in order to minimize adverse side effects (Rodman and Evans, 1991).

Labeling For Human Prescription Drug and Biological Products

In 2013, the FDA redesigned the format of the prescribing information necessary for safe and effective use of the drugs and biological products

(FDA Guidance for Industry, 2013). This design was developed to make information in prescription drug labeling easier for health care practitioners to access and read. The practitioner can use the prescribing information to make prescribing decisions. The labeling includes three sections:

- *Highlights of Prescribing Information (Highlights)*—contains selected information from the Full Prescribing Information (FPI) that health care practitioners most commonly reference and consider most important. In addition, highlights may contain any boxed warnings that give a concise summary of all of the risks described in the **Boxed Warning** section in the **FPI**.
- *Table of Contents (Contents)*—lists the sections and subsections of the FPI.
- *Full Prescribing Information (FPI)*—contains the detailed prescribing information necessary for safe and effective use of the drug.

An example of the Highlights of Prescribing Information and Table of Contents for Nexium (esomeprazole magnesium) delayed release capsules appears in Table 1-3B. The prescribing information sometimes referred to as the approved label or the package insert may be found at the FDA website, Drugs@FDA (http://www.accessdata.fda.gov/scripts/cder/drugsatfda/). Prescribing information is updated periodically as new information becomes available. The prescribing information contained in the label recommends dosage regimens for the average patient from data obtained from clinical trials. The indications and usage section are those indications that the FDA has approved and that have been shown to be effective in clinical trials. On occasion, a practitioner may want to prescribe the drug to a patient drug for a non-approved use or indication. The pharmacist must decide if there is sufficient evidence for dispensing the drug for a non-approved use (off-label indication). The decision to dispense a drug for a non-approved indication may be difficult and often made with consultation of other health professionals.

Clinical Pharmacology

Pharmacology is a science that generally deals with the study of drugs, including its mechanism, effects, and uses of drugs; broadly speaking, it includes pharmacognosy, pharmacokinetics, pharmacodynamics, pharmacotherapeutics, and toxicology. The application of pharmacology in clinical medicine including clinical trial is referred to as clinical pharmacology. For pharmacists and health professionals, it is important to know that NDA drug labels report many important study information under **Clinical Pharmacology** in Section 12 of the standard prescription label (Tables 1-3A and 1-3B).

12 CLINICAL PHARMACOLOGY

12.1 Mechanism of Action
12.2 Pharmacodynamics
12.3 Pharmacokinetics

Question

Where is toxicology information found in the prescription label for a new drug? Can I find out if a drug is mutagenic under side-effect sections?

Answer

Nonclinical toxicology information is usefully in Section 13 under **Nonclinical Toxicology** if available. Mutagenic potential of a drug is usually reported under animal studies. It is unlikely that a drug with known humanly mutagenicity will be marketed, if so, it will be labeled with special warning. Black box warnings are usually used to give warnings to prescribers in Section 5 under Warnings and Precautions.

Pharmacogenetics

Pharmacogenetics is the study of drug effect including distribution and disposition due to genetic differences, which can affect individual responses to drugs, both in terms of therapeutic effect and adverse effects. A related field is pharmacogenomics, which emphasizes different aspects of genetic effect on drug response. This important discipline is discussed in Chapter 13. Pharmacogenetics is the main reason why many new drugs still have to be further studied after regulatory approval, that is, postapproval phase 4 studies. The clinical trials prior to drug approval are generally limited such that some side effects and special responses due to genetic differences may not be adequately known and labeled.

TABLE 1-3A Highlights of Prescribing Information for Nexium (Esomeprazole Magnesium) Delayed Release Capsules

HIGHLIGHTS OF PRESCRIBING INFORMATION

These highlights do not include all the information needed to use NEXIUM safely and effectively. See full prescribing information for NEXIUM.
NEXIUM (esomeprazole magnesium) delayed-release capsules, for oral use
NEXIUM (esomeprazole magnesium) for delayed-release oral suspension
Initial U.S. Approval: 1989 (omeprazole)

RECENT MAJOR CHANGES

Warnings and Precautions. Interactions with Diagnostic
Investigations for Neuroendocrine Tumors (5.8)   03/2014

INDICATIONS AND USAGE

NEXIUM is a proton pump inhibitor indicated for the following:
• Treatment of gastroesophageal reflux disease (GERD) (1.1)
• Risk reduction of NSAID-associated gastric ulcer (1.2)
• *H. pylori* eradication to reduce the risk of duodenal ulcer recurrence (1.3)
• Pathological hypersecretory conditions, including Zollinger-Ellison syndrome (1.4)

DOSAGE AND ADMINISTRATION

Indication	Dose	Frequency
Gastroesophageal Reflux Disease (GERD)		
Adults	20 mg or 40 mg	Once daily for 4 to 8 weeks
12 to 17 years	20 mg or 40 mg	Once daily for up to 8 weeks
1 to 11 years	10 mg or 20 mg	Once daily for up to 8 weeks
1 month to less than 1 year 2.5 mg, 5 mg or 10 mg (based on weight). Once daily, up to 6 weeks for erosive esophagitis (EE) due to acid-mediated GERD only.		
Risk Reduction of NSAID-Associated Gastric Ulcer		
	20 mg or 40 mg	Once daily for up to 6 months
***H. pylori* Eradication** (*Triple Therapy*):		
NEXIUM	40 mg	Once daily for 10 days
Amoxicillin	1000 mg	Twice daily for 10 days
Clarithromycin	500 mg	Twice daily for 10 days
Pathological Hypersecretory Conditions		
	40 mg	Twice daily
See full prescribing information for administration options (2)		
Patients with severe liver impairment do not exceed dose of 20 mg (2)		

DOSAGE FORMS AND STRENGTHS

• NEXIUM Delayed-Release Capsules: 20 mg and 40 mg (3)
• NEXIUM for Delayed-Release Oral Suspension: 2.5 mg, 5 mg, 10 mg, 20 mg, and 40 mg (3)

CONTRAINDICATIONS

Patients with known hypersensitivity to proton pump inhibitors (PPIs) (angioedema and anaphylaxis have occurred) (4)

(Continued)

TABLE 1-3A   Highlights of Prescribing Information for Nexium (Esomeprazole Magnesium) Delayed Release Capsules (Continued)

HIGHLIGHTS OF PRESCRIBING INFORMATION

WARNINGS AND PRECAUTIONS

- Symptomatic response does not preclude the presence of gastric malignancy (5.1)
- Atrophic gastritis has been noted with long-term omeprazole therapy (5.2)
- PPI therapy may be associated with increased risk of *Clostriodium difficle*-associated diarrhea (5.3)
- Avoid concomitant use of NEXIUM with clopidogrel (5.4)
- Bone Fracture: Long-term and multiple daily dose PPI therapy may be associated with an increased risk for osteoporosis-related fractures of the hip, wrist, or spine (5.5)
- Hypomagnesemia has been reported rarely with prolonged treatment with PPIs (5.6)
- Avoid concomitant use of NEXIUM with St John's Wort or rifampin due to the potential reduction in esomeprazole levels (5.7,7.3)
- Interactions with diagnostic investigations for Neuroendocrine Tumors: Increases in intragastric pH may result in hypergastrinemia and enterochromaffin-like cell hyperplasia and increased chromogranin A levels which may interfere with diagnostic investigations for neuroendocrine tumors (5.8,12.2)

ADVERSE REACTIONS

Most common adverse reactions (6.1):
- Adults (≥18 years) (incidence ≥1%) are headache, diarrhea, nausea, flatulence, abdominal pain, constipation, and dry mouth
- Pediatric (1 to 17 years) (incidence ≥2%) are headache, diarrhea, abdominal pain, nausea, and somnolence
- Pediatric (1 month to less than 1 year) (incidence 1%) are abdominal pain, regurgitation, tachypnea, and increased ALT

To report SUSPECTED ADVERSE REACTIONS, contact AstraZeneca at 1-800-236-9933 or FDA at 1-800-FDA-1088 or www.fda.gov/medwatch.

DRUG INTERACTIONS

- May affect plasma levels of antiretroviral drugs – use with atazanavir and nelfinavir is not recommended: if saquinavir is used with NEXIUM, monitor for toxicity and consider saquinavir dose reduction (7.1)
- May interfere with drugs for which gastric pH affects bioavailability (e.g., ketoconazole, iron salts, erlotinib, and digoxin) Patients treated with NEXIUM and digoxin may need to be monitored for digoxin toxicity. (7.2)
- Combined inhibitor of CYP 2C19 and 3A4 may raise esomeprazole levels (7.3)
- Clopidogrel: NEXIUM decreases exposure to the active metabolite of clopidogrel (7.3)
- May increase systemic exposure of cilostazol and an active metabolite. Consider dose reduction (7.3)
- Tacrolimus: NEXIUM may increase serum levels of tacrolimus (7.5)
- Methotrexate: NEXIUM may increase serum levels of methotrexate (7.7)

USE IN SPECIFIC POPULATIONS

- Pregnancy: Based on animal data, may cause fetal harm (8.1)

See 17 for PATIENT COUNSELING INFORMATION and FDA-approved Medication Guide.

Revised: 03/2014

PRACTICAL FOCUS

Relationship of Drug Concentrations to Drug Response

The initiation of drug therapy starts with the manufacturer's recommended dosage regimen that includes the drug dose and frequency of doses (eg, 100 mg every 8 hours). Due to individual differences in the patient's genetic makeup (see Chapter 13 on pharmacogenetics) or pharmacokinetics, the recommended dosage regimen drug may not provide the desired therapeutic outcome. The measurement of plasma drug concentrations can confirm whether the drug dose was subtherapeutic due to the patient's individual pharmacokinetic profile (observed by low plasma drug concentrations) or was not responsive to drug therapy due to genetic difference in receptor response. In this case, the drug concentrations

TABLE 1-3B   Contents for Full Prescribing Information for Nexium (Esomeprazole Magnesium) Delayed Release Capsules

FULL PRESCRIBING INFORMATION: CONTENTS*

1. **INDICATIONS AND USAGE**
    1.1 Treatment of Gastroesophageal Reflux Disease (GERD)
    1.2 Risk Reduction of NSAID-Associated Gastric Ulcer
    1.3 *H. pylori* Eradication to Reduce the Risk of Duodenal Ulcer Recurrence
    1.4 Pathological Hypersecretory Conditions Including Zollinger-Ellison Syndrome
2. **DOSAGE AND ADMINISTRATION**
3. **DOSAGE FORMS AND STRENGTHS**
4. **CONTRAINDICATIONS**
5. **WARNINGS AND PRECAUTIONS**
    5.1 Concurrent Gastric Malignancy
    5.2 Atrophic Gastritis
    5.3 *Clostridium difficile* associated diarrhea
    5.4 Interaction with Clopidogrel
    5.5 Bone Fracture
    5.6 Hypomagnesemia
    5.7 Concomitant Use of NEXIUM with St John's Wort or rifampin
    5.8 Interactions with Diagnostic Investigations for Neuroendocrine Tumors
    5.9 Concomitant Use of NEXIUM with Methotrexate
6. **ADVERSE REACTIONS**
    6.1 Clinical Trials Experience
    6.2 Postmarketing Experience
7. **DRUG INTERACTIONS**
    7.1 Interference with Antiretroviral Therapy
    7.2 Drugs for Which Gastric pH Can Affect Bioavailability
    7.3 Effects on Hepatic Metabolism/Cytochrome P-450 Pathways
    7.4 Interactions with Investigations of Neuroendocrine Tumors
    7.5 Tacrolimus
    7.6 Combination Therapy with Clarithromycin
    7.7 Methotrexate
8. **USE IN SPECIFIC POPULATIONS**
    8.1 Pregnancy
    8.3 Nursing Mothers
    8.4 Pediatric Use
    8.5 Geriatric Use
10. **OVERDOSAGE**
11. **DESCRIPTION**
12. **CLINICAL PHARMACOLOGY**
    12.1 Mechanism of Action
    12.2 Pharmacodynamics
    12.3 Pharmacokinetics
    12.4 Microbiology
13. **NONCLINICAL TOXICOLOGY**
    13.1 Carcinogenesis, Mutagenesis, Impairment of Fertility
    13.2 Animal Toxicology and/or Pharmacology
14. **CLINICAL STUDIES**
    14.1 Healing of Erosive Esophagitis
    14.2 Symptomatic Gastroesophageal Reflux Disease (GERD)
    14.3 Pediatric Gastroesophageal Reflux Disease (GERD)
    14.4 Risk Reduction of NSAID-Associated Gastric Ulcer
    14.5 *Helicobacter pylori (H. Pylon)* Eradication in Patients with Duodenal Ulcer Disease
    14.6 Pathological Hypersecretory Conditions Including Zollinger-Ellison Syndrome
16. **HOW SUPPLIED/STORAGE AND HANDLING**
17. **PATIENT COUNSELING INFORMATION**

*Sections or subsections omitted from the full prescribing information are not listed.

Source: FDA Guidance for Industry (February 2013).

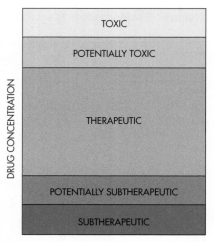

FIGURE 1-2 Relationship of drug concentrations to drug response.

are in the therapeutic range but the patient does not respond to drug treatment. Figure 1-2 shows that the concentration of drug in the body can range from subtherapeutic to toxic. In contrast, some patients respond to drug treatment at lower drug doses that result in lower drug concentrations. Other patients may need higher drug concentrations to obtain a therapeutic effect, which requires higher drug doses. It is desirable that adverse drug responses occur at drug concentrations higher relative to the therapeutic drug concentrations, but for many potent drugs, adverse effects can also occur close to the same drug concentrations as needed for the therapeutic effect.

> **Frequently Asked Questions**
> ▶ *Which is more closely related to drug response, the total drug dose administered or the concentration of the drug in the body?*
>
> ▶ *Why do individualized dosing regimens need to be determined for some patients?*

PHARMACODYNAMICS

Pharmacodynamics refers to the relationship between the drug concentration at the site of action (receptor) and pharmacologic response, including biochemical

and physiologic effects that influence the interaction of drug with the receptor. The interaction of a drug molecule with a receptor causes the initiation of a sequence of molecular events resulting in a pharmacologic or toxic response. Pharmacokinetic–pharmacodynamic models are constructed to relate plasma drug level to drug concentration at the site of action and establish the intensity and time course of the drug. Pharmacodynamics and pharmacokinetic–pharmacodynamic models are discussed more fully in Chapter 21.

DRUG EXPOSURE AND DRUG RESPONSE

Drug exposure refers to the dose (drug input to the body) and various measures of acute or integrated drug concentrations in plasma and other biological fluid (eg, C_{max}, C_{min}, C_{ss}, AUC) (FDA Guidance for Industry, 2003). *Drug response* refers to a direct measure of the pharmacologic effect of the drug. Response includes a broad range of endpoints or biomarkers ranging from the clinically remote biomarkers (eg, receptor occupancy) to a presumed mechanistic effect (eg, ACE inhibition), to a potential or accepted surrogate (eg, effects on blood pressure, lipids, or cardiac output), and to the full range of short-term or long-term clinical effects related to either efficacy or safety.

Toxicologic and efficacy studies provide information on the safety and effectiveness of the drug during development and in special patient populations such as subjects with renal and hepatic insufficiencies. For many drugs, clinical use is based on weighing the risks of favorable and unfavorable outcomes at a particular dose. For some potent drugs, the doses and dosing rate may need to be titrated in order to obtain the desired effect and be tolerated.

TOXICOKINETICS AND CLINICAL TOXICOLOGY

Toxicokinetics is the application of pharmacokinetic principles to the design, conduct, and interpretation of drug safety evaluation studies (Leal et al, 1993) and in validating dose-related exposure in animals. Toxicokinetic data aid in the interpretation of toxicologic findings in animals and extrapolation of the resulting data to humans. Toxicokinetic studies are performed in animals during preclinical drug development and may continue after the drug has been tested in clinical trials.

Clinical toxicology is the study of adverse effects of drugs and toxic substances (poisons) in the body. The pharmacokinetics of a drug in an overmedicated (intoxicated) patient may be very different from the pharmacokinetics of the same drug given in lower therapeutic doses. At very high doses, the drug concentration in the body may saturate enzymes involved in the absorption, biotransformation, or active renal secretion mechanisms, thereby changing the pharmacokinetics from linear to *nonlinear pharmacokinetics*. Nonlinear pharmacokinetics is discussed in Chapter 10. Drugs frequently involved in toxicity cases include acetaminophen, salicylates, opiates (eg, morphine), and the tricylic antidepressants (TCAs). Many of these drugs can be assayed conveniently by fluorescence immunoassay (FIA) kits.

MEASUREMENT OF DRUG CONCENTRATIONS

Because drug concentrations are an important element in determining individual or population pharmacokinetics, drug concentrations are measured in biologic samples, such as milk, saliva, plasma, and urine. Sensitive, accurate, and precise analytical methods are available for the direct measurement of drugs in biologic matrices. Such measurements are generally validated so that accurate information is generated for pharmacokinetic and clinical monitoring. In general, chromatographic and mass spectrometric methods are most frequently employed for drug concentration measurement, because chromatography separates the drug from other related materials that may cause assay interference and mass spectrometry allows detection of molecules or molecule fragments based on their mass-to-charge ratio.

Sampling of Biologic Specimens

Only a few biologic specimens may be obtained safely from the patient to gain information as to the drug concentration in the body. *Invasive methods* include sampling blood, spinal fluid, synovial fluid, tissue biopsy, or any biologic material that requires parenteral or surgical intervention in the patient. In contrast, *noninvasive methods* include sampling of urine, saliva, feces, expired air, or any biologic material that can be obtained without parenteral or surgical intervention.

The measurement of drug and metabolite concentration in each of these biologic materials yields important information, such as the amount of drug retained in, or transported into, that region of the tissue or fluid, the likely pharmacologic or toxicologic outcome of drug dosing, and drug metabolite formation or transport. Analytical methods should be able to distinguish between protein-bound and unbound parent drug and each metabolite, and the pharmacologically active species should be identified. Such distinctions between metabolites in each tissue and fluid are especially important for initial pharmacokinetic modeling of a drug.

Drug Concentrations in Blood, Plasma, or Serum

Measurement of drug and metabolite concentrations (levels) in the blood, serum, or plasma is the most direct approach to assessing the pharmacokinetics of the drug in the body. Whole blood contains cellular elements including red blood cells, white blood cells, platelets, and various other proteins, such as albumin and globulins (Table 1-4). In general, serum or plasma is most commonly used for drug measurement. To obtain serum, whole blood is allowed to clot and the serum is collected from the supernatant after centrifugation. Plasma is obtained from the supernatant of centrifuged whole blood to which an anticoagulant, such as heparin, has been added. Therefore, the protein content of serum and plasma is not the same. Plasma perfuses all the tissues of the body, including the cellular elements in the blood. Assuming that a drug in the plasma is in dynamic equilibrium with the tissues, then changes in the drug concentration in plasma will reflect changes in tissue drug concentrations. Drugs in the plasma are often bound to plasma proteins, and often plasma proteins are filtered from the plasma before drug concentrations are measured. This is the unbound

TABLE 1-4   Blood Components

Blood Component	How Obtained	Components
Whole blood	Whole blood is generally obtained by venous puncture and contains an anticoagulant such as heparin or EDTA	Whole blood contains all the cellular and protein elements of blood
Serum	Serum is the liquid obtained from whole blood after the blood is allowed to clot and the clot is removed	Serum does not contain the cellular elements, fibrinogen, or the other clotting factors from the blood
Plasma	Plasma is the liquid supernatant obtained after centrifugation of non-clotted whole blood that contains an anticoagulant	Plasma is the noncellular liquid fraction of whole blood and contains all the proteins including albumin

drug concentration. Alternatively, drug concentration may be measured from unfiltered plasma; this is the total plasma drug concentration. When interpreting plasma concentrations, it is important to understand what type of plasma concentration the data reflect.

Frequently Asked Questions

▶ Why are drug concentrations more often measured in plasma rather than whole blood or serum?

▶ What are the differences between bound drug, unbound drug, total drug, parent drug, and metabolite drug concentrations in the plasma?

Plasma Drug Concentration–Time Curve

The plasma drug concentration (level)–time curve is generated by obtaining the drug concentration in plasma samples taken at various time intervals after a drug product is administered. The concentration of drug in each plasma sample is plotted on rectangular-coordinate graph paper against the corresponding time at which the plasma sample was removed. As the drug reaches the general (systemic) circulation, plasma drug concentrations will rise up to a maximum if the drug was given by an extravascular route. Usually, absorption of a drug is more rapid than elimination. As the drug is being absorbed into the systemic circulation, the drug is distributed to all the tissues in the body and is also *simultaneously* being eliminated. Elimination of a drug can proceed by excretion, biotransformation, or a combination of both. Other elimination mechanisms may also be

involved, such as elimination in the feces, sweat, or exhaled air.

The relationship of the drug level–time curve and various pharmacologic parameters for the drug is shown in Fig. 1-3. MEC and MTC represent the *minimum effective concentration* and *minimum toxic concentration* of drug, respectively. For some drugs, such as those acting on the autonomic nervous system, it is useful to know the concentration of drug that will just barely produce a pharmacologic effect (ie, MEC). Assuming the drug concentration in the plasma is in equilibrium with the tissues, the MEC reflects the minimum concentration of drug needed

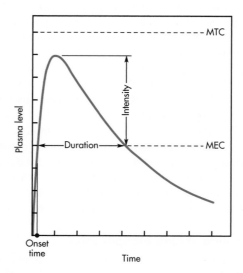

FIGURE 1-3   Generalized plasma level–time curve after oral administration of a drug.

at the receptors to produce the desired pharmacologic effect. Similarly, the MTC represents the drug concentration needed to just barely produce a toxic effect. The *onset time* corresponds to the time required for the drug to reach the MEC. The intensity of the pharmacologic effect is proportional to the number of drug receptors occupied, which is reflected in the observation that higher plasma drug concentrations produce a greater pharmacologic response, up to a maximum. The *duration of drug action* is the difference between the onset time and the time for the drug to decline back to the MEC.

The *therapeutic window* is the concentrations between the MEC and the MTC. Drugs with a wide therapeutic window are generally considered safer than drugs with a narrow therapeutic window. Sometimes the term *therapeutic index* is used. This term refers to the ratio between the toxic and therapeutic doses.

In contrast, the pharmacokineticist can also describe the plasma level–time curve in terms of such pharmacokinetic terms as *peak plasma level* (C_{max}), *time for peak plasma level* (T_{max}), and *area under the curve,* or AUC (Fig. 1-4). The time for peak plasma level is the time of maximum drug concentration in the plasma and is a rough marker of average rate of drug absorption. The peak plasma level or maximum drug concentration is related to the dose, the rate constant for absorption, and the elimination constant of the drug. The AUC is related to the amount of drug absorbed systemically. These and other pharmacokinetic parameters are discussed in succeeding chapters.

Frequently Asked Questions

▶ *At what time intervals should plasma drug concentration be taken in order to best predict drug response and side effects?*

▶ *What happens if plasma concentrations fall outside of the therapeutic window?*

Drug Concentrations in Tissues

Tissue biopsies are occasionally removed for diagnostic purposes, such as the verification of a malignancy. Usually, only a small sample of tissue is removed, making drug concentration measurement difficult. Drug concentrations in tissue biopsies may not reflect drug concentration in other tissues nor the drug concentration in all parts of the tissue from which the biopsy material was removed. For example, if the tissue biopsy was for the diagnosis of a tumor within the tissue, the blood flow to the tumor cells may not be the same as the blood flow to other cells in this tissue. In fact, for many tissues, blood flow to one part of the tissues need not be the same as the blood flow to another part of the same tissue. The measurement of the drug concentration in tissue biopsy material may be used to ascertain if the drug reached the tissues and reached the proper concentration within the tissue.

Drug Concentrations in Urine and Feces

Measurement of drug in urine is an indirect method to ascertain the bioavailability of a drug. The rate and extent of drug excreted in the urine reflects the rate and extent of systemic drug absorption. The use of urinary drug excretion measurements to establish various pharmacokinetic parameters is discussed in Chapter 4.

Measurement of drug in feces may reflect drug that has not been absorbed after an oral dose or may

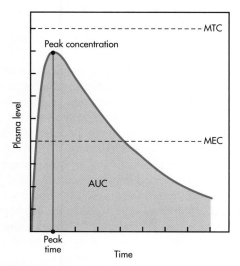

FIGURE 1-4 Plasma level–time curve showing peak time and concentration. The shaded portion represents the AUC (area under the curve).

reflect drug that has been expelled by biliary secretion after systemic absorption. Fecal drug excretion is often performed in mass balance studies, in which the investigator attempts to account for the entire dose given to the patient. For a mass balance study, both urine and feces are collected and their drug content measured. For certain solid oral dosage forms that do not dissolve in the gastrointestinal tract but slowly leach out drug, fecal collection is performed to recover the dosage form. The undissolved dosage form is then assayed for residual drug.

Drug Concentrations in Saliva

Saliva drug concentrations have been reviewed for many drugs for therapeutic drug monitoring (Pippenger and Massoud, 1984). Because only free drug diffuses into the saliva, saliva drug levels tend to approximate free drug rather than total plasma drug concentration. The saliva/plasma drug concentration ratio is less than 1 for many drugs. The saliva/plasma drug concentration ratio is mostly influenced by the pKa of the drug and the pH of the saliva. Weak acid drugs and weak base drugs with pKa significantly different than pH 7.4 (plasma pH) generally have better correlation to plasma drug levels. The saliva drug concentrations taken after equilibrium with the plasma drug concentration generally provide more stable indication of drug levels in the body. The use of salivary drug concentrations as a therapeutic indicator should be used with caution and preferably as a secondary indicator.

Forensic Drug Measurements

Forensic science is the application of science to personal injury, murder, and other legal proceedings. Drug measurements in tissues obtained at autopsy or in other bodily fluids such as saliva, urine, and blood may be useful if a suspect or victim has taken an overdose of a legal medication, has been poisoned, or has been using drugs of abuse such as opiates (eg, heroin), cocaine, or marijuana. The appearance of social drugs in blood, urine, and saliva drug analysis shows short-term drug abuse. These drugs may be eliminated rapidly, making it more difficult to prove that the subject has been using drugs of abuse. The analysis for drugs of abuse in hair samples by very sensitive assay methods, such as gas chromatography coupled with mass spectrometry, provides information regarding past drug exposure. A study by Cone et al (1993) showed that the hair samples from subjects who were known drug abusers contained cocaine and 6-acetylmorphine, a metabolite of heroin (diacetylmorphine).

Significance of Measuring Plasma Drug Concentrations

The intensity of the pharmacologic or toxic effect of a drug is often related to the concentration of the drug at the receptor site, usually located in the tissue cells. Because most of the tissue cells are richly perfused with tissue fluids or plasma, measuring the plasma drug level is a responsive method of monitoring the course of therapy.

Clinically, individual variations in the pharmacokinetics of drugs are quite common. Monitoring the concentration of drugs in the blood or plasma ascertains that the calculated dose actually delivers the plasma level required for therapeutic effect. With some drugs, receptor expression and/or sensitivity in individuals varies, so monitoring of plasma levels is needed to distinguish the patient who is receiving too much of a drug from the patient who is supersensitive to the drug. Moreover, the patient's physiologic functions may be affected by disease, nutrition, environment, concurrent drug therapy, and other factors. Pharmacokinetic models allow more accurate interpretation of the relationship between plasma drug levels and pharmacologic response.

In the absence of pharmacokinetic information, plasma drug levels are relatively useless for dosage adjustment. For example, suppose a single blood sample from a patient was assayed and found to contain 10 μg/mL. According to the literature, the maximum safe concentration of this drug is 15 μg/mL. In order to apply this information properly, it is important to know when the blood sample was drawn, what dose of the drug was given, and the route of administration. If the proper information is available, the use of pharmacokinetic equations and models may describe the blood level–time curve accurately and be used to modify dosing for that specific patient.

Monitoring of plasma drug concentrations allows for the adjustment of the drug dosage in order to individualize and optimize therapeutic drug regimens. When alterations in physiologic functions occur, monitoring plasma drug concentrations may provide a guide to the progress of the disease state and enable the investigator to modify the drug dosage accordingly. Clinically, sound medical judgment and observation are most important. Therapeutic decisions should not be based solely on plasma drug concentrations.

In many cases, the *pharmacodynamic response* to the drug may be more important to measure than just the plasma drug concentration. For example, the electrophysiology of the heart, including an electrocardiogram (ECG), is important to assess in patients medicated with cardiotonic drugs such as digoxin. For an anticoagulant drug, such as dicumarol, prothrombin clotting time may indicate whether proper dosage was achieved. Most diabetic patients taking insulin will monitor their own blood or urine glucose levels.

For drugs that act irreversibly at the receptor site, plasma drug concentrations may not accurately predict pharmacodynamic response. Drugs used in cancer chemotherapy often interfere with nucleic acid or protein biosynthesis to destroy tumor cells. For these drugs, the plasma drug concentration does not relate directly to the pharmacodynamic response. In this case, other pathophysiologic parameters and side effects are monitored in the patient to prevent adverse toxicity.

BASIC PHARMACOKINETICS AND PHARMACOKINETIC MODELS

Drugs are in a dynamic state within the body as they move between tissues and fluids, bind with plasma or cellular components, or are metabolized. The biologic nature of drug distribution and disposition is complex, and drug events often happen simultaneously. Such factors must be considered when designing drug therapy regimens. The inherent and infinite complexity of these events requires the use of mathematical models and statistics to estimate drug dosing and to predict the time course of drug efficacy for a given dose.

A *model* is a hypothesis using mathematical terms to describe quantitative relationships concisely.

The predictive capability of a model lies in the proper selection and development of mathematical function(s) that parameterizes the essential factors governing the kinetic process. The key parameters in a process are commonly estimated by fitting the model to the experimental data, known as *variables*. A *pharmacokinetic parameter* is a constant for the drug that is estimated from the experimental data. For example, estimated pharmacokinetic parameters such as k depend on the method of tissue sampling, the timing of the sample, drug analysis, and the predictive model selected.

A pharmacokinetic function relates an *independent variable* to a *dependent variable,* often through the use of parameters. For example, a pharmacokinetic model may predict the drug concentration in the liver 1 hour after an oral administration of a 20-mg dose. The independent variable is the time and the dependent variable is the drug concentration in the liver. Based on a set of time-versus-drug concentration data, a model equation is derived to predict the liver drug concentration with respect to time. In this case, the drug concentration depends on the time after the administration of the dose, where the time–concentration relationship is defined by a pharmacokinetic parameter, k, the elimination rate constant.

Such mathematical models can be devised to simulate the rate processes of drug absorption, distribution, and elimination to describe and *predict* drug concentrations in the body as a function of time. Pharmacokinetic models are used to:

1. Predict plasma, tissue, and urine drug levels with any dosage regimen
2. Calculate the optimum dosage regimen for each patient individually
3. Estimate the possible accumulation of drugs and/or metabolites
4. Correlate drug concentrations with pharmacologic or toxicologic activity
5. Evaluate differences in the rate or extent of availability between formulations (bioequivalence)
6. Describe how changes in physiology or disease affect the absorption, distribution, or elimination of the drug
7. Explain drug interactions

Simplifying assumptions are made in pharmacokinetic models to describe a complex biologic system concerning the movement of drugs within the body. For example, most pharmacokinetic models assume that the plasma drug concentration reflects drug concentrations globally within the body.

A model may be empirically, physiologically, or compartmentally based. The model that simply interpolates the data and allows an empirical formula to estimate drug level over time is justified when limited information is available. *Empirical models* are practical but not very useful in explaining the mechanism of the actual process by which the drug is absorbed, distributed, and eliminated in the body. Examples of empirical models used in pharmacokinetics are described in Chapter 25.

Physiologically based models also have limitations. Using the example above, and apart from the necessity to sample tissue and monitor blood flow to the liver *in vivo,* the investigator needs to understand the following questions. What is the clinical implication of the liver drug concentration value? Should the drug concentration in the blood within the tissue be determined and subtracted from the drug in the liver tissue? What type of cell is representative of the liver if a selective biopsy liver tissue sample can be collected without contamination from its surroundings? Indeed, depending on the spatial location of the liver tissue from the hepatic blood vessels, tissue drug concentrations can differ depending on distance to the blood vessel or even on the type of cell in the liver. Moreover, changes in the liver blood perfusion will alter the tissue drug concentration. If heterogeneous liver tissue is homogenized and assayed, the homogenized tissue represents only a hypothetical concentration that is an *average* of all the cells and blood in the liver at the time of collection. Since tissue homogenization is not practical for human subjects, the drug concentration in the liver may be estimated by knowing the liver extraction ratio for the drug based on knowledge of the physiologic and biochemical composition of the body organs.

A great number of models have been developed to estimate regional and global information about drug disposition in the body. Some physiologic pharmacokinetic models are also discussed in Chapter 25. Individual pharmacokinetic processes are discussed

in separate chapters under the topics of drug absorption, drug distribution, drug elimination, and pharmacokinetic drug interactions involving one or all of the above processes. Theoretically, an unlimited number of models may be constructed to describe the kinetic processes of drug absorption, distribution, and elimination in the body, depending on the degree of detailed information considered. Practical considerations have limited the growth of new pharmacokinetic models.

A very simple and useful tool in pharmacokinetics is *compartmentally based models*. For example, assume a drug is given by intravenous injection and that the drug dissolves (distributes) rapidly in the body fluids. One pharmacokinetic model that can describe this situation is a tank containing a volume of fluid that is rapidly equilibrated with the drug. The concentration of the drug in the tank after a given dose is governed by two parameters: (1) the fluid volume of the tank that will dilute the drug, and (2) the elimination rate of drug per unit of time. Though this model is perhaps an overly simplistic view of drug disposition in the human body, a drug's pharmacokinetic properties can frequently be described using a fluid-filled tank model called the *one-compartment open model* (see below). In both the tank and the one-compartment body model, a fraction of the drug would be continually eliminated as a function of time (Fig. 1-5). In pharmacokinetics, these parameters are assumed to be constant for a given drug. If drug concentrations in the tank are determined at various time intervals following administration of a known dose, then the volume of fluid in the tank or compartment (V_D, volume of distribution) and the rate of drug elimination can be estimated.

In practice, pharmacokinetic parameters such as k and V_D are determined experimentally from a set of drug concentrations collected over various times and

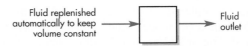

FIGURE 1-5 Tank with a constant volume of fluid equilibrated with drug. The volume of the fluid is 1.0 L. The fluid outlet is 10 mL/min. The fraction of drug removed per unit of time is 10/1000, or 0.01 min^{-1}.

known as *data*. The number of parameters needed to describe the model depends on the complexity of the process and on the route of drug administration. In general, as the number of parameters required to model the data increases, accurate estimation of these parameters becomes increasingly more difficult. With complex pharmacokinetic models, computer programs are used to facilitate parameter estimation. However, for the parameters to be valid, the number of data points should always exceed the number of parameters in the model.

Because a model is based on a hypothesis and simplifying assumptions, a certain degree of caution is necessary when relying totally on the pharmacokinetic model to predict drug action. For some drugs, plasma drug concentrations are not useful in predicting drug activity. For other drugs, an individual's genetic differences, disease state, and the compensatory response of the body may modify the response to the drug. If a simple model does not fit all the experimental observations accurately, a new, more elaborate model may be proposed and subsequently tested. Since limited data are generally available in most clinical situations, pharmacokinetic data should be interpreted along with clinical observations rather than replacing sound judgment by the clinician. Development of pharmacometric statistical models may help to improve prediction of drug levels among patients in the population (Sheiner and Beal, 1982; Mallet et al, 1988). However, it will be some time before these methods become generally accepted.

Compartment Models

If the tissue drug concentrations and binding are known, physiologic pharmacokinetic models, which are based on actual tissues and their respective blood flow, describe the data realistically. Physiologic pharmacokinetic models are frequently used in describing drug distribution in animals, because tissue samples are easily available for assay. On the other hand, tissue samples are often not available for human subjects, so most physiological models assume an average set of blood flow for individual subjects.

In contrast, because of the vast complexity of the body, drug kinetics in the body are frequently simplified to be represented by one or more tanks, or compartments, that communicate reversibly with each other. A *compartment* is not a real physiologic or anatomic region but is considered a tissue or group of tissues that have similar blood flow and drug affinity. Within each compartment, the drug is considered to be uniformly distributed. Mixing of the drug within a compartment is rapid and homogeneous and is considered to be "well stirred," so that the drug concentration represents an average concentration, and each drug molecule has an equal probability of leaving the compartment. *Rate constants* are used to represent the overall rate processes of drug entry into and exit from the compartment. The model is an *open system* because drug can be eliminated from the system. Compartment models are based on linear assumptions using linear differential equations.

Mammillary Model

A compartmental model provides a simple way of grouping all the tissues into one or more compartments where drugs move to and from the central or plasma compartment. The *mammillary model* is the most common compartment model used in pharmacokinetics. The mammillary model is a strongly connected system, because one can estimate the amount of drug in any compartment of the system after drug is introduced into a given compartment. In the one-compartment model, drug is both added to and eliminated from a central compartment. The central compartment is assigned to represent plasma and highly perfused tissues that rapidly equilibrate with drug. When an intravenous dose of drug is given, the drug enters directly into the central compartment. Elimination of drug occurs from the central compartment because the organs involved in drug elimination, primarily kidney and liver, are well-perfused tissues.

In a two-compartment model, drug can move between the central or plasma compartment to and from the tissue compartment. Although the tissue compartment does not represent a specific tissue, the mass balance accounts for the drug present in all the tissues. In this model, the total amount of drug in the body is simply the sum of drug present in the central compartment plus the drug present in the tissue compartment. Knowing the parameters of either the one-compartment or the two-compartment model, one can estimate the amount of drug left in the body and the amount of drug eliminated from the body at any time. The compartmental models are particularly useful when little information is known about the tissues.

Several types of compartment models are described in Fig. 1-6. The pharmacokinetic rate constants are represented by the letter k. Compartment 1 represents the plasma or central compartment, and compartment 2 represents the tissue compartment. The drawing of models has three functions. The model (1) enables the pharmacokineticist to write differential equations to describe drug concentration changes in each compartment, (2) gives a visual representation of the rate processes, and (3) shows how many pharmacokinetic constants are necessary to describe the process adequately.

Catenary Model

In pharmacokinetics, the mammillary model must be distinguished from another type of compartmental model called the catenary model. The *catenary model* consists of compartments joined to one another like the compartments of a train (Fig. 1-7). In contrast, the mammillary model consists of one or

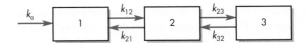

FIGURE 1-7   Example of caternary model.

more compartments around a central compartment like satellites. Because the catenary model does not apply to the way most functional organs in the body are directly connected to the plasma, it is not used as often as the mammillary model.

Physiologic Pharmacokinetic Model (Flow Model)

Physiologic pharmacokinetic models, also known as blood flow or perfusion models, are pharmacokinetic models based on known anatomic and physiologic data. The models describe the data kinetically, with the consideration that blood flow is responsible for distributing drug to various parts of the body. Uptake of drug into organs is determined by the

---

EXAMPLE ▶ ▶ ▶

Two parameters are needed to describe model 1 (Fig. 1-6): the volume of the compartment and the elimination rate constant, k. In the case of model 4, the pharmacokinetic parameters consist of the volumes of compartments 1 and 2 and the rate constants—k_a, k, k_{12}, and k_{21}—for a total of six parameters.

In studying these models, it is important to know whether drug concentration data may be sampled directly from each compartment. For models 3 and 4 (Fig. 1-6), data concerning compartment 2 cannot be obtained easily because tissues are not easily sampled and may not contain homogeneous concentrations of drug. If the amount of drug absorbed and eliminated per unit time is obtained by sampling compartment 1, then the amount of drug contained in the tissue compartment 2 can be estimated mathematically. The appropriate mathematical equations for describing these models and evaluating the various pharmacokinetic parameters are given in subsequent chapters.

MODEL 1. One-compartment open model, IV injection.

MODEL 2. One-compartment open model with first-order absorption.

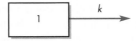

MODEL 3. Two-compartment open model, IV injection.

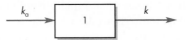

MODEL 4. Two-compartment open model with first-order absorption.

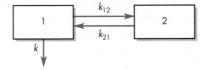

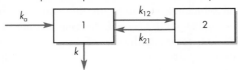

FIGURE 1-6   Various compartment models.

binding of drug in these tissues. In contrast to an estimated tissue volume of distribution, the actual tissue volume is used. Because there are many tissue organs in the body, each tissue volume must be obtained and its drug concentration described. The model would potentially predict realistic tissue drug concentrations, which the two-compartment model fails to do. Unfortunately, much of the information required for adequately describing a physiologic pharmacokinetic model is experimentally difficult to obtain. In spite of this limitation, the physiologic pharmacokinetic model does provide much better insight into how physiologic factors may change drug distribution from one animal species to another. Other major differences are described below.

First, no data fitting is required in the perfusion model. Drug concentrations in the various tissues are predicted by organ tissue size, blood flow, and experimentally determined drug tissue–blood ratios (ie, partition of drug between tissue and blood).

Second, blood flow, tissue size, and the drug tissue–blood ratios may vary due to certain pathophysiologic conditions. Thus, the effect of these variations on drug distribution must be taken into account in physiologic pharmacokinetic models.

Third, and most important of all, physiologically based pharmacokinetic models can be applied to several species, and, for some drugs, human data may be extrapolated. Extrapolation from animal data is not possible with the compartment models, because the volume of distribution in such models is a mathematical concept that does not relate simply to blood volume and blood flow. To date, numerous drugs (including digoxin, lidocaine, methotrexate, and thiopental) have been described with perfusion models. Tissue levels of some of these drugs cannot be predicted successfully with compartment models, although they generally describe blood levels well. An example of a perfusion model is shown in Fig. 1-8.

The number of tissue compartments in a perfusion model varies with the drug. Typically, the tissues or organs that have no drug penetration are excluded from consideration. Thus, such organs as the brain, the bones, and other parts of the central nervous system are often excluded, as most drugs have little penetration into these organs. To describe each organ separately with a differential equation

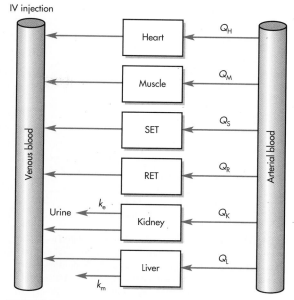

FIGURE 1-8 Pharmacokinetic model of drug perfusion. The ks represent kinetic constants: k_e is the first-order rate constant for urinary drug excretion and k_m is the rate constant for hepatic elimination. Each "box" represents a tissue compartment. Organs of major importance in drug absorption are considered separately, while other tissues are grouped as RET (rapidly equilibrating tissue) and SET (slowly equilibrating tissue). The size or mass of each tissue compartment is determined physiologically rather than by mathematical estimation. The concentration of drug in the tissue is determined by the ability of the tissue to accumulate drug as well as by the rate of blood perfusion to the tissue, represented by Q.

would make the model very complex and mathematically difficult. A simpler but equally good approach is to group all the tissues with similar blood perfusion properties into a single compartment.

A physiologic based pharmacokinetic model (PBPK) using known blood flow was used to describe the distribution of lidocaine in blood and various organs (Benowitz et el 1974) and applied in anesthesiology in man (Tucker et el 1971). In PBKB models, organs such as lung, liver, brain, and muscle were individually described by differential equations as shown in Fig. 1-8, sometimes tissues were grouped as RET (rapidly equilibrating tissue) and SET (slowly equilibrating tissue) for simplicity to account for the mass balance of the drug. A general scheme showing blood flow for typical organs is shown in Fig. 1-8.

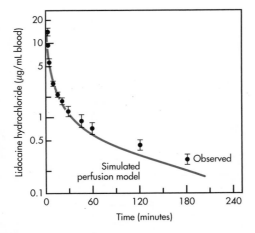

FIGURE 1-9   Observed mean (•) and simulated (—) arterial lidocaine blood concentrations in normal volunteers receiving 1 mg/kg/min constant infusion for 3 minutes. (From Tucker GT, Boas RA: Pharmacokinetic aspects of intravenous regional anesthesia. *Anesthesiology* **34**(6):538–549, 1971, with permission.)

The data showing blood concentration of lidocaine after an IV dose declining biexponentially (Fig. 1-9) was well predicted by the model. A later PBPK model was applied to model cyclosporine (Fig. 1-10). Drug level in various organs were well predicted and scaled to human based on this physiologic model (Kawai R et al, 1998). The tissue cyclosporine levels in the lung, muscle, and adipose and other organs are shown in Fig. 1-10. For lidocaine, the tissue such as adipose (fat) tissue accumulates drugs slowly because of low blood supply. In contrast, vascular tissues, like the lung, equilibrate rapidly with the blood and start to decline as soon as drug level in the blood starts to fall resulting in curvature of plasma profile. The physiologic pharmacokinetic model provides a realistic means of modeling tissue drug levels. However, drug levels in tissues are not available. A criticism of physiologic pharmacokinetic models in general has been that there are fewer data points than parameters that one tries to fit. Consequently, the projected data are not well *constrained*.

The real significance of the physiologically based model is the potential application of this model in the prediction of human pharmacokinetics from animal data (Sawada et al, 1985). The mass of various body organs or tissues, extent of protein binding, drug metabolism capacity, and blood flow in humans and other species are often known or can be determined. Thus, physiologic and anatomic parameters can be used to predict the effects of drugs on humans from the effects on animals in cases where human experimentation is difficult or restricted.

More sophisticated models are introduced as the understanding of human and animal physiology improves. For example, in Chapter 25, special compartment models that take into account transporter-mediated drug disposition are introduced for specific drugs. This approach is termed Physiologic Pharmacokinetic Model Incorporating Hepatic Transporter-Mediated Clearance. The differences between the physiologic pharmacokinetic model, the classical compartmental model, and the noncompartmental approach are discussed. It is important to note that mass transfer and balances of drug in and out of the body or body organs are fundamentally a kinetic process. Thus, the model may be named as physiologically based when all drug distributed to body organs are identified. For data analysis, parameters are obtained quantitatively with different assumptions. The model analysis may be compartmental or noncompartmental (Chapter 25). One approach is to classify models simply as empirically based models and mechanistic models. Although compartment models are critically referred to as a "black box" approach and not physiological. The versatility of compartment models and their easy application are based on simple mass transfer algorithms or a system of differential equations. This approach has allowed many body processes such as binding, transport, and metabolic clearance to be monitored. The advantage of a noncompartmental analysis is discussed in Chapter 25. In Appendix B, softwares used for various type of model analysis are discussed, for example, noncompartmental analysis is often used for pharmacokinetic and bioavailability data analysis for regulatory purpose.

1998

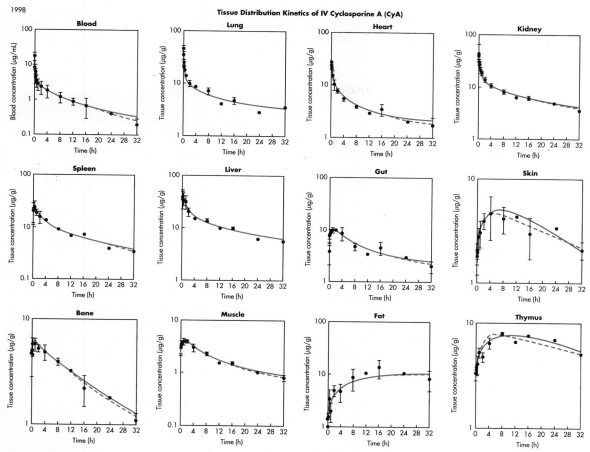

FIGURE 1-10   Measured and best fit predictions of CyA concentration in arterial blood and various organs/tissues in rat. Each plot and vertical bar represent the mean and standard deviation, respectively. Solid and dotted lines are the physiological-based pharmacokinetic (PBPK) best fit predictions based on the parameters associated with the linear or nonlinear model, respectively. (Reproduced with permission from Kawai R, Mathew D, Tanaka C, Rowland M: Physiologically based pharmacokinetics of cyclosporine A: Extension to tissue distribution kinetics in rats and scale-up to human. *JPET* **287:**457–468, 1998.)

CHAPTER SUMMARY

Drug product performance is the release of the drug substance from the drug product leading to bioavailability of the drug substance and eventually leading to one or more pharmacologic effects, both desirable and undesirable. *Biopharmaceutics* provides the scientific basis for drug product design and drug product performance by examining the interrelationship of the physical/chemical properties of the drug, the drug product in which the drug is given, and the route of administration on the rate and extent of systemic drug absorption. *Pharmacokinetics* is the science of the dynamics (kinetics) of drug absorption, distribution, and elimination (ie, excretion and metabolism), whereas *clinical pharmacokinetics* considers the applications of pharmacokinetics to drug therapy.

The quantitative measurement of drug concentrations in the plasma after dose administration is important to obtain relevant data of systemic drug exposure. The plasma drug concentration-versus-time profile provides the basic data from which various pharmacokinetic models can be developed that predict the time course of drug action, relates the

drug concentration to the pharmacodynamic effect or adverse response, and enables the development of individualized therapeutic dosage regimens and new and novel drug delivery systems.

LEARNING QUESTIONS

1. What is the significance of the plasma level–time curve? How does the curve relate to the pharmacologic activity of a drug?

2. What is the purpose of pharmacokinetic models?

3. Draw a diagram describing a three-compartment model with first-order absorption and drug elimination from compartment 1.

4. The pharmacokinetic model presented in Fig. 1-11 represents a drug that is eliminated by renal excretion, biliary excretion, and drug metabolism. The metabolite distribution is described by a one-compartment open model. The following questions pertain to Fig. 1-11.

   a. How many parameters are needed to describe the model if the drug is injected intravenously (ie, the rate of drug absorption may be neglected)?

   b. Which compartment(s) can be sampled?

   c. What would be the overall elimination rate constant for elimination of drug from compartment 1?

   d. Write an expression describing the rate of change of drug concentration in compartment 1 (dC_1/dt).

5. Give two reasons for the measurement of the plasma drug concentration, C_p, assuming (a) the C_p relates directly to the pharmacodynamic activity of the drug and (b) the C_p does not relate to the pharmacodynamic activity of the drug.

6. Consider two biologic compartments separated by a biologic membrane. Drug A is found in compartment 1 and in compartment 2 in a concentration of c_1 and c_2, respectively.

   a. What possible conditions or situations would result in concentration $c_1 > c_2$ at equilibrium?

   b. How would you experimentally demonstrate these conditions given above?

   c. Under what conditions would $c_1 = c_2$ at equilibrium?

   d. The total amount of Drug A in each biologic compartment is A_1 and A_2, respectively. Describe a condition in which $A_1 > A_2$, but $c_1 = c_2$ at equilibrium.

   Include in your discussion, how the physico-chemical properties of Drug A or the biologic properties of each compartment might influence equilibrium conditions.

7. Why is it important for a pharmacist to keep up with possible label revision in a drug newly approved? Which part of the label you expect to be mostly likely revised with more phase 4 information?

   a. The chemical structure of the drug

   b. The Description section

   c. Adverse side effect in certain individuals

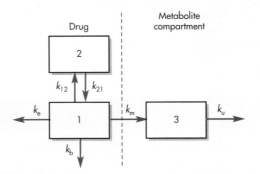

FIGURE 1-11 Pharmacokinetic model for a drug eliminated by renal and biliary excretion and drug metabolism. k_m = rate constant for metabolism of drug; k_u = rate constant for urinary excretion of metabolites; k_b = rate constant for biliary excretion of drug; and k_e = rate constant for urinary drug excretion.

8. A pharmacist wishing to find if an excipient such as aspartame in a product is mostly found under which section in the SPL drug label?
   a. How supplied
   b. Patient guide
   c. Description

9. A pregnant patient is prescribed pantoprazole sodium (Protonix) delayed release tablets for erosive gastroesophageal reflux disease (GERD). Where would you find information concerning the safety of this drug in pregnant women?

ANSWERS

Frequently Asked Questions

Why are drug concentrations more often measured in plasma rather than whole blood or serum?

- Blood is composed of plasma and red blood cells (RBCs). Serum is the fluid obtained from blood after it is allowed to clot. Serum and plasma do not contain identical proteins. RBCs may be considered a cellular component of the body in which the drug concentration in the serum or plasma is in equilibrium, in the same way as with the other tissues in the body. Whole blood samples are generally harder to process and assay than serum or plasma samples. Plasma may be considered a liquid tissue compartment in which the drug in the plasma fluid equilibrates with drug in the tissues and cellular components.

At what time intervals should plasma drug concentration be taken in order to best predict drug response and side effects?

- The exact site of drug action is generally unknown for most drugs. The time needed for the drug to reach the site of action, produce a pharmacodynamic effect, and reach equilibrium are deduced from studies on the relationship of the time course for the drug concentration and the pharmacodynamic effect. Often, the drug concentration is sampled during the elimination phase after the drug has been distributed and reached equilibrium. For multiple-dose studies, both the peak and trough drug concentrations are frequently taken.

What are the reasons to use a multicompartment model instead of a physiologic model?

- Physiologic models are complex and require more information for accurate prediction compared to compartment models. Missing information in the physiologic model will lead to bias or error in the model. Compartment models are more simplistic in that they assume that both arterial and venous drug concentrations are similar. The compartment model accounts for a rapid distribution phase and a slower elimination phase. Physiologic clearance models postulate that arterial blood drug levels are higher than venous blood drug levels. In practice, only venous blood samples are usually sampled. Organ drug clearance is useful in the treatment of cancers and in the diagnosis of certain diseases involving arterial perfusion. Physiologic models are difficult to use for general application.

Learning Questions

1. The plasma drug level–time curve describes the pharmacokinetics of the systemically absorbed drug. Once a suitable pharmacokinetic model is obtained, plasma drug concentrations may be predicted following various dosage regimens such as single oral and IV bolus doses, multiple-dose regimens, IV infusion, etc. If the pharmacokinetics of the drug relates to its pharmacodynamic activity (or any adverse drug response or toxicity), then a drug regimen based on the drug's pharmacokinetics may be designed to provide optimum drug efficacy. In lieu of a direct

pharmacokinetic–pharmacodynamic relationship, the drug's pharmacokinetics describes the
bioavailability of the drug including inter- and
intrasubject variability; this information allows
for the development of drug products that consistently deliver the drug in a predictable manner.

2. The purpose of pharmacokinetic models is to
relate the time course of the drug in the body to
its pharmacodynamic and/or toxic effects. The
pharmacokinetic model also provides a basis
for drug product design, the design of dosage
regimens, and a better understanding of the
action of the body on the drug.

3. (Figure A-1)

4. **a.** Nine parameters: V_1, V_2, V_3, k_{12}, k_{21}, k_e, k_b, k_m, k_u

   b. Compartment 1 and compartment 3 may be
   sampled.

   c. $k = k_b + k_m + k_e$

   d. $\dfrac{dC_1}{dt} = k_{21}C_2 - (k_{12} + k_m + k_e + k_b)C_1$

6.

Compartment 1	Compartment 2
C_1	C_2

   a. C_1 and C_2 are the *total* drug concentration in
   each compartment, respectively. $C_1 > C_2$ may
   occur if the drug concentrates in compartment 1 due to protein binding (compartment
   1 contains a high amount of protein or special
   protein binding), due to partitioning (compartment 1 has a high lipid content and the drug is
   poorly water soluble), if the pH is different in
   each compartment and the drug is a weak electrolyte (the drug may be more ionized in compartment 1), or if there is an active transport
   mechanism for the drug to be taken up into the

cell (eg, purine drug). Other explanations for
$C_1 > C_2$ may be possible.

   b. Several different experimental conditions are
   needed to prove which of the above hypotheses is the most likely cause for $C_1 > C_2$.
   These experiments may use *in vivo* or *in vitro*
   methods, including intracellular electrodes to
   measure pH *in vivo*, protein-binding studies
   in vitro, and partitioning of drug in chloro-
   form/water *in vitro*, among others.

   c. In the case of protein binding, the total
   concentration of drug in each compartment
   may be different (eg, $C_1 > C_2$) and, at the
   same time, the free (nonprotein-bound)
   drug concentration may be equal in each
   compartment—assuming that the free or
   unbound drug is easily diffusible. Similarly,
   if $C_1 > C_2$ is due to differences in pH and the
   nonionized drug is easily diffusible, then the
   nonionized drug concentration may be the
   same in each compartment. The total drug
   concentrations will be $C_1 = C_2$ when there
   is similar affinity for the drug and similar
   conditions in each compartment.

   d. The total amount of drug, A, in each compartment depends on the volume, V, of the
   compartment and the concentration, C, of the
   drug in the compartment. Since the amount
   of drug (A) = concentration (C) times volume
   (V), any condition that causes the product,
   $C_1V_1 \neq C_2V_2$, will result in $A_1 \neq A_2$. Thus, if
   $C_1 = C_2$ and $V_1 \neq V_2$, then $A_1 \neq A_2$.

7. A newly approved NDA generally contains
sufficient information for use labeled. However,
as more information becomes available through
postmarketing commitment studies, more
information is added to the labeling, including
Warnings and Precautions.

8. An excipient such as aspartame in a product
is mostly found under the Description section,
which describes the drug chemical structure
and the ingredients in the drug product.

9. Section 8, Use in Specific Populations, reports
information for geriatric, pediatric, renal, and
hepatic subjects. This section will report dosing
for pediatric subjects as well.

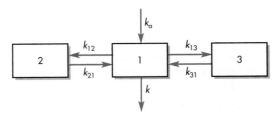

FIGURE A-1

REFERENCES

Cone EJ, Darwin WD, Wang W-L: The occurrence of cocaine, heroin and metabolites in hair of drug abusers. *Forensic Sci Int* **63:**55–68, 1993.

FDA Guidance for Industry: Exposure-Response Relationships—Study Design, Data Analysis, and Regulatory Applications, FDA, Center for Drug Evaluation and Research, April 2003 (http://www.fda.gov/cder/guidance/5341fnl.htm).

FDA Guidance for Industry: Labeling for Human Prescription Drug and Biological Products – Implementing the PLR Content and Format Requirements, February 2013.

Kawai R, Mathew D, Tanaka C, Rowland M: Physiologically based pharmacokinetics of cyclosporine.

Leal M, Yacobi A, Batra VJ: Use of toxicokinetic principles in drug development: Bridging preclinical and clinical studies. In Yacobi A, Skelly JP, Shah VP, Benet LZ (eds). *Integration of Pharmacokinetics, Pharmacodynamics and Toxicokinetics in Rational Drug Development.* New York, Plenum Press, 1993, pp 55–67.

Mallet A, Mentre F, Steimer JL, Lokiec F: Pharmacometrics: Nonparametric maximum likelihood estimation for population pharmacokinetics, with application to cyclosporine. *J Pharm Biopharm* **16:**311–327, 1988.

Pippenger CE, Massoud N: Therapeutic drug monitoring. In Benet LZ, et al (eds). *Pharmacokinetic Basis for Drug Treatment.* New York, Raven, 1984, chap 21.

Rodman JH, Evans WE: Targeted systemic exposure for pediatric cancer therapy. In D'Argenio DZ (ed). *Advanced Methods of Pharmacokinetic and Pharmacodynamic Systems Analysis.* New York, Plenum Press, 1991, pp 177–183.

Sawada Y, Hanano M, Sugiyama Y, Iga T: Prediction of the disposition of nine weakly acidic and six weakly basic drugs in humans from pharmacokinetic parameters in rats. *J Pharmacokinet Biopharm* **13:**477–492, 1985.

Sheiner LB, Beal SL: Bayesian individualization of pharmacokinetics. Simple implementation and comparison with non Bayesian methods. *J Pharm Sci* **71:**1344–1348, 1982.

Sheiner LB, Ludden TM: Population pharmacokinetics/dynamics. *Annu Rev Pharmacol Toxicol* **32:**185–201, 1992.

Tucker GT, Boas RA: Pharmacokinetic aspects of intravenous regional anesthesia.

BIBLIOGRAPHY

Benet LZ: General treatment of linear mammillary models with elimination from any compartment as used in pharmacokinetics. *J Pharm Sci* **61:**536–541, 1972.

Benowitz N, Forsyth R, Melmon K, Rowland M: Lidocaine disposition kinetics in monkey and man. *Clin Pharmacol Ther* **15:**87–98, 1974.

Bischoff K, Brown R: Drug distribution in mammals. *Chem Eng Med* **62:**33–45, 1966.

Tucker GT, Boas RA:Pharmacokinetic aspects of intravenous regional anesthesia.

Bischoff K, Dedrick R, Zaharko D, Longstreth T: Methotrexate pharmacokinetics. *J Pharm Sci* **60:**1128–1133, 1971.

Chiou W: Quantitation of hepatic and pulmonary first-pass effect and its implications in pharmacokinetic study, I: Pharmacokinetics of chloroform in man. *J Pharm Biopharm* **3:**193–201, 1975.

Colburn WA: Controversy III: To model or not to model. *J Clin Pharmacol* **28:**879–888, 1988.

Cowles A, Borgstedt H, Gilles A: Tissue weights and rates of blood flow in man for the prediction of anesthetic uptake and distribution. *Anesthesiology* **35:**523–526, 1971.

Dedrick R, Forrester D, Cannon T, et al: Pharmacokinetics of 1-β-d-arabinofurinosulcytosine (ARA-C) deamination in several species. *Biochem Pharmacol* **22:**2405–2417, 1972.

Gerlowski LE, Jain RK: Physiologically based pharmacokinetic modeling: Principles and applications. *J Pharm Sci* **72:** 1103–1127, 1983.

Gibaldi M: *Biopharmaceutics and Clinical Pharmacokinetics,* 3rd ed. Philadelphia, Lea & Febiger, 1984.

Gibaldi M: Estimation of the pharmacokinetic parameters of the two-compartment open model from post-infusion plasma concentration data. *J Pharm Sci* **58:**1133–1135, 1969.

Himmelstein KJ, Lutz RJ: A review of the applications of physiologically based pharmacokinetic modeling. *J Pharm Biopharm* **7:**127–145, 1979.

Lutz R, Dedrick RL: Physiologic pharmacokinetics: Relevance to human risk assessment. In Li AP (ed). *Toxicity Testing: New Applications and Applications in Human Risk Assessment.* New York, Raven, 1985, pp 129–149.

Lutz R, Dedrick R, Straw J, et al: The kinetics of methotrexate distribution in spontaneous canine lymphosarcoma. *J Pharm Biopharm* **3:**77–97, 1975.

Metzler CM: Estimation of pharmacokinetic parameters: Statistical considerations. *Pharmacol Ther* **13:**543–556, 1981.

Montandon B, Roberts R, Fischer L: Computer simulation of sulfobromophthalein kinetics in the rat using flow-limited models with extrapolation to man. *J Pharm Biopharm* **3:**277–290, 1975.

Rescigno A, Beck JS: The use and abuse of models. *J Pharm Biopharm* **15:**327–344, 1987.

Ritschel WA, Banerjee PS: Physiologic pharmacokinetic models: Applications, limitations and outlook. *Meth Exp Clin Pharmacol* **8:**603–614, 1986.

Rowland M, Tozer T: *Clinical Pharmacokinetics—Concepts and Applications,* 3rd ed. Philadelphia, Lea & Febiger, 1995.

Rowland M, Thomson P, Guichard A, Melmon K: Disposition kinetics of lidocaine in normal subjects. *Ann NY Acad Sci* **179:**383–398, 1971.

Segre G: Pharmacokinetics: Compartmental representation. *Pharm Ther* **17**:111–127, 1982.

Tozer TN: Pharmacokinetic principles relevant to bioavailability studies. In Blanchard J, Sawchuk RJ, Brodie BB (eds). *Principles and Perspectives in Drug Bioavailability*. New York, S Karger, 1979, pp 120–155.

Wagner JG: Do you need a pharmacokinetic model, and, if so, which one? *J Pharm Biopharm* **3**:457–478, 1975.

Welling P, Tse F: *Pharmacokinetics*. New York, Marcel Dekker, 1993.

Winters ME: *Basic Clinical Pharmacokinetics*, 3rd ed. Vancouver, WA, Applied Therapeutics, 1994.

2 Mathematical Fundamentals in Pharmacokinetics

Antoine Al-Achi

Chapter Objectives[1]

► Algebraically solve mathematical expressions related to pharmacokinetics.

► Express the calculated and theoretical pharmacokinetic values in proper units.

► Represent pharmacokinetic data graphically using Cartesian coordinates (rectangular coordinate system) and semilogarithmic graphs.

► Use the least squares method to find the best fit straight line through empirically obtained data.

► Define various models representing rates and order of reactions and calculate pharmacokinetic parameters (eg, zero- and first-order) from experimental data based on these models.

CALCULUS

Pharmacokinetic models consider drugs in the body to be in a dynamic state. Calculus is an important mathematic tool for analyzing drug movement quantitatively. Differential equations are used to relate the concentrations of drugs in various body organs over time. Integrated equations are frequently used to model the cumulative therapeutic or toxic responses of drugs in the body.

Differential Calculus

Differential calculus is a branch of calculus that involves finding the rate at which a variable quantity is changing. For example, a specific amount of drug X is placed in a beaker of water to dissolve. The rate at which the drug dissolves is determined by the rate of drug diffusing away from the surface of the solid drug and is expressed by the *Noyes–Whitney equation*:

$$\text{Dissolution rate} = \frac{dX}{dt} = \frac{DA}{l}(C_1 - C_2)$$

where d denotes a very small change; X = drug X; t = time; D = diffusion coefficient; A = effective surface area of drug; l = length of diffusion layer; C_1 = surface concentration of drug in the diffusion layer; and C_2 = concentration of drug in the bulk solution.

The derivative dX/dt may be interpreted as a change in X (or a derivative of X) with respect to a change in t.

In pharmacokinetics, the amount or concentration of drug in the body is a variable quantity (dependent variable), and time is considered to be an independent variable. Thus, we consider the amount or concentration of drug to vary with respect to time.

---

[1]It is not the objective of this chapter to provide a detailed description of mathematical functions, algebra, or statistics. Readers who are interested in learning more about these topics are encouraged to consult textbooks specifically addressing these subjects.

EXAMPLE ▶▶▶

The concentration C of a drug changes as a function of time t:

$$C = f(t) \qquad (2.1)$$

Consider the following data:

Time (hours)	Plasma Concentration of Drug C (μg/mL)
0	12
1	10
2	8
3	6
4	4
5	2

The concentration of drug C in the plasma is declining by 2 μg/mL for each hour of time. The rate of change in the concentration of the drug with respect to time (ie, the derivative of C) may be expressed as

$$\frac{dc}{dt} = 2\ \mu\text{g/mL/h}$$

Here, $f(t)$ is a mathematical equation that describes how C changes, expressed as

$$C = 12 - 2t \qquad (2.2)$$

Integral Calculus

Integration is the reverse of differentiation and is considered the summation of $f(x) \cdot dx$; the integral sign $\int$ implies summation. For example, given the function $y = ax$, plotted in Fig. 2-1, the integration is $\int ax \cdot dx$. Compare Fig. 2-1 to a second graph (Fig. 2-2), where the function $y = Ae^{-x}$ is commonly observed after an intravenous bolus drug injection. The integration process is actually a summing up of the small individual pieces under the graph. When x is specified and is given boundaries from a to b, then the expression becomes a definite integral, that is, the summing up of the area from $x = a$ to $x = b$.

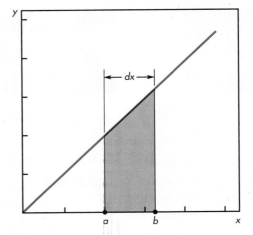

FIGURE 2-1   Integration of $y = ax$ or $\int ax \cdot dx$.

A *definite integral* of a mathematical function is the sum of individual areas under the graph of that function. There are several reasonably accurate numerical methods for approximating an area. These methods can be programmed into a computer for rapid calculation. The *trapezoidal rule* is a numerical method frequently used in pharmacokinetics to calculate the area under the plasma drug concentration-versus-time curve, called the *area under the curve* (AUC). For example, Fig. 2-2 shows a curve depicting the elimination of a drug from the plasma after a single intravenous injection. The drug plasma levels and the corresponding time intervals plotted in Fig. 2-2 are as follows:

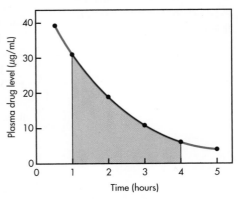

FIGURE 2-2   Graph of the elimination of drug from the plasma after a single IV injection.

Time (hours)	Plasma Drug Level (μg/mL)
0.5	38.9
1.0	30.3
2.0	18.4
3.0	11.1
4.0	6.77
5.0	4.10

The area between time intervals is the area of a trapezoid and can be calculated with the following formula:

$$[AUC]_{t_{n-1}}^{t_n} = \frac{C_{n-1} + C_n}{2}(t_n - t_{n-1}) \qquad (2.3)$$

where [AUC] = area under the curve, t_n = time of observation of drug concentration C_n, and t_{n-1} = time of prior observation of drug concentration corresponding to C_{n-1}.

To obtain the AUC from 1 to 4 hours in Fig. 2-2, each portion of this area must be summed. The AUC between 1 and 2 hours is calculated by proper substitution into Equation 2.3:

$$[AUC]_{t_1}^{t_2} = \frac{30.3 + 18.4}{2}(2-1) = 24.35 \ \mu g \cdot h/mL$$

Similarly, the AUC between 2 and 3 hours is calculated as 14.75 μg·h/mL, and the AUC between 3 and 4 hours is calculated as 8.94 μg·h/mL. The total AUC between 1 and 4 hours is obtained by adding the three smaller AUC values together.

$$[AUC]_{t_1}^{t_4} = [AUC]_{t_1}^{t_2} + [AUC]_{t_2}^{t_3} + [AUC]_{t_3}^{t_4}$$
$$= 24.3 + 14.3 + 8.94$$
$$= 48.04 \ \mu g \cdot h/mL$$

The total area under the plasma drug level–time curve from time zero to infinity (Fig. 2-2) is obtained by summation of each individual area between each pair of consecutive data points using the trapezoidal rule. The value on the y axis when time equals 0 is estimated by back extrapolation of the data points using a log linear plot (ie, log y vs x). The last plasma level–time curve is extrapolated to $t = \infty$. In this case the residual area $[AUC]_{t_n}^{t_\infty}$ is calculated as follows:

$$[AUC]_{t_n}^{t_\infty} = \frac{C_{pn}}{k} \qquad (2.4)$$

where C_{pn} = last observed plasma concentration at t_n and k = slope obtained from the terminal portion of the curve.

The trapezoidal rule written in its full form to calculate the AUC from $t = 0$ to $t = \infty$ is as follows:

$$[AUC]_0^\infty = \Sigma[AUC]_{t_{n-1}}^{t_n} + \frac{C_{pn}}{k}$$

This numerical method of obtaining the AUC is fairly accurate if sufficient data points are available. As the number of data points increases, the trapezoidal method of approximating the area becomes more accurate.

The trapezoidal rule assumes a linear or straight-line function between data points. If the data points are spaced widely, then the normal curvature of the line will cause a greater error in the area estimate.

Frequently Asked Questions

▶ *What are the units for logarithms?*

▶ *What is the difference between a common log and a natural log (ln)?*

GRAPHS

The construction of a curve or straight line by plotting observed or experimental data on a graph is an important method of visualizing relationships between variables. By general custom, the values of the independent variable (x) are placed on the horizontal line in a plane, or on the abscissa (x axis), whereas the values of the dependent variable are placed on the vertical line in the plane, or on the ordinate (y axis). The values are usually arranged so that they increase linearly or logarithmically from left to right and from bottom to top.

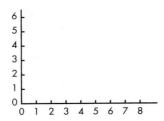

FIGURE 2-3   Rectangular coordinates.

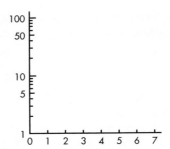

FIGURE 2-4   Semilog coordinates.

In pharmacokinetics, time is the independent variable and is plotted on the abscissa (x axis), whereas drug concentration is the dependent variable and is plotted on the ordinate (y axis). Two types of graphs or graph papers are usually used in pharmacokinetics. These are Cartesian or rectangular coordinate (Fig. 2-3) and semilogarithmic graph or graph paper (Fig. 2-4). Semilogarithmic allows placement of the data at logarithmic intervals so that the numbers need not be converted to their corresponding log values prior to plotting on the graph.

Curve Fitting

Fitting a curve to the points on a graph implies that there is some sort of relationship between the variables x and y, such as dose of drug versus pharmacologic effect (eg, lowering of blood pressure). Moreover, when using curve fitting, the relationship is not confined to isolated points but is a continuous function of x and y. In many cases, a hypothesis is made concerning the relationship between the variables x and y. Then, an empirical equation is formed that best describes the hypothesis. This empirical equation must satisfactorily fit the experimental or observed data. If the relationship between x and y is linearly related, then the relationship between the two can be expressed as a straight line.

Physiologic variables are not always linearly related. However, the data may be arranged or transformed to express the relationship between the variables as a straight line. Straight lines are very useful for accurately *predicting* values for which there are no experimental observations. The general equation of a straight line is

$$y = mx + b \qquad (2.5)$$

where m = slope and b = y intercept. Equation 2.5 could yield any one of the graphs shown in Fig. 2-5, depending on the value of m. The absolute magnitude of m gives some idea of the steepness of the curve. For example, as the value of m approaches 0, the line becomes more horizontal. As the absolute value of m becomes larger, the line slopes farther upward or downward, depending on whether m is positive or negative, respectively.

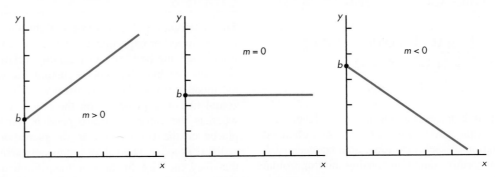

FIGURE 2-5   Graphic demonstration of variations in slope (m).

Linear Regression/Least Squares Method

This method is often encountered and used in clinical pharmacy studies to construct a linear relationship between an independent variable (also known as the input factor or the x factor) and a dependent variable (commonly known as an output variable, an outcome, or the y factor). In pharmacokinetics, the relationship between the plasma drug concentrations versus time can be expressed as a linear function. Because of the availability of computing devices (computer programs, scientific calculators, etc), the development of a linear equation has indeed become a simple task. A general format for a linear relationship is often expressed as:

$$y = mx + b \qquad (2.6)$$

where y is the dependent variable, x is the independent variable, m is the slope, and b is the y intercept. The value of the slope and the y intercept may be positive, negative, or zero. A positive linear relationship has a positive slope, and a negative slope belongs to a negative linear relationship (Gaddis and Gaddis, 1990; Munro, 2005).

The strength of the linear relationship is assessed by the correlation coefficient (r). The value of r is positive when the slope is positive and it is negative when the slope is negative. When r takes the value of either +1 or −1, a perfect relationship exists between the variables. A zero value for the slope (or for r) indicates that there is no linear relationship existing between y and x. In addition to r, the coefficient of determination (r^2) is often computed to express how much variability in the outcome is explained by the input factor. For example, if r is 0.90, then r^2 equals to 0.81. This means that the input variable explains 81% of the variability observed in y. It should be noted, however, that a high correlation between the two variables does not necessarily mean causation. For example, the passage of time is not really the cause for the drug concentration in the plasma to decrease. Rather it is the distribution and the elimination functions that cause the level of the drug to decrease over time (Gaddis and Gaddis, 1990; Munro, 2005).

The linear regression/least squares method assumes, for simplicity, that there is a linear relationship between the variables. If a linear line deviates substantially from the data, it may suggest the need for a nonlinear regression model, although several variables (multiple linear regression) may be involved. Nonlinear regression models are complex mathematical procedures that are best performed with a computer program.

> **Frequently Asked Questions**
> ▶ How is the area under the curve, AUC, calculated? What are the units for AUC?
>
> ▶ How do you know that the line that you fit to produce a curve on a graph is the line of best fit?
>
> ▶ What assumptions are made when a line is fitted to the points on a graph?

PRACTICE PROBLEM

Plot the following data and obtain the equation for the line that best fits the data by (a) using a ruler and (b) using the method of least squares. Data can be plotted manually or by using a computer spreadsheet program such as Microsoft Excel.

x (mg)	y (hours)	x (mg)	y (hours)
1	3.1	5	15.3
2	6.0	6	17.9
3	8.7	7	22.0
4	12.9	8	23.0

Solution

Many computer programs have a regression analysis, which fits data to a straight line by least squares. In the least squares method, the slope m and the y intercept b (Equation 2.7) are calculated so that the average sum of the deviations squared is minimized. The deviation, d, is defined by

$$b + mx - y = d \qquad (2.7)$$

If there are no deviations from linearity, then $d = 0$ and the exact form of Equation 2.7 is as follows:

$$b + mx - y = 0$$

To find the slope, m, and the intercept, b, the following equations are used:

$$m = \frac{\Sigma(x)\Sigma(y) - n\Sigma(xy)}{[\Sigma(x)]^2 - n\Sigma(x^2)} \qquad (2.8)$$

where n = number of data points.

$$b = \frac{\Sigma(x)\Sigma(xy) - \Sigma(x^2)\Sigma y}{[\Sigma(x)]^2 - n\Sigma(x^2)} \qquad (2.9)$$

where Σ is the sum of n data points.

The following graph was obtained by using a Microsoft Excel spreadsheet and calculating a regression line (sometimes referred to as a trendline in the computer program):

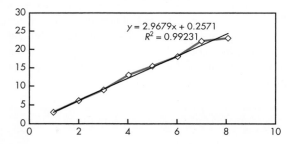

Therefore, the linear equation that best fits the data is

$$y = 2.97x + 0.257$$

Although an equation for a straight line is obtained by the least squares procedure, the reliability of the values should be ascertained. A correlation coefficient, r, is a useful statistical term that indicates the relationship of the x, y data fit to a straight line. For a perfect linear relationship between x and y, $r = +1$. Usually, $r \geq 0.95$ demonstrates good evidence or a strong correlation that there is a linear relationship between x and y.

Problems of Fitting Points to a Graph

When x and y data points are plotted on a graph, a relationship between the x and y variables is sought. Linear relationships are useful for predicting values for the dependent variable y, given values for the independent variable x.

The *linear regression* calculation using the least squares method is used for calculating a straight line through a given set of points. However, it is important to realize that, when using this method, one has already assumed that the data points are related linearly. Indeed, for three points, this linear relationship may not always be true. As shown in Fig. 2-6, Riggs (1963) calculated three different curves that fit the data accurately. Generally, one should consider the *law of parsimony*, which broadly means "keep it simple"; that is, if a choice between two hypotheses is available, choose the more simple relationship.

If a linear relationship exists between the x and y variables, one must be careful as to the estimated value for the dependent variable y, assuming a value for the independent variable x. *Interpolation*, which means filling the gap between the observed data on

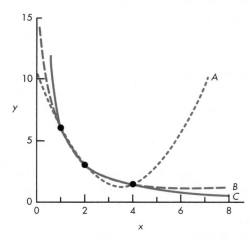

FIGURE 2-6   Three points equally well fitted by different curves. The parabola, $y = 10.5 - 5.25x + 0.75x^2$ (*curve A*); the exponential, $y = 12.93e^{-1.005}x + 1.27$ (*curve B*); and the rectangular hyperbola, $y = 6/x$ (*curve C*) all fit the three points (1,6), (2,3), and (4,1.5) perfectly, as would an infinite number of other curves. (Reprinted with permission from Riggs DS: The Mathematical Approach to Physiological Problems. Baltimore, Williams & Wilkins, 1963.)

a graph, is usually safe and assumes that the trend between the observed data points is consistent and predictable. In contrast, the process of *extrapolation* means predicting new data beyond the observed data, and assumes that the same trend obtained between two data points will extend in either direction beyond the last observed data points. The use of extrapolation may be erroneous if the regression line no longer follows the same trend beyond the measured points.

Graphs should always have the axes (abscissa and ordinate) properly labeled with units. For example, the amount of drug on the ordinate (*y* axis) is given in milligrams and the time on the abscissa (*x* axis) is given in hours. The equation that best fits the points on this curve is the equation for a straight line, or $y = mx + b$. Because the slope $m = \Delta y/\Delta x$, the units for the slope should be milligrams per hour (mg/h). Similarly, the units for the *y* intercept *b* should be the same units as those for *y*, namely, milligrams (mg).

MATHEMATICAL EXPRESSIONS AND UNITS

Mathematics is a basic science that helps to explain relationships among variables. For an equation to be valid, the units or dimensions must be constant on both sides of the equation. Many different units are used in pharmacokinetics, as listed in Table 2-1. For an accurate equation, both the integers and the units must balance. For example, a common expression for total body clearance is

$$Cl_T = kV_d \qquad (2.10)$$

After insertion of the proper units for each term in the above equation from Table 2-1,

$$\frac{\text{mL}}{\text{h}} = \frac{1}{\text{h}}\text{mL}$$

Thus, the above equation is valid, as shown by the equality mL/h = mL/h.

An important rule in using equations with different units is that the units may be added or subtracted as long as they are alike, but divided or multiplied if they are different. When in doubt, check the equation by inserting the proper units. For example,

$$\text{AUC} = \frac{FD_0}{kV_D} = \text{concentration} \times \text{time}$$

$$\frac{\mu g}{\text{mL}}\text{h} = \frac{1\,\text{mg}}{\text{h}^{-1}\,\text{L}} = \frac{\mu g \cdot \text{h}}{\text{mL}} \qquad (2.11)$$

Certain terms have no units. These terms include logarithms and ratios. Percent may have no units and is expressed mathematically as a decimal between 0 and 1 or as 0% to 100%, respectively. On occasion, percent may indicate mass/volume, volume/volume, or mass/mass. Table 2-1 lists common pharmacokinetic parameters with their symbols and units.

A constant is often inserted in an equation to quantify the relationship of the dependent variable to the independent variable. For example, *Fick's law of diffusion* relates the rate of drug diffusion, dQ/dt, to the change in drug concentration, *C*, the surface area of the membrane, *A*, and the thickness of the membrane, *h*. In order to make this relationship an equation, a diffusion constant *D* is inserted:

$$\frac{dQ}{dt} = \frac{DA}{h} \times \Delta C \qquad (2.12)$$

To obtain the proper units for *D*, the units for each of the other terms must be inserted:

$$\frac{\text{mg}}{\text{h}} = \frac{D(\text{cm}^2)}{\text{cm}} \times \frac{\text{mg}}{\text{cm}^3}$$

$$D = \text{cm}^2/\text{h}$$

The diffusion constant *D* must have the units of area/time or cm²/h if the rate of diffusion is in mg/h.

TABLE 2-1 Common Units Used in Pharmacokinetics

Parameter	Symbol	Unit	Example
Rate	$\dfrac{dD}{dt}$	$\dfrac{\text{Mass}}{\text{Time}}$	mg/h
	$\dfrac{dC}{dt}$	$\dfrac{\text{Concentration}}{\text{Time}}$	ug/mL/h
Zero-order rate constant	K_0	$\dfrac{\text{Concentration}}{\text{Time}}$	μg/mL/h
		$\dfrac{\text{Mass}}{\text{Time}}$	mg/h
First-order rate constant	k	$\dfrac{1}{\text{Time}}$	1/h or h^{-1}
Drug dose	D_0	Mass	mg
Concentration	C	$\dfrac{\text{Mass}}{\text{Volume}}$	μg/mL
Plasma drug concentration	Cp	$\dfrac{\text{Drug}}{\text{Volume}}$	μg/mL
Volume	V	Volume	mL or L
Area under the curve	AUC	Constration × time	μg·h/mL
Fraction of drug absorbed	F	No units	0 to 1
Clearance	Cl	$\dfrac{\text{Volume}}{\text{Time}}$	mL/h
Half-life	$t_{1/2}$	Time	H

UNITS FOR EXPRESSING BLOOD CONCENTRATIONS

Various units have been used in pharmacology, toxicology, and the clinical laboratory to express drug concentrations in blood, plasma, or serum. Drug concentrations or drug levels should be expressed as mass/volume. The expressions mcg/mL, μg/mL, and mg/L are equivalent and are commonly reported in the literature. Drug concentrations may also be reported as mg% or mg/dL, both of which indicate milligrams of drug per 100 mL (1 deciliter). Two older expressions for drug concentration occasionally used in veterinary medicine are the terms ppm and ppb, which indicate the number of parts of drug per million parts of blood (ppm) or per billion parts of blood (ppb), respectively. One ppm is equivalent to 1.0 μg/mL. The accurate interconversion of units is often necessary to prevent confusion and misinterpretation.

MEASUREMENT AND USE OF SIGNIFICANT FIGURES

Every measurement is performed within a certain degree of accuracy, which is limited by the instrument used for the measurement. For example, the weight of freight on a truck may be measured accurately to the nearest 0.5 kg, whereas the mass of drug in a tablet may be measured to 0.001 g (1 mg). Measuring the weight of freight on a truck to the nearest milligram is not necessary and would require a very costly balance or scale to detect a change in a milligram quantity.

Significant figures are the number of accurate digits in a measurement. If a balance measures the mass of a drug to the nearest milligram, measurements containing digits representing less than 1 mg are inaccurate. For example, in reading the weight or mass of a drug of 123.8 mg from this balance, the

0.8 mg is only approximate; the number is therefore rounded to 124 mg and reported as the observed mass.

For practical calculation purposes, all figures may be used until the final number (answer) is obtained. However, the answer should retain only the number of significant figures in the least accurate initial measurement.

PRACTICE PROBLEM

When a patient swallows a tablet containing 325 mg of aspirin (ASA), the tablet comes in contact with the contents of the gastrointestinal tract and the ASA is released from the tablet. Assuming a constant amount of the drug release over time (t), the rate of drug release is expressed as:

$$\text{Rate of drug (ASA) release (mg/min)} = \frac{d(\text{ASA})}{dt}$$
$$= k_0$$

where k_0 is a rate constant.

Integration of the rate expression above gives Equation 2.13:

$$\text{Amount of ASA released (mg)} = at + b \quad (2.13)$$

The symbol "a" represents the slope (equivalent to k_0), t is time, and b is the y intercept. Assuming that time was measured in minutes, the following mathematical expression is obtained representing Equation 2.13:

$$\text{Amount of ASA released (mg)} = 0.86t - 0.04 \quad (2.14)$$

To calculate the amount of ASA released at 180 seconds, the following algebraic manipulations are needed:

1. Convert 180 seconds to minutes: 3 minutes.
2. Replace t in Equation 2.14 by the value 3.
3. Solve the equation for the amount of ASA released.

$$\text{Amount of ASA released (mg)} = 0.86(3) - 0.04$$
$$= 2.54 \text{ mg}$$

A pharmacist is interested in learning the time needed for 90% of ASA to be released from the tablet. To answer her inquiry the following steps are taken:

1. Calculate the amount of ASA in milligrams representing 90% of the drug present in the tablet.
2. Replace the value found in step (1) in Equation 2.14 and solve for time (t):

90% of 325 = (0.9)(325 mg) = 292.5 mg
292.5 mg = 0.86t − 0.04
292.5 + 0.04 = 0.86t
Dividing both sides of the equation by 0.86:
(292.5 + 0.04)/0.86 = (0.86t)/0.86
340.07 minutes = t
Or it takes 5.7 hours for this amount of ASA (90%) to be released from the tablet.

The above calculations show that this tablet releases the drug very slowly over time and it may not be useful in practice when the need for the drug is more immediate. It should also be emphasized that only the amount of the drug released and soluble in the GI juices is available for absorption. If the drug precipitates out in the GI tract, it will not be absorbed by the GI mucosa. It is also assumed that the unabsorbed portion of the drug in the GI tract is considered to be "outside the body" because its effect cannot be exerted systematically.

To calculate the amount of ASA that was immediately released from the tablet upon contact with gastric juices, the time in Equation 2.14 is set to the value zero:

$$\text{Amount of ASA released (mg)} = 0.86(0) - 0.04$$

$$\text{Amount of ASA released (mg)} = -0.04 \text{ mg}$$

Since an amount released cannot be negative, this indicates that no amount of ASA is released from the tablet instantly upon coming in touch with the juices. Equation 2.14 may be represented graphically using Cartesian or rectangular coordinates (Fig. 2-7).

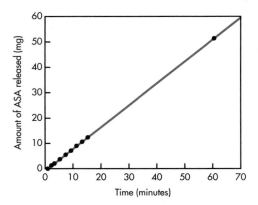

FIGURE 2-7   Amount of ASA released versus time (minutes) plotted on Cartesian coordinates.

PRACTICE PROBLEM

Briefly, C_{max} is the maximum drug concentration in the plasma and T_{max} is the time associated with C_{max}. First-order elimination rate constant signifies the fraction of the drug that is eliminated per unit time. The biological half-life of the drug is the time needed for 50% of the drug to be eliminated. The AUC term or the area under the drug plasma concentration-versus-time curve reflects the extent of absorption from the site of administration. The term AUMC is

the area under the moment curve, whereas MRT is the mean residence time, which is estimated from the ratio of AUMC(0–infinity)/AUC(0–infinity). These pharmacokinetic terms are discussed in more details throughout this textbook.

The below table (Ravi Shankar et al., 2012) shows pharmacokinetic data obtained from a study conducted in rabbits following administration of various formulations of rectal suppositories containing aspirin (600 mg each). Various formulations were prepared in a suppository base made of a mixture of gelatin and glycerin. Formulation Fas9 had the same composition as Fs9 with the exception that Fas9 contained ASA in the form of nanoparticles, whereas Fs9 had ASA in its free form (so did formulations Fs2, Fs4, and Fs11, but varied in their gelatin/glycerin composition). The authors concluded that the incorporation of ASA in the form of nanoparticles increased the T_{max}. The other pharmacokinetic parameters taken together indicate that nanoparticles produced a sustained-release profile of ASA when given in this dosage form. In this study, the plasma concentration was expressed in "micrograms per milliliter." If the $\mu g/mL$ were not specified, it would have been difficult to compare the results from this study with other similar studies. It is imperative, therefore, that pharmacokinetic parameters such as C_{max} be properly defined by units.

Pharmacokinetic Parameters	Fs2	Fs4	Fs9	Fs11	Fas9
C_{max} ($\mu g/mL$)	34.93 ± 0.60	31.16 ± 1.04	32.66 ± 1.52	35.33 ± 0.57	31.86 ± 0.41
T_{max} (hours)	1 ± 0.01	1 ± 0.03	1 ± 0.06	1 ± 0.09	6 ± 0.03
Elimination rate constant (h^{-1})	0.14 ± 0.02	0.19 ± 0.06	0.205 ± 0.03	0.17 ± 0.01	0.133 ± 0.004
Half-life (hours)	1.88 ± 0.76	1.9 ± 1.19	1.43 ± 0.56	1.99 ± 0.24	5.11 ± 0.15
AUC(0–t)	127.46 ± 8.9	126.62 ± 2.49	132.11 ± 3.88	127.08 ± 1.95	260.62 ± 4.44
AUC(0–infinity)(ng·h/mL)	138.36 ± 13.87	131.61 ± 0.27	136.89 ± 4.40	133.07 ± 2.97	300.48 ± 24.06
AUMC(0–t)(ng·h^2/mL)	524.51 ± 69.64	516.04 ± 28.25	557.84 ± 16.25	501.29 ± 26.65	2006.07 ± 38.00
AUMC(0–infinity)(ng·h^2/mL)	382.09 ± 131.45	237.74 ± 64.37	232.93 ± 28.16	257.71 ± 30.04	1494.71 ± 88.21
MRT (hours)	2.45 ± 0.36	2.31 ± 0.80	1.41 ± 0.31	2.95 ± 0.17	8.23 ± 0.06

Ravi Sankar V, Dachinamoorthi D, Chandra Shekar KB: A comparative pharmacokinetic study of aspirin suppositories and aspirin nanoparticles loaded suppositories. *Clinic Pharmacol Biopharm* **1**:105, 2012.

Expressing the C_{max} value by equivalent units is also possible. For example, converting μg/mL to mg/dL follows these steps:

1. Convert micrograms (also written as mcg) to milligrams.
2. Convert milliliters to deciliters:
   Since:
   1 mg = 1000 μg, then 31.86 μg/mL = 0.03186 mg/mL
   1 dL = 100 mL, then 31.86 μg/mL = 3186 μg/dL
   We have to divide the value of C_{max} by 1000 and multiply it by 100. The net effect is to divide the number by 10, or (31.86)(100/1000) = 3.19 mg/dL.

Expressing the C_{max} value 34.93 μg/mL in nanograms per microliter (ng/μL) is done as follows:

1. Convert the number of micrograms to nanograms.
2. Convert milliliters to microliters:

   1 μg = 1000 ng, or 34.93 μg/mL = 34,930 ng/mL
   1 mL = 1000 μL, or 34.93 μg/mL = 0.03493 μg/μL
   As 34.93 was multiplied and divided by the same number (1000), the final answer is 34.93 ng/μL.

Express the C_{max} value 35.33 μg/mL in %w/v (this is defined as the number of grams of ASA in 100 mL plasma).

(35.33 μg/mL)(100 mL) = 3533 μg/dL = 3.533 mg/dL = 0.0035 g/dL, or 0.0035% w/v (This means that there is 0.0035 g of ASA in every 100 mL plasma.)

The data (T_{max}, C_{max}) represent a maximum point on the plasma drug level-versus-time curve. This point reflects *the rate of absorption* of the drug from its site of administration. Another pharmacokinetic measure obtained from the same curve is the *area under the curve* (AUC). It reflects *the extent of absorption* for a drug from the site of administration into the circulation. The general format for the AUC

units is ([amount][time]/[volume]). Together, the rate and extent of absorption refers to the bioavailability of the drug from the site of administration. The term *"absolute bioavailability"* is used when the reference route of administration is the intravenous injection (ie, the IV route). If the reference route is different from the intravenous route, then the term *"relative bioavailability"* is used. The value for the AUC (0 to +∞) following the administration of Fs2, Fs4, and Fas9 was 138.36, 131.61, and 300.48 ng·h/mL, respectively (Ravi Sankar et al, 2012). The origin of the AUC units is based on the *trapezoidal rule*. The *trapezoidal rule* is a numerical method frequently used in pharmacokinetics to calculate the area under the plasma drug concentration-versus-time curve, called the *area under the curve* (AUC). This rule computes the average concentration value of each consecutive concentration and multiplies them by the difference in their time values. To compute the AUC (0 to time t), the sum of all these products is calculated. For example, AUC(0–t) = 127.46 ng·h/mL can be written as 127.46 (ng/mL)(h).

To convert 260.62 ng·h/mL to μg·-h/mL, divide the value by 1000 (recall that 1 μg is 1000 ng). Therefore, the AUC value becomes 0.26 μg·h/mL.

Expressing the AUC (0 to +∞) value 300.48 ng·h/mL in ng·min/mL can be accomplished by dividing 300.48 by 60 (1 hour is 60 min). Thus, the AUC value becomes 5.0 ng·min/mL.

Consider the following data:

Plasma Concentration (ng/L)	Time (hours)	AUC (ng·h/L)
0	0	0
0.05	1	0.025
0.10	2	0.075
0.18	3	0.140
0.36	5	0.540
0.13	7	0.490
0.08	9	0.210

To compute the AUC value from initial to 9 hours, sum up the values under the AUC column above (0.025 + 0.075 + ⋯ + 0.210 = 1.48 ng·h/L).

To convert the AUC value 1.48 ng·h/L to mg·min/dL, use the following steps:

1. Divide the value by 10^6 to convert the nanograms to milligrams.
2. Divide the value by 60 to convert the hours to minutes.
3. Divide the value by 10 to convert the liters to deciliters.

$$AUC = (1.48)/[(10^6)(60)(10)]$$
$$= 2.47 \times 10^{-9} \text{ mg·min/dL} \qquad (2.15)$$

Figure 2-8 represents the data in a rectangular coordinate–type graph. Time is placed on the x axis (*the abscissa*) and plasma concentration is placed on the y axis (*the ordinate*). The highest point on the graph can simply be determined by spotting it on the graph. Note that the plasma concentration declines *exponentially* from the apex point on the curve over time. Figure 2-9 shows the exponential portion of the graph on its own.

Exponential and Logarithmic Functions

These two mathematical functions are related to each other. For example, the pH of biological fluids (eg, plasma or urine) can influence all pharmacokinetic aspects including drug dissolution/release *in vitro* as well as systemic absorption, distribution, metabolism, and excretion. Since most drugs are either weak

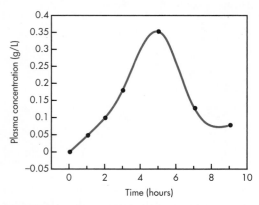

FIGURE 2-8   Plasma concentration (g/L)-versus-time (hours) curve plotted on Cartesian coordinates.

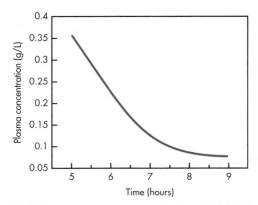

FIGURE 2-9   The exponential decline in plasma concentration over time portion in Fig. 2-8.

bases or weak acids, the pH of the biological fluid determines the degree of ionization of the drug and this in turns influences the pharmacokinetic profile of the drug. The pH scale is a logarithmic scale:

$$pH = -\log[H_3O^+] = \log(1/[H_3O^+]) \qquad (2.16)$$

where the symbol "log" is the *logarithm to base 10*. The *natural logarithm* has the symbol "ln," which is the logarithm to base e (the value of e is approximately 2.71828). The two functions are linked by the following expression:

$$\ln x = 2.303 \log x \qquad (2.17)$$

The concentration of hydronium ions $[H_3O^+]$ can be calculated from Equation 2.16 as follows:

$$[H_3O^+] = 10^{-pH} \qquad (2.18)$$

For example, the pH of a patient's plasma is 7.4 at room temperature. Therefore, the hydronium ion concentration in plasma is:

$$[H_3O^+] = 10^{-7.4} = 3.98 \times 10^{-8} \text{ M}$$

The value (3.98×10^{-8}) is the *antilogarithm* of 7.4. With the availability of scientific calculators and computers, these functions can be easily calculated.

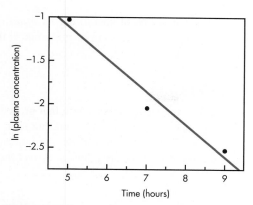

FIGURE 2-10   ln (Plasma concentration)-versus-time curve plotted on Cartesian coordinates.

Oftentimes, converting plasma concentrations to logarithmic values and plotting the logarithmic values against time would convert an exponential relationship to a linear function between the two variables. Consider, for example, Fig. 2-9. When the concentration values are converted to logarithmic values, the graph now becomes linear (Fig. 2-10). This same linear function may be obtained by plotting the *actual* values of the plasma concentration versus time using a semilogarithmic graph (Fig. 2-11). The following equation represents the straight line:

$$\ln (\text{Plasma concentration}) = 0.77 - 0.38 \; \text{Time (hours)}$$

$$(2.19)$$

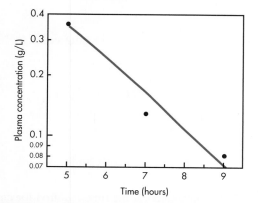

FIGURE 2-11   Plasma concentration-versus-time curve using a semilogarithmic graph.

The slope of the line is (−0.38). Thus,

$$\text{Slope} = -0.38 = -k_1$$

Multiplying both sides of the equation by (−1) results in:

$$k_1 = 0.38 \; \text{h}^{-1}$$

where k_1 is *the first-order elimination rate constant.* The units for this constant are reciprocal time, such as h^{-1} or $1/\text{h}$. The value $0.38 \; \text{h}^{-1}$ means that 38% of the concentration remaining of the drug in plasma is eliminated every hour.

Using Equation 2.17, Equation 2.19 can be converted to the following expression:

$$2.303 \, [\log (\text{Plasma concentration})] = 0.77 - 0.38 \; \text{Time (hours)}$$

Dividing both sides of the equation by 2.303:

$$2.303 \, [\log (\text{Plasma concentration})]/2.303 = [0.77 - 0.38 \; \text{Time (hours)}]/2.303$$

$$\log (\text{Plasma concentration}) = 0.334 - 0.17 \; \text{Time (hours)}$$

$$(2.20)$$

Equation 2.20 is mathematically equivalent to Equation 2.19.

The value 0.77 in Equation 2.19 equals ($\ln C_0$), where C_0 is the initial concentration of the drug in plasma. Thus,

$$\ln C_0 = 0.77$$

$$C_0 = e^{0.77} = 2.16 \; \text{g/L}$$

Once k_1 is known, the AUC from the last data point to $t_{-\text{infinity}}$ can be calculated as follows:

$$\text{AUC} = C_{\text{Last}}/k_1 \qquad (2.21)$$

Applying Equation 2.21 on the data used to obtain the AUC value in Equation 2.15 results in the following value:

$$AUC = 0.08/0.38 = 0.21 \text{ g·h/L}$$

And the total AUC ($t = 0$ to $t = $ infinity):

$$AUC_{Total} = 1.48 + 0.21 = 1.69 \text{ g·h/L}$$

The following rules may be useful in handling exponential and logarithmic functions. For this, if m and n are positive, then for the real numbers q and s (Howard, 1980):

Exponent rules:

1. $m^0 = 1$
2. $m^1 = m$
3. $m^{-1} = 1/m^1$
4. $m^q/m^s = m^{q-s}$
5. $(m^q)(m^s) = m^{q+s}$
6. $(m^q)^s = m^{qs}$
7. $(m^q/n^q) = (m/n)^q$
8. $(m^q)(n^q) = (mn)^q$

If z is any positive number other than 1 and if $z^y = x$, then following logarithmic rules apply:

Logarithm rules:

1. $y = \log_z x$ (y is the logarithm to the base z of x)
2. For $x > 1$, then $\log_e x = \ln x$ (where e is approximately 2.71828)
3. $\log_z x = (\ln x/\ln z)$
4. $\log_z mn = \log_z m + \log_z n$
5. $\log_q (m/n) = \log_q m - \log_q n$
6. $\log_z (1/m) = -\log_z m$
7. $\ln e = 1$
8. For $z = 10$, then $\log_z 1 = 0$
9. $\log_z m^h = h \log_z m$
10. For $z = 10$, then $(2.303) \log_z x = \ln x$

RATES AND ORDERS OF PROCESSES

Oftentimes a process such as drug absorption or drug elimination may be described by the *rate* by which the process proceeds. The rate of a process, in turn, may be defined in terms of specifying its *order*. In pharmacokinetics, two orders are of importance, the *zero order* and the *first order*.

Zero-Order Process

The rate of a zero-order process is one that proceeds over time (t) independent from the concentration of the drug (c). The negative sign for the rate indicates that the concentration of the drug decreases over time.

$$-dc/dt = k_0 \qquad (2.22)$$

$$dc = -k_0 \, dt$$

$$c = c_0 - k_0 t \qquad (2.23)$$

where c_0 is the initial concentration of the drug at $t = 0$ and k_0 is the zero-order rate constant. The units for k_0 are concentration per unit time (eg, [mg/mL]/h) or amount per unit time (eg, mg/h).

For example, calculate the zero-order rate constant ([ng/mL]/min) if the initial concentration of the drug is 200 ng/mL and that at $t = 30$ minutes is 35 ng/mL.

$$c = c_0 - k_0 t$$

$$35 = 200 - k_0 (30)$$

$$-k_0 = (35 - 200)/30 = -5.5$$

$$k_0 = 5.5 \text{ (ng/mL)/min}$$

When does the concentration of drug equal to 100 ng/mL?

$$100 = 200 - 5.5 t$$

$$(100 - 200)/5.5 = -t$$

$$-18.2 = -t$$

$$t = 18.2 \text{ min}$$

In pharmacokinetics, the time required for one-half of the drug concentration to disappear is known as $t_{1/2}$. Thus, for this drug the $t_{1/2}$ is 18.2 minutes.

In general, $t_{1/2}$ may be calculated as follows for a zero-order process:

$$c = c_0 - k_0 t$$

$$(0.5\,c_0) = c_0 - k_0 t_{1/2}$$

$$(0.5\,c_0) - c_0 = -k_0 t_{1/2}$$

$$-0.5\,c_0 = -k_0 t_{1/2}$$

$$t_{1/2} = (0.5\,c_0)/k_0 \qquad (2.24)$$

Applying Equation 2.24 to the example above should yield the same result:

$$t_{1/2} = (0.5\,c_0)/k_0$$

$$t_{1/2} = (0.5)(200)/5.5 = 18.2 \text{ minutes}$$

A plot of x versus time on rectangular coordinates produces a straight line with a slope equal to $(-k_0)$ and a y intercept as c_0. In a zero-order process the $t_{1/2}$ is not constant and depends upon the initial amount or concentration of drug.

First-Order Process

The rate of a first-order process is dependent upon the concentration of the drug:

$$-dc/dt = k_1 c$$

$$-dc/c = k_1 dt \qquad (2.25)$$

$$\ln c = \ln c_0 - k_1 t \qquad (2.26)$$

While the rate of the process is a function of the drug concentration, the $t_{1/2}$ is not:

$$\ln c = \ln c_0 - k_1 t$$

$$\ln (0.5\,c_0) = \ln c_0 - k_1 t_{1/2}$$

$$\ln (0.5\,c_0) - \ln c_0 = -k_1 t_{1/2}$$

$$\ln (0.5\,c_0/c_0) = -k_1 t_{1/2}$$

$$\ln 0.5/{-k_1} = t_{1/2}$$

$$t_{1/2} = -0.693/{-k_1}$$

$$t_{1/2} = 0.693/k_1 \qquad (2.27)$$

Unlike a zero-order rate process, the $t_{1/2}$ for a first-order rate process is always a constant, independent of the initial drug concentration or amount (Table 2-2, Fig. 2-12).

A plot between $\ln c$ versus t produces a straight line. A semilogarithmic graph also produces a straight line between c and t. The units of the first-order rate constant (k_1) are in reciprocal time.

TABLE 2-2   Comparison of Zero- and First-Order Reactions

	Zero-Order Reaction	First-Order Reaction
Equation	$-dC/dt = k_0$ $C = -k_0 t + C_0$	$-dC/dt = kC$ $C = C_0\,e^{-kt}$
Rate constant— units	(mg/L)/h	1/h
Half-life, $t_{1/2}$ (units = time)	$t_{1/2} = 0.5C/k_0$ (not constant)	$t_{1/2} = 0.693/k$ (constant)
Effect of time on rate	Zero-order rate is constant with respect to time	First-order rate will change with respect to time as concentration changes
Effect of time on rate constant	Rate constant with respect to time changes as the concentration changes	Rate constant remains constant with respect to time
Drug concentrations versus time—plotted on rectangular coordinates	Drug concentrations decline linearly for a zero-order rate process	Drug concentrations decline nonlinearly for a first-order rate process
Drug concentrations versus time—plotted on a semilogarithmic graph	Drug concentrations decline nonlinearly for a zero-order rate process	Drug concentrations decline linearly for a single first-order rate process

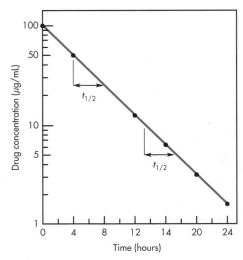

FIGURE 2-12   The $t_{1/2}$ in a first-order rate process is a constant.

For a drug with $k_1 = 0.04$ h^{-1}, find $t_{1/2}$.

$$t_{1/2} = 0.693/k_1$$

$$t_{1/2} = 0.693/0.04 = 17.3 \text{ hours}$$

The value 0.04 h^{-1} for the first-order rate constant indicates that 4% of the drug disappears every hour.

Calculate the time needed for 70% of the drug to disappear.

$$\ln c = \ln c_0 - k_1 t$$

$$\ln (0.3\, c_0) = \ln c_0 - k_1 t$$

$$\ln (0.3\, c_0) - \ln c_0 = -k_1 t$$

$$\ln 0.3/-k_1 = t$$

$$t = -1.2/-0.04 = 30 \text{ hours}$$

The value 30 hours may be written as $t_{30} = 30$ hours (it is t_{30} because 70% of the drug is eliminated).

Determination of Order

Graphical representation of experimental data provides a visual relationship between the x values (generally time) and the y axis (generally drug concentrations). Much can be learned by inspecting the line that connects the data points on a graph. The relationship between the x and y data will determine the order of the process, data quality, basic kinetics, and number of outliers, and provide the basis for an underlying pharmacokinetic model. To determine the order of reaction, first plot the data on a rectangular graph. If the data appear to be a curve rather than a straight line, the reaction rate for the data is non-zero order. In this case, plot the data on a semilog graph. If the data now appear to form a straight line with good correlation using linear regression, then the data likely follow first-order kinetics. This simple graph interpretation is true for one-compartment, IV bolus (Chapter 4). Curves that deviate from this format are discussed in other chapters in terms of route of administration and pharmacokinetic model.

> **Frequently Asked Questions**
> ▶ How is the rate and order of reaction determined graphically?
>
> ▶ What is the difference between a rate and a rate constant?

CHAPTER SUMMARY

Pharmacokinetic calculations require basic skills in mathematics. Although the availability of computer programs and scientific calculators facilitate pharmacokinetic calculations, the pharmaceutical scientist should be familiar with fundamental rules pertaining to calculus. The construction of a curve or straight line by plotting observed or experimental data on a graph is an important method of visualizing relationships between variables. The linear regression calculation using the least squares method is used for calculation of a straight line through a given set of points. However, it is important to realize that, when using this method, one has already assumed that the data points are related linearly. For all equations, both the integers and the units must balance. The rate of a process may be defined in terms of specifying its order. In pharmacokinetics, two orders are of importance, the *zero order* and the *first order*. Mathematical skills are important in pharmacokinetics in particular and in pharmacy in general.

LEARNING QUESTIONS

1. Plot the following data on both semilog graph paper and standard rectangular coordinates.

Time (minutes)	Drug A (mg)
10	96.0
20	89.0
40	73.0
60	57.0
90	34.0
120	10.0
130	2.5

   a. Does the decrease in the amount of drug *A* appear to be a zero-order or a first-order process?
   b. What is the rate constant *k*?
   c. What is the half-life $t_{1/2}$?
   d. Does the amount of drug *A* extrapolate to zero on the *x* axis?
   e. What is the equation for the line produced on the graph?

2. Plot the following data on both semilog graph paper and standard rectangular coordinates.

Time (minutes)	Drug A (mg)
4	70.0
10	58.0
20	42.0
30	31.0
60	12.0
90	4.5
120	1.7

Answer questions **a, b, c, d,** and **e** as stated in Question 1.

3. A pharmacist dissolved a few milligrams of a new antibiotic drug into exactly 100 mL of distilled water and placed the solution in a refrigerator (5°C). At various time intervals, the pharmacist removed a 10-mL aliquot from the solution and measured the amount of drug contained in each aliquot. The following data were obtained:

Time (hours)	Antibiotic (µg/mL)
0.5	84.5
1.0	81.2
2.0	74.5
4.0	61.0
6.0	48.0
8.0	35.0
12.0	8.7

   a. Is the decomposition of this antibiotic a first-order or a zero-order process?
   b. What is the rate of decomposition of this antibiotic?
   c. How many milligrams of antibiotics were in the original solution prepared by the pharmacist?
   d. Give the equation for the line that best fits the experimental data.

4. A solution of a drug was freshly prepared at a concentration of 300 mg/mL. After 30 days at 25°C, the drug concentration in the solution was 75 mg/mL.
   a. Assuming first-order kinetics, when will the drug decline to one-half of the original concentration?
   b. Assuming zero-order kinetics, when will the drug decline to one-half of the original concentration?

5. How many half-lives ($t_{1/2}$) would it take for 99.9% of any initial concentration of a drug to decompose? Assume first-order kinetics.

6. If the half-life for decomposition of a drug is 12 hours, how long will it take for 125 mg of the drug to decompose by 30%? Assume first-order kinetics and constant temperature.

7. Exactly 300 mg of a drug is dissolved into an unknown volume of distilled water. After complete dissolution of the drug, 1.0-mL samples were removed and assayed for the drug. The following results were obtained:

Time (hours)	Concentration (mg/mL)
0.5	0.45
2.0	0.3

Assuming zero-order decomposition of the drug, what was the original volume of water in which the drug was dissolved?

8. For most drugs, the overall rate of drug elimination is proportional to the amount of drug remaining in the body. What does this imply about the kinetic order of drug elimination?

9. A single cell is placed into a culture tube containing nutrient agar. If the number of cells doubles every 2 minutes and the culture tube is completely filled in 8 hours, how long does it take for the culture tube to be only half full of cells?

10. Cunha (2013) reported the following: "…CSF levels following 2 g of ceftriaxone are approximately 257 mcg/mL, which is well above the minimal inhibitory concentration (MIC) of even highly resistant (PRSP) in CSF…" What is the value of 257 mcg/mL in mg/mL?

11. Refer to Question 10 above; express the value 257 mcg/mL in mcg/dL.

12. The following information was provided by Steiner et al (2013):

"ACT-335827 hydrobromide (Actelion Pharmaceuticals Ltd., Switzerland) was freshly prepared in 10% polyethylene glycol 400/0.5% methylcellulose in water, which served as vehicle (Veh). It was administered orally at 300 mg/kg based on the weight of the free base, in a volume of 5 mL/kg, and administered daily 2 h before the onset of the dark phase."

How many milligrams of ACT-335827 hydrobromide would be given orally to a 170-g rat?

13. Refer to Question 12; how many milliliters of drug solution would be needed for the 170-g rat?

14. Refer to Question 12; express 0.5% methylcellulose (%w/v) as grams in 1 L solution.

15. The $t_{1/2}$ value for aceclofenac tablet following oral administration in Wistar male rats was reported to be 4.35 hours (Shakeel et al, 2009). Assuming a first-order process, what is the elimination rate constant value in hours^{-1}?

16. Refer to Question 15; express the value of $t_{1/2}$ in minutes.

17. Refer to Question 15; the authors reported that the relative bioavailability of aceclofenac from a transdermally applied gel is 2.6 folds higher compared to that of an oral tablet. The following equation was used by the authors to calculate the relative bioavailability:

$$F\% = \{[(AUC\ sample)(Dose\ oral)]/ [(AUC\ oral)(Dose\ sample)]\}*100 \quad (2.28)$$

where AUC/Dose sample is for the gel and AUC/Dose oral is for the tablet. *F*% is the relative bioavailability expressed in percent. If oral and transdermal doses were the same, calculate AUC sample given AUC oral of 29.1 μg·h/mL. What are the units for AUC sample in (mg·day/mL)?

18.

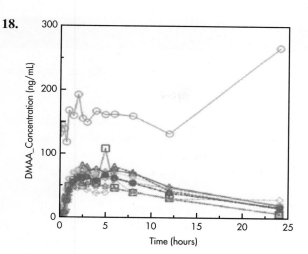

The above figure (from Basu Sarkar et al, 2013) shows the plasma concentration–time profile of DMAA (1,3-dimethylamylamine) in eight men following a single oral dose of the DMAA (25 mg).

What type of graph paper is the above graph? (Semilogarithmic or rectangular?)

19. Refer to Question 18; what are the C_{max} and T_{max} values for subject #1? (subject #1) occurred at T_{max} of _____ hour.

20. Refer to Question 18; what is the average C_{max} value for all eight subjects? Please use the correct units for your answer.

21. Refer to Question 18; what are the units for AUC obtained from the graph?

22. Refer to Question 18; for subject #3, the C_{max} value is approximately 105 ng/mL. Express this concentration in %w/v.

23. Consider the following graph (Figure 2a in the original article) presented in Schilling et al (2013):

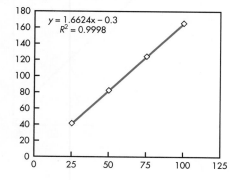

$$y = 1.6624x - 0.3$$
$$R^2 = 0.9998$$

The equation in the graph is that for the standard curve generated for progesterone using a high-performance liquid chromatography method. In the equation, y is the area under the curve of progesterone peak and x represents the concentration of the drug in μg/mL. Using this equation, predict the AUC for a drug concentration of 35 μg/mL.

24. Refer to Question 23; predict the concentration of progesterone (mg/L) for a peak area (AUC) of 145.

25. Consider the following function $dc/dt = 0.98$ with c and t being the concentration of the drug and time, respectively. This equation can also be written as _____.

a. $x = x_0 - 0.98\,t$

b. $x = 0.98 - t$

c. $x = x_0 + 0.98\,t$

d. $x = t/0.98$

ANSWERS

Learning Questions

1. a. Zero-order process (Fig. A-1).

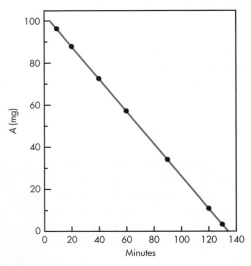

FIGURE A-1

b. Rate constant, k_0:

Method 1

Values obtained from the graph (see Fig. A-1):

t (minutes)	A (mg)
40	70
80	41

$$-k_0 = \text{slope} = \frac{\Delta Y}{\Delta X} = \frac{y_2 - y_1}{x_2 - x_1}$$

$$-k_0 = \frac{41 - 71}{80 - 40} \quad k_0 = 0.75 \text{ mg/min}$$

Notice that the negative sign shows that the slope is declining.

Method 2

By extrapolation:

$A_0 = 103.5$ at $t = 0$; $A = 71$ at $t = 40$ min

$A = k_0 t + A_0$

$71 = -40k_0 + 103.5$

$k_0 = 0.81$ mg/min

Notice that the answer differs in accordance with the method used.

c. $t_{1/2}$

For zero-order kinetics, the larger the initial amount of drug A_0, the longer the $t_{1/2}$.

Method 1

$$t_{1/2} = \frac{0.5A_0}{k_0}$$

$$t_{1/2} = \frac{0.5(103.5)}{0.78} = 66 \text{ min}$$

Method 2

The zero-order $t_{1/2}$ may be read directly from the graph (see Fig. A-1):

At $t = 0$, $A_0 = 103.5$ mg

At $t_{1/2}$, $A = 51.8$ mg

Therefore, $t_{1/2} = 66$ min.

d. The amount of drug, A, does extrapolate to zero on the x axis.

e. The equation of the line is

$$A = -k_0 t + A_0$$

$$A = -0.78t + 103.5$$

2. a. First-order process (Fig. A-2).

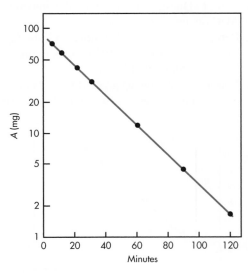

FIGURE A-2

b. Rate constant, k:

Method 1

Obtain the first-order $t_{1/2}$ from the semilog graph (see Fig. A-2):

t (minutes)	A (mg)
30	30
53	15

$t_{1/2} = 23$ min

$$k = \frac{0.693}{t_{1/2}} = \frac{0.693}{23} = 0.03 \ \text{min}^{-1}$$

Method 2

$$\text{Slope} = \frac{-k}{2.3} = \frac{\log Y_2 - \log Y_1}{X_2 - X_1}$$

$$k = \frac{-2.3(\log 15 - \log 30)}{53 - 30} = 0.03 \ \text{min}^{-1}$$

c. $t_{1/2} = 23$ min (see Method 1 above).
d. The amount of drug, A, does not extrapolate to zero on the x axis.
e. The equation of the line is

$$\log A = \frac{-kt}{2.3} + \log A_0$$

$$\log A = -\frac{0.03t}{2.3} + \log 78$$

$$A = 78e^{-0.03t}$$

On a rectangular plot, the same data show a curve (not plotted).

3. a. Zero-order process (Fig. A-3).

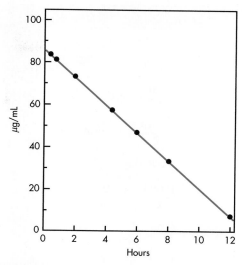

FIGURE A-3

b. $k_0 = \text{slope} = \dfrac{\Delta Y}{\Delta X}$

Values obtained from the graph (see Fig. A-3):

t (hours)	C (µg/mL)
1.2	80
4.2	60

It is always best to plot the data. Obtain a regression line (ie, the line of best fit), and then use points C and t from that line.

$$-k_0 = \frac{60 - 80}{4.2 - 1.2}$$

$$k_0 = 6.67 \ \mu g/mL/h$$

c. By extrapolation:

At t_0, $C_0 = 87.5 \ \mu g/mL$.

d. The equation (using a ruler only) is

$$A = -k_0 t + A_0 = -6.67t + 87.5$$

A better fit to the data may be obtained by using a linear regression program. Linear regression programs are available on spreadsheet programs such as Excel.

4. Given:

C (mg/mL)	t (days)
300	0
75	30

a. $\log C = -\dfrac{-kt}{2.3} + \log C_0$

$$\log 75 = -\dfrac{-30k}{2.3} + \log 300$$

$$k = 0.046 \text{ days}^{-1}$$

$$t_{1/2} = \dfrac{0.693}{k} = \dfrac{0.693}{0.046} = 15 \text{ days}$$

b. Method 1

$300 \text{ mg/mL} = C_0$ at $t = 0$

$75 \text{ mg/mL} = C$ at $t = 30$ days

$225 \text{ mg/mL} =$ difference between initial and final drug concentration

$$k_0 = \dfrac{225 \text{ mg/mL}}{30 \text{ days}} = 7.5 \text{ mg/mL/d}$$

The time, $t_{1/2}$, for the drug to decompose to one-half C_0 (from 300 to 150 mg/mL) is calculated by (assuming zero order):

$$t_{1/2} = \dfrac{150 \text{ mg/mL}}{75 \text{ mg/mL/day}} = 20 \text{ days}$$

Method 2

$$C = -k_0 t + C_0$$

$$75 = -30k_0 + 300$$

$$k_0 = 7.5 \text{ mg/mL/d}$$

At $t_{1/2}$, $C = 150$ mg/mL

$$150 = -7.5t_{1/2} + 300$$

$$t_{1/2} = 20 \text{ days}$$

Method 3

A $t_{1/2}$ value of 20 days may be obtained directly from the graph by plotting C against t on rectangular coordinates.

5. Assume the original concentration of drug to be 1000 mg/mL.

Method 1

mg/mL	No. of Half-Lives	mg/mL	No. of Half-Lives
1000	0	15.6	6
500	1	7.81	7
250	2	3.91	8
125	3	1.95	9
62.5	4	0.98	10
31.3	5		

99.9% of $1000 = 999$

Concentration of drug remaining $= 0.1\%$ of 1000

$1000 - 999 = 1$ mg/mL

It takes approximately 10 half-lives to eliminate all but 0.1% of the original concentration of drug.

Method 2

Assume any $t_{1/2}$ value:

$$t_{1/2} = \dfrac{0.693}{k}$$

Then

$$k = \dfrac{0.693}{t_{1/2}}$$

$$\log C = \dfrac{-kt}{2.3} + \log C_0$$

$$\log 1.0 = \dfrac{-kt}{2.3} + \log 1000$$

$$t = 9.96 \, t_{1/2}$$

Substituting $0.693/t_{1/2}$ for k:

$$\log 1.0 = \frac{-0.693\, t}{2.3 \times t_{1/2}} + \log 1000$$

$$t = 9.96\, t_{1/2}$$

6. $t_{1/2} = 12$ h

$$k = \frac{0.693}{t_{1/2}} = \frac{0.693}{12} = 0.058 \text{ h}^{-1}$$

If 30% of the drug decomposes, 70% is left. Then 70% of 125 mg = $(0.70)(125) = 87.5$ mg

$$A_0 = 125 \text{ mg}$$

$$A = 87.5 \text{ mg}$$

$$k = 0.058 \text{ h}^{-1}$$

$$\log A = -\frac{kt}{2.3} + \log A_0$$

$$\log 87.5 = -\frac{0.058t}{2.3} + \log 125$$

$$t = 6.1 \text{ hours}$$

7. Immediately after the drug dissolves, the drug degrades at a constant, or zero-order rate. Since concentration is equal to mass divided by volume, it is necessary to calculate the initial drug concentration (at $t = 0$) to determine the original volume in which the drug was dissolved. From the data, calculate the zero-order rate constant, k_0:

$$-k_0 = \text{slope} = \frac{\Delta Y}{\Delta X} = \frac{0.45 - 0.3}{2.0 - 0.5}$$

$$k_0 = 0.1 \text{ mg/mL/h}$$

Then calculate the initial drug concentration, C_0, using the following equation:

$$C = -k_0 t + C_0$$

At $t = 2$ hours,

$$0.3 = -0.1(2) + C_0$$

$$C_0 = 0.5 \text{ mg/mL}$$

Alternatively, at $t = 0.5$ hour,

$$0.45 = -0.1(0.5) - C_0$$

$$C_0 = 0.5 \text{ mg/mL}$$

Since the initial mass of drug D_0 dissolved is 300 mg and the initial drug concentration C_0 is 0.5 mg/mL, the original volume may be calculated from the following relationship:

$$C_0 = \frac{D_0}{V}$$

$$0.5 \text{ mg/mL} = \frac{300 \text{ mg}}{V}$$

$$V = 600 \text{ mL}$$

8. First order.
9. The volume of the culture tube is not important. In 8 hours (480 minutes), the culture tube is completely full. Because the doubling time for the cells is 2 minutes (ie, one $t_{1/2}$), then in 480 minutes less 2 minutes (478 minutes) the culture tube is half full of cells.
10. b. Since 1 mg = 1000 μg, then
$(257\ \mu\text{g/mL})/1000 = 0.257$ mg/mL.
11. c. Since 1 dL = 100 mL, then
$(257\ \mu\text{g/mL}) \times 100 = 25{,}700\ \mu\text{g/dL}$.
12. a. Since 1 kg = 1000 g, then $(170\text{ g})/1000 = 0.17$ kg.
  The oral dose was 300 mg/kg; therefore, for 0.17 kg rat, $(0.17\text{ kg})(300\text{ mg})/1\text{ kg} = 51$ mg.
13. c. The volume given was 5 mL/kg. For 0.17 kg rat, $(0.17\text{ kg})(5\text{ mL})/1\text{ kg} = 0.85$ mL.
14. d. 0.5% of methylcellulose (% w/v) means 0.5 g of methylcellulose in 100 mL solution. Or 5 g of methylcellulose in 1 L solution.
15. b. $k_{el} = 0.693/t_{1/2} = 0.693/4.35 = 0.16$ h^{-1}
16. b. 4.35 hours $\times$ 60 min/h = 261 minutes.
17. c. $F\% = \{[(\text{AUC sample})(\text{Dose oral})]/[(\text{AUC oral})(\text{Dose sample})]\} * 100$ (2.28)
  $F\% = [(\text{AUC sample})/\text{AUC oral})] * 100$
  2.6 folds higher = 260%
  $260 = [\text{AUC sample})/29.1] * 100$
  AUC sample = 75.66 μg·h/mL = 0.07566 mg·h/mL = 1.8 mg·day/mL

18. b. A rectangular coordinate graph.

19. d. According to the figure, the highest plasma concentration for subject #1 occurred at 24 hours.

20. b. From the graph, the average C_{max} was between 50 and 100 ng/mL.

21. c. It is (concentration units) × (time) = (ng/mL) × (hours) = (ng·h/mL).

22. c. 105 ng/mL = 10,500 ng/100 mL = 10.5 μg/100 mL = 0.0105 mg/100 mL = 0.0000105 g/100 mL.

23. c. $y = 1.6624 \times -0.3$
$y = 1.6624 (35) - 0.3 = 57.9 = AUC$

24. a. $y = 1.6624 \times -0.3$
$145 = 1.6624 \times -0.3$
$x = 87.4\ \mu g/mL = 87.4\ mg/L$

25. c. $dc/dt = 0.98$
$dc = 0.98\ dt$
$\int dc = 0.98 \int dt$
$c = c_0 + 0.98t$

REFERENCES

Basu Sarkar A, Kandimalla A, Dudley R: Chemical stability of progesterone in compounded topical preparations using PLO Transdermal Cream™ and HRT Cream™ base over a 90-day period at two controlled temperatures. *J Steroids Horm Sci* **4**:114, 2013. doi:10.4172/2157-7536.1000114. (© 2013 Basu Sarkar A, et al. This is an open-access article distributed under the terms of the Creative Commons Attribution License, which permits unrestricted use, distribution, and reproduction in any medium, provided the original author and source are credited.)

Cunha AB: Repeat lumbar puncture: CSF lactic acid levels are predictive of cure with acute bacterial meningitis. *J Clin Med* **2**(4):328–330, 2013. doi:10.3390/jcm2040328. (© 2013 by MDPI [http://www.mdpi.org]. Reproduction is permitted.)

Gaddis LM, Gaddis MG: Introduction to biostatistics: Part 6, Correlation and regression. *Ann Emerg Med* 19(12):1462–1468, 1990.

Howard Anton: Chapter 7: Logarithm and exponential functions. In *Calculus with Analytical Geometry*. John Wiley and Sons, 1980.

Munro HB: *Statistical Methods for Health Care Research*. Lippincott Williams & Wilkins, 2005, Philadelphia, PA.

Ravi Sankar V, Dachinamoorthi D, Chandra Shekar KB: A comparative pharmacokinetic study of aspirin suppositories and aspirin nanoparticles loaded suppositories. *Clinic Pharmacol Biopharm* **1**:105, 2012. doi:10.4172/2167-065X.1000105. (© 2012 Ravi Sankar V, et al. This is an open-access article distributed under the terms of the Creative Commons Attribution License, which permits unrestricted use, distribution, and reproduction in any medium, provided the original author and source are credited.)

Schilling et al: Physiological and pharmacokinetic effects of oral 1,3-dimethylamylamine administration in men. *BMC Pharmacol Toxicol* **14**:52, 2013. (© 2013 Schilling et al; licensee BioMed Central Ltd. This is an open-access article distributed under the terms of the Creative Commons Attribution License [http://creativecommons.org/licenses/by/2.0], which permits unrestricted use, distribution, and reproduction in any medium, provided the original work is properly cited.)

Shakeel F, Mohammed SF, Shafiq S: Comparative pharmacokinetic profile of aceclofenac from oral and transdermal application. *J Bioequiv Availab* **1**:013–017, 2009. doi:10.4172/jbb.1000003. (Permission granted under open access: The author[s] and copyright holder[s] grant to all users a free, irrevocable, worldwide, perpetual right of access and a license to copy, use, distribute, transmit, and display the work publicly and to make and distribute derivative works in any digital medium for any responsible purpose, subject to proper attribution of authorship, as well as the right to make small number of printed copies for their personal use.)

Steiner MA, Sciarretta C, Pasquali A, Jenck F: The selective orexin receptor 1 antagonist ACT-335827 in a rat model of diet-induced obesity associated with metabolic syndrome. *Front Pharmacol* **4**:165, 2013. doi: 10.3389/fphar.2013.00165. (Copyright © 2013 Steiner MA, et al. This is an open-access article distributed under the terms of the Creative Commons Attribution License [CC BY]. The use, distribution, or reproduction in other forums is permitted, provided the original author[s] or licensor is credited and that the original publication in this journal is cited, in accordance with accepted academic practice. No use, distribution, or reproduction is permitted which does not comply with these terms.)

3

Biostatistics

Charles Herring

VARIABLES[1]

Several types of variables will be discussed throughout this text. A *random variable* is "a variable whose observed values may be considered as outcomes of an experiment and whose values cannot be anticipated with certainty before the experiment is conducted" (Herring, 2014). An *independent variable* is defined as the "intervention or what is being manipulated" in a study (eg, the drug or dose of the drug being evaluated) (Herring, 2014). "The number of independent variables determines the category of statistical methods that are appropriate to use" (Herring, 2014). A *dependent variable* is the "outcome of interest within a study." In bioavailability and bioequivalence studies, examples include the maximum concentration of the drug in the circulation, the time to reach that maximum level, and the area under the curve (AUC) of drug level-versus-time curve. These are "the outcomes that one intends to explain or estimate" (Herring, 2014). There may be multiple dependent (aka outcome) variables. For example, in a study determining the half-life, clearance, and plasma protein binding of a new drug following an oral dose, the independent variable is the oral dose of the new drug. The dependent variables are the half-life, clearance, and plasma protein binding of the drug because these variables "depend upon" the oral dose given.

Discrete variables are also known as counting or nonparametric variables (Glasner, 1995). *Continuous variables* are also known as measuring or parametric variables (Glasner, 1995). We will explore this further in the next section.

TYPES OF DATA (NONPARAMETRIC VERSUS PARAMETRIC)

There are two types of *nonparametric* data, nominal and ordinal. For *nominal* data, numbers are purely arbitrary or without regard to any order or ranking of severity (Gaddis and Gaddis, 1990a; Glasner,

---

[1]The 5th edition of *Quick Stats: Basics for Medical Literature Evaluation* was utilized for the majority of the following chapter (Herring, 2014). In order to discuss basic statistics, some background terminology must be defined.

1995). Nominal data may be either dichotomous or categorical. Dichotomous (aka binary) nominal data evaluate yes/no questions. For example, patients lived or died, were hospitalized, or were not hospitalized. Examples of categorical nominal data would be things like tablet color or blood type; there is no order or inherent value for nominal, categorical data.

Ordinal data are also nonparametric and categorical, but unlike nominal data, ordinal data are scored on a continuum, without a consistent level of magnitude of difference between ranks (Gaddis and Gaddis, 1990a; Glasner, 1995). Examples of ordinal data include a pain scale, New York Heart Association heart failure classification, cancer staging, bruise staging, military rank, or Likert-like scales (poor/fair/good/very good/excellent) (Gaddis and Gaddis, 1990a; DeYoung, 2005).

Parametric data are utilized in biopharmaceutics and pharmacokinetic research more so than are the aforementioned types of nonparametric data. Parametric data are also known as continuous or measuring data or variables. There is an order and consistent level of magnitude of difference between data units. There are two types of parametric data: interval and ratio. Both interval and ratio scale parametric data have a predetermined order to their numbering and a consistent level of magnitude of difference between the observed data units (Gaddis and Gaddis, 1990a; Glasner, 1995). However, for interval scale data, there is no absolute zero, for example, Celsius or Fahrenheit (Gaddis and Gaddis, 1990a; Glasner, 1995). For ratio scale data, there is an absolute zero, for example, drug concentrations, plasma glucose, Kelvin, heart rate, blood pressure, distance, and time (Gaddis and Gaddis, 1990a; Glasner, 1995). Although the specific definitions of these two types of parametric data are listed above, their definitions are somewhat academic since all parametric data utilize the same statistical tests. In other words, regardless of whether the parametric data are interval or ratio scale, the same tests are used to detect statistical differences. Examples of parametric data include plasma protein binding, the maximum concentration of the drug in the circulation, the time to reach that maximum level, the area under the curve of drug

level-versus-time curve, drug clearance, and elimination half-life.

Frequently Asked Questions
▶ *Is it appropriate to degrade parametric data to nonparametric data for data analysis?*
▶ *What occurs if this is done?*

Data Scale Summary Example

In pharmacokinetic studies, researchers may be interested in testing the difference in the oral absorption of a generic versus a branded form of a drug. In this case, "generic or branded" is a nominal scale-type variable, whereas expressing the "rate of absorption" numerically is a ratio-type scale (Gaddis and Gaddis, 1990a; Ferrill and Brown 1994; Munro, 2005).

DISTRIBUTIONS

Normal distributions are "symmetrical on both sides of the mean" sometimes termed as a bell-shaped curve, Gaussian curve, curve of error, or normal probability curve (Shargel et al, 2012). An example of normally distributed data includes drug elimination half-lives in a specific population, as would be the case in a sample of men with normal renal and hepatic function. As will be discussed later in this chapter, parametric statistical tests like *t*-test and various types of analysis of variance (ANOVA) are utilized for normally distributed data.

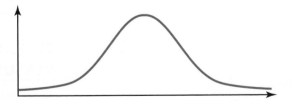

Sometimes in bioequivalence or pharmacokinetic studies, a bimodal distribution is noted. In this case two peaks of cluster or areas of high frequency occur. For example, a medication that is acetylated at different rates in humans would be a "bimodal distribution, indicating two populations consisting of fast acetylators and slow acetylators" (Gaddis and Gaddis, 1990a; Glasner, 1995; Shargel et al, 2012).

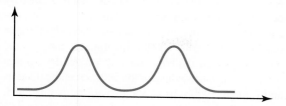

Skewed distributions occur when data are not normally distributed and tail off to either the high or the low end of measurement units. A *positive skew* occurs when data cluster on the low end of the *x* axis (Gaddis and Gaddis, 1990a; Glasner, 1995). For example, the *x* axis could be the income of patients seen in inner-city Emergency Department (ED), cost of generic medications, number of prescribed medications in patients younger than 30 years of age.

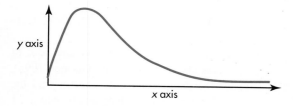

A *negative skew* occurs when data cluster on the high end of the *x* axis (Gaddis and Gaddis, 1990a; Glasner, 1995). For example, the *x* axis could be the income of patients seen in ED of an affluent area, cost of brand name medications, number of prescribed medications in patients older than 60 years of age.

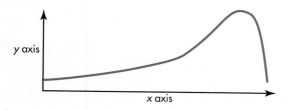

Kurtosis occurs when data cluster on both ends of the *x* axis such that the graph tails upward (ie, clusters on both ends of the graph). For example, the J-curve of hypertension treatment; with the J-curve, mortality increases if blood pressure is either too high or too low (Glasner, 1995).

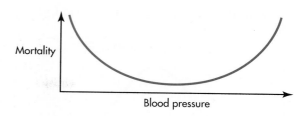

MEASURES OF CENTRAL TENDENCY

There are several *measures of central tendency* that are utilized in biopharmaceutical and pharmacokinetic research. The most common one is the *mean*, or average. It is the "sum of all values divided by the total number of values," is used for parametric data, and is affected by outliers or extreme values, which "deviate far from the majority of the data" (Gaddis and Gaddis, 1990b; Shargel et al, 2012). Mu (μ) is the population mean and *X*-bar ($\overline{X}$) is the sample mean (Gaddis and Gaddis, 1990b).

Median is also known as the 50th percentile or mid-most point (Gaddis and Gaddis, 1990b). It is "the point above which or below which half of the data points lie" (Gaddis and Gaddis, 1990b). It is not affected by outliers and may be used for ordinal and parametric data (Gaddis and Gaddis, 1990b). Median is used when outliers exist, when a data set spans a wide range of values, or "when continuous data are not normally distributed" (Gaddis and Gaddis, 1990b; DeYoung, 2005).

Mode is the most common value (Gaddis and Gaddis, 1990b). Mode is not affected by outliers and may be used for nominal, ordinal, or parametric data (Gaddis and Gaddis, 1990b). As with median, the mode is not affected by outliers (Gaddis and Gaddis, 1990b). However, the mode is not helpful when a data set contains a large range of infrequently occurring values (Gaddis and Gaddis, 1990b).

For normally distributed data, mean, median, and mode are the same. For positively skewed data, the mode is less than the median and the median is less than the mean. For negatively skewed data, the mode is greater than the median and the median is greater than the mean (Gaddis and Gaddis, 1990b; Glasner, 1995).

Normally distributed data (Gaddis and Gaddis, 1990b; Glasner, 1995)

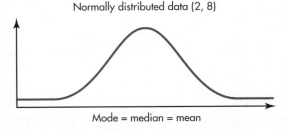

Positively skewed data (Gaddis and Gaddis, 1990b; Glasner, 1995)

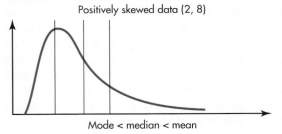

Negatively skewed data (Gaddis and Gaddis, 1990b; Glasner, 1995)

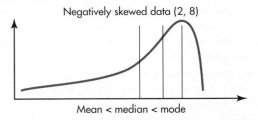

Based upon a data set's mean, median, and mode values, one can determine if the data is normally distributed or skewed when no graphical representation is provided. For biopharmaceutical and pharmacokinetic data, this is important to know so that appropriate logarithmic transformation can be performed for skewed data to restore normality.

A weakness of measures of central tendency is the data does not describe variability or spread of data.

MEASURES OF VARIABILITY

Measures of variability describe data spread and, in the case of *confidence intervals (CIs)*, can help one infer statistical significance (Gaddis and Gaddis, 1990b).

Range is the interval between lowest and highest values (Gaddis and Gaddis, 1990b; Glasner, 1995). Range only considers extreme values, so it is affected by outliers (Gaddis and Gaddis, 1990b). Range is descriptive only, so it is not used to infer statistical significance (Gaddis and Gaddis, 1990b). Interquartile range is the interval between the 25th and 75th percentiles, so it is directly related to median, or the 50th percentile (Gaddis and Gaddis, 1990b). It is not affected by outliers and, along with the median, is used for ordinal scale data (Gaddis and Gaddis, 1990b).

Variance is deviation from the mean, expressed as the square of the units used. The data are squared in the variance calculations because some deviations are negative and squaring provides a positive number (Gaddis and Gaddis, 1990b; Glasner, 1995). "As sample size (n) increases, variance decreases" (Herring, 2014). Variance equals the sum of (mean – data point) squared, divided by $n - 1$.

$$\text{Variance} = \frac{\Sigma(\overline{X} - X)^2}{n-1} \qquad (3.1)$$

Standard deviation (SD) is the square root of variance (Gaddis and Gaddis, 1990b; Glasner, 1995). SD estimates the degree of data scatter around the sample mean. Sixty-eight percent of data lie within ±1 SD of the mean and 95% of data lie within ±2 SD of the mean (Gaddis and Gaddis, 1990b; Glasner, 1995). SD is only meaningful when data are normally or near-normally distributed and, therefore, is only applicable to parametric data (Gaddis and Gaddis, 1990b; Glasner, 1995). Sigma (σ) is the population SD and S is the sample SD (Glasner, 1995).

$$\text{SD} = \sqrt{\text{Variance}} \qquad (3.2)$$

"*Coefficient of variation (or relative standard deviation)* is another measure used when evaluating dispersion from one data set to another. The coefficient of variation is the SD expressed as a percentage of the mean. This is useful in comparing the relative difference in variability between two or more samples, or which group has the largest relative variability of values from the mean" (Herring, 2014). The smaller the coefficient of variation, the less the variability in the data set.

$$\text{Coefficient of variation} = 100 \times \text{SD}/\overline{X} \qquad (3.3)$$

Standard error of the mean (SEM) is the SD divided by the square root of *n* (Gaddis and Gaddis, 1990b; Glasner, 1995). The larger *n* is, the smaller SEM is (Gaddis and Gaddis, 1990b; Glasner, 1995). SEM is always smaller than SD.

> "The mean of separate samples from a single population will give slightly different parameter estimates. The standard error (SE) is the standard deviation (SD) of the sampling distribution of a statistic and should not be confused with SEM. The distribution of means from random samples is approximately normal. The mean of this 'distribution of means' is the unknown population mean"
>
> (Glasner, 1995)

SD for the distribution of means is estimated by the SEM. One "could name the SEM as the standard deviation of means of random samples of a fixed size drawn from the original population of interest" (Herring, 2014). The SEM is the quantification of the spread of the sample means for a study that is repeated multiple times. The SEM helps to estimate how well a sample represents the population from which it was drawn (Glasner, 1995). However, the SEM should *not* be used as a measure of variability when publishing a study. Doing so is misleading. The only purpose of SEM is to calculate CIs, which contain an estimate of the true population mean from which the sample was drawn (Gaddis and Gaddis, 1990b).

$$SEM = SD/\sqrt{n} \qquad (3.4)$$

Confidence interval (CI) is a method of estimating the range of values likely to include the true value of a population parameter (Gaddis and Gaddis, 1990b). In medical literature, a 95% CI is most frequently used. The 95% CI is a range of values that "if the entire population could be studied, 95% of the time the true population value would fall within the CI estimated from the sample" (Gaddis and Gaddis, 1990b). For a 95% CI, 5 times out of 100, the true population parameter may not lie within the CI. For a 97.5% CI, 2.5 times out of 100, the true population parameter may not lie within the CI. Therefore, a 97.5% CI is more likely to include the true population value than a 95% CI (Gaddis and Gaddis, 1990b).

The true strength of a CI is that it is both descriptive and inferential. "All values contained in the CI are statistically possible" (Herring, 2014).

However, the closer the point estimate lies to the middle of the CI, the more likely the point estimate represents the population.

For example, if a point estimate and 95% CI for drug clearance are 3 L/h (95% CI: 1.5–4.5 L/h), all values including and between 1.5 and 4.5 L/h are statistically possible. However, a point estimate of 2.5 L/h is a more accurate representation of the studied population than a point estimate of 1.6 L/h since 2.5 is closer to the sample's point estimate of 3 than is 1.6. As seen in this example, CI shows the degree of certainty (or uncertainty) in each comparison in an easily interpretable way.

In addition, CIs make it easier to assess clinical significance and are less likely to mislead one into thinking that nonsignificantly different sample values imply equal population values

$$95\% \ CI = \overline{X} \pm 1.96 \ (SEM) \qquad (3.5)$$

Significance of CIs depends upon the objective of the trial being conducted or evaluated.

In superiority trials, all values within a CI are statistically possible. For *differences* like differences in half-life, differences in area under the curve (AUC), relative risk reductions/increases (RRRs/RRIs), or absolute risk reductions/increases (ARRs/ARIs), if the CI includes ZERO (0), then the results are not statistically significant (NSS). In the case of a 90% CI, if the CI includes ZERO (0) for this type of data, it can be interpreted as a $p > 0.10$. In the case of a 95% CI, if the CI includes ZERO (0) for this type of data, it can be interpreted as a $p > 0.05$. In the case of a 97.5% CI, if the CI includes ZERO (0) for this type of data, it can be interpreted as a $p > 0.025$.

For superiority trials, since all values within a CI are statistically possible, for *ratios* like relative risk (RR), odds ratio (OR), or hazards ratio (HR), if the CI includes ONE (1.0), then the results are not statistically significant (NSS). In the case of a 90% CI, if the CI includes ONE (1.0) for this type of data, it can be interpreted as a $p > 0.10$. In the case of a 95% CI, if the CI includes ONE (1.0) for this type of data, it can be interpreted as a $p > 0.05$. In the case of a 97.5% CI, if the CI includes ONE (1.0) for this type of data, it can be interpreted as a $p > 0.025$.

HYPOTHESIS TESTING

For superiority trials, the *null hypothesis* (H_0) is that no difference exists between studied populations (Gaddis and Gaddis, 1990c). For superiority trials, the *alternative hypothesis* (H_1) is that a difference does exist between studied populations (Gaddis and Gaddis, 1990c).

H_0: There is no difference in the AUC for drug formulation A relative to formulation B.

H_1 (aka H_a): There is a difference in AUC for drug formulation A relative to formulation B.

H_1 is sometimes directional. For example,

H_1: We expect AUC for drug formulation A to be 25% higher than that of formulation B.

H_0 is tested instead of H_1 because there are an infinite number of alternative hypotheses. It would be impossible to calculate the required statistics for each of the infinite number of possible magnitudes of difference between population samples H_1 hypothesizes (Gaddis and Gaddis, 1990c). H_0 is used to determine "if any observed differences between groups are due to chance alone" or sampling variation.

Statistical significance is tested (*hypothesis testing*) to indicate if H_0 should be accepted or rejected (Gaddis and Gaddis, 1990c). For superiority trials, if H_0 is "rejected," this means a statistically significant difference between groups exists (results unlikely due to chance) (Gaddis and Gaddis, 1990c). For superiority trials, if H_0 is "accepted," this means no statistically significant difference exists (Gaddis and Gaddis, 1990c). However, "failing to reject H_0 is not sufficient to conclude that groups are equal" (DeYoung, 2005).

A *type 1 error* occurs if one rejects the H_0 when, in fact, the H_0 is true (Gaddis and Gaddis, 1990c). For superiority trials this is when one concludes there is a difference between treatment groups, when in fact, no difference exists (Gaddis and Gaddis, 1990c).

Alpha (α) is *defined* as the probability of making a type 1 error (Gaddis and Gaddis, 1990c). When α level is set *a priori* (or before the trial), the H_0 is rejected when $p \leq \alpha$ (Gaddis and Gaddis, 1990c). By convention, an acceptable α is usually 0.05 (5%), which means that 1 time out of 20, a type 1 error will be committed. This is a consequence that investigators are willing to accept and is denoted in trials as a $p \leq 0.05$ (Gaddis and Gaddis, 1990c). So the *p*-value is the calculated chance that a type 1 error has occurred (Gaddis and Gaddis, 1990c). In other words, it tells us the likelihood of obtaining a statistically significant result if H_0 were true. "At $p = 0.05$, the likelihood is 5%. At $p = 0.10$, the likelihood is 10%" (Herring, 2014). A $p \leq \alpha$ means the observed treatment difference is statistically significant, it does not indicate the size or direction of the difference. The size of the *p*-value is not related to the importance of the result (Gaddis and Gaddis, 1990f; Berensen, 2000). Smaller *p*-values simply mean that "chance" is less likely to explain observed differences (Gaddis and Gaddis, 1990f; Berensen, 2000). Also, "a small *p*-value does not correct for systematic error (bias)" from a poorly designed study (DeYoung, 2005).

A *type 2 error* occurs if one accepts the H_0 when, in fact, the H_0 is false (Gaddis and Gaddis, 1990c). For superiority trials this is when one concludes there is no difference between treatment groups, when in fact, a difference does exist. *Beta* (β) is the probability of making a type 2 error (Gaddis and Gaddis, 1990c). By convention, an acceptable β is 0.2 (20%) or less (Gaddis and Gaddis, 1990c).

Regardless of the trial design (superiority, equivalence, or non-inferiority), α and β are interrelated (Gaddis and Gaddis, 1990c). All else held constant, α and β are inversely related (Gaddis and Gaddis, 1990c). In other words, as α is decreased, β is increased, and as α is increased, β is decreased (ie, as risk for a type 1 error is increased, risk for a type 2 error is decreased and vice versa) (Gaddis and Gaddis, 1990c). The most common use of β is in calculating the approximate sample size required for a study to keep α and β acceptably small (Gaddis and Gaddis, 1990c).

Frequently Asked Questions

▶ *For a superiority trial, if a statistically significant difference were detected, is there any way that the study was underpowered?*

▶ *For a superiority trial, if a statistically significant difference were detected, is there any way a type 2 error could have occurred?*

TABLE 3-1   Type 1 and 2 Error for Superiority Trials

	Reality	
	Difference Exists (H_0 False)	No Difference Exists (H_0 True)
Decision from Statistical Test		
Difference found (Reject H_0)	Correct No error	Incorrect *Type 1 error* (false positive)
No difference found (Accept H_0)	Incorrect *Type 2 error* (false negative)	Correct No error

Delta (Δ) is sometimes referred to as the "effect size" and is a measure of the degree of difference between tested population samples (Gaddis and Gaddis, 1990c). For parametric data, the value of Δ is the ratio of the clinical difference expected to be observed in the study to the standard deviation (SD) of the variable:

$$\Delta = (\mu_a - \mu_0)/SD \qquad (3.6)$$

where μ_a is the alternative hypothesis value expected for the mean and μ_0 is the null hypothesis value for the mean.

One-tailed versus two-tailed tests: It is easier to show a statistically significant difference with a *one-tailed test* than with a *two-tailed test*, because with a one-tailed test a statistical test result must *not* vary as much from the mean to achieve significance at any level of α chosen (Gaddis and Gaddis, 1990c). However, most reputable journals require that investigators perform statistics based upon a two-tailed test even if it innately makes sense that a difference would only occur unidirectionally (Al-Achi A, discussions).

Power is the ability of an experiment to detect a statistically significant difference between samples, when in fact, a significant difference truly exists (Gaddis and Gaddis, 1990c). Said another way, power is the probability of making a correct decision when H_0 is false.

$$\text{Power} = 1 - \beta \qquad (3.7)$$

As stated in the section on type 2 error risk, by convention, an acceptable β is 0.2 (20%) or less; therefore, most investigators set up their studies, and their sample sizes, based upon an estimated power of at least 80%.

For superiority trials, inadequate power may cause one to conclude that no difference exists when, in fact, a difference does exist. As described above, this would be a type 2 error (Gaddis and Gaddis, 1990c). Note that in most cases, power is an issue only if one accepts the H_0. If one rejects the H_0, there is no way that one could have made a type 2 error (see Table 3-1). Therefore, power to detect a difference would *not* be an issue in most of these cases. An exception to this general rule would be if one wanted to decrease data variability or spread. For example, if one wanted to narrow the 95% CI, increasing power by increasing sample size could help.

For research purposes, power calculations are generally used to determine the required sample size when designing a study (ie, prior to the study). Power calculations are generally based upon the primary endpoint of the study and, as is depicted in the examples below, the a priori (prespecified) α, β, Δ, SD, and whether a one-tailed or two-tailed design is used.

Parametric Data Sample Size/Power Examples

The way a study is set up will determine the required sample size. In other words, the preset α, β, Δ, SD, and tailing (one-tailed vs two-tailed) affect sample size required for a study (Drew R, discussions and provisions).

Utilizing a larger standard deviation (SD) will require a larger sample size. Also, a one-tailed test requires a smaller sample size than a two-tailed test to detect differences between groups (Drew R, discussions and provisions). This is due to the fact that given everything else is the same, a one-tailed test has more *power* to reject the null hypothesis than a two-tailed test.

Differences		Statistical Limits		Sample Size	
SD	Δ (%)	α	β	One-tailed	Two-tailed
1 (68% of data)	10	0.05	0.20	**1237**	**1570**
2 (95% of data)	10	0.05	0.20	**4947**	**6280**

Increasing the accepted type 1 (α) and type 2 (β) statistical error risks will decrease the sample size required.

Decreasing the acceptable type 1 (α) and type 2 (β) statistical error risks will increase the required sample size (Drew R, discussions and provisions).

Differences		Statistical Limits		Sample Size	
SD	Δ (%)	α	β	One-tailed	Two-tailed
2 (95% of data)	10	**0.05**	0.20	4947	6280
2 (95% of data)	10	**0.10**	0.20	3607	4947

Power = $1 - \beta$, so a larger sample size is required for smaller β and higher power (Drew R, discussions and provisions).

Differences		Statistical Limits		Sample Size	
SD	Δ (%)	α	β	One-tailed	Two-tailed
2 (95% of data)	10	0.05	**0.10**	6852	8406
2 (95% of data)	10	0.05	**0.20**	4947	6280

A smaller difference (Δ) between groups increases the sample size required to detect that difference. A larger difference (Δ) decreases the sample size required to detect that difference (Drew R, discussions and provisions).

Differences		Statistical Limits		Sample Size	
SD	Δ (%)	α	β	One-tailed	Two-tailed
2 (95% of data)	**10**	0.05	0.20	4947	6280
2 (95% of data)	**20**	0.05	0.20	1237	1570

An example for estimating the sample size for a study would be as follows:

$\alpha = 0.05$
$\beta = 0.20$
$\Delta = 0.25$
SD $= 2.0$
Statistical test = two-sided *t*-test
Single sample

From a statistics table, the total sample size needed for this study is *128, or 64 in each group*. This also indicates that the investigators are interested in *detecting* a clinically meaningful difference of 0.50 unit:

$$\Delta = (\mu_a - \mu_0)/SD$$
$$0.25 = (\mu_a - \mu_0)/2.0$$
$$(\mu_a - \mu_0) = (2.0) \times (0.25) = 0.50 \text{ unit}$$

In other words, in order for the researchers to significantly detect the difference of 0.50 units, they would need a sample size of 128 patients. This test would have an estimated power of 80% (since $\beta = 0.20$) and a confidence level of 95% (since $\alpha = 0.05$). It is important to reemphasize here that the smaller the value for Δ, the greater would be the sample size needed for the study.

STATISTICALLY VERSUS CLINICALLY SIGNIFICANT DIFFERENCES

Statistically significant differences do not necessarily translate into *clinically significant differences* (Gaddis and Gaddis, 1990c). If the sample size of a trial is large enough, nonclinically meaningful, statistically significant differences may be detected. For example, grapefruit juice induces enzymatic activity with some drugs such that their elimination $t_{1/2}$ becomes shorter. Current data support that consistent grapefruit consumption statistically *and* clinically significantly decreases the elimination $t_{1/2}$ of these drugs. However, a one-time, single glass of grapefruit juice may *statistically significantly* decrease the value of $t_{1/2}$ by only 1%, which would not be considered clinically meaningful.

Also, lack of statistical significance does not necessarily mean the results are not clinically significant; consider power, trial design, and populations studied (Gaddis and Gaddis, 1990f). A nonstatistically significant difference is more likely to be accepted as being clinically significant in the instance of safety issues (like adverse effects), than for endpoint improvements. For example, if a trial were to find a nonstatistically significant increase in the risk for invasive breast cancer with a particular medication, many clinicians would deem this as being clinically meaningful such that they would avoid using the agent until further data were obtained. Also, suppose that a study were conducted to examine the response rate for a drug in two different populations. The response rates were 55% and 72% for groups 1 and 2, respectively. This difference in response rate is 17% ($72 - 55 = 17\%$) with a 95% CI of –3% to 40%. Since the 95% CI includes zero, the difference is not statistically significant. Let's also further assume that the minimum clinically acceptable difference in response rate for the particular disease is 15%. Since the response rate is 17% (which is greater than 15%), it may very well be clinically meaningful (significant) such that another, more adequately powered study may be worth conducting.

STATISTICAL INFERENCE TECHNIQUES IN HYPOTHESIS TESTING FOR PARAMETRIC DATA

Parametric statistical methods (*t-test* and *ANOVA*) are used for analyzing normally distributed, parametric data (Gaddis and Gaddis, 1990d). Parametric data include interval and ratio data, but since the same parametric tests are used for both, knowing the

differences between these is solely academic. Parametric tests are more powerful than nonparametric tests (Gaddis and Gaddis, 1990d). Also, more information about data is generated from parametric tests (Gaddis and Gaddis, 1990d).

The *t-test (aka Student's t-test)* is the method of choice when making a single comparison between two groups. A *non-paired t-test* is used when observations between groups are independent as in the case of a parallel study as seen in the example below. E_{xp} represents the experimental group and C_{trl} represents the control group.

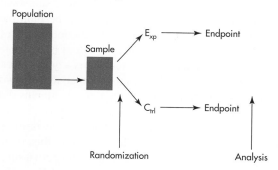

A *paired t-test* is used when observations between groups are dependent, as would be the case in a pretest/posttest study or a crossover study (Gaddis and Gaddis, 1990d). Initially in a crossover design, group A receives the experimental drug (E_{xp}) while group B receives the control (C_{trl}: placebo or gold standard treatment). After a washout period, group A receives the control (C_{trl}) and group B receives the experimental drug (E_{xp}). It is very important to ensure adequate time for washout to prevent carry-over effects.

However, when making either multiple comparisons between two groups or a single comparison between multiple groups, type 1 error risk increases if utilizing a *t-test*. For example, when rolling dice, think of rolling ones on both dice (snake eyes) as being a type 1 error. For each roll of the dice, there is a 1 in 36 chances (2.78%) of rolling snake eyes. For each statistical analysis, we generally accept a 1 in 20 chances (5%) of a type 1 error. Although the chance for snake eyes is the same for each roll and the chance for type 1 error is the same for each analysis, increasing the number of rolls and analyses increases the opportunity for snake eyes and type 1 errors, respectively. Said another way, the more times one rolls the dice, the more opportunity one has to roll snake eyes. It's the same with statistical testing. The more times one performs a statistical test on a particular data set, whether it be multiple comparisons of two groups, a single comparison of multiple groups, or multiple comparisons of multiple groups, the more likely one is to commit a type 1 error.

As an example of multiple comparisons of two groups for which the authors and/or statisticians did not make type 1 error risk corrections, a trial evaluated chlorthalidone versus placebo for the primary endpoint of blood pressure. In addition to this, there were other evaluated endpoints (including potassium concentration, serum creatinine, BUN:SCr ratio, calcium concentration, and others), and the authors did not control for these additional comparisons. Let's say there were a total of 20 comparisons including the primary endpoint of blood pressure. If the original α level were $p = 0.05$, the corrected α would be $1 - (1 - 0.05)^{20} = 0.64$. This means that if the original p-value threshold of 0.05 were used, there would be a 64% chance of inappropriately rejecting the null hypothesis (ie, committing a type 1 error) for at least one of the 20 comparisons (Gaddis and Gaddis, 1990d).

As an example of a single comparison of multiple groups for which the authors and/or statisticians did not make type 1 error risk corrections, a trial evaluated the difference in cholesterol among four lipid-lowering medications. With four groups, there were six paired comparisons. If the original α level were $p = 0.05$, the corrected α would be $1 - (1 - 0.05)^6 = 0.26$. Therefore, if the original p-value threshold of 0.05 were used, there would be a 26% chance of inappropriately rejecting the null hypothesis (type 1 error) for at least one of the six comparisons (Gaddis and Gaddis, 1990d).

Investigators should make their best effort to keep the type 1 error risk $\leq 5\%$ (ie, ≤ 0.05). The best way of doing so for multiple comparisons is by avoiding unnecessary comparisons or analyses, using the appropriate statistical test(s) for multiple comparisons, and using an alpha spending function for interim analyses. However, if investigators fail to do so, there is a crude method for adjusting the pre-set α level based upon the number of comparisons being made: the *Bonferroni* correction. This simply divides the preset α level by the number of comparisons being made (Gaddis and Gaddis, 1990d). This estimates the α level that is required to reach statistical significance (Gaddis and Gaddis, 1990d). However, Bonferroni is very conservative as the number of comparisons increases. A less conservative and more accepted way of minimizing type 1 error risk for multiple comparisons with parametric data is through utilization of one of several types of *analysis of variance (ANOVA)*.

ANOVA holds α level (type 1 error risk) constant when comparing more than two groups (Gaddis and Gaddis, 1990d). It tests for statistically significant difference(s) among a group's collective values (Gaddis and Gaddis, 1990d). In other words, intra- and intergroup variability is what is being analyzed instead of the means of the groups (Gaddis and Gaddis, 1990d). It involves calculation of an *F-ratio*, which answers the question, "is the variability between the groups large enough in comparison to the variability of data within each group to justify the conclusion that two or more of the groups differ" (Gaddis and Gaddis, 1990d)?

The most commonly used *ANOVAs are for independent (aka non-paired) samples* as is the case for a parallel design.

The first is *1-way ANOVA,* which is used if there are no confounders and at least three independent (aka non-paired) samples. For example, if investigators wanted to evaluate the excretion rate (percent of dose excreted unchanged in the urine) of different blood pressure medications, they could use a 1-way ANOVA if (1) each sample were independent (ie, a parallel design), (2) there were at least three samples (ie, at least three different blood pressure medications), and (3) the experimental groups differed in only *one* factor, which for this case would be the type of blood pressure drug being used (ie, there were no differences between the groups with regard to confounding factors like age, gender, kidney function, plasma protein binding, etc).

Multifactorial ANOVAs include any type of ANOVA that controls for at least one confounder for at least two independent (non-paired) samples as is the case for a parallel design.

A *2-way ANOVA* is used if there is one identifiable confounder and at least two independent (aka non-paired) samples. For example, if investigators wanted to evaluate the excretion rate (percent of dose excreted unchanged in the urine) of different blood pressure medications, they could use a 2-way ANOVA if (1) each sample were independent (ie, a parallel design), (2) there were at least two samples (ie, at least two different blood pressure medications), and (3) the experimental groups differed in only *two* factors, which for this case would be the type of blood pressure drug being used and one confounding variable (eg, differences between the groups' renal function).

Other types of multifactorial ANOVAs include *analyses of covariance (ANACOVA or ANCOVA)*. These are used if there are at least two confounders for at least two independent (non-paired) samples as is the case for a parallel design. These include the *3-way ANOVA, 4-way ANOVA,* etc.

A *3-way ANOVA* is used if there are two identifiable confounders and at least two independent (aka non-paired) samples. For example, if investigators wanted to evaluate the excretion rate (percent of dose excreted unchanged in the urine) of different blood pressure medications, they could use a 3-way ANOVA if (1) each sample were independent (ie, a parallel design), (2) there were at least two samples (ie, at least two different blood pressure medications), and (3) the experimental groups differed in *three* factors, which for this case would be the type of blood pressure drug being used and two confounding variables (eg, differences between the groups' renal function and plasma protein binding).

A *4-way ANOVA* is used if there are three identifiable confounders and at least two independent (aka non-paired) samples. For example, if investigators wanted to evaluate the excretion rate (percent of dose excreted unchanged in the urine) of different

blood pressure medications, they could use a 4-way ANOVA if (1) each sample were independent (ie, a parallel design), (2) there were at least two samples (ie, at least two different blood pressure medications), and (3) the experimental groups differed in *four* factors, which for this case would be the type of blood pressure drug being used and three confounding variables (eg, differences between the groups' renal function, plasma protein binding, and average patient age).

There are also *ANOVAs for related (aka paired, matched, or repeated) samples* as is the case for a crossover design. These include the *repeated measures ANOVA,* which is used if there are no confounders and at least three related (aka paired) samples. For example, if investigators wanted to evaluate the bioavailability of different cholesterol-lowering medications to determine C_{max}, they could use a *repeated measures ANOVA* if (1) each subject served as his/her own control (ie, a crossover design), (2) there were at least three samples (ie, at least three different cholesterol medications), and (3) the experimental groups differed in only *one* factor, which for this case would be the type of cholesterol drug being used (ie, there were no identified confounders like fluctuations in renal function, administration times, etc).

A second type of ANOVA for related (aka paired, matched, or repeated) samples is the *2-way repeated measures ANOVA,* which is used if there is one identifiable confounder and at least two related (aka paired) samples. For example, if investigators wanted to evaluate the bioavailability of different cholesterol-lowering medications to determine C_{max}, they could use a *2-way repeated measures ANOVA* if (1) each subject served as his/her own control (ie, a crossover design), (2) there were at least two samples (ie, at least two different cholesterol medications), and (3) the experimental groups differed in only *two* factors, which for this case would be the type of cholesterol drug being used and one confounding variable (eg, fluctuations in renal function).

Beyond that, *repeated measures regression analysis* is used if there are two or more related (aka paired) samples and two or more confounders. For example, if investigators wanted to evaluate the bioavailability of different cholesterol-lowering medications to determine C_{max}, they could use a *repeated measures regression analysis* if (1) each subject served as his/her own control (ie, a crossover design), (2) there were at least two samples (ie, at least two different cholesterol medications), and (3) the experimental groups differed in *at least three* factors, which for this case would be the type of cholesterol drug being used and at least two confounding variables (eg, fluctuations in renal function and administration times).

ANOVA will indicate if differences exist between groups, but will not indicate where these differences exist. For example, if an investigator is interested in comparing the volume of distribution of a drug among various species, both clearance and the elimination rate constant must be considered. Clearance and the elimination rate constant may be species dependent (ie, rats vs dogs vs humans) and thus, they are expected to produce different outcomes (ie, volumes of distribution). However, a statistically significant ANOVA does not point to where these differences exist. To find where the differences lie, *post hoc* multiple comparison methods must be performed.

Multiple comparison methods are types of *post hoc* tests that help determine which groups in a statistically significant ANOVA analysis differ (Gaddis and Gaddis, 1990d). These methods are based upon the *t*-test but have built-in corrections to keep α level constant when >1 comparison is being made. In other words, these help control for type 1 error rate for multiple comparisons (Gaddis and Gaddis, 1990d).

Examples include (1) *least significant difference,* which controls individual type 1 error rate for each comparison, (2) *layer (aka stepwise) methods,* which gradually adjust the type 1 error rate and include *Newman-Keuls* and *Duncan,* and (3) *experiment-wise methods,* which hold type 1 error rate constant for a set of comparisons and include *Dunnett,* which tests for contrasts with a control only; *Dunn,* which tests for small number of contrasts; *Tukey,* which tests for a large number of contrasts when no more than two means are involved; and *Scheffe,* which tests for a large number of contrasts when more than two means are involved (Gaddis and Gaddis, 1990d).

Sometimes, otherwise parametric data are not normally distributed (ie, are skewed) such that aforementioned parametric testing methods, *t*-test and the various types of ANOVA, would be inaccurate for data analysis. In these cases, investigators can logarithmically transform the data to normalize data distribution such that *t*-test or ANOVA can be used for data analysis (Shargel et al, 2012).

When performing statistical analyses of subgroup data sets, the term *interaction* or *p for interaction* is often heard (Shargel et al, 2012). *P for interaction (aka p-value for interaction)* simply detects heterogeneity or differences among subgroups. A significant *p* for interaction generally ranges from 0.05 to 0.1 depending on the analysis. In other words if a subgroup analysis finds a *p* for interaction <0.05 (or <0.1 for some studies) for half-life by male versus female patients, then there is possibly a significant difference in half-life based upon gender. This difference may be worth investigating in future analyses. Just as with other types of subgroup analyses, *p* for interaction solely detects hypothesis-generating differences. However, if multiple similar studies are available, a properly performed meta-analysis may help answer the question of gender and half-life differences.

Pharmacokinetic Study Example Incorporating Parametric Statistical Testing Principles

The $t_{1/2}$ of phenobarbital in a population is 5 days with a standard deviation of 0.5 days. A clinician observed that patients who consumed orange juice 2 hours prior to dosing with phenobarbital had a reduction in their $t_{1/2}$ by 10%. To test this hypothesis, the clinician selected a group of 9 patients who were already taking phenobarbital and asked them to drink a glass of orange juice 2 hours prior to taking the medication. The average calculated $t_{1/2}$ value from this sample of 12 patients was 4.25 days. The clinician has to decide from the results obtained from the study whether orange juice consumption decreases the value of $t_{1/2}$. Assuming that alpha was 0.05 (5%), there are several ways to reach the conclusion. Based on the statement of the null hypothesis, "drinking orange juice 2 hours prior to taking phenobarbital *does not* affect $t_{1/2}$ of the drug" (remember that H_0 is a statement of no difference, meaning that whether orange juice was or was not consumed the $t_{1/2}$ of phenobarbital is the same), the conclusion of the test is written with respect to H_0. The alternative hypothesis is that "orange juice *lowers* the $t_{1/2}$ value of phenobarbital." The alternative hypothesis has the symbol of H_1 or H_a. One way to analyze the result is to calculate a *p*-value for the test (Ferrill and Brown, 1994). The *p*-value is the exact probability of obtaining a test value of 4.25 days or less, given that H_0: $\mu_0 = 5$ days:

$$\text{Pr. } [y\text{-bar} \leq 4.25 \backslash \mu_0 = 5] \quad (3.8)$$

Equation 3.8 can be evaluated by standardizing the data using a standard normal curve (this curve has an average of $\mu = 0$ and a standard deviation of $\sigma = 1$):

$$\text{Pr. } [z \leq (y\text{-bar} - \mu)/\sigma/(n)^{0.5}] \quad (3.9)$$

$$\text{Pr. } [z \leq (4.25 - 5)/0.5/(9)^{0.5}]$$
$$= \text{Pr. } [z \leq -1.28] = 10.03\%$$

Or

$$p = 0.1003$$

Since the *p*-value for the test is greater than α of 5% ($p > 0.05$), then we conclude that drinking orange juice 2 hours prior to taking phenobarbital dose *does not* decrease the value of $t_{1/2}$. It should be noted that the value calculated from Equation 3.9 is for a *one-tailed test*. In order to calculate the *p*-value for a *two-tailed test*, the value computed from Equation 3.9 is multiplied by 2 ($p = 2 \times 0.1003 = 0.2006$).

While *z*-test and *t*-test are used for one-sample and two-sample comparisons, they cannot be used if the researcher is interested in comparing more than two samples at one time. As was explained earlier in this chapter, the parametric *analysis of variance (ANOVA) test* is used to compare two or more groups with respect to their means.

GOODNESS OF FIT

The idea of "goodness of fit" (GOF) in pharmacokinetic data analysis is an important concept to assure the reliability of proposed pharmacokinetic models.

It is a way to describe the "agreement between model and data" (Anonymous, 2003). This is done by plotting the residuals (RES; the difference between observed and predicted values) versus predicted (PRED) data points. In addition to this plot, GOF analysis includes other plots such as PRED versus observed (OBS) or PRED versus time (Brendel et al, 2007). GOF methodology is often used in population pharmacokinetic studies. For example, the pharmacokinetic profile of the antiretroviral drug nelfinavir and its active metabolite M8 was investigated with the aim of optimizing treatment in pediatric population (Hirt et al, 2006). The authors used GOF in their assessment of the proposed pharmacokinetic models to compare the population predicted versus the observed nelfinavir and M8 concentrations.

STATISTICAL INFERENCE TECHNIQUES FOR HYPOTHESIS TESTING WITH NONPARAMETRIC DATA

Nonparametric statistical methods are used for analyzing data that are not normally distributed and cannot be defined as parametric data (Gaddis and Gaddis, 1990e). For *nominal data*, the most common tests for proportions and frequencies include *chi-square* (χ^2) and *Fisher's exact*. These tests are "used to answer questions about rates, proportions, or frequencies" (Gaddis and Gaddis, 1990e). *Fisher's exact* test is only used for very small data sets ($N \leq 20$). *Chi-square* (χ^2) is used for all others. For matrices that are larger than 2×2, χ^2 tests will detect difference(s) between groups, but will not indicate where the difference(s) lie(s) (Gaddis and Gaddis, 1990e). To find this, *post hoc* tests are needed. These *post hoc* tests should only be performed if the χ^2 test was statistically significant. Doing otherwise will increase type 1 error risk.

For *ordinal data*, the most appropriate test depends upon the number of groups being compared, the number of comparisons being made, and whether the study is of parallel or crossover design. The most commonly used ordinal tests are *Mann–Whitney U, Wilcoxon Rank Sum, Kolmogorov–Smirnov, Wilcoxon Signed Rank, Kruskal–Wallis*, and *Friedman*.

The procedure for utilizing all of these tests is very similar to the example provided in the parametric data testing section:

1. State the null and alternate hypotheses at a given alpha value.
2. Calculate test statistics (a computed value for Chi-square or z, depending on the test being used).
3. Compare the calculated value with a tabulated value.
4. Build a confidence interval on the true proportion that is expected in the population.
5. Make a decision whether or not to reject the null hypothesis.

Many statistical software programs perform the above tests or other similar tests found in the literature. Computer programs calculate a p-value for the test to determine whether or not the results are significant. This is, of course, accomplished by comparing the computed p-value with a predetermined α value. In the practice of pharmacokinetics, it is recommended to have computer software for calculating pharmacokinetic parameters and another software program for statistical analysis of experimental data.

> **Frequently Asked Question**
> ▶ *How do nonparametric statistical tests differ from parametric statistical test regarding power?*

Least Squares method

Statistical testing is also applicable to the linear least squares method (Gaddis and Gaddis, 1990f; Ferrill and Brown 1994). In this instance, the analysis focuses on whether the slope of the line is different from zero as a slope of zero means that no linear relationship exists between the variables x and y. To that end, testing for the *significance* of the slope (a statistically *significant* test is that when the H_0 is rejected; an insignificant result means that the null hypothesis is not rejected) requires the use of a *Student's t-test*. This test replaces the z distribution whenever the standard deviation of the variable in the population is unknown (ie, σ is unknown). The t-test uses a bell-shaped distribution similar to that of the z distribution; however, the tails of

the t-distribution are "less pinched." The mean of the t-distribution is zero, and its standard deviation is a function of the sample size (or the degrees of freedom). The larger the sample size, the closer the value of the standard deviation is to 1 (recall that the standard deviation for the z distribution, the standard normal curve, is always 1). With the advances in computer technology and the availability of software programs that readily calculate these statistics, the function of the researcher is to enter the data in a computer database, calculate the slope, and find the p-value associated with the slope. If the p-value is less than α, then the slope is different from zero. Otherwise, do not reject the null hypothesis and declare the slope is zero. Similar analysis can be done on the y intercept using a t-test. For the significance of the regression coefficient (r), a critical value is obtained from statistics tables at a given degrees of freedom ($n - 2$), a two- or one-tailed test, and a selected α value. If the observed r value equals or exceeds the critical value, then r is significant (ie, reject H_0 of $r = 0$); otherwise, r is statistically insignificant. For example, a calculated r value of 0.75 was computed based on 30 pairs of x and y values. The following calculations are taken in the analysis:

1. State the null hypothesis and alternate hypothesis:
   H_0: $r = 0$
   H_1: r is not equal to zero
   Two-tailed test
2. State the alpha value:
   $\alpha = 0.05$
3. Find the critical value of r (tables for this may be found in statistical textbooks):
   Degrees of freedom = $n - 2 = 30 - 2 = 28$
   Critical value = 0.361
4. Since the calculated value ($r = 0.75$) is greater than 0.361, then the null hypothesis is rejected
5. A linear relationship exists between variables x and y

Another way to test the significance of r is to build a confidence interval on the true value of r in the population. The procedure for this test includes the following steps:

1. Convert the observed r value to z_r value, also known as Fisher's z:
   $r = 0.75$, then $z_r = 0.973$

2. Fisher's z distribution has a bell-shaped distribution with a mean equal to zero and a standard error of the mean (SE) equal to $[1/(n-3)^{0.5}]$:

$$SE = [1/(30-3)^{0.5}] = 0.192$$

3. Construct a confidence interval on the true value of Fisher's z in the population:

$$95\% \text{ CI}_{Z_r} = Z_r \pm 1.96 \text{ (SE)}$$
$$95\% \text{ CI}_{Z_r} = 0.973 \pm 1.96 (0.192)$$
$$95\% \text{ CI}_{Z_r} = [0.60, 1.35]$$

4. Convert the interval found in (3) above to a confidence interval on the true value of r in the population:

$$95\% \text{ CI}_r = [0.54, 0.88]$$

5. If the interval in step (4) contains the value of zero, then do not reject the null hypothesis (H_0: the true value of r in the population is zero); otherwise, reject H_0 and declare that r is statistically significantly different from zero (this indicates that a linear relationship exists between the variables x and y):

Since the 95% CI does not contain the value zero, reject the null hypothesis and conclude that r is statistically significant.

Accuracy Versus Precision

"*Accuracy* refers to the closeness of the observation to the actual or true value. *Precision (or reproducibility)* refers to the closeness of repeated measurements" (Shargel et al, 2012).

Error Versus Bias

Error occurs when mistakes that neither systematically under- nor overestimate effect size are made (Drew, 2003). This is sometimes referred to as random error. An example would be if a coin were tossed 10 times, yielding 8 "heads," leading one to conclude that the probability of heads is 80% (Drew, 2003). *Bias* refers to systematic errors or flaws in study design that lead to incorrect results (Drew, 2003). In other words, bias is "error with direction" leading to systematic under- or overestimation of effect size (Drew, 2003). There are many types of bias. *Selection*

bias occurs when investigators select included and/or excluded samples or data. *Diagnostic or detection bias* can occur when outcomes are detected more or less frequently. For example, this can be from changes in the sensitivity of instruments used to detect drug concentrations. *Observer or investigator bias* may occur when an investigator favors one sample over another. This is most problematic with "open" or unblinded study designs. *Misclassification bias* may occur when samples are inappropriately classified and may bias in favor of one group over another or in favor of finding no difference between the groups. Bias can also occur when there is a significant dropout rate or loss to follow-up such that data collection is incomplete. *Channeling bias* is sometimes called *confounding by indication* and can occur when one group or sample is "channeled" into receiving one treatment over another.

Bias is minimized through a combination of proper study design, methods, and analysis. Proper analysis *cannot* "de-flaw" a study with poor design or methodology (DeYoung, 2000). There are several means of minimizing bias. *Randomization* is sometimes referred to as allocation. In this process, samples are divided into groups by chance alone such that potential confounders are divided equally among the groups and bias is minimized. Doing so helps ensure that all within a studied sample have an equal and independent opportunity of being selected as part of the sample. This can be carried a step further in that once the subject has been selected for a sample, he/she has an equal opportunity of being selected for any of the study arms. An example of *simple randomization* would be drawing numbers from a hat. Its advantage is that it is simple. Its disadvantage is that if a study were stopped early, there is no assurance of similar numbers of subjects in each group at any given point in time. *Block randomization* involves randomizing subjects into small groups called blocks. These blocks generally range from 4 to 20 subjects. Block randomization is advantageous in that there are nearly equal numbers of subjects in each group at any point during a study. Therefore, if a study is stopped early, equal comparisons and more valid conclusions can be made.

Other means of minimizing bias include utilizing objective study endpoints, proper and accurate means of defining exposures and endpoints, accurate and complete sources of information, proper controls to allow investigators to minimize outside influences when evaluating treatments or exposures, proper selection of study subjects, which would require proper inclusion and exclusion criteria, minimizing loss of data, appropriate statistical tests for data analysis, blinding as described later in this chapter, and *matching,* which involves identifying characteristics that are a potential source of bias and matching controls based upon those characteristics (DeYoung, 2000, 2005; Drew, 2003).

CONTROLLED VERSUS NONCONTROLLED STUDIES

Uncontrolled studies do not utilize a control group such that outside influences may affect study results. Using *controls* helps minimize bias through keeping study groups as similar as possible and minimizing outside influences. Ideally, groups will differ only in the factor being studied. There are many types of controls. "Utilizing a *placebo control* is not always practical or ethical, but one or more groups receive(s) active treatment(s) while the control group receives a placebo" (Drew, 2003). *Historical control* studies are generally less expensive to perform but this design introduces problems with diagnostic, detection, and procedure biases. "Data from a group of subjects receiving the experimental drug or intervention are compared to data from a group of subjects previously treated during a different time period, perhaps in a different place" (Herring, 2014). *Crossover control* is very efficient at minimizing bias while maximizing power when used appropriately. Each subject serves as his/her own control. Initially, group A receives the experimental drug while group B receives the control (placebo or gold standard treatment). After a washout period, group A receives the control and group B receives the experimental drug. *Standard treatment (aka active treatment) control* is very practical and ethical. The control group receives "standard" treatment while the other group(s) receives experimental treatment(s). This type of control is used when the investigator wishes to demonstrate that the experimental treatment(s)

is/are equally efficacious, non-inferior, or superior to "standard" treatment.

BLINDING

Blinding limits investigators' treating or assessing one group differently from another. It is especially important if there is any degree of subjectivity associated with the outcome(s) being assessed. However, it is expensive and time consuming. There are several types of blinding but we will only discuss the three most common forms. In a *single-blind* study, someone, usually the subject, but in rare cases it may be the investigator, is unaware of what treatment or intervention the subject is receiving. In a *double-blind* study, neither the investigator nor the subject is aware of what treatment or intervention the subject is receiving. In a *double-dummy* study, if one is comparing two different dosage forms (eg, intranasal sumatriptan vs injectable sumatriptan), and doesn't want the patient or investigator to know in which arm a patient is participating, then one group would receive intranasal sumatriptan and a placebo injection and the other group would receive intranasal placebo and a sumatriptan injection. Another example would be for a trial evaluating a tablet versus an inhaler. Some trials that claim to be blinded are not. For example, a medication may have a distinctive taste, physiologic effect, or adverse effect that un-blinds patients and/or investigators.

CONFOUNDING

Confounding occurs when variables, other than the one(s) being studied, influence study results. Confounding variables are difficult to detect sometimes and are linked to study outcome(s) and may be linked to hypothesized cause(s). As discussed in more detail later in this chapter, *validity* of a study depends upon how well investigators minimize the influence of confounders (DeYoung, 2000).

For example, atherosclerosis and myocardial infarction (MI): There is an association between atherosclerosis and smoking, smoking and risk for an MI, and atherosclerosis and risk for an MI. The proposed cause is atherosclerosis and the potential confounder is smoking.

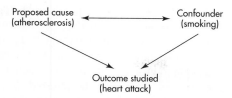

Another example of confounding is the relationship between fasting blood glucose (FBG) in patients being treated for diabetes with medication. One confounding factor on their FBG is their diet. For example, dietary cinnamon consumption can lower blood glucose. If patients regularly consume cinnamon, FBG could be lowered beyond the diabetic medication's capabilities. In this case, although cinnamon may not affect the proposed cause (type of diabetes medication that is being used), it very well may affect FBG concentrations, possibly resulting in biased results by augmenting the diabetes drug's FBG lowering effect, and therefore affecting its pharmacodynamic profile.

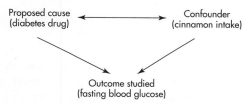

As with bias, confounding is minimized through the combination of proper study design and methodology, including randomization, proper inclusion and exclusion criteria, and matching if appropriate. However, unlike bias, confounding may also be minimized through proper statistical analysis. *Stratification* separates subjects into nonoverlapping groups called strata, where specific factors (eg, gender, ethnicity, race, smoking status, weight, diet) are evaluated for any influence on study results (DeYoung, 2000). "Stratification has limits" (Herring, 2014). As one stratifies, subgroup sample sizes decrease, so one's ability to detect meaningful influences in each subgroup will also decrease.

Multivariate (or multiple) regression analysis (MRA) is a possible solution (DeYoung, 2000). With MRA, "multiple predictor variables (aka independent variables) can be used to predict outcomes (aka dependent variables)" (Herring, 2014). For example,

the national cholesterol guidelines utilize multiple regression to help establish atherosclerotic cardiovascular disease (ASCVD) risk for patients based upon population data. A patient's ASCVD risk is the dependent variable because its estimate "depends upon" several independent variables. The independent variables include gender, race, age, total cholesterol, HDL-cholesterol, smoking status, systolic blood pressure, and whether or not a patient is being treated for hypertension, or has diabetes. All of these independent variables are used to help predict a patient's ASCVD risk. Similar factors to those listed above can influence a multitude of pharmacokinetic parameters as well.

As previously discussed, various types of ANOVAs help account for confounding: multivariate ANOVAs for non-paired data, and two-way repeated measures ANOVA for paired data.

VALIDITY

Internal validity addresses how well a study was conducted: if appropriate methods were used to minimize bias and confounding and ensure that exposures, interventions, and outcomes were measured correctly (DeYoung, 2000). This includes ensuring the study accurately tested and measured what it claims to have tested and measured (DeYoung, 2000; Anonymous, 2003). Internal validity directly affects external validity; without internal validity, a study has no external validity. Presuming internal validity, *external validity* addresses the application of study findings to other groups, patients, systems, or the general population (DeYoung, 2000; Drew, 2003). "A high degree of internal validity is often achieved at the expense of external validity" (Drew, 2003). For example, excluding diabetic hypertensive patients from a study may provide very clean statistical endpoints. However, clinicians who treat mainly diabetic hypertensive patients may be unable to utilize the results from such a trial (Drew, 2003).

Frequently Asked Question

▶ *Are there any types of statistical tests that can be used to correct for a lack of internal validity?*

BIOEQUIVALENCE STUDIES

"Statistics have wide application in bioequivalence studies for the comparison of drug bioavailability for two or more drug products. The FDA has published Guidance for Industry for the statistical determination of bioequivalence (1992, 2001) that describes the comparison between a test (T) and reference (R) drug product. These trials are needed for approval of new or generic drugs. If the drug formulation changes, bioequivalence studies may be needed to compare the new drug formulation to the previous drug formulation. For new drugs, several investigational formulations may be used at various stages, or one formulation with several strengths must show equivalency by extent and rate (eg, 2 × 250-mg tablet vs 1 × 500-mg tablet, suspension vs capsule, immediate-release vs extended-release product). The blood levels of the drug are measured for both the new and the reference formulation. The derived pharmacokinetic parameters, such as maximum concentration (C_{max}) and area under the curve (AUC), must meet accepted statistical criteria for the two drugs to be considered bioequivalent. In bioequivalence trials, a 90% confidence interval of the ratio of the mean of the new formulation to the the mean of the old formulation (Test/Reference) is calculated. That confidence interval needs to be completely within 0.80–1.25 for the drugs to be considered bioequivalent. Adequate power should be built into the design and validated methods used for analysis of the samples. Typically, both the rate (reflected by C_{max}) and the extent (AUC) are tested. The ANOVA may also reveal any sequence effects, period effects, treatment effects, or inter- and intrasubject variability. Because of the small subject population usually employed in bioequivalence studies, the ANOVA uses log-transformed data to make an inference about the difference of the two groups" (Shargel et al, 2012).

EVALUATION OF RISK FOR CLINICAL STUDIES

Risk calculations estimate the magnitude of association between exposure and outcome (DeYoung, 2000). These effect measurers are mainly used for nominal outcomes, but in rare cases may be applied to ordinal outcomes. The following calculations for cohort and randomized controlled trial (RCT) are the same, but nomenclature is different. For a cohort study, the exposed group is referred to as such. For an RCT, the exposed group may be referred to as the interventional, experimental, or treatment group. For a cohort study, the unexposed group is referred to as such. For an RCT, the unexposed group is referred to as the control group. For the following examples, the subscript "E" will refer to the exposed or experimental (treatment, interventional) group and the subscript "C" will refer to the unexposed or control group.

Absolute risk (AR) is simply another term for incidence. It is the number of *new cases* that occur during a specified time period divided by the number of subjects initially followed to detect the outcome(s) of interest (Gaddis and Gaddis, 1990c).

$$AR = \frac{\text{Number who develop the outcome of interest during a specified time period}}{\text{Number initially followed to detect the outcome of interest}}$$

(3.10)

Absolute risk reduction (ARR) is a measure of the absolute incidence differences in the event rate between the studied groups. Absolute differences are more meaningful than relative differences in outcomes when evaluating clinical trials (DeYoung, 2005). When outcomes are worse for the experimental group, the absolute risk difference is termed *absolute risk increase (ARI)*.

$$\text{ARR (or ARI)} = AR_C - AR_E \qquad (3.11)$$

Numbers needed to treat (NNT) is the "reciprocal of the ARR" (DeYoung, 2000).

$$NNT = \frac{1}{ARR} \qquad (3.12)$$

When outcomes are worse for the experimental group, there is an ARI and this calculation is referred to as *numbers needed to harm (NNH)*.

$$NNH = \frac{1}{ARI} \qquad (3.13)$$

These calculations help in understanding the magnitude of an intervention's effectiveness (DeYoung, 2000).

A weakness of these is that they "assume baseline risk is the same for all patients or that it is unrelated to relative risk" (DeYoung, 2000). Although rarely seen, "confidence intervals (CIs) may be calculated for NNT and NNH" (DeYoung, 2005).

Relative risk (RR) compares the AR (incidence) of the experimental group to that of the control group (DeYoung, 2000). It is simply a ratio of the AR for the experimental or exposed group to the AR of the control or unexposed group. RR is sometimes called *risk ratio, rate ratio,* or *incidence rate ratio.*

$$RR = \frac{AR_E}{AR_C} \qquad (31.4)$$

Relative risk differences are sometimes presented in studies and these estimate the percentage of baseline risk that is changed between the exposed or experimental group and the unexposed or control group. The relative risk difference is termed *relative risk reduction (RRR)* when risk is decreased. The relative risk difference is termed *relative risk increase (RRI)* when risk is increased. RRR and RRI can be calculated in two different ways:

$$RRR \text{ (or RRI)} = 1 - RR \qquad (3.15)$$

or

$$RRR \text{ (or RRI)} = \frac{ARR \text{ (or ARI)}}{AR_C} \qquad (3.16)$$

Hazard ratio (HR) is used with Cox proportional hazards regression analysis. It is used when a study is evaluating the length of time required for an outcome of interest to occur (Katz, 2003). HR is often used similarly to RR, and is a reasonable estimate of RR as long as adequate data are collected and outcome incidence is <15% (Katz, 2003; Shargel et al, 2012). However, whereas RR only represents the probability of having an event between the beginning and the end of a study, HR can represent the probability of having an event during a certain time interval between the beginning and the end of the study (DeYoung, 2005).

Odds ratio (OR) is mainly used in case-control studies as an estimate of RR since incidence cannot be calculated. Estimation accuracy decreases as outcome or disease incidence increases. However, OR is fairly accurate as long as disease incidence is <15%, which is usually the case since case-control studies evaluate potential risk factors for rare diseases (Katz, 2003). In addition, OR is sometimes reported for RCTs

utilizing logistic or multivariate regression analysis simply because these analyses automatically calculate OR. They do so because regression analysis is utilized to adjust for confounding and adjustments are easier to perform with OR than with RR (De Muth, 2006). OR is presented differently for case-control studies than for RCTs. For RCTs, OR is presented in the same way as RR. For example, in an RCT evaluating an association of an intervention and death rate, an OR of 0.75 would be reported as patients receiving the intervention were 25% less likely, or 75% as likely, to have died than controls. Since case-control studies identify patients based upon disease rather than intervention, OR is presented differently than for an RCT; it compares the odds that a case was exposed to a risk factor to the odds that a control was exposed to a risk factor. For example, in a case-control study evaluating an association of a rare type of cancer and exposure to pesticides, an OR of 1.5 would be reported as cases (those with the rare cancer) were 50% more likely, or 1½ times as likely, to have been exposed to pesticides than controls. CIs should always be provided for RR, OR, and HR.

These above calculations and principles are commonly utilized for interpreting data in FDA-approved package inserts. For example, in the Coreg® (carvedilol) package insert, there are several major studies that are presented. The Copernicus trial evaluated carvedilol's efficacy against that of placebo for patients with severe systolic dysfunction heart failure over a median of 10 months (GlaxoSmithKline, 2008). The primary endpoint of mortality occurred in 190 out of 1133 patients taking placebo and 130 out of 1156 patients taking carvedilol. This means that the AR for patients taking placebo was 190/1133 = 0.17 or 17% and the AR for patients taking carvedilol was 130/1156 = 0.11 or 11%. The RR would be 0.11/0.17 or 11%/17% = 0.65 or 65%. RRR would be 1 – 0.65 = 0.35 or 35%. Therefore, patients treated with carvedilol were 35% less likely to die than were patients treated with placebo. However, sometimes RR and RRR can be deceptive, so one should always calculate the ARR or ARI and NNT or NNH. In this case, carvedilol improved the death rate, so one would calculate ARR and NNT. The AAR is simply the difference between the AR of each agent: 17% – 11% = 6% or 0.17 – 0.11 = 0.06. NNT is the reciprocal of

ARR, so 1/0.06 = 17. Therefore, since the median follow-up of this trial was 10 months, one would need to treat 17 patients for 10 months with carvedilol rather than placebo to prevent 1 death.

Frequently Asked Question

▶ *Which are more important: relative or absolute differences?*

CHAPTER SUMMARY

Statistical applications are vital in conducting and evaluating biopharmaceutical and pharmacokinetic research. Utilization includes, but is not limited to, studies involving hypothesis testing, finding ways to improve a product, its safety, or performance. Proper statistics are required for experimental planning, data collection, analysis, and interpretation of results, allowing for rational decision making throughout these processes (Durham, 2008; Shargel et al, 2012).

In this chapter, we have presented very basic, practical principles in hopes of guiding the reader throughout the research process. For readers who are interested in learning about this topic in more depth, we recommend statistics textbooks or online resources and/or taking a research-based statistics course at the college or university of their choosing.

LEARNING QUESTIONS

1. The following data represent the concentration of vitamin C in infant urine:

Age (months)	Gender	Conc. (ng/mL)
1	F	2.7
3	F	2.8
4	M	2.9
6	M	2.9
7	M	2.3
9	M	2.3
12	F	1.5
15	F	1.1
16	M	1.3
17	F	1.3
18	F	1.1
24	F	1.5
25	F	1.0
29	M	0.4
30	F	0.2

The column for concentration (ng/mL) refers to the concentration of vitamin C in infant urine. Calculate the arithmetic mean for vitamin C in the urine.

2. Refer to Question 1; find the standard deviation for the concentration of vitamin C in urine for the male infants.

3. Refer to Question 1; find the coefficient of variation (%) value for the variable age.

4. Refer to Question 1; consider the following graph representing the data:

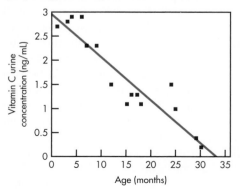

Based on the above graph, the value for the correlation coefficient is most likely_____.

5. Refer to Questions 1 and 4. The older the infant, the _____ is the concentration of vitamin C in the urine.

6. The *p*-value associated with the slope of the line in Question 4 is less than 0.0001 ($p < 0.0001$). For α of 5%, the slope value is statistically _____.

7. Find the slop value for the graph in Question 4.

8. The following results were presented by Chin KH, Sathyyasurya DR, Abu Saad H, Jan Mohamed HJB: Effect of ethnicity, dietary intake and physical activity on plasma adiponectin concentrations among Malaysian patients with type 2 diabetes mellitus. *Int J Endocrinol Metab* **11**(3):16–174, 2013. DOI:10.5812/ijem.8298.) (Copyright © 2013, Research Institute for Endocrine Sciences and Iran Endocrine Society; Licensee Kowsar Ltd. This is an Open Access article distributed under the terms of the Creative Commons Attribution License [http://creativecommons.org/licenses/by/3.0], which permits unrestricted use, distribution, and reproduction in any medium, provided the original work is properly cited):

	Malay	**Chinese**	**Indian**
Adiponectin (μg/mL)	6.85 (4.66)	6.21 (3.62)	4.98 (2.22)

(Chin KH, Sathyyasurya DR, Abu Saad H, Jan Mohamed HJB: Effect of ethnicity, dietary intake and physical activity on plasma adiponectin concentrations among Malaysian patients with type 2 diabetes mellitus. *Int J Endocrinol Metab* **11**(3):16–174, 2013.)

The concentration of adiponectin (a protein produced by adipocytes) in plasma is reported in Malaysian patients with three different ethnicities. The values in the table above are given as arithmetic mean (standard deviation). The significance of adiponectin plasma concentration is that its plasma levels correlate well with the clinical response to administered insulin in patients with type 2 diabetes. Referring to the results above, which group of patients is more variable with respect to its mean than the other two groups?

9. Which statistics did you use in answering Question 8?

10. Investigators want to perform a study comparing two doses of an investigational anticoagulant for prevention of thromboembolism. They calculate that a sample size of 400 subjects (200 in each arm) will be needed to show a difference (based upon an alpha of 0.05 and beta of 0.20). They predict that given the patient population, approximately 50% of subjects will drop out of the study. Based upon the dropout rate, how many subjects will be needed in each treatment arm?

11. A superiority trial evaluating the doses of a new cholesterol medication was performed comparing AUC. There were 200 patients in this trial and differences were statistically significant. Was this study underpowered?

12. A study is planned to evaluate differences in half-life ($t_{\frac{1}{2}}$) of three different metoprolol formulations. The investigators plan to include 150 subjects (50 in each arm) to reach statistical significance based upon a beta of 0.20 and alpha of 0.05. Which statistical test would be the most appropriate? (Hint: Assume no confounders.)

13. If you conduct a pharmacokinetic study that utilizes appropriate methodology and a broad population base for inclusion, how will this affect the strength of internal and external validity?

14. Investigators wish to study the differences in patients with subtherapeutic concentrations of vancomycin via two difference delivery systems. The results from this 2-week study are listed below:

	Formulation A (FA) ($n = 55$)	**Formulation B (FB) ($n = 62$)**
Subtherapeutic vancomycin concentrations	35	17

How should these results be reported?

ANSWERS

Learning Questions

1. Using a scientific calculator, the arithmetic mean for vitamin C in infant urine was 1.69 ng/mL.

2. Using a scientific calculator, the standard deviation of vitamin C in urine for male infants was 0.98 ng/mL.

3. The coefficient of variation (%) for age was (SD/mean) × 100 = (9.49/14.4) × 100 = 66%

4. The slope of the line depicted in the graph was negative. Therefore, the correlation coefficient must be a negative value.

5. A negative linear relationship was observed between age of infants and the concentration of vitamin C in urine. Thus, the vitamin C concentration in urine in older infants would be lower than that found in younger infants.

6. Since p-value is less than 0.05, the results were statistically significant.

7. The slope of the line is negative. The value of the slope may be obtained by a scientific calculator.

8. The coefficient of variation (%) for Malay, Chinese, and Indian patients was 68.03%, 58.29%, and 44.58%, respectively. Recall that CV (%) = (SD/mean) × 100. Since Malay patients had the highest CV (%) value, then adiponectin plasma concentration was more variable with respect to its mean than the other two values.

9. The coefficient of variation (%).

10. Sample size (corrected for drop-outs)

$$= \frac{\text{Number of patients}}{1 - \% \text{ of expected drop-outs}}$$

200 in each arm/(1 − 0.5) = 200/0.5 = 400 in each treatment arm. If the question had asked how many total subjects would be needed (ie, both arms), the answer would have been 400/(1 − 0.5) = 400/0.5 = 800.

11. Power is associated with beta: power = 1 − beta. Beta is the risk of committing a type 2 error. If a statistically significant difference is detected, a type 2 error could not occur. Therefore, the trial was not underpowered. With this scenario, there are only two possibilities: either (1) the findings were correct or (2) a type 1 error occurred.

12. Differences in half-life ($t_{1/2}$) are parametric data since they are scored on a continuum and there is a consistent level of magnitude of difference between data units. Since there are three metoprolol formulations being evaluated, and no identified confounders, a 1-way ANOVA is appropriate. If there were only two groups and no identified confounders, a t-test would be appropriate.

13. Utilizing appropriate methodology helps increase internal validity. Including a broad population helps increase external validity.

14. There are several ways the results could be reported. $AR_{FA} = 35/55 = 0.64$ or 64%, $AR_{FB} = 17/62 = 0.27$ or 27%, $ARI = AR_C − AR_E = 0.27 − 0.64 = 0.37$ or 37%, NNH = 1/0.37 = 2.7, so 3 patients over 2 weeks. In other words, one would need to treat 3 patients over 2 weeks with formulation A rather than formulation B to cause one episode of a subtherapeutic vancomycin concentration. $RR = 0.64/0.27 = 2.3$. The results could be reported as those utilizing formulation A were 2.3 times as likely to be subtherapeutic as those being given formulation B. Since $RRI = 1 − RR = 1 − 2.3 = −1.3$, another way of explaining the results would be that those utilizing formulation A were 130% more likely to have subtherapeutic vancomycin concentrations than those being given formulation B.

REFERENCES

Anonymous: SOP 13: Pharmacokinetic data analysis. *Onkologie* **26**(suppl 6):56–59, 2003.

Al-Achi A, PhD. Discussions.

Berensen NM: Biostatistics review with lecture for the MUSC/VAMC BCPS study group, Charleston, SC, July 17, 2000.

Brendel K, Dartois C, Comets E, et al: Are population pharmacokinetic-pharmacodynamic models adequately evaluated? A survey of the literature from 2002 to 2004. *Clin Pharmacokinet* **46**(3):221–234, 2007.

De Muth JE: In Chow SC (ed). *Basic Statistics and Pharmaceutical Statistical Applications*, 2nd ed. Boca Raton, London, New York, Chapman & Hall/CRC, Taylor & Francis Group, 2006.

DeYoung GR: Clinical Trial Design (handout). 2000 Updates in Therapeutics: The Pharmacotherapy Preparatory Course, 2000.

DeYoung GR: *Understanding Statistics: An Approach for the Clinician. Science and Practice of Pharmacotherapy PSAP Book 5*, 5th ed. American College of Clinical Pharmacy, Kansas City, MO, 2005.

Drew R: Clinical Research Introduction (handout). Drug Literature Evaluation/Applied Statistics Course. Campbell University School of Pharmacy, 2003.

Durham TA, Turner JR: *Introduction to Statistics in Pharmaceutical Clinical Trials*. London, UK, Pharmaceutical Press, RPS Publishing, 2008.

Ferrill JM, Brown LD: Statistics for the Nonstatistician: A Systematic Approach to Evaluating Research Reports. US Pharmacist July:H-3-H-16, 1994.

Gaddis ML, Gaddis GM: Introduction to biostatistics: Part 1, Basic concepts. *Ann Emerg Med* **19**(1):86–89, 1990a.

Gaddis ML, Gaddis GM: Introduction to biostatistics: Part 2, Descriptive statistics. *Ann Emerg Med* **19**(3):309–315, 1990b.

Gaddis ML, Gaddis GM: Introduction to biostatistics: Part 3, Sensitivity, specificity, predictive value, and hypothesis testing. *Ann Emerg Med* **19**(5):591–597, 1990c.

Gaddis ML, Gaddis GM: Introduction to biostatistics: Part 4, Statistical inference techniques in hypothesis testing. *Ann Emerg Med* **19**(7):820–825, 1990d.

Gaddis ML, Gaddis GM: Introduction to biostatistics: Part 5, Statistical inference techniques for hypothesis testing with nonparametric data. *Ann Emerg Med* **19**(9):1054–1059, 1990e.

Gaddis ML, Gaddis GM: Introduction to biostatistics: Part 6, Correlation and regression. *Ann Emerg Med* **19**(12):1462–1468, 1990f.

Glasner AN: *High Yield Biostatistics*. PA, Williams & Willkins, 1995.

GlaxoSmithKline. Coreg CR [package insert], https://www.gsk-source.com/gskprm/htdocs/documents/COREG-CR-PI-PIL.PDF. Research Triangle Park, NC, 2008.

Herring C: *Quick Stats: Basics for Medical Literature Evaluation*, 5th ed. Massachusetts, USA, Xanedu Publishing Inc., 2014.

Hirt D, Urien S, Jullien V, et al: Age-related effects on nelfinavir and M8 pharmacokinetics: A population study with 182 children. *Antimicrob Agents Chemother* **50**(3):910–916, 2006.

Katz MH: Multivariable analysis: A primer for readers of medical research. *Annal Internal Med* **138**:644–650, 2003.

Munro HB: *Statistical Methods for Health Care Research*. Lippincott Williams & Wilkins, Philadelphia, PA, 2005.

Drew R, PharmD, MS, BCPS. Discussions and provisions.

Shargel L, Wu-Pong S, Yu A: *Statistics. Applied Biopharmaceutics and Pharmacokinetics*, 6th ed. New York, NY, USA, McGraw-Hill, 2012, Appendix.

REFERENCES

4 One-Compartment Open Model: Intravenous Bolus Administration

David S.H. Lee

Chapter Objectives

▶ Describe a one-compartment model, IV bolus injection.

▶ Provide the pharmacokinetic terms that describe a one-compartment model, IV bolus injection, and the underlying assumptions.

▶ Explain how drugs follow one-compartment kinetics using drug examples that follow one-compartment kinetics.

▶ Calculate pharmacokinetic parameters from drug concentration–time data using a one-compartment model.

▶ Simulate one-compartment plasma drug level graphically using the one-compartment model equation.

▶ Calculate the IV bolus dose of a drug using the one-compartment model equation.

▶ Relate the relevance of the magnitude of the volume of distribution and clearance of various drugs to underlying processes in the body.

▶ Derive model parameters from slope and intercept of the appropriate graphs.

While the oral route of drug administration is the most convenient, intravenous (IV) administration is the most desirable for critical care when reaching desirable drug concentrations quickly is needed. Examples of when IV administration is desirable include antibiotic administration during septic infections or administration of antiarrhythmic drugs during a myocardial infarction. Because pharmacokinetics is the science of the kinetics of drug absorption, distribution, and elimination, IV administration is desirable in understanding these processes since it simplifies drug absorption, essentially making it complete and instantaneous. This leaves only the processes of drug distribution and elimination left to study. This chapter will introduce the concepts of drug distribution and elimination in the simplest model, the *one-compartment open model*.

The one-compartment open model assumes that the body can be described as a single, uniform compartment (ie, one compartment), and that drugs can enter and leave the body (ie, open model). The simplest drug administration is when the entire drug is given in a rapid IV injection, also known as an IV bolus. Thus, the one-compartment open model with IV bolus administration is the simplest pharmacokinetic model. It assumes that the drug is administered instantly into the body, it is instantaneously and rapidly distributed throughout the body, and drug elimination occurs immediately upon entering the body. This model is a simplistic representation of the processes in the body that determine drug disposition, but nonetheless, it can be useful to describe and predict drug disposition.

In reality, when a drug is administered intravenously, the drug travels through the bloodstream and distributes throughout the bloodstream in the body. While this process is not truly instantaneous, it is relatively rapid enough that we can make this assumption for most drugs. Through the bloodstream, the drug is distributed to the various tissue organs in the body. The rate and extent of distribution to the tissue organs depends on several processes and properties. Tissues in the body are presented the drug at various rates, depending on the blood flow to that organ, and the drug may have different abilities to cross from the vasculature to the organ depending on the molecular weight of the drug. Tissues also have different affinity for the drug, depending on lipophilicity and drug binding. Finally, large organs may have a large capacity for drugs to distribute to.

While drug distribution is complex, if these processes are rapid enough, we can simplify our conceptualization as if the drug uniformly distributes into a single (one) compartment of fluid. The volume of this single compartment is termed the *apparent volume of distribution*, V_D. The apparent volume of distribution is not an actual volume in the body, but is a theoretical volume that the drug uniformly distributes to immediately after being injected into the body. This uniform and instantaneous distribution is termed a *well-stirred* one-compartment model. The apparent volume of distribution is a proportion between the dose and the concentration of the drug in plasma, C_p^0, at that time immediately after being injected.

Most drugs are eliminated from the body by liver metabolism and/or renal excretion. All of the processes of drug elimination can be described by the *elimination rate constant, k*. The elimination rate constant is the proportion between the rate of drug elimination and the amount of drug in the body. Because the amount of drug in the body changes over time, the rate of drug elimination changes, but the elimination rate constant remains constant for first-order elimination. This makes it convenient to summarize drug elimination from the body independent of time or the amount of drug in the body. However, because it's difficult to measure the amount of *drug in the body, D_B*, pharmacokineticists and pharmacists also prefer to convert drug amounts to drug concentrations in the body using the apparent volume of distribution. Thus, the elimination rate constant also describes the proportion between the rate of change of drug concentration and drug concentration in the compartment.

The one-compartment open model with IV bolus dosing describes the distribution and elimination after an IV bolus administration and is shown in Fig. 4-1. The fluid that the drug is directly injected into is the blood, and generally, drug concentrations are measured in plasma since it is accessible. Therefore, this model predicts the concentrations in

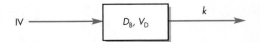

FIGURE 4-1 Pharmacokinetic model for a drug administered by rapid intravenous injection. D_B = drug in body; V_D = apparent volume of distribution; k = elimination rate constant.

the plasma, but does not predict the concentrations in tissues. However, using this model, which assumes distribution to tissues is rapid, we can assume the declines in drug concentration in the plasma and tissues will be proportional. For these reasons, the one-compartment open model is useful for predicting concentrations in the plasma, and declines in plasma concentrations will be proportional to declines in tissue concentrations.

ELIMINATION RATE CONSTANT

The rate of elimination for most drugs from a tissue or from the body is a first-order process, in which the rate of elimination at any point in time is dependent on the amount or concentration of drug present at that instance. The elimination rate constant, k, is a first-order elimination rate constant with units of time^{-1} (eg, h^{-1} or 1/h). Generally, the injected drug is measured in the blood or plasma, sometimes termed the vascular compartment. Total removal or elimination of the injected drug from this compartment is affected by metabolism (biotransformation) and excretion. The elimination rate constant represents the sum of each of these processes:

$$k = k_m + k_e \tag{4.1}$$

where k_m = first-order rate process of metabolism and k_e = first-order rate process of excretion. There may be several routes of elimination of drug by metabolism or excretion. In such a case, each of these processes has its own first-order rate constant.

A rate expression for Fig. 4-1 is

$$\frac{dD_B}{dt} = -kD_B \tag{4.2}$$

This expression shows that the rate of elimination of drug in the body is a first-order process, depending on the overall elimination rate constant, k, and the amount of drug in the body, D_B, remaining at any given time, t. Integration of Equation 4.2 gives the following expression:

$$\log D_B = \frac{-kt}{2.3} + \log D_B^0 \qquad (4.3)$$

where D_B = the drug in the body at time t and D_B^0 is the amount of drug in the body at $t = 0$. When $\log D_B$ is plotted against t for this equation, a straight line is obtained (Fig. 4-2). In practice, instead of transforming values of D_B to their corresponding logarithms, each value of D_B is placed at logarithmic intervals on semilog paper.

Equation 4.3 can also be expressed as

$$D_B = D_B^0 e^{-kt} \qquad (4.4)$$

Frequently Asked Questions

▶ *What is the difference between a rate and a rate constant?*

▶ *Why does k always have the unit 1/time (eg, h⁻¹), regardless of what concentration unit is plotted?*

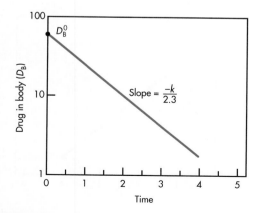

FIGURE 4-2   Semilog graph of the rate of drug elimination in a one-compartment model.

APPARENT VOLUME OF DISTRIBUTION

In general, drug equilibrates rapidly in the body. When plasma or any other biologic compartment is sampled and analyzed for drug content, the results are usually reported in units of concentration instead of amount. Each individual tissue in the body may contain a different concentration of drug due to differences in blood flow and drug affinity for that tissue. The amount of drug in a given location can be related to its concentration by a proportionality constant that reflects the apparent volume of fluid in which the drug is dissolved. The *volume of distribution* represents a volume that must be considered in estimating the amount of drug in the body from the concentration of drug found in the sampling compartment. The volume of distribution is the apparent volume (V_D) in which the drug is dissolved (Equation 4.5). Because the value of the volume of distribution does not have a true physiologic meaning in terms of an anatomic space, the term *apparent* volume of distribution is used.

The amount of drug in the body is not determined directly. Instead, blood samples are collected at periodic intervals and the plasma portion of blood is analyzed for their drug concentrations. The V_D relates the concentration of drug in plasma (C_p) and the amount of drug in the body (D_B), as in the following equation:

$$D_B = V_D C_p \qquad (4.5)$$

Substituting Equation 4.5 into Equation 4.3, a similar expression based on drug concentration in plasma is obtained for the first-order decline of drug plasma levels:

$$\log C_p = \frac{-kt}{2.3} + \log C_p^0 \qquad (4.6)$$

where C_p = concentration of drug in plasma at time t and C_p^0 = concentration of drug in plasma at $t = 0$. Equation 4.6 can also be expressed as

$$C_p = C_p^0 e^{-kt} \qquad (4.7)$$

The relationship between apparent volume, drug concentration, and total amount of drug may be better understood by the following example.

EXAMPLE ▶▶▶

Exactly 1 g of a drug is dissolved in an unknown volume of water. Upon assay, the concentration of this solution is 1 mg/mL. What is the original volume of this solution?

The original volume of the solution may be obtained by the following proportion, remembering that 1 g = 1000 mg:

$$\frac{1000\,mg}{x\,mL}=\frac{1\,mg}{mL}$$

$$x=1000\,mL$$

Therefore, the original volume was 1000 mL or 1 L. This is analogous to how the apparent volume of distribution is calculated.

If, in the above example, the volume of the solution is known to be 1 L, and the amount of drug dissolved in the solution is 1 g, what is the concentration of drug in the solution?

$$\frac{1000\,mg}{1000\,mL}=1\,mg/mL$$

Therefore, the concentration of the drug in the solution is 1 mg/mL. This is analogous to calculating the initial concentration in the plasma if the apparent volume of distribution is known.

From the preceding example, if the volume of solution in which the drug is dissolved and the drug concentration of the solution are known, then the total amount of drug present in the solution may be calculated. This relationship between drug concentration, volume in which the drug is dissolved, and total amount of drug present is given in the following equation:

$$V_D=\frac{Dose}{C_p^0}=\frac{D_B^0}{C_p^0} \tag{4.8}$$

where D = total amount of drug, V = total volume, and C = drug concentration. From Equation 4.8, which is similar to Equation 4.5, if any two parameters are known, then the third term may be calculated.

The one-compartment open model considers the body a constant-volume system or compartment. Therefore, the apparent volume of distribution for any given drug is generally a constant. If both the concentration of drug in the plasma and the apparent volume of distribution for the drug are known, then the total amount of drug in the body (at the time in which the plasma sample was obtained) may be calculated from Equation 4.5.

Calculation of Volume of Distribution

In a one-compartment model (IV administration), the V_D is calculated with the following equation:

$$V_D=\frac{Dose}{C_p^0}=\frac{D_B^0}{C_p^0} \tag{4.9}$$

When C_p^0 is determined by extrapolation, C_p^0 represents the instantaneous drug concentration after drug equilibration in the body at $t = 0$ (Fig. 4-3). The dose of drug given by IV bolus (rapid IV injection) represents the amount of drug in the body, D_B^0, at $t = 0$. Because both D_B^0 and C_p^0 are known at $t = 0$, then the

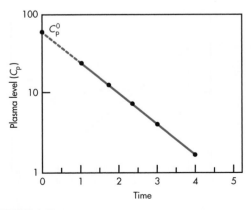

FIGURE 4-3   Semilog graph giving the value of C_p^0 by extrapolation.

apparent volume of distribution, V_D, may be calculated from Equation 4.9.

From Equation 4.2 (repeated here), the rate of drug elimination is

$$\frac{dD_B}{dt} = -kD_B$$

Substituting Equation 4.5, $D_B = V_D C_p$, into Equation 4.2, the following expression is obtained:

$$\frac{dD_B}{dt} = -kV_D C_p \qquad (4.10)$$

Rearrangement of Equation 4.10 gives

$$dD_B = -kV_D C_p dt \qquad (4.11)$$

As both k and V_D are constants, Equation 4.10 may be integrated as follows:

$$\int_0^{D_0} dD_B = -kV_D \int_0^\infty C_p dt \qquad (4.12)$$

Equation 4.12 shows that a small change in time (dt) results in a small change in the amount of drug in the body, D_B.

The integral $\int_0^\infty C_p dt$ represents the AUC_0^∞, which is the summation of the area under the curve from $t = 0$ to $t = \infty$. Thus, the apparent V_D may also be calculated from knowledge of the dose, elimination rate constant, and the area under the curve (AUC) from $t = 0$ to $t = \infty$. This is usually estimated by the trapezoidal rule (see Chapter 2). After integration, Equation 4.12 becomes

$$D_0 = kV_D [AUC]_0^\infty$$

which upon rearrangement yields the following equation:

$$V_D = \frac{D_0}{k[AUC]_0^\infty} \qquad (4.13)$$

The calculation of the apparent V_D by means of Equation 4.13 is a *model-independent* or *noncompartmental model* method, because no pharmacokinetic model is considered and the AUC is determined directly by the trapezoidal rule.

Significance of the Apparent Volume of Distribution

The apparent volume of distribution is not a true physiologic volume, but rather reflects the space the drug seems to occupy in the body. Equation 4.9 shows that the apparent V_D is dependent on C_p^0, and thus is the proportionality constant between C_p^0 and dose. Most drugs have an apparent volume of distribution smaller than, or equal to, the body mass. If a drug is highly bound to plasma proteins or the molecule is too large to leave the vascular compartment, then C_p^0 will be higher, resulting in a smaller apparent V_D. For example, the apparent volume of distribution of warfarin is small, approximately 0.14 L/kg, much less than the total body mass. This is because warfarin is highly bound to plasma proteins, making it hard to leave the vascular compartment.

For some drugs, the volume of distribution may be several times the body mass. In this case, a very small C_p^0 may occur in the body due to concentration of the drug in peripheral tissues and organs, resulting in a large V_D. Drugs with a large apparent V_D are more concentrated in extravascular tissues and less concentrated intravascularly. For example, the apparent volume of distribution of digoxin is very high, 7.0 L/kg, much greater than the body mass. This is because digoxin binds extensively to tissues, especially muscle tissues. Consequently, binding of a drug to peripheral tissues or to plasma proteins will significantly affect the V_D.

The apparent V_D is a volume term that can be expressed as a simple volume or in terms of percent of body weight. In expressing the apparent V_D in terms of percent of body weight, a 1-L volume is assumed to be equal to the weight of 1 kg. For example, if the V_D is 3500 mL for a subject weighing 70 kg, the V_D expressed as percent of body weight is

$$\frac{3.5 \text{ kg}}{70 \text{ kg}} \times 100 = 5\% \text{ of body weight}$$

In the example of warfarin above, 0.14 L/kg is estimated to be 14% of body weight.

If V_D is a very large number—that is, >100% of body weight—then it may be assumed that the drug is concentrated in certain tissue compartments. In the digoxin example above, 7.0 L/kg is estimated to be 700% of body weight. Thus, the apparent V_D is a useful parameter in considering the relative amounts of drug in the vascular and in the extravascular tissues.

Pharmacologists often attempt to conceptualize the apparent V_D as a true physiologic or anatomic fluid compartment. By expressing the V_D in terms of percent of body weight, values for the V_D may be found that appear to correspond to true anatomic volumes (Table 4-1). In the example above where the V_D is 5% of body weight, this is approximately the volume of plasma, and it would be assumed that this drug occupies the vascular compartment with very little distributing to tissues outside the vascular compartment. However, it may be only fortuitous that the value for the apparent V_D of a drug has the same value as a real anatomic volume. If a drug is to be considered to be distributed in a true physiologic volume, then an investigation is needed to test this hypothesis.

Given the apparent V_D for a particular drug, the total amount of drug in the body at any time after administration of the drug may be determined by the measurement of the drug concentration in the plasma (Equation 4.5). Because the magnitude of the apparent V_D is a useful indicator for the amount of drug outside the sampling compartment (usually the blood), the larger the apparent V_D, the greater the amount of drug in the extravascular tissues.

For each drug, the apparent V_D is a constant. In certain pathologic cases, the apparent V_D for the drug may be altered if the distribution of the drug is changed. For example, in edematous conditions, the total body water and total extracellular water increases; this is reflected in a larger apparent V_D value for a drug that is highly water soluble. Similarly, changes in total body weight and lean body mass (which normally occur with age, less lean mass, and more fat) may also affect the apparent V_D.

> **Frequently Asked Question**
> ▶ If a drug is distributed in the one-compartment model, does it mean that there is no drug in the tissue?

CLEARANCE

Clearance is a measure of drug elimination from the body without identifying the mechanism or process. Clearance is also discussed in subsequent chapters. Clearance (*drug clearance*, *systemic clearance*, *total body clearance*, Cl_T) considers the entire body or compartment (in the case of a one-compartment model) as a drug-eliminating system from which many elimination processes may occur.

Drug Clearance in the One-Compartment Model

The body may be considered a system of organs perfused by plasma and body fluids. Drug elimination from the body is an ongoing process due to both metabolism (biotransformation) and drug excretion through the kidney and other routes. The mechanisms of drug elimination are complex, but collectively drug elimination from the body may be quantitated using the concept of drug clearance. Drug clearance refers to the volume of plasma fluid that is cleared of drug per unit time. Clearance may also be considered the fraction of drug removed per unit time. The rate of drug elimination may be expressed in several ways, each of which essentially describes the same process, but with different levels of insight and application in pharmacokinetics.

TABLE 4-1   Fluid in the Body

Water Compartment	Percent of Body Weight	Percent of Total Body Water
Plasma	4.5	7.5
Total extracellular water	27.0	45.0
Total intracellular water	33.0	55.0
Total body water	60.0	100.0

Drug Elimination Expressed as Amount per Unit Time

The expression of drug elimination from the body in terms of mass per unit time (eg, mg/min, or mg/h) is simple, absolute, and unambiguous. For a zero-order elimination process, expressing the rate of drug elimination as mass per unit time is convenient because the elimination rate is constant (Fig. 4-4A). However, drug clearance is not constant for a drug that has zero-order elimination (see Chapter 6). For most drugs, the rate of drug elimination is a first-order elimination process, that is, the elimination rate is not constant and changes with respect to the drug concentration in the body. For first-order elimination, drug clearance expressed as volume per unit time (eg, L/h or mL/min) is convenient because it is a constant.

Drug Elimination Expressed as Volume per Unit Time

The concept of expressing a rate in terms of volume per unit time is common in pharmacy. For example, a patient may be dosed at the rate of 2 teaspoonfuls (10 mL) of a liquid medicine (10 mg/mL) daily, or alternatively, a dose (weight) of 100 mg of the drug daily. Many intravenous medications are administered as a slow infusion with a flow rate (30 mL/h) of a sterile solution (1 mg/mL).

Clearance is a concept that expresses "the rate of drug removal" in terms of the volume of drug in solution removed per unit time (at whatever drug concentration in the body prevailing at that time) (Fig. 4-4B). In contrast to a solution in a bottle, the drug concentration in the body will gradually decline by a first-order process such that the mass of drug removed over time is not constant. The plasma volume in the healthy state is relatively constant because water lost through the kidney is rapidly replaced with fluid absorbed from the gastrointestinal tract.

Since a constant volume of plasma (about 120 mL/min in humans) is filtered through the glomeruli of the kidneys, the rate of drug removal is dependent on the plasma drug concentration at all times. This observation is based on a first-order process governing drug elimination. For many drugs, the rate of drug elimination is dependent on the plasma drug concentration, multiplied by a constant factor ($dC/dt = kC$). When the plasma drug concentration is high, the rate of drug removal is high, and vice versa.

Clearance (volume of fluid removed of drug) for a first-order process is constant regardless of the drug concentration because clearance is expressed in volume per unit time rather than drug amount per unit time. Mathematically, the rate of drug elimination is similar to Equation 4.10:

$$\frac{dD_B}{dt} = -kC_p V_D \qquad (4.10)$$

Dividing this expression on both sides by C_p yields Equation 4.14:

$$\frac{dD_B/dt}{C_p} = \frac{-kC_p V_D}{C_p} \qquad (4.14)$$

$$\frac{dD_B/dt}{C_p} = -kV_D = -Cl \qquad (4.15)$$

where dD_B/dt is the rate of drug elimination from the body (mg/h), C_p is the plasma drug concentration (mg/L), k is a first-order rate constant (h^{-1} or 1/h), and V_D is the apparent volume of distribution (L).

A. Mass approach

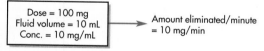

| Dose = 100 mg
Fluid volume = 10 mL
Conc. = 10 mg/mL | → | Amount eliminated/minute
= 10 mg/min |

B. Clearance (volume) approach

| Dose = 100 mg
Fluid volume = 10 mL
Conc. = 10 mg/mL | → | Volume eliminated/minute
= 1 mL/min |

C. Fractional approach

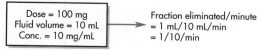

| Dose = 100 mg
Fluid volume = 10 mL
Conc. = 10 mg/mL | → | Fraction eliminated/minute
= 1 mL/10 mL/min
= 1/10/min |

FIGURE 4-4 Diagram illustrating three different ways of describing drug elimination after a dose of 100 mg injected IV into a volume of 10 mL (a mouse, for example).

Cl is clearance and has the units L/h in this example. In the example in Fig. 4-4B, Cl is in mL/min.

Clearance, Cl, is expressed as volume/time. Equation 4.15 shows that clearance is a constant because V_D and k are both constants. D_B is the amount of drug in the body, and dD_B/dt is the rate of change (of amount) of drug in the body with respect to time. The negative sign refers to the drug exiting from the body. In many ways, Cl expressed as a flow rate makes sense since drugs are presented to the eliminating organs at the flow rate of blood to that organ: 1000 mL/min to the kidneys and 1500 mL/min to the liver. Clearance is a reflection of what percentage of drug is eliminated when passing through these organs.

Drug Elimination Expressed as Fraction Eliminated per Unit Time

Consider a compartment volume, containing V_D liters. If Cl is expressed in liters per minute (L/min), then the fraction of drug cleared per minute in the body is equal to Cl/V_D.

Expressing drug elimination as the fraction of total drug eliminated is applicable regardless of whether one is dealing with an amount or a volume (Fig. 4-4C). This approach is most flexible and convenient because of its dimensionless nature in terms of concentration, volume, or amounts. Thus, it is valid to express drug elimination as a fraction (eg, one-tenth of the amount of drug in the body is eliminated or one-tenth of the drug volume is eliminated per unit time). Pharmacokineticists have incorporated this concept into the first-order equation (ie, k) that describes drug elimination from the one-compartment model. Indeed, the universal nature of many processes forms the basis of the first-order equation of drug elimination (eg, a fraction of the total drug molecules in the body will perfuse the glomeruli, a fraction of the filtered drug molecules will be reabsorbed at the renal tubules, and a fraction of the filtered drug molecules will be excreted from the body, giving an overall first-order drug elimination rate constant, k). The rate of drug elimination is the product of k and the drug concentration (Equation 4.2a). The first-order equation of drug elimination can also be based on probability and a consideration of the statistical moment theory (see Chapter 25).

Clearance and Volume of Distribution Ratio, Cl/V_D

EXAMPLE ▶▶▶

Consider that 100 mg of drug is dissolved in 10 mL of fluid and 10 mg of drug is removed in the first minute. The drug elimination process could be described as:

a. Number of mg of drug eliminated per minute (mg/min)

b. Number of mL of fluid cleared of drug per minute

c. Fraction of drug eliminated per minute

The relationship of the three drug elimination processes is illustrated in Fig. 4-4A–C. Note that in Fig. 4-4C, the fraction Cl/V_D is dependent on both the volume of distribution and the rate of drug clearance from the body. This clearance concept forms the basis of classical pharmacokinetics and is later extended to flow models in pharmacokinetic modeling. If the drug concentration is C_p, the rate of drug elimination (in terms of rate of change in concentration, dC_p/dt) is:

$$\frac{dC_p}{dt} = -(Cl/V_D) \times C_p \qquad (4.16)$$

For a first-order process,

$$\frac{dC_p}{dt} = -kC_p = \text{rate of drug elimination} \qquad (4.17)$$

Equating the two expressions yields:

$$kC_p = Cl/V_D \times C_p \qquad (4.18)$$

$$k = \frac{Cl}{V_D} \qquad (4.19)$$

Thus, a first-order rate constant is the fractional constant Cl/V_D. Some pharmacokineticists regard drug clearance and the volume of distribution as independent parameters that are necessary to describe the time course of drug elimination. They also consider k to be a secondary parameter that comes about as a result of Cl and V_D. Equation 4.19 is a rearrangement of Equation 4.15 given earlier.

One-Compartment Model Equation in Terms of Cl and V_D

Equation 4.20 may be rewritten in terms of clearance and volume of distribution by substituting Cl/V_D for k. The clearance concept may also be applied to a biologic system in physiologic modeling without the need of a theoretical compartment.

$$C_p = C_p^0 e^{-kt} \tag{4.20}$$

$$C_p = D_0/V_D e^{-(Cl/V_D)t} \tag{4.21}$$

Equation 4.21 is applied directly in clinical pharmacy to determine clearance and volume of distribution in patients. When only one sample is available, that is, C_p is known at one sample time point, t, after a given dose, the equation cannot be determined unambiguously because two unknown parameters must be solved, that is, Cl and V_D. In practice, the mean values for Cl and V_D of a drug are obtained from the population values (derived from a large population of subjects or patients) reported in the literature. The values of Cl and V_D for the patient are adjusted using a computer program. Ultimately, a new pair of Cl and V_D values that better fit the observed plasma drug concentration is found. The process is repeated through iterations until the "best" parameters are obtained. Since many mathematical techniques (algorithms) are available for iteration, different results may be obtained using different iterative programs. An objective test to determine the accuracy of the estimated clearance and V_D values is to monitor how accurately those parameters will predict the plasma level of the drug after a new dose is given to the patient. In subsequent chapters, mean predictive error will be discussed and calculated in order to determine the performance of various drug monitoring methods in practice.

The ratio of Cl/V_D may be calculated regardless of compartment model type using minimal plasma samples. Clinical pharmacists have applied many variations of this approach to therapeutic drug monitoring and drug dosage adjustments in patients.

Clearance from Drug-Eliminating Tissues

Clearance may be applied to any organ that is involved in drug elimination from the body. As long as first-order elimination processes are involved, clearance represents the sum of the clearances for both renal and nonrenal clearance, each drug-eliminating organ as shown in Equation 4.22:

$$Cl_T = Cl_R + Cl_{NR} \tag{4.22}$$

where Cl_R is renal clearance or drug clearance through the kidney, and Cl_{NR} is nonrenal clearance through other organs. Cl_{NR} is assumed to be due primarily to hepatic clearance (Cl_H) in the absence of other significant drug clearances, such as elimination through the lung or the bile, as shown in Equation 4.23:

$$Cl_T = Cl_R + Cl_H \tag{4.23}$$

Drug clearance considers that the drug in the body is uniformly dissolved in a volume of fluid (apparent volume of distribution, V_D) from which drug concentrations can be measured easily. Typically, plasma drug concentration is measured and drug clearance is then calculated as the fixed volume of plasma fluid (containing the drug) cleared of drug per unit of time. The units for clearance are volume/time (eg, mL/min, L/h).

Alternatively, Cl_T may be defined as the rate of drug elimination divided by the plasma drug concentration. Thus, clearance is expressed in terms of the volume of plasma containing drug that is eliminated per unit time. This clearance definition is equivalent to the previous definition and provides a practical way to calculate clearance based on plasma drug concentration data.

$$Cl_T = \frac{\text{Elimination rate}}{\text{Plasma concentration } (C_p)} \tag{4.24}$$

$$Cl_T = \frac{(dD_E/dt)}{C_p} = (\mu g/\text{min})/(\mu g/\text{mL}) = \text{mL}/\text{min} \tag{4.25}$$

where D_E is the amount of drug eliminated and dD_E/dt is the rate of drug elimination.

Rearrangement of Equation 4.25 gives Equation 4.26:

$$\text{Rate of Drug elimination } \frac{dD_E}{dt} = C_p Cl_T \quad (4.26)$$

Therefore, Cl_T is a constant for a specific drug and represents the slope of the line obtained by plotting dD_E/dt versus C_p, as shown in Equation 4.26.

For drugs that follow first-order elimination, the rate of drug elimination is dependent on the amount of drug remaining in the body.

$$\frac{dD_E}{dt} = kD_B = kC_p V_D \quad (4.27)$$

Substituting the elimination rate in Equation 4.26 for $kC_p V_D$ in Equation 4.27 and solving for Cl_T gives Equation 4.28:

$$Cl_T = \frac{kC_p V_D}{C_p} = kV_D \quad (4.28)$$

Equation 4.28 shows that clearance, Cl_T, is the product of V_D and k, both of which are constant. This Equation 4.28 is similar to Equation 4.19 shown earlier. As the plasma drug concentration decreases during elimination, the rate of drug elimination, dD_E/dt, will decrease accordingly, but clearance will remain constant. Clearance will be constant as long as the rate of drug elimination is a first-order process.

For some drugs, the elimination rate processes are not well known and few or no model assumptions are desirable; in this situation, a noncompartment method may be used to calculate certain pharmacokinetic parameters such as clearance, which can be determined directly from the plasma drug concentration–time curve by

$$Cl_T = \frac{D_0}{[AUC]_0^\infty} \quad (4.29)$$

where D_0 is the dose and $[AUC]_0^\infty = \int_0^\infty C_p dt$.

Because $[AUC]_0^\infty$ is calculated from the plasma drug concentration–time curve from 0 to infinity (∞) using the trapezoidal rule, no compartmental model is assumed. However, to extrapolate the data to infinity to obtain the residual $[AUC]_0^\infty$ or ($C_p t/k$), first-order elimination is usually assumed. In this case, if the drug follows the kinetics of a one-compartment model, the Cl_T is numerically similar to the product of V_D and k obtained by fitting the data to a one-compartment model.

The approach (Equation 4.29) of using $[AUC]_0^\infty$ to calculate body clearance is preferred by some statisticians/pharmacokineticists who desire an alternative way to calculate drug clearance without a compartmental model. The alternative approach is often referred to as a *noncompartmental* method of analyzing the data. The noncompartmental approach may be modified in different ways in order to avoid subjective interpolation or extrapolation (see Chapters 7 and 25 for more discussion). While the advantage of this approach is not having to make assumptions about the compartmental model, the disadvantage of the noncompartmental approach is that it does not allow for predicting the concentration at any specific time.

In the noncompartmental approach, the two model parameters, (1) clearance and (2) volume of distribution, govern drug elimination from the physiologic (plasma) fluid directly and no compartment model is assumed. The preference to replace k with Cl/V_D was prompted by Equation 4.19 as rearranged in the above section:

$$k = \frac{Cl}{V_D} \quad (4.19)$$

For a drug to be eliminated from the body fluid, the volume cleared of drug over the size of the pool indicates that k is really computed from Cl and V_D.

In contrast, the classical one-compartment model is described by two model parameters: (1) elimination constant, k, and (2) volume of distribution, V_D. Clearance is derived from $Cl = kV_D$. The classical approach considers V_D the volume in which the drug appears to dissolve, and k reflects how the drug declines due to excretion or metabolism over time. In chemical kinetics, the rate constant, k, is related to "encounters" or "collisions" of the molecules involved when a chemical reaction takes place. An ordinary hydrolysis or oxidation reaction occurring in the test tube can also occur in the body. Classical pharmacokineticists similarly realized that regardless of whether the reaction occurs in a beaker or in the body fluid, the drug molecules must *encounter* the enzyme molecule for biotransformation or the exit site (renal glomeruli) to be eliminated. The probability of getting to the glomeruli or metabolic site during systemic circulation must be first order because both events are probability or chance related (ie, a fraction of drug concentration will be eliminated). Therefore, the rate of elimination (dC/dt) is related to drug concentration and is aptly described by

$$\frac{dC}{dt} = k \times C_p \qquad (4.30)$$

The compartment model provides a useful way to track mass balance of the drug in the body. It is virtually impossible to account for all the drug in the body with a detailed quantitative model. However, keeping track of systemic concentrations and the mass balance of the dose in the body is still important to understand a drug's pharmacokinetic properties. For example, the kinetic parameters for drugs such as aspirin and acetaminophen were determined using mass balance, which indicates that both drugs are over 90% metabolized (acetaminophen urinary excretion = 3%; aspirin urinary excretion = 1.4%). It is important for a pharmacist to apply such scientific principles during drug modeling in order to optimize dosing, such as if a patient has liver failure and metabolism is decreased. Drug metabolism may be equally well described by applying clearance and first-order/saturation kinetics concepts to kinetic models.

Frequently Asked Question
▶ *How is clearance related to the volume of distribution and k?*

CLINICAL APPLICATION

IV bolus injection provides a simple way to study the pharmacokinetics of a drug. The pharmacokinetic parameters of the drug are determined from the slope and the intercept of the plasma drug concentration–time curve obtained after IV bolus injection. This approach is particularly useful for a new or investigational drug when little pharmacokinetic information is known. In practice, rapid bolus injection is often not desirable for many drugs and a slow IV drip or IV drug infusion is preferred. Rapid injection of a large drug dose may trigger adverse drug reactions (ADR) that would have been avoided if the body had sufficient time to slowly equilibrate with the drug. This is particularly true for certain classes of antiarrhythmics, anticonvulsants, antitumor, anticoagulants, oligonucleotide drugs, and some systemic anesthetics. Immediately after an intravenous injection, the concentrated drug solution/vehicle is directly exposed to the heart, lung, and other vital organs before full dilution in the entire body. During the drug's first pass through the body, some tissues may react adversely to a transient high drug concentration because of the high plasma/tissue drug concentration difference (gradients) that exists prior to full dilution and equilibration. Most intravenous drugs are formulated as aqueous solutions, lightly buffered with a suitable pH for this reason. A poorly soluble drug may precipitate from solution if injected too fast. Suspensions or drugs designed for IM injection only could cause serious injury or fatality if injected intravenously. For example, the antibiotic Bicillin intended for IM injection has a precaution that accompanies the packaging to ensure that the drug will not be injected accidentally into a vein. Pharmacists should be especially alert to verify extravascular injection when drugs are designed for IM injection.

With many drugs, the initial phase or transient plasma concentrations are not considered as important as the steady-state "trough" level during long-term drug dosing. However, drugs with the therapeutic endpoint (eg, target plasma drug concentration) that lie within the steep initial distributive phase are much harder to dose accurately and not overshoot the target endpoint. This scenario is particularly true for some drugs used in critical care where rapid responses are needed and IV bolus routes are used more often. Many new biotechnological drugs are administered intravenously because of instability or poor systemic absorption by the oral route. The choice of a proper drug dose and rate of infusion relative to the elimination half-life of the drug is an important consideration for safe drug administration. Individual patients may behave very differently with regard to drug metabolism, drug transport, and drug efflux in target cell sites. Drug receptors and enzymes may have genetic variability making some people more prone to allergic reactions, drug interactions, and side effects. Simple kinetic half-life determination coupled with a careful review of the patient's chart by a pharmacist can greatly improve drug safety and efficacy.

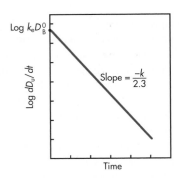

FIGURE 4-5   Graph of Equation 4.33: log rate of drug excretion versus t on regular paper.

> **Frequently Asked Question**
> ▶ If we use a physiologic model, are we dealing with actual volumes of blood and tissues? Why do volumes of distribution emerge for drugs that often are greater than the real physical volume?

CALCULATION OF k FROM URINARY EXCRETION DATA

The elimination rate constant k may be calculated from urinary excretion data. In this calculation the excretion rate of the drug is assumed to be first order. The term k_e is the renal excretion rate constant, and D_u is the amount of drug excreted in the urine.

$$\frac{dD_u}{dt} = k_e D_B \qquad (4.31)$$

From Equation 4.4, D_B can be substituted for $D_B^0 e^{-kt}$:

$$\frac{dD_u}{dt} = k_e D_B^0 e^{-kt} \qquad (4.32)$$

Taking the natural logarithm of both sides and then transforming to common logarithms, the following expression is obtained:

$$\log \frac{dD_u}{dt} = \frac{-kt}{2.3} + \log k_e D_B^0 \qquad (4.33)$$

A straight line is obtained from this equation by plotting log dD_u/dt versus time on regular paper or on semilog paper dD_u/dt against time (Figs. 4-5 and 4-6). The slope of this curve is equal to $-k/2.3$ and the y intercept is equal to $k_e D_B^0$. For rapid intravenous administration, D_B^0 is equal to the dose D_0. Therefore, if D_B^0 is known, the renal excretion rate constant (k_e) can be obtained. Because both k_e and k can be determined by this method, the nonrenal rate constant (k_{nr}) for any route of elimination other than renal excretion can be found as follows:

$$k - k_e = k_{nr} \qquad (4.34)$$

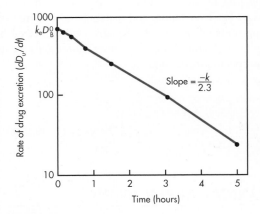

FIGURE 4-6   Semilog graph of rate of drug excretion versus time according to Equation 4.33 on semilog paper (intercept = $k_e D_B^0$).

Substitution of k_m for k_{nr} in Equation 4.34 gives Equation 4.1. Because the major routes of elimination for most drugs are renal excretion and metabolism (biotransformation), k_{nr} is approximately equal to k_m.

$$k_{nr} = k_m \qquad (4.35)$$

There are practical considerations of collecting urine for drug analysis since urine is produced at an approximate rate of 1 mL/min and collected in the bladder until voided for collection. Thus, the drug urinary excretion rate (dD_u/dt) cannot be determined experimentally for any given instant. In practice, urine is collected over a specified time interval, and the urine specimen is analyzed for drug. An average urinary excretion rate is then calculated for that collection period. Therefore, the average rate of urinary drug excretion, D_u/t, is plotted against the time corresponding to the midpoint of the collection interval, t^*, for the collection of the urine sample. The average value of dD_u/dt is plotted on a semilogarithmic scale against the time that corresponds to the midpoint (average time) of the collection period.

PRACTICE PROBLEM

A single IV dose of an antibiotic was given to a 50-kg woman at a dose level of 20 mg/kg. Urine and blood samples were removed periodically and assayed for parent drug. The following data were obtained:

Time (hours)	C_p (μg/mL)	D_u (mg)
0.25	4.2	160
0.50	3.5	140
1.0	2.5	200
2.0	1.25	250
4.0	0.31	188
6.0	0.08	46

What is the elimination rate constant, k, for this antibiotic?

Solution

Set up the following table:

Time (hours)	D_u (mg)	D_u/t	mg/h	t^* (hours)
0.25	160	160/0.25	640	0.125
0.50	140	140/0.25	560	0.375
1.0	200	200/0.5	400	0.750
2.0	250	250/1	250	1.50
4.0	188	188/2	94	3.0
6.0	46	46/2	23	5.0

Here t^* = midpoint of collection period and t = time interval for collection of urine sample.

Construct a graph on a semilogarithmic scale of D_u/t versus t^*. The slope of this line should equal $-k/2.3$. It is usually easier to determine the elimination $t_{1/2}$ directly from the curve and then calculate k from

$$k = \frac{0.693}{t_{1/2}}$$

In this problem, $t_{1/2} = 1.0$ hour and $k = 0.693$ h^{-1}. Note that the slope of the log excretion rate constant is a function of the elimination rate constant k and not of the urinary excretion rate constant k_e (Fig. 4-6).

A similar graph of the C_p values versus t should yield a curve with a slope having the same value as that derived from the previous curve. Note that this method uses the time of plasma sample collection, not the midpoint of collection.

An alternative method for the calculation of the elimination rate constant k from urinary excretion data is the *sigma-minus method*, or *the amount of drug remaining to be excreted method*. The sigma-minus method is sometimes preferred over the previous method because fluctuations in the rate of elimination are minimized.

The amount of unchanged drug in the urine can be expressed as a function of time through the following equation:

$$D_u = \frac{k_e D_0}{k}(1 - e^{-kt}) \qquad (4.36)$$

where D_u is the cumulative amount of unchanged drug excreted in the urine.

The amount of unchanged drug that is ultimately excreted in the urine, D_u^∞, can be determined by making time t equal to ∞. Thus, the term e^{-kt} becomes negligible and the following expression is obtained:

$$D_u^\infty = \frac{k_e D_0}{k} \tag{4.37}$$

Substitution of D_u^∞ for $k_e D_0/k$ in Equation 4.36 and rearrangement yields

$$D_u^\infty - D_u = D_u^\infty \, e^{-kt} \tag{4.38}$$

Equation 4.38 can be written in logarithmic form to obtain a linear equation:

$$\log(D_u^\infty - D_u) = \frac{-kt}{2.3} + \log D_u^\infty \tag{4.39}$$

Equation 4.39 describes the relationship for the amount of drug remaining to be excreted $(D_u^\infty - D_u)$ versus time.

A linear curve is obtained by graphing the logarithm scale of the amount of unchanged drug yet to be eliminated, $\log (D_u^\infty - D_u)$, versus time. On semilog paper, the slope of this curve is $-k/2.3$ and the y intercept is (D_u^∞) (Fig. 4-7).

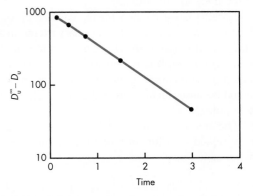

FIGURE 4-7   Sigma-minus method, or the amount of drug remaining to be excreted method, for the calculation of the elimination rate constant according to Equation 4.39.

PRACTICE PROBLEM

Using the data in the preceding problem, determine the elimination rate constant.

Solution

Construct the following table:

Time (hours)	D_u (mg)	Cumulative D_u	$D_u^\infty - D_u$
0.25	160	160	824
0.50	140	300	684
1.0	200	500	484
2.0	250	750	234
4.0	188	938	46
6.0	46	984	0

Plot $\log (D_u^\infty - D_u)$ versus time. Use a semilogarithmic scale for $(D_u^\infty - D_u)$. Evaluate k and $t_{1/2}$ from the slope.

Comparison of the Rate and the Sigma-Minus Methods

The rate method is highly dependent on the accurate measurement of drug in the urine at each time point. Fluctuations in the rate of drug elimination and experimental errors including incomplete bladder emptying for a collection period cause appreciable departure from linearity using the rate method, whereas the accuracy of the sigma-minus method is less affected. The rate method is applicable to zero-order drug elimination process, while the sigma-minus method is not. Lastly, the renal drug excretion rate constant may be obtained from the rate method but not from the sigma-minus method.

The sigma-minus method requires knowing the D_u^∞ and even a single missed urine collection will invalidate the entire urinary drug excretion study. This method also requires the collection of urine until urinary drug excretion is complete; prematurely ending the study early will invalidate the study. Finally, a small error in the assessment of D_u^∞ introduces an error in terms of curvature of the plot, because each point is based on $\log (D_u^\infty - D_u)$ versus time.

CLINICAL APPLICATION

The sigma-minus method and the excretion rate method were applied to the urinary drug excretion in subjects following the smoking of a single marijuana cigarette (Huestis et al, 1996). The urinary excretion curves of 11-nor-carboxy 9-tetrahydrocannabinol (THCCOOH), a metabolite of marijuana, in one subject from 24 to 144 hours after smoking one marijuana cigarette are shown in Figs. 4-8 and 4-9. A total of 199.7 mg of THCCOOH was excreted in the urine over 7 days, which represents 0.54% of the total 9-tetrahydrocannabinol available in the cigarette. Using either urinary drug excretion method, the elimination half-life was determined to be about 30 hours. However, the urinary drug excretion rate method data were more scattered (variable) and the correlation coefficient r was equal to 0.744 (Fig. 4-9), compared to the correlation coefficient r of 0.992 using the sigma-minus method (Fig. 4-8).

Problems in Obtaining Valid Urinary Excretion Data

Certain factors can make it difficult to obtain valid urinary excretion data. Some of these factors are as follows:

1. A significant fraction of the unchanged drug must be excreted in the urine.
2. The assay technique must be specific for the unchanged drug and must not include interference due to drug metabolites that have similar chemical structures.
3. Frequent sampling is necessary for a good curve description.
4. Urine samples should be collected periodically until almost all of the drug is excreted. A graph of the cumulative drug excreted versus time will yield a curve that approaches an asymptote at "infinite" time (Fig. 4-10). In practice, approximately seven elimination half-lives are needed for 99% of the drug to be eliminated.
5. Variations in urinary pH and volume may cause significant variation in urinary excretion rates.
6. Subjects should be carefully instructed as to the necessity of giving a complete urine specimen (ie, completely emptying the bladder).

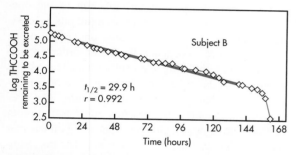

FIGURE 4-8   Amount remaining to be excreted method. The half-life of THCCOOH was calculated to be 29.9 hours from the slope of this curve; the correlation coefficient r was equal to 0.992. (Data from Huestis et al, 1996.)

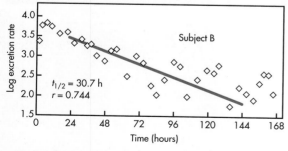

FIGURE 4-9   Excretion rate method. The half-life of THCCOOH was calculated to be 30.7 hours from the slope of this curve; the correlation coefficient r was equal to 0.744. (Data from Huestis et al, 1996.)

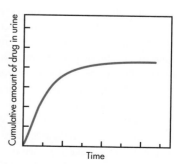

FIGURE 4-10   Graph showing the cumulative urinary excretion of drug as a function of time.

CHAPTER SUMMARY

The one-compartment model assumes that the drug is uniformly distributed within a single hypothetical compartment volume from which the drug concentration can be sampled and assayed easily. The one-compartment model, IV bolus drug injection, provides the simplest approach for estimating the apparent volume of distribution, V_D, and the elimination rate constant, k. If V_D, k, and the drug dose are known, the model equation allows drug concentration in the compartment (body) at any time to be calculated. The volumes of plasma fluid and extracellular fluid may be relatively constant under normal conditions. However, these volumes added together do not usually numerically equal to the (apparent) volume of distribution of the drug, which may be larger or smaller depending on how widely the drug distributes into tissues.

The one-compartment model may be described with the two model parameters, clearance and volume of distribution. Alternatively, the one-compartment model can also be described by two model parameters, the elimination constant, k, and volume of distribution. The latter model explains that drugs are fractionally removed at any time, whatever the initial drug concentration is, and k as a ratio of Cl/V_D. Expressing drug elimination as the fraction of total drug eliminated per time is applicable regardless of whether one is dealing with an amount or a volume.

This approach is most flexible and convenient because of its dimensionless nature in terms of amount or volume (k is expressed as h^{-1} or min^{-1}). Clearance may be computed by $Cl = kV_D$. This method is preferred by many pharmacists since it can be calculated from two concentration measurements, making it more clinically feasible than a full pharmacokinetic study. Many pharmacokineticists do not prefer this method since k is considered a secondary model parameter, while V_D and Cl are considered to be independent model parameters. That is, V_D and Cl give k its properties. Instead, many prefer the noncompartmental approach using area under the concentration-time curve to calculate Cl; this method avoids the basic assumptions inherent in the one-compartmental model but requires a full pharmacokinetic study to determine the area under the curve. Drug clearance is constant for a first-order process regardless of the drug concentration. Clearance is expressed as the apparent volume of fluid of the dissolved drug that is removed per unit time. The one-compartment model may assume either a first-order or a zero-order elimination rate depending on whether the drug follows linear kinetics or not. The disadvantage of the noncompartmental approach is that predicting concentrations at specific times may not hold true, while using a one-compartmental model allows for predicting the concentration at any time point.

LEARNING QUESTIONS

1. A 70-kg volunteer is given an intravenous dose of an antibiotic, and serum drug concentrations were determined at 2 hours and 5 hours after administration. The drug concentrations were 1.2 and 0.3 μg/mL, respectively. What is the biologic half-life for this drug, assuming first-order elimination kinetics?

2. A 50-kg woman was given a single IV dose of an antibacterial drug at a dose level of 6 mg/kg. Blood samples were taken at various time intervals. The concentration of the drug (C_p) was determined in the plasma fraction of each blood sample and the following data were obtained:

t (hours)	C_p (μg/mL)
0.25	8.21
0.50	7.87
1.00	7.23
3.00	5.15
6.00	3.09
12.0	1.11
18.0	0.40

a. What are the values for V_D, k, and $t_{1/2}$ for this drug?

b. This antibacterial agent is not effective at a plasma concentration of less than 2 μg/mL. What is the duration of activity for this drug?

c. How long would it take for 99.9% of this drug to be eliminated?

d. If the dose of the antibiotic was doubled exactly, what would be the increase in duration of activity?

3. A new drug was given in a single intravenous dose of 200 mg to an 80-kg adult male patient. After 6 hours, the plasma drug concentration of drug was 1.5 mg/100 mL of plasma. Assuming that the apparent V_D is 10% of body weight, compute the total amount of drug in the body fluids after 6 hours. What is the half-life of this drug?

4. A new antibiotic drug was given in a single intravenous bolus of 4 mg/kg to 5 healthy male adults ranging in age from 23 to 38 years (average weight 75 kg). The pharmacokinetics of the plasma drug concentration–time curve for this drug fits a one-compartment model. The equation of the curve that best fits the data is

$$C_p = 78e^{-0.46t}$$

Determine the following (assume units of μg/mL for C_p and hours for t):

a. What is the $t_{1/2}$?

b. What is the V_D?

c. What is the plasma level of the drug after 4 hours?

d. How much drug is left in the body after 4 hours?

e. Predict what body water compartment this drug might occupy and explain why you made this prediction.

f. Assuming the drug is no longer effective when levels decline to less than 2 μg/mL, when should you administer the next dose?

5. Define the term *apparent volume of distribution*. What criteria are necessary for the measurement of the apparent volume of distribution to be useful in pharmacokinetic calculations?

6. A drug has an elimination $t_{1/2}$ of 6 hours and follows first-order kinetics. If a single 200-mg dose is given to an adult male patient (68 kg) by IV bolus injection, what percent of the dose is lost in 24 hours?

7. A rather intoxicated young man (75 kg, age 21 years) was admitted to a rehabilitation center. His blood alcohol content was found to be 210 mg%. Assuming the average elimination rate of alcohol is 10 mL of ethanol per hour, how long would it take for his blood alcohol concentration to decline to less than the legal blood alcohol concentration of 100 mg%? (*Hint:* Alcohol is eliminated by zero-order kinetics.) The specific gravity of alcohol is 0.8. The apparent volume of distribution for alcohol is 60% of body weight.

8. A single IV bolus injection containing 500 mg of cefamandole nafate (Mandol, Lilly) is given to an adult female patient (63 years, 55 kg) for a septicemic infection. The apparent volume of distribution is 0.1 L/kg and the elimination half-life is 0.75 hour. Assuming the drug is eliminated by first-order kinetics and may be described by a one-compartment model, calculate the following:

a. The C_p^0

b. The amount of drug in the body 4 hours after the dose is given

c. The time for the drug to decline to 0.5 μg/mL, the minimum inhibitory concentration for streptococci

9. If the amount of drug in the body declines from 100% of the dose (IV bolus injection) to 25% of the dose in 8 hours, what is the elimination half-life for this drug? (Assume first-order kinetics.)

10. A drug has an elimination half-life of 8 hours and follows first-order elimination kinetics. If a single 600-mg dose is given to an adult female patient (62 kg) by rapid IV injection, what percent of the dose is eliminated (lost) in 24 hours assuming the apparent V_D is 400 mL/kg? What is the expected plasma drug concentration (C_p) at 24 hours postdose?

11. For drugs that follow the kinetics of a one-compartment open model, must the tissues and plasma have the same drug concentration? Why?

12. An adult male patient (age 35 years, weight 72 kg) with a urinary tract infection was given a single intravenous bolus of an antibiotic (dose = 300 mg). The patient was instructed to empty his bladder prior to being medicated. After dose administration, the patient saved his urine specimens for drug analysis. The urine specimens were analyzed for both drug content and sterility (lack of bacteriuria). The drug assays gave the following results:

t (hours)	Amount of Drug in Urine (mg)
0	0
4	100
8	26

a. Assuming first-order elimination, calculate the elimination half-life for the antibiotic in this patient.

b. What are the practical problems in obtaining valid urinary drug excretion data for the determination of the drug elimination half-life?

ANSWERS

Frequently Asked Questions

What is the difference between a rate and a rate constant?

- A rate represents the change in amount or concentration of drug in the body per time unit. For example, a rate equal to –5 mg/h means the amount of drug is decreasing at 5 mg/h. A *positive* or *negative* sign indicates that the rate is increasing or decreasing, respectively. Rates may be zero order, first order, or higher orders. For a first-order rate, the rate of change of drug in the body is determined by the *product of the elimination rate constant, k,* and the *amount of drug* remaining in the body, that is, rate = $-kD_B$, where k represents "the fraction" of the amount of drug in the body that is eliminated per hour. If $k = 0.1$ h^{-1} and $D_B = 10$ mg, then the rate = 0.1 h^{-1} × 10 mg = 1 mg/h. The rate constant in this example shows that one-tenth of the drug is eliminated per hour, whatever amount of drug is present in the body. For a first-order rate, the rate states the absolute amount eliminated per unit time (which changes with the amount of drug in the body), whereas the first-order rate constant, k, gives a constant fraction of drug that is eliminated per unit time (which does not change with the amount of drug in the body).

Why does k always have the unit 1/time (eg, h^{-1}), regardless of what concentration unit is plotted?

- The first-order rate constant k has no concentration or mass units. In the calculation of the slope, k, the unit for mass or concentration is canceled when taking the log of the number:

$$\text{Slope} = \frac{\ln y_2 - \ln y_1}{x_2 - x_1} = \frac{\ln (y_2/y_1)}{x_2 - x_1}$$

If a drug is distributed in the one-compartment model, does it mean that there is no drug in the tissue?

- The one-compartment model uses a single homogeneous compartment to represent the fluid and the vascular tissues. This model ignores the heterogeneity of the tissues in the body, so there is no merit in predicting precise tissue drug levels. However, the model provides useful insight into the mass balance of drug distribution in and out of the plasma fluid in the body. If V_D is larger than the physiologic vascular volume, the conclusion is that there is some drug outside the vascular pool, that is, in the tissues. If V_D is small, then there is little extravascular tissue drug storage, except perhaps in the lung, liver, kidney, and heart. With some knowledge about the lipophilicity of the drug and an understanding of blood flow and perfusion within the body, a postulation may be made as to which organs are involved in storing the extravascular drug. The concentration of a biopsy sample may support or refute the postulation.

How is clearance related to the volume of distribution and k?

- Clearance is the volume of plasma fluid that is cleared of drug per unit time. Clearance may also be derived for the physiologic model as the fraction of drug that is eliminated by an organ as blood flows through it. The former definition is equivalent to $Cl = kV_D$ and is readily adapted to dosing since V_D is the volume of distribution. If the drug is eliminated solely by metabolism in the liver, then $Cl_H = Cl$. Cl_H is usually estimated by the difference between Cl and Cl_R. Cl_H is directly estimated by the product of the hepatic blood flow and the extraction ratio.

If we use a physiologic model, are we dealing with actual volumes of blood and tissues? Why do volumes of distribution emerge for drugs that often are greater than the real physical volume?

- Since mass balance (ie, relating dose to plasma drug concentration) is based on volume of distribution rather than blood volume, the compartment model is used in determining dose. Generally, the total blood concentrations of most drugs are not known, since only the plasma or serum concentration is assayed. Some drugs have an RBC/plasma drug ratio much greater than 1, making the application of the physiologic model difficult without knowing the apparent volume of distribution.

Learning Questions

1. The C_p decreased from 1.2 to 0.3 μg/mL in 3 hours.

t (hours)	C_p (μg/mL)
2	1.2
5	0.3

$$\log C_p = -\frac{kt}{2.3} + \log C_P^0$$

$$\log 0.3 = -\frac{k(3)}{2.3} + \log 1.2$$

$$k = 0.462 \text{ h}^{-1}$$

$$t_{1/2} = \frac{0.693}{k} = \frac{0.693}{0.462}$$

$$t_{1/2} = 1.5 \text{ h}$$

These data may also be plotted on a semilog graph and $t_{1/2}$ obtained from the graph.

2. Dose (IV bolus) = 6 mg/kg × 50 kg = 300 mg

   a. $V_D = \dfrac{\text{dose}}{C_P^0} = \dfrac{300 \text{ mg}}{8.4 \, \mu g/\text{mL}} = \dfrac{300 \text{ mg}}{8.4 \text{ mg/L}}$

   $= 35.7 \text{ L}$

   (1) Plot the data on semilog graph paper and use two points from the line of best fit.

t (hours)	C_p (μg/mL)
2	6
6	3

   (2) $t_{1/2}$ (from graph) = 4 hours

   $$k = \frac{0.693}{4} = 0.173 \text{ h}^{-1}$$

   b. $C_P^0 = 8.4 \, \mu g/\text{mL}$ $C_p = 2 \, \mu g/\text{mL}$ $k = 0.173 \text{ h}^{-1}$

   $$\log C_p = -\frac{kt}{2.3} + \log C_P^0$$

   $$\log 2 = -\frac{0.173t}{2.3} + \log 8.4$$

   $$t = 8.29 \text{ h}$$

   Alternatively, time t may be found from a graph of C_p versus t.

   c. Time required for 99.9% of the drug to be eliminated:

   (1) Approximately 10 $t_{1/2}$

   $$t = 10(4) = 40 \text{ h}$$

   (2) $C_P^0 = 8.4 \, \mu g/\text{mL}$

   With 0.1% of drug remaining,

   $$C_p = 0.001 (8.4 \, \mu g/\text{mL}) = 0.0084 \, \mu g/\text{mL}$$

   $$k = 0.173 \text{ h}^{-1}$$

   $$\log 0.0084 = \frac{-0.173t}{2.3} + \log 8.4$$

   $$t = 39.9 \text{ h}$$

d. If the dose is doubled, then C_p^0 will also double. However, the elimination half-life or first-order rate constant will remain the same. Therefore,

$$C_p^0 = 16.8 \ \mu g/mL \quad C_p = 2 \mu g/mL \quad k = 0.173 \ h^{-1}$$

$$\log 2 = \frac{0.173t}{2.3} + \log 16.8$$

$$t = 12.3 \ h^{-1}$$

Notice that doubling the dose does not double the duration of activity.

3. $D_0 = 200$ mg

$$V_D = 10\% \text{ of body weight} = 0.1 \ (80 \text{ kg})$$

$$= 8000 \text{ mL} = 8 \text{ L}$$

At 6 hours:

$$C_p = 1.5 \text{ mg}/100 \text{ mL}$$

$$V_D = \frac{\text{drug in body } (D_B)}{C_p}$$

$$D_B = C_p V_D = \frac{1.5}{100 \text{ mL}} (8000 \text{ mL}) = 120 \text{ mg}$$

$$\log D_B = -\frac{kt}{2.3} + \log D_B^0$$

$$\log 120 = -\frac{k(6)}{2.3} + \log 200$$

$$k = 0.085 \ h^{-1}$$

$$t_{1/2} = \frac{0.693}{k} = \frac{0.693}{0.085} = 8.1 \ h$$

4. $C_p = 78e^{-0.46t}$ (the equation is in the form $C_p = C_p^0 e^{-kt}$)

$$\ln C_p = \ln 78 - 0.46t$$

$$\log C_p = -\frac{0.46t}{2.3} + \log 78$$

Thus, $k = 0.46 \ h^{-1}$, $C_p^0 = 78 \ \mu g/mL$.

a. $t_{1/2} = \dfrac{0.693}{k} = \dfrac{0.693}{0.46} = 1.5 \ h$

b. $V_D = \dfrac{\text{dose}}{C_p^0} = \dfrac{300,000 \ \mu g}{78 \ \mu g/mL} = 3846 \text{ mL}$

Dose = 4 mg/kg × 75 kg = 300 mg

c.

(1) $\log C_p = \dfrac{0.46(4)}{2.3} + \log 78 = 1.092$

$$C_p = 12.4 \ \mu g/mL$$

(2) $C_p = 78e^{-0.46(4)} = 78e^{-18.4} = 78 \ (0.165)$

$$C_p = 12.9 \ \mu g/mL$$

d. At 4 hours:

$$D_B = C_p V_D = 12.4 \ \mu g/mL \times 3846 \text{ mL}$$

$$= 47.69 \text{ mg}$$

e. $V_D = 3846$ mL

Average weight = 75 kg

Percent body wt = (3.846 kg/75 kg) × 100

$$= 5.1\%$$

The apparent V_D approximates the plasma volume.

f. $C_p = 2 \ \mu g/mL$

Find t.

$$\log 2 = -\frac{0.46t}{2.3} + \log 78$$

$$t = -\frac{2.3 \ (\log 2 - \log 78)}{0.46}$$

$$t = 7.96 \ h \approx 8 \ h$$

Alternate Method

$$2 = 78e^{-0.46t}$$

$$\frac{2}{78} = 0.0256 = e^{-0.46t}$$

$$-37 = -0.46t$$

$$t = \frac{37}{0.46} = 8 \ h$$

6. For first-order elimination kinetics, one-half of the initial quantity is lost each $t_{1/2}$. The following table may be developed:

Time (hours)	Number of $t_{1/2}$	Amount of Drug in Body (mg)	Percent of Drug in Body	Percent of Drug Lost
0	0	200	100	0
6	1	100	50	50
12	2	50	25	75
12	2	50	25	75
18	3	25	12.5	87.5
24	4	12.5	6.25	93.75

Method 1

From the above table the percent of drug remaining in the body after each $t_{1/2}$ is equal to 100% times $(1/2)^n$, where n is the number of half-lives, as shown below:

Number of $t_{1/2}$	Percent of Drug in Body	Percent of Drug Remaining in Body after $n\,t_{1/2}$
0	100	
1	50	$100 \times 1/2$
2	25	$100 \times 1/2 \times 1/2$
3	12.5	$100 \times 1/2 \times 1/2 \times 1/2$
N		$100 \times (1/2)^n$

Percent of drug remaining $\dfrac{100}{2^n}$, where n = number of $t_{1/2}$

Percent of drug lost $= 100 - \dfrac{100}{2^n}$

At 24 hours, $n = 4$, since $t_{1/2} = 6$ hours.

Percent of drug lost $= 100 - \dfrac{100}{16} = 93.75\%$

Method 2

The equation for a first-order elimination after IV bolus injection is

$$\log D_B = \frac{-kt}{2.3} + \log D_0$$

where

D_B = amount of drug remaining in the body

D_0 = dose = 200 mg

k = elimination rate constant

$$= \frac{0.693}{t_{1/2}} = 0.1155\,\text{h}^{-1}$$

$t = 24$ h

$$\log D_B = \frac{-0.1155(24)}{2.3} + \log 200$$

$$D_B = 12.47\,\text{mg} \approx 12.5\,\text{mg}$$

$$\% \text{ of drug lost} = \frac{200 - 12.5}{200} \times 100 = 93.75\%$$

7. The zero-order rate constant for alcohol is 10 mL/h. Since the specific gravity for alcohol is 0.8,

$$0.8\,\text{g/mL} = \frac{x(g)}{10\,\text{mL}}$$

$$x = 8\,\text{g}$$

Therefore, the zero-order rate constant, k_0, is 8 g/h.

Drug in body at $t = 0$:

$$D_B^0 = C_p V_D = \frac{210\,\text{mg}}{0.100\,\text{L}} \times (0.60)(75\,\text{L}) = 94.5\,\text{g}$$

Drug in body at time t:

$$D_B = C_p V_D = \frac{100\,\text{mg}}{0.100\,\text{L}} \times (0.60)(75\,\text{L}) = 45.0\,\text{g}$$

For a zero-order reaction:

$$D_B = -k_0 t + D_B^0$$

$$45 = -8t + 94.5$$

$$t = 6.19\,\text{h}$$

8. a. $C_p^0 = \dfrac{\text{dose}}{V_D} = \dfrac{500\,\text{mg}}{(0.1\,\text{L/kg})(55\,\text{kg})} = 90.9\,\text{mg/L}$

b. $\log D_B = \dfrac{-kt}{2.3} + \log D_B^0$

$$\log D_B = \frac{(0.693/0.75)(4)}{2.3} + \log 500$$

$$D_B = 12.3\,\text{mg}$$

c. $\log 0.5 = \dfrac{-(0.693/0.75)t}{2.3} + \log 90.0$

$$t = 5.62 \, h$$

9. $\log D_B = \dfrac{-kt}{2.3} + \log D_B^0$

$$\log 25 = \dfrac{-k(8)}{2.3} + \log 100$$

$$k = 0.173 \, h^{-1}$$

$$t_{1/2} = \dfrac{0.693}{0.173} = 4 \, h$$

10. $\log D_B = \dfrac{-kt}{2.3} + \log D_B^0$

$$= \dfrac{(-0.693/8)(24)}{2.3} + \log 600$$

$$D_B = 74.9 \, mg$$

$$\text{Percent drug lost} = \dfrac{600 - 74.9}{600} \times 100$$

$$= 87.5\%$$

C_p at $t = 24$ hours:

$$C_p = \dfrac{74.9 \, mg}{(0.4 \, L/kg)(62 \, kg)} = 3.02 \, mg/L$$

11. The total drug concentration in the plasma is not usually equal to the total drug concentration in the tissues. A one-compartment model implies that the drug is rapidly equilibrated in the body (in plasma and tissues). At equilibrium, the drug concentration in the tissues may differ from the drug concentration in the body because of drug protein binding, partitioning of drug into fat, differences in pH in different regions of the body causing a different degree of ionization for a weakly dissociated electrolyte drug, an active tissue uptake process, etc.

12. Set up the following table:

Time (hours)	D_u (mg)	dD_u/t	mg/h	t^*
0	0			
4	100	100/4	25	2
8	26	26/4	6.5	6

The elimination half-life may be obtained graphically after plotting mg/h versus t^*. The $t_{1/2}$ obtained graphically is approximately 2 hours.

$$\log \dfrac{dD_u}{dt} = \dfrac{-kt}{2.3} + \log k_e D_B^0$$

$$\text{Slope} = \dfrac{-k}{2.3} = \dfrac{\log Y_2 - \log Y_1}{X_2 - X_1} = \dfrac{\log 6.5 - \log 2.5}{6 - 2}$$

$$k = 0.336 \, h^{-1}$$

$$t_{1/2} = \dfrac{0.693}{k} = \dfrac{0.693}{0.336} = 2.06 \, h$$

REFERENCE

Huestis MA, Mitchell J, Cone EJ: Prolonged urinary excretion of marijuana metabolite (abstract). Committee on Problems of Drug Dependence, San Juan, PR, June 25, 1996.

BIBLIOGRAPHY

Gibaldi M, Nagashima R, Levy G: Relationship between drug concentration in plasma or serum and amount of drug in the body. *J Pharm Sci* **58:**193–197, 1969.

Riegelman S, Loo JCK, Rowland M: Shortcomings in pharmacokinetic analysis by conceiving the body to exhibit properties of a single compartment. *J Pharm Sci* **57:**117–123, 1968.

Riegelman S, Loo J, Rowland M: Concepts of volume of distribution and possible errors in evaluation of this parameter. *Science* **57:**128–133, 1968.

Wagner JG, Northam JI: Estimation of volume of distribution and half-life of a compound after rapid intravenous injection. *J Pharm Sci* **58:**529–531, 1975.

5 Multicompartment Models: Intravenous Bolus Administration

Shabnam N. Sani and Rodney C. Siwale

Chapter Objectives

▶ Define the pharmacokinetic terms used in a two- and three-compartment model.

▶ Explain using examples why drugs follow one-compartment, two-compartment, or three-compartment kinetics.

▶ Use equations and graph to simulate plasma drug concentration at various time periods after an IV bolus injection of a drug that follows the pharmacokinetics of a two- and three-compartment model drug.

▶ Relate the relevance of the magnitude of the volume of distribution and clearance of various drugs to underlying processes in the body.

▶ Estimate two-compartment model parameters by using the method of residuals.

▶ Calculate clearance and alpha and beta half-lives of a two-compartment model drug.

▶ Explain how drug metabolic enzymes, transportors, and binding proteins in the body may modify the distribution and/or elimination phase of a drug after IV bolus.

Pharmacokinetic models are used to simplify all the complex processes that occur during drug administration that include drug distribution and elimination in the body. The model simplification is necessary because of the inability to measure quantitatively all the rate processes in the body, including the lack of access to biological samples from the interior of the body. As described in Chapter 1, pharmacokinetic models are used to simulate drug disposition under different conditions/time points so that dosing regimens for individuals or groups of patients can be designed.

Compartmental models are classic pharmacokinetic models that simulate the kinetic processes of drug absorption, distribution, and elimination with little physiologic detail. In contrast, the more sophisticated physiologic model is discussed in Chapter 25. In compartmental models, drug tissue concentration, C_t, is assumed to be uniform within a given hypothetical compartment. Hence, all muscle mass and connective tissues may be lumped into one hypothetical tissue compartment that equilibrates with drug from the central (composed of blood, extracellular fluid, and highly perfused organs/tissues such as heart, liver, and kidneys) compartment. Since no data are collected on the tissue mass, the theoretical tissue concentration cannot be confirmed and used to forecast actual tissue drug levels. Only a theoretical, C_t, concentration of drug in the tissue compartment can be calculated. Moreover, drug concentrations in a particular tissue mass may not be homogeneously distributed. However, plasma concentrations, C_p, are kinetically simulated by considering the presence of a tissue or a group of tissue compartments. In reality, the body is more complex than depicted in the simple one-compartment model and the eliminating organs, such as the liver and kidneys, are much more complex than a simple extractor. Thus, to gain a better appreciation regarding how drugs are handled in the body, multicompartment models are found helpful. Contrary to the monoexponential decay in the simple one-compartment model, most drugs given by IV bolus dose decline in a biphasic fashion, that is, plasma drug concentrations rapidly decline soon after IV bolus injection, and then decline moderately as some of the drug that initially distributes (equilibrates) into the tissue moves back into the plasma. The early decline phase is commonly called the distribution phase (because distribution into tissues primarily determines the early rapid decline in plasma concentration) and the latter phase is called the terminal or elimination phase. During the distribution phase, changes in the concentration of drug in plasma primarily reflect the movement of drug within the body, rather than elimination. However, with time, distribution equilibrium is established in more and more tissues between the tissue and plasma, and eventually changes in plasma concentration reflect proportional changes in the concentrations of drug in all other tissues. During this proportionality phase, the body kinetically acts as a single compartment and because decline of the plasma concentration is now associated solely with elimination of drug from the body, this phase is often called the elimination phase.

Concentration of the drug in the tissue compartment (C_t), is not a useful parameter due to the non-homogenous tissue distribution of drugs. However, amount of the drug in the tissue compartment (D_t) is useful because it is an indication of how much drug accumulates extravascularly in the body at any given time. The two-compartment model provides a simple way to keep track of the mass balance of the drug in the body.

Multicompartment models provide answers to such questions as: (1) How much of a dose is eliminated? (2) How much drug remains in the plasma compartment at any given time? and (3) How much drug accumulates in the tissue compartment? The latter information is particularly useful for drug safety since the amount of drug in a deep tissue compartment may be harder to eliminate by renal excretion or by dialysis after drug overdose.

Multicompartment models explain the observation that, after a rapid IV bolus drug injection, the plasma level–time curve does not decline linearly, implying that the drug does not equilibrate rapidly in the body, as observed for a single first-order rate process in a one-compartment model. Instead, a biphasic or triphasic drug concentration decline is often observed. The initial decline phase represents the drug leaving the plasma compartment and entering one or more tissue compartments as well as being eliminated. Later, after drug distribution to the tissues

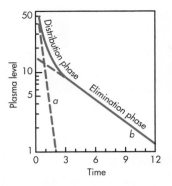

FIGURE 5-1   Plasma level–time curve for the two-compartment open model (single IV dose) described in Fig. 5-2 (model A).

is completed, the plasma drug concentrations decline more gradually when eventually plasma drug equilibrium with peripheral tissues occurs. Drug kinetics after distribution is characterized by the composite rate constant, β (or b), which can be obtained from the terminal slope of the plasma level–time curve in a semilogarithmic plot (Fig. 5-1).

Nonlinear plasma drug level–time decline occurs because some drugs distribute at various rates into different tissue groups. Multicompartment models were developed to explain and predict plasma and tissue concentrations for those types of drugs. In contrast, a one-compartment model is used when a drug appears to distribute into tissues instantaneously and uniformly or when the drug does not extensively distribute into extravascular tissues such as aminoglycosides. Extent of distribution is partially determined by the physical-chemical properties of the drug. For instance, aminoglycosides are polar molecules; therefore, their distribution is primarily limited to extracellular water. Lipophilic drugs with more extensive distribution into tissues such as the benzodiazepines or those with extensive intracellular uptake may be better described by more complex models. For both one- and multicompartment models, the drug in those tissues that have the highest blood perfusion equilibrates rapidly with the drug in the plasma. These highly perfused tissues and blood make up the *central compartment* (often called the *plasma compartment*). While this initial drug distribution is taking place, multicompartment drugs are delivered concurrently to one or more *peripheral compartments* (often considered as the *tissue compartment that includes fat, muscle, and cerebrospinal fluid*) composed of groups of tissues with lower blood perfusion and different affinity for the drug. A drug will concentrate in a tissue in accordance with the affinity of the drug for that particular tissue. For example, lipid-soluble drugs tend to accumulate in fat tissues. Drugs that bind plasma proteins may be more concentrated in the plasma, because protein-bound drugs do not diffuse easily into the tissues. Drugs may also bind with tissue proteins and other macromolecules, such as DNA and melanin.

Tissue sampling often is invasive, and the drug concentration in the tissue sample may not represent the drug concentration in the entire organ due to the nonhomogenous tissue distribution of drugs. In recent years, the development of novel experimental methods such as magnetic resonance spectroscopy (MRS), single photon emission computed tomography (SPECT), and tissue microdialysis has enabled us to study the drug distribution in the target tissues of animals and humans (Eichler and Müller, 1998, and Müller, 2009). These innovative technologies have enabled us to follow the path of the drug from the plasma compartment into anatomically defined regions or tissues. More importantly, for some classes of drugs the concentration in the interstitial fluid space of the target tissue can be measured. This also affords a means to quantify, for the first time, the inter- or intraindividual variability associated with the *in vivo* distribution process. Although these novel techniques are promising, measurement of drug or active metabolite concentrations in target tissues and the subsequent development of associated pharmacokinetic models is not a routine practice in standard drug development and certainly is not mandated by regulatory requirements. Occasionally, tissue samples may be collected after a drug overdose episode. For example, the two-compartment model has been used to describe the distribution of colchicine, even though the drug's toxic tissue levels after fatal overdoses have only been recently described (Rochdi et al, 1992). Colchicine distribution is now known to be affected by P-gp (also known as ABCB1 or MDR1, a common transport protein of the ABC [ATP-binding cassette] transporter subfamily found in the body). Drug transporters are now known to influence the curvature in the log plasma drug concentration–time graph of drugs. The drug isotretinoin has a long half-life because of substantial distribution into lipid tissues.

Kinetic analysis of a multicompartment model assumes that all transfer rate processes for the passage of drug into or out of individual compartments are first-order processes. On the basis of this assumption, the plasma level–time curve for a drug that follows a multicompartment model is best described by the summation of a series of exponential terms, each corresponding to first-order rate processes associated with a given compartment. Most multicompartment models used in pharmacokinetics are *mamillary models*. Mamillary models are well connected and dynamically exchange drug concentration between compartments making them very suitable for modeling drug distribution.

Because of all these distribution factors, drugs will generally concentrate unevenly in the tissues, and different groups of tissues will accumulate the drug at very different rates. A summary of the approximate blood flow to major human tissues is presented in Table 5-1. Many different tissues and rate processes are involved in the distribution of any drug. However, limited physiologic significance has been assigned to a few groups of tissues (Table 5-2).

The nonlinear profile of plasma drug concentration–time is the result of many factors interacting together, including blood flow to the tissues, the permeability of the drug into the tissues (fat solubility), partitioning, the capacity of the tissues to accumulate drug, and the effect of disease factors on these processes (see Chapter 11). Impaired cardiac function may produce a change in blood flow and these affect the drug distributive phase, whereas impairment of the kidney or the liver may decrease drug elimination as shown by a prolonged elimination half-life and corresponding reduction in the slope of the terminal elimination phase of the curve. Frequently, multiple factors can complicate the distribution profile in such a way that the profile can only be described clearly with the assistance of a simulation model.

TABLE 5-1   Blood Flow to Human Tissues

Tissue	Percent Body Weight	Percent Cardiac Output	Blood Flow (mL/100 g tissue per min)
Adrenals	0.02	1	550
Kidneys	0.4	24	450
Thyroid	0.04	2	400
Liver			
Hepatic	2.0	5	20
Portal		20	75
Portal-drained viscera	2.0	20	75
Heart (basal)	0.4	4	70
Brain	2.0	15	55
Skin	7.0	5	5
Muscle (basal)	40.0	15	3
Connective tissue	7.0	1	1
Fat	15.0	2	1

Data from Spector WS: Handbook of Biological Data, Saunders, Philadelphia, 1956; Glaser O: Medical Physics, Vol II, Year Book Publishers, Chicago, 1950; Butler TC: Proc First International Pharmacological Meeting, vol 6, Pergamon Press, 1962.

TABLE 5-2   General Grouping of Tissues According to Blood Supply[a]

Blood Supply	Tissue Group	Percent Body Weight
Highly perfused	Heart, brain, hepatic-portal system, kidney, and endocrine glands	9
	Skin and muscle	50
	Adipose (fat) tissue and marrow	19
Slowly perfused	Bone, ligaments, tendons, cartilage, teeth, and hair	22

[a]Tissue uptake will also depend on such factors as fat solubility, degree of ionization, partitioning, and protein binding of the drug.

Adapted with permission from Eger (1963).

TWO-COMPARTMENT OPEN MODEL

Many drugs given in a single intravenous bolus dose demonstrate a plasma level–time curve that does not decline as a single exponential (first-order) process. The plasma level–time curve for a drug that follows a two-compartment model (Fig. 5-1) shows that the plasma drug concentration declines *biexponentially* as the sum of two first-order processes—distribution and elimination. A drug that follows the pharmacokinetics of a two-compartment model does not equilibrate rapidly throughout the body, as is assumed for a one-compartment model. In this model, the drug distributes into two compartments, the central compartment and the tissue, or peripheral, compartment. The drug distributes rapidly and uniformly in the central compartment. A second compartment, known as the *tissue or peripheral compartment,* contains tissues in which the drug equilibrates more slowly. Drug transfer between the two compartments is assumed to take place by first-order processes.

There are several possible two-compartment models (Fig. 5-2). Model A is used most often and describes the plasma level–time curve observed in Fig. 5-1. By convention, compartment 1 is the central compartment and compartment 2 is the tissue

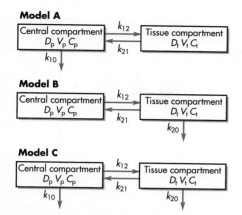

FIGURE 5-2 Two-compartment open models, intravenous injection.

compartment. The rate constants k_{12} and k_{21} represent the first-order rate transfer constants for the movement of drug from compartment 1 to compartment 2 (k_{12}) and from compartment 2 to compartment 1 (k_{21}). The transfer constants are sometimes termed *microconstants*, and their values cannot be estimated directly. Most two-compartment models assume that elimination occurs from the central compartment model, as shown in Fig. 5-2 (model A), unless other information about the drug is known. Drug elimination is presumed to occur from the central compartment, because the major sites of drug elimination (renal excretion and hepatic drug metabolism) occur in organs such as the kidney and liver, which are highly perfused with blood.

The plasma level–time curve for a drug that follows a two-compartment model may be divided into two parts, (*a*) a distribution phase and (*b*) an elimination phase. The two-compartment model assumes that, at $t = 0$, no drug is in the tissue compartment. After an IV bolus injection, drug equilibrates rapidly in the central compartment. The *distribution phase* of the curve represents the initial, more rapid decline of drug from the central compartment into the tissue compartment (Fig. 5-1, line *a*). Although drug elimination and distribution occur *concurrently* during the distribution phase, there is a net transfer of drug from the central compartment to the tissue compartment because the rate of distribution is faster than the rate of elimination. The fraction of drug in the tissue compartment during the distribution phase

increases up to a maximum in a given tissue, whose value may be greater or less than the plasma drug concentration. At maximum tissue concentrations, the rate of drug entry into the tissue equals the rate of drug exit from the tissue. The fraction of drug in the tissue compartment is now in equilibrium (*distribution equilibrium*) with the fraction of drug in the central compartment (Fig. 5-3), and the drug concentrations in both the central and tissue compartments decline in parallel and more slowly compared to the distribution phase. This decline is a first-order process and is called the *elimination phase* or the *beta* (β) *phase* (Fig. 5-1, line *b*). Since plasma and tissue concentrations decline in parallel, plasma drug concentrations provide some indication of the concentration of drug in the tissue. At this point, drug kinetics appears to follow a one-compartment model in which drug elimination is a first-order process described by β (also known as *b*). A typical tissue drug level curve after a single intravenous dose is shown in Fig. 5-3.

Tissue drug concentrations in the pharmacokinetic model are theoretical only. The drug level in the theoretical tissue compartment can be calculated once the parameters for the model are estimated. However, the drug concentration in the tissue compartment represents the *average* drug concentration in a group of tissues rather than any real anatomic tissue drug concentration. In reality, drug concentrations may vary among different tissues and possibly within an individual tissue. These varying tissue

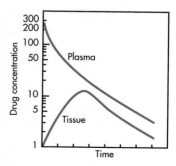

FIGURE 5-3 Relationship between tissue and plasma drug concentrations for a two-compartment open model. The maximum tissue drug concentration may be greater or less than the plasma drug concentration.

drug concentrations are due to differences in the partitioning of drug into the tissues, as discussed in Chapter 11. In terms of the pharmacokinetic model, the differences in tissue drug concentration are reflected in the k_{12}/k_{21} ratio. Thus, tissue drug concentration may be higher or lower than the plasma drug concentrations, depending on the properties of the individual tissue. Moreover, the elimination rates of drug from the tissue compartment may not be the same as the elimination rates from the central compartment. For example, if $k_{12} \cdot C_p$ is greater than $k_{21} \cdot C_t$ (rate into tissue > rate out of tissue), tissue drug concentrations will increase and plasma drug concentrations will decrease. Real tissue drug concentration can sometimes be calculated by the addition of compartments to the model until a compartment that mimics the experimental tissue concentrations is found.

In spite of the hypothetical nature of the tissue compartment, the theoretical tissue level is still valuable information for clinicians. The theoretical tissue concentration, together with the blood concentration, gives an accurate method of calculating the total amount of drug remaining in the body at any given time (see digoxin example in Table 5-5). This information would not be available without pharmacokinetic models.

In practice, a blood sample is removed periodically from the central compartment and the plasma is analyzed for the presence of drug. The drug plasma level–time curve represents a phase of initial rapid equilibration with the central compartment (the distribution phase), followed by an elimination phase after the tissue compartment has also equilibrated with drug. The distribution phase may take minutes or hours and may be missed entirely if the blood is sampled too late or at wide intervals after drug administration.

In the model depicted above, k_{12} and k_{21} are first-order rate constants that govern the rate of drug distribution into and out of the tissues and plasma:

$$\frac{dC_t}{dt} = k_{12}C_p - k_{21}C_t \qquad (5.1)$$

$$\frac{dC_p}{dt} = k_{21}C_t - k_{12}C_p - k_{10}C_p \qquad (5.2)$$

The relationship between the amount of drug in each compartment and the concentration of drug in that compartment is shown by Equations 5.3 and 5.4:

$$C_p = \frac{D_p}{V_p} \qquad (5.3)$$

$$C_t = \frac{D_t}{V_t} \qquad (5.4)$$

where D_p = amount of drug in the central compartment, D_t = amount of drug in the tissue compartment, V_p = volume of drug in the central compartment, and V_t = volume of drug in the tissue compartment.

$$\frac{dC_p}{dt} = k_{21}\frac{D_t}{V_t} - k_{12}\frac{D_p}{V_p} - k_{10}\frac{D_p}{V_d} \qquad (5.5)$$

$$\frac{dC_t}{dt} = k_{12}\frac{D_p}{V_p} - k_{21}\frac{D_t}{V_t} \qquad (5.6)$$

Solving Equations 5.5 and 5.6 using Laplace transforms and matrix algebra will give Equations 5.7 and 5.8, which describe the change in drug concentration in the blood and in the tissue with respect to time:

$$C_p = \frac{D_P^0}{V_p}\left(\frac{k_{21}-\alpha}{\beta-\alpha}e^{-\alpha t} + \frac{k_{21}-\beta}{\alpha-\beta}e^{-\beta t}\right) \qquad (5.7)$$

$$C_t = \frac{k_{21}D_P^0}{V_t(\alpha-\beta)}\left(e^{-\beta t} - e^{-\alpha t}\right) \qquad (5.8)$$

$$D_p = D_P^0\left(\frac{k_{21}-\alpha}{\beta-\alpha}e^{-\alpha t} + \frac{k_{21}-\beta}{\alpha-\beta}e^{-\beta t}\right) \qquad (5.9)$$

$$D_t = \frac{k_{21}D_P^0}{(\alpha-\beta)}\left(e^{-\beta t} - e^{-\alpha t}\right) \qquad (5.10)$$

where D_P^0 = dose given intravenously, t = time after administration of dose, and α and β are constants that depend solely on k_{12}, k_{21}, and k_{10}. The amount of drug remaining in the plasma and tissue compartments at any time may be described realistically by Equations 5.9 and 5.10.

The rate constants for the transfer of drug between compartments are referred to as *microconstants* or *transfer constants*. They relate the amount of drug being transferred per unit time from one compartment to the other. The values for these microconstants cannot be determined by direct measurement, but they can be estimated by a graphic method.

$$\alpha + \beta = k_{12} + k_{21} + k_{10} \qquad (5.11)$$

$$\alpha\beta = k_{21}k_{10} \qquad (5.12)$$

The constants α and β are hybrid first-order rate constants for the distribution phase and elimination phase, respectively. The mathematical relationships of α and β to the rate constants are given by Equations 5.11 and 5.12, which are derived after integration of Equations 5.5 and 5.6. Equation 5.7 can be transformed into the following expression:

$$C_{\mathrm{p}} = Ae^{-\alpha t} + Be^{-\beta t} \qquad (5.13)$$

The constants α and β are rate constants for the distribution phase and elimination phase, respectively. The constants A and B are intercepts on the y axis for each exponential segment of the curve in Equation 5.13. These values may be obtained graphically by the method of residuals or by computer. Intercepts A and B are actually hybrid constants, as shown in Equations 5.14 and 5.15, and do not have actual physiologic significance.

$$A = \frac{D_0(\alpha - k_{21})}{V_{\mathrm{P}}(\alpha - \beta)} \qquad (5.14)$$

$$B = \frac{D_0(k_{21} - \beta)}{V_{\mathrm{P}}(\alpha - \beta)} \qquad (5.15)$$

Please note that the values of A and B are empirical constants directly proportional to the dose administered. All the rate constants involved in two-compartment model will have units consistent with the first-order process (Jambhekar SS and Breen JP. 2009).

Method of Residuals

The *method of residuals* (also known as *feathering, peeling,* or *curve stripping*) is a commonly employed technique for resolving a curve into various exponential terms. This method allows the separation of the monoexponential constituents of a biexponential plot of plasma concentration against time and therefore, it is a useful procedure for fitting a curve to the experimental data of a drug when the drug does not clearly follow a one-compartment model. For example, 100 mg of a drug was administered by rapid IV injection to a healthy 70-kg adult male. Blood samples were taken periodically after the administration of drug, and the plasma fraction of each sample was assayed for drug. The following data were obtained:

Time (hour)	Plasma Concentration (µg/mL)
0.25	43.00
0.5	32.00
1.0	20.00
1.5	14.00
2.0	11.00
4.0	6.50
8.0	2.80
12.0	1.20
16.0	0.52

When these data are plotted on semilogarithmic graph paper, a curved line is observed (Fig. 5-4). The curved-line relationship between the logarithm of the plasma concentration and time indicates that the drug is distributed in more than one compartment. From these data a biexponential equation, Equation 5.13, may be derived, either by computer or by the method of residuals.

As shown in the biexponential curve in Fig. 5-4, the decline in the initial distribution phase is more rapid than the elimination phase. The rapid distribution phase is confirmed with the constant α being larger than the rate constant β. Therefore, at some later time (generally at a time following the attainment of distribution equilibrium), the term

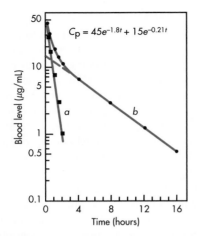

FIGURE 5-4 Plasma level–time curve for a two-compartment open model. The rate constants and intercepts were calculated by the method of residuals.

$Ae^{-\alpha t}$ will approach 0, while $Be^{-\beta t}$ will still have a finite value. At this later time Equation 5.13 will reduce to:

$$C_p = Be^{-\beta t} \qquad (5.16)$$

which, in common logarithms, is:

$$\log C_p = \log B - \frac{\beta t}{2.3} \qquad (5.17)$$

From Equation 5.17, the rate constant can be obtained from the slope ($-\beta/2.3$) of a straight line representing the terminal exponential phase (Fig. 5-4). The $t_{1/2}$ for the elimination phase (beta half-life) can be derived from the following relationship:

$$t_{1/2\beta} = \frac{0.693}{\beta} \qquad (5.18)$$

In the sample case considered here, β was found to be 0.21 h⁻¹. From this information the regression line for the terminal exponential or β phase is extrapolated to the y axis; the y intercept is equal to B, or 15 μg/mL. Values from the extrapolated line are then subtracted from the original experimental data points (Table 5-3) and a straight line is obtained. This line represents the rapidly distributed α phase (Fig. 5-4).

The new line obtained by graphing the logarithm of the residual plasma concentration ($C_p - C_p'$) against time represents the α phase. The value for α is 1.8 h⁻¹, and the y intercept is 45 μg/mL. The elimination $t_{1/2\beta}$ is computed from β by the use of Equation 5.18 and has the value of 3.3 hours.

A number of pharmacokinetic parameters may be derived by proper substitution of rate constants α and β and y intercepts A and B into the following equations:

$$k_{10} = \frac{\alpha\beta(A+B)}{A\beta + B\alpha} \qquad (5.19)$$

TABLE 5-3   Application of the Method of Residuals

Time (hour)	C_p Observed Plasma Level	C_p' Extrapolated Plasma Concentration	$C_p - C_p'$ Residual Plasma Concentration
0.25	43.0	14.5	28.5
0.5	32.0	13.5	18.5
1.0	20.0	12.3	7.7
1.5	14.0	11.0	3.0
2.0	11.0	10.0	1.0
4.0	6.5		
8.0	2.8		
12.0	1.2		
16.0	0.52		

$$k_{12} = \frac{AB(\beta - \alpha)^2}{(A+B)(A\beta + B\alpha)} \qquad (5.20)$$

$$k_{21} = \frac{A\beta + B\alpha}{A+B} \qquad (5.21)$$

When an administered drug exhibits the characteristics of a two-compartment model, the difference between the distribution rate constant α and the slow post-distribution/elimination rate constant β plays a critical role. The greater the difference between α and β, the greater is the need to apply two-compartment model. Failure to do so will result in false clinical predictions (Jambhekar SS and Breen JP. 2009). On the other hand, if this difference is small, it will not cause any significant difference in the clinical predictions, regardless of the model chosen to describe the pharmacokinetics of a drug. Then, it may be prudent to follow the principle of PARSIMONY when selecting the compartment model by choosing the simpler of the two available models (eg, one-compartment versus two) (Jambhekar SS and Breen JP. 2009).

CLINICAL APPLICATION

Digoxin in a Normal Patient and in a Renal-Failure Patient—Simulation of Plasma and Tissue Level of a Two-Compartment Model Drug

Once the pharmacokinetic parameters are determined for an individual, the amount of drug remaining in the plasma and tissue compartments may be calculated using Equations 5.9 and 5.10. The pharmacokinetic data for digoxin were calculated in a normal and in a renal-impaired, 70-kg subject using the parameters in Table 5-4 as reported in the literature. The amount of digoxin remaining in the plasma and tissue compartments is tabulated in Table 5-5 and plotted in Fig. 5-5. It can be seen that digoxin stored in the plasma declines rapidly during the initial distributive phase, while drug amount in the tissue compartment takes 3–4 hours to accumulate for a normal subject. It is interesting that clinicians have recommended that digoxin plasma samples be taken at least several hours after IV bolus dosing (3–4+ hours, Winters, 1994, and 4–8 hours, Schumacher, 1995) for a normal subject, since the equilibrated level is more representative of

TABLE 5-4   Two-Compartment Model Pharmacokinetic Parameters of Digoxin

Parameters	Unit	Normal	Renal Impaired
k_{12}	h^{-1}	1.02	0.45
k_{21}	h^{-1}	0.15	0.11
k	h^{-1}	0.18	0.04
V_p	L/kg	0.78	0.73
D	µg/kg	3.6	3.6
a	1/h	1.331	0.593
b	1/h	0.019	0.007

myocardium digoxin level. In the simulation below, the amount of the drug in the plasma compartment at any time divided by V_p (54.6 L for the normal subject) will yield the plasma digoxin level. At 4 hours after

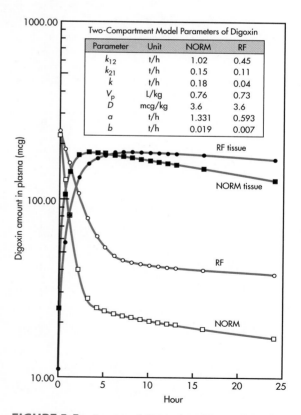

FIGURE 5-5   Amount of digoxin (simulated) in the plasma and tissue compartment after an IV dose to a normal and a renal-failure (RF) patient.

an IV dose of 0.25 mg, $C_p = D_p/V_p = 24.43$ µg/54.6 L = 0.45 ng/mL, corresponding to 3×0.45 ng/mL = 1.35 ng/mL if a full loading dose of 0.75 mg is given in a single dose. Although the initial plasma drug levels were much higher than after equilibration, the digoxin plasma concentrations are generally regarded as not toxic, since drug distribution is occurring rapidly.

The tissue drug levels were not calculated. The tissue drug concentration represents the hypothetical tissue pool, which may not represent actual drug concentrations in the myocardium. In contrast, the amount of drug remaining in the tissue pool is real,

since the amount of drug is calculated using mass balance. The rate of drug entry into the tissue in micrograms per hour at any time is $k_{12}D_p$, while the rate of drug leaving the tissue is $k_{21}D_t$ in the same units. Both of these rates may be calculated from Table 5-5 using k_{12} and k_{21} values listed in Table 5-4.

Although some clinicians assume that tissue and plasma concentrations are equal when at full equilibration, tissue and plasma drug ratios are determined by the partition coefficient (a drug-specific physical ratio that measures the lipid/water affinity of a drug) and the extent of protein binding of the drug.

TABLE 5-5   **Amount of Digoxin in Plasma and Tissue Compartment after an IV Dose of 0.252 mg in a Normal and a Renal-Failure Patient Weighing 70 kg[a]**

	Digoxin Amount				
	Normal Renal Function			**Renal Failure (RF)**	
Time (hour)	D_p (µg)	D_t (µg)		D_p (µg)	D_t (µg)
0.00	252.00	0.00		252.00	0.00
0.10	223.68	24.04		240.01	11.01
0.60	126.94	105.54		189.63	57.12
1.00	84.62	140.46		158.78	85.22
2.00	40.06	174.93		107.12	131.72
3.00	27.95	181.45		78.44	156.83
4.00	24.43	180.62		62.45	170.12
5.00	23.17	177.91		53.48	176.88
6.00	22.53	174.74		48.39	180.04
7.00	22.05	171.50		45.45	181.21
8.00	21.62	168.28		43.69	181.29
9.00	21.21	165.12		42.59	180.77
10.00	20.81	162.01		41.85	179.92
11.00	20.42	158.96		41.32	178.89
12.00	20.03	155.97		40.89	177.77
13.00	19.65	153.04		40.53	176.60
16.00	18.57	144.56		39.62	173.00
24.00	15.95	124.17		37.44	163.59

[a]D_p, drug in plasma compartment; D_t, drug in tissue compartment.

Source: Data generated from parameters published by Harron (1989).

Figure 5-5 shows that the time for the RF (renal-failure or renal-impaired) patient to reach stable tissue drug levels is longer than the time for the normal subject due to changes in the elimination and transfer rate constants. As expected, a significantly higher amount of digoxin remains in both the plasma and tissue compartments in the renally impaired subject compared to the normal subject.

PRACTICE PROBLEM

From Figure 5-5 or Table 5-4, how many hours does it take for maximum tissue concentration to be reached in the normal and the renal-impaired patient?

Solution

At maximum tissue concentration, the rate of drug entering the tissue compartment is equal to the rate of leaving (ie, at the peak of the tissue curve, where the slope $= 0$ or not changing). This occurs at about 3–4 hours for the normal patient and at 7–8 hours for the renal-impaired patient. This may be verified by examining at what time $D_p k_{12} = D_t k_{21}$ using the data from Tables 5-4 and 5-5. Before maximum C_t is reached, there is a net flux of drug into the tissue, that is, $D_p k_{12} > D_t k_{21}$, and beyond this point, there is a net flux of drug out of the tissue compartment, that is, $D_t k_{12} > D_p k_{12}$.

PRACTICAL FOCUS

The distribution half-life of digoxin is about 31 minutes $(t_{1/2}\alpha = 0.694/\alpha = 0.694/1.331 = 31$ min$)$ based on Table 5-4. Both clinical experience and simulated tissue amount in Table 5-4 recommend "several hours" for equilibration, longer than $5t_{1/2}\alpha$ or 5×32 minutes. (1) Is digoxin elimination in tissue adequately modeled in this example? (2) Digoxin was not known to be a P-gp substrate when the data were analyzed; can the presence of a transporter at the target site change tissue drug concentration, necessitating a longer equilibration time?

Generally, the ability to obtain a blood sample and get accurate data in the alpha (distribution) phase is difficult for most drugs because of its short duration. Moreover, the alpha phase may not be very reproducible because they are affected by short-term physiologic changes. For example, stress may result in short-term change of the hematocrit or plasma volume and possibly other hemodynamic factors.

> **Frequently Asked Questions**
>
> ▶ *Are "hypothetical" or "mathematical" compartment models useful in designing dosage regimens in the clinical setting? Does "hypothetical" mean "not real"?*
>
> ▶ *If physiologic models are better than compartment models, why not just use physiologic models?*
>
> ▶ *Since clearance is the term most often used in clinical pharmacy, why is it necessary to know the other pharmacokinetic parameters?*

Apparent Volumes of Distribution

As discussed in Chapter 4, the apparent V_D is a useful parameter that relates plasma concentration to the amount of drug in the body. For drugs with large extravascular distribution, the apparent volume of distribution is generally large. Conversely, for polar drugs with low lipid solubility, the apparent V_D is generally small. Drugs with high peripheral tissue binding also contribute to a large apparent V_D. In multiple-compartment kinetics, such as the two-compartment model, several types of volumes of distribution, each based on different assumptions, can be calculated. Volumes of distribution generally reflect the extent of drug distribution in the body on a relative basis, and the calculations depend on the availability of data. In general, it is important to refer to the same volume parameter when comparing kinetic changes in disease states. Unfortunately, values of apparent volumes of distribution of drugs from tables in the clinical literature are often listed without specifying the underlying kinetic processes, model parameters, or methods of calculation.

Volume of the Central Compartment

This is a proportionality constant that relates the amount or mass of drug and the plasma concentration immediately (ie, at time zero) following the administration of a drug. The volume of the central compartment is useful for determining the drug concentration directly after an IV injection into the body. In clinical pharmacy, this volume is also referred to as V_i or the initial volume of distribution as the drug distributes within the plasma and other accessible body fluids. This volume is generally smaller than the terminal volume of distribution after drug distribution to tissue is completed. The volume of the central compartment is generally greater than 3 L, which is the volume of the plasma fluid for an average adult. For many polar drugs, an initial volume of 7–10 L may be interpreted as rapid drug distribution within the plasma and some extracellular fluids. For example, the V_p of moxalactam ranges from 0.12 to 0.15 L/kg, corresponding to about 8.4–10.5 L for a typical 70-kg patient (Table 5-6). In contrast, the V_p of hydromorphone is about 24 L, possibly because of its rapid exit from the plasma into tissues even during the initial phase.

As in the case of the one-compartment model, V_p may be determined from the dose and the instantaneous plasma drug concentration, C_p^0. V_p is also useful in the determination of drug clearance if k (or $t_{1/2}$) is known, as in Chapter 4.

In the two-compartment model, V_p may also be considered a mass balance factor governed by the mass balance between dose and concentration, that is, drug concentration multiplied by the volume of the fluid must equal the dose at time = 0. At time = 0, no drug is eliminated, $D_0 = V_p C_p$. The basic model assumption is that plasma drug concentration is representative of drug concentration within the distribution fluid of plasma. If this statement is true, then the volume of distribution will be 3 L; if it is not, then distribution of drug may also occur outside the vascular pool into extra- and intracellular fluid.

$$V_p = \frac{D_0}{C_p^0} \tag{5.22}$$

At zero time ($t = 0$), the entire drug in the body is in the central compartment. C_p^0 can be shown to be equal to $A + B$ by the following equation:

$$C_p = Ae^{-\alpha t} + Be^{-\beta t} \tag{5.23}$$

At $t = 0$, $e^0 = 1$. Therefore,

$$C_p^0 = A + B \tag{5.24}$$

V_p is determined from Equation 5.25 by measuring A and B after feathering the curve, as discussed previously:

$$V_p = \frac{D_0}{A + B} \tag{5.25}$$

Alternatively, the volume of the central compartment may be calculated from the $[\text{AUC}]_0^\infty$ in a manner similar to the calculation for the apparent V_D in the one-compartment model. For a one-compartment model

$$[\text{AUC}]_0^\infty = \frac{D_0}{k V_D} \tag{5.26}$$

TABLE 5-6   **Pharmacokinetic Parameters (mean ± SD) of Moxalactam in Three Groups of Patients**

Group	A µg/mL	B µg/mL	α h⁻¹	β h⁻¹	k h⁻¹
1	138.9 ± 114.9	157.8 ± 87.1	6.8 ± 4.5	0.20 ± 0.12	0.38 ± 0.26
2	115.4 ± 65.9	115.0 ± 40.8	5.3 ± 3.5	0.27 ± 0.08	0.50 ± 0.17
3	102.9 ± 39.4	89.0 ± 36.7	5.6 ± 3.8	0.37 ± 0.09	0.71 ± 0.16

Group	Cl mL/min	V_p L/kg	V_t L/kg	$(V_D)_{ss}$ L/kg	$(V_D)_\beta$ L/kg
1	40.5 ± 14.5	0.12 ± 0.05	0.08 ± 0.04	0.20 ± 0.09	0.21 ± 0.09
2	73.7 ± 13.1	0.14 ± 0.06	0.09 ± 0.04	0.23 ± 0.10	0.24 ± 0.12
3	125.9 ± 28.0	0.15 ± 0.05	0.10 ± 0.05	0.25 ± 0.08	0.29 ± 0.09

In contrast, $[AUC]_0^\infty$ for the two-compartment model is:

$$[AUC]_0^\infty = \frac{D_0}{kV_p} \tag{5.27}$$

Rearrangement of this equation yields:

$$V_p = \frac{D_0}{k[AUC]_0^\infty} \tag{5.28}$$

Apparent Volume of Distribution at Steady State

This is a proportionality constant that relates the plasma concentration and the amount of drug remaining in the body at a time, following the attainment of practical steady state (which is reached at a time greater by at least four elimination half-lives of the drug). At steady-state conditions, the rate of drug entry into the tissue compartment from the central compartment is equal to the rate of drug exit from the tissue compartment into the central compartment. These rates of drug transfer are described by the following expressions:

$$D_t k_{21} = D_p k_{12} \tag{5.29}$$

$$D_t = \frac{k_{12}D_p}{k_{21}} \tag{5.30}$$

Because the amount of drug in the central compartment, D_p, is equal to V_pC_p, by substitution in the above equation,

$$D_t = \frac{k_{12}C_pV_p}{k_{21}} \tag{5.31}$$

The total amount of drug in the body at steady state is equal to the sum of the amount of drug in the tissue compartment, D_t, and the amount of drug in the central compartment, D_p. Therefore, the apparent volume of drug at steady state $(V_D)_{ss}$ may be calculated by dividing the total amount of drug in the body by the concentration of drug in the central compartment at steady state:

$$(V_D)_{ss} = \frac{D_p + D_t}{C_p} \tag{5.32}$$

Substituting Equation 5.31 into Equation 5.32, and expressing D_p as V_pC_p, a more useful equation for the calculation of $(V_D)_{ss}$ is obtained:

$$(V_D)_{ss} = \frac{C_pV_p + k_{12}V_pC_p/k_{21}}{C_p} \tag{5.33}$$

which reduces to

$$(V_D)_{ss} = V_p + \frac{k_{12}}{k_{21}}V_p \tag{5.34}$$

In practice, Equation 5.34 is used to calculate $(V_D)_{ss}$. The $(V_D)_{ss}$ is a function of the transfer constants, k_{12} and k_{21}, which represent the rate constants of drug going into and out of the tissue compartment, respectively. The magnitude of $(V_D)_{ss}$ is dependent on the hemodynamic factors responsible for drug distribution and on the physical properties of the drug, properties which, in turn, determine the relative amount of intra- and extravascular drug remaining in the body.

Extrapolated Volume of Distribution

The extrapolated volume of distribution $(V_D)_{exp}$ is calculated by the following equation:

$$(V_D)_{exp} = \frac{D_0}{B} \tag{5.35}$$

where B is the y intercept obtained by extrapolation of the β phase of the plasma level curve to the y axis (Fig. 5-4). Because the y intercept is a hybrid constant, as shown by Equation 5.15, $(V_D)_{exp}$ may also be calculated by the following expression:

$$(V_D)_{exp} = V_p\left(\frac{\alpha - \beta}{k_{21} - \beta}\right) \tag{5.36}$$

This equation shows that a change in the distribution of a drug, which is observed by a change in the value for V_p, will be reflected in a change in $(V_D)_{exp}$.

Volume of Distribution by Area

The volume of distribution by area $(V_D)_{area}$, also known as $(V_D)_\beta$, is obtained through calculations similar to those used to find V_p, except that the rate constant β is used instead of the overall elimination rate constant k. This volume represents a proportionality factor between plasma concentrations and amount of drug in body during the terminal or β phase of disposition. $(V_D)_\beta$ is often calculated from total body clearance divided by β and is influenced by drug elimination in the beta, or β, phase. This volume will be considered a time-dependent and clearance-dependent volume of distribution parameter. The value of $(V_D)_\beta$ is affected by elimination, and it changes as clearance is altered. Reduced drug clearance from the body may increase AUC (area under the curve), such that $(V_D)_\beta$ is either reduced or unchanged depending on the value of β, as shown by Equation 5.36.

$$(V_D)_\beta = (V_D)_{area} = \frac{D_0}{\beta[\text{AUC}]_0^\infty} \quad (4.37)$$

A slower clearance allows more time for drug equilibration between plasma and tissues yielding a smaller $(V_D)_\beta$. The lower limit of $(V_D)_\beta$ is V_{ss}:

$$\text{Lim}(V_D)_\beta = V_{ss}$$

$$\text{Cl} \rightarrow 0$$

Thus, $(V_D)_\beta$ has value in representing V_{ss} for low-clearance drugs as well as estimating terminal or β phase. Smaller $(V_D)_\beta$ values than normal are often observed in patients with renal failure because of the reduced Cl. This is a consequence of the Cl-dependent time of equilibration between plasma and tissue. Thus, V_{ss} is preferred in separating alterations in elimination from those in distribution.

Generally, reduced drug clearance is also accompanied by a decrease in the constant β (ie, an increase in the β elimination half-life). For example, in patients with renal dysfunction, the elimination half-life of the antibiotic amoxicillin is longer because renal clearance is reduced.

Because total body clearance is equal to $D_0/[\text{AUC}]_0^\infty$, $(V_D)_\beta$ may be expressed in terms of clearance and the rate constant β:

$$(V_D)_\beta = \frac{Cl}{\beta} \quad (5.38)$$

Substituting kV_p for clearance in Equation 5.38, one obtains:

$$(V_D)_\beta = \frac{kV_p}{\beta} \quad (5.39)$$

Theoretically, the value for β may remain unchanged in patients showing various degrees of moderate renal impairment. In this case, a reduction in $(V_D)_\beta$ may account for all the decrease in Cl, while β is unchanged in Equation 5.39. Within the body, a redistribution of drug between the plasma and the tissue will mask the expected decline in β. The following example in two patients shows that the β elimination rate constant remains the same, while the distributional rate constants change. Interestingly, V_p is unchanged, while $(V_D)_\beta$ would be greatly changed in the simulated example. An example of a drug showing a constant β slope while the renal function as measured by Cl_{cr} decreases from 107 to 56, 34, and 6 mL/min (see Chapter 7) has been observed with the aminoglycoside drug gentamicin in various patients after IV bolus dose (Schentag et al, 1977). Gentamicin follows polyexponential decline with a significant distributive phase. The following simulation problem may help clarify the situation by changing k and clearance while keeping β constant.

PRACTICE PROBLEM

Simulated plasma drug concentrations after an IV bolus dose (100 mg) of an antibiotic in two patients, patient 1 with a normal k, and patient 2 with a reduced k, are shown in Fig. 5-6. The data in the two patients were simulated with parameters using the two-compartment model equation. The parameters used are as follows:

Normal subject, $k = 0.3$ h^{-1}, $V_p = 10$ L, $Cl = 3$ L/h

$$k_{12} = 5 \text{ h}^{-1}, \quad k_{21} = 0.2 \text{ h}^{-1}$$

Subject with moderate renal impairment, $k = 0.1$ h^{-1}, $V_p = 10$ L, $Cl = 1$ L/h

$$k_{12} = 2 \text{ h}^{-1}, \quad k_{21} = 0.25 \text{ h}^{-1}$$

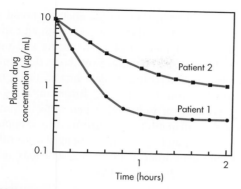

FIGURE 5-6   Simulation of plasma drug concentration after an IV bolus dose (100 mg) of an antibiotic in two patients, one with a normal k (patient 1) and the other with reduced k (patient 2).

Questions

1. Is a reduction in drug clearance generally accompanied by an increase in plasma drug concentration, regardless of which compartment model the drug follows?
2. Is a reduction in drug clearance generally accompanied by an increase in the β elimination half-life of a drug? [Find $(V_D)_\beta$ using Equation 5.38, and then β using Equation 5.39.]
3. Many antibiotics follow multiexponential plasma drug concentration profiles indicating drug distribution into tissue compartments. In clinical pharmacokinetics, the terminal half-life is often determined with limited early data. Which patient has a greater terminal half-life based on the simulated data?

Solutions

1. A reduction in drug clearance results in less drug being removed from the body per unit time. Drug clearance is model independent. Therefore, the plasma drug concentration should be higher in subjects with decreased drug clearance compared to subjects with normal drug clearance, regardless of which compartment model is used (see Fig. 5-6).
2. Clearance in the two-compartment model is affected by the elimination rate constant, β, and the volume of distribution in the β phase, which

reflects the data. A decrease in the $(V_D)_\beta$ with β unchanged is possible, although this is not the common case. When this happens, the terminal data (see Fig. 5-6) conclude that the beta elimination half-lives of patients 1 and 2 are the same due to a similar β. Actually, the real elimination half-life of the drug derived from k is a much better parameter, since k reflects the changes in renal function, but not β, which remains unchanged since it is masked by the changes in $(V_D)_\beta$.

3. Both patients have the same β value ($\beta = 0.011$ h^{-1}); the terminal slopes are identical. Ignoring early points by only taking terminal data would lead to an erroneous conclusion that the renal elimination process is unchanged, while the volume of distribution of the renally impaired patient is smaller. In this case, the renally impaired patient has a clearance of 1 L/h compared with 3 L/h for the normal subject, and yet the terminal slopes are the same. The rapid distribution of drug into the tissue in the normal subject causes a longer and steeper distribution phase. Later, redistribution of drug out of tissues masks the effect of rapid drug elimination through the kidney. In the renally impaired patient, distribution to tissue is reduced; as a result, little drug is redistributed out from the tissue in the β phase. Hence, it appears that the beta phases are identical in the two patients.

Significance of the Volumes of Distribution

From Equations 5.38 and 5.39 we can observe that $(V_D)_\beta$ is affected by changes in the overall elimination rate (ie, change in k) and by change in total body clearance of the drug. After the drug is distributed, the total amount of drug in the body during the elimination of β phase is calculated by using $(V_D)_\beta$.

V_p is sometimes called the initial volume of distribution and is useful in the calculation of drug clearance. The magnitudes of the various apparent volumes of distribution have the following relationships to each other:

$$(V_D)_{exp} > (V_D)_\beta > V_p$$

Calculation of another V_D, $(V_D)_{ss}$, is possible in multiple dosing or infusion (see Chapters 6 and 9). $(V_D)_{ss}$ is much larger than V_p; it approximates $(V_D)_\beta$ but differs somewhat in value, depending on the transfer constants.

In a study involving a cardiotonic drug given intravenously to a group of normal and congestive heart failure (CHF) patients, the average AUC for CHF was 40% higher than in the normal subjects. The β elimination constant was 40% less in CHF patients, whereas the average $(V_D)_\beta$ remained essentially the same. In spite of the edematous conditions of these patients, the volume of distribution apparently remained constant. No change was found in the V_p or $(V_D)_\beta$. In this study, a 40% increase in AUC in the CHF subjects was offset by a 40% smaller β elimination constant estimated by using computer methods. Because the dose was the same, the $(V_D)_\beta$ would not change unless the increase in AUC is not accompanied by a change in β elimination constant.

From Equation 5.38, the clearance of the drug in CHF patients was reduced by 40% and accompanied by a corresponding decrease in the β elimination constant, possibly due to a reduction in renal blood flow as a result of reduced cardiac output in CHF patients. In physiologic pharmacokinetics, clearance (Cl) and volume of distribution (V_D) are assumed to be independent parameters that explain the impact of disease factors on drug disposition. Thus, an increase in AUC of a cardiotonic in a CHF patient was assumed to be due to a reduction in drug clearance, since the volume of distribution was unchanged. The elimination half-life was reduced due to reduction in drug clearance. In reality, pharmacokinetic changes in a complex system are dependent on many factors that interact within the system. Clearance is affected by drug uptake, metabolism, binding, and more; all of these factors can also influence the drug distribution volume. Many parameters are assumed to be constant and independent for simplification of the model. Blood flow is an independent parameter that will affect both clearance and distribution. However, blood flow is, in turn, affected and regulated by many physiologic compensatory factors.

For drugs that follow two-compartment model kinetics, changes in disease states may not result in different pharmacokinetic parameters. Conversely, changes in pharmacokinetic parameters should not be attributed to physiologic changes without careful consideration of method of curve fitting and intersubject differences. Equation 5.39 shows that, unlike a simple one-compartment open model, $(V_D)_\beta$ may be estimated from k, β, and V_p. Errors in fitting are easily carried over to the other parameter estimates even if the calculations are performed by computer. The terms k_{12} and k_{21} often fluctuate due to minor fitting and experimental difference and may affect calculation of other parameters.

> **Frequently Asked Questions**
> ▶ *What is the significance of the apparent volume of distribution?*
>
> ▶ *Why are there different volumes of distribution in the multiple-compartment models?*

Drug in the Tissue Compartment

The apparent volume of the tissue compartment (V_t) is a conceptual volume only and does not represent true anatomic volumes. The V_t may be calculated from knowledge of the transfer rate constants and V_p:

$$V_t = \frac{V_p k_{12}}{k_{21}} \qquad (5.40)$$

The calculation of the amount of drug in the tissue compartment does not entail the use of V_t. Calculation of the amount of drug in the tissue compartment provides an estimate for drug accumulation in the tissues of the body. This information is vital in estimating chronic toxicity and relating the duration of pharmacologic activity to dose. Tissue compartment drug concentration is an average estimate of the tissue pool and does not mean that all tissues have this concentration. The drug concentration in a tissue biopsy will provide an estimate for drug in that tissue sample. Due to differences in blood flow and drug partitioning into the tissue, and heterogenicity, even a biopsy from the same tissue may have different drug concentrations. Together with V_p and C_p, used to calculate the amount of drug in the plasma, the compartment model provides mass balance information.

Moreover, the pharmacodynamic activity may correlate better with the tissue drug concentration–time curve. To calculate the amount of drug in the tissue compartment D_t, the following expression is used:

$$D_t = \frac{k_{12} D_p^0}{\alpha - \beta} (e^{-\beta t} - e^{-\alpha t}) \qquad (5.41)$$

PRACTICAL FOCUS

The therapeutic plasma concentration of digoxin is between 1 and 2 ng/mL; because digoxin has a long elimination half-life, it takes a long time to reach a stable, constant (steady-state) level in the body. A loading dose is usually given with the initiation of digoxin therapy. Consider the implications of the loading dose of 1 mg suggested for a 70-kg subject. The clinical source cited an apparent volume of distribution of 7.3 L/kg for digoxin in determining the loading dose. Use the pharmacokinetic parameters for digoxin in Table 5-4.

Solution

The loading dose was calculated by considering the body as one compartment during steady state, at which time the drug well penetrates the tissue compartment. The volume of distribution $(V_D)_\beta$ of digoxin is much larger than V_p, or the volume of the plasma compartment.

Using Equation (5.39),

$$(V_D)_\beta = \frac{k V_p}{\beta}$$

$$= \frac{0.18/h \times 0.78\ \text{L/kg}}{0.019/h} = 7.39\ \text{L/kg}$$

$$D_L = 7390 \frac{\text{mL}}{\text{kg}} \times 70\ \text{kg} \times 1.5 \frac{\text{ng}}{\text{mL}}$$

where $D_L = (V_D)_\beta \cdot (C_p)_{ss}$. The desired steady plasma concentration, $(C_p)_{ss}$, was selected by choosing a value in the middle of the therapeutic range. The loading dose is generally divided into two or three doses or is administered as 50% in the first dose with the remaining drug given in two divided doses

6–8 hours apart to minimize potential side effects from overdigitization. If the entire loading dose were administered intravenously, the plasma level would be about 4–5 ng/mL after 1 hour, while the level would drop to about 1.5 ng/mL at about 4 hours. The exact level after a given IV dose may be calculated using Equation 5.7 at any time desired. The pharmacokinetic parameters for digoxin are available in Table 5-4.

In addition to metabolism, digoxin distribution is affected by a number of processes besides blood flow. Digoxin and many other drugs are P-gp (P-glycoprotein) substrates, a transporter that is often located in cell membranes that efflux drug in and out of cells, and can theoretically affect k_{12} (cell uptake) and k_{21} (cell efflux). Some transporters such as P-gp or ABC transporters exhibit genetic variability and therefore can contribute to pharmacokinetic varability between patients. For example, if drug transporters avidly carry drug to metabolic sites, then metabolism would increase, and plasma levels AUC would decrease. The converse is also true; examples of drugs that are known to increase digoxin level include amidiodarone, quinidine, and verapamil. Verapamil is a potent P-gp inhibitor and a common agent used to test if an unknown substrate can be blocked by a P-gp inhibitor.

Many anticancer drugs such as taxol, vincristine, and vinblastine are P-gp substrates. P-gp can be located in GI, kidney, liver, and entry to BBB (see Chapter 11 for distribution and Chapter 13 for genetically expressed transporters). There are other organic anion and cation transporters in the body that contribute to efflux of drug into and out of cells. Efflux and translocation of a drug can cause a drug to lose efficacy (MDR resistance) in many anticancer drugs. It may not always be possible to distinquish a specific drug transporter in a specific organ or tissue *in vivo* due to ongoing perfusion and the potential for multiple transporter/carriers involved. These factors; drug binding to proteins in blood, cell, and cell membranes; and diffusion limiting processes contribute to "multiexponential" drug distribution kinetically for many drugs. Much of *in vivo* kinetics information can be learned by examining the kinetics of the IV bolus time-concentration profile when a suitable substrate probe is administered.

Drug Clearance

The definition of clearance of a drug that follows a two-compartment model is similar to that of the one-compartment model. *Clearance* is the volume of plasma that is cleared of drug per unit time. Clearance may be calculated without consideration of the compartment model. Thus, clearance may be viewed as a physiologic concept for drug removal, even though the development of clearance is rooted in classical pharmacokinetics.

Clearance is often calculated by a noncompartmental approach, as in Equation 5.37, in which the bolus IV dose is divided by the area under the plasma concentration–time curve from zero to infinity, $[AUC]_0^\infty$. In evaluating the $[AUC]_0^\infty$, early time points must be collected frequently to observe the rapid decline in drug concentrations (distribution phase) for drugs with multicompartment pharmacokinetics. In the calculation of clearance using the noncompartmental approach, underestimating the area can inflate the calculated value of clearance.

$$Cl = \frac{D_0}{[AUC]_0^\infty} \qquad (5.42)$$

Equation 5.42 may be rearranged to Equation 5.43 to show that *Cl* in the two-compartment model is the product of $(V_D)_\beta$ and β.

$$Cl = (V_D)_\beta \beta \qquad (5.43)$$

If both parameters are known, then calculation of clearance is simple and more accurate than using the trapezoidal rule to obtain area. Clearance calculations that use the two-compartment model are viewed as model dependent because more assumptions are required, and such calculations cannot be regarded as noncompartmental. However, the assumptions provide additional information and, in some sense, specifically describe the drug concentration–time profile as biphasic.

Clearance is a term that is useful in calculating average drug concentrations. With many drugs, a biphasic profile suggests a rapid tissue distribution phase followed by a slower elimination phase. Multicompartment pharmacokinetics is an important

consideration in understanding drug permeation and toxicity. For example, the plasma–time profiles of aminoglycosides, such as gentamicin, are more useful in explaining toxicity than average plasma or drug concentration taken at peak or trough time.

Elimination Rate Constant

In the two-compartment model (IV administration), the elimination rate constant, k, represents the elimination of drug from the central compartment, whereas β represents drug elimination during the beta or elimination phase, when distribution is mostly complete. Because of redistribution of drug out of the tissue compartment, the plasma drug level curve declines more slowly in the β phase. Hence β is smaller than k; thus k is a true elimination constant, whereas β is a hybrid elimination rate constant that is influenced by the rate of transfer of drug into and out of the tissue compartment. When it is impractical to determine k, β is calculated from the β slope. The $t_{1/2\beta}$ is often used to calculate the drug dose.

THREE-COMPARTMENT OPEN MODEL

The three-compartment model is an extension of the two-compartment model, with an additional deep tissue compartment. A drug that demonstrates the necessity of a three-compartment open model is distributed most rapidly to a highly perfused central compartment, less rapidly to the second or tissue compartment, and very slowly to the third or deep tissue compartment, containing such poorly perfused tissue as bone and fat. The deep tissue compartment may also represent tightly bound drug in the tissues. The three-compartment open model is shown in Fig. 5-7.

A solution of the differential equation describing the rates of flow of drug into and out of the central compartment gives the following equation:

$$C_p = Ae^{-\alpha t} + Be^{-\beta t} + Ce^{-\delta t} \qquad (5.44)$$

where A, B, and C are the y intercepts of extrapolated lines for the central, tissue, and deep tissue compartments, respectively, and α, β, and γ are first-order

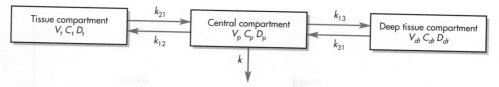

FIGURE 5-7   Three-compartment open model. This model, as with the previous two-compartment models, assumes that all drug elimination occurs via the central compartment.

rate constants for the central, tissue, and deep tissue compartments, respectively.

A three-compartment equation may be written by statisticians in the literature as

$$C_p = Ae^{-\lambda_1 t} + Be^{-\lambda_2 t} + Ce^{-\lambda_3 t} \qquad (5.44a)$$

Instead of α, β, γ, etc., λ_1, λ_2, λ_3 are substituted to express the triexponential feature of the equation. Similarly, the n-compartment model may be expressed with λ_1, λ_2, ..., λ_n. The preexponential terms are sometimes expressed as C_1, C_2, and C_3.

The parameters in Equation 5.44 may be solved graphically by the method of residuals (Fig. 5-8) or by computer. The calculations for the elimination rate constant k, volume of the central compartment, and area are shown in the following equations:

$$k = \frac{(A+B+C)\alpha\beta\delta}{A\beta\delta + B\alpha\delta + C\alpha\beta} \qquad (5.45)$$

$$V_p = \frac{D_0}{A+B+C} \qquad (5.46)$$

$$[AUC] = \frac{A}{\alpha} + \frac{B}{\beta} + \frac{C}{\delta} \qquad (5.47)$$

CLINICAL APPLICATION

Hydromorphone (Dilaudid)

Three independent studies on the pharmacokinetics of hydromorphone after a bolus intravenous injection reported that hydromorphone followed the pharmacokinetics of a one-compartment model (Vallner et al, 1981), a two-compartment model (Parab et al, 1988), or a three-compartment model (Hill et al, 1991), respectively. A comparison of these studies is listed in Table 5-7.

Comments

The adequacy of the pharmacokinetic model will depend on the sampling intervals and the drug assay. The first two studies showed a similar elimination half-life. However, both Vallner et al (1981) and Parab et al (1988) did not observe a three-compartment pharmacokinetic model due to lack of appropriate description of the early distribution phases for hydromorphone. After an IV bolus injection, hydromorphone is very rapidly distributed into the tissues. Hill et al (1991) obtained a triexponential function by closely sampling early time periods after the dose. Average distribution half-lives were 1.27 and

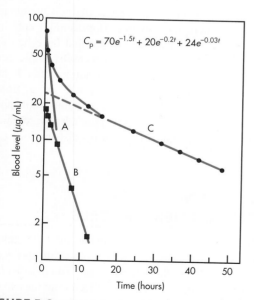

$$C_p = 70e^{-1.5t} + 20e^{-0.2t} + 24e^{-0.03t}$$

FIGURE 5-8   Plasma level–time curve for a three-compartment open model. The rate constants and intercepts were calculated by the method of residuals.

TABLE 5-7   Comparison of Hydromorphone Pharmacokinetics

Study	Timing of Blood Samples	Pharmacokinetic Parameters
6 Males, 25–29 years; mean weight, 76.8 kg Dose, 2-mg IV bolus (Vallner et al, 1981)	0, 15, 30, 45 minutes 1, 1.5, 2, 3, 4, 6, 8, 10, 12 hours	One-compartment model Terminal $t_{1/2}$ = 2.64 (± 0.88) hours
8 Males, 20–30 years; weight, 50–86 kg Dose, 2-mg IV bolus (Parab et al, 1988)	0, 3, 7, 15, 30, 45 minutes 1, 1.5, 2, 3, 4, 6, 8, 10, 12 hours	Two-compartment model Terminal $t_{1/2}$ = 2.36 (± 0.58) hours
10 Males, 21–38 years; mean weight, 72.7 kg Dose, 10, 20, and 40 μg/kg IV bolus (Hill et al, 1991)	1, 2, 3, 4, 5, 7, 10, 15, 20, 30, 45 minutes 1, 1.5, 2, 2.5, 3, 4, 5 hours	Three-compartment model Terminal $t_{1/2}$ = 3.07 (± 0.25) hours

14.7 minutes, and the average terminal elimination was 184 minutes ($t_{1/2\beta}$). The average value for systemic clearance (Cl) was 1.66 L/min; the initial dilution volume was 24.4 L. If distribution is rapid, the drug becomes distributed during the absorption phase. Thus, hydromorphone pharmacokinetics follows a one-compartment model after a single oral dose.

Hydromorphone is administered to relieve acute pain in cancer or postoperative patients. Rapid pain relief is obtained by IV injection. Although the drug is effective orally, about 50%–60% of the drug is cleared by the liver through first-pass effects. The pharmacokinetics of hydromorphone after IV injection suggests a multicompartment model. The site of action is probably within the central nervous system, as part of the tissue compartment. The initial volume or initial dilution volume, V_p, is the volume into which IV injections are injected and diluted. Hydromorphone follows linear kinetics, that is, drug concentration is proportional to dose. Hydromorphone systemic clearance is much larger than the glomerular filtration rate (GFR) of 120 mL/min (see Chapter 7), hence the drug is probably metabolized significantly by the hepatic route. A clearance of 1.66 L/min is faster than the blood flow of 1.2–1.5 L/min to the liver. The drug must be rapidly extracted or, in addition, must have extrahepatic elimination. When the distribution phase is short, the distribution phase may be disregarded provided that the targeted plasma concentration is sufficiently low and the terminal elimination phase is relatively long. If the drug has a sufficiently high target plasma drug concentration and the elimination half-life is short, the distributive phase must not be ignored. For example, lidocaine's effective target concentration often lies close to the distributive phase, since its beta elimination half-life is very short, and ignoring the alpha phase will result in a large error in dosing projection.

CLINICAL APPLICATION

Loperamide (Imodium®) is an opioid anti-diarrhea agent that is useful for illustrating the importance of understanding drug distribution. Loperamide has little central opiate effect. Loperamide is a P-gp (an efflux transporter) substrate. The presence of P-gp transporter at the blood–brain barrier allows the drug to be pumped out of the cell at the cell membrane surface without the substrate (loperamide) entering into the interior of the cell. Mice that have had the gene for P-gp removed experimentally show profound central opioid effects when administered loperamide. Hypothesizing the presence of a tissue compartment coupled with a suitable molecular probe can provide a powerful approach toward elucidating the mechanism of drug distribution and improving drug safety.

DETERMINATION OF COMPARTMENT MODELS

Models based on compartmental analysis should always use the fewest number of compartments necessary to describe the experimental data adequately. Once an empirical equation is derived from the experimental observations, it becomes necessary to examine how well the theoretical values that are calculated from the derived equation fit the experimental data.

The observed number of compartments or exponential phases will depend on (1) the route of drug administration, (2) the rate of drug absorption, (3) the total time for blood sampling, (4) the number of samples taken within the collection period, and (5) the assay sensitivity. If drug distribution is rapid, then, after oral administration, the drug will become distributed during the absorption phase and the distribution phase will not be observed. For example, theophylline follows the kinetics of a one-compartment model after oral absorption, but after intravenous bolus (given as aminophylline), theophylline follows the kinetics of a two-compartment model. Furthermore, if theophylline is given by a slow intravenous infusion rather than by intravenous bolus, the distribution phase will not be observed. Hydromorphone (Dilaudid), which follows a three-compartment model, also follows a one-compartment model after oral administration, since the first two distribution phases are rapid.

Depending on the sampling intervals, a compartment may be missed because samples may be taken too late after administration of the dose to observe a possible distributive phase. For example, the data plotted in Fig. 5-9 could easily be mistaken for those of a one-compartment model, because the distributive phase has been missed and extrapolation of the data to C_p^0 will give a lower value than was actually the case. Slower drug elimination compartments may also be missed if sampling is not performed at later sampling times, when the dose or the assay for the drug cannot measure very low plasma drug concentrations.

The total time for collection of blood samples is usually estimated from the terminal elimination half-life of the drug. However, lower drug concentrations may not be measured if the sensitivity of the assay is not adequate. As the assay for the drug becomes more sensitive in its ability to measure lower drug concentrations, then another compartment with a smaller first-order rate constant may be observed.

In describing compartments, each new compartment requires an additional first-order plot. Compartment models having more than three compartments are rarely of pharmacologic significance. In certain cases, it is possible to "lump" a few compartments together to get a smaller number of compartments, which, together, will describe the data adequately.

An adequate description of several tissue compartments can be difficult. When the addition of a compartment to the model seems necessary, it is important to realize that the drug may be retained or slowly concentrated in a deep tissue compartment.

PRACTICAL FOCUS

Two-Compartment Model: Relation Between Distribution and Apparent (Beta) Half-Life

The distribution half-life of a drug is dependent on the type of tissues the drug penetrates as well as blood supply to those tissues. In addition, the capacity of the tissue to store drug is also a factor. Distribution half-life is generally short for many drugs because of the ample blood supply to and rapid drug equilibration in the tissue compartment. However, there is some supporting evidence that a drug with a long elimination half-life is often associated with a longer distribution phase. It is conceivable that a tissue with little blood supply and affinity for the drug may not attain a sufficiently high drug concentration to exert its impact on the overall plasma drug concentration profile during rapid elimination. In contrast, drugs such as digoxin have a long elimination half-life, and drug is eliminated slowly to allow more time for distribution to tissues. Human follicle-stimulating hormone (hFSH) injected intravenously has a very long elimination

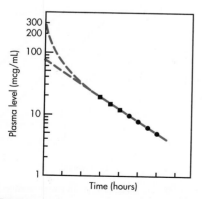

FIGURE 5-9   The samples from which data were obtained for this graph were taken too late to show the distributive phase; therefore, the value of C_p^0 obtained by extrapolation (straight broken line) is deceptively low.

half-life, and its distribution half-life is also quite long. Drugs such as lidocaine, theophylline, and milrinone have short elimination half-lives and generally relatively short distributional half-lives.

In order to examine the effect of changing k (from 0.6 to 0.2 h^{-1}) on the distributional (alpha phase) and elimination (beta phase) half-lives of various drugs, four simulations based on a two-compartment model were generated (Table 5-8). The simulations show that a drug with a smaller k has a longer beta elimination half-life. Keeping all other parameters (k_{12}, k_{21}, V_p) constant, a smaller k will result in a smaller α, or a slower distributional phase. Examples of drugs with various distribution and elimination half-lives are shown in Table 5-8.

TABLE 5-8   Comparison of Beta Half-Life and Distributional Half-Life of Selected Drugs

Drug	Beta Half-Life	Distributional Half-Life
Lidocaine	1.8 hours	8 minutes
Cocaine	1 hours	18 minutes
Theophylline	4.33 hours	7.2 minutes
Ergometrine	2 hours	11 minutes
Hydromorphone	3 hours	14.7 minutes
Milrinone	3.6 hours	4.6 minutes
Procainamide	2.5–4.7 hours	6 minutes
Quinidine	6–8 hours	7 minutes
Lithium	21.39 hours	5 hours
Digoxin	1.6 days	35 minutes
Human FSH	1 day	60 minutes
IgG1 kappa MAB	9.6 days (monkey)	6.7 hours
Simulation 1	13.26 hours	36.24 minutes
Simulation 2	16.60 hours	43.38 minutes
Simulation 3	26.83 hours	53.70 minutes
Simulation 4	213.7 hours	1.12 hours

Simulation was performed using V_p of 10 L; dose = 100 mg; k_{12} = 0.5 h^{-1}; k_{21} = 0.1 h^{-1}; k = 0.6, 0.4, 0.2, and 0.02 hour for simulations 1–4, respectively (using Equations 5.11 and 5.12).

Source: Data from manufacturer and Schumacher (1995).

CLINICAL APPLICATION

Moxalactam Disodium—Effect of Changing Renal Function in Patients with Sepsis

The pharmacokinetics of moxalactam disodium, a recently discontinued antibiotic (see Table 5-6), was examined in 40 patients with abdominal sepsis (Swanson et al, 1983). The patients were grouped according to creatinine clearances into three groups:

Group 1: Average creatinine clearance = 35.5 mL/min/1.73 m^2

Group 2: Average creatinine clearance = 67.1 ± 6.7 mL/min/1.73 m^2

Group 3: Average creatinine clearance = 117.2 ± 29.9 mL/min/1.73 m^2

After intravenous bolus administration, the serum drug concentrations followed a biexponential decline (Fig. 5-10). The pharmacokinetics at steady state (2 g every 8 hours) was also examined in these

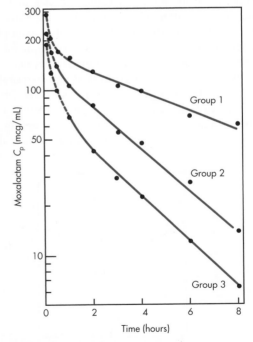

FIGURE 5-10   Moxalactam serum concentration in three groups of patients: group 1, average creatinine concentration = 35.5 mL/min/1.73 m^2; group 2, average creatinine concentration = 67.1 ± 6.7 mL/min/1.73 m^2; group 3, average creatinine concentration = 117.2 ± 29.9 mL/min/1.73 m^2.

patients. Mean steady-state serum concentrations ranged from 27.0 to 211.0 μg/mL and correlated inversely with creatinine clearance ($r = 0.91$, $p < 0.0001$). The terminal half-life ranged from 1.27 to 8.27 hours and reflected the varying renal function of the patients. Moxalactam total body clearance (Cl) had excellent correlation with creatinine clearance ($r^2 = 0.92$). Cl determined by noncompartmental data analysis was in agreement with Cl determined by nonlinear least squares regression ($r = 0.99$, $p < 0.0001$). Moxalactam total body clearance was best predicted from creatinine clearance corrected for body surface area.

Questions (Refer to Table 5-6)

1. Calculate the beta half-life of moxalactam in the most renally impaired group.
2. What indicator is used to predict moxalactam clearance in the body?
3. What is the beta volume of distribution of patients in group 3 with normal renal function?
4. What is the initial volume (V_i) of moxalactam?

Solutions

1. Mean beta half-life is $0.693/0.20 = 3.47$ hours in the most renally impaired group.
2. Creatinine is mainly filtered through the kidney, and creatinine clearance is used as an indicator of renal glomerular filtration rate. Group 3 has normal renal function (average creatinine clearance $= 117.2$ mL/min/1.73 m^2) (see Chapter 7).
3. Beta volume of distribution: Moxalactam clearance in group 3 subjects is 125.9 mL/min. From Equation 5.38,

$$(V_D)_\beta = \frac{Cl}{\beta}$$

$$= \frac{125.9 \text{ mL/min} \times 60 \text{ min/h}}{0.37 \text{ h}^{-1}}$$

$$= 20{,}416 \text{ mL or } 20.4 \text{ L}$$

4. The volume of the plasma compartment, V_p, is sometimes referred to as the initial volume. V_p ranges from 0.12 to 0.15 L/kg among the three groups and is considerably smaller than the steady-state volume of distribution.

Clinical Example—Azithromycin Pharmacokinetics

Following oral administration, azithromycin (Zithromax®) is an antibiotic that is rapidly absorbed and widely distributed throughout the body. Azithromycin is rapidly distributed into tissues, with high drug concentrations within cells, resulting in significantly higher azithromycin concentrations in tissue than in plasma. The high values for plasma clearance (630 mL/min) suggest that the prolonged half-life is due to extensive uptake and subsequent release of drug from tissues.

Plasma concentrations of azithromycin decline in a polyphasic pattern, resulting in an average terminal half-life of 68 hours. With this regimen, C_{min} and C_{max} remained essentially unchanged from day 2 through day 5 of therapy. However, without a loading dose, azithromycin C_{min} levels required 5–7 days to reach desirable plasma levels.

The pharmacokinetic parameters of azithromycin in healthy elderly male subjects (65–85 years) were similar to those in young adults. Although higher peak drug concentrations (increased by 30%–50%) were observed in elderly women, no significant accumulation occurred.

Questions

1. Do you agree with the following statements for a drug that is described by a two-compartment pharmacokinetic model? At peak C_t, the drug is well equilibrated between the plasma and the tissue compartment, $C_p = C_t$, and the rates of drug diffusion into and from the plasma compartment are equal.
2. What happens after peak C_t?
3. Why is a loading dose used?
4. What is V_i? How is this volume related to V_p?
5. What population factors could affect the concentration of azithromycin?

Solutions

1. For a drug that follows a multicompartment model, the rates of drug diffusion into the tissues from the plasma and from the tissues into the plasma are equal at peak tissue concentrations.

However, the tissue drug concentration is generally not equal to the plasma drug concentration.

2. After peak C_t, the rate out of the tissue exceeds the rate into the tissue, and C_t falls. The decline of C_t parallels that of C_p, and occurs because distribution equilibrium has occurred.

3. When drugs are given in a multiple-dose regimen, a loading dose may be given to achieve desired therapeutic drug concentrations more rapidly (see Chapter 9).

4. The volume of the plasma compartment, V_p, is sometimes referred to as the initial volume.

5. Age and gender may affect the C_{max} level of the drug.

PRACTICAL PROBLEM

Clinical Example—Etoposide Pharmacokinetics

Etoposide is a drug used for the treatment of lung cancer. Understanding the distribution of etoposide in normal and metastatic tissues is important to avoid drug toxicity. Etoposide follows a two-compartment model. The $(V_D)_\beta$ is 0.28 L/kg, and the beta elimination half-life is 12.9 hours. Total body clearance is 0.25 mL/min/kg.

Questions

1. What is the $(V_D)_\beta$ in a 70-kg subject?
2. How is the $(V_D)_\beta$ different than the volume of the plasma fluid, V_p?
3. Why is the $(V_D)_\beta$ useful if it does not represent a real tissue volume?
4. How is $(V_D)_\beta$ calculated from plasma time–concentration profile data for etoposide? Is $(V_D)_\beta$ related to total body clearance?
5. Etopside was recently shown to be a P-gp substrate. How may this affect drug tolerance in different patients?

Solutions

1. $(V_D)_\beta$ of etoposide in a 70-kg subject is 0.28 L/kg × 70 kg = 19.6 L.
2. The plasma fluid volume is about 3 L in a 70-kg subject and is much smaller than $(V_D)_\beta$. The apparent volume of distribution, $(V_D)_\beta$, is also considerably larger than the volume of the

plasma compartment (also referred to as the initial volume by some clinicians), which includes some extracellular fluid.

3. Etoposide is a drug that follows a two-compartment model with a beta elimination phase. Within the first few minutes after an intravenous bolus dose, most of the drug is distributed in the plasma fluid. Subsequently, the drug will diffuse into tissues and drug uptake may occur. Eventually, plasma drug levels will decline due to elimination, and some redistribution as etoposide in tissue diffuses back into the plasma fluid.

The real tissue drug level will differ from the plasma drug concentration, depending on the partitioning of drug in tissues and plasma. This allows the AUC, the volume distribution $(V_D)_\beta$, to be calculated, an area that has been related to toxicities associated with many cancer chemotherapy agents.

The two-compartment model allows continuous monitoring of the amount of the drug present in and out of the vascular system, including the amount of drug eliminated. This information is important in pharmacotherapy.

4. $(V_D)_\beta$ may be determined from the total drug clearance and beta:

$$Cl = \beta \times (V_D)_\beta$$

$(V_D)_\beta$ is also calculated from Equation 5.37 where

$$(V_D)_\beta = (V_D)_{area} = \frac{D_0}{\beta [AUC]_0^\infty}$$

This method for $(V_D)_\beta$ determination using $[AUC]_0^\infty$ is popular because $[AUC]_0^\infty$ is easily calculated using the trapezoidal rule. Many values for apparent volumes of distribution reported in the clinical literature are obtained using the area equation. In general, both volume terms reflect extravascular drug distribution. $(V_D)_\beta$ appears to be affected by the dynamics of drug disposition in the beta phase. In clinical practice, many potent drugs are not injected by bolus dose. Instead, these drugs are infused over a short interval, making it difficult to obtain accurate information on the distributive phase. As a result, many drugs that follow a two-compartment model are approximated using a single compartment. It should be cautioned that there are substantial deviations in some cases. When in doubt, the full equation with all parameters should be applied for comparison. A small bolus (test) dose may be injected to obtain the necessary data if a therapeutic dose injected rapidly causes side effects or discomfort to the subject.

> **Frequently Asked Questions**
> ▶ *What is the error assumed in a one-compartment model compared to a two-compartment or multi-compartment model?*
>
> ▶ *What kind of improvement in terms of patient care or drug therapy is made using the compartment model?*

CLINICAL APPLICATION

Dosing of Drugs with Different Biexponential Profiles

Drugs are usually dosed according to clearance principles with an objective of achieving a steady-state therapeutic level after multiple dosing (see Chapter 9). The method uses a simple well-stirred one-compartment or noncompartmental approach.

The distributive phase is not a major issue if the distribution phase has a short duration (Fig. 5-11) relative to the beta phase for chronic dosing. However, from the adverse reaction perspective, injury may occur even with short exposure to sensitive organs or enzyme sites. The observation of where the therapeutically effective levels are relative to the time-concentration profile presents an interesting case below.

PRACTICAL APPLICATION

Drugs A, B, and C are investigated for the treatment of arrhythmia (Fig. 5-12). Drug A has a very short distributive phase. The short distributive phase does not distort the overall kinetics when drug A is modeled by the one-compartment model. Simple one-compartment model assumptions are often made in practice and published in the literature for simplicity.

Drugs B and C have different distributive profiles. Drug B has a gradual distributive phase followed by a slower elimination (beta phase). The pharmacokinetic profile for drug C shows a longer and steeper distributive phase. Both drugs are well described by the two-compartment model.

Assuming drugs A and B both have the same effective level of 0.1 $\mu g/mL$, which drug would you prefer for dosing your patient based on the above plasma profiles provided and assuming that both

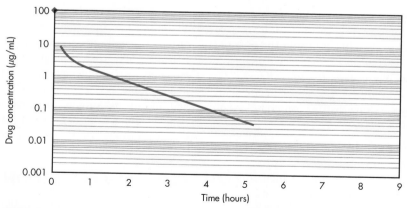

FIGURE 5-11   A two-compartment model drug showing a short distributive phase. The graph shows the log of the drug concentrations ($\mu g/mL$) versus time (hours). Drug mass rapidly distributes within the general circulation and highly vascular organs (central compartment) and is gradually distributed into other tissues or bound to cellular transporters or proteins.

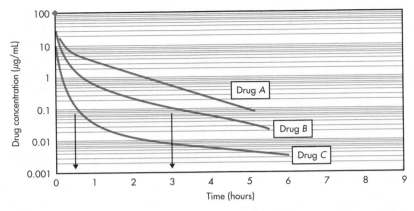

FIGURE 5-12   Plasma drug concentration profile of three drugs after IV bolus injection. Plasma drug concentration (C_p)–time profiles of three drugs (A, B, C) with different distributive (*a*) phase after single IV bolus injection are plotted on a semilogarithmic scale. Plasma concentrations are in μg/mL (*x* axis) and time in hours (*y* axis). Drugs A, B, and C are each given at a dose of 10 mg/kg to subjects by IV bolus injection, and each drug has minimum effective concentration of 0.1 μg/mL.

drugs have the same toxic endpoint (as measured by plasma drug level)?

At what time would you recommend giving a second dose for each drug? Please state your supportive reasons. Hints: Draw a line at 0.1 μg/mL and see how it intersects the plasma curve for drugs *B* and *C*.

If you ignore the distributive phase and dose a drug based only on clearance or the terminal half-life, how would this dose affect the duration above minimum effective drug concentration of 0.1 μg/mL for each drug after an IV bolus dose?

Drug *A* represents a drug that has limited tissue distribution with mostly a linear profile and is dosed by the one-compartment model. Can you recognize when the terminal phase starts for drugs *B* and *C*?

Drug *A*—short distribution, drug *B*—intermediate distribution, drug *C*—long distribution phase due to transporter or efflux.

- Which drug is acceptable to be modeled by a simple one compartment model?
- When re-dosed (ie, at 0.1 μg/mL), which drug was equilibrated with the tissue compartment?

Significance of Distribution Phase

With many drugs, the initial phase or transient concentration is not considered as important as the steady-state "trough" level during long-term drug dosing.

However, for a drug with the therapeutic endpoint (eg, target plasma drug concentration) that lies within the steep initial distributive phase, it is much harder to dose accurately and not overshoot the target endpoint. This scenario is particularly true for some drugs used in critical care where rapid responses are needed and IV bolus routes are used more often. Many new biotechnological drugs are administered intravenously because of instability by oral route. The choice of a proper dose and rate of infusion relative to the half-life of the drug is an important consideration for safe drug administration. Individual patients may behave very differently with regard to drug metabolism, drug transport, and drug efflux in target cell sites. Drug receptors can be genetically expressed differently making some people more prone to allergic reactions and side effects. Simple kinetic half-life determination coupled with a careful review of the patient's chart by a pharmacist can greatly improve drug safety.

CLINICAL APPLICATION

Lidocaine is a drug with low toxicity and a long history of use for anesthetization and for treating ventricular arrhythmias. The drug has a steep distributive phase and is biphasic. The risk of adverse effects is dose related and increases at intravenous infusion rates of above 3 mg/min. Dosage and dose rate are important for proper use (Greenspon et al, 1989). A case of inappropriate drug use was reported (Avery, 1998).

An overdose of lidocaine was given to a patient to anesthetize the airway due to bronchoscopy by an inexperienced hospital personnel. The patient was then left unobserved and subsequently developed convulsions and cardiopulmonary arrest. He survived with severe cerebral damage. His lidocaine concentration was 24 μg/mL about 1 hour after initial administration (a blood concentration over 6 μg/mL is considered to be toxic). What is the therapeutic plasma concentration range? Is the drug highly protein bound? Is V_D sufficiently large to show extravascular distribution?

A second case of adverse drug reaction (ADR) based on inappropriate use of this drug due to rapid absorption was reported by Pantuck et al (1997). A 40-year-old woman developed seizures after lidocaine gel 40 mL was injected into the ureter. Vascular absorption can apparently be very rapid depending on the site of application even if the route is not directly intravenous. It is important to note that for a drug with a steeply declining elimination plasma profile, it is harder to maintain a stable target level with dosing because a small change on the time scale (*x* axis) can greatly alter the drug concentration (*y* axis). Some drugs that have a steep distributive phase may easily cause a side effect in a susceptible subject.

Frequently Asked Questions

▶ *A new experimental drug can be modeled by a two-compartment model. What potential adverse event could occur for this drug if given by single IV bolus injection?*

▶ *A new experimental drug can be modeled by a three-compartment model. What potential adverse event could occur for this drug if given by multiple IV bolus injections?*

CHAPTER SUMMARY

Compartment is a term used in pharmacokinetic models to describe a theoreticized region within the body in which the drug concentrations are presumed to be uniformly distributed.

- A two-compartment model typically shows a biexponential plasma drug concentration–time curve with an initial distributive phase and a later terminal phase.
- One or more tissue compartments may be present in the model depending on the shape of the polyexponential curve representing log plasma drug concentration versus time.
- The central compartment refers to the volume of the plasma and body regions that are in rapid equilibrium with the plasma.
- The amount of drug within each compartment after a given dose at a given time can be calculated once the model is developed and model parameters are obtained by data fitting.

A pharmacokinetic model is a quantitative description of how drug concentrations change over time. Pharmacokinetic parameters are numerical values of model descriptors derived from data that are fitted to a model. These parameters are initially estimated and later refined using computing curve-fitting techniques such as least squares.

- Mamillary models are pharmacokinetic models that are well connected or dynamically exchange drug concentration between compartments. The two- and three-compartment models are examples.
- Compartment models are useful for estimating the mass balance of the drug in the body. As more physiological and genetic information is known, the model may be refined. Efflux and special transporters are now known to influence drug distribution and plasma profile. The well-known ABC transporters (eg, P-gp) are genetically expressed and vary among individuals. These drug transporters can be kinetically simulated using transfer constants in a compartment model designed to mimic drug efflux in and out of a cell or compartment model.

During curve fitting, simplifying the two-compartment model after an IV bolus dose and ignoring the presence of the distributive phase may cause serious errors unless the beta phase is very long relative to the distributive phase.

- An important consideration is whether the effective concentration lies near the distributive phase after the IV bolus dose is given.

LEARNING QUESTIONS

1. A drug was administered by rapid IV injection into a 70-kg adult male. Blood samples were withdrawn over a 7-hour period and assayed for intact drug. The results are tabulated below. Using the method of residuals, calculate the values for intercepts A and B and slopes α, β, k, k_{12}, and k_{21}.

Time (hours)	C_p (µg/mL)	Time (hours)	C_p (µg/mL)
0.00	70.0	2.5	14.3
0.25	53.8	3.0	12.6
0.50	43.3	4.0	10.5
0.75	35.0	5.0	9.0
1.00	29.1	6.0	8.0
1.50	21.2	7.0	7.0
2.00	17.0		

2. A 70-kg male subject was given 150 mg of a drug by IV injection. Blood samples were removed and assayed for intact drug. Calculate the slopes and intercepts of the three phases of the plasma level–time plot from the results tabulated below. Give the equation for the curve.

Time (hours)	C_p (µg/mL)	Time (hours)	C_p (µg/mL)
0.17	36.2	3.0	13.9
0.33	34.0	4.0	12.0
0.50	27.0	6.0	8.7
0.67	23.0	7.0	7.7
1.00	20.8	18.0	3.2
1.50	17.8	23.0	2.4
2.00	16.5		

3. Mitenko and Ogilvie (1973) demonstrated that theophylline followed a two-compartment pharmacokinetic model in human subjects. After administering a single intravenous dose (5.6 mg/kg) in nine normal volunteers, these investigators demonstrated that the equation best describing theophylline kinetics in humans was as follows:

$$C_p = 12e^{-.58t} + 18e^{-0.16t}$$

What is the plasma level of the drug 3 hours after the IV dose?

4. A drug has a distribution that can be described by a two-compartment open model. If the drug is given by IV bolus, what is the cause of the initial or rapid decline in blood levels (α phase)? What is the cause of the slower decline in blood levels (β phase)?

5. What does it mean when a drug demonstrates a plasma level–time curve that indicates a three-compartment open model? Can this curve be described by a two-compartment model?

6. A drug that follows a multicompartment pharmacokinetic model is given to a patient by rapid intravenous injection. Would the drug concentration in each tissue be the same after the drug equilibrates with the plasma and all the tissues in the body? Explain.

7. Park and associates (1983) studied the pharmacokinetics of amrinone after a single IV bolus injection (75 mg) in 14 healthy adult male volunteers. The pharmacokinetics of this drug followed a two-compartment open model and fit the following equation:

$$C_p = Ae^{-\alpha t} + Be^{-\beta t}$$

where
$A = 4.62 \pm 12.0 \ \mu g/mL$
$B = 0.64 \pm 0.17 \ \mu g/mL$

$\alpha = 8.94 \pm 13 \text{ h}^{-1}$

$\beta = 0.19 \pm 0.06 \text{ h}^{-1}$

From these data, calculate:

a. The volume of the central compartment
b. The volume of the tissue compartment
c. The transfer constants k_{12} and k_{21}
d. The elimination rate constant from the central compartment
e. The elimination half-life of amrinone after the drug has equilibrated with the tissue compartment

8. A drug may be described by a three-compartment model involving a central compartment and two peripheral tissue compartments. If you could sample the tissue compartments (organs), in which organs would you expect to find a drug level corresponding to the two theoretical peripheral tissue compartments?

9. A drug was administered to a patient at 20 mg by IV bolus dose and the time–plasma drug concentration is listed below. Use a suitable compartment model to describe the data and list the fitted equation and parameters. What are the statistical criteria used to describe your fit?

Hour	mg/L
0.20	3.42
0.40	2.25
0.60	1.92
0.80	1.80
1.00	1.73
2.00	1.48
3.00	1.28
4.00	1.10
6.00	0.81
8.00	0.60
10.00	0.45
12.00	0.33
14.00	0.24
18.00	0.13
20.00	0.10

10. The toxicokinetics of colchicine in seven cases of acute human poisoning was studied by Rochdi et al (1992). In three further cases, postmortem tissue concentrations of colchicine were measured. Colchicine follows the two-compartment model with wide distribution in various tissues. Depending on the time of patient admission, two disposition processes were observed. The first, in three patients, admitted early, showed a biexponential plasma colchicine decrease, with distribution half-lives of 30, 45, and 90 minutes. The second, in four patients, admitted late, showed a mono-exponential decrease. Plasma terminal half-lives ranged from 10.6 to 31.7 hours for both groups.

11. Postmortem tissue analysis of colchicine showed that colchicine accumulated at high concentrations in the bone marrow (more than 600 ng/g), testicle (400 ng/g), spleen (250 ng/g), kidney (200 ng/g), lung (200 ng/g), heart (95 ng/g), and brain (125 ng/g). The pharmacokinetic parameters of colchicine are:

> Fraction of unchanged colchicine in urine = 30%
> Renal clearance = 13 L/h
> Total body clearance = 39 L/h
> Apparent volume of distribution = 21 L/kg

a. Why is colchicine described by a mono-exponential profile in some subjects and a biexponential in others?
b. What is the range of distribution of half-life of colchicine in the subjects?
c. Which parameter is useful in estimating tissue drug level at any time?
d. Some clinical pharmacists assumed that, at steady state when equilibration is reached between the plasma and the tissue, the tissue drug concentration would be the same as the plasma. Do you agree?
e. Which tissues may be predicted by the tissue compartment?

ANSWERS

Frequently Asked Questions

Are "hypothetical" or "mathematical" compartment models useful in designing dosage regimens in the clinical setting? Does "hypothetical" mean "not real"?

- *Mathematical* and *hypothetical* are indeed vague and uninformative terms. Mathematical equations are developed to calculate how much drug is in the vascular fluid, as well as outside the vascular fluid (ie, extravascular or in the tissue pool). *Hypothetical* refers to an unproven model. The assumptions in the compartmental models simply imply that the model simulates the mass transfer of drug between the circulatory system and the tissue pool. The mass balance of drug moving out of the plasma fluid is described even though we know the tissue pool is not real (the tissue pool represents the virtual tissue mass that receives drug from the blood). While the model is a less-than-perfect representation, we can interpret it, knowing its limitations. All pharmacokinetic models need interpretation. We use a model when there are no simple ways to obtain needed information. As long as we know the model limitations (ie, that the tissue compartment is not the brain or the muscle!) and stay within the bounds of the model, we can extract useful information from it. For example, we may determine the amount of drug that is stored outside the plasma compartment at any desired time point. After an IV bolus drug injection, the drug distributes rapidly throughout the plasma fluid and more slowly into the fluid-filled tissue spaces. Drug distribution is initially rapid and confined to a fixed fluid volume known as the V_p or the initial volume. As drug distribution expands into other tissue regions, the volume of the penetrated spaces increases, until a critical point (steady state) is obtained when all penetrable tissue regions are equilibrated with the drug. Knowing that there is heterogenous drug distribution within and between tissues, the tissues are grouped into compartments to determine the amount of drugs in them. Mass balance, including drug inside and outside the vascular pool, accounts for all body drug storage ($D_B = D_t + D_p$). Assuming steady state, the tissue drug concentration is equal to the plasma drug concentration, $(C_p)_{ss}$, and one may determine size of the tissue volume using $D_t/(C_p)_{ss}$. This volume is really a "numerical factor" that is used to describe the relationship of the tissue storage drug relative to the drug in the blood pool. The sum of the two volumes is the steady-state volume of distribution. The product of the steady-state concentration, $(C_p)_{ss}$, and the $(V_D)_{ss}$ yields the amount of drug in the body at steady state. The amount of drug in the body at steady state is considered vital information in dosing drugs clinically. Students should realize that tissue drug concentrations are not predicted by the model. However, plasma drug concentration is fully predictable after any given dose once the parameters become known. Initial pharmacokinetic parameter estimation may be obtained from the literature using comparable age and weight for a specific individual.

If physiologic models are better than compartment models, why not just use physiologic models?

- A physiologic model is a detailed representation of drug disposition in the body. The model requires blood flow, extraction ratio, and specific tissue and organ size. This information is not often available for the individual. Thus, the less sophisticated compartment models are used more often.

Since clearance is the term most often used in clinical pharmacy, why is it necessary to know the other pharmacokinetic parameters?

- Clearance is used to calculate the steady-state drug concentration and to calculate the maintenance dose. However, clearance alone is not useful in determining the maximum and minimum drug concentrations in a multiple-dosing regimen.

What is the significance of the apparent volume of distribution?

- Apparent volumes of distribution are not real tissue volumes, but rather reflect the volume in which the drug is contained. For example,

V_p = initial or plasma volume

V_t = tissue volume

$(V_D)_{ss}$ = steady-state volume of distribution (most often listed in the literature).

The steady-state drug concentration multiplied by $(V_D)_{ss}$ yields the amount of drug in the body. $(V_D)_\beta$ is a volume usually determined from area under the curve (AUC), and differs from $(V_D)_{ss}$ somewhat in magnitude. $(V_D)_\beta$ multiplied by b gives clearance of the drug.

What is the error assumed in a one-compartment model compared to a two-compartment or multicompartment model?

- If the two-compartment model is ignored and the data are treated as a one-compartment model, the estimated values for the pharmacokinetic parameters are distorted. For example, during the distributive phase, the drug declines rapidly according to distribution α half-life, while in the elimination (terminal) part of the curve, the drug declines according to a β elimination half-life.

What kind of improvement in terms of patient care or drug therapy is made using the compartment model?

- Compartment models have been used to develop dosage regimens and pharmacodynamic models. Compartment models have improved the dosing of drugs such as digoxin, gentamicin, lidocaine, and many others. The principal use of compartment models in dosing is to simulate a plasma drug concentration profile based on pharmacokinetic (PK) parameters. This information allows comparison of PK parameters in patients with only two or three points to a patient with full profiles using generated PK parameters.

Learning Questions

1. Equation for the curve:

$$C_p = 52e^{-1.39t} + 18e^{-0.135t}$$

$$k = 0.41 \text{ h}^{-1} \quad k_{12} = 0.657 \text{ h}^{-1} \quad k_{21} = 0.458 \text{ h}^{-1}$$

2. Equation for the curve:

$$C_p = 28e^{-0.63t} + 10.5e^{-0.46t} + 14e^{-0.077t}$$

Note: When feathering curves by hand, a minimum of three points should be used to determine the line. Moreover, the rate constants and y intercepts may vary according to the individual's skill. Therefore, values for C_p should be checked by substitution of various times for t, using the derived equation. The theoretical curve should fit the observed data.

3. $C_p = 11.14 \ \mu g/mL$.

4. The initial decline in the plasma drug concentration is due mainly to uptake of drug into tissues. During the initial distribution of drug, some drug elimination also takes place. After the drug has equilibrated with the tissues, the drug declines at a slower rate because of drug elimination.

5. A third compartment may indicate that the drug has a slow elimination component. If the drug is eliminated by a very slow elimination component, then drug accumulation may occur with multiple drug doses or long IV drug infusions. Depending on the blood sampling, a third compartment may be missed. However, some data may fit both a two-compartment and a three-compartment model. In this case, if the fit for each compartment model is very close statistically, the simpler compartment model should be used.

6. Because of the heterogeneity of the tissues, drug equilibrates into the tissues at different rates and different drug concentrations are usually observed in the different tissues. The drug concentration in the "tissue" compartment represents an "average" drug concentration and does not represent the drug concentration in any specific tissue.

7. $C_p = Ae^{-\alpha t} + Be^{-\beta t}$

After substitution,

$$C_p = 4.62e^{-8.94t} + 0.64e^{-019t}$$

a. $V_p = \dfrac{D_0}{A + B} = \dfrac{75,000}{4.62 + 0.64} = 14,259 \text{ mL}$

b. $V_t = \dfrac{V_p k_{12}}{k_{21}} = \dfrac{(14,259)(6.52)}{(1.25)} = 74,375 \text{ mL}$

c. $k_{12} = \dfrac{AB(\beta - \alpha)^2}{(A+B)(A\beta + B\alpha)}$

$k_{12} = \dfrac{(4.62)(064)(0.19 - 8.94)^2}{(4.62 + 0.64)[(4.62)(0.19) + (0.64)(8.94)]}$

$k_{12} = 6.52 \text{ h}^{-1}$

$k_{21} = \dfrac{A\beta + B\alpha}{A+B} = \dfrac{(4.62)(0.19)(4.64)(8.94)}{4.62 + 0.64}$

$k_{21} = 1.25 \text{ h}^{-1}$

d. $k = \dfrac{\alpha\beta(A+B)}{A\beta + B\alpha}$

$= \dfrac{(8.94)(0.19)(4.62 + 0.64)}{(4.62)(0.19) + (0.64)(8.94)}$

$= 1.35 \text{ h}^{-1}$

8. The tissue compartments may not be sampled directly to obtain the drug concentration. Theoretical drug concentration, C_t, represents the average concentration in all the tissues outside the central compartment. The amount of drug in the tissue, D_t, represents the total amount of drug outside the central or plasma compartment. Occasionally C_t may be equal to a particular tissue drug concentration in an organ. However, this C_t may be equivalent by chance only.

9. The data were analyzed using computer software called RSTRIP, and found to fit a two-compartment model:

$A(1) = 2.0049 \quad A(2) = 6.0057$ (two preexponential values)

$k(1) = 0.15053 \quad k(2) = 7.0217$ (two exponential values)

The equation that describes the data is:

$C_p = 2.0049 e^{-0.15053t} + 6.0057 e^{-7.0217t}$

The coefficient of correlation = 0.999 (very good fit).
The model selection criterion = 11.27 (good model).
The sum of squared deviations = 9.3×10^{-5} (there is little deviation between the observed data and the theoretical value).

$\alpha = 7.0217 \text{ h}^{-1}, \beta = 0.15053 \text{ h}^{-1}$.

10. a. Late-time samples were taken in some patients, yielding data that resulted in a monoexponential elimination profile. It is also possible that a patient's illness contributes to impaired drug distribution.

b. The range of distribution half-lives is 30–45 minutes.

c. None. Tissue concentrations are not generally well predicted from the two-compartment model. Only the amount of drug in the tissue compartment may be predicted.

d. No. At steady state, the rate in and the rate out of the tissues are the same, but the drug concentrations are not necessarily the same. The plasma and each tissue may have different drug binding.

e. None. Only the pooled tissue is simulated by the tissue compartment.

REFERENCES

Avery JK: Routine procedure—bad outcome. *Tenn Med* **91**(7): 280–281, 1998.

Butler TC: The distribution of drugs. In LaDu BN, et al (eds). *Fundamentals of Drug Metabolism and Disposition*. Baltimore, Williams & Wilkins, 1972.

Eger E: In Papper EM and Kitz JR (eds). *Uptake and Distribution of Anesthetic Agents*. New York, McGraw-Hill, 1963, p. 76.

Eichler HG, Müller M: Drug distribution; the forgotten relative in clinical pharmacokinetics. *Clin Pharmacokinet* **34**(2): 95–99, 1998.

Greenspon AJ, Mohiuddin S, Saksena S, et al: Comparison of intravenous tocainide with intravenous lidocaine for treating ventricular arrhythmias. *Cardiovasc Rev Rep* **10**:55–59, 1989.

Harron DWG: Digoxin pharmacokinetic modelling—10 years later. *Int J Pharm* **53:**181–188, 1989.

Hill HF, Coda BA, Tanaka A, Schaffer R: Multiple-dose evaluation of intravenous hydromorphone pharmacokinetics in normal human subjects. *Anesth Analg* **72:**330–336, 1991.

Jambhekar SS, Breen JP: Two compartment model. *Basic Pharmacokinetics.* London, Chicago, Pharmaceutical Press, 2009, p. 269.

Mitenko PA, Ogilvie RI: Pharmacokinetics of intravenous theophylline. *Clin Pharmacol Ther* **14:**509, 1973.

Müller M: Monitoring tissue drug levels by clinical microdialysis. *Altern Lab Anim* **37**(suppl 1):57–59, 2009.

Pantuck AJ, Goldsmith JW, Kuriyan JB, Weiss RE: Seizures after ureteral stone manipulation with lidocaine. *J Urol* **157**(6):2248, 1997.

Parab PV, Ritschel WA, Coyle DE, Gree RV, Denson DD: Pharmacokinetics of hydromorphone after intravenous, peroral and rectal administration to human subjects. *Biopharm Drug Dispos* **9:**187–199, 1988.

Park GP, Kershner RP, Angellotti J, et al: Oral bioavailability and intravenous pharmacokinetics of amrinone in humans. *J Pharm Sci* **72:**817, 1983.

Rochdi M, Sabouraud A, Baud FJ, Bismuth C, Scherrmann JM: Toxicokinetics of colchicine in humans: Analysis of tissue, plasma and urine data in ten cases. *Hum Exp Toxicol* **11**(6):510–516, 1992.

Schentag JJ, Jusko WJ, Plaut ME, Cumbo TJ, Vance JW, Abutyn E: Tissue persistence of gentamicin in man. *JAMA* **238:**327–329, 1977.

Schumacher GE: *Therapeutic Drug Monitoring.* Norwalk, CT, Appleton & Lange, 1995.

Swanson DJ, Reitberg DP, Smith IL, Wels PB, Schentag JJ: Steady-state moxalactam pharmacokinetics in patients: Noncompartmental versus two-compartmental analysis. *J Pharmacokinet-Biopharm* **11**(4):337–353, 1983.

Vallner JJ, Stewart JT, Kotzan JA, Kirsten EB, Honiger IL: Pharmacokinetics and bioavailability of hydromorphone following intravenous and oral administration to human subjects. *J Clin Pharmacol* **21:**152–156, 1981.

Winters ME: *Basic Clinical Pharmacokinetics*, 3rd ed. Vancouver, WA, Applied Therapeutics, 1994, p. 23.

BIBLIOGRAPHY

Dvorchick BH, Vessell ES: Significance of error associated with use of the one-compartment formula to calculate clearance of 38 drugs. *Clin Pharmacol Ther* **23:**617–623, 1978.

Jusko WJ, Gibaldi M: Effects of change in elimination on various parameters of the two-compartment open model. *J Pharm Sci* **61:**1270–1273, 1972.

Loughman PM, Sitar DS, Oglivie RI, Neims AH: The two-compartment open-system kinetic model: A review of its clinical implications and applications. *J Pediatr* **88:**869–873, 1976.

Mayersohn M, Gibaldi M: Mathematical methods in pharmacokinetics, II: Solution of the two compartment open model. *Am J Pharm Ed* **35:**19–28, 1971.

Riegelman S, Loo JCK, Rowland M: Concept of a volume of distribution and possible errors in evaluation of this parameter. *J Pharm Sci* **57:**128–133, 1968.

Riegelman S, Loo JCK, Rowland M: Shortcomings in pharmacokinetics analysis by conceiving the body to exhibit properties of a single compartment. *J Pharm Sci* **57:**117–123, 1968.

6 Intravenous Infusion

HaiAn Zheng

Chapter Objectives

▶ Describe the concept of steady state and how it relates to continuous dosing.

▶ Determine optimum dosing for an infused drug by calculating pharmacokinetic parameters from clinical data.

▶ Calculate loading doses to be used with an intravenous infusion.

▶ Describe the purpose of a loading dose.

▶ Compare the pharmacokinetic outcomes and clinical implications after giving a loading dose for a drug that follows a one-compartment model to a drug that follows a two-compartment model.

Drugs may be administered to patients by oral, topical, parenteral, or other various routes of administration. Examples of parenteral routes of administration include intravenous, subcutaneous, and intramuscular. Intravenous (IV) drug solutions may be either injected as a bolus dose (all at once) or infused slowly through a vein into the plasma at a constant rate (zero order). The main advantage for giving a drug by IV infusion is that it allows precise control of plasma drug concentrations to fit the individual needs of the patient. For drugs with a narrow therapeutic window (eg, heparin), IV infusion maintains an effective constant plasma drug concentration by eliminating wide fluctuations between the peak (maximum) and trough (minimum) plasma drug concentration. Moreover, the IV infusion of drugs, such as antibiotics, may be given with IV fluids that include electrolytes and nutrients. Furthermore, the duration of drug therapy may be maintained or terminated as needed using IV infusion.

The plasma drug concentration–time curve of a drug given by constant IV infusion is shown in Fig. 6-1. Because no drug was present in the body at zero time, drug level rises from zero drug concentration and gradually becomes constant when a plateau or *steady-state* drug concentration is reached. At steady state, the rate of drug leaving the body is equal to the rate of drug (infusion rate) entering the body. Therefore, at steady state, the rate of change in the plasma drug concentration $dC_p/dt = 0$, and

$$\text{Rate of drug input} = \text{rate of drug output}$$
$$\text{(infusion rate)} \qquad \text{(elimination rate)}$$

Based on this simple mass balance relationship, a pharmacokinetic equation for infusion may be derived depending on whether the drug follows one- or two-compartment kinetics.

ONE-COMPARTMENT MODEL DRUGS

The pharmacokinetics of a drug given by constant IV infusion follows a zero-order input process in which the drug is directly infused into the systemic blood circulation. For most drugs, elimination of drug from the plasma is a first-order process. Therefore, in this one-compartment model, the infused drug follows zero-order input and first-order output. The change in the amount of drug in the body at any time (dD_B/dt) during the infusion is the rate of input minus the rate of output.

$$\frac{dD_B}{dt} = R - kD_B \qquad (6.1)$$

where D_B is the amount of drug in the body, R is the infusion rate (zero order), and k is the elimination rate constant (first order).

Integration of Equation 6.1 and substitution of $D_B = C_p V_D$ gives:

$$C_p = \frac{R}{V_D k}(1 - e^{-kt}) \qquad (6.2)$$

Equation 6.2 gives the plasma drug concentration at any time during the IV infusion, where t is the time for infusion. The graph for Equation 6.2 appears in Figs. 6-1 and 6-2. As the drug is infused, the value for certain time (t) increases in Equation 6.2. At infinite time $t = \infty$, e^{-kt} approaches zero, and Equation 6.2 reduces to Equation 6.4, as the steady-state drug concentration (C_{ss}).

$$C_p = \frac{R}{V_D k}(1 - e^{-\infty}) \qquad (6.3)$$

$$C_{ss} = \frac{R}{V_D k} \qquad (6.4)$$

The body clearance, Cl, is equal to $V_D k$, therefore:

$$C_{ss} = \frac{R}{V_D k} = \frac{R}{Cl} \qquad (6.5)$$

Steady-State Drug Concentration (C_{ss}) and Time Needed to Reach C_{ss}

Once the steady state is reached, the rate of drug leaving the body is equal to the rate of drug entering the body (infusion rate). In other words, there is no *net* change in the amount of drug in the body, D_B, as a function of time during steady state. Drug elimination occurs according to first-order elimination kinetics. Whenever the infusion stops, either before or after steady state is reached, the drug concentration always declines according to first-order kinetics. The slope of the elimination curve equals to $-k/2.3$ (Fig. 6-2). Even if the infusion is stopped before steady state is reached, the slope of the elimination curve remains the same (Fig. 6-2B).

Mathematically, the time to reach true steady-state drug concentrations, C_{ss}, would take an infinite time. The time required to reach the steady-state drug concentration in the plasma is dependent on the elimination rate constant of the drug for a constant volume of distribution, as shown in Equation 6.4. Because drug elimination is exponential (first order), the plasma drug concentration becomes asymptotic to the theoretical steady-state plasma drug concentration. For zero-order elimination processes, if rate of input is greater than rate of elimination, plasma drug concentrations will keep increasing and no steady state will be reached. This is a potentially dangerous situation that will occur when saturation of metabolic process occurs.

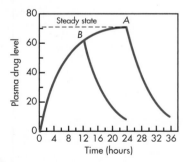

FIGURE 6-2   Plasma drug concentration–time profiles after IV infusion. IV infusion is stopped at steady state (*A*) or prior to steady state (*B*). In both cases, plasma drug concentrations decline exponentially (first order) according to a similar slope.

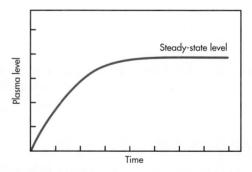

FIGURE 6-1   Plasma level–time curve for constant IV infusion.

In clinical practice, a plasma drug concentration prior to, but asymptotically approaching, the theoretical steady state is considered the steady-state plasma drug concentration (C_{ss}). In a constant IV infusion, drug solution is infused at a constant or zero-order rate, R. During the IV infusion, the plasma drug concentration increases and the rate of drug elimination increases because rate of elimination is concentration dependent (ie, rate of drug elimination $= kC_p$). C_p keeps increasing until steady state is reached at which time the rate of drug input (IV infusion rate) equals rate of drug output (elimination rate). The resulting plasma drug concentration at steady state (C_{ss}) is related to the rate of infusion and inversely related to the body clearance of the drug as shown in Equation 6.5.

In clinical practice, the drug activity will be observed when the drug concentration is close to the desired plasma drug concentration, which is usually the *target* or *desired* steady-state drug concentration. For therapeutic purposes, the time for the plasma drug concentration to reach more than 95% of the steady-state drug concentration in the plasma is often estimated. The time to reach 90%, 95%, and 99% of the steady-state drug concentration, C_{ss}, may be calculated. As detailed in Table 6-1, after IV infusion of the drug for 5 half-lives, the plasma drug concentration will be between 95% ($4.32\ t_{1/2}$) and 99% ($6.65\ t_{1/2}$) of the steady-state drug concentration. Thus, the time for a drug whose $t_{1/2}$ is 6 hours to reach 95% of the steady-state plasma drug concentration will be approximately $5\ t_{1/2}$, or 5×6 hours $= 30$ hours. The calculation of the values in Table 6-1 is given in the example that follows.

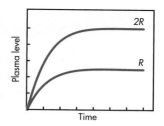

FIGURE 6-3 Plasma level–time curve for IV infusions given at rates of R and $2R$, respectively.

An increase in the infusion rate will not shorten the time to reach the steady-state drug concentration. If the drug is given at a more rapid infusion rate, a higher steady-state drug level will be obtained, but the time to reach steady state is the same (Fig. 6-3). This equation may also be obtained with the following approach. At steady state, the rate of infusion equals the rate of elimination. Therefore, the rate of change in the plasma drug concentration is equal to zero.

$$\frac{dC_p}{dt} = 0$$

$$\frac{dC_p}{dt} = \frac{R}{V_D} - kC_p = 0$$

$$(\text{Rate}_{in}) - (\text{Rate}_{out}) = 0$$

$$\frac{R}{V_D} = kC_p$$

$$C_{ss} = \frac{R}{V_D k} \qquad (6.6)$$

Equation 6.6 is the same as Equation 6.5 that shows that the steady-state concentration (C_{ss}) is dependent on the volume of distribution, the elimination rate constant, and the infusion rate. Altering any one of these factors can affect steady-state concentration.

TABLE 6-1 Number of $t_{1/2}$ to Reach a Fraction of C_{ss}

Percent of C_{ss} Reached[a]	Number of Half-Lives
90	3.32
95	4.32
99	6.65

[a]C_{ss} is the steady-state drug concentration in plasma.

EXAMPLES ▶ ▶ ▶

1. An antibiotic has a volume of distribution of 10 L and a k of 0.2 h^{-1}. A steady-state plasma concentration of 10 μg/mL is desired. The infusion rate needed to maintain this concentration can be determined as follows:

Equation 6.6 can be rewritten as

$$R = C_{ss}V_D k$$

$$= (10\ \mu g/mL)(10)(1000\ mL)(0.2\ h^{-1})$$

$$= 20\ mg/h$$

Assume the patient has a uremic condition and the elimination rate constant has decreased to 0.1 h^{-1}. To maintain the steady-state concentration of 10 μg/mL, we must determine a new rate of infusion as follows:

$$R = (10\ \mu g/mL)(10)(1000\ mL)(0.1\ h^{-1}) = 10\ mg/h$$

When the elimination rate constant decreases, then the infusion rate must decrease proportionately to maintain the same C_{ss}. However, because the elimination rate constant is smaller (ie, the elimination $t_{1/2}$ is longer), the time to reach C_{ss} will be longer.

2. An infinitely long period of time is needed to reach steady-state drug levels. However, in practice it is quite acceptable to reach 99% C_{ss} (ie, 99% steady-state level). Using Equation 6.6, we know that the steady-state level is

$$C_{ss} = \frac{R}{V_D k}$$

and 99% steady-state level would be equal to

$$99\% \frac{R}{V_D k}$$

Substituting into Equation 6.2 for C_p, we can find out the time needed to reach steady state by solving for t.

$$99\% \frac{R}{V_D k} = \frac{R}{V_D k}(1 - e^{-kt})$$

$$99\% = 1 - e^{-kt}$$

$$e^{-kt} = 1\%$$

Take the natural logarithm on both sides:

$$-kt = \ln 0.01$$

$$t_{99\%ss} = \frac{\ln 0.01}{-k} = \frac{-4.61}{-k} = \frac{4.61}{k}$$

Substituting $(0.693/t_{1/2})$ for k,

$$t_{99\%ss} = \frac{4.61}{(0.693/t_{1/2})} = \frac{4.61}{0.693}t_{1/2}$$

$$t_{99\%ss} = 6.65 t_{1/2}$$

Notice that in the equation directly above, the time needed to reach steady state is not dependent on the rate of infusion, but only on the elimination half-life. Using similar calculations, the time needed to reach any percentage of the steady-state drug concentration may be obtained (Table 6-1).

IV infusion may be used to determine total body clearance if the infusion rate and the steady-state level are known, as with Equation 6.6 repeated here:

$$C_{ss} = \frac{R}{V_D k} \tag{6.6}$$

$$V_D k = \frac{R}{C_{ss}}$$

Because total body clearance, Cl_T, is equal to $V_D k$,

$$Cl_T = \frac{R}{C_{ss}} \tag{6.7}$$

3. A patient was given an antibiotic ($t_{1/2} = 6$ hours) by constant IV infusion at a rate of 2 mg/h. At the end of 2 days, the serum drug concentration was 10 mg/L. Calculate the total body clearance Cl_T for this antibiotic.

Solution

The total body clearance may be estimated from Equation 6.7. The serum sample was taken after 2 days or 48 hours of infusion, which time represents $8 \times t_{1/2}$; therefore, this serum drug concentration approximates the C_{ss}.

$$Cl_T = \frac{R}{C_{ss}} = \frac{2\ mg/h}{10\ mg/L} = 200\ mL/h$$

INFUSION METHOD FOR CALCULATING PATIENT ELIMINATION HALF-LIFE

The C_p-versus-time relationship that occurs during an IV infusion (Equation 6.2) may be used to calculate k, or indirectly the elimination half-life of the drug in a patient. Some information about the elimination half-life of the drug in the population must be known, and one or two plasma samples must be taken at a known time after infusion. Knowing the half-life in the general population helps determine if the sample is taken at steady state in the patient. To simplify calculation, Equation 6.2 is arranged to solve for k:

$$C_p = \frac{R}{V_D k}(1 - e^{-kt}) \qquad (6.2)$$

Since

$$C_{ss} = \frac{R}{V_D k}$$

substituting into Equation 6.2:

$$C_p = C_{ss}(1 - e^{-kt})$$

Rearranging and taking the log on both sides:

$$\log\left(\frac{C_{ss} - C_p}{C_{ss}}\right) = -\frac{kt}{2.3} \quad \text{and}$$

$$k = \frac{-2.3}{t}\log\left(\frac{C_{ss} - C_p}{C_{ss}}\right) \qquad (6.8)$$

where C_p is the plasma drug concentration taken at time t, and C_{ss} is the approximate steady-state plasma drug concentration in the patient.

EXAMPLE ▶▶▶

1. An antibiotic has an elimination half-life of 3–6 hours in the general population. A patient was given an IV infusion of an antibiotic at an infusion rate of 15 mg/h. Blood samples were taken at 8 and 24 hours, and plasma drug concentrations were 5.5 and 6.5 mg/L, respectively. Estimate the elimination half-life of the drug in this patient.

Solution

Because the second plasma sample was taken at 24 hours, or 24/6 = 4 half-lives after infusion, the plasma drug concentration in this sample is approaching 95% of the true plasma steady-state drug concentration, assuming the extreme case of $t_{1/2} = 6$ hours.

By substitution into Equation 6.8:

$$\log\left(\frac{6.5 - 5.5}{6.5}\right) = -\frac{k(8)}{2.3}$$

$$k = 0.234 \text{ h}^{-1}$$

$$t_{1/2} = 0.693/0.234 = 2.96 \text{ hours}$$

The elimination half-life calculated in this manner is not as accurate as the calculation of $t_{1/2}$ using multiple plasma drug concentration time points after a single IV bolus dose or after stopping the IV infusion. However, this method may be sufficient in clinical practice. As the second blood sample is taken closer to the time for steady state, the accuracy of this method improves. At the 30th hour, for example, the plasma concentration would be 99% of the true steady-state value (corresponding to 30/6 or 5 elimination half-lives), and less error would result in applying Equation 6.8.

When Equation 6.8 was used in the example above to calculate the drug $t_{1/2}$ of the patient, the second plasma drug concentration was assumed to be the theoretical C_{ss}. As demonstrated below, when k and the corresponding values are substituted,

$$\log\left(\frac{C_{ss} - 5.5}{C_{ss}}\right) = -\frac{(0.234)(8)}{2.3}$$

$$\frac{C_{ss} - 5.5}{C_{ss}} = 0.157$$

$$C_{ss} = 6.5 \text{ mg/L}$$

(Note that C_{ss} is in fact the same as the concentration at 24 hours in the example above.)

In practice, before starting an IV infusion, an appropriate infusion rate (R) is generally calculated from Equation 6.8 using literature values for C_{ss}, k, and V_D or Cl_T. Two plasma samples are taken and the sampling times recorded. The second sample should be taken near the theoretical time for steady state. Equation 6.8 would then be used to calculate a k and then $t_{1/2}$. If the elimination half-life calculated confirms that the second sample was taken at steady state, the plasma concentration is simply assumed as the steady-state concentration and a new infusion rate may be calculated.

EXAMPLE ▶▶▶

1. If the desired therapeutic plasma concentration is 8 mg/L for the above patient (Example 1), what is the suitable infusion rate for the patient?

Solution

From Example 1, the trial infusion rate was 15 mg/h. Assuming the second blood sample is the steady-state level, 6.5 mg/mL, the clearance of the patient is

$$C_{ss} = R/Cl$$

$$Cl = R/C_{ss} = 15/6.5 = 2.31 \text{ L/h}$$

The new infusion rate should be

$$R = C_{ss} \times Cl = 8 \times 2.31 = 18.48 \text{ mg/h}$$

In this example, the $t_{1/2}$ of this patient is a little shorter, about 3 hours compared to 3–6 hours reported for the general population. Therefore, the infusion rate should be a little greater in order to maintain the desired steady-state level of 15 mg/L.

Equation 6.7 or the steady-state clearance method has been applied to the clinical infusion of drugs. The method was regarded as simple and accurate compared with other methods, including the two-point method (Hurley and McNeil, 1988).

LOADING DOSE PLUS IV INFUSION—ONE-COMPARTMENT MODEL

The loading dose D_L, or initial bolus dose of a drug, is used to obtain desired concentrations as rapidly as possible. The concentration of drug in the body for a one-compartment model after an IV bolus dose is described by

$$C_1 = C_0 e^{-kt} = \frac{D_L}{V_D} e^{-kt} \qquad (6.9)$$

and concentration by infusion at the rate R is

$$C_2 = \frac{R}{V_D k}(1 - e^{-kt}) \qquad (6.10)$$

Assume that an IV bolus dose D_L of the drug is given and that an IV infusion is started at the same time. The total concentration C_p at t hours after the start of infusion would be equal to $C_1 + C_2$ due to the sum contributions of bolus and infusion, or

$$C_p = C_1 + C_2$$

$$C_p = \frac{D_L}{V_D} e^{-kt} + \frac{R}{V_D k}(1 - e^{-kt})$$

$$= \frac{D_L}{V_D} e^{-kt} + \frac{R}{V_D k} - \frac{R}{V_D k} e^{-kt}$$

$$= \frac{R}{V_D k} + \left(\frac{D_L}{V_D} e^{-kt} - \frac{R}{V_D k} e^{-kt} \right) \qquad (6.11)$$

Let the loading dose (D_L) equal the amount of drug in the body at steady state

$$D_L = C_{ss} V_D$$

From Equation 6.4, $C_{ss} V_D = R/k$. Therefore,

$$D_L = R/k \qquad (6.12)$$

Substituting $D_L = R/k$ in Equation 6.11 makes the expression in parentheses cancel out. Equation 6.11 reduces to Equation 6.13, which is the same expression for C_{ss} or steady-state plasma concentrations (Equation 6.14 is identical to Equation 6.6):

$$C_p = \frac{R}{V_D k} \qquad (6.13)$$

$$C_{ss} = \frac{R}{V_D k} \qquad (6.14)$$

Therefore, if an IV loading dose of R/k is given, followed by an IV infusion, steady-state plasma drug concentrations are obtained immediately and maintained (Fig. 6-4). In this situation, steady state is also achieved in a one-compartment model, since the rate in = rate out ($R = dD_B/dt$).

The loading dose needed to get immediate steady-state drug levels can also be found by the following approach.

Loading dose equation:

$$C_1 = \frac{D_L}{V_D} e^{-kt}$$

Infusion equation:

$$C_2 = \frac{R}{V_D k}(1 - e^{-kt})$$

Adding up the two equations yields Equation 6.15, an equation describing simultaneous infusion after a loading dose.

$$C_p = \frac{D_L}{V_D} e^{-kt} + \frac{R}{V_D k}(1 - e^{-kt}) \qquad (6.15)$$

By differentiating this equation at steady state, we obtain:

$$\frac{dC_p}{dt} = 0 = \frac{-D_L k}{V_D} e^{-kt} + \frac{Rk}{V_D k} e^{-kt} \qquad (6.16)$$

$$0 = e^{-kt}\left(\frac{-D_L k}{V_D} + \frac{R}{V_D}\right)$$

$$\frac{D_L k}{V_D} = \frac{R}{V_D} \qquad (6.17)$$

$$D_L = \frac{R}{k} = \text{loading dose}$$

In order to maintain instant steady-state level ($[dC_p/dt] = 0$), the loading dose should be equal to R/k.

For a one-compartment drug, if the D_L and infusion rate are calculated such that C_0 and C_{ss} are the same and both D_L and infusion are started concurrently, then steady state and C_{ss} will be achieved immediately after the loading dose is administered (Fig. 6-4). Similarly, in Fig. 6-5, curve b shows the blood level after a single loading dose of R/k plus infusion from which the concentration desired at steady state is obtained. If the D_L is not equal to R/k, then steady state will not occur immediately. If the loading dose given is larger than R/k, the plasma drug concentration takes longer to decline to the concentration desired at steady state (curve a). If the loading dose is lower than R/k, the plasma drug concentrations will increase slowly to desired drug levels (curve c), but more quickly than without any loading dose.

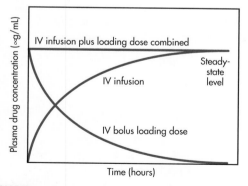

FIGURE 6-4   IV infusion with loading dose D_L. The loading dose is given by IV bolus injection at the start of the infusion. Plasma drug concentrations decline exponentially after D_L whereas they increase exponentially during the infusion. The resulting plasma drug concentration–time curve is a straight line due to the summation of the two curves.

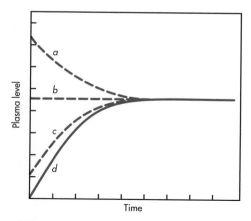

FIGURE 6-5   Intravenous infusion with loading doses a, b, and c. Curve d represents an IV infusion without a loading dose.

Another method for the calculation of loading dose D_L is based on knowledge of the desired steady-state drug concentration C_{ss} and the apparent volume of distribution V_D for the drug, as shown in Equation 6.18.

$$D_L = C_{ss}V_D \qquad (6.18)$$

For many drugs, the desired C_{ss} is reported in the literature as the effective therapeutic drug concentration. The V_D and the elimination half-life are also available for these drugs.

PRACTICE PROBLEMS

1. A physician wants to administer an anesthetic agent at a rate of 2 mg/h by IV infusion. The elimination rate constant is 0.1 h⁻¹ and the volume of distribution (one compartment) is 10 L. How much is the drug plasma concentration at the steady state? What loading dose should be recommended to reach steady state immediately?

Solution

$$C_{ss} = \frac{R}{V_D k} = \frac{2000}{(10 \times 10^3)(0.1)} = 2 \ \mu g/mL$$

To reach C_{ss} instantly,

$$D_L = \frac{R}{k} = \frac{2 \ mg/h}{0.1/h} \quad D_L = 20 \ mg$$

2. What is the concentration of a drug at 6 hours after infusion administration at 2 mg/h, with an initial loading dose of 10 mg (the drug has a $t_{1/2}$ of 3 hours and a volume of distribution of 10 L)?

Solution

$$k = \frac{0.693}{3 \ h}$$

$$C_p = \frac{D_L}{V_D}e^{-kt} + \frac{R}{V_D k}(1 - e^{-kt})$$

$$C_p = \frac{10,000}{10,000}(e^{-(0.693/3)(6)})$$

$$+ \frac{2000}{(10,000)(0.693/3)}(1 - e^{-(0.693/3)(6)})$$

$$C_p = 0.90 \ \mu g/mL$$

3. Calculate the drug concentration in the blood after infusion has been stopped.

Solution

This concentration can be calculated in two parts (see Fig. 6-2A). First, calculate the concentration of drug during infusion, and second, calculate the concentration after the stop of the infusion, C. Then use the IV bolus dose equation ($C = C_0 e^{-kt}$) for calculations for any further point in time. For convenience, the two equations can be combined as follows:

$$C_p = \frac{R}{V_D k}(1 - e^{-kb})e^{-k(t-b)} \qquad (6.19)$$

where b = length of time of infusion period, t = total time (infusion and postinfusion), and $t - b$ = length of time after infusion has stopped. Here, we assume no bolus loading dose was given.

4. A patient was infused for 6 hours with a drug ($k = 0.01$ h⁻¹; $V_D = 10$ L) at a rate of 2 mg/h. What is the concentration of the drug in the body 2 hours after cessation of the infusion?

Solution

Using Equation 6.19,

$$C_p = \frac{2000}{(0.01)(10,000)}(1 - e^{-0.01(6)})e^{-0.01(8-6)}$$

$$C_p = 1.14 \ \mu g/mL$$

Alternatively, when infusion stops, C_p' is calculated:

$$C_p' = \frac{R}{V_D k}(1 - e^{-kt})$$

$$C_p' = \frac{2000}{0.01 \times 10,000}(1 - e^{-0.01(6)})$$

$$C = C_p' e^{-0.01(2)}$$

$$C = 1.14 \ \mu g/mL$$

The two approaches should give the same answer.

5. An adult male asthmatic patient (78 kg, 48 years old) with a history of heavy smoking was given an IV infusion of aminophylline at a rate of

0.75 mg/kg/h. A loading dose of 6 mg/kg was given by IV bolus injection just prior to the start of the infusion. Two hours after the start of the IV infusion, the plasma theophylline concentration was measured and found to contain 5.8 μg/mL of theophylline. The apparent V_D for theophylline is 0.45 L/kg. (Aminophylline is the ethylenediamine salt of theophylline and contains 80% of theophylline base.)

Because the patient was responding poorly to the aminophylline therapy, the physician wanted to increase the plasma theophylline concentration in the patient to 10 μg/mL. What dosage recommendation would you give the physician? Would you recommend another loading dose?

Solution

If no loading dose is given and the IV infusion rate is increased, the time to reach steady-state plasma drug concentrations will be about 4 to 5 $t_{1/2}$ to reach 95% of C_{ss}. Therefore, a second loading dose should be recommended to rapidly increase the plasma theophylline concentration to 10 μg/mL. The infusion rate must also be increased to maintain this desired C_{ss}.

The calculation of loading dose D_L must consider the present plasma theophylline concentration.

$$D_L = \frac{V_D(C_{p,desired} - C_{p,present})}{(S)(F)} \qquad (6.20)$$

where S is the salt form of the drug and F is the fraction of drug bioavailable. For aminophylline S is equal to 0.80 and for an IV bolus injection F is equal to 1.

$$D_L = \frac{(0.45 \text{ L/kg})(78 \text{ kg})(10-5.8 \text{ mg/L})}{(0.8)(1)}$$

$$D_L = 184 \text{ mg aminophylline}$$

The maintenance IV infusion rate may be calculated after estimation of the patient's clearance, Cl_T. Because a loading dose and an IV infusion of 0.75 mg/h aminophylline

(equivalent to $0.75 \times 0.8 = 0.6$ mg theophylline) per kg was given to the patient, the plasma theophylline concentration of 5.8 mg/L is the steady-state C_{ss}. Total clearance may be estimated by

$$Cl_T = \frac{R}{C_{ss,present}} = \frac{(0.6 \text{ mg/h/kg})(78 \text{ kg})}{5.8 \text{ mg/L}}$$

$$Cl_T = 8.07 \text{ L/h or } 1.72 \text{ mL/min/kg}$$

The usual Cl_T for adult, nonsmoking patients with uncomplicated asthma is approximately 0.65 mL/min/kg. Heavy smoking is known to increase Cl_T for theophylline.

The new IV infusion rate, R' in terms of theophylline, is calculated by

$R' = C_{ss,desired} \, Cl_T$
$R' = 10 \text{ mg/L} \times 8.07 \text{ L/h} = 80.7 \text{ mg/h or}$
1.03 mg/h/kg of theophylline, which is equivalent to 1.29 mg/h/kg of aminophylline.

6. An adult male patient (43 years, 80 kg) is to be given an antibiotic by IV infusion. According to the literature, the antibiotic has an elimination $t_{1/2}$ of 2 hours and V_D of 1.25 L/kg, and is effective at a plasma drug concentration of 14 mg/L. The drug is supplied in 5-mL ampuls containing 150 mg/mL.

a. Recommend a starting infusion rate in milligrams per hour and liters per hour.

Solution

Assume the effective plasma drug concentration is the target drug concentration or C_{ss}.

$$R = C_{ss}kV_D$$

$$= (14 \text{ mg/L})(0.693/2 \text{ h})(1.5 \text{ L/kg})(80 \text{ kg})$$

$$= 485.1 \text{ mg/h}$$

Because the drug is supplied at a concentration of 150 mg/mL,

$$(485.1 \text{ mg})(\text{mL/150 mg}) = 3.23 \text{ mL}$$

Thus, $R = 3.23$ mL/h.

b. Blood samples were taken from the patient at 12, 16, and 24 hours after the start of the infusion. Plasma drug concentrations were as shown below:

t (hours)	C_p (mg/L)
12	16.1
16	16.3
24	16.5

From these additional data, calculate the total body clearance Cl_T for the drug in this patient.

Solution

Because the plasma drug concentrations at 12, 16, and 24 hours were similar, steady state has essentially been reached. (Note: The continuous increase in plasma drug concentrations could be caused by drug accumulation due to a second tissue compartment, or could be due to variation in the drug assay.) Assuming a C_{ss} of 16.3 mg/mL, Cl_T is calculated.

$$Cl_T = \frac{R}{C_{ss}} = \frac{485.1 \text{ mg/h}}{16.3 \text{ mg/L}} = 29.8 \text{ L/h}$$

c. From the above data, estimate the elimination half-life for the antibiotics in this patient.

Solution

Generally, the apparent volume of distribution (V_D) is less variable than $t_{1/2}$. Assuming that the literature value for V_D is 1.25 L/kg, then $t_{1/2}$ may be estimated from the Cl_T.

$$k = \frac{Cl_T}{V_D} = \frac{29.9 \text{ L/h}}{(1.25 \text{ L/kg})(80 \text{ kg})} = 0.299 \text{ h}^{-1}$$

$$t_{1/2} = \frac{0.693}{0.299 \text{ h}^{-1}} = 2.32 \text{ h}$$

Thus the $t_{1/2}$ for the antibiotic in this patient is 2.32 hours, which is in good agreement with the literature value of 2 hours.

d. After reviewing the pharmacokinetics of the antibiotic in this patient, should the infusion rate for the antibiotic be changed?

Solution

To properly decide whether the infusion rate should be changed, the clinical pharmacist must consider the pharmacodynamics and toxicity of the drug. Assuming the drug has a wide therapeutic window and shows no sign of adverse drug toxicity, the infusion rate of 485.1 mg/h, calculated according to pharmacokinetic literature values for the drug, appears to be correct.

$$C_p = \frac{R}{Cl}(1 - e^{-(Cl/V_D)t})$$

ESTIMATION OF DRUG CLEARANCE AND V_D FROM INFUSION DATA

The plasma concentration of a drug during constant infusion was described in terms of volume of distribution V_D and elimination constant k in Equation 6.2. Alternatively, the equation may be described in terms of clearance by substituting for k into Equation 6.2 with $k = Cl/V_D$:

$$C_p = \frac{R}{Cl}(1 - e^{-(Cl/V_D)t}) \tag{6.21}$$

The drug concentration in this physiologic model is described in terms of volume of distribution V_D and total body clearance Cl. The independent parameters are clearance and volume of distribution; k is viewed as a dependent variable that depends on Cl and V_D. In this model, the time for steady state and the resulting steady-state concentration will be dependent on both clearance and volume of distribution. When a constant volume of distribution is evident, the time for steady state is then inversely related to clearance. Thus, drugs with small clearance will take a long time to reach steady state. Although this newer approach is preferred by some clinical pharmacists, the alternative approach to parameter estimation was known for some time in classical pharmacokinetics. Equation 6.21 has been applied in population pharmacokinetics to estimate both Cl and V_D in individual patients with one or more data points. However, clearance in patients may differ greatly from subjects in the population, especially subjects with different renal functions. Unfortunately, the plasma samples taken at time equivalent to less than 1 half-life after infusion was started may not be very discriminating due to the small change in the drug concentration. Blood samples taken at 3–4 half-lives later are much more reflective of their difference in clearance.

INTRAVENOUS INFUSION OF TWO-COMPARTMENT MODEL DRUGS

Many drugs given by IV infusion follow two-compartment kinetics. For example, the respective distributions of theophylline and lidocaine in humans are described by the two-compartment open model. With two-compartment-model drugs, IV infusion requires a distribution and equilibration of the drug before a stable blood level is reached. During a constant IV infusion, drug in the tissue compartment is in distribution equilibrium with the plasma; thus, constant C_{ss} levels also result in constant drug concentrations in the tissue, that is, no *net* change in the amount of drug in the tissue occurs during steady state. Although some clinicians assume that tissue and plasma concentrations are equal when fully equilibrated, kinetic models only predict that the rates of drug transfer into and out of the compartments are equal at steady state. In other words, drug concentrations in the tissue are also constant, but may differ from plasma concentrations.

The time needed to reach a steady-state blood level depends entirely on the distribution half-life of the drug. The equation describing plasma drug concentration as a function of time is as follows:

$$C_p = \frac{R}{V_p k}\left[1 - \left(\frac{k-b}{a-b}\right)e^{-at} - \left(\frac{a-k}{a-b}\right)e^{-bt}\right] \quad (6.22)$$

where a and b are hybrid rate constants and R is the rate of infusion. At steady state (ie, $t = \infty$), Equation 6.22 reduces to

$$C_{ss} = \frac{R}{V_p k} \quad (6.23)$$

By rearranging this equation, the infusion rate for a desired steady-state plasma drug concentration may be calculated.

$$R = C_{ss} V_p k \quad (6.24)$$

Loading Dose for Two-Compartment Model Drugs

Drugs with long half-lives require a loading dose to more rapidly attain steady-state plasma drug levels. It is clinically desirable to achieve rapid therapeutic drug levels by using a loading dose. However, for a drug that follows the two-compartment pharmacokinetic model, the drug distributes slowly into extravascular tissues (compartment 2). Thus, drug equilibrium is not immediate. The plasma drug concentration of a drug that follows a two-compartment model after various loading doses is shown in Fig. 6-6. If a loading dose is given too rapidly, the drug may initially give excessively high concentrations in the plasma (central compartment), which then decreases as drug equilibrium is reached (Fig. 6-6). It is not possible to maintain an instantaneous, stable steady-state blood level for a two-compartment model drug with a zero-order rate of infusion. Therefore, a loading dose produces an initial blood level either slightly higher or lower than the steady-state blood level. To overcome this problem, several IV bolus injections given as short intermittent IV infusions may be used as a

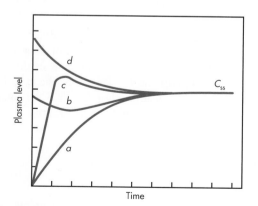

FIGURE 6-6   Plasma drug level after various loading doses and rates of infusion for a drug that follows a two-compartment model: *a*, no loading dose; *b*, loading dose = R/k (rapid infusion); *c*, loading dose = R/b (slow infusion); and *d*, loading dose = R/b (rapid infusion).

method for administering a loading dose to the patient (see Chapter 9).

Apparent Volume of Distribution at Steady State, Two-Compartment Model

After administration of any drug that follows two-compartment kinetics, plasma drug levels will decline due to elimination, and some redistribution will occur as drug in tissue diffuses back into the plasma fluid. The volume of distribution at steady state, $(V_D)_{ss}$, is the "hypothetical space" in which the drug is assumed to be distributed. The product of the plasma drug concentration with $(V_D)_{ss}$ will give the total amount of drug in the body at that time period, such that $(C_p)_{ss} \times (V_D)_{ss} =$ amount of drug in the body at steady state. At steady-state conditions, the rate of drug entry into the tissue compartment from the central compartment is equal to the rate of drug exit from the tissue compartment into the central compartment. These rates of drug transfer are described by the following expressions:

$$D_t k_{21} = D_p k_{12} \qquad (6.25)$$

$$D_t = \frac{k_{12} D_p}{k_{21}} \qquad (6.26)$$

Because the amount of drug in the central compartment D_p is equal to $V_p C_p$, by substitution in the above equation,

$$D_t = \frac{k_{12} C_p V_p}{k_{21}} \qquad (6.27)$$

The total amount of drug in the body at steady state is equal to the sum of the amount of drug in the tissue compartment, D_t, and the amount of drug in the central compartment, D_p. Therefore, the apparent volume of drug at steady state $(V_D)_{ss}$ may be calculated by dividing the total amount of drug in the body by the concentration of drug in the central compartment at steady state:

$$(V_D)_{ss} = \frac{D_p + D_t}{C_p} \qquad (6.28)$$

Substituting Equation 6.27 into Equation 6.28, and expressing D_p as $V_p C_p$, a more useful equation for the calculation of $(V_D)_{ss}$ is obtained:

$$(V_D)_{ss} = \frac{C_p V_p + k_{12} V_p C_p / k_{21}}{C_p} \qquad (6.29)$$

which reduces to

$$(V_D)_{ss} = V_p + \frac{k_{12}}{k_{21}} V_p \qquad (6.30)$$

In practice, Equation 6.30 is used to calculate $(V_D)_{ss}$. The $(V_D)_{ss}$ is a function of the transfer constants, k_{12} and k_{21}, which represent the rate constants of drug going into and out of the tissue compartment, respectively. The magnitude of $(V_D)_{ss}$ is dependent on the hemodynamic factors responsible for drug distribution and on the physical properties of the drug, properties which, in turn, determine the relative amount of intra- and extravascular drug.

Another volume term used in two-compartment modeling is $(V_D)_\beta$ (see Chapter 5). $(V_D)_\beta$ is often calculated from total body clearance divided by b, unlike the steady-state volume of distribution, $(V_D)_{ss}$, $(V_D)_\beta$ is influenced by drug elimination in the beta "β" phase. Reduced drug clearance from the body may increase AUC, such that $(V_D)_\beta$ is either reduced or unchanged depending on the value of b as shown in Equation 5.37 (see Chapter 5):

$$(V_D)_\beta = (V_D)_{area} = \frac{D_0}{b[AUC]_0^\infty} \qquad (5.37)$$

Unlike $(V_D)_\beta$, $(V_D)_{ss}$ is not affected by changes in drug elimination. $(V_D)_{ss}$ reflects the true distributional volume occupied by the plasma and the tissue pool when steady state is reached. Although this volume is not useful in calculating the amount of drug in the body during pre-steady state, $(V_D)_{ss}$ multiplied by the steady-state plasma drug concentration, C_{ss}, yields the amount of drug in the body. This volume is often used to determine the loading dose necessary to upload the body to a desired plasma drug concentration. As shown by Equation 6.30, $(V_D)_{ss}$ is several times greater than V_p, which represents the volume of the plasma compartment, but differs somewhat in value depending on the transfer constants.

PRACTICAL FOCUS

Questions

1. Do you agree with the following statements for a drug that is described by a two-compartment pharmacokinetic model? At steady state, the drug is well equilibrated between the plasma and the tissue compartment, $C_p = C_t$, and the rates of drug

diffusion into and from the plasma compartment are equal.

2. Azithromycin may be described by a plasma and a tissue compartment model (refer to Chapter 5). The steady-state volume of distribution is much larger than the initial volume, V_i, or the original plasma volume, V_p, of the central compartment. Why?

3. "Rapid distribution of azithromycin into cells causes higher concentration in the tissues than in the plasma. ..." Does this statement conflict with the steady-state concept? Why is the loading dose often calculated using the $(V_D)_{ss}$ instead of V_p.

4. Why is a loading dose used?

Solutions

1. For a drug that follows a multiple-compartment model, the rates of drug diffusion into the tissues from the plasma and from the tissues into the plasma are equal at steady state. However, the tissue drug concentration is generally not equal to the plasma drug concentration.

2. When plasma drug concentration data are used alone to describe the disposition of the drug, no information on tissue drug concentration is known, and no model will predict actual tissue drug concentrations. To account for the mass balance (drug mass/volume = body drug concentration) of drug present in the body (tissue and plasma pool) at any time after dosing, the body drug concentration is assumed to be the plasma drug concentration. In reality, azithromycin tissue concentration is much higher. Therefore, the calculated volume of the tissue compartment is much bigger (31.1 L/kg) than its actual volume.

3. The product of the steady-state apparent $(V_D)_{ss}$ and the steady-state plasma drug concentration C_{ss} estimates the amount of drug present in the body. The amount of drug present in the body may be important information for toxicity considerations, and may also be used as a therapeutic end point. In most cases, the therapeutic drug at the site of action accounts for only a small fraction of total drug in the tissue compartment. The pharmacodynamic profile may be described as a separate compartment (see effect compartment in Chapter 21). Based on pharmacokinetic and

biopharmaceutic studies, the factors that account for high tissue concentrations include diffusion constant, lipid solubility, and tissue binding to cell components. A ratio measuring the relative drug concentration in tissue and plasma is the partition coefficient, which is helpful in predicting the distribution of a drug into tissues. Ultimately, studies of tissue drug distribution using radiolabeled drug are much more useful.

The real tissue drug level will differ from the plasma drug concentration depending on the partitioning of drug in tissues and plasma. $(V_D)_\beta$ is a volume of distribution often calculated because it is easier to calculate than $(V_D)_{ss}$. This volume of distribution, $(V_D)_\beta$, allows the area under the curve to be calculated, an area which has been related to toxicities associated with many cancer chemotherapy agents. Many values for apparent volumes of distribution reported in the clinical literature are obtained using the area equation. Some early pharmacokinetic literature only includes the steady-state volume of distribution, which approximates the $(V_D)_\beta$ but is substantially smaller in many cases. In general, both volume terms reflect extravascular drug distribution. $(V_D)_\beta$ appears to be much more affected by the dynamics of drug disposition in the beta phase, whereas $(V_D)_{ss}$ reflects more accurately the inherent distribution of the drug.

4. When drugs are given in a multiple-dose regimen, a loading dose may be given to achieve steady-state drug concentrations more rapidly.

Frequently Asked Questions

▶ *What is the main reason for giving a drug by slow IV infusion?*

▶ *Why do we use a loading dose to rapidly achieve therapeutic concentration for a drug with a long elimination half-life instead of increasing the rate of drug infusion or increasing the size of the infusion dose?*

▶ *Explain why the application of a loading dose as a single IV bolus injection may cause an adverse event or drug toxicity in the patient if the drug follows a two-compartment model with a slow elimination phase.*

▶ *What are some of the complications involved with IV infusion?*

CHAPTER SUMMARY

An IV bolus injection puts the drug into the systemic circulation almost instantaneously. For some drugs, IV bolus injections can result in immediate high plasma drug concentrations and drug toxicity. An IV drug infusion slowly inputs the drug into the circulation and can provide stable drug concentrations in the plasma for extended time periods. Constant IV drug infusions are considered to have zero-order drug absorption because of direct input. Once the drug is infused, the drug is eliminated by first-order elimination. Steady state is achieved when the rate of drug infusion (ie, rate of drug absorption) equals the rate of drug elimination. Four to five elimination half-lives are needed to achieve 95% of steady state.

A loading dose given as an IV bolus injection may be used at the start of an infusion to quickly achieve the desired steady-state plasma drug concentration. For drugs that follow a two-compartment model, multiple small loading doses or intermittent IV infusions may be needed to prevent plasma drug concentrations from becoming too high. Pharmacokinetic parameters may be calculated from samples taken during the IV infusion and after the infusion is stopped, regardless of whether steady state has been achieved. These calculated pharmacokinetic parameters are then used to optimize dosing for that patient when population estimates do not provide outcomes suitable for the patient.

LEARNING QUESTIONS

1. A female patient (35 years old, 65 kg) with normal renal function is to be given a drug by IV infusion. According to the literature, the elimination half-life of this drug is 7 hours and the apparent V_D is 23.1% of body weight. The pharmacokinetics of this drug assumes a first-order process. The desired steady-state plasma level for this antibiotic is 10 $\mu g/mL$.

   a. Assuming no loading dose, how long after the start of the IV infusion would it take to reach 95% of the C_{ss}?

   b. What is the proper loading dose for this antibiotic?

   c. What is the proper infusion rate for this drug?

   d. What is the total body clearance?

   e. If the patient suddenly develops partial renal failure, how long would it take for a new steady-state plasma level to be established (assume that 95% of the C_{ss} is a reasonable approximation)?

   f. If the total body clearance declined 50% due to partial renal failure, what new infusion rate would you recommend to maintain the desired steady-state plasma level of 10 $\mu g/mL$.

2. An anticonvulsant drug was given as (a) a single IV dose and then (b) a constant IV infusion.

The serum drug concentrations are as presented in Table 6-2.

   a. What is the steady-state plasma drug level?

   b. What is the time for 95% steady-state plasma drug level?

   c. What is the drug clearance?

   d. What is the plasma concentration of the drug 4 hours after stopping infusion (infusion was stopped after 24 hours)?

TABLE 6-2   Serum Drug Concentrations for a Hypothetical Anticonvulsant Drug

TIME (hour)	Single IV dose (1 mg/kg)	Constant IV Infusion (0.2 mg/kg per hour)
0	10.0	0
2	6.7	3.3
4	4.5	5.5
6	3.0	7.0
8	2.0	8.0
10	1.35	8.6
12		9.1
18		9.7
24		9.9

e. What is the infusion rate for a patient weighing 75 kg to maintain a steady-state drug level of 10 $\mu g/mL$?

f. What is the plasma drug concentration 4 hours after an IV dose of 1 mg/kg followed by a constant infusion of 0.2 mg/kg/h?

3. An antibiotic is to be given by IV infusion. How many milliliters per hour should a sterile 25 mg/mL drug solution be given to a 75-kg adult male patient to achieve an infusion rate of 1 mg/kg/h?

4. An antibiotic drug is to be given to an adult male patient (75 kg, 58 years old) by IV infusion. The drug is supplied in sterile vials containing 30 mL of the antibiotic solution at a concentration of 125 mg/mL. What rate in milliliters per hour would you infuse this patient to obtain a steady-state concentration of 20 $\mu g/mL$? What loading dose would you suggest? Assume the drug follows the pharmacokinetics of a one-compartment open model. The apparent volume of distribution of this drug is 0.5 L/kg and the elimination half-life is 3 hours.

5. According to the manufacturer, a steady-state serum concentration of 17 mg/mL was measured when the antibiotic, cephradine (Velosef®) was given by IV infusion to 9 adult male volunteers (average weight, 71.7 kg) at a rate of 5.3 mg/kg/h for 4 hours.

a. Calculate the total body clearance for this drug.

b. When the IV infusion was discontinued, the cephradine serum concentration decreased exponentially, declining to 1.5 mg/mL at 6.5 hours after the start of the infusion. Calculate the elimination half-life.

c. From the information above, calculate the apparent volume of distribution.

d. Cephradine is completely excreted unchanged in the urine, and studies have shown that probenecid given concurrently causes elevation of the serum cephradine concentration. What is the probable mechanism for this interaction of probenecid with cephradine?

6. Calculate the excretion rate at steady state for a drug given by IV infusion at a rate of 30 mg/h. The C_{ss} is 20 $\mu g/mL$. If the rate of infusion were increased to 40 mg/h, what would be the new steady-state drug concentration, C_{ss}? Would the excretion rate for the drug at the new steady state be the same? Assume first-order elimination kinetics and a one-compartment model.

7. An antibiotic is to be given to an adult male patient (58 years, 75 kg) by IV infusion. The elimination half-life is 8 hours and the apparent volume of distribution is 1.5 L/kg. The drug is supplied in 60-mL ampules at a drug concentration of 15 mg/mL. The desired steady-state drug concentration is 20 $\mu g/mL$.

a. What infusion rate in mg/h would you recommend for this patient?

b. What loading dose would you recommend for this patient? By what route of administration would you give the loading dose? When?

c. Why should a loading dose be recommended?

d. According to the manufacturer, the recommended starting infusion rate is 15 mL/h. Do you agree with this recommended infusion rate for your patient? Give a reason for your answer.

e. If you were to monitor the patient's serum drug concentration, when would you request a blood sample? Give a reason for your answer.

f. The observed serum drug concentration is higher than anticipated. Give two possible reasons based on sound pharmacokinetic principles that would account for this observation.

8. Which of the following statements **(a–e)** is/are true regarding the time to reach steady-state for the three drugs below?

	Drug A	Drug B	Drug C
Rate of infusion (mg/h)	10	20	15
k (h^{-1})	0.5	0.1	0.05
Cl (L/h)	5	20	5

a. Drug A takes the longest time to reach steady state.

b. Drug B takes the longest time to reach steady state.

c. Drug C takes the longest time to reach steady state.

d. Drug A takes 6.9 hours to reach steady state.

e. None of the above is true.

9. If the steady-state drug concentration of a cephalosporin after constant infusion of 250 mg/h is 45 μg/mL, what is the drug clearance of this cephalosporin?

10. Some clinical pharmacists assumed that, at steady state when equilibration is reached between the plasma and the tissue, the tissue drug concentration would be the same as the plasma. Do you agree?

ANSWERS

Frequently Asked Questions

What is the main reason for giving a drug by slow IV infusion?

- Slow IV infusion may be used to avoid side effects due to rapid drug administration. For example, intravenous immune globulin (human) may cause a rapid fall in blood pressure and possible anaphylactic shock in some patients when infused rapidly. Some antisense drugs also cause a rapid fall in blood pressure when injected via rapid IV into the body. The rate of infusion is particularly important in administering antiarrhythmic agents in patients. The rapid IV bolus injection of many drugs (eg, lidocaine) that follow the pharmacokinetics of multiple-compartment models may cause an adverse response due to the initial high drug concentration in the central (plasma) compartment before slow equilibration with the tissues.

Why do we use a loading dose to rapidly achieve therapeutic concentration for a drug with a long elimination half-life instead of increasing the rate of drug infusion or increasing the size of the infusion dose?

- The loading drug dose is used to rapidly attain the target drug concentration, which is approximately the steady-state drug concentration. However, the loading dose will not maintain the steady-state level unless an appropriate IV drug infusion rate or maintenance dose is also used. If a larger IV drug infusion rate or maintenance dose is given, the resulting steady-state drug concentration will be much higher and will remain sustained at the higher level. A higher infusion rate may be

administered if the initial steady-state drug level is inadequate for the patient.

What are some of the complications involved with IV infusion?

- The common complications associated with intravenous infusion include phlebitis and infections at the infusion site caused by poor intravenous techniques or indwelling catheters.

Learning Questions

1. a. To reach 95% of C_{ss}:

$$4.32 t_{1/2} = (4.32)(7) = 30.2 \text{ hours}$$

b. $D_L = C_{ss} V_D$

$$= (10)(0.231)(65,000) = 150 \text{ mg}$$

c. $R = C_{ss} V_D k = (10)(15,000)(0.099)$

$$= 14.85 \text{ mg/h}$$

d. $Cl_T = V_D k = (15,000)(0.099) = 1485 \text{ mL/h}$

e. To establish a new C_{ss} will still take $4.32 t_{1/2}$. However, the $t_{1/2}$ will be longer in renal failure.

f. If Cl_T is decreased by 50%, then the infusion rate R should be decreased proportionately:

$$R = 10(0.50)(1485) = 7.425 \text{ mg/h}$$

2. a. The steady-state level can be found by plotting the IV infusion data. The plasma drug–time curves plateau at 10 μg/mL.

Alternatively, V_D and k can be found from the single IV dose data:

$$V_D = 100 \text{ mL/kg} \quad k = 0.2 \text{ h}^{-1}$$

b. Using equations developed in Example 2 in the first set of examples in this chapter:

$$0.95 \frac{R}{V_D k} = \frac{R}{V_D k}(1 - e^{-kt})$$

$$0.95 = 1 - e^{-0.2t}$$

$$0.05 = e^{-0.2t}$$

$$t_{95\% \text{ ss}} = \frac{\ln 0.05}{-0.2} = 15 \text{ hours}$$

c. $Cl_T = V_D k \quad V_D = \dfrac{D_0}{C_P^0}$

$$Cl_T = 100 \times 0.2 \quad V_D = \frac{1000}{10} = \frac{100 \text{ mL}}{\text{kg}}$$

$$Cl_T = 20 \text{ mL/kg} \cdot \text{h}$$

d. The drug level 4 hours after stopping the IV infusion can be found by considering the drug concentration at the termination of infusion as C_P^0. At the termination of the infusion, the drug level will decline by a first-order process.

$$C_p = C_p^0 e^{-kt}$$

$$C_p = 9.9 \, e^{-(0.2)(4)}$$

$$C_p = 4.5 \, \mu\text{g/mL}$$

e. The infusion rate to produce a C_{ss} of 10 μg/mL is 0.2 mg/kg/h. Therefore, the infusion rate needed for this patient is

$$0.2 \text{ mg/kg} \cdot \text{h} \times 75 \text{ kg} = 15 \text{ mg/h}$$

f. From the data shown, at 4 hours after the start of the IV infusion, the drug concentration is 5.5 μg/mL; the drug concentration after an IV bolus of 1 mg/kg is 4.5 μg/mL. Therefore, if a 1-mg dose is given and the drug is then infused at 0.2 mg/kg/h, the plasma drug concentration will be $4.5 + 5.5 = 10 \, \mu\text{g/mL}$.

3. Infusion rate R for a 75-kg patient:

$$R = (1 \text{ mg/kg} \cdot \text{h})(75 \text{ kg}) = 75 \text{ mg/h}$$

Sterile drug solution contains 25 mg/mL. Therefore, 3 mL contains (3 mL) $\times$ (25 mg/mL), or 75 mg. The patient should receive 3 mL (75 mg/h) by IV infusion.

4. $C_{ss} = \dfrac{R}{V_D k} \quad R = C_{ss} V_D k$

$$R = (20 \text{ mg/L})(0.5 \text{ L/kg})(75 \text{ kg})\left(\frac{0.693}{3 \text{ h}}\right)$$

$$= 173.25 \text{ mg/h}$$

Drug is supplied as 125 mg/mL. Therefore,

$$125 \text{ mg/mL} = \frac{173.25 \text{ mg}}{X} \quad X = 1.386 \text{ mL}$$

$$R = 1.386 \text{ mL/h}$$

$$D_L = C_{ss} V_D = (20 \text{ mg/L})(0.5 \text{ L/kg})(75 \text{ kg})$$

$$= 750 \text{ mg}$$

5. $C_{ss} = \dfrac{R}{k V_D} = \dfrac{R}{Cl_T}$

a. $Cl_T = \dfrac{R}{C_{ss}} = \dfrac{5.3 \text{ mg/kg} \cdot \text{h} \times 71.71 \text{ kg}}{17 \text{ mg/L}}$

$$= 22.4 \text{ L/h}$$

b. At the end of IV infusion, $C_p = 17 \, \mu$g/mL. Assuming first-order elimination kinetics:

$$C_p = C_p^0 e^{-kt}$$

$$1.5 = 17 e^{-kt(2.5)}$$

$$0.0882 = e^{-2.5k}$$

$$\ln 0.0882 = -2.5 \, k$$

$$-2.43 = -2.5 \, k$$

$$k = 0.971 \text{ h}^{-1}$$

$$t_{1/2} = \frac{0.693}{0.971} = 0.714 \text{ hour}$$

c. $Cl_T = kV_D$ $V_D = \dfrac{Cl_T}{k}$

$$V_D = \frac{22.4}{0.971} = 23.1 \text{ L}$$

d. Probenecid blocks active tubular secretion of cephradine.

6. At steady state, the rate of elimination should equal the rate of absorption. Therefore, the rate of elimination would be 30 mg/h. The C_{ss} is directly proportional to the rate of infusion R, as shown by

$$C_{ss} = \frac{R}{kV_D}   kV_D = \frac{R}{C_{ss}}$$

$$\frac{R_{old}}{C_{ss,old}} = \frac{R_{new}}{C_{ss,new}}$$

$$\frac{30 \text{ mg/h}}{20 \text{ } \mu g/mL} = \frac{40 \text{ mg/h}}{C_{ss,new}}$$

$$C_{ss,new} = 26.7 \text{ } \mu g/mL$$

The new elimination rate will be 40 mg/h.

7. a.

$$R = C_{ss}kV_D$$

$$R = (20 \text{ mg/L})(0.693/8 \text{ h})(1.5 \text{ L/kg})(75 \text{ kg})$$

$$= 194.9 \text{ mg/h}$$

$$R = \frac{195 \text{ mg/h}}{15 \text{ mg/mL}} = 13 \text{ mL/h}$$

b. $D_L = C_{ss}V_D = (20)(1.5)(75) = 2250$ mg given by IV bolus injection.

c. The loading dose is given to obtain steady-state drug concentrations as rapidly as possible.

d. 15 mL of the antibiotic solution contains 225 mg of drug. Thus, an IV infusion rate of 15 mL/h is equivalent to 225 mg/h. The C_{ss} achieved by the manufacturer's recommendation is

$$C_{ss} = \frac{R}{kV_D} = \frac{225}{(0.0866)(112.5)} = 23.1 \text{ mg/L}$$

The theoretical C_{ss} of 23.1 mg/L is close to the desired C_{ss} of 20 mg/L. Assuming a reasonable therapeutic window, the manufacturer's suggested starting infusion rate is satisfactory.

REFERENCE

Hurley SF, McNeil JJ: A comparison of the accuracy of a least-squares regression, a Bayesian, Chiou's and the steady-state clearance method of individualizing theophylline dosage. *Clin Pharmacokinet* **14**:311–320, 1988.

BIBLIOGRAPHY

Gibaldi M: Estimation of the pharmacokinetic parameters of the two-compartment open model from postinfusion plasma concentration data. *J Pharm Sci* **58**:1133–1135, 1969.

Koup J, Greenblatt D, Jusko W, et al: Pharmacokinetics of digoxin in normal subjects after intravenous bolus and infusion dose. *J Pharmacokinet Biopharm* **3**:181–191, 1975.

Loo J, Riegelman S: Assessment of pharmacokinetic constants from postinfusion blood curves obtained after IV infusion. *J Pharm Sci* **59**:53–54, 1970.

Loughnam PM, Sitar DS, Ogilvie RI, Neims AH: The two-compartment open system kinetic model: A review of its clinical implications and applications. *J Pediatr* **88**:869–873, 1976.

Mitenko P, Ogilvie R: Rapidly achieved plasma concentration plateaus, with observations on theophylline kinetics. *Clin Pharmacol Ther* **13**:329–335, 1972.

Riegelman JS, Loo JC: Assessment of pharmacokinetic constants from postinfusion blood curves obtained after IV infusion. *J Pharm Sci* **59**:53, 1970.

Sawchuk RJ, Zaske DE: Pharmacokinetics of dosing regimens which utilize multiple intravenous infusions: Gentamicin in burn patients. *J Pharmacokinet Biopharm* **4**:183–195, 1976.

Wagner J: A safe method for rapidly achieving plasma concentration plateaus. *Clin Pharmacol Ther* **16**:691–700, 1974.

7 Drug Elimination, Clearance, and Renal Clearance

Murray P. Ducharme

Chapter Objectives

▶ Describe the main routes of drug elimination from the body.

▶ Understand the importance of the role of clearance as a PK parameter.

▶ Define clearance and its relationship to a corresponding half-life and a volume of distribution.

▶ Differentiate between clearance and renal clearance.

▶ Describe the processes for renal drug excretion and explain which renal excretion process predominates in the kidney for a specific drug, given its renal clearance.

▶ Describe the renal clearance model based on renal blood flow, glomerular filtration, and drug reabsorption.

▶ Describe organ drug clearance in terms of blood flow and extraction.

▶ Calculate clearance using different methods including the physiological, noncompartmental, and compartmental approaches.

DRUG ELIMINATION

Drugs are removed from the body by various elimination processes. *Drug elimination* refers to the irreversible removal of drug from the body by all routes of elimination. The declining plasma drug concentration observed after systemic drug absorption shows that the drug is being eliminated from the body but does not necessarily differentiate between distribution and elimination, and does not indicate which elimination processes are involved.

Drug elimination is usually divided into two major components: excretion and biotransformation. *Drug excretion* is the removal of the intact drug. Nonvolatile and polar drugs are excreted mainly by renal excretion, a process in which the drug passes through the kidney to the bladder and ultimately into the urine. Other pathways for drug excretion may include the excretion of drug into bile, sweat, saliva, milk (via lactation), or other body fluids. Volatile drugs, such as gaseous anesthetics, alcohol, or drugs with high volatility, are excreted via the lungs into expired air.

Biotransformation or *drug metabolism* is the process by which the drug is chemically converted in the body to a metabolite. Biotransformation is usually an enzymatic process. A few drugs may also be changed chemically[1] by a nonenzymatic process (eg, ester hydrolysis). The enzymes involved in the biotransformation of drugs are located mainly in the liver (see Chapter 12). Other tissues such as kidney, lung, small intestine, and skin also contain biotransformation enzymes.

Drug elimination in the body involves many complex rate processes. Although organ systems have specific functions, the tissues within the organs are not structurally homogeneous, and elimination processes may vary in each organ. In Chapter 4, drug elimination was modeled by an overall first-order elimination rate process. In this chapter, drug elimination is described in terms of clearance from a hypothetical well-stirred compartment containing

---

[1] Nonenzymatic breakdown of drugs may also be referrered to as *degradation*. For example, some drugs such as aspirin (acetylsalicylic acid) may break down in the stomach due to acid hydrolysis at pH 1–3.

uniform drug distribution. The term *clearance* describes the process of drug elimination from the body or from a single organ without identifying the individual processes involved. *Clearance* may be defined as the volume of fluid removed of the drug from the body per unit of time. The units for clearance are sometimes in milliliters per minute (mL/min) but most often reported in liters per hour (L/h). The volume concept is simple and convenient, because all drugs are dissolved and distributed in the fluids of the body.

Clearance is even more important clinically than a half-life for several reasons. First and foremost, clearance directly relates to the systemic exposure of a drug (eg, AUC_{inf}), making it the most useful PK parameter clinically as it will be used to calculate doses to administer in order to reach a therapeutic goal in terms of exposure. While the terminal half-life gives information only on the terminal phase of drug disposition, clearance takes into account all processes of drug elimination regardless of their mechanism. When the PK behavior of the drug follows linear PK, clearance is a constant, whereas the *rate of drug elimination* is not. For example, first-order elimination processes consider that a certain portion or fraction (percent) of the distribution volume is cleared of drug over a given time period. This basic concept (see also Chapter 3) will be elaborated along with a review of the anatomy and physiology of the kidney.

As will be seen later on in this chapter and in the noncompartmental analysis chapter (Chapter 25), the clearance of a drug (*Cl*) is directly related to the dose administered and to the overall systemic exposure achieved with that dose as per the equation $Cl = DOSE/AUC_{0-inf}$. The overall systemic exposure (AUC_{0-inf}) of a drug resulting from an administered dose correlates with its efficacy and toxicity. The drug clearance (*Cl*) is therefore the most important PK parameter to know in a given patient. If the therapeutic goal in terms of AUC_{0-inf} is known for a drug, then the dose to administer to this patient is completely dictated by the clearance value (*Cl*).

Hence, after IV administration

$$DOSE = Cl \times AUC_{0-inf} \qquad (7.1)$$

or more generally

$$DOSE = Cl/F \times AUC_{0-inf} \qquad (7.2)$$

in which *Cl/F* can be called the "apparent clearance" when the absolute bioavailability (*F*) is unknown or simply not specified or assumed.

Frequently Asked Question
▶ *Why is clearance a useful pharmacokinetic parameter?*

DRUG CLEARANCE

Drug clearance is a pharmacokinetic term for describing drug elimination from the body without identifying the mechanism of the process. Drug clearance (also called *body clearance or total body clearance*, and abbreviated as *Cl* or Cl_T) considers the entire body as a single drug-eliminating system from which many unidentified elimination processes may occur. Instead of describing the drug elimination rate in terms of amount of drug removed per unit of time (eg, mg/h), drug clearance is described in terms of volume of fluid removed from the drug per unit of time (eg, L/h).

There are several definitions of clearance, which are similarly based on a volume removed from the drug per unit of time. The simplest concept of clearance regards the body as a space that contains a definite volume of apparent body fluid (apparent volume of distribution, *V* or V_D) in which the drug is dissolved. Drug clearance is defined as the fixed volume of fluid (containing the drug) removed from the drug per unit of time. The units for clearance are volume/time (eg, mL/min, L/h). For example, if the *Cl* of penicillin is 15 mL/min in a patient and penicillin has a V_D of 12 L, then from the clearance definition, 15 mL of the 12 L will be removed from the drug per minute.

Alternatively, *Cl* may be defined as the rate of drug elimination divided by the plasma drug concentration. This definition expresses drug elimination in terms of the volume of plasma eliminated of drug per unit time. This definition is a practical way to calculate clearance based on plasma drug concentration data.

$$Cl = \frac{\text{Elimination rate}}{\text{Plasma concentration } (C_{\text{p}})} \qquad (7.3)$$

$$Cl = \left(\frac{dD_{\text{E}}/dt}{C_{\text{p}}}\right) = \frac{\mu g/min}{\mu g/mL} = mL/min \qquad (7.4)$$

where D_{E} is the amount of drug eliminated and dD_{E}/dt is the rate of elimination.

Rearrangement of Equation 7.4 gives Equation 7.5.

$$\text{Elimination rate} = \frac{dD_{\text{E}}}{dt} = C_{\text{p}}Cl \qquad (7.5)$$

The two definitions for clearance are similar because dividing the elimination rate by the C_{p} yields the volume of plasma cleared of drug per minute, as shown in Equation 7.4.

As discussed in previous chapters, a first-order elimination rate, dD_{E}/dt, is equal to kD_{B} or $kC_{\text{p}}V_{\text{D}}$. Based on Equation 7.3, substituting elimination rate for $kC_{\text{p}}V_{\text{D}}$,

$$Cl = \frac{kC_{\text{p}}V_{\text{D}}}{C_{\text{p}}} = kV_{\text{D}} \qquad (7.6)$$

Equation 7.6 shows that clearance is the product of a volume of distribution, V_{D}, and a rate constant, k, both of which are constants when the PK is linear. As the plasma drug concentration decreases during elimination, the rate of drug elimination, dD_{E}/dt, decreases accordingly, but clearance remains constant. Clearance is constant as long as the rate of drug elimination is a first-order process.

EXAMPLE ▶ ▶ ▶

Penicillin has a Cl of 15 mL/min. Calculate the elimination rate for penicillin when the plasma drug concentration, C_{p}, is 2 μg/mL.

Solution

Elimination rate $= C_{\text{p}} \times Cl$ (from Equation 7.5)

$$\frac{dD_{\text{E}}}{dt} = 2 \; \mu g/mL \times 15 \; mL/min = 30 \; \mu g/min$$

Using the previous penicillin example, assume that the plasma penicillin concentration is 10 μg/mL.

From Equation 7.4, the rate of drug elimination is

$$\frac{dD_{\text{E}}}{dt} = 10 \; \mu g/mL \times 15 \; mL/min = 150 \; \mu g/min$$

Thus, 150 μg/min of penicillin is eliminated from the body when the plasma penicillin concentration is 10 μg/mL.

Clearance may be used to estimate the rate of drug elimination at any given concentration. Using the same example, if the elimination rate of penicillin was measured as 150 μg/min when the plasma penicillin concentration was 10 μg/mL, then the clearance of penicillin is calculated from Equation 7.4:

$$Cl = \frac{150 \; \mu g/min}{10 \; \mu g/mL} = 15 \; mL/min$$

Just as the elimination rate constant (k or k_{el}) represents the total sum of all of the different rate constants for drug elimination, including for example the renal (k_{R}) and liver (k_{H}) elimination rate constants, Cl is the total sum of all of the different clearance processes in the body that are occurring in parallel in terms of cardiac blood flow (therefore excepting lung clearance), including for example clearance through the kidney (renal clearance abbreviated as Cl_{R}), and through the liver (hepatic clearance abbreviated as Cl_{H}):

Elimination rate constant:
k or k_{el} where $\quad k = k_{\text{R}} + k_{\text{H}} + k_{\text{other}} \qquad (7.7)$
Clearance:
Cl where $\quad Cl = Cl_{\text{R}} + Cl_{\text{H}} + Cl_{\text{other}} \qquad (7.8)$

where

Renal clearance: $Cl_{\text{R}} = k_{\text{R}} \times V \qquad (7.9)$

Hepatic clearance: $Cl_{\text{H}} = k_{\text{H}} \times V \qquad (7.10)$

Total clearance:

$$Cl = k \times V = (k_{\text{R}} + k_{\text{H}} + k_{\text{other}}) \times V \qquad (7.11)$$

From Equation 7.11, for a one-compartment model (ie, where $V = V_{\text{ss}}$ and where $k = \lambda_{\text{z}}$), the total body clearance Cl of a drug is the product of two constants, λ_{z} and V_{ss}, which reflect all the distribution and elimination processes of the drug in the body.

Distribution and elimination are affected by blood flow, which will be considered below (and in Chapter 11) using a physiologic model.

For a multicompartment model (eg, where the total volume of distribution $[V_{ss}]$ includes a central volume of distribution $[V_c]$, and one $[V_p]$ or more peripheral volumes of distributions), the total body clearance of a drug will be the product of the elimination rate constant from the central compartment (k_{10}) and V_c. The equations become:

Renal clearance: $Cl_R = k_R \times V_C$ (7.12)

Hepatic clearance: $Cl_H = k_H \times V_C$ (7.13)

Total clearance:

$Cl = k_{10} \times V_C = (k_R + k_H + k_{other}) \times V_C$ (7.14)

Clearance values are often adjusted on a per-kilogram-of-actual-body-weight (ABW) or on a per-meter-square-of-surface-area basis, such as L/h per kilogram or per m², or normalized for a "typical" adult of 72 kg or 1.72 m². This approach is similar to the method for expressing V, because both pharmacokinetic parameters vary with body weight or body size. It has been found, however, that when expressing clearance between individuals of varying ABW, such as predicting Cl between children and adults, Cl varies best allometrically with ABW, meaning that Cl is best expressed with an allometric exponent (most often 0.75 is recommended) relating it to ABW as per the following expression (see also Chapter 25):

Cl (predicted in a patient)

     $= Cl_{\text{(population value for a 72-kg patient)}} \times (\text{ABW}/72)^{0.75}$

(7.15)

EXAMPLE ▶▶▶

Determine the total body clearance for a drug in a 70-kg male patient. The drug follows the kinetics of a one-compartment model and has an elimination half-life of 3 hours with an apparent volume of distribution of 100 mL/kg.

Solution

First determine the elimination rate constant (k) and then substitute properly into Equation 7.11.

$$k = \frac{0.693}{t_{1/2}} = \frac{0.693}{3} = 0.231 \text{ h}^{-1}$$

$$Cl = 0.23 \text{ h}^{-1} \times 100 \text{ mL/kg} = 23.1 \text{ mL/(kg·h)}$$

For a 70-kg patient, $Cl = 23.1 \times 70 = 1617$ mL/h

CLEARANCE MODELS

The calculation of clearance from a rate constant (eg, k or k_{10}) and a volume of distribution (eg, V or V_c) assumes (sometimes incorrectly) a defined compartmental model, whereas clearance estimated directly from the plasma drug concentration–time curve using noncompartmental PK approaches does not need one to specify the number of compartments that would describe the shape of the concentration–time curve. Although clearance may be regarded as the product of a rate constant k and a volume of distribution V, Equation 7.11 is far more general because the reaction order for the rate of drug elimination, dD_E/dt, is not specified, and the elimination rate may or may not follow first-order kinetics. The various approaches for estimating a drug clearance are described in Fig. 7-1 and will be explored one by one below:

Compartmental model

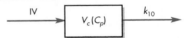

Static volume and first-order processes are assumed in simpler models. Here $Cl = k_{10} \times V_c$.

Physiologic model

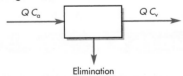

Clearance is the product of the flow through an organ (Q) and the extraction ratio of that organ (E). For example, the hepatic clearance is $Cl_H = Q_H \times E_H$.

Noncompartmental approach

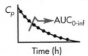

Volume of distribution does not need to be defined. $Cl = $ DOSE/AUCinf.

FIGURE 7-1   General approaches to clearance. Volume and elimination rate constant not defined.

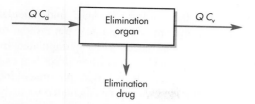

FIGURE 7-2 Drug clearance model. (Q = blood flow, C_a = incoming drug concentration [usually arterial drug concentration], C_v = outgoing drug concentration [venous drug concentration].)

Physiologic/Organ Clearance

Clearance may be calculated for any organ involved in the irreversible removal of drug from the body. Many organs in the body have the capacity for drug elimination, including drug excretion and biotransformation. The kidneys and liver are the most common organs involved in excretion and metabolism, respectively. Physiologic pharmacokinetic models are based on drug clearance through individual organs or tissue groups (Fig. 7-2).

For any organ, clearance may be defined as the fraction of blood volume containing drug that flows through the organ and is eliminated of drug per unit time. From this definition, clearance is the product of the blood flow (Q) to the organ and the extraction ratio (E). The E is the fraction of drug extracted by the organ as drug passes through.

$$Cl \text{ (organ)} = Q \text{ (organ)} \times E \text{ (organ)} \qquad (7.16)$$

If the drug concentration in the blood (C_a) entering the organ is greater than the drug concentration of blood (C_v) leaving the organ, then some of the drug has been extracted by the organ (Fig. 7-2). The E is $C_a - C_v$ divided by the entering drug concentration (C_a), as shown in Equation 7.17.

$$E = \frac{C_a - C_v}{C_a} \qquad (7.17)$$

E is a ratio with no units. The value of E may range from 0 (no drug removed by the organ) to 1 (100% of the drug is removed by the organ). An E of 0.25 indicates that 25% of the incoming drug concentration is removed by the organ as the drug passes through.

Substituting for E into Equation 7.16 yields

$$Cl \text{ (organ)} = Q \text{ (organ)} \frac{C_a - C_v}{C_a} \qquad (7.18)$$

Equation 7.16 adapted for the liver as an organ yields the hepatic clearance (Cl_H)

$$Cl_H = Q_H \times E_H \qquad (7.19)$$

Therefore, if $Cl = Cl_H + Cl_{NH}$ (where Cl_{NH} is the nonhepatic clearance), then

$$Cl = (Q_H \times E_H) + Cl_{NH} \qquad (7.20)$$

For some drugs $Cl \sim Cl_H$, and so $Cl \sim Q_H \times E_H$.

The physiologic approach to organ clearance shows that the clearance from an organ depends on its blood flow rate and its ability at eliminating the drug, whereas the total clearance is that of a constant or static fraction of the volume in which the drug is distributed or is removed from the drug per unit of time. Organ clearance measurements using the physiologic approach require invasive techniques to obtain measurements of blood flow and extraction ratio. The physiologic approach has been used to describe hepatic clearance, which is discussed further under hepatic elimination (Chapter 12). More classical definitions of clearance have been applied to renal clearance because direct measurements of plasma drug concentration and urinary drug excretion may be obtained. Details will be presented in the Renal Clearance section of this chapter.

Noncompartmental Methods

Clearance is commonly used to describe first-order drug elimination from compartment models such as the one-compartment model, $C(t) = C_p = C_p^0 e^{-kt}$ in which the distribution volume and elimination rate constant are well defined. Clearance estimated directly from the area under the plasma drug concentration–time curve using the noncompartmental method is often called a "*model-independent*" approach as it does not need any assumption to be set in terms of the number of compartments describing the kinetics or concentration–time profile of the drug under study. It is not exactly true that this method is a "model-independent" one, though, as this method still assumes that the terminal phase decreases in a log-linear fashion that is model dependent, and many of its parameters can be calculated only when one assumes PK linearity. Referring to this method as "noncompartmental" is therefore more appropriate.

The *noncompartmental* approach is based on statistical moment theory and is presented in more details in Chapter 25. The main advantages of this approach are that (1) clearance can be easily calculated without making any assumptions relating to rate constants (eg, distribution vs. elimination rate constants), (2) volume of distribution is presented in a clinically useful context as it is related to systemic exposure and the dose administered, and (3) its estimation is robust in the context of rich sampling data as very little modeling is involved, if any (eg, no modeling at steady-state data, and only very limited modeling by way of linear regression of the terminal phase after single dose administration).

Clearance can be determined directly from the time–concentration curve by

$$Cl = \int_0^\infty D \times F / C(t)\, dt \qquad (7.21)$$

where D is the dose administered, F is the bioavailability factor associated with the administration route used of the drug product, and $C(t)$ is an unknown function that describes the changing plasma drug concentrations.

Using the noncompartmental approach, the general equation therefore uses the area under the drug concentration curve, $[AUC]_0^\infty$, for the calculation of clearance.

$$Cl = \frac{F \times D}{AUC_{0\text{-inf}}} \qquad \text{(as presented before in Equation 7.2)}$$

where $AUC_{0\text{-inf}} = [AUC]_0^\infty = \int_0^\infty C_p\, dt$ and is the total systemic exposure obtained after a single dose (D) until infinity.

Because $[AUC]_0^\infty$ is calculated from the drug concentration–time curve from zero to infinity using the trapezoidal rule, no model is assumed until the terminal phase after the last detectable concentration is obtained (C_t). To extrapolate the data to infinity to obtain the residual $[AUC]_t^\infty$ or (C_{p_t}/k), first-order elimination is usually assumed.

Equation 7.2 is used to calculate clearance after administration of a single dose, and where concentrations would be obtained in a rich sampling fashion until a last detectable concentration time point, C_t. The AUC from time zero to t (AUC_{0-t}) is often described as the "observed" AUC and calculated using the linear or mixed log-linear trapezoidal rule, while the AUC that needs to be extrapolated from time t to infinity ($AUC_{t\text{-inf}}$) is often described as the "extrapolated" AUC. It is good pharmacokinetic practice for the clearance to be calculated robustly to never extrapolate the AUC_{0-t} by more than 20%. In addition, it is also good pharmacokinetic practice for the AUC_{0-t} to be calculated using a rich sampling strategy, meaning a minimum of 12 concentration–time points across the concentration–time curve from zero to C_t.

At steady state, when the concentration–time profiles between administered doses become constant, the amount of drug administered over the dosing interval is exactly equal to the amount eliminated over that dosing interval (τ). The formula for clearance therefore becomes:

$$Cl \text{ or } Cl_{(ss)} = \frac{F \times D}{AUC_{\tau(ss)}} \qquad (7.22)$$

If the drug exhibits linear pharmacokinetics in terms of time, then the clearance calculated after single dose administration (Cl) using Equation 7.2 and the clearance calculated from steady-state data ($Cl_{(ss)}$) using Equation 7.22 will be the same.

From Equation 7.22, it can be derived that following a constant intravenous infusion (see Chapter 6), the steady-state concentration (C_{ss}) will then be equal to "rate in," the administration dosing rate (R_0), divided by "rate out" or the clearance:

$$C_{(ss)} = \frac{F \times R_0}{Cl} \quad \text{or} \quad Cl = \frac{F \times R_0}{C_{ss}} \qquad (7.23)$$

where R_0 is the constant dosing rate (eg, in mg/h), C_{ss} is the steady-state concentration (eg, in mg/L), and Cl is the total body clearance (eg, in L/h).

Compartmental Methods

Clearance is a direct measure of elimination from the central compartment, regardless of the number of compartments. The central compartment consists of the plasma and highly perfused tissues in which drug equilibrates rapidly (see Chapter 5). The tissues for drug elimination, namely, kidney and liver, are considered integral parts of the central compartment.

Clearance is always the product of a rate constant and a volume of distribution. There are different clearance formulas depending on the pharmacokinetic model that would describe appropriately the concentration-versus-time profiles of a drug product. The clearance formulas depend upon whether the drug is administered intravenously or extravascularly and range from simple to more complicated scenarios:

Drug that is well described pharmacokinetically with a one-compartment model

After intravenous administration, such a drug will exhibit a concentration–time profile that decreases in a straight line when viewed on a semilog plot and would therefore be well described by a monoexponential decline. This is the simplest model that can be used and often will describe well the pharmacokinetics of drugs that are very polar and that are readily eliminated in the urine. Clinically, aminoglycoside antibiotics are relatively well characterized and predicted by a one-compartment model.

$$Cl = \lambda_z \times V_{ss}$$

where λ_z is the only rate constant describing the fate of the concentration–time profile and dividing 0.693 by its value, therefore, estimates the terminal half-life. V_{ss} is the total volume of distribution, and in this case, there is only one volume that is describing the pharmacokinetic behavior of the drug.

Calculated parameters:

The terminal half-life of the drug is $T_{1/2} = 0.693/\lambda_z$

After oral administration the formula for clearance is exactly the same but a Cl/F is calculated. There is also an absorption process in addition to an elimination one. If the absorption process is faster than the elimination, the terminal rate constant, λ_z, will describe the elimination of the drug. If the drug exhibits a "flip-flop" profile because the absorption of the drug is much slower than the elimination process (eg, often the case with modified release formulations), then the terminal rate constant, λ_z, will be reflective of the absorption and not the elimination. It is sometimes not possible to know if a drug exhibits a slower absorption than elimination. In these cases, it is always best to refer to λ_z as the "terminal"

rate constant instead of assuming it is the "elimination" rate constant.

$$\frac{Cl}{F} = \lambda_z \times \frac{V_{ss}}{F}$$

Relationship with the noncompartmental approach after IV administration:

$$Cl = \lambda_z \times V_{ss} \quad \text{and} \quad Cl = \frac{Dose}{AUC_{0\text{-inf}}}$$

$$\text{and} \quad V_{ss} = Cl \times MRT$$

Therefore, MRT (mean residence time[2]) $= 1/\lambda_z$ and $V_{ss} = Dose/(AUC_{0\text{-inf}} \times \lambda_z)$.

Relationship with the noncompartmental approach after extravascular administration:

$$\frac{Cl}{F} = \lambda_z \times \frac{V_{ss}}{F} \quad \text{and} \quad \frac{Cl}{F} = \frac{Dose}{AUC_{0\text{-inf}}}$$

MRT and V_{ss}/F are not computable directly using noncompartmental methods after extravascular administration, but only MTT (mean transit time), which is the sum of MAT (mean absorption time) and MRT.

But we have seen that MRT $= 1/\lambda_z$ and $V_{ss}/F = Dose/(AUC_{0\text{-inf}} \times \lambda_z)$. MAT can then be calculated by subtracting MRT from the MTT.

Drug that is well described pharmacokinetically with a two-compartment model

After intravenous administration, such a drug will exhibit a concentration–time profile that decreases in a profile that can be characterized by two different exponentials or two different straight lines when viewed on a semilog plot (see Chapter 5). This model will describe well the pharmacokinetics of drugs that are not so polar and distribute in a second compartment that is not so well perfused by blood or plasma. Clinically, the antibiotic vancomycin is relatively well characterized and predicted by a two-compartment model.

$$Cl = k_{10} \times V_c \qquad (7.24)$$

where k_{10} is the rate constant describing the disappearance of the drug from its central volume of distribution (V_c).

---

[2]MRT is mean residence time and is discussed more fully in Chapter 25.

The distributional clearance (Cl_d) describes the clearance occurring between the central (V_c) and the peripheral compartment (V_p), and where the central compartment includes the plasma and the organs that are very well perfused, while the peripheral compartment includes organs that are less well perfused.

The concentration–time curve profile will follow a biexponential decline on a semilog graph and the distributional rate constant (λ_1) will be describing the rapid decline after IV administration that describes the distribution process, and the second and last exponential (λ_z) will describe the terminal elimination phase.

The distribution (λ_1) and terminal elimination (λ_z) rate constants can be obtained with the following equations:

- $\lambda_1 = [((Cl + Cl_d)/V_c + Cl_d/V_p) + \text{SQRT} ((((Cl + Cl_d)/V_c + Cl_d/V_p)^2 - 4 \times Cl/V_c*Cl_d/V_p))]/2$
- $\lambda_z = [((Cl + Cl_d)/V_c + Cl_d/V_p) - \text{SQRT} ((((Cl + Cl_d)/V_c + Cl_d/V_p)^2 - 4 \times Cl/V_c*Cl_d/V_p))]/2$

The distribution and terminal elimination half-lives are therefore:

- $T_{1/2}(\lambda_1) = 0.693/\lambda_1$
- $T_{1/2}(\lambda_z) = 0.693/\lambda_z$

The total volume of distribution V_{ss} will be the sum of V_c and V_p:

$$V_{ss} = V_c + V_p \qquad (7.25)$$

Relationship with the noncompartmental approach after IV administration:

$$Cl = \frac{\text{Dose}}{\text{AUC}_{0\text{-inf}}} \quad \text{and} \quad V_{ss} = Cl \times \text{MRT}$$

(noncompartmental equations)

$$Cl = k_{10} \times V_c \quad \text{and} \quad V_{ss} = V_c + V_p$$

(compartmental equations)

Therefore, $\text{MRT} = (V_c + V_p)/(k_{10} \times V_c)$.

Relationship between Rate Constants, Volumes of Distribution, and Clearances

As seen previously in Equation 7.24, $Cl = k_{10} \times V_c$, which for a drug well described by a one-compartment model can be simplified to $Cl = \lambda_z \times V_{ss}$.

It is often stated that clearances and volumes are "independent" parameters, while rate constants are "dependent" parameters. This assumption is made in PK models to facilitate data analysis of the underlying kinetic processes. Stated differently, a change in a patient in its drug clearance may not result in a change in its volume of distribution or vice versa, while a change in clearance or in the volume of distribution will result in a change in the appropriate rate constant (eg, k_{10}, λ_z). While mostly true, this statement can be somewhat confusing, as there are clinical instances where a change can lead to both volume of distribution and clearance changes, without a resulting change in the rate constant (eg, k_{10}, λ_z). A common example is a significant abrupt change in actual body weight (ABW) as both clearances and volumes of distribution correlate with ABW. A patient becoming suddenly edematous will not see his or her liver or renal function necessarily affected. In that example, both the patient's clearance and volume of distribution will be increased, while half-life or half-lives will remain relatively unchanged. In that situation the dosing interval will not need to be changed, as the half-life will stay constant, but the dose to be given will need to be increased due to the greater volume of distribution and clearance.

Summary Regarding Clearance Calculations

Clearance can be calculated using physiologic, compartmental, or noncompartmental methods. What is important to remember is that all methods will lead to the same results if they are applied correctly and if there are enough data supporting the calculations. Clearance can therefore be calculated:

- After a single dose administration using the area under the concentration–time curve from time zero to infinity using a noncompartmental approach: $Cl = (\text{Dose} \times F)/\text{AUC}_{0\text{-inf}}$.
- At steady-state conditions using the area under the concentration–time curve during a dosing interval using a noncompartmental approach: $Cl = (\text{Dose} \times F)/\text{AUC}_{\tau(ss)}$.
- When a constant infusion is administered until steady-state concentrations (C_{ss}) are achieved: $Cl = F \times R_0/C_{ss}$.

- At any time using a compartmental approach with the appropriate volume(s) of distribution and rate constant(s):

  ○ $Cl = k_{10} \times V_c$ when the PK of a drug is well described by any compartment model when the drug displays linear pharmacokinetics.
  ○ Which equation can be simplified to $Cl = \lambda_z \times V_{ss}$ when the PK of a drug is well described by only a one-compartment model as λ_z is then equal to k_{10}, and V_{ss} to V_c.

- For an organ using its blood flow and its extraction ratio. For example, the hepatic clearance could be calculated as $Cl_H = Q_H \times E_H$. For a drug that would be only eliminated via the liver, then Cl would be equal to Cl_H.

THE KIDNEY

The liver (see Chapter 12) and the kidney are the two major drug-eliminating organs in the body, though drug elimination can also occur almost anywhere in the body. The kidney is the main excretory organ for the removal of metabolic waste products and plays a major role in maintaining the normal fluid volume and electrolyte composition in the body. To maintain salt and water balance, the kidney excretes excess electrolytes, water, and waste products while conserving solutes necessary for proper body function. In addition, the kidney has two endocrine functions: (1) secretion of renin, which regulates blood pressure, and (2) secretion of erythropoietin, which stimulates red blood cell production.

Anatomic Considerations

The kidneys are located in the peritoneal cavity. A general view is shown in Fig. 7-3 and a longitudinal view in Fig. 7-4. The outer zone of the kidney is called the *cortex*, and the inner region is called the *medulla*. The *nephrons* are the basic functional units, collectively responsible for the removal of metabolic waste and the maintenance of water and electrolyte balance. Each kidney contains 1–1.5 million nephrons. The *glomerulus* of each nephron starts in the cortex. *Cortical nephrons* have short *loops of Henle* that remain exclusively in the cortex; *juxtamedullary*

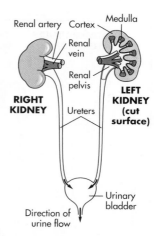

FIGURE 7-3   The general organizational plan of the urinary system. (Reproduced with permission from Guyton AC: Textbook of Medical Physiology, 8th ed. Philadelphia, Saunders, 1991.)

nephrons have long loops of Henle that extend into the medulla (Fig. 7-5). The longer loops of Henle allow for a greater ability of the nephron to reabsorb water, thereby producing more concentrated urine.

Blood Supply

The kidneys represent about 0.5% of the total body weight and receive approximately 20%–25% of the cardiac output. The kidney is supplied by blood via the renal artery, which subdivides into the interlobar

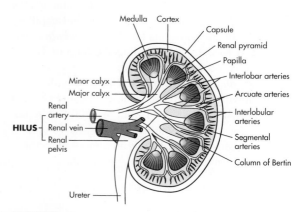

FIGURE 7-4   Longitudinal section of the kidney, illustrating major anatomical features and blood vessels. (From West, 1985, with permission.)

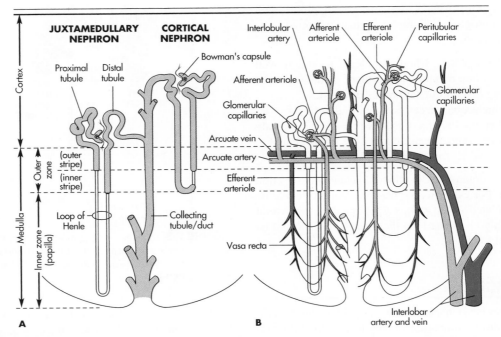

FIGURE 7-5   Cortical and juxtamedullary nephrons and their vasculature. (From West, 1985, p. 452, with permission.)

arteries penetrating within the kidney and branching further into the afferent arterioles. Each afferent arteriole carries blood toward a single nephron into the glomerular portion of the nephron (*Bowman's capsule*). The filtration of blood occurs in the glomeruli in Bowman's capsule. From the capillaries (*glomerulus*) within Bowman's capsule, the blood flows out via the efferent arterioles and then into a second capillary network that surrounds the tubules (*peritubule capillaries* and *vasa recti*), including the loop of Henle, where some water is reabsorbed.

The *renal blood flow* (RBF) is the volume of blood flowing through the renal vasculature per unit of time. RBF exceeds 1.2 L/min or 1700 L/d. *Renal plasma flow* (RPF) is the RBF minus the volume of red blood cells present. RPF is an important factor in the rate of drug filtration at the glomerulus.

$$RPF = RBF - (RBF \times Hct) \qquad (7.26)$$

where Hct is the *hematocrit*.

Hct is the fraction of blood cells in the blood, about 0.45 or 45% of the total blood volume.

The relationship of RBF to RPF is given by a rearrangement of Equation 7.26:

$$RPF = RBF\,(1 - Hct) \qquad (7.27)$$

Assuming a hematocrit of 0.45 and an RBF of 1.2 L/min and using the above equation, RPF = 1.2 − (1.2 × 0.45) = 0.66 L/min or 660 mL/min, or approximately 950 L/d. The average *glomerular filtration rate* (GFR) is about 120 mL/min in an average adult,[3] or about 20% of the RPF. The ratio GFR/RPF is the *filtration fraction*.

Regulation of Renal Blood Flow

Blood flow to an organ is directly proportional to the arteriovenous pressure difference (*perfusion pressure*) across the vascular bed and indirectly proportional to the vascular resistance. The normal renal arterial pressure (Fig. 7-6) is approximately 100 mm Hg and falls to approximately 45–60 mm Hg in the glomerulus

---

[3]GFR is often based on average body surface, 1.73 m². GFR is less in women and also decreases with age.

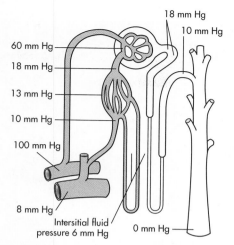

60 mm Hg
18 mm Hg
13 mm Hg
10 mm Hg
100 mm Hg
18 mm Hg
10 mm Hg
8 mm Hg
Intersitial fluid pressure 6 mm Hg
0 mm Hg

FIGURE 7-6   Approximate pressures at different points in the vessels and tubules of the functional nephron and in the interstitial fluid. (Reproduced with permission from Guyton AC: Textbook of Medical Physiology, 8th ed. Philadelphia, Saunders, 1991.)

autoregulation refers to the maintenance of a constant blood flow in the presence of large fluctuations in arterial blood pressure. Because autoregulation maintains a relatively constant blood flow, the filtration fraction (GFR/RPF) also remains fairly constant in this pressure range.

Glomerular Filtration and Urine Formation

A normal adult subject has a GFR of approximately 120 mL/min. About 180 L of fluid per day are filtered through the kidneys. In spite of this large filtration volume, the average urine volume is 1–1.5 L. Up to 99% of the fluid volume filtered at the glomerulus is reabsorbed. Besides fluid regulation, the kidney also regulates the retention or excretion of various solutes and electrolytes (Table 7-1). With the exception of proteins and protein-bound substances, most small molecules are filtered through the glomerulus from the plasma. The filtrate contains some ions, glucose, and essential nutrients as well as waste products, such as urea, phosphate, sulfate, and other substances. The essential nutrients and water are reabsorbed at various sites, including the proximal tubule, loops of Henle, and distal tubules. Both active reabsorption and secretion mechanisms are involved. The urine volume is reduced, and the urine generally contains a high concentration of metabolic wastes and eliminated drug products. Advances in molecular biology have shown that transporters such as P-glycoprotein and other efflux proteins are present in the kidney, and can influence urinary drug excretion. Further, CYP enzymes are also present in the kidney, and can impact drug clearance by metabolism.

(glomerular capillary hydrostatic pressure). This pressure difference is probably due to the increasing vasculature resistance provided by the small diameters of the capillary network. Thus, the GFR is controlled by changes in the glomerular capillary hydrostatic pressure.

In the normal kidney, RBF and GFR remain relatively constant even with large differences in mean systemic blood pressure (Fig. 7-7). The term

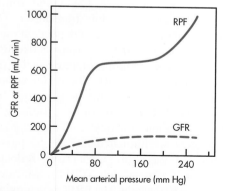

FIGURE 7-7   Schematic representation of the effect of mean arterial pressure on GFR and RPF, illustrating the phenomenon of autoregulation. (From West, 1985, p. 465, with permission.)

Renal Drug Excretion

Renal excretion is a major route of elimination for many drugs. Drugs that are nonvolatile, are water soluble, have a low molecular weight (MW), or are slowly biotransformed by the liver are eliminated by renal excretion. The processes by which a drug is excreted via the kidneys may include any combination of the following:

- Glomerular filtration
- Active tubular secretion
- Tubular reabsorption

TABLE 7-1   Quantitative Aspects of Urine Formation[a]

Substance	Per 24 Hours				
	Filtered	**Reabsorbed**	**Secreted**	**Excreted**	**Percent Reabsorbed**
Sodium ion (mEq)	26,000	25,850		150	99.4
Chloride ion (mEq)	18,000	17,850		150	99.2
Bicarbonate ion (mEq)	4,900	4,900		0	100
Urea (mM)	870	460[b]		410	53
Glucose (mM)	800	800		0	100
Water (mL)	180,000	179,000		1000	99.4
Hydrogen ion			Variable	Variable[c]	
Potassium ion (mEq)	900	900[d]	100	100	100[d]

[a]Quantity of various plasma constituents filtered, reabsorbed, and excreted by a normal adult on an average diet.

[b]Urea diffuses into, as well as out of, some portions of the nephron.

[c]pH or urine is on the acid side (4.5–6.9) when all bicarbonate is reabsorbed.

[d]Potassium ion is almost completely reabsorbed before it reaches the distal nephron. The potassium ion in the voided urine is actively secreted into the urine in the distal tubule in exchange for sodium ion.

From Levine (1990), with permission.

Glomerular filtration is a unidirectional process that occurs for most small molecules (MW < 500), including undissociated (nonionized) and dissociated (ionized) drugs. Protein-bound drugs behave as large molecules and do not get filtered at the glomerulus. The major driving force for glomerular filtration is the hydrostatic pressure within the glomerular capillaries. The kidneys receive a large blood supply (approximately 25% of the cardiac output) via the renal artery, with very little decrease in the hydrostatic pressure.

Glomerular filtration rate (GFR) is measured by using a drug that is eliminated primarily by filtration only (ie, the drug is neither reabsorbed nor secreted). Clinically inulin and creatinine are often used for this purpose, although creatinine is also secreted. The clearance of inulin is approximately equal to the GFR, which can equal 120 mL/min. The value for the GFR correlates fairly well with body surface area. Glomerular filtration of drugs is directly related to the free or nonprotein-bound drug concentration in the plasma. As the free drug concentration in the plasma increases, the glomerular filtration for the drug increases proportionately, thus increasing renal drug clearance for some drugs.

Active tubular secretion is an active transport process. As such, active renal secretion is a carrier-mediated system that requires energy input, because the drug is transported against a concentration gradient. The carrier system is capacity limited and may be saturated. Drugs with similar structures may compete for the same carrier system. Among the active renal secretion systems that have been identified, there are some for weak acids (organic anion transporter, OAT) and some for weak bases (organic cation transporter, OCT). Active tubular secretion rate is dependent on RPF. Drugs commonly used to measure active tubular secretion include *p*-amino-hippuric acid (PAH) and iodopyracet (Diodrast). These substances are both filtered by the glomeruli and secreted by the tubular cells. Active secretion is extremely rapid for these drugs, and practically all the drug carried to the kidney is eliminated in a single pass. The clearance for these drugs therefore reflects the *effective renal plasma flow* (ERPF), which varies from 425 to 650 mL/min. The ERPF is determined by both RPF and the fraction of drug that is effectively extracted by the kidney relative to the concentration in the renal artery.

For a drug that is excreted solely by glomerular filtration, the elimination half-life may change markedly in accordance with the binding affinity of the drug for plasma proteins. In contrast, drug protein binding has very little effect on the elimination half-life of the drug excreted mostly by active secretion. Because drug protein binding is reversible, drug bound to plasma protein rapidly dissociates as free drug is secreted by the kidneys. For example, some of the penicillins are extensively protein bound, but their elimination half-lives are short due to rapid elimination by active secretion.

Tubular reabsorption occurs after the drug is filtered through the glomerulus and can be an active or a passive process involving transporting back into the plasma. If a drug is completely reabsorbed (eg, glucose), then the value for the clearance of the drug is approximately zero. For drugs that are partially reabsorbed without being secreted, clearance values are less than the GFR of 120 mL/min.

The reabsorption of drugs that are acids or weak bases is influenced by the pH of the fluid in the renal tubule (ie, urine pH) and the pK_a of the drug. Both of these factors together determine the percentage of dissociated (ionized) and undissociated (nonionized) drug. Generally, the undissociated species is more lipid soluble (less water soluble) and has greater membrane permeability. The undissociated drug is easily reabsorbed from the renal tubule back into the body. This process of drug reabsorption can significantly reduce the amount of drug excreted, depending on the pH of the urinary fluid and the pK_a of the drug. The pK_a of the drug is a constant, but the normal urinary pH may vary from 4.5 to 8.0, depending on diet, pathophysiology, and drug intake. In addition, the initial morning urine generally is more acidic and becomes more alkaline later in the day. Vegetable and fruit diets (alkaline residue diet[4]) result in higher urinary pH, whereas diets rich in protein result in lower urinary pH. Drugs such as ascorbic acid and antacids such as sodium carbonate

may decrease (acidify) or increase (alkalinize) the urinary pH, respectively, when administered in large quantities. By far the most important changes in urinary pH are caused by fluids administered intravenously. Intravenous fluids, such as solutions of bicarbonate or ammonium chloride, are used in acid–base therapy to alkalinize or acidify the urine, respectively. Excretion of these solutions may drastically change urinary pH and alter drug reabsorption and drug excretion by the kidney.

The percentage of ionized weak acid drug corresponding to a given pH can be obtained from the *Henderson–Hasselbalch equation*.

$$pH = pK_a + \log \frac{\text{Ionized}}{\text{Nonionized}} \qquad (7.28)$$

Rearrangement of this equation yields:

$$\frac{\text{Ionized}}{\text{Nonionized}} = 10^{pH - pK_a} \qquad (7.29)$$

Fraction of drug ionized

$$= \frac{[\text{Ionized}]}{[\text{Ionized}] + [\text{Nonionized}]}$$

$$= \frac{10^{pH - pK_a}}{1 + 10^{pH - pK_a}} \qquad (7.30)$$

The fraction or percent of weak acid drug ionized in any pH environment may be calculated with Equation 7.30. For acidic drugs with pK_a values from 3 to 8, a change in urinary pH affects the extent of dissociation (Table 7-2). The extent of dissociation is more greatly affected by changes in urinary pH for drugs with a pK_a of 5 than with a pK_a of 3. Weak acids with

---

[4]The alkaline residue diet (also known as the alkaline ash diet) is a diet composed of foods, such as fruits and vegetables, from which the carbohydrate portion of the diet is metabolized in the body leaving an alkaline residue containing cations such as sodium, potassium, calcium, etc. These cations are excreted through the kidney and cause the urine to become alkaline.

TABLE 7-2   Effect of Urinary pH and pK_a on the Ionization of Drugs

pH of Urine	Percent of Drug Ionized: pK_a 53	Percent of Drug Ionized: pK_a 55
7.4	100	99.6
5	99	50.0
4	91	9.1
3	50	0.99

TABLE 7-3   Properties of Renal Drug Elimination Processes

Process	Active/Passive Transport	Location in Nephron	Drug Ionization	Drug Protein Binding	Influenced by
Filtration	Passive	Glomerulus	Either	Only free drug	Protein binding
Secretion	Active	Proximal tubule	Mostly weak acids and weak bases	No effect	Competitive inhibitors
Reabsorption	Passive/Active	Distal tubule	Nonionized	Not applicable	Urinary pH and flow

pK_a values of less than 2 are highly ionized at all urinary pH values and are only slightly affected by pH variations.

For a weak base drug, the Henderson–Hasselbalch equation is given as

$$pH = pK_a + \log \frac{\text{Nonionized}}{\text{Ionized}} \qquad (7.31)$$

and

$$\text{Percent of drug ionized} = \frac{10^{pK_a - pH}}{1 + 10^{pK_a - pH}} \qquad (7.32)$$

The greatest effect of urinary pH on reabsorption occurs for weak base drugs with pK_a values of 7.5–10.5.

From the Henderson–Hasselbalch relationship, a concentration ratio for the distribution of a weak acid or basic drug between urine and plasma may be derived. The urine–plasma (U/P) ratios for these drugs are as follows.

For weak acids,

$$\frac{U}{P} = \frac{1 + 10^{pH_{urine} - pK_a}}{1 + 10^{pH_{plasma} - pK_a}} \qquad (7.33)$$

For weak bases,

$$\frac{U}{P} = \frac{1 + 10^{pK_a - pH_{urine}}}{1 + 10^{pK_a - pH_{plasma}}} \qquad (7.34)$$

For example, amphetamine, a weak base, will be reabsorbed if the urine pH is made alkaline and more lipid-soluble nonionized species are formed. In contrast, acidification of the urine will cause the amphetamine to become more ionized (form a salt). The salt form is more water soluble, less likely to be reabsorbed, and tends to be excreted into the urine more quickly. In the case of weak acids (such as salicylic acid), acidification of the urine causes greater reabsorption of the drug and alkalinization of the urine causes more rapid excretion of the drug.

In summary, renal drug excretion is a composite of passive filtration at the glomerulus, active secretion in the proximal tubule, and passive and/or active reabsorption in the distal tubule (Table 7-3). Active secretion is an enzyme (transporter)-mediated process that is saturable. Although reabsorption of drugs is mostly a passive process, the extent of reabsorption of weak acid or weak base drugs is influenced by the pH of the urine and the degree of ionization of the drug. In addition, an increase in blood flow to the kidney, which may be due to diuretic therapy or large alcohol consumption, decreases the extent of drug reabsorption in the kidney and increases the rate of drug excreted in the urine.

CLINICAL APPLICATION

Both sulfisoxazole (Gantrisin) tablets and the combination product, sulfamethoxazole/trimethoprim (Bactrim) tablets, are used for urinary tract infections. Sulfisoxazole and sulfamethoxazole are sulfonamides that are well absorbed after oral administration and are excreted in high concentrations in the urine. Sulfonamides are N-acetylated to a less water-soluble metabolite. Both sulfonamides and their corresponding N-acetylated metabolite are less water soluble in acid and more soluble in alkaline conditions. In acid urine, renal toxicity can occur due to precipitation of the sulfonamides in the renal tubules. To prevent crystalluria and renal complications, patients are instructed to take these drugs with a high amount of fluid intake and to keep the urine alkaline.

PRACTICE PROBLEMS

Let $pK_a = 5$ for an acidic drug. Compare the U/P at urinary pH (**a**) 3, (**b**) 5, and (**c**) 7.

Solution

a. At pH = 3,

$$\frac{U}{P} = \frac{1+10^{3-5}}{1+10^{7.4-5}} = \frac{1.01}{1+10^{2.4}} = \frac{1.01}{252} = \frac{1}{252}$$

b. At pH = 5,

$$\frac{U}{P} = \frac{1+10^{5-5}}{1+10^{7.4-5}} = \frac{2}{1+10^{2.4}} = \frac{2}{252}$$

c. At pH = 7,

$$\frac{U}{P} = \frac{1+10^{7-5}}{1+10^{7.4-5}} = \frac{101}{1+10^{2.4}} = \frac{101}{252}$$

In addition to the pH of the urine, the rate of urine flow influences the amount of filtered drug that is reabsorbed. The normal flow of urine is approximately 1–2 mL/min. Nonpolar and nonionized drugs, which are normally well reabsorbed in the renal tubules, are sensitive to changes in the rate of urine flow. Drugs that increase urine flow, such as ethanol, large fluid intake, and methylxanthines (such as caffeine or theophylline), decrease the time for drug reabsorption and promote their excretion. Thus, forced diuresis through the use of diuretics may be a useful adjunct for removing excessive drug in an intoxicated patient, by increasing renal drug excretion.

RENAL CLEARANCE

Renal clearance, Cl_R, is defined as the volume that is removed from the drug per unit of time through the kidney. Similarly, renal clearance may be defined as a constant fraction of the central volume of distribution in which the drug is contained that is excreted by the kidney per unit of time. More simply, renal clearance is defined as the urinary drug excretion rate (dD_u/dt) divided by the plasma drug concentration (C_p).

$$Cl_R = \frac{\text{Excretion rate}}{\text{Plasma concentration}} = \frac{dD_u/dt}{C_p} \quad (7.35)$$

As seen earlier in this chapter, most clearances besides that of the lung are additive, and therefore, the total body clearance can be defined as the sum of the renal clearance (Cl_R) and the nonrenal clearance (Cl_{NR}), whatever it may consist of (eg, hepatic or other):

$$Cl = Cl_R + Cl_{NR} \quad (7.36)$$

Therefore,

$$Cl_R = f_e \times Cl \quad (7.37)$$

where f_e is the proportion of the bioavailable dose that is eliminated unchanged in the urine. Using the noncompartmental formula for Cl studied earlier (Equation 7.2), we obtain

$$Cl_R = \frac{f_e \times F \times \text{Dose}}{\text{AUC}_{0-\text{inf}}}$$

and consequently

$$Cl_R = \frac{\text{Ae}_{0-\text{inf}}}{\text{AUC}_{0-\text{inf}}} \quad (7.38)$$

where $\text{Ae}_{0-\text{inf}}$ is the amount of drug eliminated unchanged in the urine from time 0 to infinity after a single dose. In practice it is not possible to measure the amount of drug excreted unchanged in the urine until infinity, and so in order to get a reasonable estimate of the renal clearance with this noncompartmental approach formula using the amount excreted unchanged in the urine and the systemic exposure, one has to collect the urine and observe the AUC for the longest time period possible, ideally more than 3–4 terminal half-lives, so that the error made using this formula is less than 10%. So if, for example, a drug product has a terminal half-life of 12 hours, then one may need to collect the urine for 48 hours and calculate the ratio of Ae_{0-48} divided by AUC_{0-48}.

In essence for that particular drug product one could say that:

$$Cl_R = \frac{Ae_{0\text{-inf}}}{AUC_{0\text{-inf}}} \sim \frac{Ae_{0\text{-}48}}{AUC_{0\text{-}48}}$$

At steady-state conditions it is easier to calculate renal clearance, as at steady state all of the excreted drug eliminated unchanged in the urine from one dose occurs over one dosing interval. Equation 7.38 therefore becomes:

$$Cl_{R(ss)} = \frac{Ae_{\tau(ss)}}{AUC_{\tau(ss)}} \qquad (7.39)$$

where τ is the dosing interval at which the drug is administered until steady state (ss) conditions are seen, and $Ae_{\tau(ss)}$ is the amount of drug excreted unchanged in the urine during a dosing interval at steady state and $AUC_{\tau(ss)}$ is the area under the systemic concentration–time curve over the same dosing interval at steady state.

One important note is that by virtue of its method of calculation, the relative bioavailability (F) of the drug is not present in the renal clearance calculations while it always is for the total body clearance. So this means that if systemic concentrations and collected urinary excretion are only obtained after a drug product is administered extravascularly, for example orally, then only an apparent clearance will be calculated (eg, Cl/F and not Cl) while the true renal clearance will be (eg, Cl_R and not Cl_R/F).

Total clearance will be reported as an "apparent" clearance:

$$\frac{Cl}{F} = \frac{Dose}{AUC_{0\text{-inf}}} \quad \text{(after single dose administration)}$$

$$\frac{Cl}{F} = \frac{Dose}{AUC_{\tau(ss)}} \quad \text{(at steady state during a dosing interval)}$$

While the renal clearance will not be "apparent":

$Cl_R = Ae_{0\text{-}x}/AUC_{0\text{-}x}$ (after single dose administration and where x is the maximum length of time during which both urinary excreted amounts and the AUC can be observed; as mentioned earlier it should be a minimum of 3–4 terminal half-lives)

$$Cl_R = \frac{Ae_{\tau(ss)}}{AUC_{\tau(ss)}} \quad \text{(at steady state during a dosing interval)}$$

It can therefore be appreciated that the nonrenal clearance can be readily calculated when the drug product is administered intravenously, as $Cl_{NR} = Cl - Cl_R$. However, this calculation is not possible after extravascular administration if the exact relative bioavailability is not known or assumed as the exact renal clearance can be calculated (Cl_R), but only the apparent clearance can (Cl/F). The nonrenal clearance can only be estimated if the relative bioavailability is assumed. For example, if the relative bioavailability is estimated to be hypothetically between 75% and 100%, then the nonrenal clearance could be presented in the following manner:

$$\frac{Cl}{F} = 10 \text{ L/h} \quad \text{and} \quad Cl_R = 5 \text{ L/h}$$

Therefore,

If F~100%, then Cl_{NR} = 5 L/h (eg, Cl_{NR} = $(Cl/F \times 1) - Cl_R$)

But if F ~ 75%, then Cl_{NR} = 2.5 L/h (eg, Cl_{NR} = $(Cl/F \times 0.75) - Cl_R$)

An alternative approach to obtaining Equation 7.38 is to consider the mass balance of drug cleared by the kidney and ultimately excreted in the urine. For any drug cleared through the kidney, the rate of the drug passing through kidney (via filtration, reabsorption, and/or active secretion) must equal the rate of drug excreted in the urine.

Rate of drug passing through kidney = rate of drug excreted:

$$Cl_R \times C_p = Q_u \times C_u \qquad (7.40)$$

where Cl_R is renal clearance, C_p is plasma drug concentration, Q_u is the rate of urine flow, and C_u is the urine drug concentration. Rearrangement of Equation 7.40 gives

$$Cl_R = \frac{Q_u \times C_u}{C_p} = \frac{\text{Excretion rate}}{C_p} \qquad (7.41)$$

Because the excretion rate = $Q_u C_u = dD_u/dt$, Equation 7.41 is the equivalent of Equation 7.38.

Renal clearance can also be obtained using data modeling and fitting with compartmental methods. The most accurate method to obtain renal clearance as well as total clearance with this method will be to

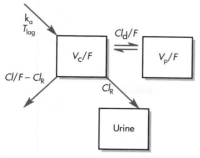

FIGURE 7-8 Schematic description of a hypothetical two-compartment PK model in which plasma concentrations and urinary excreted data would be simultaneously fitted and explained.

model simultaneously observed systemic concentrations with observed excreted urinary amounts over a period of time that allows for robust estimates, so ideally over 3–4 terminal half-lives or longer. As with any data modeling exercise, it is critical to use the simplest model that can explain all the data appropriately and to use a model that is identifiable.

So using the example of a drug administered via the oral route and where the plasma concentration profile is fitted to a two-compartment model and where the excreted urinary amounts are fitted simultaneously, a typical model would look like Fig. 7-8, where the "fitted" pharmacokinetic parameters by the model would be:

- T_{lag} would be the time elapsed after dosing before the beginning of the absorption process
- k_a would be the first-order absorption rate constant
- V_c/F would be the apparent central volume of distribution
- $(Cl/F - Cl_R)$ would be the apparent total clearance that does not include the renal clearance
- Cl_R would be the renal clearance
- Cl_d/F would be the apparent distributional clearance between the central and peripheral volumes of distribution
- V_p/F would be the apparent peripheral volume of distribution

And where the subsequently "derived" or "calculated" pharmacokinetic parameters would be:

- The apparent total clearance, Cl/F, would be the addition of Cl_R to the $(Cl/F - Cl_R)$

- The apparent total volume of distribution, V_{ss}/F, would be the addition of V_c/F to the V_p/F
- The distribution (λ_1) and terminal elimination (λ_z) rate constants would be:
  - $\lambda_1 = [((Cl + Cl_d)/V_c + Cl_d/V_p) + \text{SQRT}((((Cl + Cl_d)/V_c + Cl_d/V_p)^2 - 4 \times Cl/V_c * Cl_d/V_p))]/2$
  - $\lambda_z = [((Cl + Cl_d)/V_c + Cl_d/V_p) - \text{SQRT}((((Cl + Cl_d)/V_c + Cl_d/V_p)^2 - 4 \times Cl/V_c * Cl_d/V_p))]/2$
- The distribution and terminal elimination half-lives would be:
  - $T_{1/2}(\lambda_1) = 0.693/\lambda_1$
  - $T_{1/2}(\lambda_z) = 0.693/\lambda_z$

Comparison of Drug Excretion Methods

Renal clearance may be measured without regard to the physiologic mechanisms involved in the process. From a physiologic viewpoint, however, renal clearance may be considered the ratio of the sum of the glomerular filtration and active secretion rates less the reabsorption rate divided by the plasma drug concentration:

$$Cl_R = \frac{\text{Filtration rate} + \text{Secretion rate} - \text{Reabsorption rate}}{C_p}$$

$$(7.42)$$

The renal clearance of a drug is often related to the renal glomerular filtration rate, GFR, when reabsorption is negligible and the drug is not actively secreted. The renal clearance value for the drug is compared to that of a standard reference, such as inulin, which is cleared completely through the kidney by glomerular filtration only. The *clearance ratio,* which is the ratio of drug clearance to inulin clearance, may give an indication for the mechanism of renal excretion of the drug (Table 7-4). However, further renal drug excretion studies are necessary to confirm unambiguously the mechanism of excretion.

Filtration Only

If glomerular filtration is the sole process for drug excretion, the drug is not bound to plasma proteins, and is not reabsorbed, then the amount of drug filtered at any time (t) will always be $C_p \times$ GFR (Table 7-5). Likewise, if the Cl_R of the drug is by glomerular filtration only, as in the case of inulin, then $Cl_R = $ GFR. Otherwise, Cl_R represents all the processes by which

TABLE 7-4   Comparison of Clearance of a Sample Drug to Clearance of a Reference Drug, Inulin

Clearance Ratio	Probable Mechanism of Renal Excretion
$\dfrac{Cl_{drug}}{Cl_{inulin}} < 1$	Drug is partially reabsorbed
$\dfrac{Cl_{drug}}{Cl_{inulin}} = 1$	Drug is filtered only
$\dfrac{Cl_{drug}}{Cl_{inulin}} > 1$	Drug is actively secreted

the drug is cleared through the kidney, including any combination of filtration, reabsorption, and active secretion.

Filtration and Active Secretion

For a drug that is primarily filtered and secreted, with negligible reabsorption, the overall excretion rate will exceed GFR (Table 7-4). At low drug plasma concentrations, active secretion is not saturated, and the drug is excreted by filtration and active secretion. At high concentrations, the percentage of drug excreted by active secretion decreases due to saturation. Clearance decreases because excretion rate decreases (Fig. 7-9). Clearance decreases because the total excretion rate of the drug increases to the point where it is approximately equal to the filtration rate (Fig. 7-10).

TABLE 7-5   Urinary Drug Excretion Rate[a]

Time (minutes)	C_p (μg/mL)	Excretion Rate (μg/min) (Drug Filtered by GFR per Minute)
0	$(C_p)_0$	$(C_p)_0 \times 125$
1	$(C_p)_1$	$(C_p)_1 \times 125$
2	$(C_p)_2$	$(C_p)_2 \times 125$
T	$(C_p)_t$	$(C_p)_t = 125$

[a]Assumes that the drug is excreted by filtration only, is not plasma protein bound, and that the GFR is 125 mL/min.

Note that the quantity of drug excreted per minute is always the plasma concentration (C_p) multiplied by a constant (eg, 125 mL/min), which in this case is also the renal clearance for the drug. The glomerular filtration rate may be treated as a first-order process relating to C_p.

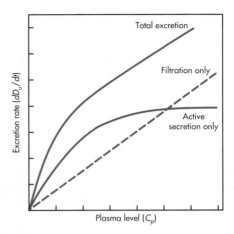

FIGURE 7-9   Excretion rate–plasma level curves for a drug that demonstrate active tubular secretion and a drug that is secreted by glomerular filtration only.

Using compartmental PK even when lacking any knowledge of GFR, active secretion, or the reabsorption process, modeling the data allows the process of drug elimination to be described quantitatively. If a change to a higher-order elimination rate process occurs, then an additional process besides GFR may be involved. The compartmental analysis aids the ultimate development of a model consistent with physiologic functions of the body.

We often relate creatinine clearance (CrCl) to the overall clearance of a drug in clinical practice. This allows clinicians to adjust dosage of drugs depending on a patient's observed renal function. As the renal clearance is the summation of filtration, secretion, and reabsorption, it can be simplified to:

$$Cl_R = \text{Slope} \times \text{CrCl} + \text{Intercept} \qquad (7.43)$$

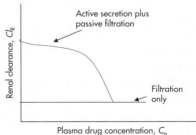

FIGURE 7-10   Graph representing the decline of renal clearance. As the drug plasma level increases to a concentration that saturates the active tubular secretion, glomerular filtration becomes the major component for renal clearance.

where the intercept reflects the reabsorption and secretion processes, assuming that the CrCl only reflects GFR.

Because $Cl = Cl_R + Cl_{NR}$, then

$$Cl = (Slope \times CrCl + Intercept) + Cl_{NR}$$

An assumption that is often made when adjusting doses based on differing renal function is that decreasing renal function does not change the nonrenal clearance (eg, hepatic and/or other clearances). This is a reasonable assumption to make until quite-severe renal impairment is observed at which point changes in protein binding capacity and affinity as well as changes in enzymatic and transporter affinity and/or activity may be seen. Because Cl_{NR} and the intercept are both constants, then overall clearance formula can therefore be simplified to:

$$Cl = (Slope \times CrCl) + Intercept_2 \qquad (7.44)$$

The intercept$_2$ is often simplified to Cl_{NR}, but in reality if CrCl is assumed to only reflect GFR function, then it is really representative of the clearance from kidney secretion and reabsorption as well as from nonrenal routes.

EXAMPLES ▶ ▶ ▶

1. Two drugs, A and B, are entirely eliminated through the kidney by glomerular filtration (125 mL/min), with no reabsorption, and are well described by a one-compartment model. Drug A has half the distribution volume of drug B, and the V_{ss} of drug B is 20 L. What are the drug clearances for each drug using both the compartmental and physiologic approaches?

Solution

Since glomerular filtration of the two drugs is the same, and both drugs are not eliminated by other means, clearance for both drugs depends on renal plasma flow and extraction by the kidney only.

Basing the clearance calculation on the physiologic definition and using Equation 7.18 results in

$$Cl = \frac{Q(C_a - C_v)}{C_a} = 125 \text{ mL/min}$$

Interestingly, known drug clearance tells little about the dosing differences of the two drugs, although it

helps identify the mechanism of drug elimination. In this example, both drugs have the same clearance.

Basing the calculation on the elimination concept and applying Equation 7.14, k_R and λ_z are easily determined, resulting in an obvious difference in the elimination $t_{1/2}$ between the two drugs—in spite of similar drug clearance.

$$k_{R(drug A)} = k_{10(drug A)} = \lambda_{z(drug A)} = \frac{Cl}{V_{ss}}$$

$$= \frac{125}{10 \times 1000} = 0.0125 \text{ min}^{-1}$$

$$k_{R(drug B)} = k_{10(drug B)} = \lambda_{z(drug B)} = \frac{Cl}{V_{ss}}$$

$$= \frac{125}{20 \times 1000} = 0.00625 \text{ min}^{-1}$$

In spite of identical drug clearances, the λ_z for drug A is twice that of drug B. Drug A has an elimination half-life of 55.44 minutes, while that of drug B is 110.88 minutes—much longer because of the bigger volume of distribution.

2. In a subject with a normal GFR (eg, a CrCl of 125 mL/min), the renal clearance of a drug is 10 L/h while the nonrenal clearance is 5 L/h. Assuming no significant secretion and reabsorption, how should we adjust the dosing regimen of the drug if the renal function and the GFR decrease in half (eg, CrCl = 62.5 mL/min)?

Solution

For a patient with "normal GFR":

$Cl = Cl_R + Cl_{NR}$, so $Cl = 15$ L/h

$Cl_R = Slope \times CrCl$, therefore,
slope = $10/(125 \times 60/1000) = 1.33$

For a patient with a GFR that decreases in half:

$Cl_R = Slope \times CrCl = 1.33 \times (62.5 \times 60/1000)$
$= 5$ L/h

$Cl = Cl_R + Cl_{NR} = 5 + 5 = 10$ L/h

The clearance therefore decreased by 33%. In order to reach the same target exposure of the drug (AUC_{inf}), the dose per day will need to be decreased by 33% as Dose = Cl/AUC_{inf}.

DETERMINATION OF RENAL CLEARANCE

Graphical Methods

Clearance is given by the slope of the curve obtained by plotting the rate of drug excretion in urine (dD_u/dt) against C_p (Equation 7.45). For a drug that is excreted rapidly, dD_u/dt is large, the slope is steeper, and clearance is greater (Fig. 7-11, line *A*). For a drug that is excreted slowly through the kidney, the slope is smaller (Fig. 7-11, line *B*).

From Equation 7.35,

$$Cl_R = \frac{dD_u/dt}{C_p}$$

Multiplying both sides by C_p gives

$$Cl_R \times C_p = dD_u/dt \tag{7.45}$$

By rearranging Equation 7.45 and integrating, one obtains

$$[D_u]_{0\text{-}t} = Cl_R \times \text{AUC}_{0\text{-}t} \tag{7.46}$$

A graph is then plotted of cumulative drug excreted in the urine versus the area under the concentration–time curve (Fig. 7-12). Renal clearance is obtained from the slope of the curve. The area under the curve can be

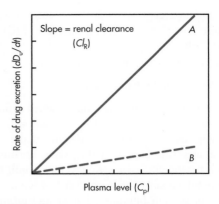

FIGURE 7-12   Rate of drug excretion versus concentration of drug in the plasma. Drug A has a higher clearance than drug B, as shown by the slopes of line *A* and line *B*.

estimated by the trapezoidal rule or by other measurement methods. The disadvantage of this method is that if a data point is missing, the cumulative amount of drug excreted in the urine is difficult to obtain. However, if the data are complete, then the determination of clearance is more accurate by this method.

By plotting cumulative drug excreted in the urine from t_1 to t_2, $(D_u)_{t_1}^{t_2}$ versus $(\text{AUC})_{t_1}^{t_2}$, one obtains an equation similar to that presented previously:

$$[D_u]_{t1\text{-}t2} = Cl_R \times \text{AUC}_{t1\text{-}t2} \tag{7.47}$$

The slope is equal to the renal clearance (Fig. 7-13).

Midpoint Method

From Equation 7.35,

$$Cl_R = \frac{dD_u/dt}{C_p}$$

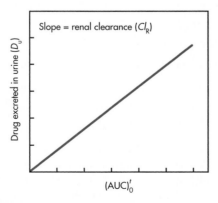

FIGURE 7-11   Cumulative drug excretion versus AUC. The slope is equal to Cl_R.

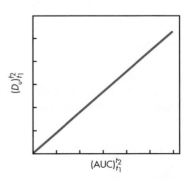

FIGURE 7-13   Drug excreted versus $(\text{AUC})_{t_1}^{t_2}$. The slope is equal to Cl_R.

which can be simplified to

$$Cl_R = \frac{X_{u(0-24)}/C_{p12}}{24} \tag{7.48}$$

where $X_{u(0-24)}$ is the 24-hour excreted urinary amount of the drug obtained by multiplying the collected 24-hour urine volume ($V_{u(0-24)}$) by the measured urinary concentration ($C_{u(0-24)}$) and C_{p12} is the midpoint plasma concentration of the drug measured at the midpoint of the collected interval, here at 12 hours.

This equation is obviously not very robust as it is based on only one measured plasma concentration, but it is often very useful in the clinic when very few plasma concentrations of drugs can be collected and measured. The overall duration of urinary collection is typically 24 hours, but different collection intervals can obviously be used.

PRACTICE PROBLEM

Consider a drug that is eliminated by first-order renal excretion and hepatic metabolism. The drug follows a one-compartment model and is given in a single intravenous or oral dose (Fig. 7-14). Working with the model presented, assume that a single dose (100 mg) of this drug is given orally. The drug has a 90% oral bioavailability. The total amount of unchanged drug recovered in the urine is 60 mg, and the total amount of metabolite recovered in the urine is 30 mg (expressed as milligram equivalents to the parent drug). According to the literature, the elimination half-life for this drug is 3.3 hours and its apparent volume of distribution is

1000 L. From the information given, find **(a)** the apparent clearance and the clearance, **(b)** the renal and nonrenal clearance, **(c)** the formation clearance of the drug to the metabolite, and **(d)** if the drug undergoes another systemic metabolic or elimination route.

Solution

a. Apparent clearance and clearance:

$$\frac{Cl}{F} = K \times \frac{V}{F}$$

$$\frac{Cl}{F} = \frac{0.693}{3.3} \times 1000 = 210 \text{ L/h}$$

$$Cl = \frac{Cl}{F} \times F = 210 \times 0.9 = 189 \text{ L/h}$$

b. Renal and nonrenal clearance:

$$Cl_R = \frac{Ae_{0\text{-inf}}}{AUC_{0\text{-inf}}}$$

and,

$$AUC_{0\text{-inf}} = \frac{DOSE}{Cl/F} = \frac{100}{210} = 0.4762 \text{ mg} \cdot \text{h/L}$$

Therefore,

$$Cl_R = \frac{60}{0.4762} = 126 \text{ L/h}$$

$$Cl_{NR} = 189 - 126 = 63 \text{ L/h}$$

c. Formation clearance of the parent drug to the metabolite:

$$Cl_f = \frac{Ae_{0\text{-inf}}}{AUC_{0\text{-inf}}} = \frac{30}{0.4762} = 63 \text{ L/h}$$

d. Does the drug undergo other elimination or metabolic routes?

$$\frac{Cl}{F} = Cl_R + Cl_{NR} = Cl_R + (Cl_f + Cl_{other})$$

Then, $Cl_{other} = Cl - Cl_R - Cl_f = 189 - 126 - 63 = 0$ L/h

The drug does not undergo additional elimination or metabolic routes.

PRACTICE PROBLEM

An antibiotic is given by IV bolus injection at a dose of 500 mg. The drug follows a one-compartment model. The total volume of distribution was 21 L and the elimination half-life was 6 hours. Urine was collected for 48 hours, and 400 mg of unchanged drug was recovered. What is the fraction of the dose excreted unchanged in the urine? Calculate k, k_R, Cl, Cl_R, and Cl_{NR}.

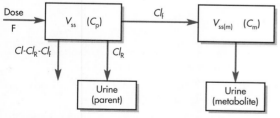

FIGURE 7-14 Model of a drug eliminated by first-order renal excretion and hepatic transformation into a metabolite also excreted in the urine. (Cl_R = renal clearance of parent drug, Cl_f = formation clearance of parent drug to metabolite, C_m = plasma concentration of the metabolite, C_p = plasma concentration of the parent drug, V_{ss} = total volume of distribution of parent drug, $V_{ss(m)}$ = apparent volume of distribution of metabolite, ($Cl - Cl_R - Cl_f$) clearance of parent drug minus the renal and formation clearances, F = absolute bioavailability of parent drug.)

Solution

Since the elimination half-life, $t_{1/2}$, for this drug is 6 hours, a urine collection for 48 hours represents $8 \times t_{1/2}$, which allows for greater than 99% of the drug to be eliminated from the body. The fraction of drug excreted unchanged in the urine, f_e, is obtained by using Equation 7.37 and recalling that $F = 1$ for drugs given by IV bolus injection.

$$f_e = \frac{400}{500} = 0.8$$

Therefore, 80% of the bioavailable dose is excreted in the urine unchanged. Calculations for k, k_R, Cl_T, Cl_R, and Cl_{NR} are given here:

$$k = \frac{0.693}{6} = 0.1155 \text{ h}^{-1}$$

$$k_R = f_e \times k = 0.8 \times 0.1155 = 0.0924 \text{ h}^{-1}$$

$$Cl = k \times V_{ss} = 0.1155 \times 21 = 2.43 \text{ L/h}$$
$$Cl_R = k_R \times V_{ss} = 0.0924 \times 21 = 1.94 \text{ L/h}$$
$$Cl_{NR} = Cl - Cl_R = 2.43 - 1.94 = 0.49 \text{ L/h}$$

RELATIONSHIP OF CLEARANCE TO ELIMINATION HALF-LIFE AND VOLUME OF DISTRIBUTION

A common area of confusion for students is the relationship between half-lives, volumes of distribution, clearances, and noncompartmental-versus-compartmental approaches.

As seen previously, clearances are always related to a rate constant (k) and a volume of distribution (V_d) but these will vary according to the mathematical model that describes appropriately the PK of the drug. Table 7-6 aims at reconciling this.

TABLE 7-6　Relationships between Clearance, Volumes of Distribution, and Half-Life

Appearance of C_p Versus Time	Compartmental Method	Noncompartmental Method
Monoexponential decline	Model after IV administration: $Cl = k_{10} \times V_c$ $V_{ss} = V_c$ as there is only one compartment $\lambda_z = k_{10}$ as there is only one compartment $Cl = Cl_R + Cl_{NR}$ $Cl_R = k_R \times V_c$ $T_{1/2} = 0.693/\lambda_z$	Single dose IV administration: AUC$_{0-t}$ typically calculated with linear or mixed linear/log-linear trapezoidal rule C_t is the last detectable concentration time point.
Biexponential decline	Model after IV administration: $Cl = k_{10} \times V_c$ $V_p = k_{12} \times V_c/k_{21}$ $V_{ss} = V_c + V_p$ $\lambda 1 = [((Cl + Cl_d)/V_c + Cl_d/V_p) + \text{SQRT}(((Cl + Cl_d)/V_c$ $\quad + Cl_d/V_p)^2 - 4 \times Cl/V_c{}^*Cl_d/V_p))]/2$ $\lambda_z = [((Cl + Cl_d)/V_c + Cl_d/V_p) - \text{SQRT}(((Cl+Cl_d)/V_c$ $\quad + Cl_d/V_p)^2 - 4 \times Cl/N_c{}^*Cl_d/V_p))]/2$ $T_{1/2}$ (distribution) $= 0.693/\lambda_1$ $T_{1/2}$ (elimination) $= 0.693/\lambda_z$	λ_z is the negative slope using linear regression of the terminal elimination log-linear phase of the concentration-versus-time profile. $Cl = \text{DOSE}/\text{AUC}_{0-\text{inf}}$ AUC$_{0-\text{inf}}$ = AUC$_{0-t}$ + C_t/λ_z MRT = AUMC$_{0-\text{inf}}$/AUC$_{0-\text{inf}}$ − (Duration of infusion/2) $V_{ss} = Cl \times \text{MRT}$ $T_{1/2}$ (elimination) $= 0.693/\lambda_z$

CHAPTER SUMMARY

Clearance refers to the irreversible removal of drug from the systemic circulation of the body by all routes of elimination. Clearance may be defined as the volume of fluid removed from the drug per unit of time. The clearance of a drug is a very clinically useful parameter as it is related to the systemic exposure of a drug, which dictates efficacy and safety, and its administered dose. Clearance is a constant when the PK behavior of a drug is linear in terms of time and dose. Clearance can be calculated by many different methods, including noncompartmental, compartmental, and physiological. Assuming a specific compartment model, clearance will be the product of an elimination rate constant and a volume of distribution. In the simplest case, a one-compartment model for drugs whose concentration–time profile decreases according to a monoexponential decline,

the clearance will be the product of the terminal elimination rate constant and the total volume of distribution. Clearance is therefore inversely related to the elimination half-life of a drug. Organ clearances are additive, except for lung, and so the total body clearance is often described in terms of renal and nonrenal clearance. The renal clearance is dependent on renal blood flow, glomerular filtration, drug secretion, and reabsorption. Reabsorption of drugs is often a passive process and the extent of reabsorption of weak acid or weak base drugs is influenced by the pH of the urine and the degree of ionization of the drug. In addition, an increase in blood flow to the kidney, which may be due to diuretic therapy or large beer consumption, decreases the extent of drug reabsorption in the kidney and increases the rate of drug excreted in the urine.

LEARNING QUESTIONS

1. Theophylline is effective in the treatment of bronchitis at a blood level of 10–20 μg/mL. At therapeutic range, theophylline follows linear pharmacokinetics. The average $t_{1/2}$ is 3.4 hours, and the range is 1.8–6.8 hours. The average volume of distribution is 30 L.

   a. What are the average upper and lower clearance limits for theophylline assuming a one-compartment model?

   b. The renal clearance of theophylline is 0.36 L/h. What are the k_{NR} and k_R?

2. A single 250-mg oral dose of an antibiotic is given to a young man (age 32 years, creatinine clearance CrCl = 122 mL/min, ABW = 78 kg). From the literature, the drug is known to have an apparent V_{ss} equal to 21% of body weight and an elimination half-life of 2 hours. The dose is normally 90% bioavailable and is not bound significantly to plasma proteins. Urinary excretion of the unchanged drug is equal to 70% of the bioavailable dose.

   a. What is the total body clearance for this drug assuming a one-compartment model?

   b. What is the renal clearance for this drug?

   c. What is the probable mechanism for renal clearance of this drug?

3. A drug with an elimination half-life of 1 hour was given to a male patient (80 kg) by intravenous infusion at a rate of 300 mg/h. At 7 hours after infusion, the plasma drug concentration was 11 μg/mL.

   a. What is the total body clearance for this drug?

   b. What is the apparent V_{ss} for this drug assuming a one-compartment model?

   c. If the drug is not metabolized and is eliminated only by renal excretion, what is the renal clearance of this drug?

   d. What would then be the probable mechanism for renal clearance of this drug?

4. In order to rapidly estimate the renal clearance of a drug in a patient, a 2-hour postdose urine sample was collected and found to contain 200 mg of drug. A midpoint plasma sample was taken (1 hour postdose) and the drug concentration in plasma was found to be 2.5 mg/L. Estimate the renal clearance for this drug in this patient.

5. According to the manufacturer, after the antibiotic cephradine (Velosef), given by IV infusion at a rate of 5.3 mg/kg/h to 9 adult male volunteers (average weight, 71.7 kg), a steady-state serum concentration of 17 μg/mL was measured. Calculate the average clearance for this drug in adults.

6. Cephradine is completely excreted unchanged in the urine, and studies have shown that probenecid given concurrently causes elevation of the serum cephradine concentration. What is the probable mechanism for the interaction of probenecid with cephradine?

7. When deciding on a dosing regimen of a drug to administer to a patient, what information can be obtained from knowing only the elimination half life? The clearance?

8. A patient was given 2500 mg of a drug by IV bolus dose, and periodic urinary data were collected. (a) Determine the renal clearance of

the drug using urinary data. (b) Determine the clearance using the noncompartmental method. (c) Is there any nonrenal clearance of the drug in this patient? What would be the nonrenal clearance, if any? How would you determine clearance using a compartmental approach and compare that with the noncompartmental method?

9. Ciprofloxacin hydrochloride (Cipro) is a fluoroquinolone antibacterial drug used to treat urinary tract infections. Ciprofloxacin contains several pK_as (basic amine and carboxylic group) and may be considered a weak acid and eliminated primarily by renal excretion, although about 15% of a drug dose is metabolized. The serum elimination half-life in subjects with normal renal function is approximately 4 hours. The renal clearance of ciprofloxacin is approximately 300 mL/min. By what processes of renal excretion would you conclude that ciprofloxacin is excreted? Why?

ANSWERS

Frequently Asked Questions

Why is clearance a useful pharmacokinetic parameter?

- Clearance is very useful clinically as it is the only PK parameter that relates to dose and the overall exposure of a drug, for example, $Cl/F = DOSE/AUC_{0\text{-inf}}$.

Which renal elimination processes are influenced by protein binding?

- Only the free drug can be filtered by the kidney, so protein binding influences the filtration of drugs, but it has no significant influences on secretion and reabsorption.

Is clearance a first-order process? Is clearance a better parameter to describe drug elimination and exposure than half-life? Why is it necessary to use both parameters in the literature?

- The clearance of a drug is a constant only if the drug exhibits linear pharmacokinetic characteristics. If the clearance changes with drug concentrations, for example, when metabolism becomes

saturated, then the clearance cannot be described by a constant.

  Clearance is related to the administered dose and the overall exposure of a drug as per the formula $Cl/F = DOSE/AUC_{0\text{-inf}}$. As the exposure of a drug correlates with its efficacy and toxicity, clearance is a much more useful parameter clinically than the terminal half-life as it will directly dictate what dose to administer to a patient in order *to reach a* certain systemic exposure. Although it will not dictate what dose to administer, the terminal half-life will be important in deciding how often to administer a drug. Both parameters are therefore important.

What is the relationship between drug clearance and creatinine clearance?

- The Cl of a drug is composed of the renal (Cl_R) and the nonrenal (Cl_{NR}) components. The Cl_R is composed of filtration, reabsorption, and secretion components. Creatinine is mostly filtrated but also secreted, so the creatinine clearance (CrCl), whether estimated by the Cockcroft and Gault formula or calculated by collecting its urinary excretion, is used in clinical practice to give us an indication of the filtration capacity (eg, GFR) of the kidney in a given patient.

Because $Cl = Cl_R + Cl_{NR}$, and because the CrCl directly correlates with Cl_R, the clearance of a drug can often be expressed as $Cl = (\text{Slope} \times \text{CrCl}) + \text{Intercept}$, where the intercept can often be assumed to mostly reflect the nonrenal clearance component.

Learning Questions

1. a. $Cl = k \times V$, where $V = 30$ L and $k = 0.693/T_{1/2}$

Average $Cl = 30 \times 0.693/3.4 = 6.11$ L/h

Upper $Cl = 30 \times 0.693/1.8 = 11.55$ L/h

Lower $Cl = 30 \times 0.693/6.8 = 3.06$ L/h

b. $Cl_R = k_R \times V$

$k_R = Cl_R/V = 0.36/30 = 0.36$ L/h

$Cl = Cl_R + Cl_{NR}$

$Cl_{NR} = Cl - Cl_R = 6.11 \times 0.36 = 5.75$ L/h

$k_{NR} = Cl_{NR}/V = 5.75/30 = 0.192$ h^{-1}

2. a. $Cl = \lambda_z \times V_{ss}$ as the drug PK is well described by a one-compartment model

$\lambda_z = 0.693/2 = 0.3465$ h^{-1}

$V_{ss} = 0.21 \times 78 = 16.38$ L

$Cl = 0.3465 \times 16.38 = 5.68$ L/h

b. $f_e = 70\%$

$Cl_R = f_e \times Cl = 0.7 \times 5.68 = 3.97$ L/h

c. $Cl_R = 3.97$ L/h $= 66.2$ mL/min

This man has a CrCl of 122 mL/min. Because the Cl_R is less than the CrCl, and because the drug is not bound to plasma protein, then we can expect that the drug is filtered but also reabsorbed with or without being secreted.

3. a. During intravenous infusion, the drug levels will reach more than 99% of the plasma steady-state concentration after 7 half-lives of the drug, 7 hours in this case. So we can assume that steady-state conditions are reached. At steady state,

$$Cl = \frac{R_0}{C_{ss}} = \frac{300}{11} = 27.27 \text{ mg/L}$$

$$Cl = \lambda_z \times V_{ss}$$

b.
$$V_{ss} = \frac{Cl}{\lambda_z} = \frac{27.27}{0.693/1} = 39.354 \text{ L}$$

c. $Cl_R \sim Cl = 27.27$ L/h

d. $Cl_R = 27.27 \times 1000/60 = 454.54$ mL/min

The binding to plasma protein is unknown (eg, only free drug is filtered), the renal function of the patient is unknown, and the molecular weight of the drug is unknown (drugs with large molecular weight are not filtered). So at this point, this drug is likely filtered but we cannot be sure based on the limited information available.

Because the $Cl_R >$ GFR, we know for sure, though, that the drug is actively secreted. It could also be reabsorbed, but we cannot be sure based on the information available.

4. The renal clearance can be calculated using the midpoint clearance formula,

$$Cl_R = \frac{C_{urine} \times \text{Volume urine}}{C_{p(midpoint)}}$$

where $(C_{urine} \times \text{Volume urine}) = 200$ mg.

$$Cl_R = \frac{200}{2.5} = 80 \text{ L per 2 hours, or } 40 \text{ L/h}$$

5. $C_{ss} = \dfrac{R_0}{Cl}$

$$Cl = \frac{R_0}{C_{ss}} = \frac{5.3 \times 71.7}{17} = 22.4 \text{ L/h}$$

6. Probenecid is likely decreasing the renal secretion of cephradine.

7. $Cl/F = \text{DOSE}/\text{AUC}_{0-inf}$, so if the target AUC_{0-inf} is known in order to achieve a desired level of efficacy without significant toxicity, then the dose to administer per day to a patient will be dictated by its Cl/F value.

For example, if the targeted AUC per day is 100 mg/L and the Cl/F in a patient is 1 L/h, then the drug has to be administered at a dose of 100 mg per day.

The elimination half-life will not help us understand what dose per day to administer, but will help us decide how frequently to administer the drug.

For example, if the minimum level of efficacy of the previous drug is seen at 1 mg/L, if its C_{max} at steady state after 100-mg dose per day is 4 mg/L, then the drug can be given every 2 half-lives in order to reach a C_{max} of 4 and a minimum concentration of 1 mg/L at steady state. If the half-life in a patient is 12 hours, then the drug can be administered as 100 mg every 24 hours.

8.

Time (hours)	Plasma Urinary Concentration (μg/mL)	Urinary Volume (mL)	Urinary Concentration (μg/mL)
0	250.00	100.00	0.00
1	198.63	125.00	2880.00
2	157.82	140.00	1901.20
3	125.39	100.00	2114.80
4	99.63	80.00	2100.35
5	79.16	250.00	534.01
6	62.89	170.00	623.96
7	49.97	160.00	526.74
8	39.70	90.00	744.03
9	31.55	400.00	133.01
10	25.06	240.00	176.13

From the data, determine urinary rate of drug excretion per time period by multiplying urinary volume by the urinary concentration for each point. Average C_p for each period by taking the mean of two consecutive points (see table). Plot dD_u/dt versus C_p to determine renal clearance from the slope. The renal clearance from the slope is 1493.4 mL/h (Fig. A-1).

To determine the total body clearance by the area method, the area under the plasma

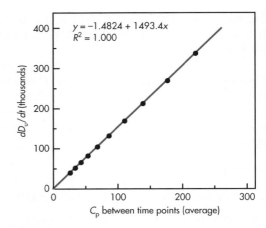

FIGURE A-1

concentration curve [AUC] must be calculated and summed. The tailpiece is extrapolated because the data are not taken to the end. A plot of log C_p versus t (Fig. A-2) yields a slope of $k = 0.23$ h^{-1}. The tailpiece of area is extrapolated using the last data point divided by k or $31.55/0.23 = 137.17$ μg/mL/h.

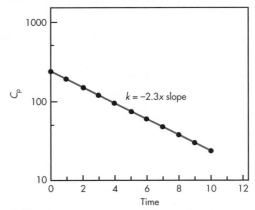

FIGURE A-2

Subtotal area	(0–9 h)	953.97
Tailpiece	(9–∞ h)	137.17
Total area	(0–∞)	1091.14

$$\text{Total clearance} = Cl_T = \frac{FD_0}{[AUC]_0^\infty} = \frac{2{,}500{,}000}{1091.14}$$

$$= 2291.2 \text{ mL/h}$$

Time (hours)	Plasma Concentration (μg/mL)	Urinary Volume (mL)	Urinary Concentration (μg/mL)	Urinary Rate, dD_u/dt (μg/h)	Average C_p
0	250.00	100.00	0	0	
1	198.63	125.00	2680.00	334,999.56	224.32
2	157.82	140.00	1901.20	266,168.41	178.23
3	125.39	100.00	2114.80	211,479.74	141.61
4	99.63	80.00	2100.35	168,027.76	112.51
5	79.16	250.00	534.01	133,503.70	89.39
6	62.89	170.00	623.96	106,073.18	71.03
7	49.97	160.00	526.74	84,278.70	56.43
8	39.70	90.00	744.03	66,962.26	44.84
9	31.55	400.00	133.01	53,203.77	35.63

Because total body clearance is much larger than renal clearance, the drug is probably also excreted by a nonrenal route.

Nonrenal clearance = 2291.2 − 1493.4

= 797.8 mL/h

The easiest way to determine clearance by a compartmental approach is to estimate k and V_D from the graph. V_D is 10 L and k is 0.23 h^{-1}. Total clearance is 2300 mL/min (a slightly different value when compared with the area method).

9. The Cl_R of Ciprofloxacin is larger than the GFR (eg, 300 mL/min) and so the drug is at least secreted in addition to be filtered. Weak acids are known to be secreted.

REFERENCES

Guyton AC: *Textbook of Medical Physiology*, 8th ed. Philadelphia, Saunders, 1991.

Levine RR: *Pharmacology: Drug Actions and Reactions*, 4th ed. Boston, Little, Brown, 1990.

West JB (ed): *Best and Taylor's Physiological Basis of Medical Practice*, 11th ed. Baltimore, Williams & Wilkins, 1985.

BIBLIOGRAPHY

Benet LZ: Clearance (née Rowland) concepts: A downdate and an update. *J Pharmacokinet Pharmacodyn* **37**:529–539, 2010.

Cafruny EJ: Renal tubular handling of drugs. *Am J Med* **62**: 490–496, 1977.

Hewitt WR, Hook JB: The renal excretion of drugs. In Bridges VW, Chasseaud LF (eds.), *Progress in Drug Metabolism*, vol. 7. New York, Wiley, 1983, chap 1.

Holford N, Heo YA, Anderson B. A pharmacokinetic standard for babies and adults. *J Pharm Sci* **102**(9):2941–2952, 2013.

Renkin EM, Robinson RR: Glomerular filtration. *N Engl J Med* **290**:785–792, 1974.

Rowland M, Benet LZ, Graham GG: Clearance concepts in pharmacokinetics. *J Pharm Biopharm* **1**:123–136, 1973.

Smith H: *The Kidney: Structure and Function in Health and Disease.* New York, Oxford University Press, 1951.

Thomson P, Melmon K, Richardson J, et al: Lidocaine pharmacokinetics in advanced heart failure, liver disease and renal failure in humans. *Ann Intern Med* **78**:499–508, 1973.

Tucker GT: Measurement of the renal clearance of drugs. *Br J Clin Pharm* **12**:761–770, 1981.

Weiner IM, Mudge GH: Renal tubular mechanisms for excretion and organic acids and bases. *Am J Med* **36**:743–762, 1964.

Wilkinson GR: Clearance approaches in pharmacology. *Pharmacol Rev* **39**:1–47, 1987.

8 Pharmacokinetics of Oral Absorption

John Z. Duan

Chapter Objectives

▶ Define oral drug absorption and describe the absorption process.

▶ Introduce two general approaches used for studying absorption kinetics and their similarities and differences.

▶ Understand the basic principles for physiologically based absorption kinetics.

▶ Describe the oral one-compartment model and explain how this model simulates drug absorption from the gastrointestinal tract.

▶ Calculate the pharmacokinetic parameters of a drug that follows the oral one-compartment model.

▶ Calculate the fraction of drug absorbed in a one-compartment model using the Wagner–Nelson method.

▶ Calculate the fraction of drug absorbed in a two-compartment model using the Loo–Riegelman method.

▶ Describe the conditions that may lead to flip-flop of k_a and k during pharmacokinetics (PK) data analysis.

INTRODUCTION

Extravascular delivery routes, particularly oral dosing, are important and popular means of drug administration. Unlike intravenous administration, in which the drug is injected directly into the general circulation (see Chapters 4–7), pharmacokinetic models after extravascular drug administration must consider drug absorption from the site of administration, for example, the gut, the lung, etc.

The aim of this chapter is to study the kinetics of absorption. Before delving into the details, it is important to clarify the definition of absorption.

There are three different definitions of absorption in existence. Traditionally, absorption occurs when drug reaches the systemic circulation, or sometimes when it reaches the portal vein blood stream. In recent years, a new definition is presented, in which drug is assumed to be absorbed when it leaves the lumen and crosses the apical membrane of the enterocytes lining the intestine (GastroPlus manual). It is important to distinguish among these definitions when the kinetics study is performed, especially during comparisons of the study results.

Drug absorption from the gastrointestinal (GI) tract or any other extravascular site is dependent on (1) the physicochemical properties of the drug and the environment in the small intestine, (2) the dosage form used, and (3) the anatomy and physiology of the absorption site, such as surface area of the GI tract, stomach-emptying rate, GI mobility, and blood flow to the absorption site. Extravascular drug delivery is further complicated by variables at the absorption site, including possible drug degradation and significant inter- and intrapatient differences in the rate and extent of absorption. The variability in drug absorption can be minimized to some extent by proper biopharmaceutical design of the dosage form to provide predictable and reliable drug therapy (Chapters 15–18). Although this chapter will focus primarily on oral dosing, the concepts discussed here may be easily extrapolated to other extravascular routes.

There are generally two methodologies to study the kinetics of absorption. Pharmacokinetic models can be built based mainly on

▶ Describe the model parameters that form the foundation of drug absorption and bioavailability of oral dosage forms.

▶ Discuss how k_a and k may influence C_{max}, t_{max}, and AUC and how changes in these parameters may affect drug safety in a clinical situation.

the observed clinical data ("top-down" approach) or based on the broader understanding of the human body and its mechanisms ("bottom-up" approach) (Jamei et al, 2009). A top-down model is often specified with the assistance of "black boxes" (such as the compartment model). In a bottom-up approach the elements of the system are first specified in great detail. These elements are then linked together to form larger subsystems, which in turn are linked, sometimes in many levels, until a complete top-level system is formed. The goals of the two approaches are the same: to make physiologically plausible predictions.

This chapter will introduce the basic concept of the physiologically based absorption kinetics (the bottom-up approach) with some examples followed by the detailed explanation of the traditional top-down approach, and finally, the combination of the two approaches is proposed.

BASIC PRINCIPLES OF PHYSIOLOGICALLY BASED ABSORPTION KINETICS (BOTTOM-UP APPROACH)

The physiologically based absorption models provide a quantitative mechanistic framework by which scaled drug-specific parameters can be used to predict the plasma and, importantly, tissue concentration–time profiles of drugs following oral administration. The main advantage of *physiology-based pharmacokinetic* (PBPK) models is that they can be used to extrapolate outside the studied population and experimental conditions. For example, PBPK can be used to extrapolate the absorption process in healthy volunteers to that in a disease population if the relevant physiological properties of the target population are available. The trade-off for this advantage is a complex system of differential equations with a considerable number of model parameters. When these parameters cannot be informed from *in vitro* or *in silico*[1] experiments, PBPK models are usually optimized with respect to observed clinical data. Parameter estimation in complex models is a challenging task associated with many methodological issues.

Historically, PBPK approach stemmed from a natural thinking for elucidating the kinetics of absorption. The first pharmacokinetic model described in the scientific literature was in fact a PBPK model (Teorell, 1937). However, this model led to great difficulty in computations due to lack of computers. Additionally, the *in vitro* science was not advanced enough to obtain the necessary key information. Therefore, the lack of *in vitro* and *in silico* techniques hindered the development of PBPK approach for many

---

[1]*In silico* refers to computer-based models.

years. Recently, PBPK development has been accelerated mainly due to the explosion of computer science and the increasing availability of *in vitro* systems that act as surrogates for *in vivo* reactions relevant to absorption.

Parameter estimation in PBPK models is challenging because of the large number of parameters involved and the relative small amount of observed data usually available. An absorption model consists of a set of values for the absorption scale factors, transit times, pH assignments, compartment geometries (individual compartment radii and lengths, and volume), and pharmacokinetic parameters that provide the best predictions for a compound in human. For example, an advanced absorption transit model developed in *GastroPlus*[TM2] contains nine compartments, which represent the five segments of the GI tract—stomach, duodenum, jejunum, ileum, and colon. The fluid content, carrying dissolved and undissolved compound, passes from one compartment to the next, simulating the action of peristaltic motion. Within each compartment, the dynamic interconversion between dissolved and undissolved compound is modeled. Dissolved compound can be absorbed across the GI tract epithelium. The volume of each compartment, which represents the fluid content, is modeled dynamically, simulating the following processes:

- Transit of the fluid with characteristic rate constants through each compartment
- Gastric secretion into the stomach, and biliary and pancreatic secretions into the duodenum
- Absorption of fluid from duodenum, jejunum, ileum, and large intestine

Figure 8-1 shows the graphic representation of this model. As seen, each of the nine compartments is divided into four subcompartments: unreleased, undissolved, dissolved, and enterocyte.

In the figure, the compartments and subcompartments in GI tract are connected to each other by arrows. These arrows are of either one direction or two directions, indicating the drug transit among these compartments. Each transit process, represented by an arrow in Fig. 8-1, can be expressed by a differential equation. The model equations follow the principles of mass transport, fluid dynamics, and biochemistry in order to simulate the fate of a substance in the body. Most of the equations involve linear kinetics. For example, for non-eliminating tissues, the following principles are followed: the "rate of change of drug in the tissue" is equal to the "rate in" ($Q_T \cdot C_A$) minus the "rate out" ($Q_T \cdot C_{vT}$) as shown in Equation 8.1.

$$V_T \frac{dC_T}{dt} = Q_T C_A - Q_T C_{vT} \qquad (8.1)$$

where Q = blood flow (L/h), C = concentration (mg/L), V = volume (L), T = tissues, A = arterial, v = venous, $C_{vT} = C_T/(K_p/\text{B:P})$, B:P = blood-to-plasma ratio. On the other hand, Michaelis–Menten nonlinear kinetics is used to describe saturable metabolism and carrier-mediated transport.

The PBPK approach can specifically define the absorption for a specific drug product. Figure 8-2 shows the simulation results using PBPK software *GastroPlus* for several drugs with different physicochemical properties. The first column lists the drug names and the second column is the pK_a of the compound. The solubility factor (Sol Factor) is the ratio of the solubility of the completely ionized form of an ionizable group to the completely unionized form. The figure also lists the solubility and logD pH profiles for each drug (two green vertical lines indicate pH 1.2 and 7.5, respectively). Notice that the color of the cells for dose number (Dose No), absorption number (Abs No), and dissolution number (Dis No) changes depending on the physicochemical and biopharmaceutical properties of the drug selected. The colors approximate the four Biopharmaceutical Classification System (BCS) categories. All green indicates high permeability, high solubility, and rapid dissolution (BCS Class I). Red absorption number and green dose number may indicate low permeability and high solubility (BCS Class III). All red may indicate low permeability and low solubility (BCS Class VI). These color systems are not perfect cutoffs for the BCS, but they represent most drugs.

[2]GastroPlus is a mechanistically based simulation software package that simulates absorption, pharmacokinetics, and pharmacodynamics in human and animals (http://www.simulations-plus.com/Products.aspx?GastroPlus&grpID=3&cID=16&pID=11).

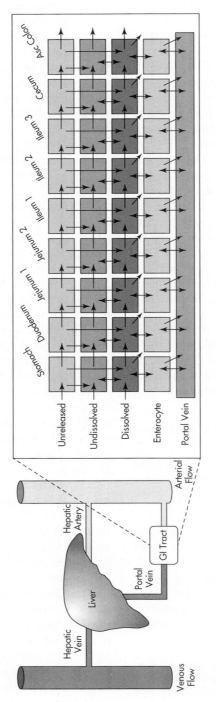

FIGURE 8-1 A graphic representation of drug absorption from the GI tract.

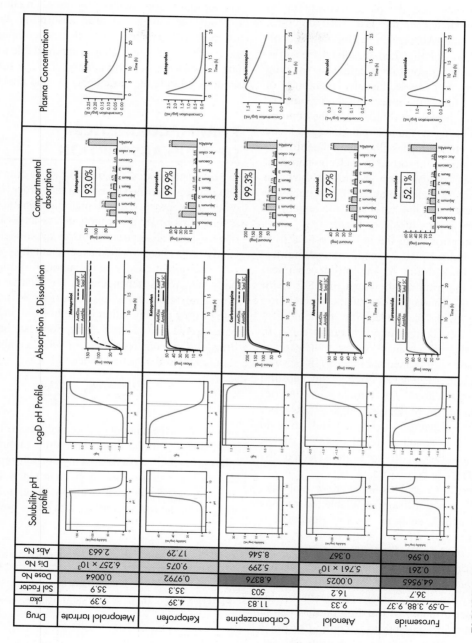

FIGURE 8-2 The modeling results for several drugs using GastroPlus software.

181

Based on the *in vitro* properties and assuming a set of general physiological conditions, the absorption profiles, the absorption amount in each of the nine compartments, and the plasma concentration profiles are predicted in the last three columns, respectively. In the "Absorption & Dissolution" column, the profiles for the total dissolved (red), the absorbed (cyan, the absorption is defined as the drug leaves the lumen and crosses the apical membrane of the enterocytes lining the intestine), the cumulative amount entering portal vein (blue), and the cumulative amount entering systemic circulation (green) are characterized. These profiles along with the information about the amount absorbed in each compartment give the plasma concentration profiles as shown in the last column. As seen, due to the physicochemical property differences, the rate and the extent of absorption vary among the drugs listed.

Drug absorption from the gastrointestinal tract is a highly complex process dependent upon numerous factors. In addition to the physicochemical properties of the drug as shown in Fig. 8-2 (with limited extents), characteristics of the formulation and interplay with the underlying physiological properties of the GI tract play important roles. In GastroPlus, the formulation types that can be selected include both immediate release (IR) formulations (solution, suspension, tablet, and capsule) and controlled release (CR) formulations (enteric-coated or other form of delayed release [DR]). For CR, release of either dissolved material (drug in solution) or undissolved material (solid particles, which then dissolve according to the selected dissolution model) can be evoked.

In addition to GastroPlus, there are several other physiologically based softwares available for studying absorption kinetics, such as *SimCyp* (http://www.simcyp.com/) and *PK-Sim* (http://www.systems-biology.com/products/pk-sim.html).

The major advantage of the PBPK approach is that if adequate information of physicochemical properties of a drug is available, a reasonable prediction for the performance of the drug product can be made with certain assumptions according to previous experience. With little or no human PK data generated, the predictions would be very valuable for further drug development.

ABSOROPTION KINETICS (THE TOP-DOWN APPROACH)

The top-down approach is a traditional methodology to study the kinetics of drug absorption. With the advances of statistical methods and computer science, many software packages are available to calculate the pharmacokinetic parameters. The following sections provide the basic concepts and rationales.

PHARMACOKINETICS OF DRUG ABSORPTION

In pharmacokinetics, the overall rate of drug absorption may be described as either a first-order or a zero-order input process. Most pharmacokinetic models assume first-order absorption unless an assumption of zero-order absorption improves the model significantly or has been verified experimentally.

The rate of change in the amount of drug in the body, dD_B/dt, is dependent on the relative rates of drug absorption and elimination (Fig. 8-3). The net rate of drug accumulation in the body at any time is equal to the rate of drug absorption less the rate of drug elimination, regardless of whether absorption rate is zero-order or first-order.

$$\frac{dD_B}{dt} = \frac{dD_{GI}}{dt} - \frac{dD_E}{dt} \qquad (8.2)$$

where D_{GI} is the amount of drug in the gastrointestinal tract and D_E is the amount of drug eliminated. A plasma level–time curve showing drug absorption and elimination rate processes is given in Fig. 8-4. During the *absorption phase* of a plasma level–time curve (Fig. 8-4), the rate of drug absorption[3] is greater than

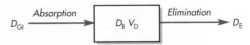

FIGURE 8-3   Model of drug absorption and elimination.

---

[3]The rate of drug absorption is dictated by the product of the drug in the gastrointestinal tract, D_{GI} times the first-order absorption rate constant, k_a.

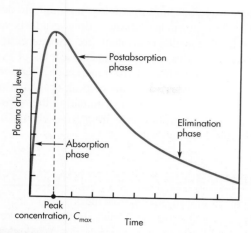

FIGURE 8-4   Plasma level–time curve for a drug given in a single oral dose. The drug absorption and elimination phases of the curve are shown.

the rate of drug elimination.[4] Note that during the absorption phase, elimination occurs *whenever* drug is present in the plasma, even though absorption predominates.

$$\frac{dD_{GI}}{dt} > \frac{dD_E}{dt} \qquad (8.3)$$

At the *peak drug concentration* in the plasma (Fig. 8-4), the rate of drug absorption just equals the rate of drug elimination, and there is no net change in the amount of drug in the body.

$$\frac{dD_{GI}}{dt} = \frac{dD_E}{dt} \qquad (8.4)$$

Immediately after the time of peak drug absorption, some drug may still be at the absorption site (ie, in the GI tract or other site of administration). However, the rate of drug elimination at this time is faster than the rate of absorption, as represented by the *postabsorption phase* in Fig. 8-4.

$$\frac{dD_{GI}}{dt} < \frac{dD_E}{dt} \qquad (8.5)$$

When the drug at the absorption site becomes depleted, the rate of drug absorption approaches zero,

---

[4]The rate of drug elimination is dictated by the product of the amount of drug in the body, D_B times the first-order elimination rate constant, k.

or $dD_{GI}/dt = 0$. The plasma level–time curve (now the *elimination phase*) then represents only the elimination of drug from the body, usually a first-order process. Therefore, during the elimination phase the rate of change in the amount of drug in the body is described as a first-order process:

$$\frac{dD_B}{dt} = -kD_B \qquad (8.6)$$

where k is the first-order elimination rate constant.

Clinical Application

Manini et al (2005) reported a case of adverse drug reaction in a previously healthy young man who ingested a recommended dose of an over-the-counter (OTC) cold remedy containing pseudoephedrine. Forty-five minutes later, he had an acute myocardial infarction (MI). Elevations of cardiac-specific creatinine kinase and cardiac troponin I confirmed the diagnosis. Cardiac magnetic resonance imaging (MRI) confirmed a regional MI. Cardiac catheterization 8 hours later revealed normal coronary arteries, suggesting a mechanism of vasospasm.

1. Could rapid drug absorption (large k_a) contribute to high-peak drug concentration of pseudoephedrine in this subject?
2. Can an adverse drug reaction (ADR) occur before absorption is complete or, before C_{max} is reached?
3. What is the effect of a small change in k on the time and magnitude of C_{max} (maximum plasma concentration)? (Remember to correctly assign k_a and k values when computing k_a and k from patient data. See Flip-flop in oral absorption model in the next section.) In addition, see Chapter 13 for reasons why some subjects may have a smaller k.
4. Do you believe that *therapeutic drug concentration* and *toxic plasma concentration* are always clearly defined for individual subjects as introduced in Fig. 1-2 (see Chapter 1)?

Discussion

From past experience, generally transient high plasma drug concentrations are not considered unsafe as long as the steady-state plasma concentration is within a recommended range. This is generally true for OTC drugs. This case highlights a potential danger of some sympathomimetic drugs such as pseudoephedrine and should alert the pharmacist that even drugs with a long history of safe use may still exhibit dangerous ADRs in some susceptible subjects.

Do you believe that pseudoephedrine can be sold safely without advice from a pharmacist? What other types of medication are important to monitor where a large k_a may present transient high drug concentrations in the blood?

A small elimination rate constant, k may be caused by reduced renal drug excretion as discussed in Chapter 7, but a small k may also be due to reduced hepatic clearance caused by relatively inactive metabolic enzymes such as CYPs for some patients (see Chapter 12). What are the kinetic tools that will allow one to make this differentiation?

The pharmacokinetic concepts presented in this chapter will allow you to decide whether an unusual peak plasma drug concentration, C_{max} is caused by a large k_a, a small k (or Cl), both, or neither.

SIGNIFICANCE OF ABSORPTION RATE CONSTANTS

The overall rate of systemic drug absorption from an orally administered solid dosage form encompasses many individual rate processes, including dissolution of the drug, GI motility, blood flow, and transport of the drug across the capillary membranes and into the systemic circulation. The rate of drug absorption represents the net result of all these processes. The selection of a model with either first-order or zero-order absorption is generally empirical.

The actual drug absorption process may be zero-order, first-order, or a combination of rate processes that is not easily quantitated. For many immediate-release dosage forms, the absorption process is first-order due to the physical nature of drug diffusion. For certain controlled-release drug products, the rate of drug absorption may be more appropriately described by a zero-order rate constant.

The calculation of k_a is useful in designing a multiple-dosage regimen. Knowledge of the k_a and k values allows for the prediction of peak and trough

plasma drug concentrations following multiple dosing. In bioequivalence studies, drug products are given in chemically equivalent (ie, pharmaceutical equivalents) doses, and the respective rates of systemic absorption may not differ markedly. Therefore, for these studies, t_{max}, or time of peak drug concentration, can be very useful in comparing the respective rates of absorption of a drug from chemically equivalent drug products.

ZERO-ORDER ABSORPTION MODEL

Zero-order drug absorption from the dosing site into the plasma usually occurs when either the drug is absorbed by a saturable process or a zero-order controlled-release delivery system is used (see Chapter 19). The pharmacokinetic model assuming zero-order absorption is described in Fig. 8-5. In this model, drug in the gastrointestinal tract, D_{GI}, is absorbed systemically at a constant rate, k_0. Drug is simultaneously and immediately eliminated from the body by a first-order rate process defined by a first-order rate constant, k. This model is analogous to that of the administration of a drug by intravenous infusion (see Chapter 6).

The rate of first-order elimination at any time is equal to $D_B k$. The rate of input is simply k_0. Therefore, the net change per unit time in the body can be expressed as

$$\frac{dD_B}{dt} = k_0 - kD_B \qquad (8.7)$$

Integration of this equation with substitution of $V_D C_p$ for D_B produces

$$C_p = \frac{k_0}{V_D k}(1 - e^{-kt}) \qquad (8.8)$$

The rate of drug absorption is constant until the amount of drug in the gut, D_{GI}, is depleted. The time for complete drug absorption to occur is equal to D_{GI}/k_0. After this time, the drug is no longer available

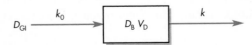

FIGURE 8-5 One-compartment pharmacokinetic model for zero-order drug absorption and first-order drug elimination.

for absorption from the gut, and Equation 8.7 no longer holds. The drug concentration in the plasma subsequently declines in accordance with a first-order elimination rate process.

CLINICAL APPLICATION— TRANSDERMAL DRUG DELIVERY

The stratum corneum (horny layer) of the epidermis of the skin acts as a barrier and rate-limiting step for systemic absorption of many drugs. After application of a transdermal system (patch), the drug dissolves into the outer layer of the skin and is absorbed by a pseudo first-order process due to high concentration and is eliminated by a first-order process. Once the patch is removed, the residual drug concentrations in the skin continues to decline by a first-order process.

Ortho Evra is a combination transdermal contraceptive patch with a contact surface area of 20 cm². Each patch contains 6.00 mg norelgestromin (NGMN) and 0.75 mg ethinyl estradiol (EE) and is designed to deliver 0.15 mg of NGMN and 0.02 mf EE to the systemic circulation daily. As shown in Fig. 8-6, serum EE (ethinyl estradiol) is absorbed from the patch at a zero-order rate.

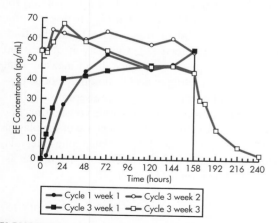

FIGURE 8-6   Mean serum EE concentrations (pg/mL) in healthy female volunteers following application of Ortho Evra on the buttock for three consecutive cycles (vertical arrow indicates time of patch removal). (Adapted from approved label for Ortho Evra, September, 2009.)

FIRST-ORDER ABSORPTION MODEL

Although zero-order drug absorption can occur, systemic drug absorption after oral administration of a drug product (eg, tablet, capsule) is usually assumed to be a first-order process. This model assumes a first-order input across the gut wall and first-order elimination from the body (Fig. 8-7). This model applies mostly to the oral absorption of drugs in solution or rapidly dissolving dosage (immediate release) forms such as tablets, capsules, and suppositories. In addition, drugs given by intramuscular or subcutaneous aqueous injections may also be described using a first-order process.

After oral administration of a drug product, the drug is relased from the drug product and dissolves into the fluids of the GI tract. In the case of an immediate-release compressed tablet, the tablet first disintegrates into fine particles from which the drug then dissolves into the fluids of the GI tract. Only drug in solution is absorbed into the body. The rate of disappearance of drug from the gastrointestinal tract is described by

$$\frac{dD_{GI}}{dt} = -k_a D_{GI} F \tag{8.9}$$

where k_a is the first-order absorption rate constant from the GI tract, F is the fraction absorbed, and D_{GI} is the amount of drug in solution in the GI tract at any time t. Integration of the differential Equation (8.8) gives

$$dD_{GI} = D_0 e^{-k_a t} \tag{8.10}$$

where D_0 is the dose of the drug.

The rate of drug elimination is described by a first-order rate process for most drugs and is equal to $-kD_B$. The rate of drug change in the body, dD_B/dt,

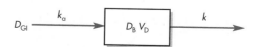

FIGURE 8-7   One-compartment pharmacokinetic model for first-order drug absorption and first-order elimination.

is therefore the rate of drug in, minus the rate of drug out—as given by the differential equation, Equation 8.10:

$$\frac{dD_B}{dt} = \text{rate in} - \text{rate out}$$

(8.11)

$$\frac{dD_B}{dt} = Fk_a D_{GI} - kD_B$$

where F is the fraction of drug absorbed systemically. Since the drug in the gastrointestinal tract also follows a first-order decline (ie, the drug is absorbed across the gastrointestinal wall), the amount of drug in the gastrointestinal tract at any time t is equal to $D_0 e^{-k_a t}$.

$$\frac{dD_B}{dt} = Fk_a D_0 e^{-k_a t} - kD_B$$

The value of F may vary from 1 for a fully absorbed drug to 0 for a drug that is completely unabsorbed. This equation can be integrated to give the general oral absorption equation for calculation of the drug concentration (C_p) in the plasma at any time t, as shown below.

$$C_p = \frac{Fk_a D_0}{V_D(k_a - k)}(e^{-kt} - e^{-k_a t})$$

(8.12)

A typical plot of the concentration of drug in the body after a single oral dose is presented in Fig. 8-8.

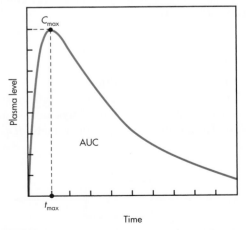

FIGURE 8-8 Typical plasma level–time curve for a drug given in a single oral dose.

The maximum plasma concentration after oral dosing is C_{max}, and the time needed to reach maximum concentration is t_{max}. The t_{max} is independent of dose and is dependent on the rate constants for absorption (k_a) and elimination (k) (Equation 8.13). At C_{max}, sometimes called *peak concentration*, the rate of drug absorbed is equal to the rate of drug eliminated. Therefore, the net rate of concentration change is equal to zero. At C_{max}, the rate of concentration change can be obtained by differentiating Equation 8.11, as follows:

$$\frac{dC_p}{dt} = \frac{Fk_a D_0}{V_D(k_a - k)}(-ke^{-kt} + k_a e^{-k_a t}) = 0 \quad (8.13)$$

This can be simplified as follows:

$$-ke^{-kt} + k_a e^{-k_a t} = 0 \quad \text{or} \quad ke^{-kt} = k_a e^{-k_a t}$$

$$\ln k - kt = \ln k_a - k_a t$$

$$t_{max} = \frac{\ln k_a - \ln k}{k_a - k} = \frac{\ln (k_a / k)}{k_a - k}$$

$$t_{max} = \frac{2.3 \log (k_a / k)}{k_a - k}$$

(8.14)

As shown in Equation 8.13, the time for maximum drug concentration, t_{max}, is dependent only on the rate constants k_a and k. In order to calculate C_{max}, the value for t_{max} is determined via Equation 8.13 and then substituted into Equation 8.11, solving for C_{max}. Equation 8.11 shows that C_{max} is directly proportional to the dose of drug given (D_0) and the fraction of drug absorbed (F). Calculation of t_{max} and C_{max} is usually necessary, since direct measurement of the maximum drug concentration may not be possible due to improper timing of the serum samples.

The first-order elimination rate constant may be determined from the elimination phase of the plasma level–time curve (Fig. 8-4). At later time intervals, when drug absorption has been completed, that is, $e^{-k_a t} \approx 0$, Equation 8.11 reduces to

$$C_p = \frac{Fk_a D_0}{V_D(k_a - k)} e^{-kt}$$

(8.15)

Taking the natural logarithm of this expression,

$$\ln C_p = \ln \frac{Fk_a D_0}{V_D(k_a - k)} - kt$$

(8.16)

Substitution of common logarithms gives

$$\log C_p = \log \frac{Fk_a D_0}{V_D(k_a - k)} - \frac{kt}{2.3} \quad (8.17)$$

With this equation, a graph constructed by plotting $\log C_p$ versus time will yield a straight line with a slope of $-k/2.3$ (Fig. 8-9A).

With a similar approach, urinary drug excretion data may also be used for calculation of the first-order elimination rate constant. The rate of drug excretion after a single oral dose of drug is given by

$$\frac{dD_u}{dt} = \frac{Fk_a k_e D_0}{k_a - k} - (e^{-kt} - e^{-k_a t}) \quad (8.18)$$

where dD_u/dt = rate of urinary drug excretion, k_e = first-order renal excretion constant, and F = fraction of dose absorbed.

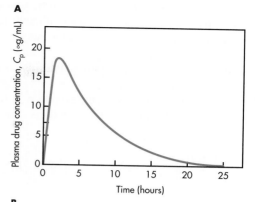

A

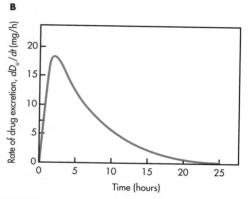

B

FIGURE 8-10   A. Plasma drug concentration versus time, single oral dose. B. Rate of urinary drug excretion versus time, single oral dose.

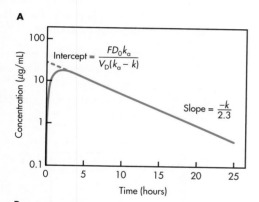

A

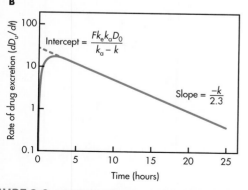

B

FIGURE 8-9   A. Plasma drug concentration versus time, single oral dose. B. Rate of urinary drug excretion versus time, single oral dose.

A graph constructed by plotting dD_u/dt versus time will yield a curve identical in appearance to the plasma level–time curve for the drug (Fig. 8-10B). After drug absorption is virtually complete, $-e^{-k_a t}$ approaches zero, and Equation 8.18 reduces to

$$\frac{dD_u}{dt} = \frac{Fk_a k_e D_0}{k_a - k} e^{-kt} \quad (8.19)$$

Taking the natural logarithm of both sides of this expression and substituting for common logarithms, Equation 8.19 becomes

$$\log \frac{dD_u}{dt} = \log \frac{Fk_a k_e D_0}{k_a - k} - \frac{kt}{2.3} \quad (8.20)$$

When $\log(dD_u/dt)$ is plotted against time, a graph of a straight line is obtained with a slope of

−$k/2.3$ (Fig. 8-9B). Because the rate of urinary drug excretion, dD_u/dt, cannot be determined directly for any given time point, an average rate of urinary drug excretion is obtained (see also Chapter 4), and this value is plotted against the midpoint of the collection period for each urine sample.

To obtain the cumulative drug excretion in the urine, Equation 8.18 must be integrated, as shown below.

$$D_u = \frac{Fk_a k_e D_0}{k_a - k}\left(\frac{-e^{-k_a t}}{k_a} - \frac{e^{-kt}}{k}\right) + \frac{Fk_e D_0}{k} \qquad (8.21)$$

A plot of D_u versus time will give the urinary drug excretion curve described in Fig. 8-11. When all of the drug has been excreted, at $t = \infty$, Equation 8.21 reduces to

$$D_u^\infty = \frac{Fk_e D_0}{k} \qquad (8.22)$$

where D_u^∞ is the maximum amount of active or parent drug excreted.

Determination of Absorption Rate Constants from Oral Absorption Data

Method of Residuals

Assuming $k_a \gg k$ in Equation 8.12, the value for the second exponential will become insignificantly small with time (ie, $e^{-k_a t} \approx 0$) and can therefore be omitted. When this is the case, drug absorption is

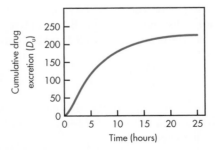

FIGURE 8-11 Cumulative urinary drug excretion versus time, single oral dose. Urine samples are collected at various time periods after the dose. The amount of drug excreted in each sample is added to the amount of drug recovered in the previous urine sample (cumulative addition). The total amount of drug recovered after all the drug is excreted is D_u^∞.

virtually complete. Equation 8.12 then reduces to Equation 8.23.

$$C_p = \frac{Fk_a D_0}{V_D(k_a - k)}e^{-kt} \qquad (8.23)$$

From this, one may also obtain the intercept of the y axis (Fig. 8-12).

$$\frac{Fk_a D_0}{V_D(k_a - k)} = A$$

where A is a constant. Thus, Equation 8.23 becomes

$$C_p = Ae^{-kt} \qquad (8.24)$$

This equation, which represents first-order drug elimination, will yield a linear plot on semilog paper. The slope is equal to $-k/2.3$. The value for k_a can be obtained by using the method of residuals or a feathering technique, as described in Chapter 5. The value of k_a is obtained by the following procedure:

1. Plot the drug concentration versus time on semilog paper with the concentration values on the logarithmic axis (Fig. 8-12).
2. Obtain the slope of the terminal phase (line BC, Fig. 8-12) by extrapolation.

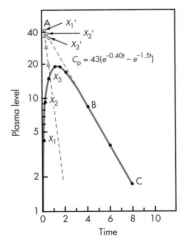

FIGURE 8-12 Plasma level–time curve for a drug demonstrating first-order absorption and elimination kinetics. The equation of the curve is obtained by the method of residuals.

3. Take any points on the upper part of line BC (eg, x'_1, x'_2, x'_3, ...) and drop vertically to obtain corresponding points on the curve (eg, x_1, x_2, x_3, ...).

4. Read the concentration values at x_1 and x'_1, x_2 and x'_2, x_3 and x'_3, and so on. Plot the values of the differences at the corresponding time points Δ_1, Δ_2, Δ_3, ... A straight line will be obtained with a slope of $-k_a/2.3$ (Fig. 8-12).

When using the method of residuals, a minimum of three points should be used to define the straight line. Data points occurring shortly after t_{max} may not be accurate, because drug absorption is still continuing at that time. Because this portion of the curve represents the postabsorption phase, only data points from the elimination phase should be used to define the rate of drug absorption as a first-order process.

If drug absorption begins immediately after oral administration, the residual lines obtained by feathering the plasma level–time curve (as shown in Fig. 8-12) will intersect on the y axis at point A. The value of this y intercept, A, represents a hybrid constant composed of k_a, k, V_D, and FD_0. The value of A has no direct physiologic meaning (see Equation 8.24).

$$A = \frac{Fk_a D_0}{V_D(k_a - k)}$$

The value for A, as well as the values for k and k_a, may be substituted back into Equation 8.11 to obtain a general theoretical equation that will describe the plasma level–time curve.

Lag Time

In some individuals, absorption of drug after a single oral dose does not start immediately, due to such physiologic factors as stomach-emptying time and intestinal motility. The time delay prior to the commencement of first-order drug absorption is known as *lag time*.

The lag time for a drug may be observed if the two residual lines obtained by feathering the oral absorption plasma level–time curve intersect at a point greater than $t = 0$ on the x axis. The time at the point of intersection on the x axis is the lag time (Fig. 8-13).

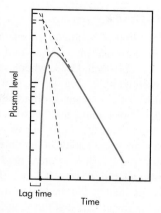

FIGURE 8-13   The lag time can be determined graphically if the two residual lines obtained by feathering the plasma level–time curve intersect at a point where $t > 0$.

The lag time, t_0, represents the beginning of drug absorption and should not be confused with the pharmacologic term *onset time*, which represents latency, that is, the time required for the drug to reach minimum effective concentration.

Two equations can adequately describe the curve in Fig. 8-13. In one, the lag time t_0 is subtracted from each time point, as shown in Equation 8.25.

$$C_p = \frac{Fk_a D_0}{V_D(k_a - k)}(e^{-k(t-t_0)} - e^{-k_a(t-t_0)}) \qquad (8.25)$$

where $Fk_a D_0/V_D(k_a - k)$ is the y value at the point of intersection of the residual lines in Fig. 8-13.

The second expression that describes the curve in Fig. 8-13 omits the lag time, as follows:

$$C_p = Be^{-kt} - Ae^{-k_a t} \qquad (8.26)$$

where A and B represent the intercepts on the y axis after extrapolation of the residual lines for absorption and elimination, respectively.

Frequently Asked Question

▶ *If drug absorption is simulated using the oral one-compartment model, would a larger absorption rate constant result in a greater amount of drug absorbed?*

Flip-Flop of k_a and k

In using the method of residuals to obtain estimates of k_a and k, the terminal phase of an oral absorption curve is usually represented by k, whereas the steeper slope is represented by k_a (Fig. 8-14). In a few cases, the elimination rate constant k obtained from oral absorption data does not agree with that obtained after intravenous bolus injection. For example, the k obtained after an intravenous bolus injection of a bronchodilator was 1.72 h^{-1}, whereas the k calculated after oral administration was 0.7 h^{-1} (Fig. 8-14). When k_a was obtained by the method of residuals, the rather surprising result was that the k_a was 1.72 h^{-1}.

Apparently, the k_a and k obtained by the method of residuals have been interchanged. This phenomenon is called *flip-flop* of the absorption and elimination rate constants. Flip-flop, or the reversal of the rate constants, may occur whenever k_a and k are estimated from oral drug absorption data. Use of computer methods does not ensure against flip-flop of the two constants estimated.

In order to demonstrate unambiguously that the steeper curve represents the elimination rate for a drug given extravascularly, the drug must be given by intravenous injection into the same patient. After intravenous injection, the decline in plasma drug levels over time represents the true elimination rate. The relationship between k_a and k on the shape of the plasma drug concentration–time curve for a constant dose of drug given orally is shown in Fig. 8-14.

Most of the drugs observed to have flip-flop characteristics are drugs with fast elimination (ie, $k > k_a$). Drug absorption of most drug solutions or fast-dissolving products is essentially complete or at least half-complete within an hour (ie, absorption half-life of 0.5 or 1 hour, corresponding to a k_a of 1.38 h^{-1} or 0.69 h^{-1}). Because most of the drugs used orally have longer elimination half-lives compared to absorption half-lives, the assumption that the smaller slope or smaller rate constant (ie, the terminal phase of the curve in Fig. 8-14) should be used as the elimination constant is generally correct.

For drugs that have a large elimination rate constant ($k > 0.69$ h^{-1}), the chance for flip-flop of k_a and k is much greater. The drug isoproterenol, for example, has an oral elimination half-life of only a few minutes, and flip-flop of k_a and k has been noted (Portmann, 1970). Similarly, salicyluric acid was flip-flopped when oral data were plotted. The k for salicyluric acid was much larger than its k_a (Levy et al, 1969). Many experimental drugs show flip-flop of k and k_a, whereas few marketed oral drugs do. Drugs with a large k are usually considered to be unsuitable for an oral drug product due to their large elimination rate constant, corresponding to a very short elimination half-life. An extended-release drug product may slow the absorption of a drug, such that the k_a is smaller than the k and producing a flip-flop situation.

> **Frequently Asked Question**
> ▶ *How do you explain that k_a is often greater than k with most drugs?*

Determination of k_a by Plotting Percent of Drug Unabsorbed Versus Time (Wagner–Nelson Method)

The Wagner–Nelson method may be used as an alternative means of calculating k_a. This method estimates the loss of drug from the GI over time, whose slope is inversely proportional to k_a. After a single oral dose of a drug, the total dose should be completely accounted for for the amount present in the body, the amount present in the urine, and the amount present in the GI tract. Therefore, dose (D_0) is expressed as follows:

$$D_0 = D_{GI} + D_B + D_u \qquad (8.27)$$

Let Ab $= D_B + D_u =$ amount of drug absorbed and let Ab$^\infty =$ amount of drug absorbed at $t = \infty$. At any given time the fraction of drug absorbed is Ab/Ab$^\infty$,

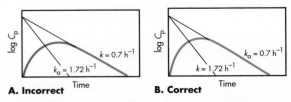

FIGURE 8-14   Flip-flop of k_a and k. Because $k > k_a$, the right-hand figure and slopes represent the correct values for k_a and k.

and the fraction of drug unabsorbed is $1 - (Ab/Ab^\infty)$. The amount of drug excreted at any time t can be calculated as

$$D_u = kV_D[AUC]_0^t \qquad (8.28)$$

The amount of drug in the body (D_B) at any time $= C_pV_D$. At any time t, the amount of drug absorbed (Ab) is

$$Ab = C_pV_D + kV_D[AUC]_0^t \qquad (8.29)$$

At $t = \infty$, $C_p^\infty = 0$ (ie, plasma concentration is negligible), and the total amount of drug absorbed is

$$Ab^\infty = 0 + kV_D[AUC]_0^\infty \qquad (8.30)$$

The fraction of drug absorbed at any time is

$$\frac{Ab}{Ab^\infty} = \frac{C_pV_D + kV_D[AUC]_0^t}{kV_D[AUC]_0^\infty} \qquad (8.31)$$

$$\frac{Ab}{Ab^\infty} = \frac{C_p + k[AUC]_0^t}{k[AUC]_0^\infty} \qquad (8.32)$$

The fraction unabsorbed at any time t is

$$1 - \frac{Ab}{Ab^\infty} = 1 - \frac{C_p + k[AUC]_0^t}{k[AUC]_0^\infty} \qquad (8.33)$$

The drug remaining in the GI tract at any time t is

$$D_{GI} = D_0 e^{-k_a t} \qquad (8.34)$$

Therefore, the fraction of drug remaining is

$$\frac{D_{GI}}{D_0} = e^{-k_a t} \quad \log \frac{D_{GI}}{D_0} = \frac{-k_a t}{2.3} \qquad (8.35)$$

Because D_{GI}/D_0 is actually the fraction of drug *unabsorbed*—that is, $1 - (Ab/Ab^\infty)$—a plot of $1 - (Ab/Ab^\infty)$ versus time gives $-k_a/2.3$ as the slope (Fig. 8-15).

The following steps should be useful in determination of k_a:

1. Plot log concentration of drug versus time.
2. Find k from the terminal part of the slope when the slope $= -k/2.3$.
3. Find $[AUC]_0^t$ by plotting C_p versus t.
4. Find $k[AUC]_0^t$ by multiplying each $[AUC]_0^t$ by k.

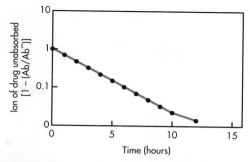

FIGURE 8-15 Semilog graph of data in Table 8-2, depicting the fraction of drug unabsorbed versus time using the Wagner–Nelson method.

5. Find k by adding up all the $[AUC]$ pieces, from $t = 0$ to $t = \infty$.
6. Determine the $1 - (Ab/Ab^\infty)$ value corresponding to each time point t by using Table 8-1.
7. Plot $1 - (Ab/Ab^\infty)$ versus time on semilog paper, with $1 - (Ab/Ab^\infty)$ on the logarithmic axis.

If the fraction of drug unabsorbed, $1 - Ab/Ab^\infty$, gives a linear regression line on a semilog graph, then the rate of drug absorption, dD_{GI}/dt, is a first-order process. Recall that $1 - Ab/Ab^\infty$ is equal to dD_{GI}/dt (Fig. 8-15).

As the drug approaches 100% absorption, C_p becomes very small and difficult to assay accurately. Consequently, the terminal part of the line described by $1 - Ab/Ab^\infty$ versus time tends to become scattered or nonlinear. This terminal part of the curve is excluded, and only the initial linear segment of the curve is used for the estimate of the slope.

PRACTICE PROBLEM

Drug concentrations in the blood at various times are listed in Table 8-1. Assuming the drug follows a one-compartment model, find the k_a value, and compare it with the k_a value obtained by the method of residuals.

Solution

The AUC is approximated by the trapezoidal rule. This method is fairly accurate when there are sufficient data points. The area between each time point

TABLE 8-1   Blood Concentrations and Associated Data for a Hypothetical Drug

Time t_n (h)	Concentration C_p ($\mu g/mL$)	$[AUC]_{t_{n-1}}^{t_n}$	$[AUC]_0^t$	$k[AUC]_0^t$	$C_p + k[AUC]_0^t$	$\dfrac{Ab}{Ab^\infty}$	$\left(1 - \dfrac{Ab}{Ab^\infty}\right)$
0	0	0	0				1.000
1	3.13	1.57	1.57	0.157	3.287	0.328	0.672
2	4.93	4.03	5.60	0.560	5.490	0.548	0.452
3	5.86	5.40	10.99	1.099	6.959	0.695	0.305
4	6.25	6.06	17.05	1.705	7.955	0.794	0.205
5	6.28	6.26	23.31	2.331	8.610	0.856	0.140
6	6.11	6.20	29.51	2.951	9.061	0.905	0.095
7	5.81	5.96	35.47	3.547	9.357	0.934	0.066
8	5.45	5.63	41.10	4.110	9.560	0.955	0.045
9	5.06	5.26	46.35	4.635	9.695	0.968	0.032
10	4.66	4.86	51.21	5.121			
12	3.90	8.56	59.77	5.977			
14	3.24	7.14	66.91	6.691			
16	2.67	5.92	72.83	7.283			
18	2.19	4.86	77.69	7.769			
24	1.20	10.17	87.85	8.785			
28	0.81	4.02	91.87	9.187			
32	0.54	2.70	94.57	9.457			
36	0.36	1.80	96.37	9.637			
48	0.10	2.76	99.13	9.913			

$k = 0.1$ h^{-1}.

is calculated as

$$[AUC]_{t_{n-1}}^{t_n} = \frac{C_{n-1} + C_n}{2}(t_n - t_{n-1}) \qquad (8.36)$$

where C_n and C_{n-1} are concentrations. For example, at $n = 6$, the [AUC] is

$$\frac{6.28 + 6.11}{2}(6 - 5) = 6.20$$

To obtain $[AUC]_0^\infty$, add all the area portions under the curve from zero to infinity. In this case, 48 hours is long enough to be considered infinity, because the blood concentration at that point already

has fallen to an insignificant drug concentration, 0.1 $\mu g/mL$. The rest of the needed information is given in Table 8-1. Notice that k is obtained from the plot of log C_p versus t; k was found in this example to be 0.1 h^{-1}. The plot of $1 - (Ab/Ab^\infty)$ versus t on semilog paper is shown in Fig. 8-15.

A more complete method of obtaining k_a is to estimate the residual area from the last observed plasma concentration, C_p at t_n to time equal to infinity. This equation for the residual AUC from C_p to time equal to infinity is

$$[AUC]_t^\infty = \frac{C_{p_n}}{k} \qquad (8.37)$$

The total $[AUC]_0^\infty$ is the sum of the areas obtained by the trapezoidal rule, $[AUC]_0^t$, and the residual area $[AUC]_t^\infty$, as described in the following expression:

$$[AUC]_0^\infty = [AUC]_0^t + [AUC]_t^\infty \qquad (8.38)$$

Estimation of k_a from Urinary Data

The absorption rate constant may also be estimated from urinary excretion data, using a plot of percent of drug unabsorbed versus time. For a one-compartment model:

Ab = total amount of drug absorbed—that is, the amount of drug in the body plus the amount of drug excreted

D_B = amount of drug in the body

D_u = amount of unchanged drug excreted in the urine

C_p = plasma drug concentration

D_E = total amount of drug eliminated (drug and metabolites)

$$Ab = D_B + D_E \qquad (8.39)$$

The differential of Equation 8.39 with respect to time gives

$$\frac{dAb}{dt} = \frac{dD_B}{dt} + \frac{dD_E}{dt} \qquad (8.40)$$

Assuming first-order elimination kinetics with renal elimination constant k_e,

$$\frac{dD_u}{dt} = k_e D_B = k_e V_D C_p \qquad (8.41)$$

Assuming a one-compartment model,

$$V_D C_p = D_B$$

Substituting $V_D C_p$ into Equation 8.40,

$$\frac{dAb}{dt} = V_D \frac{dC_p}{dt} + \frac{dD_E}{dt} \qquad (8.42)$$

And rearranging Equation 8.41,

$$C_p = \frac{1}{k_e V_D} \left(\frac{dD_u}{dt} \right) \qquad (8.43)$$

$$\frac{dC_p}{dt} = \frac{d(dD_u/dt)}{dt \, k_e V_D} \qquad (8.44)$$

Substituting for dC_p/dt into Equation 8.42 and kD_u/k_e for D_E,

$$\frac{dAb}{dt} = \frac{d(dD_u/dt)}{k_e \, dt} + \frac{k}{k_e} \left(\frac{dD_u}{dt} \right) \qquad (8.45)$$

When the above expression is integrated from zero to time t,

$$Ab_t = \frac{1}{k_e} \left(\frac{dD_u}{dt} \right)_t + \frac{k}{k_e} (D_u)_t \qquad (8.46)$$

At $t = \infty$, all the drug that is ultimately absorbed is expressed as Ab^∞ and $dD_u/dt = 0$. The total amount of drug absorbed is

$$Ab^\infty = \frac{k}{k_e} D_u^\infty$$

where D_u^∞ is the total amount of unchanged drug excreted in the urine.

The fraction of drug absorbed at any time t is equal to the amount of drug absorbed at this time, Ab_t, divided by the total amount of drug absorbed, Ab^∞.

$$\frac{Ab_t}{Ab^\infty} = \frac{(dD_u/dt)_t + k(D_u)_t}{kD_u^\infty} \qquad (8.47)$$

A plot of the fraction of drug unabsorbed, $1 - Ab/Ab^\infty$, versus time gives $-k_a/2.3$ as the slope from which the absorption rate constant is obtained (Fig. 8-15; refer to Equation 8.35).

When collecting urinary drug samples for the determination of pharmacokinetic parameters, one should obtain a valid urine collection as discussed in Chapter 4. If the drug is rapidly absorbed, it may be difficult to obtain multiple early urine samples to describe the absorption phase accurately. Moreover, drugs with very slow absorption will have low concentrations, which may present analytical problems.

Effect of k_a and k on C_{max}, t_{max}, and AUC

Changes in k_a and k may affect t_{max}, C_{max}, and AUC as shown in Table 8-2. If the values for k_a and k are reversed, then the same t_{max} is obtained, but the C_{max} and AUC are different. If the elimination rate constant is kept at 0.1 h^{-1} and the k_a changes from 0.2 to 0.6 h^{-1} (absorption rate increases), then the t_{max} becomes shorter (from 6.93 to 3.58 hours), the C_{max} increases

TABLE 8-2   Effects of the Absorption Rate Constant and Elimination Rate[a]

Absorption Rate Constant, k_a (h⁻¹)	Elimination Rate Constant, k (h⁻¹)	t_{max} (h)	C_{max} (μg/mL)	AUC (μg · h/mL)
0.1	0.2	6.93	2.50	50
0.2	0.1	6.93	5.00	100
0.3	0.1	5.49	5.77	100
0.4	0.1	4.62	6.29	100
0.5	0.1	4.02	6.69	100
0.6	0.1	3.58	6.99	100
0.3	0.1	5.49	5.77	100
0.3	0.2	4.05	4.44	50
0.3	0.3	3.33	3.68	33.3
0.3	0.4	2.88	3.16	25
0.3	0.5	2.55	2.79	20

[a]t_{max} = peak plasma concentration, C_{max} = peak drug concentration, AUC = area under the curve. Values are based on a single oral dose (100 mg) that is 100% bioavailable ($F = 1$) and has an apparent V_D of 10 L. The drug follows a one-compartment open model. t_{max} is calculated by Equation 8.14 and C_{max} is calculated by Equation 8.12. The AUC is calculated by the trapezoidal rule from 0 to 24 hours.

(from 5.00 to 6.99 μg/mL), but the AUC remains constant (100 μg h/mL). In contrast, when the absorption rate constant is kept at 0.3 h⁻¹ and k changes from 0.1 to 0.5 h⁻¹ (elimination rate increases), then the t_{max} decreases (from 5.49 to 2.55 hours), the C_{max} decreases (from 5.77 to 2.79 μg/mL), and the AUC decreases (from 100 to 20 μg h/mL). Graphical representations for the relationships of k_a and k on the time for peak absorption and the peak drug concentrations are shown in Figs. 8-16 and 8-17.

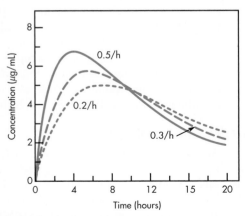

FIGURE 8-16   Effect of a change in the absorption rate constant, k_a, on the plasma drug concentration–time curve. Dose of drug is 100 mg, V_D is 10 L, and k is 0.1 h⁻¹.

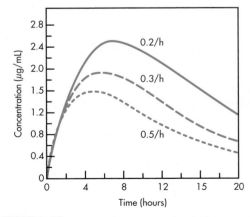

FIGURE 8-17   Effect of a change in the elimination rate constant, k, on the plasma drug concentration–time curve. Dose of drug is 100 mg, V_D is 10 L, and k_a is 0.1 h⁻¹.

Modified Wagner–Nelson Method

Hayashi et al (2001) introduced a modified Wagner–Nelson method to study the subcutaneous absorption of a drug with nonlinear kinetics from the central compartment. Nonlinear kinetics occurs in some drugs where the kinetic parameter such as k change with dose. The method was applicable to a biotechnological drug (recombinant human granulocyte-colony stimulating factors, rhG-CSF) which is eliminated nonlinearly. The drug was absorbed into the blood from the dermal site after subcutaneous injection. Because of nonlinear kinetics the extent of absorption was not easily determined. The amount of drug absorbed, Ab for each time sample, t_n, is given by Equation 8.48. V_1 and V_{ss} are central compartment and steady-state volume of distribution, respectively.

V_{max} and K_m are Michaelis–Menten parameters that describe the saturable elimination (see Chapter 10) of the drug. t_i is the sample time which = 0,1,2,4... 48 hours in this example, and $C(t)$ is the average serum drug concentraton between time points, that is, t_i and t_{i+1}.

$$A_{ab}(t_n) = \sum_{i=1}^{n-1} \int_{t_i}^{t_{i+1}} \left[\frac{V_{max}C(t)}{C(t)+K_m} + kV_1C(t) \right] dt + V_{ss}C(t_n)$$

(8.48)

From the mass balance of the above equation, the authors did account for the amount of drug present in the tissue compartment. (Note the authors stated that the central compartment V_1 is 4.56 L and that of V_{ss} is 4.90 L.) To simplify the model, the authors used convolution to show that the contribution of the tissue compartment is not significant and therefore may be neglected. Thus, the Loo–Riegelman method which requires a tissue compartment was not used by the authors. Convolution is an analytical method that predicts plasma time drug concentration using input and disposition functions for drugs with linear kinetics. The disposition function may be first obtained by deconvolution of simple IV plasma drug concentration data or from the terminal phase of an oral solution. Alternatively, the method of Lockwood and Gillespie (1996) abbreviated the need for the simple solution.

Models for Estimation of Drug Absorption

There are many models and approaches that have been used to predict drug absorption since the introduction of the classical approaches by John Wagner (1967) and Jack Loo. Deconvolution and convolution approaches are used to predict plasma drug concentration of oral dosage forms. Several commercial software (eg, GastroPlus, iDEA, Intellipharm PK, and PK-Sim) are now available for formulation and drug development or to determine the extent of drug absorption. The new software allows the characteristics of the drug, physiologic factors, and the dosage form to be inputed into the software. An important class of programs involves the **C**ompartmental **A**bsorption and **T**ransit (CAT) models. This model integrates the effect of solubility, permeability, as well as gastric emptying and GI transit time in the estimation of *in vivo* drug absorption. CAT models were successfully used to predict the fraction of drug oral absorption of 10 common drugs based on a small intestine transit time (Yu, 1999). The CAT models compared well overall with other plausible models such as the dispersion model, the single mixing tank model, and some flow models. It is important to note that the models discussed earlier in this chapter are used to compute extent of absorption after the plasma drug concentrations are measured. In contrast, the later models/software allow a comprehensive way to simulate or predict drug (product) performance *in vivo*. The subjects of dissolution, dosage form design, and drug absorption will be discussed in more detail in Chapters 14 and 15.

Determination of k_a from Two-Compartment Oral Absorption Data (Loo–Riegelman Method)

Plotting the percent of drug unabsorbed versus time to determine k_a may also be calculated for a drug exhibiting a two-compartment kinetic model. As in the method used previously to obtain an estimate of the k_a, no limitation is placed on the order of the absorption process. However, this method does require that the drug be given intravenously as well as orally to obtain all the necessary kinetic constants.

After oral administration of a dose of a drug that exhibits two-compartment model kinetics, the amount

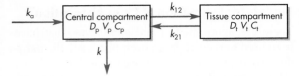

FIGURE 8-18   Two-compartment pharmacokinetic mode. Drug absorption and elimination occur from the central compartment.

of drug absorbed is calculated as the sum of the amounts of drug in the central compartment (D_p), in the tissue compartment (D_t), and the amount of drug eliminated by all routes (D_u) (Fig. 8-18).

$$Ab = D_p + D_t + D_u \qquad (8.49)$$

Each of these terms may be expressed in terms of kinetics constants and plasma drug concentrations, as follows:

$$D_p = V_p C_p \qquad (8.50)$$

$$D_t = V_t C_t \qquad (8.51)$$

$$\frac{dD_u}{dt} = k V_p C_p \qquad (8.52)$$

$$D_u = k V_p [AUC]_0^t$$

Substituting the above expression for D_p and D_u into Equation 8.49,

$$Ab = V_p C_p + D_t + k V_p [AUC]_0^t \qquad (8.53)$$

By dividing this equation by V_p to express the equation on drug concentrations, we obtain

$$\frac{Ab}{V_p} = C_p + \frac{D_t}{V_p} + k[AUC]_0^t \qquad (8.54)$$

At $t = \infty$, this equation becomes

$$\frac{Ab}{V_p} = k[AUC]_0^\infty \qquad (8.55)$$

Equation 8.54 divided by Equation 8.55 gives the fraction of drug absorbed at any time as shown in Equation 8.56.

$$\frac{Ab}{Ab^\infty} = \frac{C_p + \left(\dfrac{D_t}{V_p}\right) + k[AUC]_0^t}{k[AUC]_0^\infty} \qquad (8.56)$$

A plot of the fraction of drug unabsorbed, $1 - Ab/Ab^\infty$, versus time gives $-k_a/2.3$ as the slope from which the value for the absorption rate constant is obtained (refer to Equation 8.35).

The values for $k[AUC]_0^t$ are calculated from a plot of C_p versus time. Values for (D_t/V_p) can be approximated by the Loo–Riegelman method, as follows:

$$(C_t)_{t_n} = \frac{k_{12}\Delta C_p \Delta t}{2} + \frac{k_{12}}{k_{21}} (C_p)_{t_{n-1}} (1 - e^{-k_{21}\Delta t}) + (C_t)_{t_{n-1}} e^{-k_{21}\Delta t}$$

$$(8.57)$$

where C_t is D_t/V_p, or apparent tissue concentration; t = time of sampling for sample n; t_{n-1} = time of sampling for the sampling point preceding sample n; and $(C_p)_{t_{n-1}}$ = concentration of drug at central compartment for sample $n - 1$.

Calculation of C_t values is shown in Table 8-3, using a typical set of oral absorption data. After calculation of C_t values, the percent of drug unabsorbed is calculated with Equation 8.56, as shown in Table 8-4. A plot of percent of drug unabsorbed versus time on semilog graph paper gives a k_a of approximately 0.5 h^{-1}.

For calculation of k_a by this method, the drug must be given intravenously to allow evaluation of the distribution and elimination rate constants. For drugs that cannot be given by the IV route, the k_a cannot be calculated by the Loo–Riegelman method. For drugs that are given by the oral route only, the Wagner–Nelson method, which assumes a one-compartment model, may be used to provide an initial estimate of k_a. If the drug is given intravenously, there is no way of knowing whether there is any variation in the values for the elimination rate constant, k and the distributive rate constants, k_{12} and k_{21}. Such variations alter the rate constants. Therefore, a one-compartment model is frequently used to fit the plasma curves after an oral or intramuscular dose. The plasma level predicted from the k_a obtained by this method does deviate from the actual plasma level. However, in many instances, this deviation is not significant.

Cumulative Relative Fraction Absorbed

The fraction of drug absorbed at any time t (Equation 8.32) may be summed or cumulated for each time period for which a plasma drug sample was obtained.

TABLE 8-3   Calculation of C_t Values[a]

$(C_p)t_n$	$(t)t_n$	$\Delta(C_p)$	Δt	$\dfrac{(k_{12}\Delta C_p \Delta t)}{2}$	$(C_p)_{t_{n-1}}$	$(k_{12}/k_{21})\times$ $(1-e^{-k_{21}\Delta t})$	$(C_p)_{t_{n-1}}(k_{12}/k_{21})\times$ $(1-e^{-k_{21}\Delta t})$	$(C_t)_{t_{n-1}}e^{-k_{21}\Delta t}$	$(C_t)t_n$
3.00	0.5	3.0	0.5	0.218	0	0.134	0	0	0.218
5.20	1.0	2.2	0.5	0.160	3.00	0.134	0.402	0.187	0.749
6.50	1.5	1.3	0.5	0.094	5.20	0.134	0.697	0.642	1.433
7.30	2.0	0.8	0.5	0.058	6.50	0.134	0.871	1.228	2.157
7.60	2.5	0.3	0.5	0.022	7.30	0.134	0.978	1.849	2.849
7.75	3.0	0.15	0.5	0.011	7.60	0.134	1.018	2.442	3.471
7.70	3.5	−0.05	0.5	−0.004	7.75	0.134	1.039	2.976	4.019
7.60	4.0	−0.10	0.5	−0.007	7.70	0.134	1.032	3.444	4.469
7.10	5.0	−0.50	1.0	−0.073	7.60	0.250	1.900	3.276	5.103
6.60	6.0	−0.50	1.0	−0.073	7.10	0.250	1.775	3.740	5.442
6.00	7.0	−0.60	1.0	−0.087	6.60	0.250	1.650	3.989	5.552
5.10	9.0	−0.90	2.0	−2.261	6.00	0.432	2.592	2.987	5.318
4.40	11.0	−0.70	2.0	−0.203	5.10	0.432	2.203	2.861	4.861
3.30	15.0	−1.10	4.0	−0.638	4.40	0.720	3.168	1.361	3.891

[a]Calculated with the following rate constants: $k_{12} = 0.29$ h^{-1}, $k_{21} = 0.31$ h^{-1}.

Adapted with permission from Loo and Riegelman (1968).

From Equation 8.32, the term Ab/Ab$^\infty$ becomes the *cumulative relative fraction absorbed* (CRFA).

$$\text{CRFA} = \frac{C_p + k[\text{AUC}]_0^t}{k[\text{AUC}]_0^\infty} \tag{8.58}$$

where C_p is the plasma concentration at time t.

In the Wagner–Nelson equation, Ab/Ab$^\infty$ or CRFA will eventually equal unity, or 100%, even though the drug may not be 100% systemically bioavailable. The percent of drug absorbed is based on the total amount of drug absorbed (Ab$^\infty$) rather than the dose D_0. Because the amount of drug ultimately absorbed, Ab$^\infty$ in fractional term, is analogous to $k[\text{AUC}]_0^\infty$, the numerator will always equal the denominator at time infinity, whether the drug is 10%, 20%, or 100% bioavailable. The percent of drug absorbed based on Ab/Ab$^\infty$ is therefore different from the real percent of drug absorbed unless $F = 1$. However, for the calculation of k_a, the method is acceptable.

To determine the real percent of drug absorbed, a modification of the Wagner–Nelson equation was suggested by Welling (1986). A reference drug product was administered and plasma drug concentrations were determined over time. CRFA was then estimated by dividing Ab/Ab$^\infty_{\text{ref}}$, where Ab is the cumulative amount of drug absorbed from the drug product and Ab$^\infty_{\text{ref}}$ is the cumulative final amount of drug absorbed from a reference dosage form. In this case, the denominator of Equation 8.58 is modified as follows:

$$\text{CRFA} = \frac{C_p + k[\text{AUC}]_0^\infty}{k_{\text{ref}}[\text{AUC}]_{\text{ref}}^\infty} \tag{8.59}$$

where k_{ref} and $[\text{AUC}]_{\text{ref}}^\infty$ are the elimination constant and the area under the curve determined from the reference product, respectively. The terms in the numerator of Equation 8.59 refer to the product, as in Equation 8.58.

TABLE 8-4   Calculation of Percentage Unabsorbed[a]

Time (h)	$(C_p)t_n$	$[AUC]_{t_{n-1}}^{t_n}$	$[AUC]_{t_0}^{t_n}$	$k[AUC]_{t_0}^{t_n}$	$(C_t)t_n$	Ab/V_p	$\%Ab/V_p$	$100\% - Ab/V_p\%$
0.5	3.00	0.750	0.750	0.120	0.218	3.338	16.6	83.4
1.0	5.20	2.050	2.800	0.448	0.749	6.397	31.8	68.2
1.5	6.50	2.925	5.725	0.916	1.433	8.849	44.0	56.0
2.0	7.30	3.450	9.175	1.468	2.157	10.925	54.3	45.7
2.5	7.60	3.725	12.900	2.064	2.849	12.513	62.2	37.8
3.0	7.75	3.838	16.738	2.678	3.471	13.889	69.1	30.9
3.5	7.70	3.863	20.601	3.296	4.019	15.015	74.6	25.4
4.0	7.60	3.825	24.426	3.908	4.469	15.977	79.4	20.6
5.0	7.10	7.350	31.726	5.084	5.103	17.287	85.9	14.1
6.0	6.60	6.850	38.626	6.180	5.442	18.222	90.6	9.4
7.0	6.00	6.300	44.926	7.188	5.552	18.740	93.1	6.9
9.0	5.10	11.100	56.026	8.964	5.318	19.382	96.3	3.7
11.0	4.40	9.500	65.526	10.484	4.861	19.745	98.1	1.9
15.0	3.30	15.400	80.926	12.948	3.891	20.139	100.0	0

[a] $Ab/V_p = (C_p) + k[AUC]_{t_0}^{t_n} + (C_t)_{t_n}$

$(C_t)_{t_n} = k_{12}\Delta C_p \Delta t/2 + k_{12}/k_{21}(C_p)_{t_{n-1}}(1-e^{-k_{21}\Delta t}) + (C_t)_{t_{n-1}}e^{-k_{21}\Delta t}$

$k = 0.16; k_{12} = 0.29; k_{21} = 0.31$

Each fraction of drug absorbed is calculated and plotted against the time interval in which the plasma drug sample was obtained (Fig. 8-19). An example of the relationship of CRFA versus time for the absorption of tolazamide from four different drug products is shown in Fig. 8-20. The data for Fig. 8-21 were obtained from the serum tolazamide levels–time curves in Fig. 8-20. The CRFA–time graph provides a visual image of the relative rates of drug absorption from various drug products. If the CRFA–time

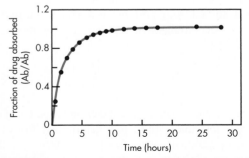

FIGURE 8-19   Fraction of drug absorbed. (Wagner–Nelson method.)

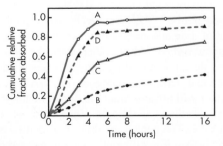

FIGURE 8-20   Mean cumulative relative fractions of tolazamide absorbed as a function of time. (From Welling et al, 1982, with permission.)

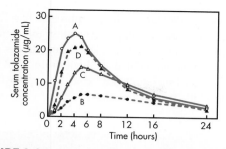

FIGURE 8-21   Mean serum tolazamide levels as a function of time. (From Welling et al, 1982, with permission.)

curve is a straight line, then the drug was absorbed from the drug product at an apparent zero-order absorption rate.

The calculation of k_a is useful in designing a multiple-dosage regimen. Knowledge of the k_a and k allows for the prediction of peak and trough plasma drug concentrations following multiple dosing. In bioequivalence studies, drug products are given in chemically equivalent (ie, pharmaceutical equivalents) doses, and the respective rates of systemic

absorption may not differ markedly. Therefore, for these studies, t_{max}, or time of peak drug concentration, can be very useful in comparing the respective rates of absorption of a drug from chemically equivalent drug products.

Frequently Asked Questions

▶ *Can the Wagner–Nelson method be used to calculate k_a for an orally administered drug that follows the pharmacokinetics of a two-compartment model?*

▶ *What is the absorption half-life of a drug and how is it determined?*

▶ *In switching a drug from IV to oral dosing, what is the most important consideration?*

▶ *Drug clearance is dependent on dose and area under the time–drug concentration curve. Would drug clearance be affected by the rate of absorption?*

▶ *Does a larger absorption rate constant affect C_{max}, t_{max}, and AUC if the dose and elimination rate constant, k remains constant?*

CHAPTER SUMMARY

Pharmacokinetic absorption models range from being entirely "exploratory" and empirical, to semi-mechanistic and ultimately complex physiologically based pharmacokinetic (PBPK) models. This choice is conditional on the modeling purpose as well as the amount and quality of the available data.

Empirically, the pharmacokinetics of drug absorption may be described by zero-order or first-order kinetics. Drug elimination from the body is generally described by first-order kinetics. Using the compartment model, various important pharmacokinetics parameters about drug absorption such as k_a, k, C_{max}, t_{max}, and other parameters may be computed from data by the method of residuals (feathering) or by computer modeling. The pharmacokinetic parameters are important in evaluating drug absorption and understanding how these parameters affect drug concentrations in the body. The fraction of drug absorbed may be computed in a one-compartment model using the Wagner–Nelson method or in a

two-compartment model using the Loo–Riegelman method. The determination of the fraction of drug absorbed is an important tool in evaluating drug dosage form and design. The Wagner–Nelson method and Loo–Reigelman method are classical methods for determinating absorption rate constants and fraction of drug absorbed. Convolution and deconvolution are powerful alternative tools used to predict a plasma drug concentration–time profile from dissolution of data during drug development.

The empirical models presented in this chapter are very basic with simple assumptions. More sophisticated methods based on these basic concepts may be extended to include physiological factors such as GI transit in the physiologically based models that represent the advance drug absorption model development. These models are useful to predict drug absorption over time curves in designing oral dosage forms (see Chapters 14 and 15).

Although the current development of *in vitro* studies and computer science have allowed rapid advances of PBPK models, the combination of physiologically based modeling with parameter estimation techniques seems to be the way forward and its impact on the drug development progressively increases. Although such an approach has limitations, further methodology research in this field and the advances in computer science can address many of them. It is apparent that "bottom-up" and "top-down" modeling strategies need to approach and borrow skills from each other.

ANSWERS

Frequently Asked Questions

If drug absorption is simulated using the oral one-compartment model, would a larger absorption rate constant result in a greater amount of drug absorbed?

- The fraction of drug absorbed, F, and the absorption rate constant, k_a, are independent parameters. A drug in an oral solution may have a more rapid rate of absorption compared to a solid drug product. If the drug is released from the drug product slowly or is formulated so that the drug is absorbed slowly, the drug may be subjected to first-pass effects, degraded in the gastrointestinal tract, or eliminated in the feces so that less drug (smaller F) may be absorbed systemically compared to the same drug formulated to be absorbed more rapidly from the drug product.

How do you explain that k_a is often greater than k with most drugs?

- A drug with a rate of absorption slower than its rate of elimination will not be able to obtain optimal systemic drug concentrations to achieve efficacy. Such drugs are generally not developed into products. However, the apartment k_a for drugs absorbed from controlled-release products (Chapter 18) may be smaller, but the initial rate of absorption from the GI tract is faster than the rate of drug elimination since, $dD_{GI}/dt = -k_a D_{GI}$.

What is the absorption half-life of a drug and how is it determined?

- For drugs absorbed by a first-order process, the absorption half-life is $0.693/k_a$. Although drug absorption involves many stochastic (system-based random) steps, the overall rate process is often approximated by a first-order process, especially with oral solutions and immediate-release drug products such as compressed tablets or capsules. The determination of the absorption rate constant, k_a, is most often calculated by the Wagner–Nelson method for drugs, which follows a one-compartment model with first-order absorption and first-order elimination.

In switching a drug from IV to oral dosing, what is the most important consideration?

- The fraction of drug absorbed may be less than 1 (ie, 100% bioavailable) after oral administration. In some cases, there may be a different salt form of the drug used for IV infusion compared to the salt form of the drug used orally. Therefore, a correction is needed for the difference in MW of the two salt forms.

Drug clearance is dependent on dose and area under the time–drug concentration curve. Would drug clearance be affected by the rate of absorption?

- Total body drug clearance and renal drug clearance are generally not affected by drug absorption from most absorption sites. In the gastrointestinal tract, a drug is absorbed via the hepatic portal vein to the liver and may be subject to hepatic clearance.

Learning Questions

1. **a.** The elimination rate constant is 0.1 h^{-1} ($t_{1/2}$ = 6.93 h).
   b. The absorption rate constant, k_a, is 0.3 h^{-1} (absorption half-life = 2.31 h).

$$\text{The calculated } t_{max} = \frac{\ln(k_a/k)}{k_a - k} = 5.49 \text{ h}$$

c. The y intercept was observed to be 60 ng/mL. Therefore, the equation that fits the observed data is

$$C_p = 60(e^{-0.1t} - e^{-0.3t})$$

Note: Answers obtained by "hand" feathering the data on semilog graph paper may vary somewhat depending on graphing skills and skill in reading data from a graph.

2. By direct observation of the data, the t_{max} is 6 hours and the C_{max} is 23.01 ng/mL. The apparent volume of distribution, V_D, is obtained from the intercept, I, of the terminal elimination phase, and substituting $F = 0.8$, $D = 10,000,000$ ng, $k_a = 0.3$ h^{-1}, $k = 0.1$ h^{-1}:

$$I = \frac{Fk_a D_0}{V_D(k_a - k)}$$

$$60 = \frac{(0.8)(0.3)(10,000,000)}{V_D(0.3 - 0.1)}$$

$$V_D = 200 \text{ L}$$

3. The percent-of-drug-unabsorbed method is applicable to any model with first-order elimination, regardless of the process of drug input. If the drug is given by IV injection, the elimination rate constant, k, may be determined accurately. If the drug is administered orally, k and k_a may *flip-flop*, resulting in an error unless IV data are available to determine k. For a drug that follows a two-compartment model, an IV bolus injection is used to determine the rate constants for distribution and elimination.

4. After an IV bolus injection, a drug such as theophylline follows a two-compartment model with a rapid distribution phase. During oral absorption, the drug is distributed during the absorption phase, and no distribution phase is observed. Pharmacokinetic analysis of the plasma drug concentration data obtained after oral drug administration will show that the drug follows a one-compartment model.

5. The equations for a drug that follows the kinetics of a one-compartment model with first-order absorption and elimination are

$$C_p = \frac{FD_0 k_a}{VD(k_a - k)}(e^{kt} - e^{-k_a t}) \qquad t_{max} = \frac{\ln(k_a/k)}{k_a - k}$$

As shown by these equations:

a. t_{max} is influenced by k_a and k and not by F, D_0, or V_D.

b. C_p is influenced by F, D_0, V_D, k_a, and k.

6. A drug product that might provide a zero-order input is an oral controlled-release tablet or a transdermal drug delivery system (patch). An IV drug infusion will also provide a zero-order drug input.

7. The general equation for a one-compartment open model with oral absorption is

$$C_p = \frac{FD_0 k_a}{V_D(k_a - k)}(e^{-kt} - e^{-k_a t})$$

From $C_p = 45(e^{-0.17t} - e^{-1.5t})$

$$\frac{FD_0 k_a}{V_D(k_a - k)} = 45$$

$$k = 0.17 \text{ h}^{-1}$$

$$k_a = 1.5 \text{ h}^{-1}$$

a. $t_{max} = \dfrac{\ln(k_a/k)}{k_a - k} = \dfrac{\ln(1.5/0.17)}{1.5 - 0.17} = 1.64$ h

b. $C_{max} = 45(e^{-(0.17)(1.64)} - e^{-(1.5)(1.64)})$

$$= 30.2 \ \mu g/mL$$

c. $t_{1/2} = \dfrac{0.693}{k} = \dfrac{0.693}{0.17} = 4.08$ h

8. a. Drug A $\quad t_{max} = \dfrac{\ln(1.0/0.2)}{1.0 - 1.2} = 2.01$ h

Drug B $\quad t_{max} = \dfrac{\ln(0.2/1.0)}{0.2 - 1.0} = 2.01$ h

b. $C_{max} = \dfrac{FD_0 k_a}{V_D(k_a - k)}(e^{-kt_{max}} - e^{-k_a t_{max}})$

Drug A $C_{max} = \dfrac{(1)(500)(1)}{(10)(1 - 0.2)}(e^{-(0.2)(2)} - e^{-(1)(2)})$

$$C_{max} = 33.4 \ \mu g/mL$$

$$\text{Drug B } C_{max} = \frac{(1)(500)(0.2)}{(20)(0.2 - 1.0)}$$

$$= (e^{-1(2)} - e^{-(0.2)(2)})$$

$$C_{max} = 33.4 \ \mu g/mL$$

9. a. The method of residuals using manual graphing methods may give somewhat different answers depending on personal skill and the quality of the graph paper. Values obtained by the computer program ESTRIP gave the following estimates:

$$k_a = 2.84 \ h^{-1} \quad k = 0.186 \ h^{-1} \quad t_{1/2} = 3.73 \ h$$

b. A drug in an aqueous solution is in the most absorbable form compared to other oral dosage forms. The assumption that $k_a > k$ is generally true for drug solutions and immediate-release oral dosage forms such as compressed tablets and capsules. Drug absorption from extended-release dosage forms may have $k_a < k$. To demonstrate unequivocally which slope represents the true k, the drug must be given by IV bolus or IV infusion, and the slope of the elimination curve obtained.

c. The Loo–Riegelman method requires IV data. Therefore, only the Wagner–Nelson method may be used on these data.

d. Observed t_{max} and C_{max} values are taken directly from the experimental data. In this example, C_{max} is 85.11 ng/mL, which occurred at a t_{max} of 1 hour. The theoretical t_{max} and C_{max} are obtained as follows:

$$t_{max} = \frac{2.3\log(k_a/k)}{k_a - k}$$

$$= \frac{2.3\log(2.84/0.186)}{2.84 - 0.186} = 1.03 \ h$$

$$C_{max} = \frac{FD_0 k_a}{V_D(k_a - k)}(e^{-kt_{max}} - e^{-k_a t_{max}})$$

where $FD_0 k_a/V_D(k_a - k)$ is the y intercept equal to 110 ng/mL and $t_{max} = 1.03$ h.

$$C_{max} = (110)(e^{-(1.186)(1.0)} - e^{-(2.84)(1.03)})$$

$$C_{max} = 85 \ \text{ng/mL}$$

e. A more complete model-fitting program, such as WINNONLIN, is needed to fit the data statistically to a one-compartment model.

APPLICATION QUESTIONS

1. Plasma samples from a patient were collected after an oral bolus dose of 10 mg of a new benzodiazepine solution as follows:

Time (hours)	Concentration (ng/mL)
0.25	2.85
0.50	5.43
0.75	7.75
1.00	9.84
2.00	16.20
4.00	22.15
6.00	23.01
10.00	19.09
14.00	13.90
20.00	7.97

From the given data:

a. Determine the elimination constant of the drug.

b. Determine k_a by feathering.

c. Determine the equation that describes the plasma drug concentration of the new benzodiazepine.

2. Assuming that the drug in Question 1 is 80% absorbed, find **(a)** the absorption constant, k_a; **(b)** the elimination half-life, $t_{1/2}$; **(c)** the t_{max}, or time of peak drug concentration; and **(d)** the volume of distribution of the patient.

3. Contrast the percent of drug-unabsorbed methods for the determination of rate constant for absorption, k_a, in terms of **(a)** pharmacokinetic model, **(b)** route of drug administration, and **(c)** possible sources of error.

4. What is the error inherent in the measurement of k_a for an orally administered drug that follows a two-compartment model when a one-compartment model is assumed in the calculation?

5. What are the main pharmacokinetic parameters that influence **(a)** time for peak drug concentration and **(b)** peak drug concentration?

6. Name a method of drug administration that will provide a zero-order input.

7. A single oral dose (100 mg) of an antibiotic was given to an adult male patient (43 years, 72 kg). From the literature, the pharmacokinetics of this drug fits a one-compartment open model. The equation that best fits the pharmacokinetics of the drug is

$$C_p = 45(e^{-0.17t} - e^{-1.5t})$$

From the equation above, calculate **(a)** t_{max}, **(b)** C_{max}, and **(c)** $t_{1/2}$ for the drug in this patient. Assume C_p is in $\mu g/mL$ and the first-order rate constants are in h^{-1}.

8. Two drugs, A and B, have the following pharmacokinetic parameters after a single oral dose of 500 mg:

Drug	k_a (h⁻¹)	k (h⁻¹)	V_D (mL)
A	1.0	0.2	10,000
B	0.2	1.0	20,000

Both drugs follow a one-compartment pharmacokinetic model and are 100% bioavailable.
a. Calculate the t_{max} for each drug.
b. Calculate the C_{max} for each drug.

9. The bioavailability of phenylpropanolamine hydrochloride was studied in 24 adult male subjects. The following data represent the mean blood phenylpropanolamine hydrochloride concentrations (ng/mL) after the oral administration of a single 25-mg dose of phenylpropanolamine hydrochloride solution:

Time (hours)	Concentration (ng/mL)	Time (hours)	Concentration (ng/mL)
0	0	3	62.98
0.25	51.33	4	52.32
0.5	74.05	6	36.08
0.75	82.91	8	24.88
1.0	85.11	12	11.83
1.5	81.76	18	3.88
2	75.51	24	1.27

a. From the above data, obtain the rate constant for absorption, k_a, and the rate constant for elimination, k, by the method of residuals.

b. Is it reasonable to assume that $k_a > k$ for a drug in a solution? How would you determine unequivocally which rate constant represents the elimination constant k?

c. From the data, which method, Wagner–Nelson or Loo–Riegelman, would be more appropriate to determine the order of the rate constant for absorption?

d. From your values, calculate the theoretical t_{max}. How does your value relate to the observed t_{max} obtained from the subjects?

e. Would you consider the pharmacokinetics of phenylpropanolamine HCl to follow a one-compartment model? Why?

REFERENCES

Jamei M, Dickinson GL, Rostami-Hodjegan A. A framework for assessing inter-individual variability in pharmacokinetics using virtual human populations and integrating general knowledge of physical chemistry, biology, anatomy, physiology and genetics: A tale of "bottom-up" vs "top-down" recognition of covariates. *Drug Metab Pharmacokinet* **24**:53–75, 2009.

Hayashi N, Aso H, Higashida M, et al: Estimation of rhG-CSF absorption kinetics after subcutaneous administration using a modified Wagner–Nelson method with a nonlinear elimination model. *J Pharm Sci* **13**:151–158, 2001.

Lockwood P, Gillespie WR: A convolution approach to in vivo:in vitro correlation (IVIVC) that does not require an IV or solution reference dose. *Pharm Res* **34**:369, 1996.

Loo JCK, Riegelman S: New method for calculating the intrinsic absorption rate of drugs. *J Pharm Sci* **57:**918–928, 1968.

Levy G, Amsel LP, Elliot HC: Kinetics of salicyluric acid elimination in man. *J Pharm Sci* **58:**827–829, 1969.

Manini AF, Kabrhel C, Thomsen TW: Acute myocardial infarction after over-the-counter use of pseudoephedrine. *Ann Emerg Med* **45**(2):213–216, Feb 2005.

Portmann G: Pharmacokinetics. In Swarbrick J (ed), *Current Concepts in the Pharmaceutical Sciences*, vol 1. Philadelphia, Lea & Febiger, 1970, Chap 1.

Teorell T: Kinetics of distribution of substances administered to the body. *Archives Internationales de Pharmacodynamie et de Thérapie* **57:**205–240, 1937.

Wagner JG: Use of computers in pharmacokinetics. *Clin Pharmacol Ther* **8:**201–218, 1967.

Welling PG: *Pharmacokinetics: Processes and Mathematics*. ACS monograph 185. Washington, DC, American Chemical Society, 1986, pp 174–175.

Welling PG, Patel RB, Patel UR, et al: Bioavailability of tolazamide from tablets: Comparison of in vitro and in vivo results. *J Pharm Sci* **71:**1259, 1982.

Yu LX, Amidon GL: A compartmental absorption and transit model for estimating oral drug absorption. *Int J Pharm* **186:**119–125, 1999.

BIBLIOGRAPHY

Boxenbaum HG, Kaplan SA: Potential source of error in absorption rate calculations. *J Pharmacokinet Biopharm* **3:**257–264, 1975.

Boyes R, Adams H, Duce B: Oral absorption and disposition kinetics of lidocaine hydrochloride in dogs. *J Pharmacol Exp Ther* **174:**1–8, 1970.

Dvorchik BH, Vesell ES: Significance of error associated with use of the one-compartment formula to calculate clearance of 38 drugs. *Clin Pharmacol Ther* **23:**617–623, 1978.

Veng-Pedersena P, Gobburub JVS, Meyer MC, Straughn AB: Carbamazepine level-A in vivo–in vitro correlation (IVIVC): A scaled convolution based predictive approach. *Biopharm Drug Dispos* **21:**1–6, 2000.

Wagner JG, Nelson E: Kinetic analysis of blood levels and urinary excretion in the absorptive phase after single doses of drug. *J Pharm Sci* **53:**1392, 1964.

9

Multiple-Dosage Regimens

Rodney C. Siwale and Shabnam N. Sani

Chapter Objectives

▶ Define the index for measuring drug accumulation.

▶ Define drug accumulation and drug accumulation $t_{1/2}$.

▶ Explain the principle of superposition and its assumptions in multiple-dose regimens.

▶ Calculate the steady-state C_{max} and C_{min} after multiple IV bolus dosing of drugs.

▶ Calculate k and V_D of aminoglycosides in multiple-dose regimens.

▶ Adjust the steady-state C_{max} and C_{min} in the event the last dose is given too early, too late, or totally missed following multiple IV dosing.

Earlier chapters of this book discussed single-dose drug and constant-rate drug administration. By far though, most drugs are given in several doses, for example, multiple doses to treat chronic disease such as arthritis, hypertension, etc. After single-dose drug administration, the plasma drug level rises above and then falls below the *minimum effective concentration* (MEC), resulting in a decline in therapeutic effect. To treat chronic disease, multiple-dosage or IV infusion regimens are used to maintain the plasma drug levels within the narrow limits of the therapeutic window (eg, plasma drug concentrations above the MEC but below the *minimum toxic concentration* or MTC) to achieve optimal clinical effectiveness. These drugs may include antibacterials, cardiotonics, anticonvulsants, hypoglycemics, antihypertensives, hormones, and others. Ideally, a dosage regimen is established for each drug to provide the correct plasma level without excessive fluctuation and drug accumulation outside the therapeutic window.

For certain drugs, such as antibiotics, a desirable MEC can be determined. For drugs that have a narrow therapeutic range (eg, digoxin and phenytoin), there is a need to define the therapeutic minimum and maximum nontoxic plasma concentrations (MEC and MTC, respectively). In calculating a multiple-dose regimen, the desired or *target* plasma drug concentration must be related to a therapeutic response, and the multiple-dose regimen must be designed to produce plasma concentrations within the therapeutic window.

There are two main parameters that can be adjusted in developing a dosage regimen: (1) the size of the drug dose and (2) τ, the frequency of drug administration (ie, the time interval between doses).

DRUG ACCUMULATION

To calculate a multiple-dose regimen for a patient or patients, pharmacokinetic parameters are first obtained from the plasma level–time curve generated by single-dose drug studies. With these pharmacokinetic parameters and knowledge of the size of the dose and dosage interval (τ), the complete plasma level–time curve or the plasma level may be predicted at any time after the beginning of the dosage regimen.

For calculation of multiple-dose regimens, it is necessary to decide whether successive doses of drug will have any effect on the previous dose. The principle of *superposition* assumes that early doses of drug do not affect the pharmacokinetics of subsequent doses. Therefore, the blood levels after the second, third, or *n*th dose will overlay or superimpose the blood level attained after the $(n-1)$th dose. In addition, the $\mathrm{AUC} = (\int_0^\infty C_p \, dt)$ for the first dose is equal to the steady-state area between doses, that is, $(\int_{t_1}^{t_2} C_p \, dt)$ as shown in Fig. 9-1.

The principle of *superposition* allows the pharmacokineticist to project the plasma drug concentration–time curve of a drug after multiple consecutive doses based on the plasma drug concentration–time curve obtained after a single dose. The basic assumptions are (1) that the drug is eliminated by first-order kinetics and (2) that the pharmacokinetics of the drug after a single dose (first dose) are not altered after taking multiple doses.

The plasma drug concentrations after multiple doses may be predicted from the plasma drug concentrations obtained after a single dose. In Table 9-1, the plasma drug concentrations from 0 to 24 hours are measured after a single dose. A constant dose of drug is given every 4 hours and plasma drug concentrations after each dose are generated using the data after the first dose. Thus, the *predicted* plasma drug concentration in the patient is the total drug concentration obtained by adding the residual drug concentration obtained after each previous dose. The superposition principle may be used to predict drug concentrations after multiple doses of many drugs. Because the superposition principle is an overlay method, it may be used to predict drug concentrations after multiple doses given at either *equal* or *unequal* dosage intervals. For example, the plasma drug concentrations may be predicted after a drug dose is given every 8 hours, or 3 times a day before meals at 8 AM, 12 noon, and 6 PM.

There are situations, however, in which the superposition principle does not apply. In these cases, the pharmacokinetics of the drug change after multiple dosing due to various factors, including changing pathophysiology in the patient, saturation of a drug carrier system, enzyme induction, and enzyme inhibition. Drugs that follow nonlinear pharmacokinetics (see Chapter 10) generally do not have predictable plasma drug concentrations after multiple doses using the superposition principle.

If the drug is administered at a fixed dose and a fixed dosage interval, as is the case with many multiple-dose regimens, the amount of drug in the body will increase and then plateau to a mean plasma level higher than the peak C_p obtained from the initial dose (Figs. 9-1 and 9-2). When the second dose is given after a time interval shorter than the time required to "completely" eliminate the previous dose, *drug accumulation* will occur in the body. In other words, the plasma concentrations following the second dose will be higher than corresponding plasma concentrations immediately following the first dose. However, if the second dose is given after a time interval longer than the time required to eliminate the previous dose, drug will not accumulate (see Table 9-1).

As repetitive equal doses are given at a constant frequency, the plasma level–time curve plateaus and a steady state is obtained. At steady state, the plasma drug levels fluctuate between $C_{\max}^\infty$ and $C_{\min}^\infty$. Once steady state is obtained, $C_{\max}^\infty$ and $C_{\min}^\infty$ are constant and remain unchanged from dose to dose. In addition, the AUC between $(\int_{t_1}^{t_2} C_p \, dt)$ is constant during a dosing interval at steady state (see Fig. 9-1). The $C_{\max}^\infty$ is important in determining drug safety. The $C_{\max}^\infty$ should always remain below the MTC. The $C_{\max}^\infty$

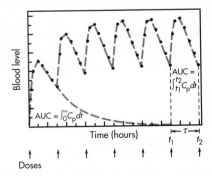

FIGURE 9-1   Simulated data showing blood levels after administration of multiple doses and accumulation of blood levels when equal doses are given at equal time intervals.

TABLE 9-1   Predicted Plasma Drug Concentrations for Multiple-Dose Regimen Using the Superposition Principle[a]

Dose Number	Time (h)	Plasma Drug Concentration (μg/mL)						
		Dose 1	Dose 2	Dose 3	Dose 4	Dose 5	Dose 6	Total
1	0	0						0
	1	21.0						21.0
	2	22.3						22.3
	3	19.8						19.8
2	4	16.9	0					16.9
	5	14.3	21.0					35.3
	6	12.0	22.3					34.3
	7	10.1	19.8					29.9
3	8	8.50	16.9	0				25.4
	9	7.15	14.3	21.0				42.5
	10	6.01	12.0	22.3				40.3
	11	5.06	10.1	19.8				35.0
4	12	4.25	8.50	16.9	0			29.7
	13	3.58	7.15	14.3	21.0			46.0
	14	3.01	6.01	12.0	22.3			43.3
	15	2.53	5.06	10.1	19.8			37.5
5	16	2.13	4.25	8.50	16.9	0		31.8
	17	1.79	3.58	7.15	14.3	21.0		47.8
	18	1.51	3.01	6.01	12.0	22.3		44.8
	19	1.27	2.53	5.06	10.1	19.8		38.8
6	20	1.07	2.13	4.25	8.50	16.9	0	32.9
	21	0.90	1.79	3.58	7.15	14.3	21.0	48.7
	22	0.75	1.51	3.01	6.01	12.0	22.3	45.6
	23	0.63	1.27	2.53	5.06	10.1	19.8	39.4
	24	0.53	1.07	2.13	4.25	8.50	16.9	33.4

[a]A single oral dose of 350 mg was given and the plasma drug concentrations were measured for 0–24 h. The same plasma drug concentrations are assumed to occur after doses 2–6. The total plasma drug concentration is the sum of the plasma drug concentrations due to each dose. For this example, $V_D = 10$ L, $t_{1/2} = 4$ h, and $k_a = 1.5$ h^{-1}. The drug is 100% bioavailable and follows the pharmacokinetics of a one-compartment open model.

is also a good indication of drug accumulation. If a drug produces the same C_{max}^{∞} at steady state, compared with the $(C_{n-1})_{max}$ after the first dose, then there is no drug accumulation. If C_{max}^{∞} is much larger than $(C_{n-1})_{max}$, then there is significant accumulation during the multiple-dose regimen. Accumulation is affected by the elimination half-life of the drug and the dosing interval. The index for measuring drug accumulation R is

$$R = \frac{(C^{\infty})_{max}}{(C_{n=1})_{max}} \quad (9.1)$$

Substituting for C_{max} after the first dose and at steady state yields

$$R = \frac{D_0/V_D[1/(1-e^{-k\tau})]}{D_0/V_D} \quad (9.2)$$

$$R = \frac{1}{1-e^{-k\tau}}$$

Equation 9.2 shows that drug accumulation measured with the R index depends on the elimination constant and the dosing interval and is independent of the dose. For a drug given in repetitive oral doses, the time required to reach steady state is dependent on the elimination half-life of the drug and is independent of the size of the dose, the length of the dosing interval, and the number of doses. For example, if the dose or dosage interval of the drug is altered as shown in Fig. 9-2, the time required for the drug to reach steady state is the same, but the final steady-state plasma level changes proportionately.

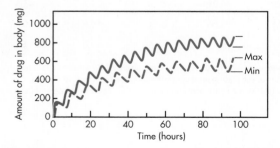

FIGURE 9-2 Amount of drug in the body as a function of time. Equal doses of drug were given every 6 hours (upper curve) and every 8 hours (lower curve). k_a and k remain constant.

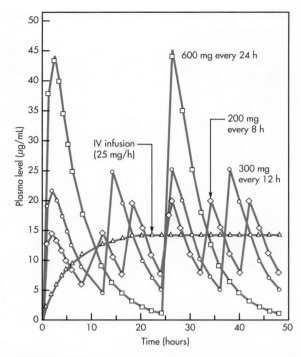

FIGURE 9-3 Simulated plasma drug concentration–time curves after IV infusion and oral multiple doses for a drug with an elimination half-life of 4 hours and apparent V_D of 10 L. IV infusion given at a rate of 25 mg/h, oral multiple doses are 200 mg every 8 hours, 300 mg every 12 hours, and 600 mg every 24 hours.

Furthermore, if the drug is given at the same dosing rate but as an infusion (eg, 25 mg/h), the average plasma drug concentrations will (C_{av}^{∞}) be the same but the fluctuations between C_{max}^{∞} and C_{min}^{∞} will vary (Fig. 9-3). An average steady-state plasma drug concentration is obtained by dividing the area under the curve (AUC) for a dosing period (ie, $\int_{t_1}^{t_2} C_p\, dt$) by the dosing interval τ, at steady state.

An equation for the estimation of the time to reach one-half of the steady-state plasma levels or the accumulation half-life has been described by van Rossum and Tomey (1968).

$$\text{Accumulation } t_{1/2} = t_{1/2}\left(1+3.3\log\frac{k_a}{k_a - k}\right) \quad (9.3)$$

For IV administration, k_a is very rapid (approaches ∞); k is very small in comparison to k_a and can be omitted in the denominator of Equation 9.3. Thus, Equation 9.3 reduces to

$$\text{Accumulation } t_{1/2} = t_{1/2}\left(1 + 3.3\log\frac{k_a}{k_a}\right) \quad (9.4)$$

Since $k_a/k_a = 1$ and $\log 1 = 0$, the accumulation $t_{1/2}$ of a drug administered intravenously is the elimination $t_{1/2}$ of the drug. From this relationship, the time to reach 50% steady-state drug concentrations is dependent only on the elimination $t_{1/2}$ and not on the dose or dosage interval.

As shown in Equation 9.4, the accumulation $t_{1/2}$ is directly proportional to the elimination $t_{1/2}$. Table 9-2 gives the accumulation $t_{1/2}$ of drugs with various elimination half-lives given by multiple oral doses (see Table 9-2).

From a clinical viewpoint, the time needed to reach 90% of the steady-state plasma concentration is 3.3 times the elimination half-life, whereas the time required to reach 99% of the steady-state plasma concentration is 6.6 times the elimination half-life (Table 9-3). It should be noted from Table 9-3 that at a constant dose size, the shorter the dosage interval, the larger the dosing rate (mg/h), and the higher the steady-state drug level.

The number of doses for a given drug to reach steady state is dependent on the elimination half-life of the drug and the dosage interval τ (see Table 9-3). If the drug is given at a dosage interval equal to the half-life of the drug, then 6.6 doses are required to reach 99% of the theoretical steady-state plasma drug concentration. The number of doses needed to reach steady state is $6.6t_{1/2}/\tau$, as calculated in the far right column of Table 9-3. As discussed in Chapter 6, Table 6-1, it takes 4.32 half-lives to reach 95% of steady state.

CLINICAL EXAMPLE

Paroxetine (Prozac) is an antidepressant drug with a long elimination half-life of 21 hours. Paroxetine is well absorbed after oral administration and has a t_{max} of about 5 hours, longer than most drugs. Slow elimination may cause the plasma curve to peak slowly. The t_{max} is affected by k and k_a, as discussed in Chapter 8. The C_{max} for paroxetine after multiple dosing of 30 mg of paroxetine for 30 days in one study ranged from 8.6 to 105 ng/mL among 15 subjects. Clinically it is important to achieve a stable steady-state level in multiple dosing that does not "underdose" or overdose the patient. The pharmacist should advise the patient to follow the prescribed dosing interval and dose as accurately as possible. Taking a dose too early or too late contributes to

TABLE 9-2   Effect of Elimination Half-Life and Absorption Rate Constant on Accumulation Half-Life after Oral Administration[a]

Elimination Half-life (h)	Elimination Rate constant (1/h)	Absorption Rate Constant (1/h)	Accumulation Half-life (h)
4	0.173	1.50	4.70
8	0.0866	1.50	8.67
12	0.0578	1.50	12.8
24	0.0289	1.50	24.7
4	0.173	1.00	5.09
8	0.0866	1.00	8.99
12	0.0578	1.00	13.0
24	0.0289	1.00	25.0

[a]Accumulation half-life is calculated by Equation 8.3, and is the half-time for accumulation of the drug to 90% of the steady-state plasma drug concentration.

TABLE 9-3 **Interrelation of Elimination Half-Life, Dosage Interval, Maximum Plasma Concentration, and Time to Reach Steady-State Plasma Concentration**[a]

Elimination Half-Life (h)	Dosage Interval, τ(h)	C_{max}^{∞} (μg/mL)	Time for $C_{av}^{\infty b}$ (h)	NO. Doses to Reach 99% Steady State
0.5	0.5	200	3.3	6.6
0.5	1.0	133	3.3	3.3
1.0	0.5	341	6.6	13.2
1.0	1.0	200	6.6	6.6
1.0	2.0	133	6.6	3.3
1.0	4.0	107	6.6	1.65
1.0	10.0	100[c]	6.6	0.66
2.0	1.0	341	13.2	13.2
2.0	2.0	200	13.2	6.1

[a]A single dose of 1000 mg of three hypothetical drugs with various elimination half-lives but equal volumes of distribution ($V_D = 10$ L) were given by multiple IV doses at various dosing intervals. All time values are in hours; C_{max}^{∞} = maximum steady-state concentration; (C_{av}^{∞}) = average steady-state plasma concentration; the maximum plasma drug concentration after the first dose of the drug is ($C_{n=1})_{max} = 100 \, \mu$g/mL.

[b]Time to reach 99% of steady-state plasma concentration.

[c]Since the dosage interval, τ, is very large compared to the elimination half-life, no accumulation of drug occurs.

variation. Individual variation in metabolism rate can also cause variable blood levels, as discussed later in Chapter 13.

REPETITIVE INTRAVENOUS INJECTIONS

The maximum amount of drug in the body following a single rapid IV injection is equal to the dose of the drug. For a one-compartment open model, the drug will be eliminated according to first-order kinetics.

$$D_B = D_0 e^{-k\tau} \qquad (9.5)$$

If τ is equal to the dosage interval (ie, the time between the first dose and the next dose), then the amount of drug remaining in the body after several hours can be determined with

$$D_B = D_0 e^{-k\tau} \qquad (9.6)$$

The fraction (f) of the dose remaining in the body is related to the elimination constant (k) and the dosage interval (τ) as follows:

$$f = \frac{D_B}{D_0} = e^{-k\tau} \qquad (9.7)$$

With any given dose, f depends on k and τ. If τ is large, f will be smaller because D_B (the amount of drug remaining in the body) is smaller.

EXAMPLES ▶▶▶

1. A patient receives 1000 mg every 6 hours by repetitive IV injection of an antibiotic with an elimination half-life of 3 hours. Assume the drug is distributed according to a one-compartment model and the volume of distribution is 20 L.
   a. Find the maximum and minimum amounts of drug in the body.
   b. Determine the maximum and minimum plasma concentrations of the drug.

Solution

a. The fraction of drug remaining in the body is estimated by Equation 9.7. The concentration of the drug declines to one-half after 3 hours ($t_{1/2} = 3$ h), after which the amount of drug will again decline by one-half at the end of the next 3 hours. Therefore, at the end of 6 hours, only one-quarter, or 0.25, of the original dose remains in the body. Thus f is equal to 0.25. To use Equation 9.7, we must first find the value of k from the $t_{1/2}$.

$$k = \frac{0.693}{t_{1/2}} = \frac{0.693}{3} = 0.231\,\text{h}^{-1}$$

The time interval τ is equal to 6 hours. From Equation 9.7,

$$f = e^{-(0.231)(6)}$$

$$f = 0.25$$

In this example, 1000 mg of drug is given intravenously, so the amount of drug in the body is immediately increased by 1000 mg. At the end of the dosage interval (ie, before the next dose), the amount of drug remaining in the body is 25% of the amount of drug present just after the previous dose, because $f = 0.25$. Thus, if the value of f is known, a table can be constructed relating the fraction of the dose in the body before and after rapid IV injection (Table 9-4).

From Table 9-4 the maximum amount of drug in the body is 1333 mg and the minimum amount of drug in the body is 333 mg. The difference between the maximum and minimum values, D_0, will always equal the injected dose.

$$D_{max} - D_{min} = D_0 \tag{9.8}$$

In this example,

$$1333 - 333 = 1000\,\text{mg}$$

D_{max}^{∞} can also be calculated directly by the relationship

$$D_{max}^{\infty} = \frac{D_0}{1-f} \tag{9.9}$$

TABLE 9-4 Fraction of the Dose in the Body before and after Intravenous Injections of a 1000-mg Dose[a]

Number of Doses	Amount of Drug in Body	
	Before Dose	After Dose
1	0	1000
2	250	1250
3	312	1312
4	328	1328
5	332	1332
6	333	1333
7	333	1333
∞	333	1333

[a]$f = 0.25$.

Substituting known data, we obtain

$$D_{max}^{\infty} = \frac{1000}{1-0.25} = 1333\,\text{mg}$$

Then, from Equation 9.8,

$$D_{min}^{\infty} = 1333 - 1000 = 333\,\text{mg}$$

The average amount of drug in the body at steady state, D_{av}^{∞}, can be found by Equation 9.10 or Equation 9.11. F is the fraction of dose absorbed. For an IV injection, F is equal to 1.0.

$$D_{av}^{\infty} = \frac{FD_0}{k\tau} \tag{9.10}$$

$$D_{av}^{\infty} = \frac{FD_0 1.44 t_{1/2}}{\tau} \tag{9.11}$$

Equations 9.10 and 9.11 can be used for repetitive dosing at constant time intervals and for any route of administration as long as elimination occurs from the central compartment. Substitution of values from the example into Equation 9.11 gives

$$D_{av}^{\infty} = \frac{(1)(1000)(1.44)(3)}{6} = 720\,\text{mg}$$

Since the drug in the body declines exponentially (ie, first-order drug elimination), the value D_{av}^{∞} is not the arithmetic mean of D_{max}^{∞} and D_{min}^{∞}. The limitation of using D_{av}^{∞} is that the fluctuations of D_{max}^{∞} and D_{min}^{∞} are not known.

b. To determine the concentration of drug in the body after multiple doses, divide the amount of drug in the body by the volume in which it is dissolved. For a one-compartment model, the maximum, minimum, and steady-state concentrations of drug in the plasma are found by the following equations:

$$C_{max}^{\infty} = \frac{D_{max}^{\infty}}{V_D} \tag{9.12}$$

$$C_{min}^{\infty} = \frac{D_{min}^{\infty}}{V_D} \tag{9.13}$$

$$C_{av}^{\infty} = \frac{D_{av}^{\infty}}{V_D} \tag{9.14}$$

A more direct approach to finding C_{max}^{∞}, and C_{min}^{∞}, is C_{av}^{∞}:

$$C_{max}^{\infty} = \frac{C_p^0}{1 - e^{-k\tau}} \tag{9.15}$$

where C_p^0 is equal to D_0/V_D.

$$C_{min}^{\infty} = \frac{C_p^0 e^{-k\tau}}{1 - e^{-k\tau}} \tag{9.16}$$

$$C_{av}^{\infty} = \frac{FD_0}{V_D k \tau} \tag{9.17}$$

For this example, the values for C_{max}^{∞}, C_{min}^{∞}, and C_{av}^{∞} are 66.7, 16.7, and 36.1 $\mu g/mL$, respectively.

As mentioned, C_{av}^{∞} is not the arithmetic mean of C_{max}^{∞} and C_{min}^{∞} because plasma drug concentration declines exponentially. The C_{av}^{∞} is equal to $[AUC]_{t_1}^{t_2}$ or $(\int_{t_1}^{t_2} C_p \, dt)$ for a dosage interval at steady state divided by the dosage interval τ.

$$C_{av}^{\infty} = \frac{[AUC]_{t_1}^{t_2}}{\tau} \tag{9.18}$$

C_{av}^{∞} gives an estimate of the mean plasma drug concentration at steady state. The C_{av}^{∞} is often the target drug concentration for optimal therapeutic effect and gives an indication as to how long this plasma drug concentration is maintained during the dosing interval (between doses). The C_{av}^{∞}

is dependent on both AUC and τ. The C_{av}^{∞} reflects drug exposure after multiple doses. Drug exposure is often related to drug safety and efficacy as discussed later in Chapter 21. For example, drug exposure is closely monitored when a cytotoxic or immunosuppressive, anticancer drug is administered during therapy. AUC may be estimated by sampling several plasma drug concentrations over time. Theoretically, AUC is superior to sampling just the C_{max} or C_{min}. For example, when cyclosporine dosing is clinically evaluated using AUC, the AUC is approximately estimated by two or three points. Dosing error is less than using AUC compared to the trough method alone (Primmett et al, 1998). In general, C_{min} or trough level is more frequently used than C_{max}^{∞}. C_{min} is the drug concentration just before the next dose is given and is less variable than peak drug concentration, C_{max}^{∞}. The sample time for C_{max}^{∞} is approximated and the true C_{max}^{∞} may not be accurately estimated. In some cases, the plasma trough level, C_{min}^{∞} is considered by some investigators as a more reliable sample since the drug is equilibrated with the surrounding tissues, although this may also depend on other factors.

The AUC is related to the amount of drug absorbed divided by total body clearance (Cl), as shown in the following equation:

$$[AUC]_{t_1}^{t_2} = \frac{FD_0}{Cl} = \frac{FD_0}{kV_D} \tag{9.19}$$

Substitution of FD_0/kV_D for AUC in Equation 9.18 gives Equation 9.17. Equation 9.17 or 9.18 can be used to obtain C_{av}^{∞} after a multiple-dose regimen regardless of the route of administration.

It is sometimes desirable to know the plasma drug concentration at any time after the administration of n doses of drug. The general expression for calculating this plasma drug concentration is

$$C_p = \frac{D_0}{V_D}\left(\frac{1 - e^{-nk\tau}}{1 - e^{-k\tau}}\right)e^{-kt} \tag{9.20}$$

where n is the number of doses given and t is the time after the nth dose.

At steady state, $e^{-nk\tau}$ approaches zero and Equation 9.20 reduces to

$$C_p^{\infty} = \frac{D_0}{V_D}\left(\frac{1}{1-e^{-k\tau}}\right)e^{-kt} \qquad (9.21)$$

where C_p^{∞} is the steady-state drug concentration at time t after the dose.

2. The patient in the previous example received 1000 mg of an antibiotic every 6 hours by repetitive IV injection. The drug has an apparent volume of distribution of 20 L and elimination half-life of 3 hours. Calculate **(a)** the plasma drug concentration, C_p at 3 hours after the second dose, **(b)** the steady-state plasma drug concentration, C_p^{∞} at 3 hours after the last dose, **(c)** C_{max}^{∞}, **(d)** C_{min}^{∞}, and **(e)** C_{ss}.

Solution

a. The C_p at 3 hours after the second dose—use Equation 9.20 and let $n = 2$, $t = 3$ hours, and make other appropriate substitutions.

$$C_p = \frac{1000}{20}\left(\frac{1-e^{-(2)(0.231)(6)}}{1-e^{-(0.231)(6)}}\right)e^{-0.231(3)}$$

$$C_p = 31.3 \text{ mg/L}$$

b. The C_p^{∞} at 3 hours after the last dose—because steady state is reached, use Equation 9.21 and perform the following calculation:

$$C_p^{\infty} = \frac{1000}{20}\left(\frac{1}{1-e^{-0.231(6)}}\right)e^{-0.231(3)}$$

$$C_p^{\infty} = 33.3 \text{ mg/L}$$

c. The C_{max}^{∞} is calculated from Equation 9.15.

$$C_{max}^{\infty} = \frac{1000/20}{1-e^{-(0.231)(6)}} = 66.7 \text{ mg/L}$$

d. The C_{min}^{∞} may be estimated as the drug concentration after the dosage interval τ, or just before the next dose.

$$C_{min}^{\infty} = C_{max}^{\infty}e^{-kt} = 66.7e^{-(0.231)(6)} = 16.7 \text{ mg/L}$$

e. The C_{av}^{∞} is estimated by Equation 9.17—because the drug is given by IV bolus injections, $F = 1$.

$$C_{av}^{\infty} = \frac{1000}{(0.231)(20)(6)} = 36.1 \text{ mg/L}$$

C_{av}^{∞} is represented as C_{ss} in some references.

Problem of a Missed Dose

Equation 9.22 describes the plasma drug concentration t hours after the nth dose is administered; the doses are administered τ hours apart according to a multiple-dose regimen:

$$C_p = \frac{D_0}{V_D}\left(\frac{1-e^{-nk\tau}}{1-e^{-k\tau}}\right)e^{-kt} \qquad (9.22)$$

Concentration contributed by the missing dose is

$$C_p' = \frac{D_0}{V_D}e^{-kt_{miss}} \qquad (9.23)$$

in which t_{miss} = time elapsed since the scheduled dose was missed. Subtracting Equation 9.23 from Equation 9.20 corrects for the missing dose as shown in Equation 9.24.

$$C_p = \frac{D_0}{V_D}\left[\left(\frac{1-e^{-nk\tau}}{1-e^{-k\tau}}\right)e^{-kt} - e^{-kt_{miss}}\right] \qquad (9.24)$$

Note: If steady state is reached (ie, either n = large or after many doses), the equation simplifies to Equation 9.25. Equation 9.25 is useful when steady state is reached.

$$C_p = \frac{D_0}{V_D}\left(\frac{e^{-kt}}{1-e^{-kt}}\right) - e^{-kt_{miss}} \qquad (9.25)$$

Generally, if the missing dose is recent, it will affect the present drug level more. If the missing dose is several half-lives later ($>5t_{1/2}$), the missing dose may be omitted because it will be very small. Equation 9.24 accounts for one missing dose, but several missing doses can be subtracted in a similar way if necessary.

EXAMPLE ▶ ▶ ▶

A cephalosporin ($k = 0.2$ h⁻¹, $V_D = 10$ L) was administered by IV multiple dosing; 100 mg was injected every 6 hours for 6 doses. What was the plasma drug concentration 4 hours after the sixth dose (ie, 40 hours later) if **(a)** the fifth dose was omitted, **(b)** the sixth dose was omitted, and **(c)** the fourth dose was omitted?

Solution

Substitute $k = 0.2$ h^{-1}, $V_D = 10$ L, $D = 100$ mg, $n = 6$, $t = 4$ hours, and $\tau = 6$ hours into Equation 9.20 and evaluate:

$$C_p = 6.425 \text{ mg/L}$$

If no dose was omitted, then 4 hours after the sixth injection, C_p would be 6.425 mg/L.

a. Missing the fifth dose, its contribution must be subtracted off, $t_{miss} = 6 + 4 = 10$ hours (the time elapsed since missing the dose) using the steady-state equation:

$$C_p' = \frac{D_0}{V_D}e^{-kt_{miss}} = \frac{100}{10}e^{-(0.2 \times 10)}$$

Drug concentration correcting for the missing dose = 6.425 − 1.353 = 5.072 mg/L.

b. If the sixth dose is missing, $t_{miss} = 4$ hours:

$$C_p' = \frac{D_0}{V_D}e^{-kt_{miss}} = \frac{100}{10}e^{-(0.2 \times 4)} = 4.493 \text{ mg/L}$$

Drug concentration correcting for the missing dose = 6.425 − 4.493 = 1.932 mg/L.

c. If the fourth dose is missing, $t_{miss} = 12 + 4 = 16$ hours:

$$C_p' = \frac{D_0}{V_D}e^{-kt_{miss}} = \frac{100}{10}e^{-(0.2 \times 16)} = 0.408 \text{ mg/L}$$

The drug concentration corrected for the missing dose = 6.425 − 0.408 = 6.017 mg/L.

Note: The effect of a missing dose becomes less pronounced at a later time. A strict dose regimen compliance is advised for all drugs. With some drugs, missing a dose can have a serious effect on therapy. For example, compliance is important for the anti-HIV1 drugs such as the protease inhibitors.

Early or Late Dose Administration during Multiple Dosing

When one of the drug doses is taken earlier or later than scheduled, the resulting plasma drug concentration can still be calculated based on the principle of superposition. The dose can be treated as missing, with the late or early dose added back to take into account the actual time of dosing, using Equation 9.26.

$$C_p = \frac{D_0}{V_D}\left(\frac{1 - e^{-nkt}}{1 - e^{-kt}}e^{-kt} - e^{-kt_{miss}} + e^{-kt_{actual}}\right) \quad (9.26)$$

in which t_{miss} = time elapsed since the dose (late or early) is scheduled, and t_{actual} = time elapsed since the dose (late or early) is actually taken. Using a similar approach, a second missed dose can be subtracted from Equation 9.20. Similarly, a second late/early dose may be corrected by subtracting the scheduled dose followed by adding the actual dose. Similarly, if a different dose is given, the regular dose may be subtracted and the new dose added back.

EXAMPLE ▶▶▶

Assume the same drug as above (ie, $k = 0.2$ h^{-1}, $V_D = 10$ L) was given by multiple IV bolus injections and that at a dose of 100 mg every 6 hours for 6 doses. What is the plasma drug concentration 4 hours after the sixth dose, if the fifth dose were given an hour late?

Substitute into Equation 9.26 for all unknowns: $k = 0.2$ h^{-1}, $V_D = 10$ L, $D = 100$ mg, $n = 6$, $t = 4$ h, $\tau = 6$ h, $t_{miss} = 6 + 4 = 10$ hours, $t_{actual} = 9$ hours (taken 1 hour late, ie, 5 hours before the sixth dose).

$$C_p = \frac{D_0}{V_D}\left(\frac{1 - e^{-nk\tau}}{1 - e^{-k\tau}}e^{-k\tau} - e^{-kt_{miss}} + e^{-kt_{actual}}\right)$$

$$C_p = 6.425 - 1.353 + 1.653 = 6.725 \text{ mg/L}$$

Note: 1.353 mg/L was subtracted and 1.653 mg/mL was added because the fifth dose was not given as planned, but was given 1 hour later.

INTERMITTENT INTRAVENOUS INFUSION

Intermittent IV infusion is a method of successive short IV drug infusions in which the drug is given by IV infusion for a short period of time followed by a drug elimination period, then followed by another

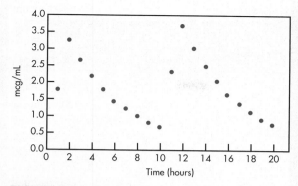

FIGURE 9-4 Plasma drug concentration after two doses by IV infusion. Data from Table 9-5.

short IV infusion (Fig. 9-4). In drug regimens involving short IV infusion, the drug may not reach steady state. The rationale for intermittent IV infusion is to prevent transient high drug concentrations and accompanying side effects. Many drugs are better tolerated when infused slowly over time compared to IV bolus dosing.

Administering One or More Doses by Constant Infusion: Superposition of Several IV Infusion Doses

For a continuous IV infusion (see Chapter 7):

$$C_p = \frac{R}{Cl}(1 - e^{-kt}) = \frac{R}{kV_D}(1 - e^{-kt}) \quad (9.27)$$

Equation 9.27 may be modified to determine drug concentration after one or more short IV infusions for a specified time period (Equation 9.28).

$$C_p = \frac{D}{t_{inf}V_D k}(1 - e^{-kt}) \quad (9.28)$$

where R = rate of infusion = D/t_{inf}, D = size of infusion dose, and t_{inf} = infusion period.

After the infusion is stopped, the drug concentration post-IV infusion is obtained using the first-order equation for drug elimination:

$$C_p = C_{stop} e^{-kt} \quad (9.29)$$

where C_{stop} = concentration when infusion stops, and t = time elapsed since infusion stopped.

EXAMPLE ▶▶▶

An antibiotic was infused with a 40-mg IV dose over 2 hours. Ten hours later, a second dose of 40 mg was infused, again over 2 hours. **(a)** What is the plasma drug concentration 2 hours after the start of the first infusion? **(b)** What is the plasma drug concentration 5 hours after the second dose infusion was started? Assume $k = 0.2$ h^{-1} and $V_D = 10$ L for the antibiotic.

Solution

The predicted plasma drug concentrations after the first and second IV infusions are shown in Table 9-5. Using the principle of superposition, the total plasma drug concentration is the sum of the residual drug concentrations due to the first IV infusion (column 3) and the drug concentrations due to the second IV infusion (column 4). A graphical representation of these data is shown in Fig. 9-4.

a. The plasma drug concentration at 2 hours after the first IV infusion starts is calculated from Equation 9.28.

$$C_p = \frac{40/2}{10 \times 0.2}(1 - e^{-0.2/2}) = 3.30 \text{ mg/L}$$

b. From Table 9-5, the plasma drug concentration at 15 hours (ie, 5 hours after the start of the second IV infusion) is 2.06 μg/mL. At 5 hours after the second IV infusion starts, the plasma drug concentration is the sum of the residual plasma drug concentrations from the first 2-hour infusion according to first-order elimination and the residual plasma drug concentrations from the second 2-hour IV infusion as shown in the following scheme:

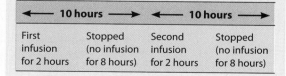

← 10 hours →		← 10 hours →	
First infusion for 2 hours	Stopped (no infusion for 8 hours)	Second infusion for 2 hours	Stopped (no infusion for 8 hours)

The plasma drug concentration is calculated using the first-order elimination equation, where C_{stop} is the plasma drug concentration at the stop of the 2-hour IV infusion.

TABLE 9-5   Drug Concentration after Two Intravenous Infusions[a]

	Time(h)	Plasma Drug Concentration after Infusion 1	Plasma Drug Concentration after Infusion 2	Total Plasma Drug Concentration
Infusion 1 begins	0	0		0
	1	1.81		1.81
Infusion 1 stopped	2	3.30		3.30
	3	2.70		2.70
	4	2.21		2.21
	5	1.81		1.81
	6	1.48		1.48
	7	1.21		1.21
	8	0.99		0.99
	9	0.81		0.81
Infusion 2 begins	10	0.67	0	0.67
	11	0.55	1.81	2.36
Infusion 2 stopped	12	0.45	3.30	3.74
	13	0.37	2.70	3.07
	14	0.30	2.21	2.51
	15	0.25	1.81	2.06

[a]Drug is given by a 2-hour infusion separated by a 10-hour drug elimination interval. All drug concentrations are in μg/mL. The declining drug concentration after the first infusion dose and the drug concentration after the second infusion dose give the total plasma drug concentration.

The plasma drug concentration after the completion of the first IV infusion when $t = 15$ hours is

$$C_p = C_{stop}e^{-kt} = 3.30e^{-0.2 \times 15} = 0.25 \ \mu g/L$$

The plasma drug concentration 5 hours after the second IV infusion is

$$C_p = C_{stop}e^{-kt} = 3.30e^{-0.2 \times 3} = 1.81 \ \mu g/mL$$

The total plasma drug concentration 5 hours after the start of the second IV infusion is

$$0.25 \ mg/L + 1.81 \ mg/L = 2.06 \ mg/L.$$

CLINICAL EXAMPLE

Gentamicin sulfate was given to an adult male patient (57 years old, 70 kg) by intermittent IV infusions. One-hour IV infusions of 90 mg of gentamicin was given at 8-hour intervals. Gentamicin clearance is similar to creatinine clearance and was estimated as 7.2 L/h with an elimination half-life of 3 hours.

a. What is the plasma drug concentration after the first IV infusion?

b. What is the peak plasma drug concentration, C_{max}, and the trough plasma drug concentration, C_{min}, at steady state?

Solution

a. The plasma drug concentration directly after the first infusion is calculated from Equation 9.27, where $R = 90$ mg/h, $Cl = 7.2$ L/h, and $k = 0.231$ h^{-1}. The time for infusion, t_{int}, is 1 hour.

$$C_p = \frac{90}{7.2}(1 - e^{-(0.231)(1)}) = 2.58 \text{ mg/L}$$

b. The C_{max}^{∞} at steady state may be obtained from Equation 9.30.

$$C_{max}^{\infty} = \frac{R(1 - e^{-kt_{inf}})}{Cl} \frac{1}{(1 - e^{-k\tau})} \qquad (9.30)$$

where C_{max} is the peak drug concentration following the nth infusion, at steady state, t_{inf} is the time period of infusion, and τ is the dosage interval. The term $1/(1 - e^{-k\tau})$ is the accumulation factor for repeated drug administration. Substitution in Equation 9.30 gives

$$C_{max}^{\infty} = \frac{90(1 - e^{-(0.231)(1)})}{7.2} \times \frac{1}{(1 - e^{-(0.231)(8)})}$$

$$= 3.06 \text{ mg/L}$$

The plasma drug concentration C_p^{∞} at any time t after the last infusion ends when steady state is obtained by Equation 9.31 and assumes that plasma drug concentrations decline according to first-order elimination kinetics.

$$C_p^{\infty} = \frac{R(1 - e^{-kt_{inf}})}{Cl} \times \frac{1}{(1 - e^{-k\tau})} \times e^{-k(t)} \qquad (9.31)$$

where t_{inf} is the time for infusion and t is the time period after the end of the infusion.

The trough plasma drug concentration, C_{min}^{∞}, at steady state is the drug concentration just before the start of the next IV infusion or after a dosage interval equal to 8 hours after the last infusion stopped. Equation 9.31 can be used to determine the plasma drug concentration at any time after the last infusion is stopped (after steady state has been reached).

$$C_{min}^{\infty} = \frac{90(1 - e^{-(0.231)(1)})}{7.2} \times \frac{e^{-(0.231)(8)}}{(1 - e^{-(0.231)(8)})}$$

$$= 0.48 \text{ mg/L}$$

ESTIMATION OF k AND V_D OF AMINOGLYCOSIDES IN CLINICAL SITUATIONS

As illustrated above, antibiotics are often infused intravenously by multiple doses, so it is desirable to adjust the recommended starting dose based on the patient's individual k and V_D values. According to Sawchuk and Zaske (1976), individual parameters for aminoglycoside pharmacokinetics may be determined in a patient by using a limited number of plasma drug samples taken at appropriate time intervals. The equation was simplified by replacing an elaborate model with the one-compartment model to describe drug elimination and appropriately avoiding the distributive phase. The plasma sample should be collected 15–30 minutes postinfusion (with infusion lasting about 60 minutes) and, in patients with poor renal function, 1–2 hours postinfusion, to allow adequate tissue distribution. The second and third blood samples should be collected about 2–3 half-lives later, in order to get a good estimation of the slope. The data may be determined graphically or by regression analysis using a scientific calculator or computer program.

$$V_D = \frac{R(1 - e^{-kt_{inf}})}{[C_{max}^{\infty} - C_{min}^{\infty} e^{-kt_{inf}}]} \qquad (9.32)$$

The dose of aminoglycoside is generally fixed by the desirable peak, C_{max}^{∞}, and trough plasma concentration, C_{min}^{∞}. For example, C_{max}^{∞} for gentamicin may be set at 6–10 μg/mL with the steady-state trough level, C_{min}^{∞}, generally about 0.5–2 μg/mL, depending on the severity of the infection and renal considerations. The upper range is used only for life-threatening infections. The infusion rate for any desired peak drug concentration may be calculated using Equation 9.33.

$$R = \frac{V_D k C_{max}^{\infty}(1 - e^{-k\tau})}{(1 - e^{-kt_{inf}})} \qquad (9.33)$$

The dosing interval τ between infusions may be adjusted to obtain a desired concentration.

MULTIPLE-ORAL-DOSE REGIMEN

Figures 9-1 and 9-2 present typical cumulation curves for the concentration of drug in the body after multiple oral doses given at a constant dosage interval. The plasma concentration at any time during an oral or extravascular multiple-dose regimen, assuming a one-compartment model and constant doses and dose interval, can be determined as follows:

$$C_p = \frac{F k_a D_0}{V_D(k - k_a)} \left[\left(\frac{1 - e^{-nk_a\tau}}{1 - e^{-k_a\tau}} \right) e^{-k_a t} - \left(\frac{1 - e^{-nk\tau}}{1 - e^{-k\tau}} \right) e^{-kt} \right]$$

where n = number of doses, τ = dosage interval, F = fraction of dose absorbed, and t = time after administration of n doses.

The mean plasma level at steady state, C_{av}^∞, is determined by a similar method to that employed for repeat IV injections. Equation 9.17 can be used for finding C_{av}^∞ for any route of administration.

$$C_{av}^\infty = \frac{FD_0}{V_D k \tau} \qquad (9.17)$$

Because proper evaluation of F and V_D requires IV data, the AUC of a dosing interval at steady state may be substituted in Equation 9.17 to obtain

$$C_{av}^\infty = \frac{\int_0^\infty C_p\, dt}{\tau} = \frac{[AUC]_0^\infty}{\tau} \qquad (9.35)$$

One can see from Equation 9.17 that the magnitude of C_{av}^∞ is directly proportional to the size of the dose and the extent of drug absorbed. Furthermore, if

the dosage interval (τ) is shortened, then the value for C_{av}^∞ will increase. The C_{av}^∞ will be predictably higher for drugs distributed in a small V_D (eg, plasma water) or that have long elimination half-lives than for drugs distributed in a large V_D (eg, total body water) or that have very short elimination half-lives. Because body clearance (Cl_T) is equal to kV_D, substitution into Equation 9.17 yields

$$C_{av}^\infty = \frac{FD_0}{Cl_T \tau} \qquad (9.36)$$

Thus, if Cl_T decreases, C_{av}^∞ will increase.

The C_{av}^∞ does not give information concerning the fluctuations in plasma concentration (C_{max}^∞ and C_{min}^∞). In multiple-dose regimens, C_p at any time can be obtained using Equation 9.34, where $n = n$th dose. At steady state, the drug concentration can be determined by letting n equal infinity. Therefore, $e^{-nk\tau}$ becomes approximately equal to zero and Equation 9.22 becomes

$$C_p^\infty = \frac{k_a FD_0}{V_D(k_a - k)} \left[\left(\frac{1}{1 - e^{-k\tau}} \right) e^{-kt} - \left(\frac{1}{1 - e^{-k_a\tau}} \right) e^{-k_a t} \right]$$

$$(9.37)$$

The maximum and minimum drug concentrations (C_{max}^∞ and C_{min}^∞) can be obtained with the following equations:

$$C_{max}^\infty = \frac{FD_0}{V_D} \left(\frac{1}{1 - e^{-k\tau}} \right) e^{-kt_p} \qquad (9.38)$$

$$C_{min}^\infty = \frac{k_a FD_0}{V_D(k_a - k)} \left(\frac{1}{1 - e^{-k\tau}} \right) e^{-k\tau} \qquad (9.39)$$

The time at which maximum (peak) plasma concentration (or t_{max}) occurs following a single oral dose is

$$t_{max} = \frac{2.3}{k_a - k} \log \frac{k_a}{k} \qquad (9.40)$$

whereas the peak plasma concentration, t_p, following multiple doses is given by Equation 9.41.

$$t_p = \frac{1}{k_a - k} \ln \left[\frac{k_a(1 - e^{-k\tau})}{k(1 - e^{-k_a\tau})} \right] \qquad (9.41)$$

Large fluctuations between C_{max}^∞ and C_{min}^∞ can be hazardous, particularly with drugs that have a narrow therapeutic index. The larger the number of divided doses, the smaller the fluctuations in the plasma drug concentrations. For example, a 500-mg dose of drug given every 6 hours will produce the same C_{av}^{∞} value as a 250-mg dose of the same drug given every 3 hours, while the C_{max}^{∞} and C_{min}^{∞} fluctuations for the latter dose will be decreased by one-half (see Fig. 9-3). With drugs that have a narrow therapeutic index, the dosage interval should not be longer than the elimination half-life.

EXAMPLE ▶ ▶ ▶

An adult male patient (46 years old, 81 kg) was given 250 mg of tetracycline hydrochloride orally every 8 hours for 2 weeks. From the literature, tetracycline hydrochloride is about 75% bioavailable and has an apparent volume of distribution of 1.5 L/kg. The elimination half-life is about 10 hours. The absorption rate constant is 0.9 h^{-1}. From this information, calculate **(a)** C_{max} after the first dose, **(b)** C_{min} after the first dose, **(c)** plasma drug concentration C_p at 4 hours after the seventh dose, **(d)** maximum plasma drug concentration at steady state, C_{max}^{∞}, **(e)** minimum plasma drug concentration at steady state, C_{min}^{∞}, and **(f)** average plasma drug concentration at steady state, C_{av}^{∞}.

Solution

a. C_{max} after the first dose occurs at t_{max}—therefore, using Equation 9.40,

$$t_{max} = \frac{2.3}{0.9-0.07} \log\left(\frac{0.9}{0.07}\right)$$

$$t_{max} = 3.07$$

Then substitute t_{max} into the following equation for a single oral dose (one-compartment model) to obtain C_{max}.

$$C_{max} = \frac{FD_0 k_a}{V_D(k_a-k)}(e^{-kt_{max}} - e^{-k_a t_{max}})$$

$$C_{max} = \frac{(0.75)(250)(0.9)}{(121.5)(0.9-0.07)}(e^{-0.07(3.07)} - e^{-0.9(3.07)})$$

$$C_{max} = 1.28 \text{ mg/L}$$

b. C_{min} after the first dose occurs just before the administration of the next dose of drug—therefore, set $t = 8$ hours and solve for C_{min}.

$$C_{min} = \frac{(0.75)(250)(0.9)}{(121.5)(0.9-0.07)}(e^{-0.07(8)} - e^{-0.9(8)})$$

$$C_{min} = 0.95 \text{ mg/L}$$

c. C_p at 4 hours after the seventh dose may be calculated using Equation 9.34, letting $n = 7$, $t = 4$, $\tau = 8$, and making the appropriate substitutions.

$$C_p = \frac{(0.75)(250)(0.9)}{(121.5)(0.07-0.9)}$$

$$\times \left[\left(\frac{1-e^{-(7)(0.9)(8)}}{1-e^{-0.9(8)}}\right)e^{-0.9(4)} - \left(\frac{1-e^{-(7)(0.07)(8)}}{1-e^{-(0.07)(8)}}\right)e^{-0.07(4)}\right]$$

$$C_p = 2.86 \text{ mg/L}$$

d. C_{max}^{∞} at steady state: t_p at steady state is obtained from Equation 9.41.

$$t_p = \frac{1}{k_a-k}\ln\left[\frac{k_a(1-e^{-k\tau})}{k(1-e^{-k_a\tau})}\right]$$

$$t_p = \frac{1}{0.9-0.07}\ln\left[\frac{0.9(1-e^{-(0.07)(8)})}{0.07(1-e^{-(0.9)(8)})}\right]$$

$$t_p = 2.05 \text{ hours}$$

Then C_{max}^{∞} is obtained using Equation 9.38.

$$C_{max}^{\infty} = \frac{0.75(250)}{121.5}\left(\frac{1}{1-e^{-0.07(8)}}\right)e^{-0.07(2.05)}$$

$$C_{min}^{\infty} = 3.12 \text{ mg/L}$$

e. C_{min}^{∞} at steady state is calculated from Equation 9.39.

$$C_{min}^{\infty} = \frac{(0.9)(0.75)(250)}{(121.5)(0.9-0.07)}\left(\frac{1}{1-e^{-0.07(8)}}\right)e^{-(0.7)(8)}$$

$$C_{max}^{\infty} = 2.23 \text{ mg/L}$$

f. C_{av}^{∞} at steady state is calculated from Equation 9.17.

$$C_{av}^{\infty} = \frac{(0.75)(250)}{(121.5)(0.07)(8)}$$

$$C_{av}^{\infty} = 2.76 \text{ mg/L}$$

LOADING DOSE

Since extravascular doses require time for absorption into the plasma to occur, therapeutic effects are delayed until sufficient plasma concentrations are achieved. To reduce the onset time of the drug—that is, the time it takes to achieve the minimum effective concentration (assumed to be equivalent to the C_{av}^{∞})—a loading (priming) or initial dose of drug is given. The main objective of the loading dose is to achieve desired plasma concentrations, C_{av}^{∞}, as quickly as possible. If the drug follows one-compartment pharmacokinetics, then in theory, steady state is also achieved immediately following the loading dose. Thereafter, a maintenance dose is given to maintain C_{av}^{∞} and steady state so that the therapeutic effect is also maintained. In practice, a loading dose may be given as a bolus dose or a short-term loading IV infusion.

As discussed earlier, the time required for the drug to accumulate to a steady-state plasma level is dependent mainly on its elimination half-life. The time needed to reach 90% of C_{av}^{∞} is approximately 3.3 half-lives, and the time required to reach 99% of C_{av}^{∞} is equal to approximately 6.6 half-lives. For a drug with a half-life of 4 hours, it will take approximately 13 and 26 hours to reach 90% and 99% of C_{av}^{∞}, respectively.

For drugs absorbed rapidly in relation to elimination ($k_a \gg k$) and that are distributed rapidly, the loading dose D_L can be calculated as follows:

$$\frac{D_L}{D_0} = \frac{1}{(1-e^{-k_a\tau})(1-e^{-k\tau})} \tag{9.42}$$

For extremely rapid absorption, as when the product of $k_a\tau$ is large or in the case of IV infusion, $e^{-k_a\tau}$ becomes approximately zero and Equation 9.42 reduces to

$$\frac{D_L}{D_0} = \frac{1}{1-e^{-k\tau}} \tag{9.43}$$

The loading dose should approximate the amount of drug contained in the body at steady state. The dose ratio is equal to the loading dose divided by the maintenance dose.

$$\text{Dose ratio} = \frac{D_L}{D_0} \tag{9.44}$$

As a general rule of thumb, if the selected dosage interval is equal to the drug's elimination half-life, then the dose ratio calculated from Equation 9.44 should be equal to 2.0. In other words, the loading dose will be equal to double the initial drug dose. Figure 9-5 shows the plasma level–time curve for dosage regimens with equal maintenance doses but

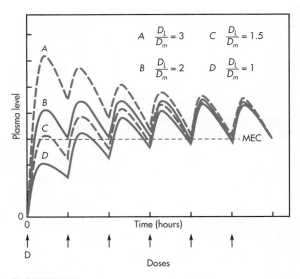

FIGURE 9-5   Concentration curves for dosage regimens with equal maintenance doses (*D*) and dosage intervals (*τ*) and different dose ratios. (From Kruger-Thiemer, 1968, with permission.)

different loading doses. A rapid approximation of loading dose, D_L, may be estimated from

$$D_L = \frac{V_D C_{av}^{\infty}}{(S)(F)} \tag{9.45}$$

where C_{av}^{∞} is the desired plasma drug concentration, S is the salt form of the drug, and F is the fraction of drug bioavailability.

Equation 9.45 assumes very rapid drug absorption from an immediate-release dosage form. The D_L calculated by this method has been used in clinical situations for which only an approximation of the D_L is needed.

These calculations for loading doses are not applicable to drugs that demonstrate multicompartment kinetics. Such drugs distribute slowly into extravascular tissues, and drug equilibration and steady state may not occur until after the apparent plateau is reached in the vascular (central) compartment.

DOSAGE REGIMEN SCHEDULES

Predictions of steady-state plasma drug concentrations usually assume the drug is given at a constant dosage interval throughout a 24-hour day. Very often,

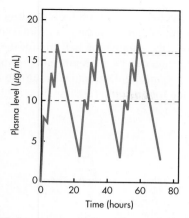

FIGURE 9-6   Plasma level–time curve for theophylline given in doses of 160 mg 3 times a day. Dashed lines indicate the therapeutic range. (From Niebergall et al, 1974, with permission.)

however, the drug is given only during the waking hours (Fig. 9-6). Niebergall et al (1974) discussed the problem of scheduling dosage regimens and particularly warned against improper timing of the drug dosage. For drugs with a narrow therapeutic index such as theophylline (Fig. 9-6), large fluctuation between the maximum and minimum plasma levels are undesirable and may lead to subtherapeutic plasma drug concentrations and/or to high, possibly toxic, drug concentrations. These wide fluctuations occur if larger doses are given at wider dosage intervals (see Fig. 9-3). For example, Fig. 9-7 shows

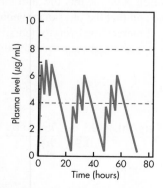

FIGURE 9-7   Plasma level–time curve for procainamide given in an initial dose of 1.0 g followed by doses of 0.5 g 4 times a day. Dashed lines indicate the therapeutic range. (From Niebergall et al, 1974, with permission.)

procainamide given with a 1.0-g loading dose on the first day followed by maintainence doses of 0.5-g four times a day. On the second, third, and subsequent days, the procainamide plasma levels did not reach the therapeutic range until after the second dose of drug.

Ideally, drug doses should be given at evenly spaced intervals. However, to improve patient compliance, dosage regimens may be designed to fit with the lifestyle of the patient. For example, the patient is directed to take a drug such as amoxicillin four times a day (QID), before meals and at bedtime, for a systemic infection. This dosage regimen will produce unequal dosage intervals during the day, because the patient takes the drug before breakfast, at 0800 hours (8 AM); before lunch, at 1200 hours (12 noon); before dinner, at 1800 hours (6 PM); and before bedtime, at 2300 hours (11 PM). For these drugs, evenly spaced dosage intervals are not that critical to the effectiveness of the antibiotic as long as the plasma drug concentrations are maintained above the *minimum inhibitory concentration* (MIC) for the microorganism. In some cases, a drug may be given at a larger dose allowing for a longer duration above MIC if fluctuation is less critical. In Augmentin Bid-875 (amoxicillin/clavulanate tablets), the amoxicillin/clavulanate tablet is administered twice daily.

Patient compliance with multiple-dose regimens may be a problem for the patient in following the prescribed dosage regimen. Occasionally, a patient may miss taking the drug dose at the prescribed dosage interval. For drugs with long elimination half-lives (eg, levothyroxine sodium or oral contraceptives), the consequences of one missed dose are minimal, since only a small fraction of drug is lost between daily dosing intervals. The patient should either take the next drug dose as soon as the patient remembers or continue the dosing schedule starting at the next prescribed dosing period. If it is almost time for the next dose, then the skipped dose should not be taken and the regular dosing schedule should be maintained. Generally, the patient should not double the dose of the medication. For specific drug information on missed doses, USP DI II, *Advice for the Patient*, published annually by the United States Pharmacopeia, is a good source of information.

The problems of widely fluctuating plasma drug concentrations may be prevented by using a controlled-release formulation of the drug, or a drug in the same therapeutic class that has a long elimination half-life. The use of extended-release dosage forms allows for less frequent dosing and prevents under-medication between the last evening dose and the first morning dose. Extended-release drug products may improve patient compliance by decreasing the number of doses within a 24-hour period that the patient needs to take. Patients generally show better compliance with a twice-a-day (BID) dosage regimen compared to a three-times-a-day (TID) dosage schedule.

CLINICAL EXAMPLE

Bupropion hydrochloride (Wellbutrin) is a noradren-ergic/dopaminergic antidepressant. Jefferson et al, 2005, have reviewed the pharmacokinetic properties of bupropion and its various various formulations and clinical applications, the goal of which is optimization of major depressive disorder treatment. Bupropion hydrochloride is available in three oral formulations. The immediate-release (IR) tablet is given three times a day, the sustained-release tablet (Wellbutrin SR) is given twice a day, and the extended-release tablet (Wellbutrin XL) is given once a day.

The total daily dose was 300 mg bupropion HCl. The area under the curve, AUC, for each dose treatment was similar showing that the formulations were bio-equivalent based on extent of absorption. The fluctua-tions between peak and trough levels were greatest for the IR product given three times a day and least for the once-a-day XL product. According to the manufac-turer, all three dosage regimens provide equivalent clinical efficacy. The advantage of the extended-release product is that the patient needs only to take the drug once a day. Often, immediate-release drug products are less expensive compared to an extended-release drug product. In this case, the fluctuating plasma drug levels for buproprion IR tablet given three times a day are not a safety issue and the tablet is equally efficacious as the 150-mg SR tablet given twice a day or the 300-mg XL tablet given once a day. The patient may also consider the cost of the medication.

PRACTICE PROBLEMS

1. Patient C.S. is a 35-year-old man weighing 76.6 kg. The patient is to be given multiple IV bolus injections of an antibiotic every 6 hours.

The effective concentration of this drug is 15 μg/mL. After the patient is given a single IV dose, the elimination half-life for the drug is determined to be 3.0 hours and the apparent V_D is 196 mL/kg. Determine a multiple IV dose regimen for this drug (assume drug is given every 6 hours).

Solution

$$C_{av}^{\infty} = \frac{FD_0}{V_D k \tau}$$

For IV dose, $F = 1$,

$$D_0 = (15 \ \mu g/mL)\left(\frac{0.693}{3 \ h}\right)(196 \ mL/kg)(6 \ h)$$

$$D_0 = 4.07 \ mg/kg \ every \ 6 \ hours$$

Since patient C.S. weighs 76.6 kg, the dose should be as shown:

$$D_0 = (4.07 \ mg/kg)(76.6 \ kg)$$
$$D_0 = 312 \ mg \ every \ 6 \ hours$$

After the condition of this patient has stabilized, the patient is to be given the drug orally for con-venience of drug administration. The objective is to design an oral dosage regimen that will produce the same steady-state blood level as the mul-tiple IV doses. The drug dose will depend on the bioavailability of the drug from the drug product, the desired therapeutic drug level, and the dosage interval chosen. Assume that the antibiotic is 90% bioavailable and that the physician would like to continue oral medication every 6 hours.

The average or steady-state plasma drug level is given by

$$C_{av}^{\infty} = \frac{FD_0}{V_D k \tau}$$

$$D_0 = \frac{(15 \ \mu g/mL)(193 \ mL/kg)(0.693)(6 \ h)}{(0.9)(3 \ h)}$$

$$D_0 = 454 \ mg/kg$$

Because patient C.S. weighs 76.6 kg, he should be given the following dose:

$$D_0 = (4.54 \ mg/kg)(76.6 \ kg)$$
$$D_0 = 348 \ mg \ every \ 6 \ hours$$

For drugs with equal absorption but slower absorption rates (F is the same but k_a is smaller), the initial dosing period may show a lower blood level; however, the steady-state blood level will be unchanged.

2. In practice, drug products are usually commercially available in certain specified strengths. Using the information provided in the preceding problem, assume that the antibiotic is available in 125-, 250-, and 500-mg tablets. Therefore, the pharmacist or prescriber must now decide which tablets are to be given to the patient. In this case, it may be possible to give the patient 375 mg (eg, one 125-mg tablet and one 250-mg tablet) every 6 hours. However, the C_{av}^{∞} should be calculated to determine if the plasma level is approaching a toxic value. Alternatively, a new dosage interval might be appropriate for the patient. It is very important to design the dosage interval and the dose to be as simple as possible, so that the patient will not be confused and will be able to comply with the medication program properly.

   a. What is the new C_{av}^{∞} if the patient is given 375 mg every 6 hours?

Solution

$$C_{av}^{\infty} = \frac{(0.9)(375,000)(3)}{(196)(76.6)(6)(0.693)}$$

$$C_{av}^{\infty} = 16.2 \ \mu g/mL$$

Because the therapeutic objective was to achieve a minimum effective concentration (MEC) of 15 μg/mL, a value of 16.2 μg/mL is reasonable.

   b. The patient has difficulty in distinguishing tablets of different strengths. Can the patient take a 500-mg dose (eg, two 250-mg tablets)?

Solution

The dosage interval (τ) for the 500-mg tablet would have to be calculated as follows:

$$\tau = \frac{(0.9)(500,000)(3)}{(196)(76.6)(15)(0.693)}$$

$$\tau = 8.63 \ h$$

   c. A dosage interval of 8.63 hours is difficult to remember. Is a dosage regimen of 500 mg every 8 hours reasonable?

Solution

$$C_{av}^{\infty} = \frac{(0.9)(500,000)(3)}{(196)(76.6)(8)(0.693)}$$

$$C_{av}^{\infty} = 16.2 \ \mu g/mL$$

Notice that a larger dose is necessary if the drug is given at longer intervals.

In designing a dosage regimen, one should consider a regimen that is practical and convenient for the patient. For example, for good compliance, the dosage interval should be spaced conveniently for the patient. In addition, one should consider the commercially available dosage strengths of the prescribed drug product.

The use of Equation 9.17 to estimate a dosage regimen initially has wide utility. The C_{av}^{∞} is equal to the dosing rate divided by the total body clearance of the drug in the patient:

$$C_{av}^{\infty} = \frac{FD_0}{\tau} \frac{1}{Cl_T} \tag{9.47}$$

where FD_0/τ is equal to the dosing rate R, and $1/Cl_T$ is equal to $1/kV_D$.

In designing dosage regimens, the dosing rate D_0/τ is adjusted for the patient's drug clearance to obtain the desired C_{av}^{∞}. For an IV infusion, the zero-order rate of infusion (R) is used to obtain the desired steady-state plasma drug concentration C_{SS}. If R is substituted for FD_0/τ in Equation 9.47, then the following equation for estimating C_{SS} after an IV infusion is obtained:

$$C_{SS} = \frac{R}{Cl_T} \tag{9.48}$$

From Equations 9.47 and 9.48, all dosage schedules having the same dosing rate D_0/τ, or R, will have the same C_{av}^{∞} or C_{SS}, whether the drug is given by multiple doses or by IV infusion. For example, dosage schedules of 100 mg every 4 hours, 200 mg every 8 hours, 300 mg every 12 hours, and 600 mg every 24 hours will yield the same C_{av}^{∞} in the patient. An IV infusion rate of 25 mg/h in the same patient will give a C_{SS} equal to the C_{av}^{∞} obtained with the multiple-dose schedule (see Fig. 9-3; Table 9-6).

TABLE 9-6   Effect of Dosing Schedule on Predicted Steady-State Plasma Drug Concentrations[a]

Dosing Schedule			Steady-State Drug Concentration (μg/mL)		
Dose (mg)	1 (h)	Dosing Rate, D_0/τ (mg/h)	C_{max}^{∞}	C_{av}^{∞}	C_{min}^{∞}
—	—	25[b]	14.5	14.5	14.5
100	4	25	16.2	14.5	11.6
200	8	25	20.2	14.5	7.81
300	12	25	25.3	14.5	5.03
600	24	25	44.1	14.5	1.12
400	8	50	40.4	28.9	15.6
600	8	75	60.6	43.4	23.4

[a]Drug has an elimination half-life of 4 hours and an apparent V_D of 10 L.
[b]Drug given by IV infusion. The first-order absorption rate constant k_a is 1.2 h^{-1} and the drug follows a one-compartment open model.

Frequently Asked Questions

▶ Why is the steady-state peak plasma drug concentration measured sometime after an IV dose is given in a clinical situation?

▶ Why is the C_{min} value at steady state less variable than the C_{max} value at steady state?

▶ Is it possible to take a single blood sample to measure the C_{av} value at steady state?

CHAPTER SUMMARY

The purpose of giving a loading dose is to achieve desired (therapeutic) plasma concentrations as quickly as possible. For a drug with long elimination half-life, it may take a long time (several half-lives) to achieve steady-state levels. The loading dose must be calculated appropriately based on pharmacokinetic parameters to avoid overdosing. When several doses are administered for a drug with linear kinetics, drug accumulation may occur according to the principle of superposition. Superposition allows the derivation of equations that predict the plasma drug peak and trough concentrations of a drug at steady state and the theoretical drug concentrations at any time after the dose is given. The principle of superposition is used to examine the effect of an early, late, or missing dose on steady-state drug concentration.

C_{max}^{∞}, C_{min}^{∞}, and C_{av}^{∞} are useful parameters for monitoring the safety and efficacy of a drug during multiple dosing. A clinical example of multiple dosing using short, intermittent intravenous infusions has been applied to the aminoglycosides and is based on pharmacokinetics and clinical factors for safer dosing. The index for measuring drug accumulation during multiple dosing, R, is related to the dosing interval and the half-life of the drug, but not the dose. This parameter compares the steady-state concentration with drug concentration after the initial dose. The plasma concentration at any time during an oral or extravascular multiple-dose regimen, for a one-compartment model and constant doses and dose interval, is dependent on n = number of doses, τ = dosage interval, F = fraction of dose absorbed, and t = time after administration of n doses.

$$C_p = \frac{Fk_a D_0}{V_D(k-k_a)}\left[\left(\frac{1-e^{-nk_a\tau}}{1-e^{-k_a\tau}}\right)e^{-k_a\tau} - \left(\frac{1-e^{-nk_a\tau}}{1-e^{-k\tau}}\right)e^{-kt}\right]$$

The trough steady-state concentration after multiple oral dosing is

$$C_{min}^{\infty} = \frac{k_a F D_0}{V_D (k_a - k)} \left(\frac{1}{1 - e^{-k\tau}} \right) e^{-k\tau}$$

The relationship between average steady-state concentration, the AUC, and dosing interval is

$$C_{av}^{\infty} = \frac{\int_0^{\infty} C_p \, dt}{\tau} = \frac{[AUC]_0^{\infty}}{\tau}$$

This parameter is a good measure of drug exposure.

LEARNING QUESTIONS

1. Gentamicin has an average elimination half-life of approximately 2 hours and an apparent volume of distribution of 20% of body weight. It is necessary to give gentamicin, 1 mg/kg every 8 hours by multiple IV injections, to a 50-kg woman with normal renal function. Calculate **(a)** C_{max}, **(b)** C_{min}, and **(c)** C_{av}^{∞}.

2. A physician wants to give theophylline to a young male asthmatic patient (age 29 years, 80 kg). According to the literature, the elimination half-life for theophylline is 5 hours and the apparent V_D is equal to 50% of the body weight. The plasma level of theophylline required to provide adequate airway ventilation is approximately 10 μg/mL.

   a. The physician wants the patient to take medication every 6 hours around the clock. What dose of theophylline would you recommend (assume theophylline is 100% bioavailable)?

   b. If you were to find that theophylline is available to you only in 225-mg capsules, what dosage regimen would you recommend?

3. What pharmacokinetic parameter is most important in determining the time at which the steady-state plasma drug level (C_{av}^{∞}) is reached?

4. Name two ways in which the fluctuations of plasma concentrations (between C_{max}^{∞} and C_{min}^{∞}) can be minimized for a person on a multiple-dose drug regimen without altering the C_{av}^{∞}.

5. What is the purpose of giving a loading dose?

6. What is the loading dose for an antibiotic ($k = 0.23$ h^{-1}) with a maintenance dose of 200 mg every 3 hours?

7. What is the main advantage of giving a potent drug by IV infusion as opposed to multiple IV injections?

8. A drug has an elimination half-life of 2 hours and a volume of distribution of 40 L. The drug is given at a dose of 200 mg every 4 hours by multiple IV bolus injections. Predict the plasma drug concentration at 1 hour after the third dose.

9. The elimination half-life of an antibiotic is 3 hours and the apparent volume of distribution is 20% of the body weight. The therapeutic window for this drug is from 2 to 10 μg/mL. Adverse toxicity is often observed at drug concentrations above 15 μg/mL. The drug will be given by multiple IV bolus injections.

   a. Calculate the dose for an adult male patient (68 years old, 82 kg) with normal renal function to be given every 8 hours.

   b. Calculate the anticipated C_{max}^{∞} and C_{min}^{∞} values.

   c. Calculate the C_{av}^{∞} value.

   d. Comment on the adequacy of your dosage regimen.

10. Tetracycline hydrochloride (Achromycin V, Lederle) is prescribed for a young adult male patient (28 years old, 78 kg) suffering from gonorrhea. According to the literature, tetracycline HCl is 77% orally absorbed, is 65% bound to plasma proteins, has an apparent volume of distribution of 0.5 L/kg, has an elimination half-life of 10.6 hours, and is 58% excreted unchanged in the urine. The minimum inhibitory drug concentration (MIC) for gonorrhea is 25–30 μg/mL.

    a. Calculate an *exact* maintenance dose for this patient to be given every 6 hours around the clock.

    b. Achromycin V is available in 250- and 500-mg capsules. How many capsules (state dose) should the patient take every 6 hours?

    c. What loading dose using the above capsules would you recommend for this patient?

11. The body clearance of sumatriptan (Imitrex) is 250 mL/min. The drug is about 14% bioavailable. What would be the average plasma drug concentration after 5 doses of 100 mg PO every 8 hours in a patient? (Assume steady state was reached.)

12. Cefotaxime has a volume of distribution of 0.17 L/kg and an elimination half-life of 1.5 hours. What is the peak plasma drug concentration in a patient weighing 75 kg after receiving 1 g IV of the drug 3 times daily for 3 days?

ANSWERS

Frequently Asked Questions

Is the drug accumulation index (R) applicable to any drug given by multiple doses or only to drugs that are eliminated slowly from the body?

- *Accumulation index*, R, is a ratio that indicates steady-state drug concentration to the drug concentration after the first dose. The accumulation index does not measure the absolute size of overdosing; it measures the amount of drug cumulation that can occur due to frequent drug administration. Factors that affect R are the elimination rate constant, k, and the dosing interval, τ. If the first dose is not chosen appropriately, the steady-state level may still be incorrect. Therefore, the first dose and the dosing interval must be determined correctly to avoid any significant drug accumulation. The accumulation index is a good indication of accumulation due to frequent drug dosing, applicable to any drug, regardless of whether the drug is bound to tissues.

What are the advantages/disadvantages for giving a drug by constant IV infusion, intermittent IV infusion, or multiple IV bolus injections? What drugs would most likely be given by each route of administration? Why?

- Some of the advantages of administering a drug by constant IV infusion include the following: (1) A drug may be infused continuously for many hours without disturbing the patient. (2) Constant infusion provides a stable blood drug level for drugs that have a narrow therapeutic index. (3) Some drugs are better tolerated when infused slowly. (4) Some drugs may be infused simultaneously with electrolytes or other infusion media in an acute-care setting. Disadvantages of administering a drug by constant IV infusion include the following: (1) Some drugs

are more suitable to be administered as an IV bolus injection. For example, some reports show that an aminoglycoside given once daily resulted in fewer side effects compared with dividing the dose into two or three doses daily. Due to drug accumulation in the kidney and adverse toxicity, aminoglycosides are generally not given by prolonged IV infusions. In contrast, a prolonged period of low drug level for penicillins and tetracyclines may not be so efficacious and may result in a longer cure time for an infection. The pharmacodynamics of the individual drug must be studied to determine the best course of action. (2) Drugs such as nitroglycerin are less likely to produce tolerance when administered intermittently versus continuously.

Why is the steady-state peak plasma drug concentration often measured sometime after an IV dose is given in a clinical situation?

- After an IV bolus drug injection, the drug is well distributed within a few minutes. In practice, however, an IV bolus dose may be administered slowly over several minutes or the drug may have a slow distribution phase. Therefore, clinicians often prefer to take a blood sample 15 minutes or 30 minutes after IV bolus injection and refer to that drug concentration as the peak concentration. In some cases, a blood sample is taken an hour later to avoid the fluctuating concentration in the distributive phase. The error due to changing sampling time can be large for a drug with a short elimination half-life.

Is a loading dose always necessary when placing a patient on a multiple-dose regimen? What are the determining factors?

- A loading or priming dose is used to rapidly raise the plasma drug concentration to therapeutic drug levels to obtain a more rapid pharmacodynamic response. In addition, the loading dose along with the maintenance dose allows the drug to reach steady-state concentration quickly, particularly for drugs with long elimination half-lives.

An alternative way of explaining the loading dose is based on clearance. After multiple IV dosing, the maintenance dose required is based on Cl, C_{ss}, and τ.

$$C_{SS} = \frac{\text{Dose}}{\tau Cl}$$

$$\text{Dose} = C_{SS}\tau Cl$$

If C_{ss} and τ are fixed, a drug with a smaller clearance requires a smaller maintenance dose. In practice, the dosing interval is adjustable and may be longer for drugs with a small Cl if the drug does not need to be dosed frequently. The steady-state drug level is generally determined by the desired therapeutic drug.

Does a loading dose significantly affect the steady-state concentration of a drug given by a constant multiple-dose regimen?

- The loading dose will affect only the initial drug concentrations in the body. Steady-state drug levels are obtained after several elimination half-lives (eg, $4.32t_{1/2}$ for 95% steady-state level). Only 5% of the drug contributed by the loading dose will remain at 95% steady state. At 99% steady-state level, only 1% of the loading dose will remain.

Learning Questions

1. $V_D = 0.20(50 \text{ kg}) = 10,000 \text{ mL}$

   a. $D_{max} = \frac{D_0}{1-f} = \frac{50 \text{ mg}}{1 - e^{-(0.693/2)(8)}} = 53.3 \text{ mg}$

   $C_{max} = \frac{D_{max}}{V_D} = \frac{53.3 \text{ mg}}{10,000 \text{ mL}} = 5.33 \text{ }\mu\text{g/mL}$

   b. $D_{min} = 53.3 - 50 = 3.3 \text{ mg}$

   $C_{min} = \frac{3.3 \text{ mg}}{10,000 \text{ mL}} = 0.33 \text{ }\mu\text{g/mL}$

   c. $C_{av}^{\infty} = \frac{FD_0 1.44 t_{1/2}}{V_D \tau}$

   $= \frac{(50)(1.44)(2)}{(10,000)(8)} = 1.8 \text{ }\mu\text{g/mL}$

2. a. $D_0 = \frac{C_{av}^{\infty} V_D \tau}{1.44 t_{1/2}}$

   $= \frac{(10)(40,000)(6)}{(1.44)(5)}$

   $= 333 \text{ mg every 6 h}$

   b. $\tau = \frac{FD_0 1.44 t_{1/2}}{V_D C_{av}^{\infty}}$

   $= \frac{(225,000)(1.44)(5)}{(40,000)(10)} = 4.05 \text{ h}$

6. Dose the patient with 200 mg every 3 hours.

   $$D_L = \frac{D_0}{1 - e^{-k\tau}} = \frac{200}{1 - e^{-(0.23)(3)}} = 400 \text{ mg}$$

   Notice that D_L is twice the maintenance dose, because the drug is given at a dosage interval equal approximately to the $t_{1/2}$ of 3 hours.

8. The plasma drug concentration, C_p, may be calculated at any time after n doses by Equation 9.21 and proper substitution.

   $$C_p = \frac{D_0}{V_D}\left(\frac{1 - e^{-nk\tau}}{1 - e^{-k\tau}}\right)e^{-kt}$$

   $$C_p = \frac{200}{40}\left(\frac{1 - e^{-(3)(0.347)(4)}}{1 - e^{-(0.347)(4)}}\right)e^{-(0.347)(1)}$$

   $$= 4.63 \text{ mg/L}$$

   Alternatively, one may conclude that for a drug whose elimination $t_{1/2}$ is 2 hours, the predicted plasma drug concentration is approximately at steady state after 3 doses or 12 hours. Therefore, the above calculation may be simplified to the following:

   $$C_p = \frac{D_0}{V_D}\left(\frac{1}{1 - e^{-k\tau}}\right)e^{-k\tau}$$

   $$C_p = \left(\frac{200}{40}\right)\left(\frac{1}{1 - e^{-(0.347)(4)}}\right)e^{-(0.347)(1)}$$

   $$= 4.71 \text{ mg/L}$$

9. $C_{max}^{\infty} = \dfrac{D_0/V_D}{1-e^{-k\tau}}$

where

$V_D = 20\% \text{ of } 82 \text{ kg} = (0.2)(82) = 16.4 \text{ L}$

$k = (0.693/3) = 0.231 \text{ h}^{-1}$

$D_0 = V_D C_{max}^{\infty}(1-e^{-k\tau}) = (16.4)(10)(1-e^{-(0.231)(8)})$

a. $D_0 = 138.16$ mg to be given every 8 hours

b. $C_{min}^{\infty} = C_{max}^{\infty}(e^{-k\tau}) = (10)(e^{-(0.231)(8)})$

$= 1.58 \text{ mg/L}$

c. $C_{av}^{\infty} = \dfrac{D_0}{kV_D\tau} = \dfrac{138.16}{(0.231)(16.4)(8)}$

$= 4.56 \text{ mg/L}$

d. In the above dosage regimen, the C_{min}^{∞} of 1.59 mg/L is below the desired C_{min}^{∞} of 2 mg/L. Alternatively, the dosage interval, τ, could be changed to 6 hours.

$D_0 = V_D C_{max}^{\infty}(1-e^{-k\tau}) = (16.4)(10)(1-e^{-(0.231)(6)})$

$D_0 = 123$ mg to be given every 6 h

$C_{min}^{\infty} = C_{max}^{\infty}(e^{-k\tau}) = (10)(e^{-(0.231)(6)}) = 2.5 \text{ mg/L}$

$C_{av}^{\infty} = \dfrac{D_0}{kV_D\tau} = \dfrac{123}{(0.231)(16.4)(6)} = 5.41 \text{ mg/L}$

10. a. $C_{av}^{\infty} = \dfrac{FD_0}{kV_D\tau}$

Let $C_{av}^{\infty} = 27.5 \text{ mg/L}$

$D_0 = \dfrac{C_{av}^{\infty}kV_D\tau}{F} = \dfrac{(27.5)(0.693/10.6)(0.5)(78)(6)}{0.77}$

$= 546.3 \text{ mg}$

$D_0 = 546.3$ mg every 6 h

b. If a 500-mg capsule is given every 6 hours,

$C_{av}^{\infty} = \dfrac{FD_0}{kV_D\tau} = \dfrac{(0.77)(500)}{(0.693/10.6)(0.5)(78)(6)}$

$= 25.2 \text{ mg/L}$

c. $D_L = \dfrac{D_M}{1-e^{-k\tau}} = \dfrac{500}{1-e^{(0.654)(6)}} = 1543 \text{ mg}$

$D_L = 3 \times 500 \text{ mg capsules} = 1500 \text{ mg}$

REFERENCES

Jefferson JW, Pradko JF, Muir KT: Bupropion for major depressive disorder: Pharmacokinetic and formulation considerations. *Clin Ther* 27(11):1685–1695, 2005.

Kruger-Thiemer E: Pharmacokinetics and dose-concentration relationships. In Ariens EJ (ed.), *Physico-Chemical Aspects of Drug Action.* New York, Pergamon, 1968, p 97.

Niebergall PJ, Sugita ET, Schnaare RC: Potential dangers of common drug dosing regimens. *Am J Hosp Pharm* 31:53–59, 1974.

Primmett D, Levine M, Kovarik, J, Mueller E, Keown, P: Cyclosporine monitoring in patients with renal transplants: Two- or three-point methods that estimate area under the curve are superior to trough levels in predicting drug exposure, therapeutic drug monitoring 20(3):276–283, June 1998.

Sawchuk RJ, Zaske DE: Pharmacokinetics of dosing regimens which utilize multiple intravenous infusions: Gentamycin in burn patients. *J Pharmacokin Biopharm* 4(2):183–195, 1976.

van Rossum JM, Tomey AHM: Rate of accumulation and plateau concentration of drugs after chronic medication. *J Pharm Pharmacol* 30:390–392, 1968.

BIBLIOGRAPHY

Gibaldi M, Perrier D: *Pharmacokinetics,* 2nd ed. New York, Marcel Dekker, 1962, pp 451–457.

Levy G: Kinetics of pharmacologic effect. *Clin Pharmacol Ther* 7:362, 1966.

van Rossum JM: Pharmacokinetics of accumulation. *J Pharm Sci* 75:2162–2164, 1968.

Wagner JG: Kinetics of pharmacological response, I: Proposed relationship between response and drug concentration in the intact animal and man. *J Theor Biol* 20:173, 1968.

Wagner JG: Relations between drug concentrations and response. *J Mond Pharm* 14:279–310, 1971.

10

Nonlinear Pharmacokinetics

Andrew B.C. Yu and Leon Shargel

Chapter Objectives

▶ Describe the differences between linear pharmacokinetics and nonlinear pharmacokinetics.

▶ Illustrate nonlinear pharmacokinetics with drug disposition examples.

▶ Discuss some potential risks in dosing drugs that follow nonlinear kinetics.

▶ Explain how to detect nonlinear kinetics using AUC-versus-doses plots.

▶ Apply the appropriate equation and graphical methods, to calculate the V_{max} and K_M parameters after multiple dosing in a patient.

▶ Describe the use of the Michaelis–Menten equation to simulate the elimination of a drug by a saturable enzymatic process.

▶ Estimate the dose for a nonlinear drug such as phenytoin in multiple-dose regimens.

▶ Describe chronopharmacokinetics, time-dependent pharmacokinetics, and its influence on drug disposition.

▶ Describe how transporters may cause uneven drug distribution at cellular level; and understand that capacity-limited or concentration-dependent kinetics may occur at the local level within body organs.

Previous chapters discussed linear pharmacokinetic models using simple first-order kinetics to describe the course of drug disposition and action. These linear models assumed that the pharmacokinetic parameters for a drug would not change when different doses or multiple doses of a drug were given. With some drugs, increased doses or chronic medication can cause deviations from the linear pharmacokinetic profile previously observed with single low doses of the same drug. This *nonlinear* pharmacokinetic behavior is also termed *dose-dependent pharmacokinetics.*

Many of the processes of drug absorption, distribution, biotransformation, and excretion involve enzymes or carrier-mediated systems. For some drugs given at therapeutic levels, one of these specialized processes may become saturated. As shown in Table 10-1, various causes of nonlinear pharmacokinetic behavior are theoretically possible. Besides saturation of plasma protein-binding or carrier-mediated systems, drugs may demonstrate nonlinear pharmacokinetics due to a pathologic alteration in drug absorption, distribution, and elimination. For example, aminoglycosides may cause renal nephrotoxicity, thereby altering renal drug excretion. In addition, gallstone obstruction of the bile duct will alter biliary drug excretion. In most cases, the main pharmacokinetic outcome is a change in the apparent elimination rate constant.

A number of drugs demonstrate *saturation* or *capacity-limited metabolism* in humans. Examples of these saturable metabolic processes include glycine conjugation of salicylate, sulfate conjugation of salicylamide, acetylation of *p*-aminobenzoic acid, and the elimination of phenytoin (Tozer et al, 1981). Drugs that demonstrate saturation kinetics usually show the following characteristics:

1. Elimination of drug does not follow simple first-order kinetics—that is, elimination kinetics are nonlinear.
2. The elimination half-life changes as dose is increased. Usually, the elimination half-life increases with increased dose due to saturation of an enzyme system. However, the elimination half-life might decrease due to "self"-induction of liver biotransformation enzymes, as is observed for carbamazepine.

TABLE 10-1   Examples of Drugs Showing Nonlinear Kinetics

Cause[a]	Drug
GI Absorption	
Saturable transport in gut wall	Riboflavin, gebapentin, L-dopa, baclofen, ceftibuten
Intestinal metabolism	Salicylamide, propranolol
Drugs with low solubility in GI but relatively high dose	Chorothiazide, griseofulvin, danazol
Saturable gastric or GI decomposition	Penicillin G, omeprazole, saquinavir
Distribution	
Saturable plasma protein binding	Phenylbutazone, lidocaine, salicylic acid, ceftriaxone, diazoxide, phenytoin, warfarin, disopyramide
Cellular uptake	Methicillin (rabbit)
Tissue binding	Imiprimine (rat)
CSF transport	Benzylpenicillins
Saturable transport into or out of tissues	Methotrexate
Renal Elimination	
Active secretion	Mezlocillin, para-aminohippuric acid
Tubular reabsorption	Riboflavin, ascorbic acid, cephapirin
Change in urine pH	Salicylic acid, dextroamphetamine
Metabolism	
Saturable metabolism	Phenytoin, salicyclic acid, theophylline, valproic acid[b]
Cofactor or enzyme limitation	Acetaminophen, alcohol
Enzyme induction	Carbamazepine
Altered hepatic blood flow	Propranolol, verapamil
Metabolite inhibition	Diazepam
Biliary Excretion	
Biliary secretion	Iodipamide, sulfobromophthalein sodium
Enterohepatic recycling	Cimetidine, isotretinoin

[a]Hypothermia, metabolic acidosis, altered cardiovascular function, and coma are additional causes of dose and time dependencies in drug overdose.
[b]In guinea pig and probably in some younger subjects.
Data from Evans et al (1992).

3. The area under the curve (AUC) is not proportional to the amount of bioavailable drug.
4. The saturation of capacity-limited processes may be affected by other drugs that require the same enzyme or carrier-mediated system (ie, competition effects).
5. The composition and/or ratio of the metabolites of a drug may be affected by a change in the dose.

Because these drugs have a changing apparent elimination constant with larger doses, prediction of drug concentration in the blood based on a single small dose is difficult. Drug concentrations in the blood can increase rapidly once an elimination process is saturated. In general, metabolism (biotransformation) and active tubular secretion of drugs by the kidney are the processes most usually saturated. Figure 10-1 shows plasma level–time curves for a drug that exhibits *saturable* kinetics. When a large dose is given, a curve is obtained with an initial slow elimination phase followed by a much more rapid elimination at lower blood concentrations (curve *A*). With a small dose of the drug, apparent first-order kinetics is observed, because no saturation kinetics occurs (curve *B*). If the pharmacokinetic data were estimated only from the blood levels described by curve *B*, then a twofold increase in the dose would give the blood profile presented in curve *C*, which considerably underestimates the drug concentration as well as the duration of action.

In order to determine whether a drug is following dose-dependent kinetics, the drug is given at various dosage levels and a plasma level–time curve is obtained for each dose. The curves should exhibit parallel slopes if the drug follows dose-independent kinetics. Alternatively, a plot of the areas under the plasma level–time curves at various doses should be linear (Fig. 10-2).

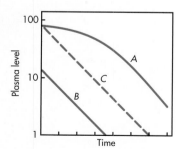

FIGURE 10-1   Plasma level–time curves for a drug that exhibits a saturable elimination process. Curves *A* and *B* represent high and low doses of drug, respectively, given in a single IV bolus. The terminal slopes of curves *A* and *B* are the same. Curve *C* represents the normal first-order elimination of a different drug.

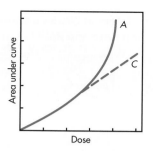

FIGURE 10-2   Area under the plasma level–time curve versus dose for a drug that exhibits a saturable elimination process. Curve *A* represents dose-dependent or saturable elimination kinetics. Curve *C* represents dose-independent kinetics.

SATURABLE ENZYMATIC ELIMINATION PROCESSES

The elimination of drug by a saturable enzymatic process is described by *Michaelis–Menten kinetics*. If C_p is the concentration of drug in the plasma, then

$$\text{Elimination rate} = \frac{dC_p}{dt} = \frac{V_{max}C_p}{K_M + C_p} \qquad (10.1)$$

where V_{max} is the maximum elimination rate and K_M is the Michaelis constant that reflects the *capacity* of the enzyme system. It is important to note that K_M is not an elimination constant, but is actually a hybrid rate constant in enzyme kinetics, representing both the forward and backward reaction rates and equal to the drug concentration or amount of drug in the body at $0.5V_{max}$. The values for K_M and V_{max} are dependent on the nature of the drug and the enzymatic process involved.

The elimination rate of a hypothetical drug with a K_M of 0.1 μg/mL and a V_{max} of 0.5 μg/mL per hour is calculated in Table 10-2 by using Equation 10.1. Because the ratio of the elimination rate to drug concentration changes as the drug concentration changes (ie, dC_p/dt is not constant, Equation 10.1), the rate of drug elimination also changes and is not a first-order or linear process. In contrast, a first-order elimination process would yield the same elimination rate constant at all plasma drug concentrations. At drug

TABLE 10-2   Effect of Drug Concentration on the Elimination Rate and Rate Constant[a]

Drug Concentration (μg/mL)	Elimination Rate (μg/mL/h)	Elimination Rate/ Concentration[b] (h^{-1})
0.4	0.400	1.000
0.8	0.444	0.556
1.2	0.462	0.385
1.6	0.472	0.294
2.0	0.476	0.238
2.4	0.480	0.200
2.8	0.483	0.172
3.2	0.485	0.152
10.0	0.495	0.0495
10.4	0.495	0.0476
10.8	0.495	0.0459
11.2	0.496	0.0442
11.6	0.496	0.0427

[a]$K_M = 0.1$ μg/mL, $V_{max} = 0.5$ μg/mL/h.

[b]The ratio of the elimination rate to the concentration is equal to the rate constant.

concentrations of 0.4–10 μg/mL, the enzyme system is not saturated and the rate of elimination is a mixed or nonlinear process (Table 10-2). At higher drug concentrations, 11.2 μg/mL and above, the elimination rate approaches the maximum velocity (V_{max}) of approximately 0.5 μg/mL per hour. At V_{max}, the elimination rate is a constant and is considered a zero-order process.

Equation 10.1 describes a nonlinear enzyme process that encompasses a broad range of drug concentrations. When the drug concentration C_p is large in relation to K_M ($C_p \gg K_M$), saturation of the enzymes occurs and the value for K_M is negligible. The rate of elimination proceeds at a fixed or constant rate equal to V_{max}. Thus, elimination of drug becomes a zero-order process and Equation 10.1 becomes:

$$-\frac{dC_p}{dt} = \frac{V_{max} C_p}{C_p} = V_{max} \qquad (10.2)$$

PRACTICE PROBLEM

Using the hypothetical drug considered in Table 10-2 ($V_{max} = 0.5$ μg/mL per hour, $K_M = 0.1$ μg/mL), how long would it take for the plasma drug concentration to decrease from 20 to 12 μg/mL?

Solution

Because 12 μg/mL is above the saturable level, as indicated in Table 10-2, elimination occurs at a zero-order rate of approximately 0.5 μg/mL per hour.

Time needed for the drug to decrease to

$$12 \ \mu\text{g/mL} = \frac{20 - 12 \ \mu\text{g}}{0.5 \ \mu\text{g/h}} = 16 \text{ h}$$

A saturable process can also exhibit linear elimination when drug concentrations are much less than enzyme concentrations. When the drug concentration C_p is small in relation to the K_M, the rate of drug elimination becomes a first-order process. The data generated from Equation 10.2 ($C_p \leq 0.05$ μg/mL, Table 10-3) using $K_M = 0.8$ μg/mL and $V_{max} = 0.9$ μg/mL per hour shows that enzymatic drug elimination can change from a nonlinear to a linear process over a restricted

TABLE 10-3   Effect of Drug Concentration on the Elimination Rate and Rate Constant[a]

Drug Concentration (C_p) (μg/mL)	Elimination Rate (μg/mL/h)	Elimination Rate Concentration (h^{-1})[b]
0.01	0.011	1.1
0.02	0.022	1.1
0.03	0.033	1.1
0.04	0.043	1.1
0.05	0.053	1.1
0.06	0.063	1.0
0.07	0.072	1.0
0.08	0.082	1.0
0.09	0.091	1.0

[a]$K_M = 0.8$ μg/mL, $V_{max} = 0.9$ μg/mL/h.

[b]The ratio of the elimination rate to the concentration is equal to the rate constant.

concentration range. This is evident because the rate constant (or elimination rate/drug concentration) values are constant. At drug concentrations below 0.05 μg/mL, the ratio of elimination rate to drug concentration has a constant value of 1.1 h^{-1}. Mathematically, when C_p is much smaller than K_M, C_p in the denominator is negligible and the elimination rate becomes first order.

$$-\frac{dC_p}{dt} = \frac{V_{max}C_p}{C_p + K_M} = \frac{V_{max}}{K_M}C_p$$

$$-\frac{dC_p}{dt} = k'C_p \qquad (10.3)$$

The first-order rate constant for a saturable process, k', can be calculated from Equation 10.3:

$$k' = \frac{V_{max}}{K_M} = \frac{0.9}{0.8} = \sim 1.1 \text{ h}^{-1}$$

This calculation confirms the data in Table 10-3, because enzymatic drug elimination at drug concentrations below 0.05 μg/mL is a first-order rate process with a rate constant of 1.1 h^{-1}. Therefore, the $t_{1/2}$ due to enzymatic elimination can be calculated:

$$t_{1/2} = \frac{0.693}{1.1} = 0.63 \text{ h}$$

PRACTICE PROBLEM

How long would it take for the plasma concentration of the drug in Table 10-3 to decline from 0.05 to 0.005 μg/mL?

Solution

Because drug elimination is a first-order process for the specified concentrations,

$$C_p = C_p^0 e^{-kt}$$

$$\log C_p = C_p^0 - \frac{kt}{2.3}$$

$$t = \frac{\log C - \log C_p^0}{k}$$

Because $C_p^0 = 0.05$ μg/mL, $k = 1.1$ h^{-1}, and $C_p = 0.005$ μg/mL.

$$t = \frac{2.3(\log 0.05 - \log 0.005)}{1.1}$$

$$= \frac{2.3(-1.30 + 2.3)}{1.1}$$

$$= \frac{2.3}{1.1} = 2.09 \text{ h}$$

When given in therapeutic doses, most drugs produce plasma drug concentrations well below K_M for all carrier-mediated enzyme systems affecting the pharmacokinetics of the drug. Therefore, most drugs at normal therapeutic concentrations follow first-order rate processes. Only a few drugs, such as salicylate and phenytoin, tend to saturate the hepatic mixed-function oxidases at higher therapeutic doses. With these drugs, elimination kinetics is first order with very small doses, is mixed order at higher doses, and may approach zero order with very high therapeutic doses.

Frequently Asked Questions
▶ *What kinetic processes in the body can be considered saturable?*

▶ *Why is it important to monitor drug levels carefully for dose dependency?*

DRUG ELIMINATION BY CAPACITY-LIMITED PHARMACOKINETICS: ONE-COMPARTMENT MODEL, IV BOLUS INJECTION

The rate of elimination of a drug that follows capacity-limited pharmacokinetics is governed by the V_{max} and K_M of the drug. Equation 10.1 describes the elimination of a drug that distributes in the body as a single compartment and is eliminated by Michaelis–Menten or capacity-limited pharmacokinetics. If a single IV bolus injection of drug (D_0) is given at $t = 0$, the drug concentration (C_p) in the plasma at any time t may be calculated by an integrated form of Equation 10.1 described by

$$\frac{C_0 - C_p}{t} = V_{max} - \frac{K_M}{t} \ln \frac{C_0}{C_p} \qquad (10.4)$$

Alternatively, the amount of drug in the body after an IV bolus injection may be calculated by the following relationship. Equation 10.5 may be used to simulate the decline of drug in the body after various size doses are given, provided the K_M and V_{max} of drug are known.

$$\frac{D_0 - D_t}{t} = V_{max} - \frac{K_M}{t} \ln \frac{D_0}{D_t} \qquad (10.5)$$

where D_0 is the amount of drug in the body at $t = 0$. In order to calculate the time for the dose of the drug to decline to a certain amount of drug in the body, Equation 10.5 must be rearranged and solved for time t:

$$t = \frac{1}{V_{max}} \left(D_0 - D_t + K_M \ln \frac{D_0}{D_t} \right) \qquad (10.6)$$

The relationship of K_M and V_{max} to the time for an IV bolus injection of drug to decline to a given amount of drug in the body is illustrated in Figs. 10-3 and 10-4. Using Equation 10.6, the time for a single 400-mg dose given by IV bolus injection to decline to 20 mg

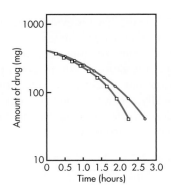

FIGURE 10-4   Amount of drug in the body versus time for a capacity-limited drug following an IV dose. Data generated using K_M of 38 mg/L ($\square$) and 76 mg/L (O). V_{max} is kept constant.

was calculated for a drug with a K_M of 38 mg/L and a V_{max} that varied from 200 to 100 mg/h (Table 10-4). With a V_{max} of 200 mg/h, the time for the 400-mg dose to decline to 20 mg in the body is 2.46 hours, whereas when the V_{max} is decreased to 100 mg/h, the time for the 400-mg dose to decrease to 20 mg is increased to 4.93 hours (see Fig. 10-3). Thus, there is an inverse relationship between the time for the dose to decline to a certain amount of drug in the body and the V_{max} as shown in Equation 10.6.

Using a similar example, the effect of K_M on the time for a single 400-mg dose given by IV bolus injection to decline to 20 mg in the body is described in Table 10-5 and Fig. 10-4. Assuming V_{max} is constant at 200 mg/h, the time for the drug to decline from 400 to 20 mg is 2.46 hours when K_M is 38 mg/L, whereas when K_M is 76 mg/L, the time for the drug dose to decline to 20 mg is 3.03 hours. Thus, an increase in K_M (with no change in V_{max}) will increase the time for the drug to be eliminated from the body.

The one-compartment open model with capacity-limited elimination pharmacokinetics adequately describes the plasma drug concentration–time profiles for some drugs. The mathematics needed to describe nonlinear pharmacokinetic behavior of drugs that follow two-compartment models and/or have both combined capacity-limited and first-order kinetic profiles are very complex and have little practical application for dosage calculations and therapeutic drug monitoring.

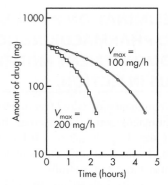

FIGURE 10-3   Amount of drug in the body versus time for a capacity-limited drug following an IV dose. Data generated using V_{max} of 100 (O) and 200 mg/h ($\square$). K_M is kept constant.

TABLE 10-4 Capacity-Limited Pharmacokinetics: Effect of V_{max} on the Elimination of Drug[a]

Amount of Drug in Body (mg)	Time for Drug Elimination (h)	
	$V_{max} =$ 200 mg/h	$V_{max} =$ 100 mg/h
400	0	0
380	0.109	0.219
360	0.220	0.440
340	0.330	0.661
320	0.442	0.884
300	0.554	1.10
280	0.667	1.33
260	0.781	1.56
240	0.897	1.79
220	1.01	2.02
200	1.13	2.26
180	1.25	2.50
160	1.37	2.74
140	1.49	2.99
120	1.62	3.25
100	1.76	3.52
80	1.90	3.81
60	2.06	4.12
40	2.23	4.47
20	2.46	4.93

[a]A single 400-mg dose is given by IV bolus injection. The drug is distributed into a single compartment and is eliminated by capacity-limited pharmacokinetics. K_M is 38 mg/L. The time for drug to decline from 400 to 20 mg is calculated from Equation 9.6 assuming the drug has $V_{max} =$ 200 mg/h or $V_{max} =$ 100 mg/h.

TABLE 10-5 Capacity-Limited Pharmacokinetics: Effects of K_M on the Elimination of Drug[a]

Amount of Drug in Body (mg)	Time for Drug Elimination (h)	
	$K_M =$ 38 mg/L	$K_M =$ 76 mg/L
400	0	0
380	0.109	0.119
360	0.220	0.240
340	0.330	0.361
320	0.442	0.484
300	0.554	0.609
280	0.667	0.735
260	0.781	0.863
240	0.897	0.994
220	1.01	1.12
200	1.13	1.26
180	1.25	1.40
160	1.37	1.54
140	1.49	1.69
120	1.62	1.85
100	1.76	2.02
80	1.90	2.21
60	2.06	2.42
40	2.23	2.67
20	2.46	3.03

[a]A single 400-mg dose is given by IV bolus injection. The drug is distributed into a single compartment and is eliminated by capacity-limited pharmacokinetics. V_{max} is 200 mg/h. The time for drug to decline from 400 to 20 mg is calculated from Equation 9.6 assuming the drug has $K_M =$ 38 mg/L or $K_M =$ 76 mg/L.

PRACTICE PROBLEMS

1. A drug eliminated from the body by capacity-limited pharmacokinetics has a K_M of 100 mg/L and a V_{max} of 50 mg/h. If 400 mg of the drug is given to a patient by IV bolus injection, calculate the time for the drug to be 50% eliminated. If 320 mg of the drug is to be given by IV bolus injection, calculate the time for 50% of the dose to be eliminated. Explain why there is a difference in the time for 50% elimination of a 400-mg dose compared to a 320-mg dose.

Solution

Use Equation 10.6 to calculate the time for the dose to decline to a given amount of drug in the body. For this problem, D_t is equal to 50% of the dose D_0.

If the dose is 400 mg,

$$t = \frac{1}{50}\left(400 - 200 + 100 \ln\frac{400}{200}\right) = 5.39 \text{ h}$$

If the dose is 320 mg,

$$t = \frac{1}{50}\left(320 - 160 + 100 \ln\frac{320}{160}\right) = 4.59 \text{ h}$$

For capacity-limited elimination, the elimination half-life is dose dependent, because the drug elimination process is partially saturated. Therefore, small changes in the dose will produce large differences in the time for 50% drug elimination. The parameters K_M and V_{max} determine when the dose is saturated.

2. Using the same drug as in Problem 1, calculate the time for 50% elimination of the dose when the doses are 10 and 5 mg. Explain why the times for 50% drug elimination are similar even though the dose is reduced by one-half.

Solution

As in Practice Problem 1, use Equation 10.6 to calculate the time for the amount of drug in the body at zero time (D_0) to decline 50%.

If the dose is 10 mg,

$$t = \frac{1}{50}\left(10 - 5 + 100 \ln\frac{10}{5}\right) = 1.49 \text{ h}$$

If the dose is 5 mg,

$$t = \frac{1}{50}\left(5 - 2.5 + 100 \ln\frac{5}{2.5}\right) = 1.44 \text{ h}$$

Whether the patient is given a 10-mg or a 5-mg dose by IV bolus injection, the times for the amount of drug to decline 50% are approximately the same. For 10- and 5-mg doses, the amount of drug in the body is much less than the K_M of 100 mg. Therefore, the amount of drug in the body is well below saturation of the elimination process and the drug declines at a first-order rate.

Determination of K_M and V_{max}

Equation 10.1 relates the rate of drug biotransformation to the concentration of the drug in the body. The same equation may be applied to determine

the rate of enzymatic reaction of a drug *in vitro* (Equation 10.7). When an experiment is performed with solutions of various concentration of drug C, a series of reaction rates (v) may be measured for each concentration. Special plots may then be used to determine K_M and V_{max} (see also Chapter 12).

Equation 10.7 may be rearranged into Equation 10.8.

$$v = \frac{V_{max}C}{K_M + C} \tag{10.7}$$

$$\frac{1}{v} = \frac{K_M}{V_{max}}\frac{1}{C} + \frac{1}{V_{max}} \tag{10.8}$$

Equation 10.8 is a linear equation when $1/v$ is plotted against $1/C$. The y intercept for the line is $1/V_{max}$, and the slope is K_M/V_{max}. An example of a drug reacting enzymatically with rate (v) at various concentrations C is shown in Table 10-6 and Fig. 10-5. A plot of $1/v$ versus $1/C$ is shown in Fig. 10-6. A plot of $1/v$ versus $1/C$ is linear with an intercept of 0.33 mmol. Therefore,

$$\frac{1}{V_{max}} = 0.33 \text{ min} \cdot \text{mL}/\mu\text{mol}$$

$$V_{max} = 3 \ \mu\text{mol/mL} \cdot \text{min}$$

because the slope = 1.65 = K_M/V_{max} = $K_M/3$ or K_M = 3 × 1.65 μmol/mL = 5 μmol/mL. Alternatively, K_M may be found from the x intercept, where $-1/K_M$ is equal to the x intercept. (This may be seen by extending the graph to intercept the x axis in the negative region.)

With this plot (Fig. 10-6), the points are clustered. Other methods are available that may spread the points more evenly. These methods are derived from rearranging Equation 10.8 into Equations 10.9 and 10.10.

$$\frac{C}{v} = \frac{1}{V_{max}}C + \frac{K_M}{V_{max}} \tag{10.9}$$

$$v = -K_M\frac{v}{C} + V_{max} \tag{10.10}$$

A plot of C/v versus C would yield a straight line with $1/V_{max}$ as slope and K_M/V_{max} as intercept (Equation 10.9). A plot of v versus v/C would yield a slope of $-K_M$ and an intercept of V_{max} (Equation 10.10).

TABLE 10-6   Information Necessary for Graphic Determination of V_{max} and K_M

Observation Number	C (μM/mL)	V (μM/mL/min)	1/V (mL/min/μM)	1/C (mL/μM)
1	1	0.500	2.000	1.000
2	6	1.636	0.611	0.166
3	11	2.062	0.484	0.090
4	16	2.285	0.437	0.062
5	21	2.423	0.412	0.047
6	26	2.516	0.397	0.038
7	31	2.583	0.337	0.032
8	36	2.63	0.379	0.027
9	41	2.673	0.373	0.024
10	46	2.705	0.369	0.021

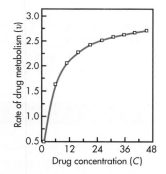

FIGURE 10-5   Plot of rate of drug metabolism at various drug concentrations. ($K_M = 0.5$ μmol/mL, $V_{max} = 3$ μmol/mL/min.)

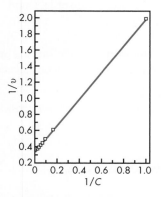

FIGURE 10-6   Plot of $1/v$ versus $1/C$ for determining K_M and V_{max}.

The necessary calculations for making the above plots are shown in Table 10-7. The plots are shown in Figs. 10-7 and 10-8. It should be noted that the data are spread out better by the two latter plots. Calculations from the slope show that the same K_M and V_{max} are obtained as in Fig. 10-6. When the data are more scattered, one method may be more accurate than the other. A simple approach is to graph the

TABLE 10-7   Calculations Necessary for Graphic Determination of K_M and V_{max}

C (μM/mL)	v (μM/mL/min)	C/v (min)	v/C (1/min)
1	0.500	2.000	0.500
6	1.636	3.666	0.272
11	2.062	5.333	0.187
16	2.285	7.000	0.142
21	2.423	8.666	0.115
26	2.516	10.333	0.096
31	2.583	12.000	0.083
36	2.634	13.666	0.073
41	2.673	15.333	0.065
46	2.705	17.000	0.058

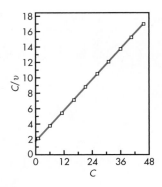

FIGURE 10-7   Plot of C/v versus C for determining K_M and V_{max}.

data and examine the linearity of the graphs. The same basic type of plot is used in the clinical literature to determine K_M and V_{max} for individual patients for drugs that undergo capacity-limited kinetics.

Determination of K_M and V_{max} in Patients

Equation 10.7 shows that the rate of drug metabolism (v) is dependent on the concentration of the drug (C). This same basic concept may be applied to the rate of drug metabolism of a capacity-limited drug in the body (see Chapter 12). The body may be regarded as a single compartment in which the drug is dissolved. The rate of drug metabolism will vary depending on the concentration of drug C_p as well as on the metabolic rate constants K_M and V_{max} of the drug in each individual.

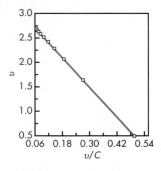

FIGURE 10-8   Plot of v versus v/C for determining K_M and V_{max}.

An example for the determination of K_M and V_{max} is given for the drug phenytoin. Phenytoin undergoes capacity-limited kinetics at therapeutic drug concentrations in the body. To determine K_M and V_{max}, two different dose regimens are given at different times, until steady state is reached. The steady-state drug concentrations are then measured by assay. At steady state, the rate of drug metabolism (v) is assumed to be the same as the rate of drug input R (dose/day). Therefore, Equation 10.11 may be written for drug metabolism in the body similar to the way drugs are metabolized *in vitro* (Equation 10.7). However, steady state will not be reached if the drug input rate, R, is greater than the V_{max}; instead, drug accumulation will continue to occur without reaching a steady-state plateau.

$$R = \frac{V_{max} C_{ss}}{K_M + C_{ss}} \qquad (10.11)$$

where R = dose/day or dosing rate, C_{ss} = steady-state plasma drug concentration, V_{max} = maximum metabolic rate constant in the body, and K_M = Michaelis–Menten constant of the drug in the body.

EXAMPLE ▶ ▶ ▶

Phenytoin was administered to a patient at dosing rates of 150 and 300 mg/d, respectively. The steady-state plasma drug concentrations were 8.6 and 25.1 mg/L, respectively. Find the K_M and V_{max} of this patient. What dose is needed to achieve a steady-state concentration of 11.3 mg/L?

Solution

There are three methods for solving this problem, all based on the same basic equation (Equation 10.11).

Method A
Inverting Equation 10.11 on both sides yields

$$\frac{1}{R} = \frac{K_M}{V_{max}} \frac{1}{C_{ss}} + \frac{1}{V_{max}} \qquad (10.12)$$

Multiply both sides by $C_{ss} V_{max}$,

$$\frac{V_{max} C_{ss}}{R} = K_M + C_{ss}$$

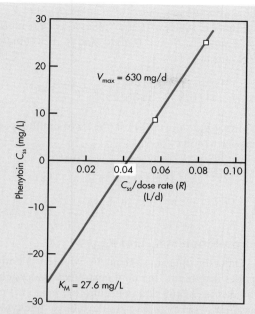

FIGURE 10-9 Plot of C_{ss} versus C_{ss}/R (method A). (From Witmer and Ritschel, 1984, with permission.)

Rearranging

$$C_{ss} = \frac{V_{max}C_{ss}}{R} - K_M \qquad (10.13)$$

A plot of C_{ss} versus C_{ss}/R is shown in Fig. 10-9. V_{max} is equal to the slope, 630 mg/d, and K_M is found from the y intercept, 27.6 mg/L (note the negative intercept).

Method B

From Equation 10.11,

$$RK_M + RC_{ss} = V_{max}C_{ss}$$

Dividing both sides by C_{ss} yields

$$R = V_{max} - \frac{K_M R}{C_{ss}} \qquad (10.14)$$

A plot of R versus R/C_{ss} is shown in Fig. 10-10. The K_M and V_{max} found are similar to those calculated by the previous method (Fig. 10-9).

Method C

A plot of R versus C_{ss} is shown in Fig. 10-11. To determine K_M and V_{max}:

1. Mark points for R of 300 mg/d and C_{ss} of 25.1 mg/L as shown. Connect with a straight line.

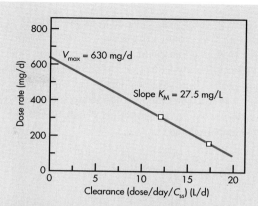

FIGURE 10-10 Plot of R versus R/C_{ss} or clearance (method B). (From Witmer and Ritschel, 1984, with permission.)

2. Mark points for R of 150 mg/d and C_{ss} of 8.6 mg/L as shown. Connect with a straight line.
3. The point where lines from the first two steps cross is called point A.
4. From point A, read V_{max} on the y axis and K_M on the x axis. (Again, V_{max} of 630 mg/d and K_M of 27 mg/L are found.)

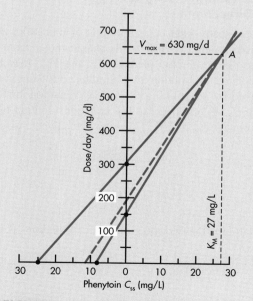

FIGURE 10-11 Plot of R versus C_{ss} (method C). (From Witmer and Ritschel, 1984, with permission.)

This V_{max} and K_M can be used in Equation 10.11 to find an R to produce the desired C_{ss} of 11.3 mg/L. Alternatively, join point A on the graph to meet 11.3 mg/L on the x axis; R can be read where this line meets the y axis (190 mg/d).

To calculate the dose needed to keep steady-state phenytoin concentration of 11.3 mg/L in this patient, use Equation 10.7.

$$R = \frac{(630 \text{ mg/d})(11.3 \text{ mg/L})}{27 \text{ mg/L} + 11.3 \text{ mg/L}}$$

$$= \frac{7119}{38.3} = 186 \text{ mg/d}$$

This answer compares very closely with the value obtained by the graphic method. All three methods have been used clinically. Vozeh et al (1981) introduced a method that allows for an estimation of phenytoin dose based on steady-state concentration resulting from one dose. This method is based on a statistically compiled nomogram that makes it possible to project a most likely dose for the patient.

Determination of K_M and V_{max} by Direct Method

When steady-state concentrations of phenytoin are known at only two dose levels, there is no advantage in using the graphic method. K_M and V_{max} may be calculated by solving two simultaneous equations formed by substituting C_{ss} and R (Equation 10.11) with C_1, R_1, C_2, and R_2. The equations contain two unknowns, K_M and V_{max}, and may be solved easily.

$$R_1 = \frac{V_{max} C_1}{K_M + C_1}$$

$$R_2 = \frac{V_{max} C_2}{K_M + C_2}$$

Combining the two equations yields Equation 10.15.

$$K_M = \frac{R_2 - R_1}{(R_1/C_1) - (R_2/C_2)} \tag{10.15}$$

where C_1 is steady-state plasma drug concentration after dose 1, C_2 is steady-state plasma drug concentration after dose 2, R_1 is the first dosing rate, and R_2

is the second dosing rate. To calculate K_M and V_{max}, use Equation 10.15 with the values $C_1 = 8.6$ mg/L, $C_2 = 25.1$ mg/L, $R_1 = 150$ mg/d, and $R_2 = 300$ mg/d. The results are

$$K_M = \frac{300 - 150}{(150/8.6) - (300/25.1)} = 27.3 \text{ mg/L}$$

Substitute K_M into either of the two simultaneous equations to solve for V_{max}.

$$150 = \frac{V_{max}(8.6)}{27.3 + 8.6}$$

$$V_{max} = 626 \text{ mg/d}$$

Interpretation of K_M and V_{max}

An understanding of Michaelis–Menten kinetics provides insight into the nonlinear kinetics and helps avoid dosing a drug at a concentration near enzyme saturation. For example, in the above phenytoin dosing example, since K_M occurs at $0.5 V_{max}$, $K_M = 27.3$ mg/L, the implication is that at a plasma concentration of 27.3 mg/L, enzymes responsible for phenytoin metabolism are eliminating the drug at 50% V_{max}, that is, 0.5×626 mg/d or 313 mg/d. When the subject is receiving 300 mg of phenytoin per day, the plasma drug concentration of phenytoin is 8.6 mg/L, which is considerably below the K_M of 27.3 mg/L. In practice, the K_M in patients can range from 1 to 15 mg/L, and V_{max} can range from 100 to 1000 mg/d. Patients with a low K_M tend to have greater changes in plasma concentrations during dosing adjustments. Patients with a smaller K_M (same V_{max}) will show a greater change in the rate of elimination when plasma drug concentration changes compared to subjects with a higher K_M. A subject with the same V_{max}, but different K_M, is shown in Fig. 10-12. (For another example, see the slopes of the two curves generated in Fig. 10-4.)

Dependence of Elimination Half-Life on Dose

For drugs that follow linear kinetics, the elimination half-life is constant and does not change with dose or drug concentration. For a drug that follows nonlinear kinetics, the elimination half-life and drug clearance both change with dose or drug concentration. Generally,

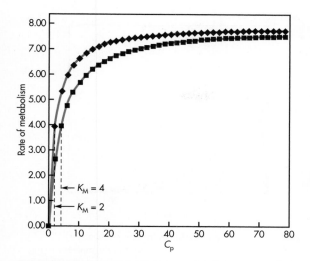

FIGURE 10-12 Diagram showing the rate of metabolism when V_{max} is constant (8 $\mu g/mL/h$) and K_M is changed ($K_M = 2$ $\mu g/mL$ for top curve and $K_M = 4$ $\mu g/mL$ for bottom curve). Note the rate of metabolism is faster for the lower K_M, but saturation starts at lower concentration.

the elimination half-life becomes longer, clearance becomes smaller, and the area under the curve becomes disproportionately larger with increasing dose. The relationship between elimination half-life and drug concentration is shown in Equation 10.16. The elimination half-life is dependent on the Michaelis–Menten parameters and concentration.

$$t_{1/2} = \frac{0.693}{V_{max}}(K_M + C_p) \qquad (10.16)$$

Some pharmacokineticists prefer not to calculate the elimination half-life of a nonlinear drug because the elimination half-life is not constant. Clinically, if the half-life is increasing as plasma concentration increases, and there is no apparent change in metabolic or renal function, then there is a good possibility that the drug may be metabolized by nonlinear kinetics.

Dependence of Clearance on Dose

The total body clearance of a drug given by IV bolus injection that follows a one-compartment model with Michaelis–Menten elimination kinetics changes with respect to time and plasma drug concentration.

Within a certain drug concentration range, an average or mean clearance (Cl_{av}) may be determined. Because the drug follows Michaelis–Menten kinetics, Cl_{av} is dose dependent. Cl_{av} may be estimated from the area under the curve and the dose given (Wagner et al, 1985).

According to the Michaelis–Menten equation,

$$\frac{dC_p}{dt} = \frac{V_{max}C_p}{K_M + C_p} \qquad (10.17)$$

Inverting Equation 10.17 and rearranging yields

$$C_p dt = \frac{K_M}{V'_{max}}dC_p - \frac{C_p}{V'_{max}}dC_p \qquad (10.18)$$

The area under the curve, $[AUC]_0^\infty$, is obtained by integration of Equation 10.18 (ie, $[AUC]_0^\infty = \int_0^\infty C_p\,dt$).

$$\int_0^\infty C_p dt = \int_{C_p^0}^\infty \frac{K_M}{V'_{max}}dC_p + \int_{C_p^0}^\infty \frac{C_p}{V'_{max}}dC_p \qquad (10.19)$$

where V'_{max} is the maximum velocity for metabolism. Units for V'_{max} are mass/compartment volume per unit time. $V'_{max} = V_{max}/V_D$; Wagner et al (1985) used V_{max} in Equation 10.20 as mass/time to be consistent with biochemistry literature, which considers the initial mass of the substrate reacting with the enzyme.

Integration of Equation 10.18 from time 0 to infinity gives Equation 10.20.

$$[AUC]_0^\infty = \frac{C_p^0}{V_{max}/V_D}\left(\frac{C_p^0}{2} + K_M\right) \qquad (10.20)$$

where V_D is the apparent volume of distribution.

Because the dose $D_0 = C_p^0 V_D$, Equation 10.20 may be expressed as

$$[AUC]_0^\infty = \frac{D_0}{V_{max}}\left(\frac{C_p^0}{2} + K_M\right) \qquad (10.21)$$

To obtain mean body clearance, Cl_{av} is then calculated from the dose and the AUC.

$$Cl_{av} = \frac{D_0}{[AUC]_0^\infty} = \frac{V_{max}}{(C_p^0/2) + K_M} \qquad (10.22)$$

$$Cl_{av} = \frac{V_{max}}{(D_0/2V_D) + K_M} \qquad (10.23)$$

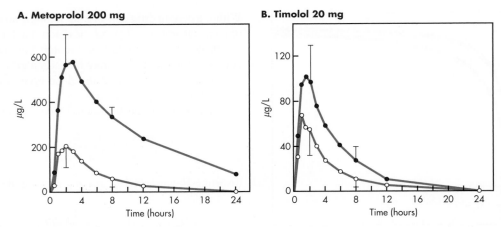

FIGURE 10-13 Mean plasma drug concentration-versus-time profiles following administration of single oral doses of **(A)** metoprolol tartrate 200 mg to 6 extensive metabolizers (EMs) and 6 poor metabolizers (PMs) and **(B)** timolol maleate 20 mg to six EMs (O) and four PMs (•). (Data from Lennard MS, et al: Oxidation phenotype—A major determinant of metoprolol metabolism and response. *NEJM* **307:**1558–1560, 1982; Lennard MS, et al: The relationship between debrisoquine oxidation phenotype and the pharmacokinetics and pharmacodynamics of propranolol. *Br J Clin Pharmac* **17**(6):679–685, 1984; Lewis RV: Timolol and atenolol: Relationships between oxidation phenotype, pharmacokinetics and pharmacodynamics. *Br J Clin Pharmac* **19**(3):329–333, 1985.)

Alternatively, dividing Equation 10.17 by C_p gives Equation 10.24, which shows that the clearance of a drug that follows nonlinear pharmacokinetics is dependent on the plasma drug concentration C_p, K_M, and V_{max}.

$$Cl = \frac{V_D(dC_p/dt)}{C_p} = \frac{V_{max}}{K_M + C_p} \qquad (10.24)$$

Equation 10.22 or 10.23 calculates the average clearance Cl_{av} for the drug after a single IV bolus dose over the entire time course of the drug in the body. For any time period, clearance may be calculated (see Chapters 7 and 12) as

$$Cl_T = \frac{dD_E/dt}{C_p} \qquad (10.25)$$

In Chapter 12, the physiologic model based on blood flow and intrinsic clearance is used to describe drug metabolism. The extraction ratios of many drugs are listed in the literature. Actually, extraction ratios are dependent on dose, enzymatic system, and blood flow, and for practical purposes, they are often assumed to be constant at normal doses.

Except for phenytoin, there is a paucity of K_M and V_{max} data defining the nature of nonlinear drug elimination in patients. However, abundant information is

available supporting variable metabolism due to genetic polymorphism (Chapter 12). The clearance (apparent) of many of these drugs in patients who are slow metabolizers changes with dose, although these drugs may exhibit linear kinetics in subjects with the "normal" phenotype. Metoprolol and many β-adrenergic antagonists are extensively metabolized. The plasma levels of metoprolol in slow metabolizers (Lennard et al, 1986) were much greater than other patients, and the AUC, after equal doses, is several times greater among slow metabolizers of metoprolol (Fig. 10-13). A similar picture is observed with another β-adrenergic antagonist, timolol. These drugs have smaller clearance than normal.

CLINICAL FOCUS

The dose-dependent pharmacokinetics of sodium valproate (VPA) was studied in guinea pigs at 20, 200, and 600 mg/kg by rapid intravenous infusion. The area under the plasma concentration–time curve increased out of proportion at the 600-mg/kg dose level in all groups (Yu et al, 1987). The total clearance (Cl_T) was significantly decreased and the beta elimination half-life ($t_{1/2}$) was significantly increased at the 600-mg/kg dose level. The dose-dependent kinetics of VPA were due to saturation of metabolism. Metabolic capacity was greatly reduced in young guinea pigs.

Clinically, similar enzymatic saturation may be observed in infants and in special patient populations, whereas drug metabolism may be linear with dose in normal subjects. These patients have lower V_{max} and longer elimination half-life. Variability in drug metabolism is described in Chapters 12 and 13.

Frequently Asked Questions

▶ *What is the Michaelis–Menten equation? How are V_{max} and K_M obtained? What are the units for V_{max} and K_M? What is the relevance of V_{max} and K_M?*

▶ *What are the main differences in pharmacokinetic parameters between a drug that follows linear pharmacokinetics and a drug that follows nonlinear pharmacokinetics?*

CLINICAL FOCUS

Paroxetine hydrochloride (Paxil) is an orally administered psychotropic drug. Paroxetine is extensively metabolized and the metabolites are considered to be inactive. Nonlinearity in pharmacokinetics is observed with increasing doses. Paroxetine exhibits autoinhibition. The major pathway for paroxetine metabolism is by CYP2D6. The elimination half-life is about 21 hours. Saturation of this enzyme at clinical doses appears to account for the nonlinearity of paroxetine kinetics with increasing dose and increasing duration of treatment. The role of this enzyme in paroxetine metabolism also suggests potential drug–drug interactions. Clinical drug interaction studies have been performed with substrates of CYP2D6 and show that paroxetine can inhibit the metabolism of drugs metabolized by CYP2D6 including itself, desipramine, risperidone, and atomoxetine.

Paroxetine hydrochloride is known to inhibit metabolism of selective serotonin reuptake inhibitors (SSRIs) and monoamine oxidase inhibitors (MAOIs) producing "serotonin syndrome" (hyperthermia, muscle rigidity, and rapid changes in vital signs). Three cases of accidental overdosing with paroxetine hydrochloride were reported (Vermeulen, 1998). In the

case of overdose, high liver drug concentrations and an extensive tissue distribution (large V_D) made the drug difficult to remove. Vermeulen (1998) reported that saturation of CYP2D6 could result in a disproportionally higher plasma level than could be expected from an increase in dosage. These high plasma drug concentrations may be outside the range of 20–50 mg normally recommended. Since publication of this article, more is known about genotype CYP2D6*10 (Yoon et al, 2000), which may contribute to intersubject variability in metabolism of this drug (see also Chapter 13).

Frequently Asked Questions

▶ *What does autoinhibition mean? Would you expect paroxetine (Paxil) plasma drug concentrations, C_p, to be higher or lower after multiple doses? Would the C_p change be predictable among different subjects?*

▶ *Name an example of SSRI and MAOI drug. Read Chapter 13 to learn how another CYP2D6 drug may greatly change the C_p of a drug such as Paxil.*

DRUGS DISTRIBUTED AS ONE-COMPARTMENT MODEL AND ELIMINATED BY NONLINEAR PHARMACOKINETICS

The equations presented thus far in this chapter have been for drugs given by IV bolus, distributed as a one-compartment model, and eliminated only by nonlinear pharmacokinetics. The following are useful equations describing other possible routes of drug administration and including mixed drug elimination, by which the drug may be eliminated by both nonlinear (Michaelis–Menten) and linear (first-order) processes.

Mixed Drug Elimination

Drugs may be metabolized to several different metabolites by parallel pathways. At low drug doses corresponding to low drug concentrations at the site of the biotransformation enzymes, the rates of formation of metabolites are first order. However, with higher doses of drug, more drug is absorbed and higher drug concentrations are presented to the biotransformation enzymes. At higher drug concentrations, the enzyme involved in metabolite formation may become saturated, and the rate of metabolite formation becomes nonlinear and approaches zero order. For example, sodium salicylate is metabolized to both a glucuronide and a glycine conjugate (hippurate). The rate of formation of the glycine conjugate is limited by the amount of glycine available. Thus, the rate of formation of the glucuronide continues as a first-order process, whereas the rate of conjugation with glycine is capacity limited.

The equation that describes a drug that is eliminated by both first-order and Michaelis–Menten kinetics after IV bolus injection is given by

$$-\frac{dC_\mathrm{p}}{dt} = kC_\mathrm{p} + \frac{V'_\mathrm{max}C_\mathrm{p}}{K_\mathrm{M}+C_\mathrm{p}} \qquad (10.26)$$

where k is the first-order rate constant representing the sum of all first-order elimination processes, while the second term of Equation 10.26 represents the saturable process. V'_max is simply V_max expressed as concentration by dividing by V_D.

CLINICAL FOCUS

The pharmacokinetic profile of niacin is complicated due to extensive first-pass metabolism that is dosing-rate specific. In humans, one metabolic pathway is through a conjugation step with glycine to form nicotinuric acid (NUA). NUA is excreted in the urine, although there may be a small amount of reversible metabolism back to niacin. The other metabolic pathway results in the formation of nicotinamide adenine dinucleotide (NAD). It is unclear whether nicotinamide is formed as a precursor to, or following the synthesis of, NAD. Nicotinamide is further metabolized to at least N-methylnicotinamide (MNA) and nicotinamide-N-oxide (NNO). MNA is further metabolized to two other compounds, N-methyl-2-pyridone-5-carboxamide (2PY) and N-methyl-4-pyridone-5-carboxamide (4PY). The formation of 2PY appears to predominate over 4PY in humans. At doses used to treat hyperlipidemia, these metabolic pathways are saturable, which explains

the nonlinear relationship between niacin dose and plasma drug concentrations following multiple doses of Niaspan (niacin) extended-release tablets (Niaspan, FDA-approved label, 2009).

Zero-Order Input and Nonlinear Elimination

The usual example of zero-order input is constant IV infusion. If the drug is given by constant IV infusion and is eliminated only by nonlinear pharmacokinetics, then the following equation describes the rate of change of the plasma drug concentration:

$$\frac{dC_\mathrm{p}}{dt} = \frac{k_0}{V_\mathrm{D}} - \frac{V'_\mathrm{max}C_\mathrm{p}}{K_\mathrm{M}+C_\mathrm{p}} \qquad (10.27)$$

where k_0 is the infusion rate and V_D is the apparent volume of distribution.

First-Order Absorption and Nonlinear Elimination

The relationship that describes the rate of change in the plasma drug concentration for a drug that is given extravascularly (eg, orally), absorbed by first-order absorption, and eliminated only by nonlinear pharmacokinetics, is given by the following equation. C_GI is concentration in the GI tract.

$$\frac{dC_\mathrm{p}}{dt} = k_\mathrm{a}C_\mathrm{GI}e^{-k_\mathrm{a}t} - \frac{V'_\mathrm{max}C_\mathrm{p}}{K_\mathrm{M}+C_\mathrm{p}} \qquad (10.28)$$

where k_a is the first-order absorption rate constant.

If the drug is eliminated by parallel pathways consisting of both linear and nonlinear pharmacokinetics, Equation 10.28 may be extended to Equation 10.29.

$$\frac{dC_\mathrm{p}}{dt} = k_\mathrm{a}C_\mathrm{GI}e^{-k_\mathrm{a}t} - \frac{V'_\mathrm{max}C_\mathrm{p}}{K_\mathrm{M}+C_\mathrm{p}} - kC_\mathrm{p} \qquad (10.29)$$

where k is the first-order elimination rate constant.

Two-Compartment Model with Nonlinear Elimination

RhG-CSF is a glycoprotein hormone (recombinant human granulocyte-colony stimulating factors, rhG-CSF, MW about 20,000) that stimulates the growth of neutropoietic cells and activates mature neutrophils.

The drug is used in neutropenia occurring during chemotherapy or radiotherapy. Similar to many biotechnological drugs, RhG-CSF is administered by injection. The drug is administered subcutaneously and absorbed into the blood from the dermis site. This drug follows a two-compartment model with two elimination processes: (1) a saturable process of receptor-mediated elimination in the bone marrow and (2) a nonsaturable process of elimination. The model is described by two differential equations as shown below:

$$\frac{dC_1}{dt} = -\left(k_{12} + k + \frac{V_{max}}{V_1(C_1 + K_M)}\right)C_1 + \frac{k_{21}X_2}{V_1} \quad (10.29a)$$

$$\frac{dX_2}{dt} = k_{12}C_1V_1 - k_{21}X_2 \quad (10.29b)$$

where k_{12} and k_{21} are first-order transfer constants between the central and peripheral comparments; k is the first-order elimination constant from the central compartment; V_1 is the volume of the central compartment and the steady-state volume of distribution is V_{ss}; X_2 is the amount in the peripheral compartment; C_1 is the drug concentration in the central compartments at time t; and V_{max} and K_M are Michaelis–Menten parameters that describe the saturable elimination.

The pharmacokinetics of this drug was described by Hayashi et al (2001). Here, α is a function of dose with no dimensions, and granulocyte colony-stimulating factor (G-CSF) takes a value from 0 to 1. When the dose approaches 0, $\alpha = 1$; when the dose approaches ∞, $\alpha = 0$.

According to Hayashi et al (2001), the drug clearance may be considered as two parts as shown below:

$$\text{Dose/AUC} = \alpha Cl_{int} + Cl_n = Cl \quad (10.29c)$$

$$\text{Dose/AUC} = \frac{\int_0^\infty \frac{CK_M}{C + K_M} dt}{\int_0^\infty C\, dt} Cl_{int} + Cl_n \quad (10.29d)$$

where Cl_{int} is intrinsic clearance for the saturable pathway; Cl_n is nonsaturable clearance; and C is serum concentration.

CHRONOPHARMACOKINETICS AND TIME-DEPENDENT PHARMACOKINETICS

Chronopharmacokinetics broadly refers to a temporal change in the rate process (such as absorption or elimination) of a drug. The temporal changes in drug absorption or elimination can be cyclical over a constant period (eg, 24-hour interval), or they may be noncyclical, in which drug absorption or elimination changes over a longer period of time. Chronopharmacokinetics is an important consideration during drug therapy.

Time-dependent pharmacokinetics generally refers to a noncyclical change in the drug absorption or drug elimination rate process over a period of time. Time-dependent pharmacokinetics leads to nonlinear pharmacokinetics. Unlike dose-dependent pharmacokinetics, which involves a change in the rate process when the dose is changed, time-dependent pharmacokinetics may be the result of alteration in the physiology or biochemistry in an organ or a region in the body that influences drug disposition (Levy, 1983).

Time-dependent pharmacokinetics may be due to autoinduction or autoinhibition of biotransformation enzymes. For example, Pitlick and Levy (1977) have shown that repeated doses of carbamazepine induce the enzymes responsible for its elimination (ie, auto-induction), thereby increasing the clearance of the drug. Auto-inhibition may occur during the course of metabolism of certain drugs (Perrier et al, 1973). In this case, the metabolites formed increase in concentration and further inhibit metabolism of the parent drug. In biochemistry, this phenomenon is known as *product inhibition*. Drugs undergoing time-dependent pharmacokinetics have variable clearance and elimination half-lives. The steady-state concentration of a drug that causes auto-induction may be due to increased clearance over time. Some anticancer drugs are better tolerated at certain times of the day; for example, the antimetabolite drug fluorouracil (FU) was least toxic when given in the morning to rodents (Von Roemeling, 1991). A list of drugs that demonstrate time dependence is shown in Table 10-8.

TABLE 10-8   Drugs Showing Circadian or Time-Dependent Disposition

Cefodizime	Fluorouracil	Ketoprofen	Theophylline
Cisplatin	Heparin	Mequitazine	

Data from Reinberg (1991).

In pharmacokinetics, it is important to recognize that many isozymes (CYPs) are involved in drug metabolisms. A drug may competitively influence the metabolism of another drug within the same CYP subfamily. Sometimes, an unrecognized effect from the presence of another drug may be misjudged as a time-dependent pharmacokinetics. Drug metabolism and pharmacogenetics are discussed more extensively in Chapter 13.

Circadian Rhythms and Influence on Drug Response

Circadian rhythms are rhythmic or cyclical changes in plasma drug concentrations that may occur daily, due to normal changes in body functions. Some rhythmic changes that influence body functions and drug response are controlled by genes and subject to modification by environmental factors. The mammalian circadian clock is a self-sustaining oscillator, usually within a period of ~24 hours, that cyclically controls many physiological and behavioral systems. The biological clock attempts to synchronize and respond to changes in length of the daylight cycle and optimize body functions.

Circadian rhythms are regulated through periodic activation of transcription by a set of clock genes. For example, melatonin onset is associated with onset of the quiescent period of cortisol secretion that regulates many functions. Some well-known circadian physiologic parameters are core body temperature (CBT), heart rate (HR), and other cardiovascular parameters. These fundamental physiologic factors can affect disease states, as well as toxicity and therapeutic response to drug therapy. The toxic dose of a drug may vary as much as several-fold, depending on the time of drug administration—during either sleep or wake cycle.

For example, the effects of timing of aminoglycoside administration on serum aminoglycoside levels and the incidence of nephrotoxicity were studied in 221 patients (Prins et al, 1997). Each patient received an IV injection of 2–4 mg/kg gentamicin or tobramycin once daily: (1) between midnight and 7:30 AM, (2) between 8 AM and 3:30 PM, or (3) between 4 PM and 11:30 PM. In this study, no statistically significant differences in drug trough levels (0–4.2 mg/L) or peak drug levels (3.6–26.8 mg/L) were found for the three time periods of drug administration. However, nephrotoxicity occurred significantly more frequently when the aminoglycosides were given during the rest period (midnight–7:30 AM). Many factors contributing to nephrotoxicity were discussed; the time of administration was considered to be an independent risk factor in the multivariate statistical analysis. Time-dependent pharmacokinetics/pharmacodynamics is important, but it may be difficult to detect the clinical difference in drug concentrations due to multivariates.

Another example of circadian changes on drug response involves observations with chronic obstructive pulmonary disease (COPD) patients. Symptoms of hypoxemia may be aggravated in some COPD patients due to changes in respiration during the sleep cycle. Circadian variations have been reported involving the incidence of acute myocardial infarction, sudden cardiac death, and stroke. Platelet aggregation favoring coagulation is increased after arising in the early morning hours, coincident with the peak incidence of these cardiovascular events, although much remains to be elucidated.

Time-dependent pharmacokinetics and physiologic functions are important considerations in the treatment of certain hypertensive subjects, in whom early-morning rise in blood pressure may increase the risk of stroke or hypertensive crisis. Verapamil is a commonly used antihypertensive. The diurnal pattern of forearm vascular resistance (FVR) between hypertensive and normotensive volunteers was studied at 9 PM on 24-hour ambulatory blood pressure monitoring, and the early-morning blood pressure rise was studied in 23 untreated hypertensives and 10 matched, normotensive controls. The diurnal pattern of FVR differed between hypertensives and normotensives, with normotensives exhibiting an FVR decline between 2 PM and 9 PM, while FVR rose at 9 PM in hypertensives. Verapamil appeared to minimize the diurnal variation in FVR in hypertensives, although there were no significant differences at any single time point. Verapamil effectively reduced ambulatory blood pressure throughout the 24-hour period, but it did not blunt the early-morning rate of blood pressure rise despite peak S-verapamil concentrations in the early morning (Nguyen et al, 2000).

CLINICAL FOCUS

Hypertensive patients are sometimes characterized as "dippers" if their nocturnal blood pressure drops below their daytime pressure. Non-dipping patients appear to be at an increased risk of cardiovascular morbidity. Blood pressure and cardiovascular events have a diurnal rhythm, with a peak of both in the morning hours, and a decrease during the night. The circadian variation of blood pressure provides assistance in predicting cardiovascular outcome (de la Sierra et al, 2011).

The pharmacokinetics of many cardiovascular acting drugs have a circadian phase dependency (Lemmer, 2006). Examples include β-blockers, calcium channel blockers, oral nitrates, and ACE inhibitors. There is clinical evidence that antihypertensive drugs should be dosed in the early morning in patients who are hypertensive "dippers," whereas for patients who are non-dippers, it may be necessary to add an evening dose or even to use a single evening dose not only to reduce high blood pressure (BP) but also to normalize a disturbed non-dipping 24-hour BP profile. However, for practical purposes, some investigators found diurnal BP monitoring in many individuals too variable to distinguish between dippers and non-dippers (Lemmer, 2006).

The issue of time-dependent pharmacokinetics/pharmacodynamics (PK/PD) may be an important issue in some antihypertensive care. Pharmacists should recognize drugs that exhibit this type of time-dependant PK/PD.

Another example of time-dependent pharmacokinetics involves ciprofloxacin. Circadian variation in the urinary excretion of ciprofloxacin was investigated in a crossover study in 12 healthy male volunteers, ages 19–32 years. A significant decrease in the rate and extent of the urinary excretion of ciprofloxacin was observed following administrations at

2200 versus 1000 hours, indicating that the rate of excretion during the night time was slower (Sarveshwer Rao et al, 1997).

Clinical and Adverse Toxicity Due to Nonlinear Pharmacokinetics

The presence of nonlinear or dose-dependent pharmacokinetics, whether due to saturation of a process involving absorption, first-pass metabolism, binding, or renal excretion, can have significant clinical consequences. However, nonlinear pharmacokinetics may not be noticed in drug studies that use a narrow dose range in patients. In this case, dose estimation may result in disproportionate increases in adverse reactions but insufficient therapeutic benefits. Nonlinear pharmacokinetics can occur anywhere above, within, or below the therapeutic window.

The problem of a nonlinear dose relationship in population pharmacokinetics analysis has been investigated using simulations (Hashimoto et al, 1994, 1995; Jonsson et al, 2000). For example, nonlinear fluvoxamine pharmacokinetics was reported (Jonsson et al, 2000) to be present even at subtherapeutic doses. By using simulated data and applying nonlinear mixed-effect models using NONMEM, the authors also demonstrated that use of nonlinear mixed-effect models in population pharmacokinetics had an important application in the detection and characterization of nonlinear processes (pharmacokinetic and pharmacodynamic). Both first-order (FO) and FO conditional estimation (FOCE) algorithms were used for the population analyses. Population pharmacokinetics is discussed further in Chapter 25.

BIOAVAILABILITY OF DRUGS THAT FOLLOW NONLINEAR PHARMACOKINETICS

The bioavailability of drugs that follow nonlinear pharmacokinetics is difficult to estimate accurately. As shown in Table 10-1, each process of drug absorption, distribution, and elimination is potentially saturable. Drugs that follow linear pharmacokinetics follow the principle of superposition (Chapter 9). The assumption in applying the rule of superposition is that each dose of drug superimposes on the previous dose. Consequently, the bioavailability of subsequent doses is predictable and not affected by the previous dose. In the presence of a saturable pathway for drug absorption, distribution, or elimination, drug bioavailability will change within a single dose or with subsequent (multiple) doses. An example of a drug with dose-dependent absorption is chlorothiazide (Hsu et al, 1987).

The extent of bioavailability is generally estimated using $[AUC]_0^\infty$. If drug absorption is saturation limited in the gastrointestinal tract, then a smaller fraction of drug is absorbed systemically when the gastrointestinal drug concentration is high. A drug with a saturable elimination pathway may also have a concentration-dependent AUC affected by the magnitude of K_M and V_{max} of the enzymes involved in drug elimination (Equation 10.21). At low C_p, the rate of elimination is first order, even at the beginning of drug absorption from the gastrointestinal tract. As more drug is absorbed, either from a single dose or after multiple doses, systemic drug concentrations increase to levels that saturate the enzymes involved in drug elimination. The body drug clearance changes and the AUC increases disproportionately to the increase in dose (see Fig. 10-2).

NONLINEAR PHARMACOKINETICS DUE TO DRUG–PROTEIN BINDING

Protein binding may prolong the elimination half-life of a drug. Drugs that are protein bound must first dissociate into the free or nonbound form to be eliminated by glomerular filtration. The nature and extent of drug–protein binding affects the magnitude of the deviation from normal linear or first-order elimination rate process.

For example, consider the plasma level–time curves of two hypothetical drugs given intravenously in equal doses (Fig. 10-14). One drug is 90% protein bound, whereas the other drug does not bind plasma protein. Both drugs are eliminated solely by glomerular filtration through the kidney.

The plasma curves in Fig. 10-14 demonstrate that the protein-bound drug is more concentrated in the plasma than a drug that is not protein bound, and

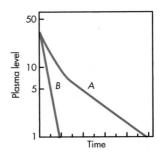

FIGURE 10-14   Plasma curve comparing the elimination of two drugs given in equal IV doses. Curve *A* represents a drug 90% bound to plasma protein. Curve *B* represents a drug not bound to plasma protein.

the protein-bound drug is eliminated at a slower, nonlinear rate. Because the two drugs are eliminated by identical mechanisms, the characteristically slower elimination rate for the protein-bound drug is due to the fact that less free drug is available for glomerular filtration in the course of renal excretion.

The concentration of free drug, C_f, can be calculated at any time, as follows:

$$C_f = C_p(1 - \text{fraction bound}) \qquad (10.30)$$

For any protein-bound drug, the free drug concentration (C_f) will always be less than the total drug concentration (C_p).

A careful examination of Fig. 10-14 shows that the slope of the bound drug decreases gradually as the drug concentration decreases. This indicates that the percent of drug bound is not constant. *In vivo*, the percent of drug bound usually increases as the plasma drug concentration decreases (see Chapter 11). Since protein binding of drug can cause nonlinear elimination rates, pharmacokinetic fitting of protein-bound drug data to a simple one-compartment model without accounting for binding results in erroneous estimates of the volume of distribution and elimination half-life. Sometimes plasma drug data for drugs that are highly protein bound have been inappropriately fitted to two-compartment models.

Valproic acid (Depakene) shows nonlinear pharmacokinetics that may be due partially to nonlinear protein binding. The free fraction of valproic acid is 10% at a plasma drug concentration of 40 $\mu g/mL$ and 18.5% at a plasma drug level of 130 $\mu g/mL$. In addition, higher-than-expected plasma drug concentrations occur in the elderly patients, and in patients with hepatic or renal disease.

One-Compartment Model Drug with Protein Binding

The process of elimination of a drug distributed in a single compartment with protein binding is illustrated in Fig. 10-15. The one compartment contains both free drug and bound drug, which are dynamically interconverted with rate constants k_1 and k_2. Elimination of drug occurs only with the free drug, at a first-order rate. The bound drug is not eliminated. Assuming a saturable and instantly reversible drug-binding process, where P = protein concentration in plasma, C_f = plasma concentration of free drug, $k_d = k_2/k_1$ = dissociation constant of the protein drug complex, C_p = total plasma drug concentration, and C_b = plasma concentration of bound drug,

$$\frac{C_b}{P} = \frac{(1/k_d)C_f}{1+(1/k_d)C_f} \tag{10.31}$$

This equation can be rearranged as follows:

$$C_b = \frac{PC_f}{k_d + C_f} = C_p - C_f \tag{10.32}$$

Solving for C_f,

$$C_f = \frac{1}{2}\left[-(P+k_d-C_p)+\sqrt{(P+k_d-C_p)^2+4k_dC_p}\right] \tag{10.33}$$

Because the rate of drug elimination is dC_p/dt,

$$\frac{dC_p}{dt} = -kC_f$$

$$\frac{dC_p}{dt} = \frac{-k}{2}\left[-(P+k_d-C_p)+\sqrt{(P+k_d-C_p)^2+4k_dC_p}\right] \tag{10.34}$$

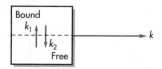

FIGURE 10-15   One-compartment model with drug–protein binding.

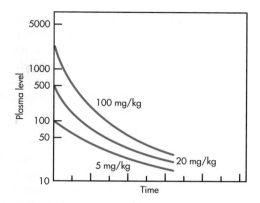

FIGURE 10-16   Plasma drug concentrations for various doses of a one-compartment model drug with protein binding. (Adapted from Coffey et al, 1971, with permission.)

This differential equation describes the relationship of changing plasma drug concentrations during elimination. The equation is not easily integrated but can be solved using a numerical method. Figure 10-16 shows the plasma drug concentration curves for a one-compartment protein-bound drug having a volume of distribution of 50 mL/kg and an elimination half-life of 30 minutes. The protein concentration is 4.4% and the molecular weight of the protein is 67,000 Da. At various doses, the pharmacokinetics of elimination of the drug, as shown by the plasma curves, ranges from linear to nonlinear, depending on the total plasma drug concentration.

Nonlinear drug elimination pharmacokinetics occurs at higher doses. Because more free drug is available at higher doses, initial drug elimination occurs more rapidly. For drugs demonstrating nonlinear pharmacokinetics, the free drug concentration may increase slowly at first, but when the dose of drug is raised beyond the protein-bound saturation point, free plasma drug concentrations may rise abruptly. Therefore, the concentration of free drug should always be calculated to make sure the patient receives a proper dose.

Determination of Linearity in Data Analysis

During new drug development, the pharmacokinetics of the drug is examined for linear or nonlinear pharmacokinetics. A common approach is to give several graded doses to human volunteers and obtain plasma drug concentration curves for each dose. From these data, a graph of AUC versus dose is generated as shown in Fig. 10-2. The drug is considered to follow linear kinetics if AUC versus dose for various doses is proportional (ie, linear relationship). In practice, the experimental data presented may not be very clear, especially when oral drug administration data are presented and there is considerable variability in the data. For example, the AUC versus three-graded doses of a new drug is shown in Fig. 10-17. A linear regression line was drawn through the three data points. The conclusion is that the drug follows dose-independent (linear) kinetics based upon a linear regression line through the data and a correlation coefficient, $R^2 = 0.97$.

- Do you agree with this conclusion after inspecting the graph?

The conclusion for linear pharmacokinetics in Fig. 10-17 seems reasonable based on the estimated regression line drawn through the data points.

However, another pharmacokineticist noticed that the regression line in Fig. 10-17 does not pass through the origin point (0,0). This pharmacokineticist considered the following questions:

- Are the patients in the study receiving the drug doses well separated by a washout period during the trial such that no residual drug remained in the body and carried to the present dose when plasma samples are collected?
- Is the method for assaying the samples validated? Could a high sample blank or interfering material be artificially adding to elevate 0 time drug concentrations?
- How does the trend line look if the point (0,0) is included?

When the third AUC point is above the trend line, it is risky to draw a conclusion. One should verify that the high AUC is not due to a lower elimination or clearance due to saturation.

In Fig. 10-18, a regression line was obtained by forcing the same data through point (0,0). The linear regression analysis and estimated R^2 appears to show that the drug followed nonlinear pharmacokinetics. The line appears to have a curvature upward and the possibility of some saturation at higher doses. This pharmacokineticist recommends additional study by adding a higher dose to more clearly check for dose dependency.

- What is your conclusion?

Considerations

- The experimental data are composed of three different drug doses.
- The regression line shows that the drug follows linear pharmacokinetics from the low dose to the high dose.
- The use of a (0.0) value may provide additional information concerning the linearity of the pharmacokinetics. However, extrapolation of curves beyond the actual experimental data can be misleading.
- The conclusion in using the (0.0) time point shows that the pharmacokinetics is nonlinear below the lowest drug dose. This may occur after oral dosing because at very low drug doses some of the drug is decomposed in the gastrointestinal tract or metabolized prior to systemic absorption. With higher doses, the small amount of drug loss is not observed systemically.

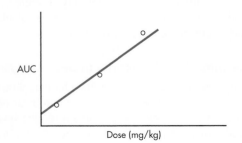

FIGURE 10-17   Plot of AUC versus dose to determine linearity. The regression line is based on the three doses of the drug.

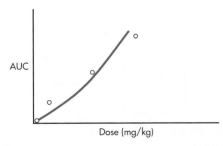

FIGURE 10-18   Plot of AUC versus dose to determine linearity.

TABLE 10-9   Some Common Issues during Data Analysis for Linearity

Oral Data	Issues during Data Analysis	Comments
	Last data point may be below the LOD or limit of detection. What should the AUC tailpiece be?	Last sample point scheduled too late in the study protocol.
	Last data point still very high, much above the LOD. What should be the AUC tailpiece?	Last sample point scheduled too early. A substantial number of data points may be incorrectly estimated by the tailpiece method.
	Incomplete sample spacing around peak.	Total AUC estimated may be quite variable or unreliable.
	Oral AUC data are influenced by F, D, and Cl.	When examining D_0/Cl vs D_0, F must be held constant. Any factor causing change in F during the trial will introduce uncertainty to AUC.
	F may be affected by efflux, transporters (see Chapter 13), and GI CYP enzymes. An increase in F and decrease in Cl or vice versa over doses may mask each other.	Nonlinearity of AUC vs D_0 may not be evident and one may incorrectly conclude a drug follows linear kinetics when it does not.
IV data	AUC data by IV are influenced by D_0 and Cl only.	When examining D_0/Cl vs D_0, F is always constant. Therefore, it is easier to see changes in AUC when Cl changes by IV route.

LOD, limit of detection.

Note if V_D of the drug is known, determining k from the terminal slope of the oral data provides another way of calculating $Cl (Cl = V_D k)$ to check whether clearance has changed at higher doses due to saturation. Some common issues during data analysis for linearity are listed in Table 10-9.

Note: In some cases, with certain drugs, the oral absorption mechanism is quite unique and drug clearance by the oral route may involve absorption site-specific enzymes or transporters located on the brush border. Extrapolating pharmacokinetic information from IV dose data should be done cautiously only after a careful consideration of these factors. It is helpful to know whether nonlinearity is caused by distribution, or absorption factors.

Unsuspected nonlinear drug disposition is one of the biggest issues concerning drug safety. Although pharmacokinetic tools are useful, nonlinearity can be easily missed during data analysis when there are outliners or extreme data scattering due to individual patient factors such as genetics, age, sex, and other unknown factors in special populations. While statistical analysis can help minimize this, it is extremely helpful to survey for problems (eg, epidemiological surveillance) and have a good understanding of how drugs are disposed in various parts of the body in the target populations.

POTENTIAL REASONS FOR UNSUSPECTED NONLINEARITY[1]

1. Nonlinearity caused by membrane resident transporters
2. Nonlinearity caused by membrane CYPs
3. Nonlinearity caused by cellular proteins
4. Nonlinearity caused by transporter proteins at the GI tract
5. Nonlinearity caused by bile acid transport (apical/bile canaliculus)

Frequently Asked Questions

▶ *What is the cause of nonlinear pharmacokinetics that is not dose related?*

▶ *For drugs that have several metabolic pathways, must all the metabolic pathways be saturated for the drug to exhibit nonlinear pharmacokinetics?*

[1]Source: Evaluation of hepatotoxic potential of drugs using transporter-based assays. Jasminder Sahi AAPS Transporter Meeting, 2005 at Parsippanny, New Jersey.

DOSE-DEPENDENT PHARMACOKINETICS

Role of Transporters

Classical pharmacokinetics studied linear pharmacokinetics of a drug by examining the area under plasma drug concentration curve at various doses given intravenously. The method is simple and definitive. The method is useful revealing the kinetics in the body as a whole. However, more useful information must now be obtained through studies based on *regional pharmacokinetics* by studying the roles of transporters in individual organs. Over the last few decades, transporters have been characterized in individual cells or in various types of cells (Chapters 11 and 13). These transporters may critically enhance or reduce local cell drug concentrations, allowing influx of drugs into the cell or removing drug from the cell by efflux transporters, a defensive mechanism of the body. Many of the cells express transporters genetically, which may also be triggered on or turned off in disease state. Whether the overall pharmacokinetic process is linear or nonlinear must be determined locally. The knowledge of the local effects of transporters on pharmacokinetics can improve safe and effective drug dosing. The impact of transporters are discussed by various authors in a review book edited by You and Morris (2007). Table 10-10 summarizes some of the transporters that play an important role in drug distribution and how they may impact drug linearity.

TABLE 10-10   Drug Transports and Comments on Roles in Altering Linearity of Absorption or Elimination

Transporters	Comments
Xenobiotic transporter expression	Transporters may be age and gender related. These differences may change the linearity of a drug through saturation.
Polymorphisms of drug transporters	Polymorphisms may have a clinical relevance affecting toxicity and efficacy in a similar way through change in pharmacokinetics.
Interplay of drug transporters and enzymes in liver	The role of transporters on hepatic drug is profound and may greatly change the overall linearity of a drug systemically.
	The concept of drug clearance, Cl, and intrinsic clearance has to be reexamined as a result of the translocation of transporters, at cellular membranes as suggested in a recent review.
Drug–drug interaction change due to transporters	Clinical relevance, pharmacokinetics, pharmacodynamics, and toxicity may decrease or increase if a drug is a transporter substrate or inhibitor. Less clear is the change from linear to nonlinear kinetics due to drug–drug interaction.
Drug transporters in the intestine	ABC transporters are very common and this can alter the absorption nature of a drug product, for example, the bioavailability and linearity of drug absorption. Bile acid transporters affect drug movement and elimination by biliary excretion. The nature of the process must be studied.
Drug transport in the kidney	Various organic anion and cation drug transporters have been described. These transporters may alter the linearity of systemic drug elimination if present in large quantity.
Multidrug resistance protein: P-glycoprotein	These proteins may affect drug concentration in a cell or group of cells. Hence, they are important elements in determining PK linearity.
Mammalian oligopeptide transporters	These transporters play a role in drug absorption and distribution.
Breast cancer resistance protein	These transporters play a role in drug linearity and dosing in cancer therapy.

CLINICAL EXAMPLE

Zmax® (Pfizer) is an extended-release microsphere formulation of the antibiotic azithromycin in an oral suspension. According to the approved label,[2] based on data obtained from studies evaluating the pharmacokinetics of azithromycin in healthy adult subjects, a higher peak serum concentration (C_{max}) and greater systemic exposure (AUC 0–24) of azithromycin are achieved on the day of dosing following a single 2-g dose of Zmax versus 1.5 g of azithromycin tablets administered over 3 days (500 mg/d) or 5 days (500 mg on day 1, 250 mg/d on days 2–5) (Table 10-11). Consequently, due to these different pharmacokinetic profiles, Zmax is not interchangeable with azithromycin tablet 3-day and 5-day dosing regimens.

Absorption

The bioavailability of Zmax relative to azithromycin immediate release (IR) (powder for oral suspension) was 83%. On average, peak serum concentrations were achieved approximately 2.5 hours later following Zmax administration and were lower by 57%, compared to 2 g azithromycin IR. Thus, single 2-g doses of Zmax and azithromycin IR are not bioequivalent and are not interchangeable.

Effect of food on absorption: A high-fat meal increased the rate and extent of absorption of a 2-g dose of Zmax (115% increase in C_{max}, and 23%

---

[2]http://labeling.pfizer.com/ShowLabeling.aspx?id=650#section-12.3.

increase in AUC_{0-72}) compared to the fasted state. A standard meal also increased the rate of absorption (119% increase in C_{max}), with less effect on the extent of absorption (12% increase in AUC_{0-72}) compared to administration of a 2-g Zmax dose in the fasted state.

Distribution

The serum protein binding of azithromycin is concentration dependent, decreasing from 51% at 0.02 μg/mL to 7% at 2 μg/mL. Following oral administration, azithromycin is widely distributed throughout the body with an apparent steady-state volume of distribution of 31.1 L/kg.

Azithromycin concentrates in fibroblasts, epithelial cells, macrophages, and circulating neutrophils and monocytes. Higher azithromycin concentrations in tissues than in plasma or serum have been observed. Following a 2-g single dose of Zmax, azithromycin achieved higher exposure (AUC_{0-120}) in mononuclear leukocytes (MNL) and polymorphonuclear leukocytes (PMNL) than in serum. The azithromycin exposure (AUC_{0-72}) in lung tissue and alveolar cells (AC) was approximately 100 times than in serum, and the exposure in epithelial lining fluid (ELF) was also higher (approximately 2–3 times) than in serum. The clinical significance of this distribution data is unknown.

Metabolism

In vitro and *in vivo* studies to assess the metabolism of azithromycin have not been performed.

TABLE 10-11 Mean (SD) Pharmacokinetic Parameters for Azithromycin on Day 1 Following the Administration of a Single Dose of 2 g Zmax or 1.5 g of Azithromycin Tablets Given over 3 Days (500 mg/d) or 5 Days (500 mg on Day 1 and 250 mg on Days 2–5) to Healthy Adult Subjects

Pharmacokinetic Parameter*	Azithromycin Regimen		
	Zmax (N = 41)	3-Day (N = 12)	5-Day (N = 12)
C_{max} (μg/mL)	0.821 (0.281)	0.441 (0.223)	0.434 (0.202)
T_{max}§ (h)	5.0 (2.0–8.0)	2.5 (1.0–4.0)	2.5 (1.0–6.0)
AUC_{0-24} (μg·h/mL)	8.62 (2.34)	2.58 (0.84)	2.60 (0.71)
$AUC_{0-\infty}$¶ (μg·h/mL)	20.0 (6.66)	17.4 (6.2)	14.9 (3.1)
$t_{1/2}$ (h)	58.8 (6.91)	71.8 (14.7)	68.9 (13.8)

*Zmax, 3-day and 5-day regimen parameters obtained from separate pharmacokinetic studies

Adapted from Zmax approved label, October 2013.

Excretion

Serum azithromycin concentrations following a single 2-g dose of Zmax declined in a polyphasic pattern with a terminal elimination half-life of 59 hours. The prolonged terminal half-life is thought to be due to a large apparent volume of distribution.

Biliary excretion of azithromycin, predominantly as unchanged drug, is a major route of elimination. Over the course of a week, approximately 6% of the administered dose appears as unchanged drug in urine.

Based on the information,

1. The bioavailability of this drug may be quite different for different dosage forms due to absorption profile.
2. Absorption is likely to be affected by GI residence time of the product and the type of dosage form.
3. The drug is widely distributed.
4. Drug binding may be nonlinear resulting in different free drug concentrations at different serum drug concentrations.

CHAPTER SUMMARY

Nonlinear pharmacokinetics refers to kinetic processes that result in disproportional changes in plasma drug concentrations when the dose is changed. This is also referred to as dose-dependent pharmacokinetics or saturation pharmacokinetics. Clearance and half-life are usually not constant with dose-dependent pharmacokinetics. Carrier-mediated processes and processes that depend on the binding of the drug to a macromolecule resulting in drug metabolism, protein binding, active absorption, and some transporter-mediated processes can potentially exhibit dose-dependent kinetics, especially at higher doses. The Michaelis–Menten kinetic equation may be applied *in vitro* or *in vivo* to describe drug disposition, for example, phenytoin.

An approach to determine nonlinear pharmacokinetics is to plot AUC versus doses and observe for nonlinearity curving. A common cause of overdosing in clinical practice is undetected saturation of a metabolic enzyme due to genotype difference in a subject, for example, CYP2D6. A second common cause of overdosing in clinical practice is undetected saturation of a metabolic enzyme due to coadministration of a second drug/agent that alters the original linear elimination process. Drug transporters play an important role in the body. Membrane-located transporters may cause uneven drug distribution at cellular level, and hiding concentration-dependent kinetics may occur at the local level within body organs. These processes include absorption and elimination and are important in drug therapy. Some transporters are triggered by disease or expressed differently in individuals and should be recognized by pharmacists during dosing regimen recommendation.

LEARNING QUESTIONS

1. Define *nonlinear pharmacokinetics*. How do drugs that follow nonlinear pharmacokinetics differ from drugs that follow linear pharmacokinetics?
   a. What is the rate of change in the plasma drug concentration with respect to time, dC_p/dt, when $C_p \ll K_M$?
   b. What is the rate of change in the plasma drug concentration with respect to time, dC_p/dt, when $C_p \gg K_M$?

2. What processes of drug absorption, distribution, and elimination may be considered "capacity limited," "saturated," or "dose dependent"?
3. Drugs, such as phenytoin and salicylates, have been reported to follow dose-dependent elimination kinetics. What changes in pharmacokinetic parameters, including $t_{1/2}$, V_D, AUC, and C_p, could be predicted if the amounts of these drugs administered were increased from low pharmacologic doses to high therapeutic doses?

4. A given drug is metabolized by capacity-limited pharmacokinetics. Assume K_M is 50 μg/mL, V_{max} is 20 μg/mL per hour, and the apparent V_D is 20 L/kg.

   a. What is the reaction order for the metabolism of this drug when given in a single intravenous dose of 10 mg/kg?

   b. How much time is necessary for the drug to be 50% metabolized?

5. How would induction or inhibition of the hepatic enzymes involved in drug biotransformation theoretically affect the pharmacokinetics of a drug that demonstrates nonlinear pharmacokinetics due to saturation of its hepatic elimination pathway?

6. Assume that both the active parent drug and its inactive metabolites are excreted by active tubular secretion. What might be the consequences of increasing the dosage of the drug on its elimination half-life?

7. The drug isoniazid was reported to interfere with the metabolism of phenytoin. Patients taking both drugs together show higher phenytoin levels in the body. Using the basic principles in this chapter, do you expect K_M to increase or decrease in patients taking both drugs? (*Hint:* see Fig. 10-4.)

8. Explain why K_M sometimes has units of mM/mL and sometimes mg/L.

9. The V_{max} for metabolizing a drug is 10 mmol/h. The rate of metabolism (v) is 5 μmol/h when drug concentration is 4 μmol. Which of the following statements is/are true?

   a. K_M is 5 μmol for this drug.

   b. K_M cannot be determined from the information given.

   c. K_M is 4 μmol for this drug.

10. Which of the following statements is/are true regarding the pharmacokinetics of diazepam (98% protein bound) and propranolol (87% protein bound)?

   a. Diazepam has a long elimination half-life because it is difficult to be metabolized due to extensive plasma–protein binding.

   b. Propranolol is an example of a drug with high protein binding but unrestricted (unaffected) metabolic clearance.

   c. Diazepam is an example of a drug with low hepatic extraction.

   d. All of the above.

   e. a and c.

   f. b and c.

11. Which of the following statements describe(s) correctly the properties of a drug that follows nonlinear or capacity-limited pharmacokinetics?

   a. The elimination half-life will remain constant when the dose changes.

   b. The area under the plasma curve (AUC) will increase proportionally as dose increases.

   c. The rate of drug elimination $= C_p \times K_M$.

   d. All of the above.

   e. a and b.

   f. None of the above.

12. The hepatic intrinsic clearances of two drugs are

   drug *A*: 1300 mL/min

   drug *B*: 26 mL/min

   Which drug is likely to show the greatest increase in hepatic clearance when hepatic blood flow is increased from 1 L/min to 1.5 L/min?

   a. Drug *A*

   b. Drug *B*

   c. No change for both drugs

ANSWERS

Frequently Asked Questions

Why is it important to monitor drug levels carefully for dose dependency?

- A patient with concomitant hepatic disease may have decreased biotransformation enzyme activity. Infants and young subjects may have immature hepatic enzyme systems. Alcoholics may have liver cirrhosis and lack certain coenzymes. Other patients may experience enzyme saturation at normal doses due to genetic polymorphism. Pharmacokinetics provides a simple way to identify nonlinear kinetics in these patients and to estimate an appropriate dose. Finally, concomitant use of other drugs may cause nonlinear pharmacokinetics at lower drug doses due to enzyme inhibition.

What are the main differences in pharmacokinetic parameters between a drug that follows linear pharmacokinetics and a drug that follows nonlinear pharmacokinetics?

- A drug that follows linear pharmacokinetics generally has a constant elimination half-life and a constant clearance with an increase in the dose. The steady-state drug concentrations and AUC are proportional to the size of the dose. Nonlinear pharmacokinetics results in dose-dependent Cl, $t_{1/2}$, and AUC. Nonlinear pharmacokinetics are often described in terms of V_{max} and K_M.

What is the cause of nonlinear pharmacokinetics that is not dose related?

- *Chronopharmacokinetics* is the main cause of nonlinear pharmacokinetics that is not dose related. The time-dependent or temporal process of drug elimination can be the result of rhythmic changes in the body. For example, nortriptyline and theophylline levels are higher when administered between 7 and 9 AM compared to between 7 and 9 PM after the same dose. Biological rhythmic differences in clearance cause a lower elimination rate in the morning compared to the evening. Other factors that cause nonlinear pharmacokinetics may result from enzyme induction (eg, carbamazepine) or enzyme inhibition after multiple doses of the drug. Furthermore, the drug or a metabolite may accumulate following multiple dosing and affect the metabolism or renal elimination of the drug.

What are the main differences between a model based on Michaelis–Menten kinetic (V_{max} and K_M) and the physiologic model that describes hepatic metabolism based on clearance?

- The physiologic model based on organ drug clearance describes nonlinear drug metabolism in terms of blood flow and intrinsic hepatic clearance (Chapter 12). Drugs are extracted by the liver as they are presented by blood flow. The physiologic model accounts for the sigmoid profile with changing blood flow and extraction, whereas the Michaelis–Menten model simulates

the metabolic profile based on V_{max} and K_M. The Michaelis–Menten model was applied mostly to describe *in vitro* enzymatic reactions. When V_{max} and K_M are estimated in patients, blood flow is not explicitly considered. This semiempirical method was found by many clinicians to be useful in dosing phenytoin. The organ clearance model was more useful in explaining clearance change due to impaired blood flow. In practice, the physiologic model has limited use in dosing patients because blood flow data for patients are not available.

Learning Questions

2. Capacity-limited processes for drugs include:
   - Absorption
     Active transport
     Intestinal metabolism by microflora
   - Distribution
     Protein binding
   - Elimination
     Hepatic elimination
     Biotransformation
     Active biliary secretion
   - Renal excretion
     Active tubular secretion
     Active tubular reabsorption

4. $C_p^0 = \dfrac{\text{dose}}{V_D} = \dfrac{10{,}000\ \mu g}{20{,}000\ \text{mL}} = 0.5\ \mu g/mL$

From Equation 10.1,

$$\text{Elimination rate} = -\frac{dC_p}{dt} = \frac{V_{max}C_p}{K_M + C_p}$$

Because $K_M = 50\ \mu g/mL$, $C_p \ll K_M$ and the reaction rate is first order. Thus, the above equation reduces to Equation 10.3.

$$-\frac{dC_p}{dt} = \frac{V_{max}C_p}{K_M} = k'C_p$$

$$k' = \frac{V_{max}}{K_M} = \frac{20\ \mu g/h}{50\ \mu g} = 0.4\ \text{h}^{-1}$$

For first-order reactions,

$$t_{1/2} = \frac{0.693}{k'} = \frac{0.693}{0.4} = 1.73\ \text{h}$$

The drug will be 50% metabolized in 1.73 hours.

7. When INH is coadminstered, plasma phenytoin concentration is increased due to a reduction in metabolic rate v. Equation 10.1 shows that v and K_M are inversely related (K_M in denominator). An increase in K_M will be accompanied by an increase in plasma drug concentration. Figure 10-4 shows that an increase in K_M is accompanied by an increase in the amount of drug in the body at any time t. Equation 10.4 relates drug concentration to K_M, and it can be seen that the two are proportionally related, although they are not linearly proportional to each other due to the complexity of the equation. An actual study in the literature shows that k is increased severalfold in the presence of INH in the body.

8. The K_M has the units of concentration. In laboratory studies, K_M is expressed in moles per liter, or micromoles per milliliter, because reactions are expressed in moles and not milligrams. In dosing, drugs are given in milligrams and plasma drug concentrations are expressed as milligrams per liter or micrograms per milliliter. The units of K_M for pharmacokinetic models are estimated from *in vivo* data. They are therefore commonly expressed as milligrams per liter, which is preferred over micrograms per milliliter because dose is usually expressed in milligrams. The two terms may be shown to be equivalent and convertible. Occasionally, when simulating amount of drug metabolized in the body as a function of time, the amount of drug in the body has been assumed to follow Michaelis–Menten kinetics, and K_M assumes the unit of D_0 (eg, mg). In this case, K_M takes on a very different meaning.

REFERENCES

Coffey J, Bullock FJ, Schoenemann PT: Numerical solution of nonlinear pharmacokinetic equations: Effect of plasma protein binding on drug distribution and elimination. *J Pharm Sci* **60:**1623, 1971.

de la Sierra A, Segura J, Banegas JR, Gorostidi M, de la Cruz JJ, Armario P, Oliveras A, Ruilope LM. Clinical features of 8295 patients with resistant hypertension classified on the basis of ambulatory blood pressure monitoring. *Hypertension* **57**(5):898–902, 2011.

Evans WE, Schentag JJ, Jusko WJ. 1992. Applied Pharmacokinetics, 3rd ed., Applied Therapeutics, Vancouver, WA.

Hashimoto Y, Odani A, Tanigawara Y, Yasuhara M, Okuno T, Hori R: Population analysis of the dose-dependent pharmacokinetics of zonisamide in epileptic patients. *Biol Pharm Bull* **17:**323–326, 1994.

Hashimoto Y, Koue T, Otsuki Y, Yasuhara M, Hori R, Inui K: Simulation for population analysis of Michaelis–Menten kinetics. *J Pharmacokinet Biopharmacol* **23:**205–216, 1995.

Hayashi N, Aso H, Higashida M, et al: Estimation of rhG-CSF absorption kinetics after subcutaneous administration using a modified Wagner–Nelson method with a nonlinear elimination model. *European J Pharm Sci* **13:**151–158, 2001.

Hsu F, Prueksaritanont T, Lee MG, Chiou WL: The phenomenon and cause of the dose-dependent oral absorption of chlorothiazide in rats: Extrapolation to human data based on the body surface area concept. *J Pharmacokinet Biopharmacol* **15:**369–386, 1987.

Jonsson EN, Wade JR, Karlsson MO: Nonlinearity detection: Advantages of nonlinear mixed-effects modeling. *AAPS Pharmsci* **2**(3), article 32, 2000.

Lemmer B: The importance of circadian rhythms on drug response in hypertension and coronary heart disease—From mice and man. *Pharmacol Ther* **111**(3):629–651, 2006.

Lennard MS, Tucker GT, Woods HF: The polymorphic oxidation of beta-adrenoceptor antagonists—Clinical pharmacokinetic considerations. *Clin Pharmacol* **11:**1–17, 1986.

Levy RH: Time-dependent pharmacokinetics. *Pharmacol Ther* **17:**383–392, 1983.

Muxfeldt ES, Cardoso CRL, Salles F: Prognostic value of nocturnal blood pressure reduction in resistant hypertension. *Arch Intern Med* **169**(9):874–880, 2009.

Nguyen BN, Parker RB, Noujedehi M, Sullivan JM, Johnson JA: Effects of coerverapamil on circadian pattern of forearm vascular resistance and blood pressure. *J Clin Pharmacol* **40** (suppl):1480–1487, 2000.

Perrier D, Ashley JJ, Levy G: Effect of product inhibition in kinetics of drug elimination. *J Pharmacokinet Biopharmacol* **1:**231, 1973.

Pitlick WH, Levy RH: Time-dependent kinetics, I. Exponential autoinduction of carbamazepine in monkeys. *J Pharm Sci* **66:**647, 1977.

Prins JM, Weverling GJ, Van Ketel RJ, Speelman P: Circadian variations in serum levels and the renal toxicity of aminoglycosides in patients. *Clin Pharmacol Ther* **62:**106–111, 1997.

Reinberg AE: Concepts of circadian chronopharmacology. In Hrushesky WJM, Langer R, Theeuwes F (eds). *Temporal Control of Drug Delivery*. New York, Annals of the Academy of Science, 1991, vol 618, p 102.

Sarveshwer Rao VV, Rambhau D, Ramesh Rao B, Srinivasu P: Circadian variation in urinary excretion of ciprofloxacin after a single dose oral administration at 1000 and 2200 hours in human subjects. *India Antimicrob Agents Chemother (USA)* **41:**1802–1804, 1997, Kakatiya Univ., Warangal-506 009.

Vermeulen T: Distribution of paroxetine in three postmortem cases. *J Analytical Toxicology* **22:**541–544, 1998.

Von Roemeling R: The therapeutic index of cytotoxic chemotherapy depends upon circadian drug timing. In Hrushesky WJM, Langer R, Theeuwes F (eds). *Temporal Control of Drug Delivery.* New York, Annals of the Academy of Science, 1991, vol 618, pp 292–311.

Vozeh S, Muir KT, Sheiner LB: Predicting phenytoin dosage. *J Pharm Biopharm* **9:**131–146, 1981.

Wagner JG, Szpunar GJ, Ferry JJ: Michaelis–Menten elimination kinetics: Areas under curves, steady-state concentrations, and clearances for compartment models with different types of input. *Biopharm Drug Disp* **6:**177–200, 1985.

Witmer DR, Ritschel WA: Phenytoin isoniazid interaction: A kinetic approach to management. *Drug Intell Clin Pharm* **18:**483–486, 1984.

Yoon YR, Cha IJ, Shon JH, et al: Relationship of paroxetine disposition to metoprolol metabolic ratio and CYP2D6*10 genotype of Korean subjects. *Clin Pharmacol Ther* **67**(5):567–576, 2000 May.

You G, Morris ME: *Drug Transporters: Molecular Characterization and Role in Drug Disposition.* John Wiley and Sons Ltd, Sep 2007.

Yu HY, Shen YZ, Sugiyama Y, Hanano M: Dose-dependent pharmacokinetics of valproate in guinea pigs of different ages. *Epilepsia* **28**(6):680–687, 1987.

BIBLIOGRAPHY

Amsel LP, Levy G: Drug biotransformation interactions in man, II. A pharmacokinetic study of the simultaneous conjugation of benzoic and salicylic acids with glycine. *J Pharm Sci* **58:**321–326, 1969.

Dutta S, Matsumoto Y, Ebling WF: Is it possible to estimate the parameters of the sigmoid E_{max} model with truncated data typical of clinical studies? *J Pharm Sci* **85:**232–239, 1996.

Gibaldi M: Pharmacokinetic aspects of drug metabolism. *Ann NY State Acad Sci* **179:**19, 1971.

Kruger-Theimer E: Nonlinear dose concentration relationships. *Il Farmaco* **23:**718–756, 1968.

Levy G: Pharmacokinetics of salicylate in man. *Drug Metab Rev* **9:**3–19, 1979.

Levy G, Tsuchiya T: Salicylate accumulation kinetics in man. *N Engl J Med* **287:**430–432, 1972.

Ludden TM: Nonlinear pharmacokinetics. Clinical applications. *Clin Pharmacokinet* **20:**429–446, 1991.

Ludden TM, Hawkins DW, Allen JP, Hoffman SF: Optimum phenytoin dosage regimen. *Lancet* **1:**307–308, 1979.

Mehvar R: Principles of nonlinear pharmacokinetics: *Am J Pharm Edu* **65:**178–184, 2001.

Mullen PW: Optimal phenytoin therapy: A new technique for individualizing dosage. *Clin Pharm Ther* **23:**228–232, 1978.

Mullen PW, Foster RW: Comparative evaluation of six techniques for determining the Michaelis–Menten parameters relating phenytoin dose and steady state serum concentrations. *J Pharm Pharmacol* **31:**100–104, 1979.

Tozer TN, et al: In Breimer DD, Speiser P (eds). *Topics in Pharmaceutical Sciences.* New York, Elsevier, 1981, p 4.

Tozer TN, Rubin GM: Saturable kinetics and bioavailability determination. In Welling PG, Tse FLS (eds). *Pharmacokinetics: Regulatory, Industrial, Academic Perspectives.* New York, Marcel Dekker, 1988.

Van Rossum JM, van Lingen G, Burgers JPT: Dose-dependent pharmacokinetics. *Pharmacol Ther* **21:**77–99, 1983.

Wagner J: Properties of the Michaelis–Menten equation and its integrated form which are useful in pharmacokinetics. *J Pharm Biopharm* **1:**103, 1973.

11

Physiologic Drug Distribution and Protein Binding

He Sun and Hong Zhao

Chapter Objectives

▶ Describe the physiology of drug distribution in the body.

▶ Explain how drug distribution is affected by blood flow, protein, and tissue binding.

▶ Describe how drug distribution can affect the apparent volume of distribution.

▶ Explain how volume of distribution, drug clearance, and half-life can be affected by protein binding.

▶ Determine drug–protein binding constants using *in vitro* methods.

▶ Evaluate the impact of change in drug–protein binding or displacement on free drug concentration.

PHYSIOLOGIC FACTORS OF DISTRIBUTION

After a drug is absorbed systemically from the site of administration, the drug molecules are distributed throughout the body by the systemic circulation. The location, extent, and distribution are dependent on the drug's physicochemical properties and individual patient characteristics such as organ perfusion and blood flow. The drug molecules are carried by the blood to the target site (receptor) for drug action and to other (nonreceptor) tissues as well, where side effects or adverse reactions may occur. These sites may be intra- and/or extracellular. Drug molecules are distributed to eliminating organs, such as the liver and kidney, and to noneliminating tissues, such as the brain, skin, and muscle. In pregnancy, drugs cross the placenta and may affect the developing fetus. Drugs can also be secreted in milk via the mammillary glands, into the saliva and into other secretory pathways. A substantial portion of the drug may be bound to proteins in the plasma and/or in the tissues. Lipophilic drugs deposit in fat, from which the drug may be slowly released.

Drug distribution throughout the body occurs primarily via the circulatory system, which consists of a series of blood vessels that carry the drug in the blood; these include the arteries that carry blood to tissues, and the veins that return the blood back to the heart. An average subject (70 kg) has about 5 L of blood, which is equivalent to about 3 L of plasma (Fig. 11-1). About 50% of the blood is in the large veins or venous sinuses. The volume of blood pumped by the heart per minute—the cardiac output—is the product of the stroke volume of the heart and the number of heartbeats per minute. An average cardiac output is 0.08 L/69 left ventricular contractions (heart beats)/min, or approximately 5.5 L/min in subjects at rest. The cardiac output may be five to six times higher during exercise. Left ventricular contraction may produce a systolic blood pressure of 120 mm Hg, and moves blood at a linear speed of 300 mm/s through the aorta. Mixing of a drug solution in the blood occurs rapidly at this flow rate. Drug molecules rapidly diffuse through a network of fine capillaries to the tissue spaces

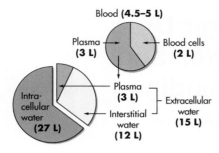

FIGURE 11-1   Major water volumes (L) in a 70-kg human.

filled with interstitial fluid (Fig. 11-2). The interstitial fluid plus the plasma water is termed *extracellular water,* because these fluids reside outside the cells. Drug molecules may further diffuse from the interstitial fluid across the cell membrane into the cell cytoplasm.

Drug distribution is generally rapid, and most small drug molecules permeate capillary membranes easily. The passage of drug molecules across a cell membrane depends on the physicochemical nature of both the drug and the cell membrane. Cell membranes are composed of protein and a bilayer of phospholipid, which act as a lipid barrier to drug uptake. Thus, lipid-soluble drugs generally diffuse across cell membranes more easily than highly polar or water-soluble drugs. Small drug molecules generally diffuse more rapidly across cell membranes than large drug molecules. If the drug is bound to a plasma protein such as albumin, the drug–protein complex becomes too large for easy diffusion across the cell or even capillary membranes. A comparison of diffusion rates for water-soluble molecules is given in Table 11-1.

Diffusion and Hydrostatic Pressure

The processes by which drugs transverse capillary membranes into the tissue include passive diffusion and hydrostatic pressure. Passive diffusion is the main process by which most drugs cross cell membranes. *Passive diffusion* (see Chapter 14) is the process by which drug molecules move from an area of high concentration to an area of low

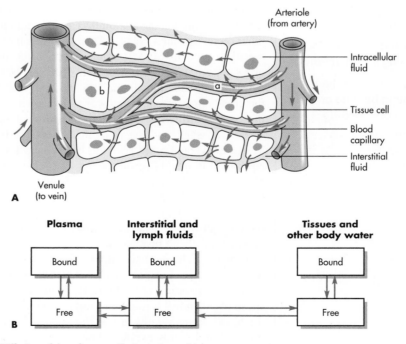

FIGURE 11-2   Diffusion of drug from capillaries to interstitial spaces.

TABLE 11-1   Permeability of Molecules of Various Sizes to Capillaries

	Molecular Weight	Radius of Equivalent Sphere A (0.1 mm)	Diffusion Coefficient	
			In Water (cm²/s) × 10⁵	Across Capillary (cm²/s × 100 g)
Water	18		3.20	3.7
Urea	60	1.6	1.95	1.83
Glucose	180	3.6	0.91	0.64
Sucrose	342	4.4	0.74	0.35
Raffinose	594	5.6	0.56	0.24
Inulin	5,500	15.2	0.21	0.036
Myoglobin	17,000	19	0.15	0.005
Hemoglobin	68,000	31	0.094	0.001
Serum albumin	69,000		0.085	<0.001

Data from Pappenheimer, JR: Passage of molecules through capillary walls, *Physiol Rev* **33**(3):387–423, July 1953; Renkin EM: Transport of large molecules across capillary walls, *Physiologist* **60**:13–28, February 1964.

concentration. Passive diffusion is described by *Fick's law of diffusion:*

$$\text{Rate of drug diffusion } \frac{dQ}{dt} = \frac{-DKA(C_p - C_t)}{h}$$

$$(11.1)$$

where $C_p - C_t$ is the difference between the drug concentration in the plasma (C_p) and in the tissue (C_t); A is the surface area of the membrane; h is the thickness of the membrane; K is the lipid–water partition coefficient; and D is the diffusion constant. The negative sign denotes net transfer of drug from inside the capillary lumen into the tissue and extracellular spaces. Diffusion is spontaneous and temperature dependent. Diffusion is distinguished from blood flow–initiated mixing, which involves hydrostatic pressure.

Hydrostatic pressure represents the pressure gradient between the arterial end of the capillaries entering the tissue and the venous capillaries leaving the tissue. Hydrostatic pressure is responsible for penetration of water-soluble drugs into spaces between endothelial cells and possibly into lymph. In the kidneys, high arterial pressure creates a filtration

pressure that allows small drug molecules to be filtered in the glomerulus of the renal nephron (see Chapter 7).

Blood flow–facilitated drug distribution is rapid and efficient, but requires pressure. As blood pressure gradually decreases when arteries branch into the small arterioles, the speed of flow slows and diffusion into the interstitial space becomes diffusion or concentration driven and facilitated by the large surface area of the capillary network. The average pressure of the blood capillary is higher (+18 mm Hg) than the mean tissue pressure (−6 mm Hg), resulting in a net total pressure of 24 mm Hg higher in the capillary over the tissue. This pressure difference is offset by an average osmotic pressure in the blood of 24 mm Hg, pulling the plasma fluid back into the capillary. Thus, on average, the pressures in the tissue and most parts of the capillary are equal, with no net flow of water.

At the arterial end, as the blood newly enters the capillary (Fig. 11-2A), the pressure of the capillary blood is slightly higher (about 8 mm Hg) than that of the tissue, causing fluid to leave the capillary and enter the tissues. This pressure is called *hydrostatic or filtration pressure*. This filtered fluid (filtrate) is later returned to the venous capillary (Fig. 11-2B) due to a lower venous pressure of about the same magnitude. The lower pressure of the venous blood compared with the tissue fluid is termed as *absorptive pressure*. A small amount of fluid returns to the circulation through the lymphatic system.

Distribution Half-Life, Blood Flow, and Drug Uptake by Organs

Because the process of drug transfer from the capillary into the tissue fluid is mainly diffusional, according to Fick's law, the membrane thickness, diffusion coefficient of the drug, and concentration gradient across the capillary membrane are important factors in determining the rate of drug diffusion. Kinetically, if a drug diffuses rapidly across the membrane in such a way that blood flow is the rate-limiting step in the distribution of drug, then the process is *perfusion* or *flow limited*. A person with congestive heart failure has a decreased cardiac output, resulting in impaired blood flow, which may reduce renal clearance through reduced filtration pressure and blood flow. In contrast, if drug distribution is limited by the slow diffusion of drug across the membrane in the tissue, then the process is termed *diffusion* or *permeability limited* (Fig. 11-3). Drugs that are permeability limited may have an increased distribution volume in disease conditions that cause inflammation and increased capillary membrane permeability. The delicate osmotic pressure balance may be altered due to changes in albumin level and/or blood loss or due to changes in electrolyte levels in renal and hepatic diseases, resulting in net flow of plasma water into the interstitial space (edema). This change in fluid distribution may partially explain the increased extravascular drug distribution during some disease states.

Blood flow, tissue size, and tissue storage (partitioning and binding) are also important in determining the time it takes the drug to become completely distributed. Table 11-2 lists the blood flow and tissue mass for many tissues in the human body. *Drug affinity* for a tissue or organ refers to the partitioning and accumulation of the drug in the tissue. The time for drug distribution is generally measured by the *distribution half-life* or the time for 50% drug distribution. The factors that determine the distribution constant of a drug into an organ are the blood flow to the organ, the volume of the organ, and the

TABLE 11-2   Blood Flow to Human Tissues

Tissue	Percent Body Weight	Percent Cardiac Output	Blood Flow (mL/100 g tissue/min)
Adrenals	0.02	1	550
Kidneys	0.4	24	450
Thyroid	0.04	2	400
Liver			
Hepatic	2.0	5	20
Portal		20	75
Portal-drained viscera	2.0	20	75
Heart (basal)	0.4	4	70
Brain	2.0	15	55
Skin	7.0	5	5
Muscle (basal)	40.0	15	3
Connective tissue	7.0	1	1
Fat	15.0	2	1

Data from Spector WS: Handbook of Biological Data, Saunders, Philadelphia, 1956; Glaser O: Medical Physics, Vol 11, Year Book Publishers, Chicago, 1950; Butler TC: Proc First International Pharmacological Meeting, Vol 6, Pergamon Press, 1962.

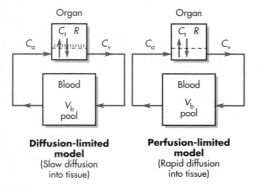

FIGURE 11-3   Drug distribution to body organs by blood flow (perfusion). Right panel for tissue with rapid permeability; Left panel for tissue with slow permeability.

partitioning of the drug into the organ tissue, as shown in Equation 11.2.

$$k_d = \frac{Q}{VR} \tag{11.2}$$

where k_d is first-order distribution constant, Q is blood flow to the organ, V is volume of the organ, R is ratio of drug concentration in the organ tissue to drug concentration in the blood (venous). The *distribution half-life* of the drug to the tissue, $t_{d1/2}$, may easily be determined from the distribution constant in the equation of $t_{d1/2} = 0.693/k_d$.

The ratio R is determined experimentally from tissue samples. With many drugs, however, only animal tissue data are available. The ratio R is usually estimated based on knowledge of the partition coefficient of the drug. The *partition coefficient* is a physical property that measures the ratio of the solubility of the drug in the oil phase to solubility in aqueous phase. The partition coefficient ($P_{o/w}$) is defined as a ratio of the drug concentration in the oil phase (usually represented by octanol) to the drug concentration in the aqueous phase measured at equilibrium under specified temperature *in vitro* in an oil/water two-layer system (Fig. 11-4). The partition coefficient is one of the most important factors that determine the tissue distribution of a drug.

If each tissue has the same ability to store the drug, then the distribution half-life is governed by the blood flow, Q, and volume (size), V, of the organ. A large blood flow, Q, to the organ decreases the distribution time, whereas a large organ size or volume, V, increases the distribution time because a

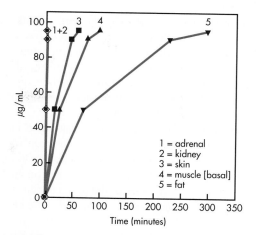

FIGURE 11-5   Drug distribution in five groups of tissues at various rates of equilibration.

longer time is needed to fill a large organ volume with drug. Figure 11-5 illustrates the distribution time (for 0%, 50%, 90%, and 95% distribution) for the adrenal gland, kidney, muscle (basal), skin, and fat tissue in an average human subject (ideal body weight, IBW = 70 kg). In this illustration, the blood drug concentration is equally maintained at 100 μg/mL, and the drug is assumed to have equal distribution between all the tissues and blood, i.e., when fully equilibrated, the partition or drug concentration ratio (R) between the tissue and the plasma will equal 1. Vascular tissues such as the kidneys and adrenal glands achieve 95% distribution in less than 2 minutes. In contrast, drug distribution time in fat tissues takes 4 hours, while less in vascular tissues, such as the skin and muscles, take between 2 and 4 hours (Fig. 11-5). When drug partition of the tissues is the same, the distribution time is dependent only on the tissue volume and its blood flow.

Blood flow is an important factor in determining how rapid and how much drug reaches the receptor site. Under normal conditions, limited blood flow reaches the muscles. During exercise, the increase in blood flow may change the fraction of drug reaching the muscle tissues. Diabetic patients receiving intramuscular injection of insulin may experience the effects of changing onset of drug action during exercise. Normally, the blood reserve

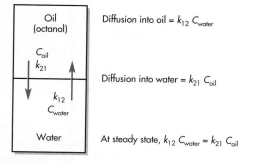

FIGURE 11-4   Diagram showing equilibration of drug between oil and water layer *in vitro*.

of the body stays mostly in the large veins and sinuses in the abdomen. During injury or when blood is lost, constriction of the large veins redirects more blood to needed areas, and therefore, affects drug distribution. Accumulation of carbon dioxide may lower the pH of certain tissues and may affect the level of drugs reaching those tissues.

Figure 11-6 illustrates the distribution of a drug to three different tissues when the partition of the drug for each tissue varies. For example, the drug partition shows that the drug concentration in the adrenal glands is five times of the drug concentration in the plasma, while the drug partition for the kidney is $R = 3$, and for basal muscle, $R = 1$. In this illustration, the adrenal gland and kidney take 5 and 3 times as long to be equilibrated with drug in the plasma. Thus, it can be seen that, even for vascular tissues, high drug partition can take much more time for the tissue to become fully equilibrated. In the example in Fig. 11-6, drug administration is continuous (as in IV infusion), since tissue drug levels remain constant after equilibrium.

Some tissues have great ability to store and accumulate drug, as shown by large R values. For example, the anti-androgen drug, flutamide and its active metabolite are highly concentrated in the prostate. The prostate drug concentration is 20 times that

of the plasma drug concentration; thus, the anti-androgen effect of the drug may not be fully achieved until distribution to this receptor site is complete. Digoxin is highly bound to myocardial membranes. Digoxin has a high tissue/plasma concentration ratio ($R = 60 - 130$) in the myocardium. This high R ratio for digoxin leads to a long distributional phase (see Chapter 5) despite abundant blood flow to the heart. It is important to note that if a tissue has a long distribution half-life, a long time is needed for the drug to leave the tissue as the blood level decreases. Understanding drug distribution is important because the activities of many drugs are not well correlated with plasma drug levels. Kinetically, both drug–protein binding and drug lipid solubility in the tissue site lead to longer distribution times.

Chemical knowledge in molecular structure often helps estimate the lipid solubility of a drug. A drug with large oil/water partition coefficient tends to have high R values *in vivo*. A reduction in the partition coefficient of a drug often reduces the rate of drug uptake into the brain. This may decrease drug distribution into the central nervous system and decrease undesirable central nervous system side effects. Extensive tissue distribution is kinetically evidenced by a large volume of distribution. A secondary effect is a prolonged drug elimination half-life, since the drug is distributed within a larger volume (thus, the drug is more diluted) and therefore, less efficiently removed by the kidney or the liver. For example, etretinate (a retinoate derivative) for acne treatment has an unusual long elimination half-life of about 100 days (Chien et al, 1992), due to its extensive distribution to body fats. Newly synthesized agents have been designed to reduce the lipophilicity and drug distribution. These new agents have less accumulation in the tissue and less potential for teratogenicity.

Drug Accumulation

The deposition or uptake of the drug into the tissue is generally controlled by the diffusional barrier of the capillary membrane and other cell membranes. For example, the brain is well perfused with blood, but many drugs with good aqueous solubility have

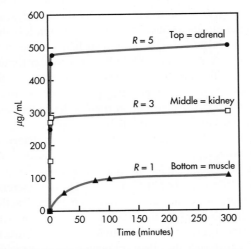

FIGURE 11-6   Drug distribution in three groups of tissues with various abilities to store drug (R).

high drug concentrations in the kidney, liver, and lung and yet little or negligible drug concentration in the brain. The brain capillaries are surrounded by a layer of tightly joined *glial* cells that act as a lipid barrier to impede the diffusion of polar or highly ionized drugs. A diffusion-limited model can be used to describe the pharmacokinetics of these drugs that are not adequately described by perfusion models.

Tissues receiving high blood flow equilibrate quickly with the drug in the plasma. However, at steady state, the drug may or may not accumulate (concentrate) within the tissue. The accumulation of drug into tissues is dependent on both the blood flow and the affinity of the drug for the tissue. Drug affinity for the tissue depends on partitioning and also binding to tissue components, such as receptors. Drug uptake into a tissue is generally reversible. The drug concentration in a tissue with low capacity equilibrates rapidly with the plasma drug concentration and then declines rapidly as the drug is eliminated from the body.

In contrast, drugs with high tissue affinity tend to accumulate or concentrate in the tissue. Drugs with a high lipid/water partition coefficient are very lipid soluble and tend to accumulate in lipid or adipose (fat) tissue. In this case, the lipid-soluble drug partitions from the aqueous environment of the plasma into the fat. This process is reversible, but the extraction of drug out of the tissue is so slow that the drug may remain for days or even longer in adipose tissues, long after the drug is depleted from the blood. Because the adipose tissue is poorly perfused with blood, drug accumulation is slow. However, once the drug is concentrated in fat tissue, drug removal from fat may also be slow. For example, the insecticide, chlorinated hydrocarbon DDT (dichlorodiphenyltrichloroethane) is highly lipid soluble and remains in fat tissue for years.

In addition to partitioning, drugs may accumulate in tissues by other processes. For example, drugs may accumulate by binding to proteins or other macromolecules in a tissue. Digoxin is highly bound to proteins in cardiac tissue, leading in a large volume of distribution (440 L/70 kg) and long elimination $t_{1/2}$ (approximately 40 hours). Some drugs may complex with melanin in the skin and eye, as observed after long-term administration of high doses of phenothiazine to chronic schizophrenic patients. The antibiotic tetracycline forms an insoluble chelate with calcium. In growing teeth and bones, tetracycline complexes with the calcium and remain in these tissues.

Some tissues have enzyme systems that actively transport natural biochemical substances into the tissues. For example, various adrenergic tissues have a specific uptake system for catecholamines, such as norepinephrine. Thus, amphetamine, which has a phenylethylamine structure similar to norepinephrine, is actively transported into adrenergic tissue. Other examples of drug accumulation are well documented. For some drugs, the actual mechanism for drug accumulation may not be clearly understood.

In a few cases, the drug is irreversibly bound into a particular tissue. Irreversible binding of drug may occur when the drug or a reactive intermediate metabolite becomes covalently bound to a macromolecule within the cell, such as to a tissue protein. Many purine and pyrimidine drugs used in cancer chemotherapy are incorporated into nucleic acids, causing destruction of the cell.

Permeability of Cells and Capillary Membranes

Cellular and plasma membranes vary in their permeability characteristics, depending on the tissue. For example, capillary membranes in the liver and kidneys are more permeable to transmembrane drug movement than capillaries in the brain. The sinusoidal capillaries of the liver are very permeable and allow the passage of large-size molecules. In the brain and spinal cord, the capillary endothelial cells are surrounded by a layer of glial cells, which have tight intercellular junctions. This added layer of cells around the capillary membranes acts effectively to slow the rate of drug diffusion into the brain by acting as a thicker lipid barrier. This lipid barrier, which slows the diffusion and penetration of water-soluble and polar drugs into the brain and spinal cord, is called the *blood–brain barrier*.

Under certain pathophysiologic conditions, the permeability of cell membranes, including capillary cell membranes, may be altered. For example, burns will alter the permeability of skin and allow drugs and larger molecules to permeate inward or outward. In meningitis, which involves inflammation of the membranes of the spinal cord and/or brain, drug uptake into the brain will be enhanced.

The diameters of the capillaries are very small and the capillary membranes are very thin. The high blood flow within a capillary allows for intimate contact of the drug molecules with the plasma membrane, providing for rapid drug diffusion. For capillaries that perfuse the brain and spinal cord, the layer of *glial* cells functions effectively to increase the thickness (term h in Equation 11.1), thereby slowing the diffusion and penetration of water-soluble and polar drugs into the brain and spinal cord.

Drug Distribution within Cells and Tissues

Pharmacokinetic models generally provide a good estimation of plasma drug concentrations in the body based on dose, volume of distribution, and clearance. However, drug concentrations within the cell or within a special region in the body are also governed by special efflux and metabolizing enzyme systems that prevent and detoxify foreign agents entering the body. Some proteins are receptors on cell surfaces that react specifically with a drug. The transporters are specialized proteins in the body that can associate transiently with a substrate drug through the hydrophobic region in the molecule, for example, P-glycoprotein, P-gp. Drug-specific transporters are very important in preventing drug accumulation in cells and may cause drug tolerance or drug resistance. Transporters can modulate drug absorption and disposition (see Chapters 13 and 14). Special families of transporters are important and well documented (You and Morris, 2007). For example, monocarboxylate transporters, organic cation transporters, organic anion transporters, oligopeptide transporters, nucleoside transporters, bile acid transporters, and multidrug resistance protein (eg, P-gp) that modulate distribution of many types of drugs. Drug transporters in the liver, kidney, brain, and gastrointestinal are discussed by You and Morris (2007) (see also Chapter 13 and Fig. 14-1 in Chapter 14). When considering drug utilization and drug–drug interactions, it is helpful to know whether the drug is a substrate for any of the transporters or enzyme systems. It is also important to determine whether the pharmacokinetic models have adequately taken transporter information into consideration.

Drug Distribution to Cerebral Spinal Fluid, CSF, and Brain: Blood–Brain Barrier

The blood–brain barrier permits selective entry of drugs into the brain and spinal cord due to (1) anatomical features (as mentioned above) and (2) the presence of cellular transporters. Anatomically, the layer of cells around the capillary membranes of the brain acts effectively as a thicker lipid barrier that slows the diffusion and penetration of water-soluble and polar drugs into the brain and spinal cord. However, some small hydrophilic molecules may cross the blood–brain barrier by simple diffusion. Efflux transporter is often found at the entry point into vital organs in the body. P-glycoprotein expression in the endothelial cells of human capillary blood vessels at the blood–brain was detected by special antibodies against the human multidrug-resistance gene product. P-gp may have a physiological role in regulating the entry of certain molecules into the central nervous system and other organs (Cordoncardo et al, 1989). P-gp substrate examples include doxorubicin, inmervectin, and others. Knocking out P-gp expression can increase brain toxicity with inmervectin in probe studies. Kim et al (1998) studied transport characteristics of protease inhibitor drugs, indinavir, nelfinavir, and saquinavir *in vitro* using the model P-gp expressing cell lines and *in vivo* administration in the mouse model. After IV administration, plasma concentrations of the drug in mdr1a (−/−) mice, the brain concentrations were elevated 7 to 36-fold. These data demonstrate that P-gp can limit the penetration of these drugs into the brain. Efflux transporters (ie, P-gp) effectively prevent certain small drug substances from entering into the brain, whereas influx transporters enable small nutrient molecules such as glucose to be actively taken into the brain. There is now much interest in understanding the mechanisms for drug uptake into brain in order to deliver therapeutic and diagnostic agents to specific regions of the brain.

CLINICAL FOCUS

Jaundice is a condition marked by high levels of bilirubin in the blood. New born infants with jaundice are particularly sensitive to the effects of bilirubin since their blood–brain barrier is not well formed at birth. The increased bilirubin, if untreated, may cause jaundice, and damage the brain centers of infants caused by increased levels of unconjugated, indirect bilirubin which is free (not bound to albumin). This syndrome is also known as kernicterus. Depending on the level of exposure to bilirubin, the effects range from unnoticeable to severe brain damage. Treatment in some cases may require phototherapy that requires special blue lights that work by helping to break down bilirubin in the skin.

Frequently Asked Questions

▶ *How does a physical property, such as partition coefficient, affect drug distribution?*

▶ *Why do some tissues rapidly take up drugs, whereas for other tissues, drug uptake is slower?*

▶ *Does rapid drug uptake into a tissue mean that the drug will accumulate into that tissue?*

▶ *What physical and chemical characteristics of a drug that would increase or decrease the uptake of the drug into the brain or cerebral spinal fluid?*

APPARENT VOLUME DISTRIBUTION

The concentration of drug in the plasma or tissues depends on the amount of drug systemically absorbed and the volume in which the drug is distributed. The *apparent volume of distribution*, V_D in a pharmacokinetic model, is used to estimate the extent of drug distribution in the body (see Chapters 3 and 5). Although the apparent volume of distribution does not represent a true anatomical or physical volume, the V_D represents the result of dynamic drug distribution between the plasma and the tissues and accounts for the mass balance of the drug in the body. To illustrate the use of V_D, consider a drug dissolved in a simple solution. A volume term is needed to relate drug concentration in the system (or human body) to the amount of drug present in

that system. The volume of the system may be estimated if the amount of drug added to the system and the drug concentration after equilibrium in the system are known.

Volume (L)

$$= \frac{\text{amount (mg) of drug added to system}}{\text{drug concentration (mg/L) in system after equilibrium}}$$

(11.3)

Equation 11.3 describes the relationship of concentration, volume, and mass, as shown in Equation 11.4.

$$\text{Concentration (mg/L)} \times \text{volume (L)} = \text{mass (mg)}$$

(11.4)

Considerations in the Calculation of Volume of Distribution: A Simulated Example

The objective of this exercise is to calculate the fluid volume in each beaker and to compare the calculated volume to the real volume of water in the beaker. Assume that three beakers are each filled with 100 mL of aqueous fluid. Beaker 1 contains water only; beakers 2 and 3 each contain aqueous fluid and a small compartment filled with cultured cells. The cells in beaker 2 can bind the drug, while the cells in beaker 3 can metabolize the drug. The three beakers represent the following, respectively:

Beaker 1. Drug distribution in a fluid (water) compartment only, without drug binding and metabolism

Beaker 2. Drug distribution in a fluid compartment containing cell clusters that reversibly bind drugs

Beaker 3. Drug distribution in a fluid compartment containing cell clusters (similar to tissues *in vivo*) in which the drug may be metabolized and the metabolites bound to cells

Suppose 100 mg of drug is then added to each beaker (Fig. 11-7). After the fluid concentration of drug in each beaker is at equilibration, and the concentration of drug in the water (fluid) compartment has been sampled and assayed, the volume of water may be computed.

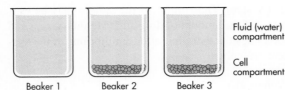

Fluid (water) compartment

Cell compartment

Beaker 1   Beaker 2   Beaker 3

FIGURE 11-7   Experiment simulating drug distribution in the body. Three beakers, each contains 100 mL of water (fluid compartment) and 100 mg of a water-soluble drug. Beakers 2 and 3 also contain 5 mL of cultured cell clusters.

Case 1

The volume of water in beaker 1 is calculated from the amount of drug added (100 mg) and the equilibrated drug concentration using Equation 11.3. After equilibration, the drug concentration was measured to be 1 mg/mL.

$$\text{Volume} = 100 \text{ mg}/1 \text{ mg/mL} = 100 \text{ mL}$$

The calculated volume in beaker 1 confirms that the system is a simple, homogeneous system and, in this case, represents the "true" fluid volume of the beaker.

Case 2

Beaker 2 contains cell clusters stuck to the bottom of the beaker. Binding of drug to the proteins of the cells occurs on the surface and within the cytoplasmic interior. This case represents a heterogeneous system consisting of a *well-stirred* fluid compartment and a tissue (cell). To determine the volume of this system, more information is needed than in Case 1:

1. The amount of drug dissolved in the fluid compartment must be determined. Because some of the drug will be bound within the cell compartment, the amount of drug in the fluid compartment will be less than the 100 mg placed in the beaker.
2. The amount of drug taken up by the cell cluster must be known to account for the entire amount of drug in the beaker. Therefore, both the cell and the fluid compartments must be sampled and assayed to determine the drug concentration in each compartment.
3. The volume of the cell cluster must be determined.

Assume that the above measurements were made and that the following information was obtained:

- Drug concentration in fluid compartment = 0.5 mg/mL
- Drug concentration in cell cluster = 10 mg/mL
- Volume of cell cluster = 5 mL
- Amount of drug added = 100 mg
- Amount of drug taken up by the cell cluster = 10 mg/mL × 5 mL = 50 mg
- Amount of drug dissolved in fluid (water) compartment = 100 mg (total) − 50 mg (in cells) = 50 mg (in water)

Using the above information, the true volume of the fluid (water) compartment is calculated using Equation 11.3.

$$\text{Volume of fluid compartment} = \frac{50 \text{ mg}}{0.5 \text{ mg/mL}} = 100 \text{ mL}$$

The value of 100 mL agrees with the volume of fluid we put into the beaker.

If the tissue cells were not accessible for sampling as in the case of *in vivo* drug administration, the volume of the fluid (water) compartment is calculated using Equation 11.3, assuming the system is homogenous and that 100 mg drug was added to the system.

$$\text{Apparent volume} = \frac{100 \text{ mg}}{0.5 \text{ mg/mL}} = 200 \text{ mL}$$

The value of 200 mL is a substantial overestimation of the true volume (100 mL) of the system.

When a heterogeneous system is involved, the real or true volume of the system may not be accurately calculated by monitoring only one compartment. Therefore, an apparent volume of distribution is calculated and the infrastructure of the system is ignored. The term *apparent volume of distribution* refers to the lack of true volume characteristics. The apparent volume of distribution is used in pharmacokinetics because the tissue (cellular) compartments are not easily sampled and the true volume is not known. When the experiment in beaker 2 is performed with an equal volume of cultured cells that have different binding affinity for the drug, then the apparent volume of distribution is very much affected by the extent of cellular drug binding (Table 11-3).

TABLE 11-3 Relationship of Volume of Distribution and Amount of Drug in Tissue (Cellular) Compartment[a]

Total Drug (mg)	Volume of Cells (mL)	Drug in Cells (mg)	Drug in Water (mg)	Drug Concentration in Water (mg/mL)	V_D in Water (mL)
100	15	75	25	0.25	400
100	10	50	50	0.50	200
100	5	25	75	0.75	133
100	1	5	95	0.95	105

[a]For each condition, the true water (fluid) compartment is 100 mL. Apparent volume of distribution (V_D) is calculated according to Equation 11.3.

As shown in Table 11-3, as the amount of drug in the cell compartment increases (column 3), the apparent V_D of the fluid compartment increases (column 6). Extensive cellular drug binding effectively pulls drug molecules out of the fluid compartment, decreases the drug concentration in the fluid compartment, and increases V_D. In biological systems, the quantity of cells, cell compartment volume, and extent of drug binding within the cells affect V_D. A large cell volume and/or extensive drug binding in the cells reduce the drug concentration in the fluid compartment and increase the apparent volume of distribution.

In this example, the fluid compartment is comparable to the *central compartment* and the cell compartment is analogous to the peripheral or *tissue compartment*. If the drug is distributed widely into the tissues or concentrated unevenly in the tissues, the V_D for a drug may exceed the physical volume of the body (about 70 L of total volume or 42 L of body water for a 70-kg subject). Besides cellular protein binding, partitioning of drug into lipid cellular components may greatly inflate V_D. Many drugs have oil/water partition coefficients above 10,000. These lipophilic drugs are mostly concentrated in the lipid phase of adipose tissue, resulting in a very low drug concentration in the extracellular water. Generally, drugs with very large V_D values have very low drug concentrations in plasma.

A large V_D is often interpreted as broad drug distribution for a drug, even though many other factors also lead to the calculation of a large apparent volume of distribution. A true V_D that exceeds the volume of the body is physically impossible. Only if the drug concentrations in both the tissue and plasma compartments are sampled, and the volumes of each compartment are clearly defined, can a true physical volume be calculated.

Case 3

The drug in the cell compartment in beaker 3 decreases due to undetected metabolism because the metabolite formed is bound to be inside the cells. Thus, the apparent volume of distribution is also greater than 100 mL. Any unknown source that decreases the drug concentration in the fluid compartment will increase the V_D, resulting in an overestimated apparent volume of distribution. This is illustrated with the experiment in beaker 3. In beaker 3, the cell cluster metabolizes the drug and binds the metabolite to the cells. Therefore, the drug is effectively removed from the fluid. The data for this experiment (note that metabolite is expressed as equivalent intact drug) are as follows:

- Total drug placed in beaker = 100 mg
- Cell compartment:
  Drug concentration = 0.2 mg/mL
  Metabolite-bound concentration = 9.71 mg/mL
  Metabolite-free concentration = 0.29 mg/mL
  Cell volume = 5 mL
- Fluid (water) compartment:
  Drug concentration = 0.2 mg/mL
  Metabolite concentration = 0.29 mg/mL

To calculate the total amount of drug and metabolite in the cell compartment, Equation 11.3 is rearranged as shown:

Total drug and metabolite in cells = 5 mL
× (0.2 + 9.96 + 0.29 mg/mL) = 52.45 mg

Therefore, the total drug and metabolite in the fluid compartment is 100 − 52.45 mg = 47.55 mg.

If only the intact drug is considered, V_D is calculated using Equation 11.3.

$$V_D = \frac{100 \text{ mg}}{0.2 \text{ mg/mL}} = 500 \text{ mL}$$

Considering that only 100 mL of water was placed into beaker 3, the calculated apparent volume of distribution of 500 mL is an overestimate of the true fluid volume of the system.

The following conclusions can be drawn from this beaker exercise:

1. Drug must be at equilibrium in the system before any drug concentration is measured. In nonequilibrium conditions, the sample removed from the system for drug assay does not represent all parts of the system.
2. Drug binding distorts the true physical volume of distribution when all components in the system are not properly sampled and assayed. Extravascular drug binding increases the apparent V_D.
3. Both intravascular and extravascular drug binding must be determined to calculate meaningful volumes of distribution.
4. The apparent V_D is essentially a measure of the relative extent of drug distribution outside the plasma compartment. Greater tissue drug binding and drug accumulation increases V_D, whereas greater plasma protein drug binding decreases the V_D distribution.
5. Undetected cellular drug metabolism increases V_D.
6. An apparent V_D larger than the combined volume of plasma and body water is indicative of (4) and (5), or both, above.
7. Although the V_D is not a true physiologic volume, the V_D is useful to relate the plasma

drug concentration to the amount of drug in the body (Equation 11.3). Equation 11.3 relating the total mass of drug to drug concentration and volume of distribution is important in pharmacokinetics.

PRACTICE PROBLEM

The amount of drug in the system calculated from V_D and the drug concentration in the fluid compartment is shown in Table 11-3. Calculate the amount of drug in the system using the true volume and the drug concentration in the fluid compartment.

Solution

In each case, the product of the drug concentration (column 5) and the apparent volume of distribution (column 6) yields 100 mg of drug, accurately accounting for the total amount of drug present in the system. For example, 0.25 mg/mL × 400 mL = 100 mg. Notice that the total amount of drug present cannot be determined using the true volume and the drug concentration (column 5).

The physiologic approach requires detailed information, including (1) cell drug concentration, (2) cell compartment volume, and (3) fluid compartment volume. Using the physiologic approach, the total amount of drug is equal to the amount of drug in the cell compartment and the amount of drug in the fluid compartment.

$$(15 \text{ mg/mL} \times 5 \text{ mL}) + (100 \text{ mL} \times 0.25 \text{ mg/mL})$$
$$= 100 \text{ mg}$$

The two approaches shown above each account correctly for the amount of drug present in the system. However, the second approach requires more information than is commonly available. The second approach does, however, make more physiologic sense. Most physiologic compartment spaces are not clearly defined for measuring drug concentrations.

Complex Biological Systems and V_D

The above example illustrates how the V_D represents the *apparent* volume into which a drug appears to distribute, whether into a beaker of fluid or the human body. The human body is a much more complex system than a beaker of water containing drug metabolizing cells. Many components within cells, tissues, or organs can bind to or metabolize drug, thereby influencing the apparent V_D. Only free, unbound drug diffuses between the plasma and tissue fluids. The tissue fluid, in turn, equilibrates with the intracellular water inside the tissue cells. The tissue drug concentration is influenced by the partition coefficient (lipid/water affinity) of the drug and tissue protein drug binding. The distribution of drug in a biological system is illustrated by Fig. 11-8.

Apparent Volume of Distribution

The apparent volume of distribution, in general, relates the plasma drug concentration to the amount of drug present in the body. In classical compartment models, V_{DSS} is the volume of distribution determined at steady state when the drug concentration in the tissue compartment is at equilibrium with

the drug concentration in the plasma compartment (Fig. 11-9A). In a physiological system involving a drug distributed to a given tissue from the plasma fluid (Fig. 11-9B), the two-compartment model is not assumed, and drug distribution from the plasma to a tissue is equilibrated by perfusion with arterial blood and returned by venous blood. The model parameter V_{app} is used to represent the apparent distribution volume in this model, which is different from V_{DSS} used in the compartment model. Similar to the apparent volume simulated in the beaker experiment in Equation 11.3, V_{app} is defined by Equation 11.5, and the amount of drug in the body is given by Equation 10.6.

$$V_{app} = \frac{D_B}{C_p} \tag{11.5}$$

$$D_B = V_p C_p + V_t C_t \tag{11.6}$$

where D_B is the amount of drug in the body, V_p is the plasma fluid volume, V_t is the tissue volume, C_p is

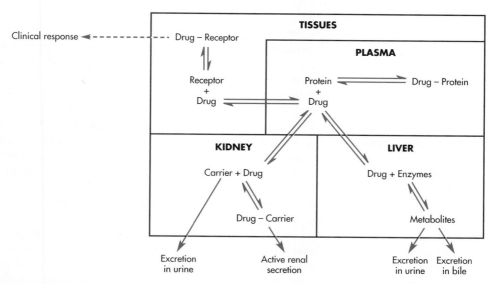

FIGURE 11-8   Effect of reversible drug–protein binding on drug distribution and elimination. Drugs may bind reversibly with proteins. Free (nonbound) drugs penetrate cell membranes, distributing into various tissues including those tissues involved in drug elimination, such as kidney and liver. Active renal secretion, which is a carrier-mediated system, may have a greater affinity for free drug molecules compared to plasma proteins. In this case, active renal drug excretion allows for rapid drug excretion despite drug–protein binding. If a drug is displaced from the plasma proteins, more free drug is available for distribution into tissues and interaction with the receptors responsible for the pharmacologic response. Moreover, more free drug is available for drug elimination.

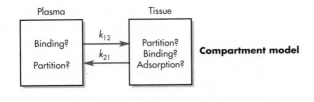

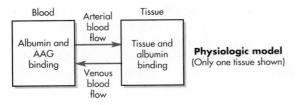

FIGURE 11-9   A diagram showing (upper panel) a two-compartment model approach to drug distribution; (lower panel) a physiologic approach to drug distribution.

the plasma drug concentration, and C_t is the tissue drug concentration.

For many protein-bound drugs, the ratio of D_B/C_p is not constant over time, and this ratio depends on the nature of dissociation of the protein–drug complex and how the free drug is distributed; the ratio is best determined at steady state. Protein binding to tissue has an apparent effect of increasing the apparent volume of distribution. Several V_D terms were introduced in the classical compartment models (see Chapter 5). However, protein binding was not introduced in those models.

Equation 11.6 describes the amount of drug in the body at any time point between a tissue and the plasma fluid. Instead of assuming that the drug distributes to a hypothetical compartment, it is assumed that, after injection, the drug diffuses from the plasma to the extracellular fluid/water, where it further equilibrates with the given tissue. One or more tissue types may be added to the model if needed. If the drug penetrates inside the cell, distribution into the intracellular water may occur. If the volume of body fluid and the protein level are known, this information may be incorporated into the model. Such a model may be more compatible with the physiology and anatomy of the human body.

When using pharmacokinetic parameters from the literature, it is important to note that most

calculations of steady-state V_D involve some assumptions on how and where the drug distributes in the body; it could involve a physiologic or a compartmental approach.

For a drug that involves protein binding, some models assume that the drug distributes from the plasma water into extracellular tissue fluids, where the drug binds to extravascular proteins, resulting in a larger V_D due to extravascular protein binding. However, drug binding and distribution to lipoid tissues are generally not distinguishable. If the pharmacokineticist suspects distribution to body lipids because the drug involved is very lipophilic, he or she may want to compare results simulated with different models before making a final conclusion.

Figure 11-10 lists the steady-state volume of distribution of 10 common drugs in ascending order. Most of these drugs follow multicompartment kinetics with various tissue distribution phases. The physiologic volumes of an ideal 70-kg subject are also plotted for comparison: (1) the plasma (3 L), (2) the extracellular fluid (15 L), and (3) the intracellular fluid (27 L). Drugs such as penicillin, cephalosporin, valproic acid, and furosemide are polar compounds that stay mostly within the plasma and extracellular fluids and therefore have a relatively low V_D.

In contrast, drugs with low distribution to the extracellular water are more extensively distributed inside the tissues and tend to have a large V_D. An excessively high volume of distribution (greater than the body volume of 70 L) is due mostly to special tissue storage, tissue protein binding, carrier, or efflux system which removes drug from the plasma fluid. Digoxin, for example, is bound to myocardial membrane that has drug levels that are 60 and 130 times the serum drug level in adults and children, respectively (Park et al, 1982). The high tissue binding is responsible for the large steady-state volume of distribution (see Chapter 5). The greater drug affinity also results in longer distribution half-life despite the heart's great vascular blood perfusion. Imipramine is a drug that is highly protein bound and concentrated in the plasma, yet its favorable tissue partition and binding accounts for a large volume of distribution. Several tricyclic antidepressants (TCAs) also have large volumes of distribution due to tissue (CNS) penetration and binding.

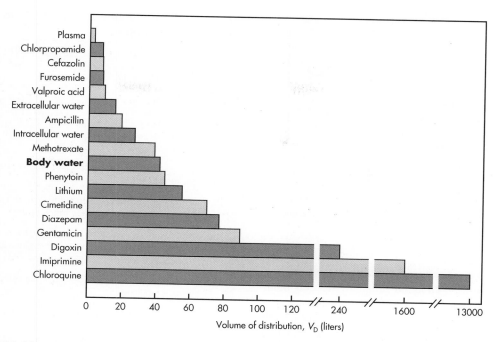

FIGURE 11-10   Lists of steady-state volumes of distribution of 10 common drugs in ascending order showing various factors that affect V_D. Drugs with high V_D generally have high tissue affinity or low binding to serum albumin. Polar or hydrophilic drugs tend to have V_D similar to the volume of extracellular water.

Frequently Asked Questions

▶ *Why is the volume of distribution, V_D, considered an "apparent" volume and not a "true" anatomic or physiologic volume?*

▶ *Can the V_D have a volume equal to a true anatomic volume in the body?*

PROTEIN BINDING OF DRUGS

Many drugs interact with plasma or tissue proteins or with other macromolecules, such as melanin and DNA, to form a *drug–macromolecule complex*. The formation of a drug–protein complex is often named *drug–protein binding*. Drug–protein binding may be a reversible or an irreversible process. *Irreversible drug–protein binding* is usually a result of chemical activation of the drug, which then attaches strongly to the protein or macromolecule by covalent chemical bonding. Irreversible drug binding accounts for certain types of drug toxicity that may occur over a long time period, as in the case of chemical carcinogenesis, or within a relatively short time period, as in the case of drugs that form reactive chemical intermediates. For example, the hepatotoxicity of high doses of acetaminophen is due to the formation of reactive metabolite intermediates that interact with liver proteins.

Most drugs bind or complex with proteins by a reversible process. *Reversible drug–protein binding* implies that the drug binds the protein with weaker chemical bonds, such as hydrogen bonds or van der Waals forces. The amino acids that compose the protein chain have hydroxyl, carboxyl, or other sites available for reversible drug interactions.

Reversible drug–protein binding is of major interest in pharmacokinetics. The protein-bound drug is a large complex that cannot easily transverse the capillary wall and therefore has a restricted distribution (Fig. 11-11). Moreover, the protein-bound

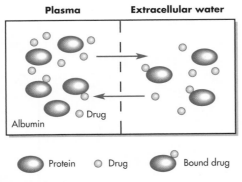

Plasma   **Extracellular water**

Albumin   ○ Drug

● Protein   ○ Drug   ◑ Bound drug

FIGURE 11-11   Diagram showing that bound drugs will not diffuse across membrane but free drug will diffuse freely between the plasma and extracellular water.

drug is usually pharmacologically inactive. In contrast, the free or unbound drug crosses cell membranes and is therapeutically active. Studies that critically evaluate drug–protein binding are usually performed *in vitro* using a purified protein such as albumin. Methods for studying protein binding, including equilibrium dialysis and ultrafiltration, make use of a semipermeable membrane that separates the protein and protein-bound drug from the free or unbound drug (Table 11-4). By these *in vitro* methods, the concentrations of bound drug, free drug, and total protein may be determined. Each method for the investigation of drug–protein binding *in vitro* has advantages and disadvantages in terms of cost, ease of measurement, time, instrumentation, and other considerations. Various experimental factors for the measurement of protein binding are listed in Table 11-5.

Drugs may bind to various macromolecular components in the blood, including albumin, α_1-acid

TABLE 11-4   Methods for Studying Drug–Protein Binding

Equilibrium dialysis	Gel chromatography
Dynamic dialysis	Spectrophotometry
Diafiltration	Electrophoresis
Ultrafiltration	Optical rotatory dispersion and circulatory dichroism

TABLE 11-5   Considerations in the Study of Drug–Protein Binding

Equilibrium between bound and free drug must be maintained.
The method must be valid over a wide range of drug and protein concentrations.
Extraneous drug binding or drug adsorption onto the apparatus walls, membranes, or other components must be avoided or considered in the method.
Denaturation of the protein or contamination of the protein must be prevented.
The method must consider pH and ionic concentrations of the media and Donnan effects due to the protein.
The method should be capable of detecting both reversible and irreversible drug binding, including fast- and slow-phase associations and dissociations of drug and protein.
The method should not introduce interfering substances, such as organic solvents.
The results of the *in vitro* method should allow extrapolation to the *in vivo* situation.

Data from Bridges and Wilson (1976).

glycoprotein, lipoproteins, immunoglobulins (IgG), and erythrocytes (RBC).

Albumin is a protein with a molecular weight of 65,000 to 69,000 Da that is synthesized in the liver and is the major component of plasma proteins responsible for reversible drug binding (Table 11-6). In the body, albumin is distributed in the plasma and in the extracellular fluids of skin, muscle, and various

TABLE 11-6   Major Proteins to Which Drugs Bind in Plasma

Protein	Molecular Weight (Da)	Normal Range of Concentrations	
		(g/L)	(mol/L)
Albumin	65,000	35–50	$5–7.5 \times 10^{-4}$
α_1-Acid glycoprotein	44,000	0.4–1.0	$0.9–2.2 \times 10^{-5}$
Lipoproteins	200,000–3,400,000	Variable	

From Tozer (1984), with permission.

other tissues. Interstitial fluid albumin concentration is about 60% of that in the plasma. The elimination half-life of albumin is 17 to 18 days. Normally, albumin concentration is maintained at a relatively constant level of 3.5% to 5.5% (weight per volume) or 4.5 mg/dL. Albumin is responsible for maintaining the osmotic pressure of the blood and for the transport of endogenous and exogenous substances in the plasma. Albumin complexes with endogeneous substances such as free fatty acids (FFAs), bilirubin, various hormones (eg, cortisone, aldosterone, thyroxine, tryptophan), and other compounds. Many weak acidic (anionic) drugs bind to albumin by electrostatic and hydrophobic bonds. Weak acidic drugs such as salicylates, phenylbutazone, and penicillins are highly bound to albumin. However, the strength of the drug binding is different for each drug.

Alpha-1-acid glycoprotein (AAG), also known as *orosomucoid*, is a globulin with a molecular weight of about 44,000 Da. The plasma concentration of AAG is low (0.4%–1%) and it binds primarily basic (cationic) drugs such as saquinavir, propranolol, imipramine, and lidocaine (see below).

Globulins (α-, β-, γ-globulins) may be responsible for the plasma transport of certain endogenous substances such as corticosteroids. These globulins have a low capacity but high affinity for the binding of these endogenous substances.

CLINICAL EXAMPLES

Case 1

Dexmedetomidine hydrochloride injection (Precedex®) is an α-2-adrenergic agonist with sedative and analgesic properties that is given intravenously using a controlled infusion device. The pharmacokinetics of dexmedetomidine was studied in volunteers with and without severe renal impairment (De Wolf et al, 2001). The pharmacokinetics of dexmedetomidine differed little in the two groups and there were no significant differences in the hemodynamic responses. The elimination half-life in subjects with severe renal impairment was significantly shorter than in normal subjects: (113 ± 11 minutes versus 136 ± 13 minutes; $p < 0.05$). However, dexmedetomidine resulted in more prolonged sedation in subjects

with severe renal impairment. The authors postulated that reduced protein binding in the renal disease subjects may be responsible for the prolonged sedation. The drug is mainly cleared by hepatic metabolism and is highly protein bound. The example indicates that simple kinetic extrapolation may be inappropriate in many clinical situations.

- Could reduced protein binding change the concentration of the active drug in the central nervous system, CNS?
- Is the drug a substrate for a transporter?

Case 2

Diazepam (Valium) is a benzodiazepine derivative for anxiolytic, sedative, muscle-relaxant, and anticonvulsant effects. Diazepam is highly protein bound (98.7%) in plasma. Ochs et al (1981) examined the effect of changing protein binding on diazepam distribution in subjects with normal renal function versus patients with renal failure. The authors found no significant change in clearance of unbound drug in the subjects with renal failure. Previous studies have suggested that changes in protein binding may be associated with altered drug disposition for some drugs. Ochs et al (1981) also studied diazepam disposition in hyperthyroidism and found no significant difference in diazepam disposition in hyperthyroid patients versus matched controls.

It is important to remember that each drug has a unique molecular structure. Although one drug may have comparable protein binding, the capacity to bind proteins and the drug–protein binding constant may be different among similar drugs as discussed later in this chapter. Individual patient characteristics and kinetic parameters are also very important. Qin et al (1999) reported great variation in clearance of diazepam among extensive and poor metabolizers due to polymorphism of the cytochrome gene (see Chapter 13) that regulates CYP2C19, which is responsible for variation in the half-life of this drug.

Lipoproteins are macromolecular complexes of lipids and proteins and are classified according to their density and separation in the ultracentrifuge. The terms VLDL, LDL, and HDL are abbreviations for very-low-density, low-density, and high-density lipoproteins, respectively. Lipoproteins are responsible for the transport of plasma lipids to the liver and may be responsible for the binding of drugs if the albumin sites become saturated.

Erythrocytes, or red blood cells (RBCs), may bind both endogenous and exogenous compounds. RBCs consist of about 45% of the volume of the blood. Phenytoin, pentobarbital, and amobarbital are known to have an RBC/plasma water ratio of 4 to 2, indicating preferential binding of drug to the erythrocytes over plasma water. Penetration into RBC is dependent on the free concentration of the drug in the plasma. In the case of phenytoin, RBC drug concentrations increase linearly with an increase in the plasma-free drug concentration (Borondy et al, 1973). Increased drug binding to plasma albumin reduces RBC drug concentration. With most drugs, however, binding of drug to RBCs generally does not significantly affect the volume of distribution, because the drug is often bound to albumin reversibly in the plasma water. Even though phenytoin has a great affinity for RBCs, only about 25% of the blood drug concentration is present in the blood cells, and 75% is present in the plasma because the drug is also strongly bound to albumin. For drugs with strong erythrocyte binding, the hematocrit will influence the total drug concentration in the blood. For these drugs, the total whole-blood drug concentration should be measured.

Frequently Asked Questions

▶ *Should drug transporter proteins be considered as a type of "drug–protein binding" in assessing its role in the drug's pharmacokinetics?*

▶ *How does a protein transporter modulate drug distribution in the body?*

Gender Differences in Drug Distribution

Gender differences in drug distribution are now known for many drugs (Anderson, 2005). For example, Meibohm et al (2002) discussed the physiologic impact of P-glycoprotein (P-gp) binding to substrate drugs. The human multidrug-resistance gene 1 (MDR1) gene product P-gp are now known to play a major role in absorption, distribution, and/or renal and hepatic excretion of therapeutic agents.

The hepatic expression of MDR1 in females was reported as about one-third to one-half of the hepatic P-gp level measured in men. However, another study reported no difference in MDR1 between females and males. Low P-gp activity in the liver was suggested to increase hepatic CYP3A metabolism in some cases. The important point is that a protein such as P-gp can translocate a drug away or closer to the site of the hepatic enzyme and therefore affecting the rate of metabolism. A similar situation can occur within the gastrointestinal (GI) tract. This situation explains why first-pass effect is often quite erratic. Pharmacokineticists now use *in vitro* methods to study both "apical to basolateral" and "basolateral to apical" drug transport to determine if the drug favors mucosal to serosal movement or vice versa.

EFFECT OF PROTEIN BINDING ON THE APPARENT VOLUME OF DISTRIBUTION

The extent of drug protein binding in the plasma or tissue affects V_D. Drugs that are highly bound to plasma proteins have a low fraction of free drug (f_u = unbound or free drug fraction) in the plasma water. The plasma protein-bound drug does not diffuse easily and is therefore less extensively distributed to tissues (see Fig. 11-11). Drugs with low plasma protein binding have larger f_u, generally diffuse more easily into tissues, and have a greater volume of distribution. Although the apparent volume of distribution is influenced by lipid solubility in addition to protein binding, there are some exceptions to this rule. However, when several drugs are selected from a single family with similar physical and lipid partition characteristics, the apparent volume of distribution may be explained by the relative degree of drug binding to tissue and plasma proteins.

The V_D of four cephalosporin antibiotics (Fig. 11-12) in humans and mice (Sawada et al, 1984) demonstrates that the differences in volume of distribution of cefazolin, cefotetan, moxalactam, and cefoperazone are due mostly to differences in the degree of protein binding. For example, the fraction of unbound drug, f_u, in the plasma is the highest

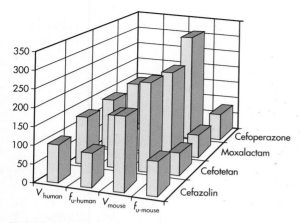

FIGURE 11-12 Plot of V_D of four cephalosporin antibiotics in humans and mice showing the relationship between the fraction of unbound drug (f_u) and the volume of distribution. (Data from Sawada et al, 1984.)

for cefoperazone in humans and mice, and the volume of distribution is also the highest among the four drugs in both humans and mice. Conversely, cefazolin has the lowest f_u in humans and is corresponding to the lowest volume of distribution. Interestingly, the volume of distribution per kilogram in humans (V_{human}) is generally higher than that in mouse (V_{mouse}) because the fraction of unbound drug is also greater, resulting in a greater volume of distribution. Differences in drug-protein binding contribute to the differences seen in V_d and $t_{1/2}$ among various species. An equation (Equation 11.12) relating quantitatively the effect of protein binding on apparent volume of distribution is derived in the next section.

Drugs such as furosemide, sulfisoxazole, tolbutamide, and warfarin are bound greater than 90% to plasma proteins and have a V_D value ranging from 7.7 to 11.2 L per 70-kg body weight. Basic drugs such as imipramine, nortriptyline, and propranolol are extensively bound to both tissue and plasma proteins and have very large V_D values. Displacement of drugs from plasma proteins can affect the pharmacokinetics of a drug in several ways: (1) directly increase the free (unbound) drug concentration as a result of reduced binding in the blood; (2) increase the free drug concentration that reaches the receptor sites directly, causing a more

intense pharmacodynamic (or toxic) response; (3) increase the free drug concentration, causing a transient increase in V_D and decreasing partly some of the increase in free plasma drug concentration; (4) increase the free drug concentration, resulting in more drug diffusion into tissues of eliminating organs, particularly the liver and kidney, resulting in a transient increase in drug elimination. The ultimate drug concentration reaching the target depends on one or more of these four factors dominating in the clinical situation. The effect of drug–protein binding must be evaluated carefully before dosing changes are made (see below).

Effect of Changing Plasma Protein Level: An Example

The effect of increasing the plasma α_1-acid glycoprotein (AAG) level on drug penetration into tissues may be verified with cloned transgenic animals that have 8.6 times the normal AAG levels. In an experiment investigating the activity of the tricyclic antidepressant drug imipramine, equal drug doses were administered to both normal and transgenic mice. Since imipramine is highly bound to AAG, the steady-state imipramine serum level was greatly increased in the blood due to protein binding.

Mouse Model	Imipramine Level (ng/mL)	
	Serum	Brian
Normal	319.9	7307.7
Transgenic	859	3862.6

However, the imipramine concentration was greatly reduced in the brain tissue because of higher degree of binding to AAG in the serum, resulting in reduced drug penetration into the brain tissue. The volume of distribution of the drug was reported to be reduced in the transgenic mice. The antidepressant effect was observed to be lower in the transgenic mouse due to lower brain imipramine levels. This experiment illustrates that high drug–protein binding in the serum can reduce drug penetration to tissue receptors for some drugs (Holladay et al, 1996).

Saquinavir mesylate (Invirase®) is an inhibitor of the human immunodeficiency virus (HIV) protease. Saquinavir is approximately 98% bound to plasma proteins over a concentration range of 15 to 700 ng/mL. Saquinavir binding in human plasma and control mouse plasma are similar and approximately 2% to 3% unbound. Saquinavir is highly bound to AAG and has reduced free drug concentrations in transgenic mice that express elevated AAG (Holladay et al, 2001). In this study, the drug was bound to both albumin and AAG (2.1% to AAG vs 11.5% to albumin). Elevated AAG caused saquinavir's volume of distribution to be reduced in this study. In AAG-overexpressing transgenic mice, AAG is genetically increased such that most saquinavir is bound in plasma and only 1.5% is free to be metabolized. The result is a decrease in systemic clearance of saquinavir. This conclusion is consistent with the observations that systemic exposure to saquinavir in HIV-1 subjects is greater than that in healthy subjects and that AAG levels increase with the degree of HIV infection. According to the approved label, HIV-infected patients administered Invirase (600-mg TID) had AUC and maximum plasma concentration (C_{max}) values approximately 2 to 2.5 times those observed in healthy volunteers receiving the same dosing regimen.

For a drug that distributes into the plasma and a given tissue in the body, the amount of drug bound may be found by Equation 11.7. Because drug may bind to both plasma and tissue proteins, the bound and unbound drug concentrations must be considered. At steady state, unbound drug in plasma and tissue are in equilibration.

$$D_B = V_p C_p + V_t C_t \qquad (11.7)$$

$$C_u = C_{ut}$$

Alternatively,

$$C_p f_u = C_t f_{ut} \qquad (11.8)$$

or

$$C_t = C_p \frac{f_u}{f_{ut}} \qquad (11.9)$$

where all terms refer to steady-state conditions: f_u is the unbound (free) drug fraction in the plasma,

f_{ut} is the unbound drug fraction in the tissue, C_u is the unbound drug concentration in the plasma, and C_{ut} is the unbound drug concentration in the tissues. Substituting for C_t in Equation 11.7 using Equation 11.9 results in

$$D_B = V_p C_p + V_t \left[C_p \left(\frac{f_u}{f_{ut}} \right) \right] \qquad (11.10)$$

Rearranging,

$$\frac{D_B}{C_p} = V_p + V_t \left(\frac{f_u}{f_{ut}} \right) \qquad (11.11)$$

Because $D_B/C_p = V_{app}$, by substitution into Equation 11.11, V_{app} may be estimated by Equation 11.12:

$$V_{app} = V_p + V_t \left(\frac{f_u}{f_{ut}} \right) \qquad (11.12)$$

Equation 11.12 relates the amount of drug in the body to plasma volume, tissue volume, and fraction of free plasma and tissue drug in the body. Equation 11.12 may be expanded to include several tissue organs with V_{ti} each with unbound tissue fraction f_{uti}.

$$V_{app} = V_p + \sum V_{ti} \left(\frac{f_u}{f_{uti}} \right)$$

where V_{ti} = tissue volume of the ith organ and f_{uti} = unbound fraction of the ith organ.

The following are important considerations in the calculation of V_{app}.

1. The volume of distribution is a constant only when the drug concentrations are in equilibrium between the plasma and tissue.
2. Values of f_u and f_{ut} are concentration dependent and must also be determined at equilibrium conditions.
3. V_{app} is an indirect measure of drug binding in the tissues rather than a measurement of a true anatomic volume.
4. When f_u and f_{ut} are unity, Equation 11.12 is simplified to

$$\frac{D_B}{C_p} = V_p + V_t$$

When no drug binding occurs in tissue and plasma, the volume of distribution will not exceed the real anatomic volume. Only at steady state are the unbound plasma drug concentration, C_u, and the tissue drug concentration, C_{ut}, equal. At any other time, C_u may not equal to C_{ut}. The amount of drug in the body, D_B, cannot be calculated easily from V_{app} and C_p under nonequilibrium conditions. For simplicity, some models assume that the drug distributed to a tissue is approximated by the drug present in the fluid of that tissue. The tissue fluid volume is then represented by the volume of the extracellular/intracellular fluid, depending on drug penetration. Such a model fails to consider drug partition into fatty tissues/lipids, and simulates extravascular drug distribution based solely on protein binding. A number of drugs have a large volume of distribution despite high protein binding to plasma proteins. Some possible reasons for this large volume of distribution could be due to strong tissue drug partition and/or high intracellular or receptor binding within the tissue. Under these situations, the model discussed above does not adequately describe the *in vivo* drug distribution.

In contrast, when the data are analyzed by the compartmental model, no specific binding interpretation is made. The analyst may interpret a large apparent volume due to either partition to fatty tissues or extravascular binding based on other observations. Compartment models are based on mass balance and focus on the amount of drug in each compartment and not on the tissue volume or tissue drug concentration. The tissue volume and drug concentrations are theoretical and do not necessarily reflect true physiologic values. Even the C_t may not be uniform in local tissues and under disease conditions.

> **Frequently Asked Questions**
> ▶ Is it possible for V_D to exceed a patient's actual physiologic volume? If so, why?
>
> ▶ How does protein binding influence V_D?
>
> ▶ What are f_{ut} and f_{up}? Are they constant?

PRACTICE PROBLEM

Drug A and drug B have V_{app} of 20 and 100 L, respectively. Both drugs have a V_p of 4 L and a V_t of 10 L, and they are 60% bound to plasma protein.

What is the fraction of tissue binding of the two drugs? Assume that V_p is 4 L and V_t is 10 L.

Solution

Drug A

Applying Equation 11.12,

$$V_{app} = V_p + V_t\left(\frac{f_u}{f_{ut}}\right)$$

Because drug A is 60% bound, the drug is 40% free, or $f_u = 0.4$.

$$20 = 4 + 10\left(\frac{0.4}{f_{ut}}\right)$$

$$f_{ut} = \frac{4}{16} = 0.25$$

The fraction of drug bound to tissues is $1 - 0.25 = 0.75$ or 75%.

Drug B

$$100 = 4 + 10\left(\frac{0.4}{f_{ut}}\right)$$

$$f_{ut} = 0.042$$

The fraction of drug bound to tissues is $1 - 0.042 = 0.958 = 95.8\%$.

In this problem, the percent free (unbound) drug for drug A is 25% and the percent free drug for drug B is 4.2% in plasma fluid. Drug B is more highly bound to tissue, which results in a larger apparent volume of distribution. This approach assumes a pooled tissue group because it is not possible to identify physically the tissue group to which the drug is bound.

Equation 11.12 may explain the wide variation in the apparent volumes of distribution for drugs observed in the literature (Tables 11-7–11-9). Drugs in Table 11-7 have small apparent volumes of distribution due to plasma drug binding (less than 10 L when extrapolated to a 70-kg subject). Drugs in Table 11-8 show that, in general, as the fraction of unbound drug, f_u, in the plasma increases, the apparent volume increases. Reduced drug binding in the plasma results in increased free drug concentration, which diffuses into the extracellular water. Drugs showing exceptionally large volumes of distribution

TABLE 11-7　Relationship between Affinity for Serum Albumin and Volume of Distribution for Some Acidic Drugs

Drug	Plasma Fraction Bound (%)	Affinity Constant (M^{-1})	V_D (L/kg)
Clofibric acid	97	300,000	0.09
Fluorophenindione	95	3,000,000	0.09
Phenylbutazone	99	230,000	0.09
Warfarin	97	230,000	0.13

From Houin (1985), with permission.

TABLE 11-9　Examples of Drugs with Tissue Distribution Apparently Independent of Plasma Protein Binding

Drug	Plasma Fraction Bound (%)	V_D (L/kg)
Desipramine	92	40
Imipramine	95	30
Nortriptyline	94	39
Vinblastine	70	35
Vincristine	70	11

From Houin (1985), with permission.

TABLE 11-8　Examples of Drugs with Diffusion Limited by Binding to Protein

Drug	Plasma Fraction Unbound (%)	V_D (L/kg)
Carbenoxolone	1	0.10
Ibuprofen	1	0.14
Phenylbutazone	1	0.10
Naproxen	2	0.09
Fusidic acid	3	0.15
Clofibrate	3	0.09
Warfarin	3	0.10
Bumetanide	4	0.18
Dicloxacillin	4	0.29
Furosemide	4	0.20
Tolbutamide	4	0.14
Nalidixic acid	5	0.35
Cloxacillin	5	0.34
Sulfaphenazole	5	0.29
Chlorpropramide	8	0.20
Oxacillin	8	0.44
Nafcillin	10	0.63

From Houin (1985), with permission.

may have unusual tissue binding. Some drugs move into the interstitial fluid but are unable to diffuse across the plasma membrane into the intracellular fluids, thereby reducing the volume of distribution.

Drugs in Table 11-9 apparently do not obey the general binding rule, because their volumes of distribution are not related to plasma drug binding. These drugs have very large volumes of distribution and may have undiscovered tissue binding or tissue metabolism. Based on their pharmacologic activities, presumably all these drugs penetrate into the intracellular space.

CLINICAL EXAMPLE

The serum protein binding of azithromycin is concentration dependent, ranging from 51% at 0.02 μg/mL to 7% at 2.0 μg/mL as reported in the literature. Following oral administration, azithromycin is widely distributed throughout the body with an apparent steady-state volume of distribution of 31.1 L/kg. Higher azithromycin concentrations in tissues than in plasma or serum have been observed.

- What is the apparent V_D for a subject weighing 70 kg?
- Is the apparent V_D greater or lower than the plasma volume of the body for this subject?
- Do you think protein binding affect the distribution of this drug?

Solution

V_D for a subject weighing 70 kg = 70 × 31.1 = 2191 L

Electrolyte Balance

Electrolyte balance affects the movement of fluid in the body. The kidney is the main regulator of electrolyte balance. Albumin is synthesized in the liver and is the main component of plasma proteins. The plasma albumin concentration contributes to osmotic pressure in the blood. Plasma albumin concentration may be increased during hypovolemia (loss of plasma volume due to movement fluid into extracellular fluid and other various factors such as dehydration, shocks, excessive blood loss, etc) or decreased during hypervolemia (increase in plasma volume due to various causes such as excessive fluid intake, sodium retention, congestive heart failure, etc). Changes in plasma protein concentration and in plasma drug–protein binding may occur to various degree, thus affecting drug disposition. Disease conditions may cause changes in protein concentration and drug–protein binding, thus altering the protein distribution in the body. An altered protein concentration and binding may result in more nonprotein-bound drug leading to a more intense pharmacodynamic effect and a change in the rate of drug elimination.

RELATIONSHIP OF PLASMA DRUG–PROTEIN BINDING TO DISTRIBUTION AND ELIMINATION

In general, drugs that are highly bound to plasma protein have reduced overall drug clearance. For a drug that is metabolized mainly by the liver, binding to plasma proteins prevents the drug from entering the hepatocytes, resulting in reduced hepatic drug metabolism. In addition, bound drugs may not be available as substrates for liver enzymes, thereby further reducing the rate of metabolism.

Protein-bound drugs act as larger molecules that cannot diffuse easily through the capillary membranes in the glomeruli. The elimination half-lives of some drugs such as the cephalosporins, which are excreted mainly by renal excretion, are generally increased when the percent of drug bound to plasma proteins increases (Table 11-10). Drug protein binding are usually measured in plasma and sometimes in serum. The effect of serum protein binding on the renal clearance and elimination half-life on several tetracycline analogs is shown in Table 11-11. For example, doxycycline, which is 93% bound to serum

TABLE 11-10 **Influence of Protein Binding on the Pharmacokinetics of Primarily Glomerular Filtrated Cephalosporins**

	Protein Bound (%)	$t_{1/2}$ (h)	Renal Clearance (mL/min/1.73 m²)
Ceftriaxone	96	8.0	10
Cefoperazone	90	1.8	19
Cefotetan	85	3.3	28
Ceforanide	81	3.0	44
Cefazolin	70	1.7	56
Moxalactam	52	2.3	64
Cefsulodin	26	1.5	90
Ceftazidime	22	1.9	85
Cephaloridine	21	1.5	125

From Houin (1985), with permission.

TABLE 11-11 Comparison of Serum Protein Binding of Several Tetracycline Analogs with Their Half-Lives in Serum Renal Clearance and Urinary Recovery after Intravenous Injection

Tetracycline Analogs	Serum Binding (%)	Half-Life (h)	Renal Clearance (mL/min)	Urinary Recovery (%)
Oxytetracycline	35.4	9.2	98.6	70
Tetracycline	64.6	8.5	73.5	60
Demeclocycline	90.8	12.7	36.5	45
Doxycycline	93.0	15.1	16.0	45

proteins, has an elimination half-life of 15.1 hours, whereas oxytetracycline, which is 35.4% bound to serum proteins, has an elimination half-life of 9.2 hours. On the other hand, a drug that is both extensively bound and actively secreted by the kidneys, such as penicillin, has a short elimination half-life, because active secretion takes preference in removing or stripping the drug from the proteins as the blood flows through the kidney.

Some cephalosporins are excreted by both renal and biliary secretion. The half-lives of drugs that are significantly excreted in the bile do not correlate well with the extent of plasma protein binding.

Relationship between V_D and Drug Elimination Half-Life

Drug elimination is governed mainly by renal and other metabolic processes in the body. However, extensive drug distribution has the effect of diluting the drug in a large volume, making it harder for the kidney to filter the drug by glomerular filtration. Thus, the $t_{1/2}$ of the drug is prolonged if clearance (Cl) is constant and V_D is increased according to Equation 11.14. Cl is related to apparent volume of distribution, V_D, and the elimination constant k, as shown in Equation 11.13 (see also Chapter 3).

$$Cl = kV_D \tag{11.13}$$

$$t_{1/2} = 0.693 \frac{V_D}{Cl} \tag{11.14}$$

For a first-order process, Cl is the product of V_D and the elimination rate constant, k, according to Equation 11.13. The equation is derived for a given drug dose distributed in a single volume of body

fluid without protein binding. The equation basically describes the empirical observation that either a large clearance or large volume of distribution leads to low plasma drug concentrations after a given dose. Mechanistically, a relatively low plasma drug concentration from a given dose may be resulted from (1) extensive distribution into tissues due to favorable lipophilicity, (2) extensive distribution into tissues due to protein binding in peripheral tissues, and/or (3) lack of drug plasma protein binding.

Two drug examples are selected to illustrate further the relationship between elimination half-life, clearance, and the volume of distribution. Although the kinetic relationship is straightforward, there is more than one way of explaining the observations.

CLINICAL EXAMPLES

Drug with a Large Volume of Distribution and a Long Elimination $t_{1/2}$

The macrolide antibiotic dirithromycin is extensively distributed in tissues, resulting in a large steady-state volume of distribution of about 800 L (range 504–1041 L). The elimination $t_{1/2}$ in humans is about 44 hours (range 16–65 h). The drug has a relatively large total body clearance of 226 to 1040 mL/min (13.6–62.4 L/hours) and is given once daily. In this case, clearance is large due to a large V_D, whereas k is relatively small. In this case, Cl is large but the elimination half-life is long because of the large V_D. Intuitively, the drug will take a long time to be removed when the drug is distributed extensively over a large volume; despite a relatively large clearance, $t_{1/2}$ accurately describes drug elimination alone.

Drug with a Small Volume of Distribution and a Long Elimination $t_{1/2}$

Tenoxicam is a nonsteroidal anti-inflammatory drug (Nilsen, 1994) that is about 99% bound to human plasma protein. The drug has low lipophilicity, is highly ionized (approximately 99%), and is distributed in blood. Because tenoxicam is very polar, the drug penetrates cell membranes slowly. The synovial fluid peak drug level is only one-third that of the plasma drug concentration and occurs 20 hours (range 10–34 h) later than the peak plasma drug level. In addition, the drug is poorly distributed to body tissues and has an apparent volume of distribution, V_D, of 9.6 L (range 7.5–11.5 L). Tenoxicam has a low total plasma clearance of 0.106 L/h (0.079–0.142 L/h) and an elimination half-life of 67 hours (range 49–81 hours), undoubtedly related to the extensive drug binding to plasma proteins.

According to Equation 11.13, drug clearance from the body is low if V_D is small and k is not too large. This relationship is consistent with a small Cl and a small V_D observed for tenoxicam. Equation 11.4, however, predicts that a small V_D would result in a short elimination $t_{1/2}$. In this case, the actual elimination half-life is long (67 hours) because the plasma tenoxicam clearance is so low that it dominates in Equation 11.4. The long elimination half-life of tenoxicam is better explained by restrictive drug clearance due to its binding to plasma proteins, making it difficult for the drug to clear rapidly.

Clearance

Pharmacokineticists regard Cl and V_D as independent model variables based on Equation 11.14. Equation 11.13 and its equivalent, Equation 11.14, are rooted in classical pharmacokinetics. Initially, it may be difficult to understand why a drug such as dirithromycin, with a rapid clearance of 226 to 1040 mL/min, has a long half-life. In pharmacokinetics, the elimination constant $k = 0.0156$ h^{-1} implies that 1/64 (ie, 0.0156 h^{-1} = 1/64) of the drug is cleared per hour (a low-efficiency elimination factor). From the elimination rate constant k, one can estimate that it takes 44 hours ($t_{1/2}$ = 44 hours) to eliminate half the drug in the body, regardless of V_D. While $t_{1/2}$ is dependent on clearance and V_D as shown

by Equation 11.4, clearance is clearly affected by the volume of distribution and by many variables of the drug in the biological system. In patients with ascites, clearance is increased but with no increase in half-life, reflecting the increase in volume of distribution in ascitic patients (Stoeckel et al, 1983).

Frequently Asked Questions

▶ *Does a large value for clearance always result in a short half-life? Explain.*

▶ *What are the causes of a long distribution half-life for a body organ if blood flow to the tissue is rapid?*

▶ *How long does it take for a tissue organ to be fully equilibrated with the plasma? How long for a tissue organ to be half-equilibrated?*

▶ *When a body organ is equilibrated with drug from the plasma, the drug concentration in that organ should be the same as that of the plasma. True or false?*

▶ *What is the parameter that tells when half of the protein-binding sites are occupied?*

Elimination of Protein-Bound Drug: Restrictive Versus Nonrestrictive Elimination

When a drug is tightly bound to a protein, only the unbound drug is assumed to be metabolized; drugs belonging to this category are described as *restrictively eliminated*. On the other hand, some drugs may be eliminated even when they are protein bound; drugs in this category are described as *nonrestrictively eliminated*. Nonrestrictively cleared drugs are normally rapidly eliminated since protein binding does not impede the elimination process. Examples of nonrestrictively cleared drugs include morphine, metoprolol, and propranolol. Para-aminohippacuric acid is also nonrestrictively cleared by the kidney and useful as a marker for renal blood flow.

If a clinician fails to consider the role of restrictive versus nonrestrictive elimination, serious dosage miscalculations may be made with regard to response to the addition of inhibitors or changes in protein concentration. Nonrestrictively cleared drugs are less influenced by changes in protein binding since drug elimination is not affected. However, free drug diffusion may be affected by a change in free fraction.

Therefore, when drugs with varying fractions of plasma protein binding are compared, the expected reduction in clearance for drugs with low protein binding is sometimes absent or very minor. However, restrictively cleared drugs will exhibit a relationship between *total* drug concentration and protein concentration, though the *free* drug concentration may not change because of the resulting proportional changes in elimination. Therefore, whether a drug is restrictively or nonrestrictively eliminated must be considered when determining the role of changes in protein binding or inhibitors. The effect of protein binding on the kinetics of drug clearance in an organ system is discussed in detail in Chapter 12.

In practice, the molecular effect of protein binding on elimination is not always predictable. Drugs with restrictive elimination are recognized by very small plasma clearances and extensive plasma protein binding. The hepatic extraction ratios (ERs) for drugs that are restrictively eliminated are generally small, because of strong protein binding. Their hepatic extraction ratios are generally smaller than their unbound fractions in plasma (ie, ER < f_u). For example, phenylbutazone and the oxicams, including piroxicam, isoxicam, and tenoxicam, all have hepatic extraction ratios smaller than their unbound fraction in plasma (Verbeeck and Wallace, 1994). The hepatic elimination for these drugs is therefore restrictive. A series of nonsteroid anti-inflammatory drugs (NSAIDs) were reported by the same authors to be nonrestrictive with the following characteristics: (1) drug elimination is exclusively hepatic, (2) bioavailability of the drug from an oral dosage form is complete, and (3) these drugs do not undergo extensive reversible biotransformation or enterohepatic circulation.

Propranolol is a drug that has low bioavailability with a hepatic extraction ratio, ER, of 0.7 to 0.9. Propranolol is 89% bound, that is, 11% free (or $f_u = 0.11$) so that ER > f_u. Thus, propranolol is considered to be *nonrestrictively* eliminated. The bioavailability of propranolol is very low because of the large first-pass effect, and its elimination half-life is relatively short.

In contrast, highly bound drugs such as warfarin (99% bound) and diazepam (98% bound) each has an average long half-life of about 37 hours (see Appendix E). Reasons for a long half-life drug in the body may include a high degree of protein binding, a lower fraction of drug metabolised, and having drug molecular properties (eg, lipophilicity) that favor extravascular partitioning into tissues.

CLINICAL EXAMPLE

Diazepam (Valium®) has an average elimination half-life of 37 hours and V_D of 77 L and is mainly eliminated by demethylation.

- Is diazepam slowly eliminated due to the extensive binding to protein, a large V_D or simply because diazepam has a low metabolic rate (or low extraction ratio, ER)?

Recent studies with CYP 2C9 have shown that drug protein binding is not the only reason for small clearance and a long $t_{1/2}$ of diazepam (Qin et al, 1999). Diazepam demethylation varies greatly among individuals due to genetic polymorphism (see Chapter 13). In some subjects, slow metabolism is the main cause for a longer elimination half-life. The half-lives of diazepam ranged from 20 to 84 hours (Qin et al, 1999). Clearance ranged from 2.8 ± 0.9 mL/min (slow metabolizer) to 19.5 ± 9.8 mL/min (fast metabolizers). The long half-life is, in part, due to the small ER in some subjects. The elimination half-lives are shorter in subjects who are fast metabolizers, although the elimination half-lives are still quite long due to the large volume of distribution of this drug (small k and large V_D). It is important to keep in mind that *free drug concentration* and how it sustains ultimately determines pharmacologic effect and duration of action. Based on a *well-stirred venous equilibrium model* (Benet and Hoener, 2002), and a given set of assumptions, one can predict that the free AUC or systemic exposure of an orally administered drug will not be affected by protein binding despite its high degree of binding since the free AUC is not affected by f_u. In general, the approach is quite useful for many drugs with receptor sites within the plasma compartment discussed earlier. In the case of diazepam, pharmacological effect occurs in the brain and penetration across the central nervous system (CNS) may not be adequately considered by the equations of one-compartment model. The risk of unknown metabolism or uptake within cells outside the plasma compartment is always present. (See illustrated *in vitro* examples for V_D in the beginning of this chapter.)

Schmidt et al (2010) recently reviewed the effect of protein binding of various drugs and they characterized various situations in which steady-state free drug concentrations may or may not be affected by protein binding. The article discussed a group of benzodiazepines with different degrees of protein binding and reported that penetration into CNS is better related to the free drug concentration, that is, after correcting for protein binding. The benzodiazepines studied were (1) flunitrazepam, 85% bound, (2) midazolam, 96%, (3) oxazepam, 91%, and (4) clobazam, 69%. The authors concluded that for each drug, the pharmacokinetics and pharmacodynamics should be considered instead of a generalized "one-size-fit-all" approach. Schmidt et al (2010) also discuss various situations that may cause changes in half-life as a result of changes in protein–drug binding. Furthermore, Schmidt et al (2010) conclude that "plasma protein binding can have multiple effects on the pharmacokinetics and pharmacodynamics of a drug and a simple, generalized guideline for the evaluation of the clinical significance of protein binding frequently cannot be applied." These authors propose that a careful analysis of protein-binding effects must be made on a drug-by-drug basis.

Frequently Asked Question

▶ *Why is it important to report detailed information of the pharmacokinetics of a drug including the number and demographics of the subjects and the nature of drug elimination when citing mean clearance or half-life data from a table in the literature?*

DETERMINANTS OF PROTEIN BINDING

Drug–protein binding is influenced by a number of important factors, including the following:

1. The drug
   - Physicochemical properties of the drug
   - Total concentration of the drug in the body

2. The protein
   - Quantity of protein available for drug–protein binding
   - Quality or physicochemical nature of the protein synthesized
3. The affinity between drug and protein
   - The magnitude of the association constant
4. Drug interactions
   - Competition for the drug by other substances at a protein-binding site
   - Alteration of the protein by a substance that modifies the affinity of the drug for the protein; for example, aspirin acetylates lysine residues of albumin
5. The pathophysiologic condition of the patient
   - For example, drug–protein binding may be reduced in uremic patients and in patients with hepatic disease

Plasma drug concentrations are generally reported as the total drug concentration in the plasma, including both protein-bound drug and unbound (free) drug. Most literature values for the therapeutic effective drug concentrations refer to the total plasma or serum drug concentration. For therapeutic drug monitoring, the total plasma drug concentrations are generally used in the development of the appropriate drug dosage regimen for the patient. In the past, measurement of free drug concentration was not routinely performed in the laboratory. More recently, free drug concentrations may be measured quickly using ultrafiltration thereby allowing the measure of the drug concentration available to the drug receptor. Because of the high plasma protein binding of phenytoin and the narrow therapeutic index of the drug, more hospital laboratories are measuring both free and total phenytoin plasma levels.

CLINICAL EXAMPLE

Macfie et al (1992) studied the disposition of intravenous dosing of alfentanil in six patients who suffered 10% to 30% surface area burns compared a control group of six patients matched for age, sex, and weight. Alfentanil binding to plasma proteins was measured by equilibrium dialysis. The burn patients had significantly greater concentrations of AAG and smaller concentrations of albumin. The mean protein binding of alfentanil was 94.2% ± 0.05 (SEM) in the burn group and 90.7% ± 0.4 in the control group ($p = 0.004$). A good correlation was found between AAG concentration and protein binding. The greater AAG concentrations in the burn group corresponded with significantly reduced volume of distribution and total clearance of alfentanil. The clearance of the unbound fraction and the elimination half-life of alfentanil were not decreased significantly.

KINETICS OF PROTEIN BINDING

The kinetics of reversible drug–protein binding for a protein with one simple binding site can be described by the *law of mass action*, as follows:

$$\text{Protein} + \text{drug} \Leftrightarrow \text{drug–protein complex}$$

or

$$[P] + [D] \Leftrightarrow [PD] \tag{11.15}$$

From Equation 11.15 and the law of mass action, an association constant, K_a (also called the affinity constant), can be expressed as the ratio of the molar concentration of the products and the molar concentration of the reactants. This equation assumes only one binding site per protein molecule.

$$K_a = \frac{[PD]}{[P][D]} \tag{11.16}$$

The extent of the drug–protein complex formed is dependent on the association binding constant, K_a. The magnitude of K_a yields information on the degree of drug–protein binding. Drugs strongly bound to protein have a very large K_a and exist mostly as the drug–protein complex. With such drugs, a large dose may be needed to obtain a reasonable therapeutic concentration of free drug.

Most kinetic studies *in vitro* use purified albumin as a standard protein source because this protein is responsible for the major portion of plasma drug–protein binding. Experimentally, both the free drug $[D]$ and the protein-bound drug $[PD]$, as well as the total protein concentration $[P] + [PD]$, may be determined.

To study the binding behavior of drugs, a determinable ratio r is defined, as follows:

$$r = \frac{\text{moles of drug bound}}{\text{total moles of protein}}$$

As moles of drug bound is $[PD]$ and the total moles of protein is $[P] + [PD]$, this equation becomes

$$r = \frac{[PD]}{[PD]+[P]} \tag{11.17}$$

According to Equation 11.16, $[PD] = K_a [P] [D]$; by substitution into Equation 11.17, the following expression is obtained:

$$r = \frac{K_a[P][D]}{K_a[P][D]+[P]}$$
$$r = \frac{K_a[D]}{1+K_a[D]} \tag{11.18}$$

This equation describes the simplest situation, in which 1 mole of drug binds to 1 mole of protein in a 1:1 complex. This case assumes only one independent binding site for each molecule of drug. If there are n identical independent binding sites per protein molecule, then the following equation is used:

$$r = \frac{nK_a[D]}{1+K_a[D]} \tag{11.19}$$

In terms of K_d, which is $1/K_a$, Equation 11.19 reduces to

$$r = \frac{n[D]}{K_d +[D]} \tag{11.20}$$

Protein molecules are quite large compared to drug molecules and may contain more than one type of binding site for the drug. If there is more than one type of binding site and the drug binds independently to each binding site with its own association constant, then Equation 11.20 expands to

$$r = \frac{n_1K_1[P]}{1+K_1[D]} + \frac{n_2K_2[P]}{1+K_2[D]} +\dots \tag{11.21}$$

where the numerical subscripts represent different types of binding sites, the Ks represent the binding constants, and the ns represent the number of binding sites per molecule of albumin.

These equations assume that each drug molecule binds to the protein at an independent binding site, and the affinity of a drug for one binding site does not influence binding to other sites. In reality, drug–protein binding sometimes exhibits a phenomenon of *cooperativity*. For these drugs, the binding of the first drug molecule at one site on the protein molecule influences the successive binding of other drug molecules. The binding of oxygen to hemoglobin is an example of drug cooperativity.

Each method for the investigation of drug–protein binding *in vitro* has advantages and disadvantages in terms of cost, ease of measurement, time, instrumentation, and other considerations. Various experimental factors for the measurement of protein binding are listed in Table 11-10. Drug–protein binding kinetics yield valuable information concerning proper therapeutic use of the drug and predictions of possible drug interactions.

When $n = 1$ and the unbound (free) drug concentration is equal to K_d, the protein binding of the drug is half-saturated. Interestingly, when $[D]$ is much greater than K_d, K_d is negligible in Equation 11.21, and $r = n$ (that is, r is independent of concentration or fully saturated).

When $K_d > [D]$, $[D]$ is negligible in the denominator of Equation 11.21, and r is dependent on $n/K_d[D]$, or $nK_a[D]$. In this case, the number of sites bound is directly proportional to n, K_a, and the free drug concentration $[D]$. This relationship also explains why a drug with a higher K_a may not necessarily have a higher percent of drug bound, because the number of binding sites, n, may be different from one drug to another. At higher $[D]$, the relationship between $[PD]$ and $[D]$ may no longer be linear.

DETERMINATION OF BINDING CONSTANTS AND BINDING SITES BY GRAPHIC METHODS

In Vitro Methods (Known Protein Concentration)

A plot of the ratio of r (moles of drug bound per mole of protein) versus free drug concentration $[D]$ is shown in Fig. 11-13. Equation 11.20 shows that as free drug concentration increases, the number of moles of drug bound per mole of protein becomes saturated and plateaus. Thus, drug protein binding

PRACTICAL FOCUS

1. How is r related to the fraction of drug bound (f_u), a term that is often of clinical interest?

   Solution

   r is the ratio of number of moles of drug bound/ number of moles of albumin. r determines the fraction of drug binding sites that are occupied. f_u is based on the fraction of drug which is free in the plasma. The value of f_u is often assumed to be fixed. However, f_u may change, especially with drugs that have therapeutic levels close to K_d. (See examples on diazoxide.)

2. At maximum drugs binding, the number of binding sites is n (see Equation 11.21). The drug disopyramide has a $K_d = 1 \times 10^{-6}$ M/L. How close to saturation is the drug when the free drug concentration is 1×10^{-6} M/L?

   Solution

   Substitution for $[D] = 1 \times 10^{-6}$ M/L and $K_d = 1 \times 10^{-6}$ M/L in Equation 11.21 gives

   $$r = \frac{n}{2}$$

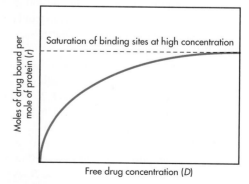

FIGURE 11-13   Graphical representation of Equation 11.20, showing saturation of protein at high drug concentrations.

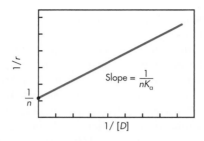

FIGURE 11-14   Hypothetical binding of drug to protein. The line was obtained with the double reciprocal equation.

resembles a *Langmuir* adsorption isotherm, which is also similar to the process where adsorption of a drug to an adsorbent becomes saturated as the drug concentration increases. Because of nonlinearity in drug–protein binding, Equation 11.20 is rearranged for the estimation of n and K_a.

The values for the association constants and the number of binding sites are obtained by various graphic methods. The reciprocal of Equation 11.20 gives the following equation:

$$\frac{1}{r} = \frac{1 + K_a[D]}{nK_a[D]}$$

$$\frac{1}{r} = \frac{1}{nK_a[D]} + \frac{1}{n}$$

(11.22)

A graph of $1/r$ versus $1/[D]$ is called a *double reciprocal plot*. The y intercept is $1/n$ and the slope is $1/nK_a$. From this graph (Fig. 11-14), the number of binding sites may be determined from the y intercept, and the association constant may be determined from the slope, if the value for n is known.

If the graph of $1/r$ versus $1/[D]$ does not yield a straight line, then the drug–protein binding process is probably more complex. Equation 11.20 assumes one type of binding site and no interaction among the binding sites. Frequently, Equation 11.22 is used to estimate the number of binding sites and binding constants, using computerized iteration methods.

Another graphic technique called the *Scatchard plot*, is a rearrangement of Equation 11.20. The Scatchard plot spreads the data to give a better line

for the estimation of the binding constants and binding sites. From Equation 11.20, we obtain

$$r = \frac{nK_a[D]}{1 + K_a[D]}$$

$$r + rK_a[D] = nK_a[D]$$

$$r = nK_a[D] - rK_a[D]$$

(11.23)

$$\frac{r}{D} = nK_a - rK_a$$

A graph constructed by plotting $r/[D]$ versus r yields a straight line with the intercepts and slope shown in Figs. 11-15 and 11-16.

Some drug–protein binding data produce Scatchard graphs of curvilinear lines (Figs. 11-17 and 11-18). The curvilinear line represents the summation of two straight lines that collectively form the curve. The binding of salicylic acid to albumin is an example of this type of drug–protein binding in which there are at least two different, independent binding sites (n_1 and n_2), each with its own independent association constant (k_1 and k_2). Equation 11.21 best describes this type of drug–protein interaction.

In Vivo Methods (Unknown Protein Concentration)

Reciprocal and Scatchard plots cannot be used if the exact nature and amount of protein in the experimental system are unknown. The percent of drug bound is often used to describe the extent of drug–protein binding in the plasma. The fraction of drug bound, β, can be determined experimentally and is equal to the ratio of the concentration of bound drug, $[D_\beta]$, and

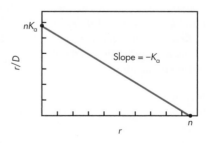

FIGURE 11-15   Hypothetical binding of drug to protein. The line was obtained with the Scatchard equation.

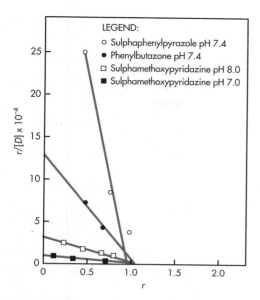

FIGURE 11-16   Graphic determination of number of binding sites and association constants for interaction of sulfonamides and phenylbutazone with albumin. (From Thorp, 1964, with permission.)

the total drug concentration, $[D_T]$, in the plasma, as follows:

$$\beta = \frac{[D_\beta]}{[D_T]} \qquad (11.24)$$

The value of the association constant, K_a, can be determined, even though the nature of the plasma proteins binding the drug is unknown, by rearranging

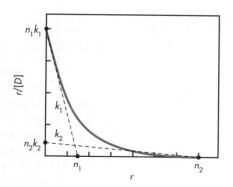

FIGURE 11-17   Hypothetical binding of drug to protein. The k's represent independent binding constants and the n's represent the number of binding sites per molecule of protein.

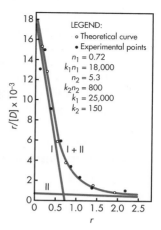

FIGURE 11-18   Binding curves for salicylic acid to crystalline bovine serum albumin. Curve I, plot for one class, $n_1 = 0.72$, $k_1 = 25,000$. Curve II, plot for second class, $n_2 = 5.3$, $k_2 = 150$. Curve I + II, plot for both binding sites, sum of the above. (From Davison, 1971, with permission.)

Equation 11.24 into Equation 11.25:

$$r = \frac{[D_\beta]}{[P_T]} = \frac{nK_a[D]}{1 + K_a[D]} \qquad (11.25)$$

where $[D_\beta]$ is the bound drug concentration; $[D]$ is the free drug concentration; and $[P_T]$ is the total protein concentration. Rearrangement of this equation gives the following expression, which is analogous to the Scatchard equation:

$$\frac{[D_\beta]}{[D]} = nK_a[P_T] - K_a[D_\beta] \qquad (11.26)$$

Concentrations of both free and bound drug may be measured experimentally, and a graph obtained by plotting $[D_\beta]/[D]$ versus $[D_\beta]$ will yield a straight line for which the slope is the association constant K_a. Equation 11.26 shows that the ratio of bound C_p to free C_p is influenced by the affinity constant, the protein concentration, $[P_T]$, which may change during disease states, and the drug concentration in the body.

The values for n and K_a give a general estimate of the affinity and binding capacity of the drug, as plasma contains a complex mixture of proteins. The drug–protein binding in plasma may be influenced by competing substances such as ions, free fatty acids, drug metabolites, and other drugs. Measurements of drug–protein binding should be obtained over a wide drug concentration range, because at low drug concentrations a high-affinity, low-capacity binding site might be missed or, at a higher drug concentration, saturation of protein-binding sites might occur.

Relationship between Protein Concentration and Drug Concentration in Drug–Protein Binding

The drug concentration, the protein concentration, and the association (affinity) constant, K_a, influence the fraction of drug bound (Equation 11.24). With a constant concentration of protein, only a certain number of binding sites are available for a drug. At low drug concentrations, most of the drug may be bound to the protein, whereas at high drug concentrations, the protein-binding sites may become saturated, with a consequent rapid increase in the free drug concentrations (Fig. 11-19).

To demonstrate the relationship of the drug concentration, protein concentration, and K_a, the following expression can be derived from Equations 11.24 and 11.25.

$$\beta = \frac{1}{1 + ([D]/n[P_T]) + (1/nK_a[P_T])} \quad (11.27)$$

From Equation 11.27, both the free drug concentration, $[D]$, and the total protein concentration, $[P_T]$,

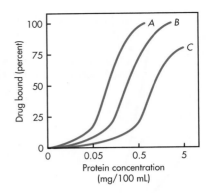

FIGURE 11-20　Effect of protein concentration on the percentage of drug bound. *A*, *B*, and *C* represent hypothetical drugs with respective decreasing binding affinity.

have important effects on the fraction of drug bound. Any factors that suddenly increase the fraction of free drug concentration in the plasma will cause a change in the pharmacokinetics of the drug.

Because protein binding is nonlinear in most cases, the percent of drug bound is dependent on the concentrations of both the drug and proteins in the plasma. In disease situations, the concentration of protein may change, thus affecting the percent of drug bound. As the protein concentration increases, the percent of drug bound increases to a maximum. The shapes of the curves are determined by the association constant of the drug–protein complex and the drug concentration. The effect of protein concentration on drug binding is demonstrated in Fig. 11-20.

CLINICAL SIGNIFICANCE OF DRUG–PROTEIN BINDING

Most drugs bind reversibly to plasma proteins to some extent. When the clinical significance of the fraction of drug bound is considered, it is important to know whether the study was performed using pharmacologic or therapeutic plasma drug concentrations. As mentioned previously, the fraction of drug bound can change with plasma drug concentration and dose of drug administered. In addition, the patient's plasma protein concentration should be considered. If a patient has a low plasma protein concentration, then, for any given dose of drug, the

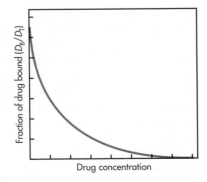

FIGURE 11-19　Fraction of drug bound versus drug concentration at constant protein concentration.

TABLE 11-12   Factors That Decrease Plasma Protein Concentration

Mechanism	Disease State
Decreased protein synthesis	Liver disease
Increased protein catabolism	Trauma, surgery
Distribution of albumin into extravascular space	Burns
Excessive elimination of protein	Renal disease

concentration of free (unbound) bioactive drug may be higher than anticipated. The plasma protein concentration is controlled by a number of variables, including (1) protein synthesis, (2) protein catabolism, (3) distribution of the protein between intravascular and extravascular space, and (4) excessive elimination of plasma protein, particularly albumin. A number of diseases, age, trauma, and related circumstances affect the plasma protein concentration (Tables 11-12–11-14).

For example, liver disease results in a decrease in plasma albumin concentration due to decreased protein synthesis. In nephrotic syndrome, an accumulation of waste metabolites, such as urea and uric acid, as well as an accumulation of drug metabolites, may alter protein binding of drugs. Severe burns may cause an increased distribution of albumin into the extracellular fluid, resulting in a smaller plasma albumin concentration. In certain genetic diseases, the quality of the protein that is synthesized in the plasma may be altered due to a change in the amino acid sequence. Both chronic liver disease and renal disease, such as uremia, may cause an alteration in the quality of plasma protein synthesized. An alteration in the protein quality may be demonstrated by an alteration in the association constant or affinity of the drug for the protein.

Drug Interactions—Competition for Binding Sites

When a highly protein-bound drug is displaced from binding by a second drug or agent, a sharp increase in the free drug concentration in the plasma may occur, leading to toxicity. For example, an increase in free warfarin level was responsible for an increase in bleeding when warfarin was coadministered with phenylbutazone, which competes for the same protein-binding site (O'Reilly, 1973; Udall, 1970; Sellers and Koch-Weser, 1971). Recently, studies and reviews have shown that the clinical significance of warfarin protein binding and its impact on bleeding are less prominent, adding other factors and explanations (Sands et al, 2002; Chan, 1995; Benet and Hoener, 2002). Since protein binding and metabolism both occur *in vivo* and can both influence the rate of metabolism in a patient, it is not always clear whether to attribute the cause of a change in metabolism based on kinetic observations alone. Change in CYP enzymes may occur in genetic polymorphism and at the same time change in protein may occur due to a number of causes. Van Steeg et al (2009) recently reviewed the effect of protein binding on drug pharmacokinetics and pharmacodynamics. The authors discussed many important aspects of protein binding and drug disposition using beta-blocker as examples. Schmidt et al (2010) reviewed many examples of drug–protein binding and concluded that appropriate analysis requires careful consideration of both pharmacokinetic and pharmacodynamic processes, as they both contribute to the safety and efficacy of drugs. Ideally, the free drug concentrations at the receptor site should be used for making inferences about a drug's pharmacological activity.

Albumin has two known binding sites that share the binding of many drugs (MacKichan, 1992). Binding site I is shared by phenylbutazone, sulfonamides, phenytoin, and valproic acid. Binding site II is shared by the semisynthetic penicillins, probenecid, medium-chain fatty acids, and the benzodiazepines. Some drugs bind to both sites. Displacement occurs when a second drug is taken that competes for the same binding site in the protein as the initial drug.

Although it is generally assumed that binding sites are preformed, there is some evidence pointing to the *allosteric* nature of protein binding. This means that the binding of a drug modifies the conformation of protein in such a way that the drug binding influences the nature of binding of further molecules of the drug. The binding of oxygen to hemoglobin is a well-studied biochemical example

TABLE 11-13   Physiologic and Pathologic Conditions Altering Protein Concentrations in Plasma^a

	Albumin	α_1-Glycoprotein	Lipoprotein
Decreasing	Age (geriatric, neonate)	Fetal concentrations	Hyperthyroidism
	Bacterial pneumonia	Nephrotic syndrome	Injury
	Burns	Oral contraceptives	Liver disease?
	Cirrhosis of liver		Trauma
	Cystic fibrosis		
	GI disease		
	Histoplasmosis		
	Leprosy		
	Liver abscess		
	Malignant neoplasms		
	Malnutrition (severe)		
	Multiple myeloma		
	Nephrotic syndrome		
	Pancreatitis (acute)		
	Pregnancy		
	Renal failure		
	Surgery		
	Trauma		
Increasing	Benign tumor	Age (geriatric)	Diabetes
	Exercise	Celiac disease	Hypothyroidism
	Hypothyroidism	Crohn's disease	Liver disease?
	Neurological disease?	Injury	Nephrotic syndrome
	Neurosis	Myocardial infarction	
	Paranoia	Renal failure	
	Psychosis	Rheumatoid arthritis	
	Schizophrenia	Stress	
		Surgery	
		Trauma	

^{a}In the conditions listed, the protein concentrations are altered, on average, by 30% or more, and in some cases by more than 100%. Data compiled from Jusko WJ, Gretch M: Plasma and tissue protein binding of drugs in pharmacokinetics, *Drug Metab Rev* **5:**43–10, 1976, and Friedman RB, et al: Effects of diseases on clinical laboratory tests, *Clin Chem* **26**, 1980.

TABLE 11-14   Protein Binding in Normal (Norm) Renal Function, End-Stage Renal Disease (ESRD), during Hemodialysis (HD), and in Nephrotic Syndrome (NS)

	Norm (% Bound)	ESRD (% Bound)	HD (% Bound)	NS (% Bound)
Azlocillin	28	25		
Bilirubin		Decreased		
Captopril	24	18		
Cefazolin	84	73	22	
Cefoxitin	73	20		
Chloramphenicol	53	45	30	
Chlorpromazine	98	98		
Clofibrate	96		89	
Clonidine	30	30		
Congo red		Decreased		
Dapsone		Normal		
Desipramine	80	Normal		
N-Desmethyldiazepam	98	94		
Desmethylimipramine	89	88		
Diazepam	99	94		
Diazoxide (30 μg/mL)	92	86	83	
(300 μg/mL)	77	72		
Dicloxacillin	96	91		
Diflunisal	88	56		39
Digitoxin	97	96	90	96
Digoxin	25		22	
Doxycycline	88	71		
Erythromycin	75	77		
Etomidate	75	57		
Fluorescein	86	Decreased		
Furosemid	96	94		93
Indomethacin		Normal		
Maprotiline	90	Normal		
β-Methyldigoxin	30		19	
Methyl orange		Decreased		
Methyl red		Decreased		
Morphine	35	31		
Nafcillin	88	81		

(Continued)

TABLE 11-14 **Protein Binding in Normal (Norm) Renal Function, End-Stage Renal Disease (ESRD), during Hemodialysis (HD), and in Nephrotic Syndrome (NS) (Continued)**

	Norm (% Bound)	ESRD (% Bound)	HD (% Bound)	NS (% Bound)
Naproxen	75	21		
Oxazepam	95	88		
Papaverine	97	94		
Penicillin G	72	36		
Pentobarbital	66	59		
Phenobarbital	55	Decreased		
Phenol red		Decreased		
Phenylbutazone	97	88		
Phenytoin	90	80	93	81
Pindolol	41	Normal		
Prazosin	95	92		
Prednisolone (50 mg)	74		65	64
(15 mg)	87	88		85
D-Propoxyphene	76	80		
Propranolol	88	89	90	
Quinidine	88	86	88	
Salicylate	94	85		
Sulfadiazine		Decreased		
Sulfamethoxazole	74	50		
Sulfonamides		Decreased		
Strophantin	1		2	
Theophylline	60	Decreased		
Thiopental	72	44		
Thyroxine		Decreased		
Triamterene	81	61		
Trimethoprim	70	68		70
Tryptophan	75	Decreased		
D-Tubocurarine	44	41		
Valproic acid	85	Decreased		
Verapamil	90	Normal		
Warfarin	99	98		

From Keller et al (1984), with permission.

in which the initial binding of other oxygen to the iron in the heme portion influences the binding of other oxygen molecules.

Effect of Change in Protein Binding

Most studies of the kinetics of drug–protein binding consider binding to plasma proteins. However, certain drugs may also bind specific tissue proteins or other macromolecules, such as melanin or DNA, drug receptors or transiently to transport proteins. Most literature exclude drug binding to other macromolecules and are limited to discussing the effect of drug binding to plasma albumin and AAG only. Since many drugs are eliminated by the liver, it is relevant to discuss the effect of protein binding after oral drug administration or by parenteral administration, after which the drug bypasses first-pass hepatic elimination.

After IV drug administration, displacement of drugs from plasma protein binding causing an increase in f_u or increased free drug concentration may potentially facilitate extravascular drug distribution and an increase in the apparent volume of distribution. The increased distribution results in a smaller plasma C_p due to wider distribution, making drug elimination more difficult ($k = Cl/V_D$). This is analogous to reducing the fraction of free drug presented for elimination per unit time based on a one-compartment model. Consequently, a longer elimination half-life is expected due to wider tissue drug distribution. The relationship is expressed by Equation 11.28 in order to assess the distribution effect due to protein binding.

$$Cl = \frac{0.693\, V_D}{t_{1/2}} = kV_D \qquad (11.28)$$

Drug clearance may remain unaffected or only slightly changed if the decrease in the elimination rate constant is not compensated by an increase in V_D as shown by Equation 11.28. The mean steady-state total drug concentration will remain unchanged based on no change in Cl or kV_D. Whether the change in plasma drug–protein binding has pharmacodynamic significance depends on whether the drug is

highly potent and has a narrow therapeutic window. Protein–drug binding has the buffering effect of preventing an abrupt rise in free drug concentration in the body. For orally administered drugs, the liver provides a good protection against drug toxicity because of hepatic portal drug absorption and metabolism. For a highly extracted drug orally administered, an increase in f_u (more free drug) causes hepatic clearance to increase (ie, $f_u Cl_{int}$), thus reducing total AUC_{oral} but not changing free drug AUC^u_{oral} due to the compensatory effect of $f_u\, AUC_{oral}$ (ie, decrease in AUC_{oral} is compensated by the same increase in free $AUC_u = f_u\, AUC_{oral}$) (see derivation of Equation 11.34 based on Benet and Hoener [2002] under *Protein Binding and Drug Exposure*).

The assumptions and derivation should be carefully observed before applying the concept to individual drugs. Most important of all, the model assumes a simple well-stirred hepatic model and excludes drugs involving transporters, which is now known to be common. A recent review (Schmidt et al, 2010) further discussed the issue of protein binding and its effect on pharmacokinetics and pharmacodynamics. The author discussed the effect of changing V_D on the elimination half-life of drugs using Equation 11.14, which is shown by rearranging to be the same as Equation 11.28

$$t_{1/2} = \ln 2\left[\frac{V_D}{Cl}\right] = \frac{V_D\; 0.693}{Cl} \qquad (11.14)$$

Drug Distribution, Drug Binding, Displacement, and Pharmacodynamics

The relationship of reversible drug–protein binding in the plasma and drug distribution and elimination is shown in Fig. 11-8. A decrease in protein binding that results in an increased free drug concentration will allow more drug to cross cell membranes and distribute into all tissues, as discussed above. More drug will therefore be available to interact at a receptor site to produce a more intense pharmacologic effect, at least temporarily. The increased free concentration also may cause an increased rate of metabolism and decreased half-life which then may produce a lower total steady-state drug concentration but similar steady-state free drug concentration (see additional discussion below).

Clinically, the pharmacodynamic response is influenced by both the distribution of the drug and the concentration of the unbound drug fraction. The drug dose and the dosage form must be chosen to provide sufficiently high unbound drug concentrations so that an adequate amount of drug reaches the site of drug action (receptor). The onset of drug action depends on the rate of the free (unbound) drug that reaches the receptor and provides a *minimum effective concentration* (MEC) to produce a pharmacodynamic response (see Chapters 1 and 21). The onset time is often dependent on the rate of drug uptake and distribution to the receptor site. The intensity of a drug action depends on the total drug concentration of the receptor site and the number of receptors occupied by drug. To achieve a pharmacodynamic response with the initial (priming) dose, the amount (mass) of drug when dissolved in the volume of distribution must give a drug concentration ≥ MEC at the receptor site. Subsequent drug doses maintain the pharmacodynamic effect by sustaining the drug concentration at the receptor site. Subsequent doses are given at a dose rate (eg, 250 mg every 6 hours) that replaces drug loss from the receptor site, usually by elimination. However, redistributional factors may also contribute to the loss of drug from the receptor site.

A less understood aspect of protein binding is the effect of binding on the intensity and pharmacodynamics of the drug after intravenous administration. Rapid IV injection may increase the free drug concentration of some highly protein-bound drugs and therefore increase its intensity of action. Sellers and Koch-Weser (1973) reported a dramatic increase in hypotensive effect when diazoxide was injected rapidly IV in 10 seconds versus a slower injection of 100 seconds. Diazoxide was 9.1% and 20.6% free when the serum levels were 20 and 100 μg/mL, respectively. Figure 11-21 shows a transient high free diazoxide concentration that resulted after a rapid IV injection, causing maximum arterial dilation and hypotensive effect due to initial saturation of the protein-binding sites. In contrast, when diazoxide was injected slowly over 100 seconds, free diazoxide serum level was low, due to binding and drug distribution. The slower injection of diazoxide produced a smaller fall in blood pressure, even though the total

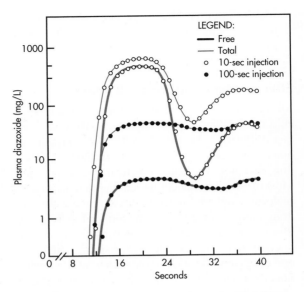

FIGURE 11-21   Calculated time course of total and free diazoxide concentrations in arterioles. (From Sellers and Koch-Weser, 1973, with permission.)

drug dose injected was the same. Although most drugs have linear binding at their therapeutic doses, in some patients, free drug concentration can increase rapidly with rising drug concentration as binding sites become saturated. An example is illustrated in Fig. 11-22 for lidocaine (MacKichan, 1992).

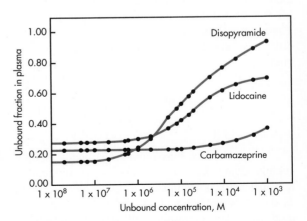

FIGURE 11-22   Simulation showing changes in fraction of free (unbound) drug over various molar drug concentrations for three drugs with protein binding. (From MacKichan, 1992, with permission.)

The nature of drug–drug and drug–metabolite interactions is also important in drug–protein binding. In this case, one drug may displace a second bound drug from the protein, causing a sudden increase in pharmacologic response due to an increase in free drug concentration.

Frequently Asked Questions

▶ *What happens to the pharmacokinetic parameters of a drug when a displacing agent is given?*

▶ *What kind of drugs are most susceptible to clinically relevant changes in pharmacokinetics? Does the rate of administration matter?*

EXAMPLE ▶ ▶ ▶

Compare the percent of change in free drug concentration when two drugs, *A* (95% bound) and *B* (50% bound), are displaced by 5% from their respective binding sites by the administration of another drug (Table 11-15). For a highly bound drug *A*, a displacement of 5% of free drug is actually a 100% increase in free drug level. For a weakly bound drug like drug *B*, a change of 5% in free concentration due to displacement would cause only a 10% increase in free drug level over the initially high (50%) free drug concentration. For a patient medicated with drug *B*, a 10% increase in free drug level would probably not affect the therapeutic outcome. However, a 100% increase in active drug, as occurs with drug *A*, might be toxic. Although

this example is based on one drug displacing another drug, nutrients, physiologic products, and the waste products of metabolism may cause displacement from binding in a similar manner.

As illustrated by this example, displacement is most important with drugs that are more than 95% bound and has a narrow therapeutic index. Under normal circumstances, only a small proportion of the total drug is active. Consequently, a small displacement of bound drug causes a disproportionate increase in the free drug concentration, which may cause drug intoxication.

With drugs that are not as highly bound to plasma proteins, a small displacement from the protein causes a transient increase in the free drug concentration, which may cause a transient increase in pharmacologic activity. However, more free drug is available for both renal excretion and hepatic biotransformation, which may be demonstrated by a transient decreased elimination half-life. Drug displacement from protein by a second drug can occur by competition of the second drug for similar binding sites. Moreover, any alteration of the protein structure may also change the capacity of the protein to bind drugs. For example, aspirin acetylates the lysine residue of albumin, which changes the binding capacity of this protein for certain other anti-inflammatory drugs, such as phenylbutazone.

The displacement of endogenous substances from plasma proteins by drugs is usually of little consequence. Some hormones, such as

TABLE 11-15   **Comparison of Effects of 5% Displacement from Binding on Two Hypothetical Drugs**

	Before Displacement	After Displacement	Percent Increase in Free Drug
Drug *A*			
Percent drug bound	95	90	
Percent drug free	5	10	+100
Drug *B*			
Percent drug bound	50	45	
Percent drug free	50	55	+10

thyroid and cortisol, are normally bound to specific plasma proteins. A small displacement of these hormones rarely causes problems because physiologic feedback control mechanisms take over. However, in infants, the displacement of bilirubin by drugs can cause mental retardation and even death, due to the difficulty of bilirubin elimination in newborns.

Finally, the binding of drugs to proteins can affect the duration of action of the drug. A drug that is extensively but reversibly bound to protein may have a long duration of action due to a depot effect of the drug–protein complex.

While a change in free drug concentration due to changing protein binding can potentially change the pharmacologic response of a drug, many drugs with a change in protein binding did not show a significant change in clinical effect (Benet and Hoener, 2002), as discussed in the next section. The important question to ask is: Will the increase in free drug concentration due to reduced binding elicit a rapid pharmacologic response before the temporary increase in free drug is diluted by a rapid distribution and/or elimination due to a greater fraction of free drug? Kruger and Figg (2001) observed that the angiogenesis activity of suramin, an inhibitor of blood vessel proliferation, is greatly altered by protein binding. In biological assays with aorta rings of rats, the effect was measured *ex vivo* at the site directly, and the degree of protein binding was reported to be important. In the body, the pathways to reach the receptor, distribution, and elimination are factors that complicate the effect of a rise in free drug due to displacement from binding. In general, the outcome of a change in protein binding *in vivo* may be harder to measure depending on where the site of action is located. The onset of a drug, and its distribution half-life to the site of action, may need to be considered. In the next section, this subject is further discussed based on the recent concept of drug exposure. The concept of drug exposure is important because adverse reactions in many organs are related to their exposure to plasma drug concentration.

Protein Binding and Drug Exposure

The impact of protein binding on clinical drug efficacy and safety has long been recognized (Koch-Weser and Sellers, 1976; Greenblatt et al, 1982) but has received renewed literature discussion recently (Sands et al, 2002; Chan, 1995; Benet and Hoener, 2002, van Steeg et al, 2009, Schmidt et al, 2010). Free plasma drug concentration or free drug concentration at the site of action is generally considered to be more relevant than total plasma drug concentration. When considering drug safety, how high and how long the free plasma drug level will be sustained are also important to a toxicokineticist. This is often measured by the AUC for the free plasma drug concentration.

Based on the well-stirred venous equilibration model incorporating protein binding (Benet and Hoener, 2002), organ clearance for a drug (Cl) is expressed as

$$Cl = \frac{Q_{organ} f_u Cl_{int}}{Q_{organ} + f_u Cl_{int}} \qquad (11.29)$$

For a low-extraction drug, where Q is blood flow, f_u is fraction of drug unchanged and Cl_{int} is intrinsic clearance, $Q_{organ} \gg f_u Cl_{int}$, the equation simplifies to

$$Cl = f_u Cl_{int} \qquad (11.30)$$

Clearance depends on f_u and intrinsic clearance. Intrinsic clearance is flow independent; whereas hepatic clearance, Cl_H, is flow dependent for a high extraction drug.

Hepatic bioavailability of a drug, F_H, is expressed as

$$F_H = \frac{Q_H}{Q_H + f_u Cl_{int}} \qquad (11.31)$$

Let F_{abs} be the fraction of drug absorbed to the gut wall and F_G be the fraction that gets through the gut wall unchanged (ie, $F_{oral} = F_{abs} F_G F_H$). The systemic AUC after an oral dose is

$$AUC_{oral} = \frac{F_{abs} F_G \text{Dose}}{f_u Cl_{int}} \qquad (11.32)$$

For an unbound drug, $AUC^u_{oral} = [f_u]AUC_{oral}$

$$\qquad (11.33)$$

When substituted for AUC_{oral} using Equation 11.32 into Equation 11.33, f_u cancels out, and the equation becomes

$$AUC_{oral}^u = \frac{F_{abs}F_G Dose}{Cl_{int}} \qquad (11.34)$$

Equation 11.34 above shows that for low-extraction drugs, unbound drug exposure as measured by unbound plasma drug area under the curve (AUC_{oral}^u) is independent of f_u.

For a low-extraction drug, both IV and oral, changes in protein binding are generally not important. For a high-extraction drug after IV administration, changes in protein binding are clinically important whether metabolism is hepatic or nonhepatic. For a drug that is administered IV and is highly extracted by the liver ($Q_{organ} \ll f_u\, Cl_{int}$), AUC_{IV}^u or unbound drug systemic exposure is expressed by

$$AUC_{IV}^u = f_u AUC_{IV} \approx \frac{f_u Dose}{Q_H} \qquad (11.35)$$

In this case, changes in binding may be clinically important, as shown by the change of f_u in Equation 11.35.

The derivation of Equation 11.33 into Equation 11.34 is dependent on the fact that f_u is constant as a function of t. If unbound drug concentration C_u is changing at various C_p, that is, concentration-dependent binding, then $C_u = F(t)$ is time dependent, and in fact, AUC will be nonlinear with dose and Equation 11.34 will be different for different doses (see Chapter 10). Within therapeutic drug concentrations, the effect of changes in f_u is apparently not sufficient to change the efficacy of most drugs and therefore is not of clinical concern. However, as more potent drugs with short elimination half-lives are used, plasma drug concentrations may potentially fall several fold and f_u may change significantly at various plasma concentrations. An anatomic-physiologic approach to evaluate drug concentrations (Mather, 2001) may be helpful in understanding how drug efficacy and safety change in protein binding and clearances in local tissues (see Chapter 13).

Frequently Asked Questions

▶ Do all drugs that bind proteins lead to clinically significant interactions?

▶ What macromolecules participate in drug–protein binding?

▶ How does drug–protein binding affect drug elimination?

▶ What are the factors to consider when adjusting the drug dose for a patient whose plasma protein concentration decreases to half that of normal?

▶ f_u is used to represent the fraction of free drug in the plasma (Equations 11.30 and 11.33). Is f_u always a constant?

▶ Can a protein-bound drug be metabolized?

CLINICAL EXAMPLE

Protein concentration may change during some acute disease states. For example, plasma AAG levels in patients may increase due to the host's acute-phase response to infection, trauma, inflammatory processes, and some malignant diseases. The acute-phase response is a change in various plasma proteins that is observed within hours or days following the onset of infection or injury. The acute-phase changes may be also indicative of chronic disease (Kremer et al, 1988).

As many basic drugs bind to AAG, a change in AAG protein concentration can contribute to more fluctuation in free drug concentrations among patients during various stages of infection or disease. Amprenavir (Agenerase), a protease inhibitor of human immunodeficiency virus type 1 (HIV-1), is highly bound to human plasma proteins, mostly to AAG (approximately 90%). AAG levels are known to vary with infection, including HIV disease. Sadler et al (2001) showed a significant inverse linear relationship between AAG levels and amprenavir clearance as estimated by Cl/F. Unbound, or free, amprenavir concentrations were not affected by AAG concentrations even though the apparent total drug clearance was increased. The intrinsic clearance of the drug was not changed. The authors cautioned that incorrect conclusions could be drawn about the pharmacokinetics of highly protein-bound drugs if AAG concentration is not included in the analysis.

In addition, race, age, and weight were also found to affect AAG levels. African American subjects had significantly lower AAG concentrations than Caucasian subjects. AAG in African-Americans was 77.2 ± 13.8 mg/dL versus 90 ± 20.2 mg/dL in Caucasians ($p < 0.0001$). Pharmacokinetic analysis showed that AAG correlated significantly with age and race and was a significant predictor of amprenavir Cl/F. Interestingly, in spite of a statistically significant difference in total plasma amprenavir level, a dose adjustment for racial differences was not indicated, because the investigators found the unbound amprenavir concentrations to be similar.

Protein binding can lead to *nonlinear* or *dose-dependent* kinetics. It was interesting to note that amprenavir Cl/F was dose dependent in the analysis without AAG data, but that no dose dependence was observed when AAG concentration was considered in the analysis. The higher doses of amprenavir, which produce the greatest antiviral activity, resulted in the largest decrease in AAG concentration, which led to the greatest changes in total drug concentration.

In evaluating change in protein binding and its impact on free plasma drug, it is important to realize that protein changes or displacement often results in changes in free plasma drug concentration. Nonetheless, the free drug is not necessarily increasingly eliminated unless the change in free drug concentration facilitates metabolism, accompanied by a change in Cl_{int} (Cl_{int} measures the inherent capacity to metabolize the drug; see Chapter 12). For some drugs, the change in protein binding may be sufficiently compensated by a redistribution of the drug from one tissue to another within the body. In contrast, a change in drug protein binding accompanied by metabolism (Cl_{int}) will invariably result in an increased amount of drug needed to maintain a steady-state level because the total drug concentration is continuously being eliminated. The maintenance of an adequate

therapeutic free drug level through re-equilibration is difficult in such a case.

The understanding of the molecular interactions of drug binding to proteins is essential to explain the clinical pharmacology and toxicology in the body. Drug–protein binding is generally assumed to be reversible as modeled in later sections of this chapter. Taheri et al (2003) studied the binding and displacement of several local anesthetics, such as lidocaine, mepivacaine, and bupivacaine with human α_1-acid glycoprotein (AAG). These investigators used a special molecular probe to see how local anesthetics behave during equilibrium-competitive displacement from AAG. The change in recovery of AAG's fluorescence as the quenching probe was displaced from its high-affinity site was used to observe change in dissociation constants for the various local anesthetics. The study demonstrated that the AAG-binding site has a strong positive correlation between hydrophobicity of the local anesthetics and their free energies of dissociation. The effect of pH and electrostatic forces on binding was also explored. Studies by other investigators of these molecular factors' influence on binding were done previously with albumin binding to different agents. More sophisticated models may be needed as the understanding of molecular interactions of a drug with a substrate protein improves. Theoretically, a change in molecular conformation or allosteric binding may change the activity of a drug but requires clinical demonstration.

CLINICAL EXAMPLE

A drug–drug interaction derived from the displacement of lidocaine from tissue binding sites by mexiletine that resulted in the increased plasma lidocaine concentrations was reported by Maeda et al (2002). A case of an unexpected increase in plasma lidocaine concentration accompanied with severe side effects was observed when mexiletine was administered to a patient with dilated cardiomyopathy. Maeda et al (2002) further studied this observation in rabbits and *in vitro*. Mexiletine significantly reduced the tissue distribution of lidocaine to the kidneys and lungs. Lidocaine plasma levels were higher. Mexiletine had a strong displacing effect of lidocaine binding to the membrane component phosphatidylserine.

- Should loading doses of lidocaine be used in the concurrent therapy of lidocaine and mexiletine?
- Would you consider the lung and kidney to be "well equilibrated" tissues based on blood flow?

MODELING DRUG DISTRIBUTION

Drug distribution may change in many disease and physiologic states, making it difficult to predict the concentration of drug that reaches the site of drug action (receptor). Pharmacokinetic models can be used to predict these pharmacokinetic changes due to changes in physiologic states. The model should consider free and bound drug equilibration and metabolism at the apparent site of action, and transient changes due to disease state (eg, pH change or impaired perfusion).

In pharmacokinetics, perfusion and rapid equilibration within a region form the basis for the *well-stirred models* that are used in many classical compartment models as well as some physiologic pharmacokinetic models. The concept of body or organ drug clearance assumes that uniform drug concentration is rapidly established within a given biological region (C_{organ} or C_{plasma}) at a given time point. The model also allows: (1) the mass of drug present in the region can be calculated by multiplying the concentration with its volume at a given time; and (2) the rate of drug elimination from the site can be calculated by the product of clearance times drug concentration.

Model simplicity using the well-stirred approach has advanced the concept of drug clearance and allowed practical drug concentration to be estimated based on body clearance and drug dose. The approach has generally provided more accurate dosing for many drugs for which drug action is determined mostly by steady-state concentration, and a transient change in concentration of short duration is not critical. However, caution should be exercised in interpreting model-predicted concentration to drug concentration at a given site in the body.

Arterial and Venous Differences in Drug Concentrations

Most pharmacokinetic studies are modeled based on blood samples drawn from various venous sites after either IV or oral dosing. Physiologists have long recognized the unique difference between arterial and venous blood. For example, arterial tension (pressure) of oxygen drives the distribution of oxygen to vital organs. Chiou (1989) and Mather (2001) have discussed the pharmacokinetic issues when differences in drug concentrations C_p in arterial and venous are observed. They question the validity of the assumption of the well-stirred condition or rapid mixing within the blood or plasma pool when there is gradual permeation into tissues in which the drug may then be metabolized. Indeed, some drug markers have shown that rapid mixing may not be typical, except when the drug is essentially confined to the blood pool due to protein binding.

Differences in arterial and venous blood levels ranging as high as several hundred fold for griseofulvin have been reported. Forty compounds have been shown to exhibit marked site dependence in plasma or blood concentration after dosing in both humans and animals. In some cases, differences are due mostly to large extraction of drug in poorly perfused local tissues, such as with nitroglycerin (3.8-fold arteriovenous difference) and procainamde (234% arteriovenous difference, venous being higher). The classical assumption in pharmacokinetics of rapid mixing within minutes in the entire blood circulation therefore may not be applicable to some drugs. Would the observed sampling differences result in significant difference in the AUCs between arterial and venous blood, or in prediction of toxicity or adverse effects of drugs? No such differences were observed in the reviews by Chiou and Mather, although the significance of these differences on drug therapy and toxicity has not been fully explored.

Frequently Asked Questions

▶ *Why are most of the plasma drug concentration data reported without indicating the sampling site when there is a substantial difference in arterial and venous blood drug concentrations for many drugs?*

▶ *Does the drug concentration in the terminal phase of the curve show less dependency on site of sampling?*

CHAPTER SUMMARY

The processes by which drugs transverse capillary membranes include passive diffusion and hydrostatic pressure. *Passive diffusion* is generally governed by Fick's law of diffusion. *Hydrostatic pressure* represents the pressure gradient between the arterial end of the capillaries entering the tissue and the venous capillaries leaving the tissue. Not all tissues have the same drug permeability. In addition, permeability of tissues may change under various disease states, such as inflammation.

Drug distribution can be *perfusion/flow limited* or diffusion/*permeability limited depending on the nature of the drug*. Drug distribution into cells is also controlled by efflux and influx transporters for some drugs. The factors that determine the distribution constant, k_d, of a drug into an organ are related to the blood flow to the organ, the volume of the organ, and the partitioning of the drug into the organ tissue, that is, $k_d = Q/VR$. The distribution half-life is inversely related to k_d.

The equation $t_{1/2} = 0.693(V_D/Cl)$ relates the elimination half-life to the apparent volume of distribution and clearance. A large apparent volume of distribution leads to low plasma drug concentrations making it harder to remove the drug by the kidney or liver. Mechanistically, a low plasma drug concentration may be due to (1) extensive distribution into tissues due to favorable lipophilicity, (2) extensive distribution into tissues due to protein binding in peripheral tissues, or (3) lack of drug plasma protein binding. The equation is the basis for considering that Cl and V_D are both independent variables in contrast to $Cl = kV_D$ which depicts Cl as proportional to V_D with a constant, k, specific for the drug.

Protein binding of a drug generally serves to retain the drug intravascularly, whereas tissue binding generally pulls the drug away from the vascular compartment. The two main proteins in the plasma that are involved in drug–protein binding are albumin and α_1-acid glycoprotein, AAG. AAG tends to bind mostly basic drugs. Protein-bound drugs are generally not considered to be pharmacodynamically active. Protein-bound drugs are slower to diffuse and are not eliminated easily. For highly extractable drugs, the bound drug may be dissociated

to the unbound drug in the liver for metabolism or in the kidney for excretion. These drugs are observed to have an ER $\gg f_u$.

The pathophysiologic condition of the patient can affect drug–protein binding. Drug–protein binding may be reduced in uremic patients and in patients with hepatic disease. During infection, stress, trauma, and severe burn, AAG levels may change and affect drug disposition.

Lipophilic (hydrophobic) drugs may accumulate in adipose or other tissues which have a good affinity for the drug.

The equation $V_{app} = V_p + V_t(f_u/f_{ut})$ defines V_{app} which is related to plasma volume, tissue volume, and fraction of free plasma and tissue drug in the body. The term V_{app} allows the amount of drug in the body to be calculated.

When a drug is tightly bound to a protein, only the unbound drug is assumed to be metabolized; drugs belonging to this category are described as restrictively eliminated. Some drugs may be eliminated even when they are protein bound and are described as nonrestrictively eliminated.

The extent of drug binding to protein may be determined by two common *in vitro* methods, ultrafiltration and equilibrium dialysis. The number of binding sites and the binding constant can be determined using a graphic technique called the Scatchard plot. A drug tightly bound to protein has a large association binding constant which is derived based on the law of mass action.

Based on a "well-stirred venous equilibration" model and hepatic clearance during absorption, many orally given drugs do not result in clinically significant changes in drug exposure when protein binding (ie, f_u) changes. The drug elimination rate increases in the liver when f_u (free drug fraction) is increased for many drugs given orally at doses below saturation. In contrast, drugs administered by IV injection and a few orally administered drugs can have significant changes in free drug concentration when protein binding changes. The clinical significance of changes in protein binding must be considered on individual drug basis and cannot be over generalized.

An important consideration regarding the effect of change in drug–protein binding is the pharmacodynamics (PD) of the individual drug involved, that is, how and where the drug exerts its action because drug penetration to the site of action is important. Recent reviews indicate that simple hepatic flow/intrinsic clearance-based analysis may sometimes be inadequate to predict drug effect due to protein-binding changes.

LEARNING QUESTIONS

1. Why is the zone of inhibition in an antibiotic disc assay larger for the same drug concentration ($10 \, \mu g/mL$) in water than in serum? See Fig. 11-23.
2. Determine the number of binding sites (n) and the association constant (K_a) from the following data using the Scatchard equation.

r	$(D \times 10^{-4} \, M)$	r/D
0.40	0.33	
0.80	0.89	
1.20	2.00	
1.60	5.33	

Can n and K_a have fractional values? Why?

3. Discuss the clinical significance of drug–protein binding on the following:
   a. Drug elimination
   b. Drug–drug interactions
   c. "Percent of drug-bound" data
   d. Liver disease
   e. Kidney disease
4. Vallner (1977) reviewed the binding of drugs to albumin or plasma proteins. The following data were reported:

Drug	Percent Drug Bound
Tetracycline	53
Gentamycin	70
Phenytoin	93
Morphine	38

Which drug listed above might be predicted to cause an adverse response due to the concurrent administration of a second drug such as sulfisoxazole (Gantrisin)? Why?

5. What are the main factors that determine the uptake and accumulation of a drug into tissues? Which tissues would have the most rapid drug uptake? Explain your answer.
6. As a result of edema, fluid may leave the capillary into the extracellular space. What effect does edema have on osmotic pressure in the blood and on drug diffusion into extracellular space?
7. Explain the effects of plasma drug–protein binding and tissue drug–protein binding on (a) the apparent volume of distribution and (b) drug elimination.
8. Naproxen (Naprosyn, Syntex) is a nonsteroidal anti-inflammatory drug (NSAID) that is highly bound to plasma proteins, >99%. Explain why the plasma concentration of free (unbound) naproxen increases in patients with chronic alcoholic liver disease and probably other forms of cirrhosis, whereas the total plasma drug concentration decreases.
9. Most literature references give an average value for the percentage of drug bound to plasma proteins.
   a. What factors influence the percentage of drug bound?

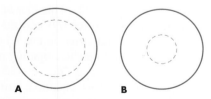

FIGURE 11-23   Antibiotic disc assay. **A.** Antibiotic in water ($10 \, \mu g/mL$). **B.** Antibiotic in serum ($10 \, \mu g/mL$).

b. How does renal disease affect the protein binding of drugs?

c. How does hepatic disease affect the protein binding of drugs?

10. It is often assumed that linear binding occurs at therapeutic dose. What are the potential risks of this assumption?

11. When a drug is 99% bound, it means that there is a potential risk of saturation. True or false?

12. Adenosine is a drug used for termination of tachycardia. The $t_{1/2}$ after IV dose is only 20 to 30 seconds according to product information. Suggest a reason for such a short half-life based on your knowledge of drug distribution and elimination.

ANSWERS

Frequently Asked Questions

How does a physical property, such as partition coefficient, affect drug distribution?

- *Partitioning* refers to the relative distribution of a drug in the lipid and aqueous phases. Generally, a high partition coefficient ($P_{oil/water}$) favors tissue distribution and leads to a larger volume of distribution. Partitioning is a major factor that, along with protein binding of a drug, determines drug distribution.

What are the causes of a long distribution half-life for a body organ if blood flow to the tissue is rapid?

- Generally, the long distribution half-life is caused by a tissue/organ that has a high drug concentration, due to either intracellular drug binding or high affinity for tissue distribution. Alternatively, the drug may be metabolized slowly within the tissue or the organ may be large and have a high capacity for organ uptake.

How long does it take for a tissue organ to be fully equilibrated with the plasma? How long for a tissue organ to be half-equilibrated?

- The distribution half-life determines the time it takes for a tissue organ to be equilibrated. It takes 4.32 distribution half-lives for the tissue organ to be 95% equilibrated and one distribution half-life for the drug to be 50% equilibrated. The concept is analogous to reaching steady state during drug infusion (see Chapter 5).

When a body organ is equilibrated with drug from the plasma, the drug concentration in that organ should be the same as that of the plasma. True or false?

- The answer is **False**. The free drug concentrations in the tissue and plasma are the same after equilibration, but the total drug concentration in the tissue is not the same as the total drug concentration in the plasma. The bound drug concentration may vary depending on local tissue binding or the lipid solubility of the drug. Many drugs have a long distributive phase due to tissue drug binding or lipid solubility. Drugs may equilibrate slowly into these tissues and then be slowly eliminated. Drugs with limited tissue affinity are easily equilibrated. Some examples of drugs with a long distributive phase are discussed in relation to the two-compartment model (see Chapter 5).

What is the parameter that tells when half of the protein-binding sites are occupied?

- The ratio, r, is defined as the ratio of the number of moles of drug bound to the number of moles of protein in the system. For a simple case of one binding site, r reflects the proportion of binding sites occupied; r is affected by (1) the association binding constant, (2) the free drug concentration, and (3) the number of binding sites per mole of protein. When $[D]$, or free drug concentration, is equal to 1 (or the dissociation constant K), the protein is 50% occupied for a drug with 1:1 binding according to Equation 11.19. (This can be verified easily by substituting for $[D]$ into the right side of the equation and determining r.) For a drug with n similar binding sites, binding occurs at the extent of 1:2 of bound drug:protein when $[D] = 1/[K_a(2n - 1)]$. This equation, however, reflects binding *in vitro* when drug concentration is not changing; therefore, its conclusions are somewhat limited.

Do all drugs that bind proteins lead to clinically significant interactions?

- No. For some drugs, protein binding does not affect the overall distribution of other drugs. Typically, if a drug is highly bound, there is an increased chance of a significant change in the fraction of free drug when binding is altered.

Which macromolecules participate in drug–protein binding?

- Albumin, α_1-acid glycoprotein, and lipoprotein. For some drugs and hormones, there may be a specific binding protein.

How does drug–protein binding affect drug elimination?

- Most drugs are assumed to be *restrictively bound,* and binding reduces drug clearance and elimination. However, some *nonrestrictively bound* drugs may be cleared easily. Changes in binding do not affect the rate of elimination of these drugs. Some drugs, such as some semisynthetic penicillins that are bound to plasma protein, may be actively secreted in the kidney. The elimination rates of these drugs are not affected by protein binding.

What are the factors to consider when adjusting the drug dose for a patient whose plasma protein concentration decreases to half that of normal?

- It is important to examine why the albumin level is reduced in the patient. For example, is the reduced albumin level due to uremia or hepatic dysfunction? In general, reduced protein binding will increase free drug concentration. Any change in drug clearance should be considered before reducing the dose, since the volume of distribution may be increased, partially offsetting the increase in free drug concentration.

How does one distinguish between the distribution phase and the elimination phase after an IV injection of a drug?

- In general, the early phase after an IV bolus dose is the distributive phase. The elimination phase occurs in the later phase, although distribution may continue for some drugs, especially for a drug with a long elimination half-life. The elimination phase is generally more gradual, since some drug may be returned to the blood from the tissues as drug is eliminated from the body.

Learning Questions

1. The zone of inhibition for the antibiotic in serum is smaller due to drug–protein binding.
2. Calculate $r/(D)$ versus r; then graph the results on rectangular coordinates.

r	$r/(D \times 10^4)$
0.4	1.21
0.8	0.90
1.2	0.60
1.6	0.30

The y intercept $= nK_a = 1.5 \times 10^4$.

The x intercept $= n = 2$.

Therefore,

$$K_a = 1.5 \times 10^4/2 = 0.75 \times 10^4$$

K_a may also be found from the slope.

8. The liver is important for the synthesis of plasma proteins. In chronic alcoholic liver disease or cirrhosis, fewer plasma proteins are synthesized in the liver, resulting in a lower plasma protein concentration. Thus, for a given dose of naproxen, less drug is bound to the plasma proteins, and the total plasma drug concentration is smaller.

10. Protein binding may become saturated at any drug concentration in patients with defective proteins or when binding sites are occupied by metabolic wastes generated during disease states (eg, renal disease). Diazoxide is an example of nonlinear binding at therapeutic dose.

11. The answer is **False**. The percent bound refers to the percent of total drug that is bound. The percent bound may be ≥99% for some drugs. Saturation may be better estimated using the Scatchard plot approach and by examining "r," which is the number of moles of drug bound divided by the number of moles of protein. When r is 0.99, most of the binding sites are occupied. The f_b, or fraction of bound drug, is useful for determining f_u, $f_u = 1 - f_b$.

12. Adenosine is extensively taken up by cells including the blood elements and the vascular endothelium. Adenosine is rapidly metabolized by deamination and/or is used as AMP in phosphorylation. Consequently, adenosine has a short elimination half-life.

REFERENCES

Anderson GD: Sex and racial differences in pharmacological response: Where is the evidence? Pharmacogenetics, pharmacokinetics, and pharmacodynamics. *J Women's Health* **14**(1), 19–29, 2005.

Andrew JD, Jeffrey L, Renae D, et al. Tissue accumulation of cephalothin in burns: A comparative study by microdialysis of subcutaneous interstitial fluid cephalothin concentrations in burn patients and healthy volunteers. *Antimicrobial Agents Chemotherapy* **53**(1): 210–215, January 2009.

Benet LZ, Hoener BA: Commentary: Changes in plasma protein binding have little clinical relevance. *Clin Pharm Ther* **71**:115–121, 2002.

Meibohm B, Beierle I, Derendorf H: How important are gender differences in pharmacokinetics? *Clin Pharmacokinet* **41**(5): 329–342, 2002.

Borondy P, Dill WA, Chang T, et al: Effect of protein binding on the distribution of 5,5-diphenylhydantoin between plasma and red cells. *Ann N Y Acad Sci* **226**:293, 1973.

Butler TC: The distribution of drugs. In LaDu BN, Mandel HG, Way EL (eds). *Fundamentals of Drug Metabolism and Disposition*. Baltimore, Williams & Wilkins, 1972.

Chan TY: Adverse interactions between warfarin and nonsteroidal anti-inflammatory drugs: Mechanism, clinical significance, and avoidance. *Ann Pharmacother* **29**:1274–1283, 1995.

Chien DS, Sandri RB, Tang-Liu DS: Systemic pharmacokinetics of acitretin, etretinate, isotretinoin, and acetylenic retinoids in guinea pigs. *Drug Metab Dispos* **20**(2):211–217, 1992.

Chiou WL: The phenomenon and rationale of marked dependence of drug concentration on blood sampling site: Implication in pharmacokinetics, pharmacodynamics, toxicology and therapeutics (Part I). *Clin Pharmacokinet* **17**(3):175–199; 275–290, 1989; Part II.

Cordoncardo C, O'Brien JP, Casals D, et al: Multidrug-resistance gene (P-glycoprotein) is expressed by endothelial cells at blood-brain barrier sites. *Proc Natl Acad Sci* **86**:695–698, January 1989.

Davison C: Protein binding. In LaDu BN, Mandel HG, Way EL (eds). *Fundamentals of Drug Metabolism and Drug Disposition*. Baltimore, Williams & Wilkins, 1971.

De Wolf AM, Fragen RJ, Avram MJ, Fitzgerald PC, Rahimi-Danesh F: The pharmacokinetics of dexmedetomidine in volunteers with severe renal impairment. *Anesth Analg* **93**: 1205–1209, 2001.

Goldstein A, Aronow L, Kalman SM: *Principles of Drug Action. The Basis of Pharmacology*, 2nd ed. New York, Wiley, 1974, p 166.

Greenblatt DJ, Sellers EM, Koch-Weser J: Importance of protein binding for the interpretation of serum or plasma drug concentration. *J Clin Pharmacol* **22**:259–263, 1982.

Holladay JW, Dewey MJ, Yoo SD: Steady state kinetics of imipramine in transgenic mice with elevated serum AAG levels. *Pharm Res* **13**(9):1313–1316, 1996.

Holladay JW, Dewey MJ, Michniak BB, et al: Elevated alpha-1-acid glycoprotein reduces the volume of distribution and systemic clearance of saquinavir. *Drug Metab Dispos* **29**(3): 299–303, 2001.

Houin G: Drug binding and apparent volume of distribution. In Tillement JP, Lindenlaub E (eds). *Protein Binding and Drug Transport*. Stuttgart, Schattauer, 1985.

Keller F, Maiga M, Neumayer HH, et al: Pharmacokinetic effects of altered plasma protein binding of drugs in renal disease. *Eur J Drug Metab Pharmacokinet* **9**:275–282, 1984.

Kim RB, Fromm MF, Wandel C, et al: The drug transporter P-glycoprotein limits oral absorption and brain entry of HIV-1 protease inhibitors. *J Clin Invest* **101**(2):289–294, 1998.

Kremer JMH, Wilting J, Janssen LHM: Drug binding to human alpha-1-acid glycoprotein in health and disease. *Pharmacol Rev* **40**:1–47, 1988.

Kruger EA, Figg WD: Protein binding alters the activity of Suramin, carboxyamidotriazole, and UCN-01 in an ex vivo rat aortic ring angiogenesis assay. *Clin Cancer Res* **7**:1867–1872, 2001.

Kuroha M, Son DS, Shimoda M: Effects of altered plasma alpha-1-acid glycoprotein levels on pharmacokinetics of some basic antibiotics in pigs: simulation analysis, *J Vet Pharmacol Ther* **24**(6):423–431, 2001.

Macfie AG, Magides AD, Reilly CS: Disposition of alfentanil in burns patients. *Br J Anaesth* **69**(5):447–450, 1992.

MacKichan JJ: Influence of protein binding. In Evans WE, Schentag JJ, Jusko WJ (eds). *Applied Pharmacokinetics—Principles of Drug Monitoring*, 3rd ed. Vancouver, WA, Applied Therapeutics, 1992, Chap 5.

Maeda Y, Funakoshi S, Nakamura M, et al: Possible mechanism for pharmacokinetic interaction between lidocaine and mexiletine. *Clin Pharmacol Ther* **71**(5):389–397, May 2002.

Mather LE: Anatomical-physioloical approach in pharmacokinetics and pharmacodynamics. *Clin Pharacokinet* **40**:707–722, 2001

Nilsen OG: Clinical pharmacokinetics of tenoxicam. *Clin Pharmacokinet* **26**(1):16–43, 1994.

Ochs HR, Greenblatt DJ, Kaschell HJ, Klehr U, Divoll M, Abernethy DR: Diazepam kinetics in patients with renal insufficiency or hyperthyroidism. *Br J Clin Pharmac* **12**:829–832, 1981.

O'Reilly RA: The binding of sodium warfarin to plasma albumin and its displacement by phenylbutazone. *Ann N Y Acad Sci* **226**:319–331, 1973.

Park MK, Ludden T, Arom KV, et al: Myocardial vs serum concentration in infants and children. *J Dis Child* **136:**418–420, 1982.

Qin XP, Xie HG, Wang W, et al: Effect of the gene dosage of CYP2C19 on diazepam metabolism in Chinese subjects. *Clinical Pharmacology and Therapeutics* **66:**642–646, 1999.

Reifell JA, Leahy EB, Drusin RE, et al: A previously unrecognized drug interaction between quinidine and digoxin. *Clin Cardiol* **2:**40–42, 1979.

Sadler BM, Gillotin C, Lou Y, Stein DS: In vivo effect of alpha(1)-acid glycoprotein on pharmacokinetics of amprenavir, a human immunodeficiency virus protease inhibitor. *Antimicrob Agents Chemother* **45:**852–856, 2001.

Sands CD, Chan ES, Welty TE: Revisiting the significance of warfarin protein-binding displacement interactions. *Ann Pharmacother* **36:**1642–1645, 2002.

Sawada Y, Hanano M, Sugiyama Y, Iga T: Prediction of the disposition of b-lactam antibiotics in human from pharmacokinetic parameters in animals. *J Pharmacokinet Biopharm* **12:**241–261, 1984.

Schmidt S, Gonzalez D, Derendorf H: Significance of protein binding in pharmacokinetics and pharmacodynamics. *J Pharm Sci* **99**(3):1107–1122, 2010.

Sellers EM, Koch-Weser J: Kinetics and clinical importance of displacement of warfarin from albumin by acidic drugs. *Ann N Y Acad Sci* **179:**213–223, 1971.

Sellers EM, Koch-Weser J: Influence of intravenous injection rate on protein binding and vascular activity of diazoxide. *Ann N Y Acad Sci* **226:**214–224, 1973.

Stoeckel K, Trueb V, Tuerk H: Minor changes in biological half-life of ceftriaxone in functionally anephric and liver diseased patients: Explanations and consequences. In Armengaud, Fernex (eds). *Long-Acting Cephalosporins: Ceftriaxone, Part 28. Proceedings of the 13th International Congress of Chemotherapy,* Vienna, 1983, pp 9–13.

Taheri S, Cogswell LP 3rd, Gent A, Strichartz GR: Hydrophobic and ionic factors in the binding of local anesthetics to the major variant of human alpha1-acid glycoprotein. *J Pharmacol Exp Ther* **304**(1):71–80, 2003.

Thorp JM: The influence of plasma proteins on the action of drugs. In Binns TB (ed). *Absorption and Distribution of Drugs.* Baltimore, Williams & Wilkins, 1964.

Tozer TN: Implications of altered plasma protein binding in disease states. In Benet LZ, Massoud N, Gambertoglio JG (eds). *Pharmacokinetic Basis for Drug Treatment.* New York, Raven, 1984.

Udall JA: Drug interference with warfarin therapy. *Clin Med* **77:**20, 1970.

Vallner JJ: Binding of drugs by albumin and plasma proteins. *J Pharm Sci* **66:**447–465, 1977.

Verbeeck RK, Wallace SM: Non-steroidal anti-inflammatory drugs: Restrictive or non-restrictive clearance? *Arzneim-Forsch* **44:**683–685 [Medline], 1994.

You G, Morris ME: *Drug Transporters: Molecular Characterization and Role in Drug Disposition.* Hoboken, NJ, John Wiley and Sons Ltd, Sep 2007.

BIBLIOGRAPHY

Anton AH, Solomon HM (eds): Drug protein binding. *Ann N Y Acad Sci* **226:**1–362, 1973.

Barza M, Samuelson T, Weinstein L: Penetration of antibiotics into fibrin loci in vivo, II. Comparison of nine antibiotics: Effect of dose and degree of protein binding. *J Infect Dis* **129:**66, 1974.

Bergen T: Pharmacokinetic properties of the cephalosporins. *Drugs* **34**(suppl 2):89–104, 1987.

Birke G, Liljedahl SO, Plantin LO, Wetterfors J: Albumin catabolism in burns and following surgical procedures. *Acta Chir Scand* **118:**353–366, 1959–1960.

Bridges JW, Wilson AGE: Drug–serum protein interactions and their biological significance. In Bridges JW, Chasseaud LF (eds). *Progress in Drug Research, Vol 1.* New York, Wiley, 1976.

Coffey CJ, Bullock FJ, Schoenemann PT: Numerical solution of nonlinear pharmacokinetic equations: Effect of plasma protein binding on drug distribution and elimination. *J Pharm Sci* **60:**1623, 1971.

D'Arcy PF, McElnay JC: Drug interactions involving the displacement of drugs from plasma protein and tissue binding sites. *Pharm Ther* **17:**211–220, 1982.

Gibaldi M, Levy G, McNamara PJ: Effect of plasma protein and tissue binding on the biologic half-life of drugs. *Clin Pharmacol Ther* **24:**1–4, 1978.

Gillette JR: Overview of drug-protein binding. *Ann N Y Acad Sci* **226:**6, 1973.

Grainger-Rousseau TJ, McElnay JC, Collier PS: The influence of disease on plasma protein binding of drugs. *Int J Pharm* **54:**1–13, 1989.

Hildebrandt P, Birch K, Mehlsen J: The relationship between the subcutaneous blood flow and the absorption of Lente type insulin. *Acta Endocrinol* **112**(suppl):275, 1986.

Holladay JW, Dewey MJ, Yoo SD: Pharmacokinetics and antidepressant activity of fluoxetine in transgenic mice with elevated serum alpha-1-acid glycoprotein levels. *Drug Metab Dispos* **26:**20–24, 1998.

Holladay JW, Dewey MJ, Yoo SD: Kinetic interaction between fluoxetine and imipramine as a function of elevated serum alpha-1-acid glycoprotein levels. *J Pharm Pharmacol* **50:**419–424, 1998.

Jusko WJ: Pharmacokinetics in disease states changing protein binding. In Benet LZ (ed). *The Effects of Disease States on Drug Pharmacokinetics.* Washington, DC, American Pharmaceutical Association, 1976.

Jusko WJ, Gretch M: Plasma and tissue protein binding of drugs in pharmacokinetics. *Drug Metab Rev* **5:**43–140, 1976.

Koch-Weser J, Sellers EM: Binding of drugs to serum albumin. *N Engl J Med* **294:**311, 1976.

Koch-Weser J, Sellers EM: Drug interactions with coumarin anticoagulants. *N Engl J Med* **285:**547–558, 1971.

Kunin CM, Craig WA, Kornguth M, Monson R: Influence of binding on the pharmacologic activity of antibiotics. *Ann N Y Acad Sci* **226:**214–224, 1973.

Levy RH, Moreland TA: Rationale for monitaring free drug levels. *Clin Pharmacokinet* **9**(suppl 1):1–91,1984.

Limbert M, Siebert G: Serum protein binding and pharmacokinetics of cephalosporins. In Tillement JP, Lindenlaub E (eds). *Protein Binding and Drug Transport*. Stuttgart, Schattauer, 1985.

MacKichan JJ: Pharmacokinetic consequences of drug displacement from blood and tissue proteins. *Clin Pharmacokinet* **9**(suppl 1):32–41, 1984.

Meijer DKF, van der Sluijs P: Covalent and noncovalent protein binding of drugs: Implication for hepatic clearance, storage and cell-specific drug delivery. *Pharm Res* **6:**105–118, 1989.

Meyer MC, Gutlman DE: The bindings of drugs by plasma proteins. *J Pharm Sci* **57:**895–918, 1968.

Oie S: Drug distribution and binding. *J Clin Pharmacol* **26:** 583–586, 1986.

Pardridge WM: Recent advances in blood–brain barrier transport. *Annu Rev Pharmacol Toxicol* **26:**25–39, 1988.

Rothschild MA, Oratz M, Schreiber SS: Albumin metabolism. *Gastroenterology* **64:**324–331, 1973.

Rowland M: Plasma protein binding and therapeutic monitoring. *Ther Drug Monitor* **2:**29–37, 1980.

Rowland M, Tozer TN: *Clinical Pharmacokinetics*. New York, Marcel Dekker, 1985, Chap 25.

Schmidt S, Gonzalez D, Derendorf H: Significance of protein binding in pharmacokinetics and pharmacodynamics. *J Pharm Sci* **99**(3):1107–1122, 2010.

Schuetz EG, Furuya KN, Schuetz JD. Interindividual variation in expression of P-glycoprotein in normal human liver and secondary hepatic neoplasms. *J Pharmacol Exp Ther* **275**(2): 1011–1018, 1995.

van Steeg TJ, Boralli VB, Krekels EH, et al: Influence of plasma protein binding on pharmacodynamics: Estimation of in vivo receptor affinities of beta blockers using a new mechanism-based PK-PD modelling approach. *J Pharm Sci* **98**(10):3816–3828, 2009.

Tillement JP, Houin G, Zini R, et al: The binding of drugs to blood plasma macromolecules: Recent advances and therapeutic significance. *Adv Drug Res* **13:**59–94, 1984.

Tillement JP, Lhoste F, Guidicelli JF: Diseases and drug protein binding. *Clin Pharmacokinet* **3:**144–154, 1978.

Tillement JP, Zini R, d'Athier P, Vassent G: Binding of certain acidic drugs to human albumin: Theoretical and practical estimation of fundamental parameters. *Eur J Clin Pharmacol* **7:**307–313, 1974.

Upton RN: Regional pharmacokinetics, I. Physiological and physicochemical basis. *Biopharm Drug Dispos* **11:**647–662, 1990.

Wandell M, Wilcox-Thole WL: Protein binding and free drug concentrations. In Mungall DR (ed). *Applied Clinical Pharmacokinetics*. New York, Raven, 1983, pp 17–48.

Zini R, Riant P, Barre J, Tillement JP: Disease-induced variations in plasma protein levels. Implications for drug dosage regimens (Parts 1 and 2). *Clin Pharmacokinet* **19:**147–159; 218–229, 1990.

12 Drug Elimination and Hepatic Clearance

He Sun and Hong Zhao

Chapter Objectives

▶ Describe the pathways for drug elimination in the body.

▶ Compare the clinical implications of hepatic and renal disease on drug therapy.

▶ Describe the role of hepatic blood flow, drug protein binding, and intrinsic clearance on hepatic clearance.

▶ Explain how the rate of drug elimination may change from first-order elimination to zero-order elimination and the clinical implications of this occurrence.

▶ Describe the biotransformation of drugs in the liver and which enzymatic processes are considered "phase I reactions" and "phase II reactions."

▶ List the organs involved in drug elimination and the significance of each.

▶ Discuss the relationship between metabolic pathways and enzyme polymorphisms on intrasubject variability and drug–drug interactions.

▶ Describe how the exposure of a drug is changed when coadministered with another drug that shares the same metabolic pathway.

ROUTE OF DRUG ADMINISTRATION AND EXTRAHEPATIC DRUG METABOLISM

The decline from peak plasma concentrations after drug administration results from drug elimination or removal by the body. The elimination of most drugs from the body involves the processes of both metabolism (biotransformation) and renal excretion (see Chapter 7). For many drugs, the principal site of metabolism is the liver. However, other tissues or organs, especially those tissues associated with portals of drug entry into the body, may also be involved in drug metabolism. These sites include the lung, skin, gastrointestinal mucosal cells, microbiological flora in the distal portion of the ileum, and large intestine. The kidney may also be involved in certain drug metabolism reactions.

Whether a change in drug elimination is more likely to be affected by renal disease, hepatic disease, or a drug–drug interaction may be predicted by measuring the fraction of the drug that is eliminated by either metabolism or excretion. Drugs that are highly metabolized (such as phenytoin, theophylline, and lidocaine) often demonstrate large intersubject variability in elimination half-lives and are dependent on the intrinsic activity of the biotransformation enzymes, which may vary by genetic and environmental factors. Intersubject variability in elimination half-lives is less for drugs that are eliminated primarily by renal drug excretion. Renal drug excretion is highly dependent on the *glomerular filtration rate* (GFR) and blood flow to the kidney. Since GFR is relatively constant among individuals with normal renal function, the elimination of drugs that are primarily excreted unchanged in the urine is also less variable.

First-Order Elimination

The rate constant of elimination (k) is the sum of the first-order rate constant for metabolism (k_m) and the first-order rate constant for excretion (k_e):

$$k = k_e + k_m \tag{12.1}$$

- ▶ Define Michaelis–Menton kinetics and capacity-mediated metabolism.

- ▶ Calculate drug and metabolite concentrations for drugs that undergo both hepatic and biliary elimination.

- ▶ Define first-pass metabolism and describe the relationship between first-pass metabolism and oral drug bioavailability.

- ▶ Use urine data to calculate fraction of drug excreted and metabolized.

- ▶ Explain how Michaelis–Menton kinetics can be used to determine the mechanism of enzyme inhibition and transporter inhibition.

- ▶ Describe biliary drug excretion and define enterohepatic drug elimination.

- ▶ Discuss the reasons why bioavailability is variable and can be less than 100%.

- ▶ Describe BDDCS—Biological Drug Disposition Classification System.

In practice, the excretion rate constant (k_e) is easily evaluated for drugs that are primarily renally excreted. Nonrenal drug elimination is usually assumed to be due for the most part to hepatic metabolism, though metabolism or degradation can occur in any organ or tissue that contains metabolic enzymes or is in a degradative condition. Therefore, the rate constant for metabolism (k_m) is difficult to measure directly and is usually obtained from the difference between k and k_e.

$$k_m = k - k_e$$

A drug may be biotransformed to several metabolites (metabolite A, metabolite B, metabolite C, etc); thus, the metabolism rate constant (k_m) is the sum of the rate constants for the formation of each metabolite:

$$k_m = k_{mA} + k_{mB} + k_{mC} + \cdots + k_{mI} \tag{12.2}$$

The relationship in this equation assumes that the process of metabolism is first order and that the substrate (drug) concentration is very low. Drug concentrations at therapeutic plasma levels for most drugs are much lower than the Michaelis–Menten constant, K_M, and do not saturate the enzymes involved in metabolism. Nonlinear Michaelis–Menten kinetics must be used when drug concentrations saturate metabolic enzymes (see also Chapter 21).

Because these rates of elimination at low drug concentration are considered first-order processes, the percentage of total drug metabolized may be obtained by the following expression:

$$\% \text{ drug metabolized} = \frac{k_m}{k} \times 100 \tag{12.3}$$

Fraction of Drug Excreted Unchanged (f_e) and Fraction of Drug Metabolized ($1 - f_e$)

For most drugs, the *fraction of dose eliminated unchanged* (f_e) and the fraction of dose eliminated as metabolites can be determined. For example, consider a drug that has two major metabolites and is also eliminated by renal excretion (Fig. 12-1). Assume that 100 mg of the drug was given to a patient and the drug was completely absorbed (bioavailability factor $F = 1$). A complete (cumulative) urine collection was obtained, and the quantities in parentheses in Fig. 12-1 indicate the amounts of each metabolite and unchanged drug that were recovered. The overall elimination half-life ($t_{1/2}$) for this drug was 2.0 hours ($k = 0.347$ h^{-1}).

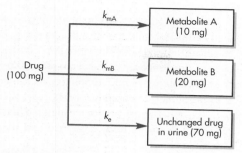

FIGURE 12-1 Model of a drug that has two major metabolites and is also eliminated by renal excretion.

To determine the renal excretion rate constant, the following relationship is used:

$$\frac{k_e}{k} = \frac{\text{total dose excreted in urine}}{\text{total dose absorbed}} = \frac{D_u^\infty}{FD_0} \quad (12.4)$$

where D_u^∞ is the total amount of unchanged drug recovered in the urine. In this example, k_e is found by proper substitution into Equation 12.4:

$$k_e = (0.347)\frac{70}{100} = 0.243 \text{ h}^{-1}$$

To find the percent of drug eliminated by renal excretion, the following approach may be used:

$$\% \text{ drug excretion} = \frac{k_e}{k} \times 100 = \frac{0.243}{0.347} \times 100 = 70\%$$

Alternatively, because 70 mg of unchanged drug was recovered from a total dose of 100 mg, the percent of drug excretion may be obtained by

$$\% \text{ drug excretion} = \frac{70}{100} \times 100 = 70\%$$

Therefore, the percent of drug metabolized is 100%–70%, or 30%.

For many drugs, the literature has approximate values for the fraction of drug (f_e) excreted unchanged in the urine. In this example, the value of k_e may be estimated from the literature values for the elimination half-life of the drug and f_e. Assuming that the elimination half-life of the drug is 2 hours and f_e is 0.7, then k_e is estimated by Equation 12.5.

$$k_e = f_e k \quad (12.5)$$

Because $t_{1/2}$ is 2 hours, k is 0.693/2 h = 0.347 h^{-1}, and k_e is

$$k_e = (0.7)(0.347) = 0.243 \text{ h}^{-1}$$

PRACTICAL FOCUS

The percentages of drug excreted and metabolised are clinically useful information. If the renal excretion pathway becomes impaired, as in certain kidney disorders, then less drug will be excreted renally and hepatic metabolism may become the primary drug elimination route. The reverse is true if liver function declines. For example, if in the above situation renal excretion becomes totally impaired ($k_e \approx 0$), the elimination $t_{1/2}$ can be determined as follows:

$$k = k_m + k_e$$

but

$$k_e \approx 0$$

Therefore,

$$k \approx k_m \approx 0.104 \text{ h}^{-1}$$

The new $t_{1/2}$ (assuming complete renal shutdown) is

$$t_{1/2} = \frac{0.693}{0.104} = 6.7 \text{ h}$$

In this example, renal impairment caused the drug elimination $t_{1/2}$ to be prolonged from 2 to 6.7 hours. Clinically, the dosage of this drug must be lowered to prevent the accumulation of toxic drug levels. Methods for adjusting the dose for renal impairment are discussed in Chapter 24.

HEPATIC CLEARANCE

The clearance concept may be applied to any organ and is used as a measure of drug elimination by the organ (see Chapter 7). *Hepatic clearance* may be defined as the volume of blood that perfuses the liver which is cleared of drug per unit of time. As discussed in Chapter 7, total body clearance is composed of all the clearances in the body:

$$Cl_T = Cl_{nr} + Cl_r \qquad (12.6)$$

where Cl_T is total body clearance, Cl_{nr} is nonrenal clearance (often equated with hepatic clearance, Cl_h), and Cl_r is renal clearance. Hepatic clearance (Cl_h) is also equal to total body clearance (Cl_T) minus renal clearance (Cl_R) assuming no other organ metabolism, as shown by rearranging Equation 12.6 to

$$Cl_h = Cl_T - Cl_R \qquad (12.6a)$$

EXAMPLES ▶▶▶

1. The total body clearance for a drug is 15 mL/min/kg. Renal clearance accounts for 10 mL/min/kg. What is the hepatic clearance for the drug?

Solution

Hepatic clearance = 15 – 10 = 5 mL/min/kg

Sometimes the renal clearance is not known, in which case hepatic clearance and renal clearance may be calculated from the percent of intact drug recovered in the urine.

2. The total body clearance of a drug is 10 mL/min/kg. The renal clearance is not known. From a urinary drug excretion study, 60% of the drug is recovered intact and 40% is recovered as metabolites. What is the hepatic clearance for the drug, assuming that metabolism occurs in the liver?

Solution

Hepatic clearance = total body clearance $\times (1 - f_e)$
$$(12.7)$$

where f_e = fraction of intact drug recovered in the urine.

Hepatic clearance = $10 \times (1 - 0.6) = 4$ mL/min/kg

In this example, the metabolites are recovered completely and hepatic clearance may be calculated as total body clearance times the percent of dose recovered as metabolites. Often, the metabolites are not completely recovered, thus precluding the accuracy of this approach. In this case, hepatic clearance is estimated as the difference between body clearance and renal clearance.

Extrahepatic Metabolism

A few drugs (eg, nitroglycerin) are metabolized extensively outside the liver. This is known as *extrahepatic metabolism*. A simple way to assess extrahepatic metabolism is to calculate hepatic (metabolic) and renal clearance of the drug and compare these clearances to total body clearance.

EXAMPLES ▶▶▶

1. Morphine clearance, Cl_T, for a 75-kg male patient is 1800 mL/min. After an oral dose, 4% of the drug is excreted unchanged in the urine ($f_e = 0.04$). The fraction of drug absorbed after an oral dose of morphine sulfate is 24% ($F = 0.24$). Hepatic blood flow is about 1500 mL/min. Does morphine have any extrahepatic metabolism?

Solution

Since $f_e = 0.04$, renal clearance $Cl_r = 0.04\ Cl_T$ and nonrenal clearance $Cl_{nr} = (1 - 0.04)\ Cl_T = 0.96\ Cl_T$. Therefore, $Cl_{nr} = 0.96 \times 1800$ mL/min = 1728 mL/min. Since hepatic blood flow is about 1500 mL/min, the drug appears to be metabolized faster than the rate of hepatic blood flow. Thus, at least some of the drug must be metabolized outside the liver. The low fraction of drug absorbed after an oral dose indicates that much of the drug is metabolized before reaching the systemic circulation.

2. Flutamide (Eulexin®, Schering), used to treat prostate cancer, is rapidly metabolized in humans to an active metabolite, α-hydroxyflutamide. The steady-state level is 51 ng/mL (range 24–78 ng/mL) after oral multiple doses of 250 mg of flutamide given 3 times daily or every 8 hours (maufacturer's approved label)*. Calculate the total body clearance and hepatic clearance assuming that flutamide is 90% metabolized, and is completely (100%) absorbed.

Solution

From Chapters 7 and 9, total body clearance, Cl_T, can be calculated by

$$Cl_T = \frac{FD_0}{C_{av}^{\infty}\tau}$$

$$Cl_T = \frac{250 \times 1,000,000}{51 \times 8}$$

$$= 6.127 \times 10^5 \text{ mL/h}$$

$$= 10,200 \text{ mL/min}$$

$$Cl_{nr} = 10,200 \text{ mL/min} \times 0.9$$

$$= 9180 \text{ mL/min}$$

The Cl_{nr} of flutamide is far greater than the rate of hepatic blood flow (about 1500 mL/min), indicating extensive extrahepatic clearance.

Frequently Asked Questions

▶ *How does the route of drug administration affect drug elimination?*

▶ *Why does the rate of drug elimination for some drugs change from first-order elimination to zero-order elimination?*

▶ *What organs are involved in drug elimination?*

▶ *How is zero- or first-order elimination processes related to either linear or nonlinear drug metabolism?*

ENZYME KINETICS—MICHAELIS–MENTEN EQUATION

The process of *biotransformation* or *metabolism* is the enzymatic conversion of a drug to a metabolite. In the body, the metabolic enzyme concentration is constant at a given site, and the drug (substrate) concentration may vary. When the drug concentration is low relative to the enzyme concentration, there are abundant enzymes to catalyze the reaction, and the rate of metabolism is a first-order process. Saturation of the enzyme usually occurs when the plasma drug concentration is relatively high, all the enzyme molecules become complexed with drug, and the reaction rate is at a maximum rate; the rate process then becomes a zero-order process (Fig. 12-2). The *maximum reaction rate* is known as V_{max}, and the substrate or drug concentration at which the reaction occurs at half the maximum rate corresponds to a composite parameter K_M. These two parameters determine the profile of a simple enzyme reaction rate at various drug concentrations. The relationship of these parameters is described by the *Michaelis–Menten* equation (see Chapter 13).

Enzyme kinetics generally considers that 1 mole of drug interacts with 1 mole of enzyme to form an enzyme–drug (ie, enzyme–substrate) intermediate. The enzyme–drug intermediate further reacts to yield a reaction product or a drug metabolite (Fig. 12-3). The rate process for drug metabolism is described by the Michaelis–Menten equation which assumes that the rate of an enzymatic reaction is dependent on

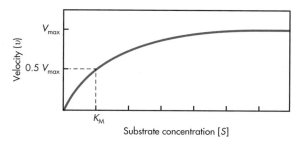

FIGURE 12-2 Michaelis–Menten enzyme kinetics. The hyperbolic relationship between enzymatic reaction velocity and the drug substrate concentration is described by Michaelis–Menten enzyme kinetics. The K_M is the substrate concentration when the velocity of the reaction is at $0.5V_{max}$.

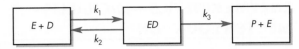

FIGURE 12-3 $[D]$ = drug; $[E]$ = enzyme; $[ED]$ = drug–enzyme intermediate; $[P]$ = metabolite or product; k_1, k_2, and k_3 = first-order rate constants. Brackets denote concentration.

the concentrations of both the enzyme and the drug and that an energetically favored drug–enzyme intermediate is initially formed, followed by the formation of the product and regeneration of the enzyme.

Each rate constant in Fig. 12-3 is a first-order reaction rate constant. The following rates may be denoted:

Rate of intermediate $[ED]$ formation = $k_1[E][D]$

Rate of intermediate $[ED]$ decomposition = $k_2[ED]$
$+ k_3[ED]$

$$\frac{d[ED]}{dt} = k_1[E][D] - k_2[ED] - k_3[ED]$$
$$\frac{d[ED]}{dt} = k_1[E][D] - (k_2 + k_3)[ED] \tag{12.8}$$

By mass balance, the total enzyme concentration $[E_t]$ is the sum of the free enzyme concentration $[E]$ and the enzyme–drug intermediate concentration $[ED]$:

$$[E_t] = [E] + [ED] \tag{12.9}$$

Rearranging,

$$[E] = [E_t] - [ED] \tag{12.10}$$

Substituting for $[E]$ in Equation 12.8,

$$\frac{d[ED]}{dt} = k_1([E_t] - [ED])[D] - (k_2 + k_3)[ED] \tag{12.11}$$

At steady state, the concentration $[ED]$ is constant with respect to time, because the rate of formation of the drug–enzyme intermediate equals the rate of decomposition of the drug–enzyme intermediate. Thus, $d[ED]/dt = 0$, and

$$k_1[E_t][D] = [ED](k_1[D] + (k_2 + k_3)) \tag{12.12}$$

$$[E_t][D] = [ED]\left([D] + \frac{k_2 + k_3}{k_1}\right) \tag{12.13}$$

Let

$$K_M = \frac{k_2 + k_3}{k_1} \tag{12.14}$$

$$[E_t][D] = [ED]([D] + K_M) \tag{12.15}$$

Solving for $[ED]$,

$$[ED] = \frac{[D][E_t]}{[D] + K_M} \tag{12.16}$$

Multiplying by k_3 on both sides,

$$\frac{k_3[E_t][D]}{[D] + K_M} = k_3[ED] \tag{12.17}$$

The *velocity* or rate (v) of the reaction is the rate for the formation of the product (metabolite) of the reaction, which is also the forward rate of decomposition of the enzyme–drug $[ED]$ intermediate (see Fig. 12-3).

$$v = k_3[ED] \tag{12.18}$$

When all the enzyme is saturated (ie, all the enzyme is in the form of the ED intermediate due to the large drug concentration), the reaction rate is dependent on the availability of free enzyme, and the reaction rate proceeds at zero-order maximum velocity, V_{max}.

$$V_{max} = k_3[E_t] \tag{12.19}$$

Therefore, the velocity of metabolism is given by the equation

$$v = \frac{V_{max}[D]}{[D] + K_M} \tag{12.20}$$

Equation 12.20 describes the rate of metabolite formation, or the *Michaelis–Menten equation*. The maximum velocity (V_{max}) corresponds to the rate when all available enzymes are in the form of the drug–enzyme (ED) intermediate. At V_{max}, the drug (substrate) concentration is in excess, and the forward reaction,

$k_3[ED]$, is dependent on the availability of more free enzyme molecules. The *Michaelis constant, K_M*, is defined as the substrate concentration when the velocity (v) of the reaction is equal to one-half the maximum velocity, or $0.5V_{max}$ (see Fig. 12-2). The K_M is a useful parameter that reveals the concentration of the substrate at which the reaction occurs at half V_{max}. In general, for a drug with a large K_M, a higher concentration will be necessary before saturation is reached.

The Michaelis–Menten equation assumes that one drug molecule is catalyzed sequentially by one enzyme at a time. However, enzymes may catalyze more than one drug molecule (multiple sites) at a time, which may be demonstrated *in vitro*. In the body, drug may be eliminated by enzymatic reactions (metabolism) to one or more metabolites and by the excretion of the unchanged drug via the kidney. In Chapter 13, the Michaelis–Menton equation is used for modeling drug conversion in the body.

The relationship of the rate of metabolism to the drug concentration is a nonlinear, hyperbolic curve (see Fig. 12-2). To estimate the parameters V_{max} and K_M, the reciprocal of the Michaelis–Menten equation is used to obtain a linear relationship.

$$\frac{1}{v} = \frac{K_M}{V_{max}} \frac{1}{[D]} + \frac{1}{V_{max}} \tag{12.21}$$

Equation 12.21 is known as the *Lineweaver–Burk equation*, in which K_M and V_{max} may be estimated from a plot of $1/v$ versus $1/[D]$ (Fig. 12-4). Although the Lineweaver–Burk equation is widely used, other rearrangements of the Michaelis–Menten equation have been used to obtain more accurate estimates of V_{max} and K_M. In Chapter 13, drug concentration [D] is replaced by C, which represents drug concentration in the body.

Frequently Asked Questions

▶ *How does one determine whether a drug follows Michaelis–Menton kinetics?*

▶ *When does the rate of drug metabolism approach V_{max}?*

▶ *What is the difference between v and V_{max}?*

Kinetics of Enzyme Inhibition

Many compounds (eg, cimetidine) may inhibit the enzymes that metabolize other drugs in the body. An inhibitor may decrease the rate of drug metabolism by several different mechanisms. The inhibitor may combine with a cofactor such as $NADPH_2$ needed for enzyme activity, interact with the drug or substrate, or interact directly with the enzyme. Enzyme inhibition may be reversible or irreversible. The mechanism of enzyme inhibition is usually classified by enzyme kinetic studies and observing changes in the K_M and V_{max} (see Fig. 12-4).

A
Competitive enzyme inhibition

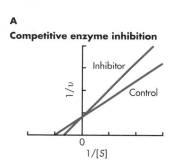

Noncompetitive enzyme inhibition

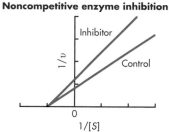

Uncompetitive enzyme inhibition

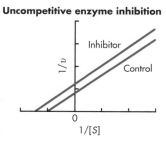

FIGURE 12-4 Relationship of substrate concentration alone or in the presence of an inhibitor. Lineweaver–Burk plots. The Lineweaver–Burk equation, which is the reciprocal of the Michaelis–Menten equation, is used to obtain estimates of V_{max} and K_M and to distinguish between various types of enzyme inhibition. [S] is the substrate concentration equal to [D] or drug concentration.

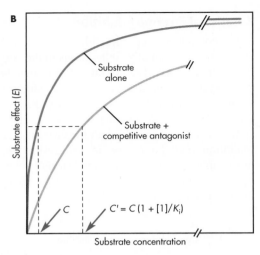

FIGURE 12-4   (*Continued*)

In the case of *competitive enzyme inhibition*, the inhibitor and drug–substrate compete for the same active site on the enzyme. The drug and the inhibitor may have similar chemical structures. An increase in the drug (substrate) concentration may displace the inhibitor from the enzyme and partially or fully reverse the inhibition. Competitive enzyme inhibition is usually observed by a change in the K_M, but the V_{max} remains the same.

The equation for competitive inhibition is, in the presence of an inhibitor, the reaction velocity V_I given by Equation 12.22.

$$V_I = \frac{V_{max}[D]}{[D] + K_M(1 + [I]/K_i)} \qquad (12.22)$$

where $[I]$ is the inhibitor concentration and is the dissociation constant of the inhibitor which can be determined experimentally. For a competitive reaction as shown in Fig. 12-5, K_i is k_{-1}/k_{+I}.

In *noncompetitive enzyme inhibition*, the inhibitor may inhibit the enzyme by combining at a site on the enzyme that is different from the active site (ie, an *allosteric site*). In this case, enzyme inhibition depends only on the inhibitor concentration. In noncompetitive enzyme inhibition, K_M is not altered, but V_{max} is lower. Noncompetitive enzyme inhibition

cannot be reversed by increasing the drug concentration, because the inhibitor will interact strongly with the enzyme and will not be displaced by the drug. The reaction velocity in the presence of a noncompetitive inhibitor is given by Equation 12.23

For a Noncompetitive reaction,

$$V_i = \frac{V_{max}[D]}{(1 + [I]/K_i)([D] + K_M)} \qquad (12.23)$$

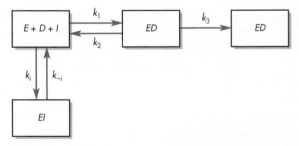

FIGURE 12-5   Diagram showing competitive inhibition of an enzyme [E] or a macromolecule (eg, a transport protein) with an inhibitor [I], respectively, $K_i = k_{-i}/k_i$, or [D] refers to the substrate concentration (ie, [D]). In the case of an interaction with a macromolecule, [D] is referred to as ligand concentration [E] would correspond to the macromolecule concentration.

Equation (12.23b) relates K_i to $[D]$, K_M and $[I]$ for a general competitive reaction. V_i and V are the reaction velocity with and without inhibitor present.

$$K_i = \frac{[I]}{\left(\dfrac{[D]}{K_M}+1\right)\left(\dfrac{V}{V_i}-1\right)} \qquad (12.23a)$$

Experimentally, IC_{50} is determined at 50% inhibition. V_i and V are the velocity with and without inhibitor, ie, $V_i/V = 2/1$. Substituting into Equation (12.23a) for $V_i/V = 2/1$ yields the familiar Chang–Prusoff equation in the next section.

$$K_i = \frac{IC_{50}}{\left(\dfrac{[D]}{K_M}+1\right)} \qquad (12.23b)$$

Other types of enzyme inhibition, such as mixed enzyme inhibition and enzyme uncompetitive inhibition, have been described by observing changes in K_M and V_{max}.

CLINICAL EXAMPLE

Pravastatin sodium (Pravachol®) is an HMG-CoA reductase inhibitor ("statin") which reduces cholesterol biosynthesis, thereby reducing cholesterol. The FDA-approved label states, "The risk of myopathy during treatment with another HMG-CoA reductase inhibitor is increased with concurrent therapy with either erythromycin, cyclosporine, niacin, or fibrates." However, neither myopathy nor significant increases in CPK levels have been observed in three reports involving a total of 100 post-transplant patients (24 renal and 76 cardiac) treated for up to 2 years concurrently with pravastatin 10–40 mg and cyclosporine." Pravastatin, like other HMG-CoA reductase inhibitors, has variable bioavailability. The coefficient of variation (CV), based on between-subject variability, was 50% to 60% for AUC. Based on urinary recovery of radiolabeled drug, the average oral absorption of pravastatin is 34% and absolute bioavailability is 17%. Pravastatin undergoes extensive first-pass extraction in the liver (extraction ratio 0.66), which is its primary site of action, and the primary site of cholesterol synthesis and of LDL-C clearance.

- How does cyclosporine change the pharmacokinetics of pravastatin?
- Is pravastatin uptake involved?

Solution

Pravastatin and other statins have variable inter- and intraindividual pharmacokinetics after oral dosing due to a large first-pass effect. A drug that is metabolized and also subject to the efflux effect of hepatic transporters can affect overall plasma drug concentrations and liver drug concentrations. It is important to examine the drug dose used in the patient and carefully assess if the dose range is adequately documented by clinical data in a similar patient population, especially if an inhibitor is involved. Finally, it is important to understand the pharmacokinetics, pharmacodynamics, and risk-benefit involved for the drug. Plasma drug concentrations are **NOT** the only consideration. An oversimplification is often assumed by considering only AUC and C_{max} (ie, drug bioavailability). In this example, the site of action is in the liver. The therapeutic goal should always be to optimize drug concentrations at the site of action and to avoid or minimize drug exposure at unintended sites where adverse effects occur. In this case, adverse drug reaction, ADR, occurs at the heart (eg, myopathy)*. Whenever possible, a critical drug–drug interaction, DDI, should be avoided or minimized with a washout period during drug coadministration. Alternative therapeutic agents with less liability for DDI may be recommended to clinicians if feasible. A very useful integrated approach and model was recently published about hepatic drug level of pravastatin. Watanabe et al (2009) discussed the simulated plasma concentrations of pravastatin with a detailed physiological model in human and animals. Sensitivity analyses showed that changes in the hepatic uptake ability altered the plasma concentration of pravastatin markedly but had a minimal effect on the liver concentration, whereas changes in canalicular efflux altered the liver concentration of pravastatin markedly but had a small

---

*Myopathy is not necessarily limited to the heart. In medicine, a *myopathy* is a muscular disease in which the muscle fibers do not function for any one of many reasons, resulting in muscular weakness.

effect on the plasma concentration. In conclusion, the model allowed the prediction of the disposition of pravastatin in humans.

This study suggested that changes in the OATP1B1 (transporter) activities may have a small impact on the therapeutic efficacy and a large impact on the side effect (myopathy) of pravastatin, respectively, whereas changes in MRP2 activities may have opposite impacts (ie, large effect on efficacy and small impact on side effect).

Kinetics of Enzymatic Inhibition or Macromolecule-Binding Inhibition *In Vitro*

When an interaction involves competitive inhibition of an enzyme $[E]$ or a macromolecule (eg, a transport protein with an inhibitor $[I]$ as shown in Fig. 12-5), *in vitro* screening assays are commonly used to evaluate potential inhibitors of enzymatic activity or macromolecule-ligand binding. IC_{50} is the total inhibitor concentration that reduces enzymatic or macromolecule-ligand binding activities by 50% (IC_{50}). However, measured IC_{50} values depend on concentrations of the enzyme (or target macromolecule), the inhibitor, and the substrate (or ligand) along with other experimental conditions. An accurate determination of the K_i value requires an intrinsic, thermodynamic quantity that is independent of the substrate (ligand) but depends on the enzyme and inhibitor. The relationship for various types of drug binding may be complex. Cer et al (2009) developed a software for computation of K_i for various types of inhibitions from IC_{50} measurements.

IC_{50} and Affinity

The relationship between the 50% inhibition concentration and the inhibition constant is given by the *Cheng–Prusoff* equation below:

$$K_i = \frac{IC_{50}}{\left(\dfrac{[D]}{K_M}+1\right)} \qquad (12.23b)$$

where K_i shows the binding affinity of the inhibitor, IC_{50} is the functional strength of the inhibitor, $[D]$ is substrate (drug) concentration. Equation 12.23b was published by Cheng and Prusoff in 1973. From Equation 12.23b, when $[D]$ is $<< K_M$, $K_i = IC_{50}$. When $[D] = K_M$, $K_i = IC_{50}/2$.

Whereas the IC_{50} value for a compound may vary between experiments depending on experimental conditions, the K_i is an absolute value. K_i is the inhibition constant of the inhibitor; the concentration of competing ligand in a competition assay which would occupy 50% of the enzyme if no ligand was present. Pharmacologists often use this relationship to determine the K_i of a competitive inhibitor on an enzyme or a macromolecule such as a transporter. Since there are many drug inhibition interactions, it is important to consider the ratio of inhibition concentration (eg, steady-state plasma concentration *in vivo* to the IC_{50}). In general, if $[I]/IC_{50} > 0.1$, the interaction involved should be investigated during early drug development in order to understand the important interaction issue and assess how significant the potential interaction might be clinically. Information on how to study drug metabolism inhibition/induction during development is available on the FDA web. Sub-class of CYP enzymes and transporters are also updated for DDI information (see FDA reference).

Metabolite Pharmacokinetics for Drugs That Follow a One-Compartment Model

The one-compartment model may be used to estimate simultaneously both metabolite formation and drug decline in the plasma. For example, a drug is given by intravenous bolus injection and then metabolized by parallel pathways (Fig. 12-6). Assume that both metabolite formation and metabolite and parent drug elimination follow linear (first-order) pharmacokinetics at therapeutic concentrations. The elimination rate constant and the volume of distribution for each metabolite and the parent drug are obtained from curve fitting of the plasma drug concentration–time and each metabolite concentration–time curve. If purified metabolites are available, each metabolite

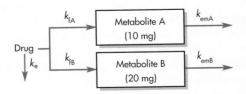

FIGURE 12-6   Parallel pathway for the metabolism of a drug to metabolite A and metabolite B. Each metabolite may be excreted and/or further metabolized.

should be administered IV separately, to verify the pharmacokinetic parameters independently.

The rate of elimination of the metabolite may be faster or slower than the rate of formation of the metabolite from the drug. Generally, metabolites such as glucuronide, sulfate, or glycine conjugates are more polar or more water soluble than the parent drug and will be eliminated more rapidly than the parent drug. Therefore, the rate of elimination of each of these metabolites is relatively more rapid than the rate of formation. In contrast, if the drug is acetylated or metabolized to a less polar or less water-soluble metabolite, then the rate of elimination of the metabolite is relatively slower than the rate of formation of the metabolite. In this case, metabolite accumulation will occur.

Compartment modeling of drug and metabolites is relatively simple and practical. The major shortcoming of compartment modeling is the lack of realistic physiologic information when compared to more sophisticated models that take into account spatial location of enzymes and flow dynamics. However, compartment models are useful for predicting drug and metabolite plasma levels.

For a drug given by IV bolus injection, the metabolite concentration exhibiting linear pharmacokinetics may be predicted from the following equation:

$$C_m = \frac{k_f D_0}{V_m (k_f - k_{em})} (e^{-k_{em}t} - e^{-k_f t}) \qquad (12.24)$$

where C_m is the metabolite concentration in plasma, k_{em} is the metabolite elimination rate constant, k_f is the metabolite formation rate constant, V_m is the metabolite volume of distribution, D_0 is the dose of drug, and V_D is the apparent volume of distribution of drug. All rate constants are first order.

PRACTICE PROBLEM

A drug is eliminated primarily by biotransformation (metabolism) to a glucuronide conjugate and a sulfate conjugate. A single dose (100 mg) of the drug is given by IV bolus injection, and all elimination processes of the drug follow first-order kinetics. The V_D is 10 L and the elimination rate constant for the drug is 0.9 h⁻¹. The rate constant (k_f) for the formation of the glucuronide conjugate is 0.6 h⁻¹, and the rate constant for the formation of the sulfate conjugate is 0.2 h⁻¹.

a. Predict the drug concentration 1 hour after the dose.

b. Predict the concentration of glucuronide and sulfate metabolites 1 hour after the dose, if the V_m for both metabolites is the same as for the parent drug and the k_{em} for both metabolites is 0.4 h⁻¹. (*Note:* V_m and k_{em} usually differ between metabolites and parent drug.) In this example, V_m and k_{em} are assumed to be the same for both metabolites, so that the concentration of the two metabolites may be compared by examining the formation constants.

Solution

The plasma drug concentration 1 hour after the dose may be estimated using the following equation for a one-compartment model, IV bolus administration:

$$C_p = C_p^0 e^{-kt} = \frac{D_0}{V_D} e^{-kt}$$

$$C_p = \frac{100}{10} e^{-(0.9)(1)} = 4.1 \text{ mg/L}$$

The plasma concentrations for the glucuronide and sulfate metabolites 1 hour postdose are estimated after substitution into Equation 12.24.

Glucuronide: $C_m = \frac{(0.6)(100)}{10(0.6 - 0.4)} (e^{-(0.4)(1)} - e^{-(0.6)(1)})$

$$C_m = 3.6 \text{ mg/L}$$

Sulfate: $C_m = \frac{(0.2)(100)}{10(0.2 - 0.4)} (e^{-(0.4)(1)} - e^{-(0.2)(1)})$

$$C_m = 1.5 \text{ mg/L}$$

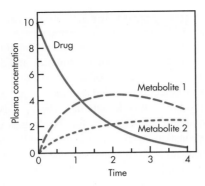

FIGURE 12-7   Simulation showing an IV bolus with formation of two metabolites.

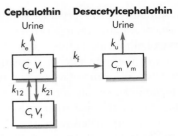

FIGURE 12-8   Pharmacokinetic model of cephalothin and desacetylcephalothin (metabolite) after an IV bolus dose.

After an IV bolus dose of a drug, the equation describing metabolite concentration formation and elimination by first-order processes is kinetically analogous to drug absorption after oral administration (see Chapter 8). Simulated plasma concentration–time curves were generated using Equation 12.24 for the glucuronide and sulfate metabolites, respectively (Fig. 12-7). The rate constant for the formation of the glucuronide is faster than the rate constant for the formation of the sulfate. Therefore, the time for peak plasma glucuronide concentrations is shorter compared to the time for peak plasma sulfate conjugate concentrations. Equation 12.24 cannot be used if drug metabolism is nonlinear because of enzyme saturation (ie, if metabolism follows Michaelis–Menten kinetics).

Metabolite Pharmacokinetics for Drugs That Follow a Two-Compartment Model

Cephalothin is an antibiotic drug that is metabolized rapidly by hydrolysis in both humans and rabbits. The metabolite desacetylcephalothin has less antibiotic activity than the parent drug. In urine, 18% to 33% of the drug was recovered as desacetylcephalothin metabolite in a human. The time course of both the drug and the metabolite may be predicted after a given dose from the distribution kinetics of both the drug and the metabolite. Cephalothin follows a two-compartment model after IV bolus injection in a rabbit, whereas the desacetylcephalothin metabolite follows a one-compartment model (Fig. 12-8).

After a single IV bolus dose of cephalothin (20 mg/kg) to a rabbit, cephalothin declines as a result of excretion and metabolism to desacetylcephalothin. The plasma levels of both cephalothin and desacetylcephalothin may be calculated using equations based on a model with linear metabolism and excretion.

The equations for cephalothin plasma and tissue levels are the same as those derived in Chapter 5 for a simple two-compartment model, except that the elimination constant k for the drug now consists of $k_e + k_f$, representing the rate constants for parent drug excretion and metabolite formation constant, respectively.

$$C_p = D_0 \left[\frac{k_{21} - a}{V_p(b-a)} e^{-at} + \frac{k_{21} - b}{V_p(a-b)} e^{-bt} \right] \quad (12.25)$$

$$C_t = D_0 \left[\frac{k_{12}}{V_t(b-a)} e^{-at} + \frac{k_{12}}{V_t(a-b)} e^{-bt} \right] \quad (12.26)$$

$$a + b = k + k_{12} + k_{21} \quad (12.27)$$

$$ab = kk_{21} \quad (12.28)$$

$$k = k_f + k_e \quad (12.29)$$

The equation for metabolite plasma concentration, C_m, is triexponential, with three preexponential coefficients (C_5, C_6, and C_7) calculated from the various kinetic constants, V_m, and the dose of the drug.

$$C_m = C_5 e^{-k_u t} + C_6 e^{-at} + C_7 e^{-bt} \quad (12.30)$$

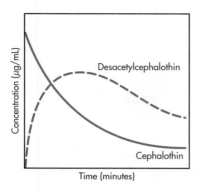

FIGURE 12-9 Formation of desacetylcephalothin from cephalothin in the rabbit after an IV bolus dose of cephalothin.

TABLE 12-1 Distribution of Cytochrome P-450 and Glutathione S-Transferase in the Rat

Tissue	CYT P-450[a]	GSH Transferase[b]
Liver	0.73	599
Lung	0.046	61
Kidney	0.135	88
Small intestine	0.042	103
Colon	0.016	—[c]
Skin	0.12	—[c]
Adrenal gland	0.5	308

[a]Cytochrome P-450, nmole/mg microsome protein.

[b]Glutathione S-transferase, nmole conjugate formed/min/mg cytosolic protein.

[c]Values not available.

Data from Wolf (1984).

$$C_5 = \frac{k_f D_0 k_{21} - k_f D_0 k_u}{V_m (b - k_u)(a - k_u)} \qquad (12.31)$$

$$C_6 = \frac{k_f D_0 k_{21} - k_f D_0 a}{V_m (b - a)(k_u - a)} \qquad (12.32)$$

$$C_7 = \frac{k_f D_0 k_{21} - k_f D_0 b}{V_m (k_u - b)(a - b)} \qquad (12.33)$$

For example, after the IV administration of cephalothin to a rabbit, both metabolite and plasma cephalothin concentration may be fitted to Equations 12.25 and 12.30 simultaneously (Fig. 12-9), with the following parameters obtained using a regression computer program (all rate constants in min^{-1}).

$k_{12} = 0.052$	$k_{21} = 0.009$	$V_m = 285$ mL/kg
$k_u = 0.079$	$k = 0.067$	$D_0 = 20$ mg/kg
$k_f = 0.045$	$V_p = 548$ mL/kg	$k_e = 0.022$

ANATOMY AND PHYSIOLOGY OF THE LIVER

The liver is the major organ responsible for drug metabolism. However, intestinal tissues, lung, kidney, and skin also contain appreciable amounts of biotransformation enzymes, as reflected by animal data (Table 12-1). Metabolism may also occur in other tissues to a lesser degree depending on drug properties and route of drug administration.

The liver is both a synthesizing and an excreting organ. The basic anatomical unit of the liver is the liver lobule, which contains parenchymal cells in a network of interconnected lymph and blood vessels. The liver consists of large right and left lobes that merge in the middle. The liver is perfused by blood from the hepatic artery; in addition, the large hepatic portal vein that collects blood from various segments of the GI tract also perfuses the liver (Fig. 12-10). The hepatic artery carries oxygen to the liver and accounts for about 25% of the liver blood supply. The hepatic portal vein carries nutrients to the liver and accounts for about 75% of liver blood flow. The terminal branches of the hepatic artery and portal vein fuse within the liver and mix with the large vascular capillaries known as *sinusoids* (Fig. 12-11). Blood leaves the liver via the hepatic vein, which empties into the vena cava (see Fig. 12-10). The liver also secretes bile acids within the liver lobes, which flow through a network of channels and eventually empty into the common bile duct (Figs. 12-11 and 12-12). The common bile duct drains bile and biliary excretion products from both lobes into the gallbladder.

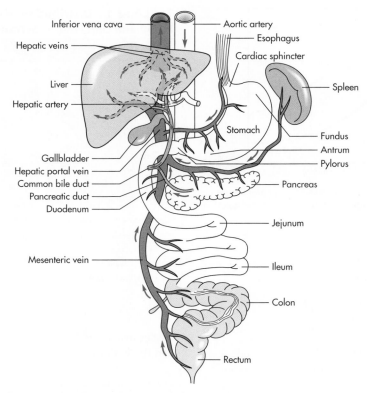

FIGURE 12-10   The large hepatic portal vein that collects blood from various segments of the GI tract also perfuses the liver.

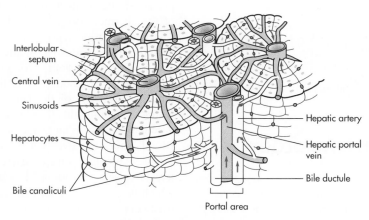

FIGURE 12-11   Intrahepatic distribution of the hepatic and portal veins.

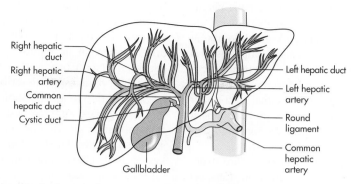

FIGURE 12-12   Intrahepatic distribution of the hepatic artery, portal vein, and biliary ducts. (From Lindner HH. *Clinical Anatomy.* Norwalk, CT, Appleton & Lange, 1989, with permission.)

Although the principal sites of liver metabolism are the hepatocytes, drug transporters are also present in the hepatocyte besides CYP isoenzymes. Transporters can efflux drug either in or out of the hepatocytes, thus influencing the rate of metabolism. In addition, drug transporters are also present in the bile canaliculi which can eliminate drug by efflux.

Sinusoids are blood vessels that form a large reservoir of blood, facilitating drug and nutrient removal before the blood enters the general circulation. The sinusoids are lined with endothelial cells, or *Kupffer cells.* Kupffer cells are phagocytic tissue macrophages that are part of the *reticuloendothelial system* (RES). Kupffer cells engulf worn-out red blood cells and foreign material.

Drug metabolism in the liver has been shown to be *flow* and *site dependent.* Some enzymes are reached only when blood flow travels from a given direction. The quantity of enzyme involved in metabolizing drug is not uniform throughout the liver. Consequently, changes in blood flow can greatly affect the fraction of drug metabolized. Clinically, hepatic diseases, such as cirrhosis, can cause tissue fibrosis, necrosis, and hepatic shunt, resulting in changing blood flow and changing bioavailability of drugs (see Chapter 24). For this reason, and in part because of genetic differences in enzyme levels among different subjects and environmental factors, the half-lives of drugs eliminated by drug metabolism are generally very variable.

A pharmacokinetic model simulating hepatic metabolism should involve several elements, including the heterogenicity of the liver, the hydrodynamics of hepatic blood flow, the nonlinear kinetics of drug metabolism, and any unusual or pathologic condition of the subject. Most models in practical use are simple or incomplete models, however, because insufficient information is available about an individual patient. For example, the average hepatic blood flow is usually cited as 1.3–1.5 L/min. Hepatic arterial blood flow and hepatic venous (portal) blood enter the liver at different flow rates, and their drug concentrations are different. It is possible that a toxic metabolite may be transiently higher in some liver tissues and not in others. The pharmacokinetic challenge is to build models that predict regional (organ) changes from easily accessible data, such as plasma drug concentration.

HEPATIC ENZYMES INVOLVED IN THE BIOTRANSFORMATION OF DRUGS

Mixed-Function Oxidases

The liver is the major site of drug metabolism, and the type of metabolism is based on the reaction involved. Oxidation, reduction, hydrolysis, and conjugation are the most common reactions, as discussed under phase I and phase II reactions in the next two sections. The enzymes responsible for oxidation and reduction of drugs (*xenobiotics*) and certain natural metabolites, such as steroids, are monoxygenase enzymes known as *mixed-function oxidases* (MFOs). The hepatic parenchymal cells contain MFOs in association with the *endoplasmic reticulum,* a network of lipoprotein membranes within the cytoplasm and continuous with the cellular and nuclear membranes. If hepatic parenchymal cells are fragmented and differentially centrifuged in an ultracentrifuge, a microsomal fraction, or *microsome,* is obtained from the postmitochondrial supernatant. The microsomal fraction contains fragments of the endoplasmic reticulum.

The mixed-function oxidase enzymes are structural enzymes that constitute an electron-transport system that requires reduced NADPH ($NADPH_2$), molecular oxygen, cytochrome P-450, NADPH–cytochrome P-450 reductase, and phospholipid. The phospholipid is involved in the binding of the drug molecule to the cytochrome P-450 and coupling the NADPH–cytochrome P-450 reductase to the cytochrome P-450. Cytochrome P-450 is a heme protein with iron protoporphyrin IX as the prosthetic group. Cytochrome P-450 is the terminal component of an electron-transfer system in the endoplasmic reticulum and acts as both an oxygen- and a substrate-binding locus for drugs and endogenous substrates in conjunction with a flavoprotein reductase, NADPH–cytochrome P-450 reductase. Many lipid-soluble drugs

bind to cytochrome P-450, resulting in oxidation (or reduction) of the drugs. Cytochrome P-450 consists of closely related isoenzymes (*isozymes*) that differ somewhat in amino acid sequence and drug specificity (see Chapter 13). A general scheme for MFO drug oxidation is described in Fig. 12-13.

In addition to the metabolism of drugs, the CYP monooxygenase enzyme system catalyzes the biotransformation of various endogenous compounds such as steroids. The CYP monooxygenase enzyme system is also located in other tissues such as kidney, GI tract, skin, and lungs.

A few enzymatic oxidation reactions involved in biotransformation do not include the CYP monooxygenase enzyme system. These include monoamine oxidase (MAO) that deaminates endogenous substrates including neurotransmitters (dopamine, serotonin, norepinephrine, epinephrine, and various drugs with a similar structure); alcohol and aldehyde dehydrogenase in the soluble fraction of liver are involved in the metabolism of ethanol and xanthine oxidase which converts hypoxanthine to xanthine and then to uric acid. Drug substrates for xanthine oxidase include theophylline and 6-mercaptopurine. Allopurinol is a substrate and inhibitor of xanthine oxidase and also delays metabolism of other substrates used in the treatment of gout.

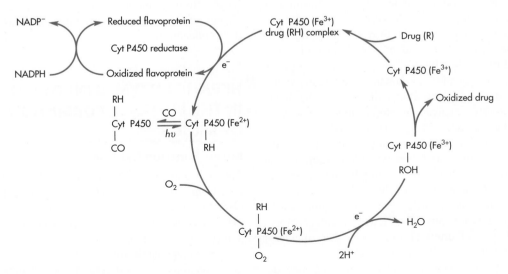

FIGURE 12-13   Electron flow pathway in the microsomal drug-oxidizing system. (From Alvares and Pratt, 1990, with permission.)

DRUG BIOTRANSFORMATION REACTIONS

The hepatic biotransformation enzymes play an important role in the inactivation and subsequent elimination of drugs that are not easily cleared through the kidney. For these drugs—theophylline, phenytoin, acetaminophen, and others—there is a direct relationship between the rate of drug metabolism (*biotransformation*) and the elimination half-life for the drug.

For most biotransformation reactions, the metabolite of the drug is more polar than the parent compound. The conversion of a drug to a more polar metabolite enables the drug to be eliminated more quickly than if the drug remained lipid soluble. A lipid-soluble drug crosses cell membranes and is easily reabsorbed by the renal tubular cells, exhibiting a consequent tendency to remain in the body. In contrast, the more polar metabolite does not cross cell membranes easily, is filtered through the glomerulus, is not readily reabsorbed, and is more rapidly excreted in the urine.

Both the nature of the drug and the route of administration may influence the type of drug metabolite formed. For example, isoproterenol given orally forms a sulfate conjugate in the gastrointestinal mucosal cells, whereas after IV administration, it forms the 3-*O*-methylated metabolite via *S*-adenosylmethionine and catechol-*O*-methyltransferase. Azo drugs such as sulfasalazine are poorly absorbed after oral administration. However, the azo group of sulfasalazine is cleaved by the intestinal microflora, producing 5-aminosalicylic acid and sulfapyridine, which is absorbed in the lower bowel.

The biotransformation of drugs may be classified according to the pharmacologic activity of the metabolite or according to the biochemical mechanism for each biotransformation reaction. For most drugs, biotransformation results in the formation of a more polar metabolite(s) that is pharmacologically inactive and is eliminated more rapidly than the parent drug (Table 12-2).

TABLE 12-2   Biotransformation Reactions and Pharmacologic Activity of the Metabolite

Reaction		Example
Active Drug to Inactive Metabolite		
Amphetamine	Deamination →	Phenylacetone
Phenobarbital	Hydroxylation →	Hydroxyphenobarbital
Active Drug to Active Metabolite		
Codeine	Demethylation →	Morphine
Procainamide	Acetylation →	*N*-acetylprocainamide
Phenylbutazone	Hydroxylation →	Oxyphenbutazone
Inactive Drug to Active Metabolite		
Hetacillin	Hydrolysis →	Ampicillin
Sulfasalazine	Azoreduction →	Sulfapyridine + 5-aminosalicylic acid
Active Drug to Reactive Intermediate		
Acetaminophen	Aromatic Hydroxylation →	Reactive metabolite (hepatic necrosis)
Benzo[a]pyrene	Aromatic Hydroxylation →	Reactive metabolite (carcinogenic)

For some drugs the metabolite may be pharmacologically active or produce toxic effects. *Prodrugs* are inactive and must be biotransformed in the body to metabolites that have pharmacologic activity. Initially, prodrugs were discovered by serendipity, as in the case of prontosil, which is reduced to the antibacterial agent sulfanilamide. More recently, prodrugs have been intentionally designed to improve drug stability, increase systemic drug absorption, or to prolong the duration of activity. For example, the antiparkinsonian agent levodopa crosses the blood–brain barrier and is then decarboxylated in the brain to L-dopamine, an active neurotransmitter. L-Dopamine does not easily penetrate the blood–brain barrier into the brain and therefore cannot be used as a therapeutic agent.

PATHWAYS OF DRUG BIOTRANSFORMATION

Pathways of drug biotransformation may be divided into two major groups of reactions, phase I and phase II reactions. *Phase I,* or *asynthetic reactions,* include oxidation, reduction, and hydrolysis. *Phase II,* or *synthetic reactions,* include conjugations. A partial list of these reactions is presented in Table 12-3. In addition, a number of drugs that resemble natural biochemical molecules are able to utilize the metabolic pathways for normal body compounds. For example, isoproterenol is methylated by catechol *O*-methyl transferase (COMT), and amphetamine is deaminated by monamine oxidase (MAO). Both COMT and MAO are enzymes involved in the metabolism of noradrenaline.

Phase I Reactions

Usually, phase I biotransformation reactions occur first and introduce or expose a functional group on the drug molecules. For example, oxygen is introduced into the phenyl group on phenylbutazone by aromatic hydroxylation to form oxyphenbutazone, a more polar metabolite. Codeine is demethylated to form morphine. In addition, the hydrolysis of esters, such as aspirin or benzocaine, yields more polar products, such as salicylic acid and *p*-aminobenzoic acid, respectively. For some compounds, such as acetaminophen,

TABLE 12-3   Some Common Drug Biotransformation Reactions

Phase I Reactions	Phase II Reactions
Oxidation	Glucuronide conjugation
Aromatic hydroxylation	Ether glucuronide
Side chain hydroxylation	Ester glucuronide
N-, O-, and S-dealkylation	Amide glucuronide
Deamination	
Sulfoxidation, N-oxidation	Peptide conjugation
N-hydroxylation	
Reduction	Glycine conjugation (hippurate)
Azoreduction	
Nitroreduction	Methylation
Alcohol dehydrogenase	N-methylation
Hydrolysis	O-methylation
Ester hydrolysis	
Amide hydrolysis	Acetylation
	Sulfate conjugation
	Mercapturic acid synthesis

benzo[a]pyrene, and other drugs containing aromatic rings, reactive intermediates, such as epoxides, are formed during the hydroxylation reaction. These aromatic epoxides are highly reactive and will react with macromolecules, possibly causing liver necrosis (acetaminophen) or cancer (benzo[a]pyrene). The biotransformation of salicylic acid (Fig. 12-14) demonstrates the variety of possible metabolites that may be formed. It should be noted that salicylic acid is also conjugated directly (phase II reaction) without a preceding phase I reaction.

Conjugation (Phase II) Reactions

Once a polar constituent is revealed or placed into the molecule, a phase II or conjugation reaction may occur. Common examples include the conjugation of salicyclic acid with glycine to form salicyluric acid or glucuronic acid to form salicylglucuronide (see Fig. 12-14).

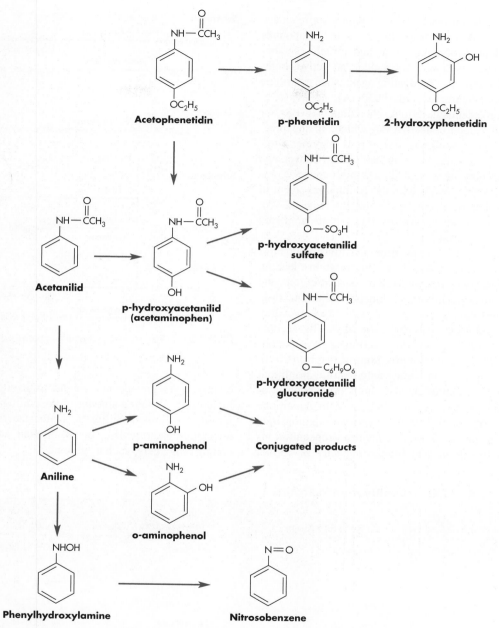

FIGURE 12-14 Biotransformation of salicylic acid. (From Hucker et al, 1980, with permission.)

Conjugation reactions use conjugating reagents, which are derived from biochemical compounds involved in carbohydrate, fat, and protein metabolism. These reactions may include an active, high-energy form of the conjugating agent, such as uridine diphosphoglucuronic acid (UDPGA), acetyl CoA, 3′-phosphoadenosine-5′-phosphosulfate (PAPS), or S-adenosylmethionine (SAM), which, in the presence of the appropriate transferase enzyme, combines with the drug to form the conjugate. Conversely, the drug may be activated to a high-energy compound that then reacts with the conjugating agent in the presence of a transferase enzyme (Fig. 12-15). The major conjugation (phase II) reactions are listed in Tables 12-3 and 12-4.

Some of the conjugation reactions may have limited capacity at high drug concentrations, leading to nonlinear drug metabolism. In most cases, enzyme activity follows first-order kinetics with low drug (substrate) concentrations. At high doses, the drug concentration may rise above the Michaelis–Menten rate constant (K_M), and the reaction rate approaches zero order (V_{max}). Glucuronidation reactions have a high capacity and may demonstrate nonlinear (saturation) kinetics at very high drug concentrations. In contrast, glycine, sulfate, and glutathione conjugations show lesser capacity and demonstrate nonlinear kinetics at therapeutic drug concentrations (Caldwell, 1980). The limited capacity of certain

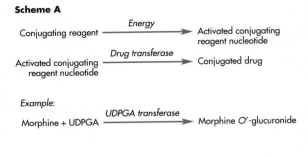

Scheme A

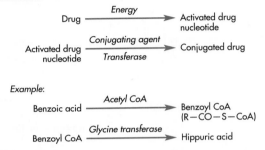

Scheme B

FIGURE 12-15   General scheme for phase II reactions.

conjugation pathways may be due to several factors, including (1) limited amount of the conjugate transferase, (2) limited ability to synthesize the active nucleotide intermediate, or (3) limited amount of conjugating agent, such as glycine.

TABLE 12-4   Phase II Conjugation Reactions

Conjugation Reaction	Conjugating Agent	High-Energy Intermediate	Functional Groups Combined with
Glucuronidation	Glucuronic acid	UDPGA[a]	—OH, —COOH, —NH₂, SH
Sulfation	Sulfate	PAPS[b]	—OH, —NH₂
Amino acid conjugation	Glycine[c]	Coenzyme A thioesters	—COOH
Acetylation	Acetyl CoA	Acetyl CoA	—OH, —NH₂
Methylation	CH₃ from S-adenosylmethionine	S-adenosylmethionine	—OH, —NH₂
Glutathione (mercapturine acid conjugation)	Glutathione	Arene oxides, epoxides	Aryl halides, epoxides, arene oxides

[a]UDPGA = uridine diphosphoglucuronic acid.

[b]PAPS = 3′-phosphoadenosine-5′-phosphosulfate.

[c]Glycine conjugates are also known as hippurates.

In addition, the *N*-acetylated conjugation reaction shows genetic polymorphism: for certain drugs, the human population may be divided into fast and slow acetylators. Finally, some of these conjugation reactions may be diminished or defective in cases of inborn errors of metabolism.

Glucuronidation and sulfate conjugation are very common phase II reactions that result in water-soluble metabolites being rapidly excreted in bile (for some high-molecular-weight glucuronides) and/or urine. Acetylation and mercapturic acid synthesis are conjugation reactions that are often implicated in the toxicity of the drug; they will now be discussed more fully.

Acetylation

The acetylation reaction is an important conjugation reaction for several reasons. First, the acetylated product is usually less polar than the parent drug. The acetylation of such drugs as sulfanilamide, sulfadiazine, and sulfisoxazole produces metabolites that are less water soluble and that in sufficient concentration precipitate in the kidney tubules, causing kidney damage and crystaluria. In addition, a less polar metabolite is reabsorbed in the renal tubule and has a longer elimination half-life. For example, procainamide (elimination half-life of 3 to 4 hours) has an acetylated metabolite, *N*-acetylprocainamide, which is biologically active and has an elimination half-life of 6 to 7 hours. Lastly, the *N*-acetyltransferase enzyme responsible for catalyzing the acetylation of isoniazid and other drugs demonstrates a genetic polymorphism. Two distinct subpopulations have been observed to inactivate isoniazid, including the "slow inactivators" and the "rapid inactivators" (Evans, 1968). Therefore, the former group may demonstrate an adverse effect of isoniazide, such as peripheral neuritis, due to the longer elimination half-life and accumulation of the drug.

Glutathione and Mercapturic Acid Conjugation

Glutathione (GSH) is a tripeptide of glutamyl-cysteine-glycine that is involved in many important biochemical reactions. GSH is important in the detoxification of reactive oxygen intermediates into nonreactive metabolites and is the main intracellular molecule for protection of the cell against reactive electrophilic compounds. Through the nucleophilic sulfhydryl group of the cysteine residue, GSH reacts nonenzymatically and enzymatically via the enzyme glutathione *S*-transferase, with reactive electrophilic oxygen intermediates of certain drugs, particularly aromatic hydrocarbons formed during oxidative biotransformation. The resulting GSH conjugates are precursors for a group of drug conjugates known as mercapturic acid (*N*-acetylcysteine) derivatives. The formation of a mercapturic acid conjugate is shown in Fig. 12-16.

The enzymatic formation of GSH conjugates is saturable. High doses of drugs such as acetaminophen (APAP) may form electrophilic intermediates and deplete GSH in the cell. The reactive intermediate covalently bonds to hepatic cellular macromolecules, resulting in cellular injury and necrosis. The suggested antidote for intoxication (overdose) of acetaminophen is the administration of *N*-acetylcysteine (Mucomyst), a drug molecule that contains available sulfhydryl (R–SH) groups.

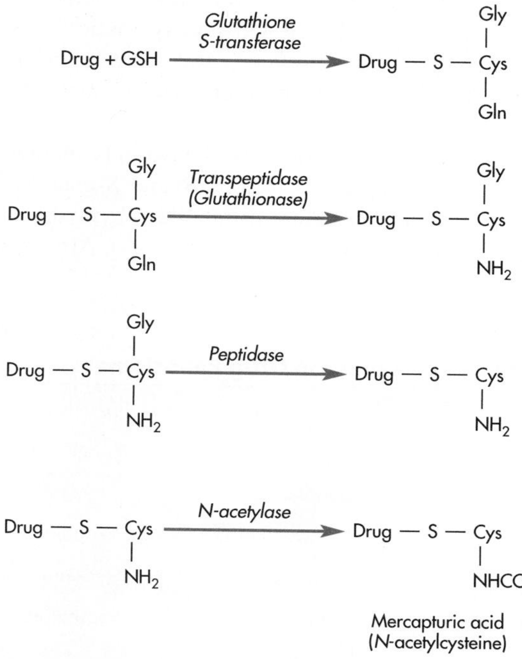

FIGURE 12-16   Mercapturic acid conjugation.

Metabolism of Enantiomers

Many drugs are given as mixtures of stereoisomers. Each isomeric form may have different pharmacologic actions and different side effects. For example, the natural thyroid hormone is *l*-thyroxine, whereas the synthetic *d* enantiomer, *d*-thyroxine, lowers cholesterol but does not stimulate basal metabolic rate like the *l* form. Since enzymes as well as drug receptors demonstrate stereoselectivity, isomers of drugs may show differences in biotransformation and pharmacokinetics (Tucker and Lennard, 1990). With improved techniques for isolating mixtures of enantiomers, many drugs are now available as pure enantiomers. The rate of drug metabolism and the extent of drug protein binding are often different for each stereoisomer. For example, (S)-(+)disopyramide is more highly bound in humans than (R)-(−)disopyramide. Carprofen, a nonsteroidal anti-inflammatory drug, also exists in both an S and an R configuration. The predominate activity lies in the S configuration. The clearance of the S-carprofen glucuronide through the kidney was found to be faster than that of the R form, 36 versus 26 mL/min (Iwakawa et al, 1989). A list of some common drugs with enantiomers is given in Table 12-5. A review (Ariens and Wuis, 1987) shows that of 475 semisynthetic drugs derived from natural sources, 469 were enantiomers, indicating that the biologic systems are very stereospecific.

The anticonvulsant drug mephenytoin is another example of a drug that exists as R and S enantiomers. Both enantiomers are metabolized by hydroxylation in humans (Wilkinson et al, 1989). After an oral dose of 300 mg of the racemic or mixed form, the plasma concentration of the S form in most subjects was only about 25% of that of the R form. The elimination half-life of the S form (2.13 hours) was much faster than that of the R form (76 hours) in these subjects (Fig. 12-17A). The severity of the sedative side effect of this drug was also less in subjects with rapid metabolism. Hydroxylation reduces the lipophilicity of the metabolite and may reduce the partition of the metabolite into the CNS. Interestingly, some subjects do not metabolize the S form of mephenytoin well, and the severity of sedation in these subjects was increased. The plasma level of the S form was much higher in these subjects (Fig. 12-17B). The variation in metabolic rate was attributed to genetically controlled enzymatic differences within the population.

Regioselectivity

In addition to stereoselectivity, biotransformation enzymes may also be regioselective. In this case, the enzymes catalyze a reaction that is specific for a particular region in the drug molecule. For example, isoproterenol is methylated via catechol-*O*-methyltransferase and *S*-adenosylmethionine primarily in the meta position, resulting in a 3-*O*-methylated metabolite. Very little methylation occurs at the hydroxyl group in the para position.

Species Differences in Hepatic Biotransformation Enzymes

The biotransformation activity of hepatic enzymes can be affected by a variety of factors (Table 12-6). During the early preclinical phase of drug development, drug metabolism studies attempt to identify the major metabolic pathways of a new drug through the use of animal models. For most drugs, different animal species may have different metabolic pathways. For example, amphetamine is mainly hydroxylated in rats, whereas in humans and dogs it is largely deaminated. In many cases, the rates of metabolism may differ among different animal species even though the biotransformation pathways are the same. In other cases, a specific pathway may be absent in a particular species. Generally, the researcher tries to find the best

TABLE 12-5   Common Drug Enantiomers

Atropine	Brompheniramine	Cocaine
Disopyramide	Doxylamine	Ephedrine
Propranolol	Nadolol	Verapamil
Tocainide	Propoxyphene	Morphine
Warfarin	Thyroxine	Flecainide
Ibuprofen	Atenolol	Subutamol
Metoprolol	Terbutaline	

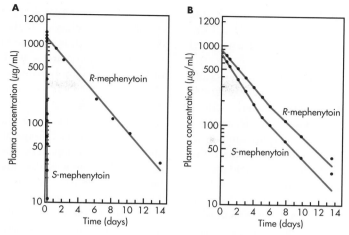

FIGURE 12-17   Plasma level of mephenytoin after 300-mg oral dose of the recemic drug. **A.** Efficient metabolizer. **B.** Poor metabolizer. The plasma levels of the R and S form are different due to different rates of metabolism of the two isomers. (Adapted from Wilkinson et al, 1989, with permission.)

animal model that will be predictive of the metabolic profile in humans.

In recent years, *in vitro* drug screening with human liver microsomes or with hepatocytes has helped confirm whether a given CYP isoenzyme is important in human drug metabolism. Animal models also provide some supportive evidence.

TABLE 12-6   Sources of Variation in Intrinsic Clearance

Genetic factors
Genetic differences within population
Racial differences among different populations
Environmental factors and drug interactions
Enzyme induction
Enzyme inhibition
Physiologic conditions
Age
Gender
Diet/nutrition
Pathophysiology
Drug dosage regimen
Route of drug administration
Dose-dependent (nonlinear) pharmacokinetics

DRUG INTERACTION EXAMPLE

Lovastatin (Mevacor®) is a cholesterol-lowering agent and was found to be metabolized by human liver microsomes to two major metabolites: 6′β-hydroxy (Michaelis-Menten constant $[K_M]$: 7.8 ± 2.7 μM) and 6′-exomethylene lovastatin (K_M, 10.3 ± 2.6 μM). 6′β-Hydroxylovastatin formation in the liver was inhibited by the specific CYP3A inhibitors cyclosporine (K_i, 7.6 ± 2.3 μM), ketoconazole (K_i, 0.25 ± 0.2 μM), and troleandomycin (K_i, 26.6 ± 18.5 μM).

Hydroxylation of lovastatin is a phase I reaction and catalyzed by a specific cytochrome P-450 enzyme commonly referred to as CYP3A. Ketoconazole and cyclosporine are CYP3A inhibitors and therefore affect lovastatin metabolism. Lovastatin is referred to as a substrate. Substrate concentrations are expressed as $[S]$ ($[D]$ in Fig. 12-4A), preferably in (μM). The Michaelis–Menten constant (K_M) of the enzyme is expressed in micromoles (μM) because most new drugs have different MW, making it easier to compare by expressing them in moles. Cyclosporine would be expected to produce a significant drug–drug interaction in the body based on a review of the K_i values. In addition to inhibiting the cytochrome P-450 enzyme pathway, an efflux transporter can deplete the drug before significant biotransformaton occurs. Efflux inhibition would have the opposite effect. Thus, location (time and place) issues are important when DDI involves a CYP and a transporter.

A systems biology approach that takes into account all aspects of ADME processes integrated with pharmacogenetics is needed to properly address various pharmacokinetic, pharmacodynamic, and clinical issues of risk/benefit. The interplay among the various processes including influx and efflux transporters may sometimes overweigh any single process when complex drug–drug interactions are involved. For most drugs, metabolism has multiple pathways which are inherently complicated. Many pharmacodynamic drug actions in patients encounter the issue of responder and nonresponder, which may be genetically defined or totally obscured.

Knowledge of drug transport of drug from one site can make the hepatic intrinsic clearance concept obsolete in some simple physiological blood flow models. Macro models based on mass balance are kinetically based and the amount of drug in the plasma pool can still be computed and properly tracked. A drug–drug interaction between lovastatin and cyclosporine occurs because cyclosporine is a CYP3A and transport inhibitor in the liver.

Frequently Asked Questions

▶ *Why is a compartment referred to as a black box?*

▶ *What are the problems about modeling a real system in drug therapy?*

Variation of Biotransformation Enzymes

Variation in metabolism may be caused by a number of biologic and environmental variables (see Table 12-6). *Pharmacogenetics* is the study of genetic differences in pharmacokinetics and pharmacodynamics, including drug elimination (see Chapter 13). For example, the *N*-acetylation of isoniazid is genetically determined, with at least two identifiable groups, including rapid and slow acetylators (Evans et al, 1968). The difference is referred to as *genetic polymorphism*. Individuals with slow acetylation are prone to isoniazid-induced neurotoxicity. Procainamide and hydralazine are other drugs that are acetylated and demonstrate genetic polymorphism.

Another example of genetic differences in drug metabolism is glucose 6-phosphate-dehydrogenase deficiency, which is observed in approximately 10% of African Americans. A well-documented example of genetic polymorphism with this enzyme was observed with phenytoin (Wilkinson et al, 1989). Two phenotypes, EM (efficient metabolizer) and PM (poor metabolizer), were identified in the study population. The PM frequency in Caucasians was about 4% and in Japanese was about 16%. Variation in metabolic rate was also observed with mephobarbital. The incidence of side effects was higher in Japanese subjects, possibly due to a slower oxidative metabolism. Variations in propranolol metabolism due to genetic difference among Chinese populations were also reported (Lai et al, 1995). Some variations in metabolism may also be related to geographic rather than racial differences (Bertilsson, 1995).

Besides genetic influence, the basal level of enzyme activity may be altered by environmental factors and exposure to chemicals. Shorter theophylline elimination half-life due to smoking was observed in smokers. Apparently, the aromatic hydrocarbons, such as benzpyrene, that are released during smoking stimulate the enzymes involved in theophylline metabolism. Young children are also known to eliminate theophylline more quickly. Phenobarbital is a potent inducer of a wider variety of hepatic enzymes. Polycyclic hydrocarbons such as 3-methylcholanthrene and benzpyrene also induce hepatic enzyme formation. These compounds are carcinogenic.

Hepatic enzyme activity may also be inhibited by a variety of agents including carbon monoxide, heavy metals, and certain imidazole drugs such as cimetidine. Enzyme inhibition by cimetidine may lead to higher plasma levels and longer elimination of coadministered phenytoin or theophylline. The physiologic condition of the host—including age, gender, nutrition, diet, and pathophysiology—also affects the level of hepatic enzyme activities.

Genetic Variation of Cytochrome P-450 (CYP) Isozymes

The most important enzymes accounting for variation in phase I metabolism of drugs is the cytochrome P-450 enzyme group, which exists in many forms among individuals because of genetic differences

(May, 1994; Tucker, 1994; Parkinson, 1996; see also Chapter 13). Initially, the cytochrome P-450 enzymes were identified according to the substrate that was biotransformed. More recently, the genes encoding many of these enzymes have been identified. Multiforms of cytochrome P-450 are referred to as *isozymes,* and are classified into families (originally denoted by Roman numerals: I, II, III, etc) and sub-families (denoted by A, B, C, etc) based on the similarity of the amino acid sequences of the isozymes. If an isozyme amino acid sequence is 60% similar or more, it is placed within a family. Within the family, isozymes with amino acid sequences of 70% or more similarity are placed into a subfamily, and an Arabic number follows for further classification. Further information on the CYP enzymes including drug interactions, classification, table of substrates, inhibitors, and inducers have been published by Nelson, (2009) and the US FDA. Nebert et al (1989) and Hansch and Zhang (1993) have reviewed the nomenclature of the P-450 family of enzymes. A new nomenclature starts with CYP as the root denoting cytochrome P-450, and an Arabic number now replaces the Roman numeral (Table 12-7). The CYP3A subfamily of CYP3 appears to be responsible for the metabolism of a large number of structurally diverse endogenous agents (eg, testosterone, cortisol, progesterone, estradiol) and xenobiotics (eg, nifedipine, lovastatin, midazolam, terfenadine, erythromycin).

TABLE 12-7 **Comparison of P-450 Nomenclatures Currently in Use**

P-450 Gene Family/Subfamily	New Nomenclature
P-450I	CYP1
P-450IIA	CYP2A
P-450IIB	CYP2B
P-450IIC	CYP2C
P-450IID	CYP2D
P-450IIE	CYP2E
P-450III	CYP3
P-450IV	CYP4

Sources: Nebert et al (1989) and Hansch and Zhang (1993).

The substrate specificities of the P-450 enzymes appear to be due to the nature of the amino acid residues, the size of the amino acid side chain, and the polarity and charge of the amino acids (Negishi et al, 1996). The individual gene is denoted by an Arabic number (last number) after the subfamily. For example, cytochrome P-450 1A2 (CYP1A2) is involved in the oxidation of caffeine and CYP2D6 is involved in the oxidation of drugs, such as codeine, propranolol, and dextromethorphan. The well-known CYP2D6 is responsible for debrisoquine metabolism among individuals showing genetic polymorphism. The vinca alkaloids used in cancer treatment have shown great inter- and intraindividual variabilities. CYP3A enzymes are known to be involved in the metabolism of vindesine, vinblastine, and other vinca alkaloids (Rahmani and Zhou, 1993). Failing to recognize variations in drug clearance in cancer chemotherapy may result in greater toxicity or even therapeutic failure.

There are now at least eight families of cytochrome isozymes known in humans and animals. CYP 1–3 are best known for metabolizing clinically useful drugs in humans. Variation in isozyme distribution and content in the hepatocytes may affect intrinsic hepatic clearance of a drug. The levels and activities of the cytochrome P-450 isozymes differ among individuals as a result of genetic and environmental factors. Clinically, it is important to look for evidence of unusual metabolic profiles in patients before dosing. Pharmacokinetic experiments using a "marker" drug such as the antipyrine or dextromethorphan may be used to determine if the intrinsic hepatic clearance of the patient is significantly different from that of an average subject.

The metabolism of debrisoquin is polymorphic in the population, with some individuals having extensive metabolism (EM) and other individuals having poor metabolism (PM). Those individuals who are PM lack functional CYP2D6 (P-450IID6). In EM individuals, quinidine will block CYP2D6 so that genotypic EM individuals appear to be phenotypic PM individuals (Caraco et al, 1996). Some drugs metabolized by CYP2D6 (P-450IID6) are codeine, flecainide, dextromethorphan, imipramine, and other cyclic antidepressants that undergo ring hydroxylation. The inability to metabolize substrates for CYP2D6 results in increased plasma concentrations of the parent drug in PM individuals.

Drug Interactions Involving Drug Metabolism

The enzymes involved in the metabolism of drugs may be altered by diet and the coadministration of other drugs and chemicals. *Enzyme induction* is a drug- or chemical-stimulated increase in enzyme activity, usually due to an increase in the amount of enzyme present. Enzyme induction usually requires some onset time for the synthesis of enzyme protein. For example, rifampin induction occurs within 2 days, while phenobarbital induction takes about 1 week to occur. Enzyme induction for carbamazepine begins after 3 to 5 days and is not complete for approximately 1 month or longer. Smoking can change the rate of metabolism of many cyclic antidepressant drugs (CAD) through enzyme induction (Toney and Ereshefsky, 1995). Agents that induce enzymes include aromatic hydrocarbons (such as benzopyrene, found in cigarette smoke), insecticides (such as chlordane), and drugs such as carbamazepine, rifampin, and phenobarbital (see also Chapter 22). *Enzyme inhibition* may be due to substrate competition or due to direct inhibition of drug-metabolizing enzymes, particularly one of several of the cytochrome P-450 enzymes. Many widely prescribed antidepressants generally known as selective serotonin reuptake inhibitors (SSRIs) have been reported to inhibit the CYP2D6 system, resulting in significantly elevated plasma concentration of coadministered psychotropic drugs. Fluoxetine causes a ten-fold decrease in the clearance of imipramine and desipramine because of its inhibitory effect on hydroxylation (Toney and Ereshefsky, 1995).

A few clinical examples of enzyme inhibitors and inducers are listed in Table 12-8. Diet also affects drug-metabolizing enzymes. For example, plasma theophylline concentrations and theophylline clearance in patients on a high-protein diet are lower than in subjects whose diets are high in carbohydrates. Sucrose or glucose plus fructose decrease the activity of mixed-function oxidases, an effect related to a slower metabolism rate and a prolongation in hexobarbital sleeping time in rats. Chronic administration of 5% glucose was suggested to affect sleeping time in subjects receiving barbiturates. A decreased intake of fatty acids may lead to decreased basal MFO activities (Campbell, 1977) and affect the rate of drug metabolism.

The protease inhibitor saquinavir mesylate (Invirase®, Roche) has very low bioavailability—only about 4%. In studies conducted by Hoffmann-La Roche, the area under the curve (AUC) of saquinavir was increased to 150% when the volunteers took a 150-mL glass of grapefruit juice with the saquinavir, and then another 150-mL glass an hour later. Concentrated grapefruit juice increased the AUC up to 220%. Naringin, a bioflavonoid in grapefruit juice, was found to be at least partially responsible for the

TABLE 12-8   Examples of Drug Interactions Affecting Mixed Function Oxidase Enzymes

Inhibitors of Drug Metabolism	Example	Result
Acetaminophen	Ethanol	Increased hepatotoxicity in chronic alcoholics
Cimetidine	Warfarin	Prolongation of prothrombin time
Erythromycin	Carbamazepine	Decreased carbazepine clearance
Fluoxetine	Imipramine (IMI)	Decreased clearance of CAD
Fluoxetine	Desipramine (DMI)	Decreased clearance of CAD
Inducers of Drug Metabolism	**Example**	**Result**
Carbamazepine	Acetaminophen	Increased acetaminophen metabolism
Rifampin	Methadone	Increased methadone metabolism, may precipitate opiate withdrawal
Phenobarbital	Dexamethasone	Decreased dexamethasone elimination half-life
Rifampin	Prednisolone	Increased elimination of prednisolone

TABLE 12-9 Change in Drug Availability Due to Oral Coadministration of Grapefruit Juice

Drug	Study
Triazolam	Hukkinen et al, 1995
Midazolam	Kupferschmidt et al, 1995
Cyclosporine	Yee et al, 1995
Coumarin	Merkel et al, 1994
Nisoldipine	Baily DG et al, 1993a
Felodipine	Baily DG et al, 1993b

inhibition of saquinavir metabolism by CYP3A4, present in the liver and the intestinal wall, which metabolizes saquinavir, resulting in an increase in its AUC. Ketoconazole and ranitidine (Zantac®) may also increase the AUC of saquinavir by inhibition of the cytochrome P-450 enzymes. In contrast, rifampin greatly reduces the AUC of saquinavir, apparently due to enzymatic stimulation. Other drugs recently shown to have increased bioavailability when taken with grapefruit juice include several sedatives and the anticoagulant coumarin (Table 12-9). Increases in drug levels may be dangerous, and the pharmacokinetics of drugs with potential interactions should be closely monitored. More complete tabulations of the cytochrome P-450s are available (Flockhart, 2003; Parkinson, 1996; Cupp and Tracy, 1998); some examples are given in Table 12-10.

TABLE 12-10 Cytochrome P450 Isoforms and Examples

CYP1A2	Substrates—amitriptyline, imipramine, theophylline (other enzymes also involved); induced by smoking
	Fluvoxamine, some quinolones, and grapefruit juice are inhibitors
CYP2B6	Substrates—cyclophosphamide, methadone
CYP2C9	Metabolism of S-warfarin and tolbutamide by CYP2C9
	Substrates—NSAIDs—ibuprofen, diclofenac
CYP2C19	Omeprazole, S-mephenytoin, and propranolol
	Diazepam (mixed), and imipramine (mixed)
	Inhibitors: cimetidine, fluoxetine, and ketoconazole
CYP2D6	Many antidepressants, β-blockers are metabolized by CYP2D6
	SRIIs, cimetidine are inhibitors
	Substrates—amitriptyline, imipramine, fluoxetine, antipsychotics (haloperidol, thioridazine)
	Inhibitors—paroxetine, fluoxetine, sertraline, fluvoxamine, cimetidine, haloperidol
CYP2E1	Substrates—acetaminophen, ethanol, halothane
	Induced by INH and disulfiram
CYP3A4, 5, 6	CYP3A subfamilies are the most abundant cytochrome enzymes in humans and include many key therapeutic and miscellaneous groups:
	Ketoconazole, atorvastatin, lovastatin
	Azithromycin, clarithromycins, amitriptyline
	Benzodiazepines—alprazolam, triazolam, midazolam
	Calcium blockers—verapamil, diltiazem
	Protease inhibitors—ritonavir, saquinavir, indinavir

Examples based on Flockhart (2003), Cupp and Tracy (1998), and Desta et al (2002).

Auto-Induction and Time-Dependent Pharmacokinetics

Many drugs enhance the activity of cytochrome P-450 (CYP) enzymes and thereby change their own metabolism (*auto-induction*) or the metabolism of other compounds. When assessing induction, the enzyme activity is usually measured before and after a period of treatment with the inducing agent. Thus, the induction magnitude of various CYP enzymes is well known for several inducing agents.

The *time-dependent pharmacokinetics* have been described with a model where the production rates of the affected enzymes were proportional to the amounts of the inducing agents and the time course of the induction process was described by the turnover model. An example of a drug with time-dependent pharmacokinetics is carbamazepine.

For new drugs, the potential for drug metabolism/ interaction is studied *in vitro* and/or *in vivo* by identifying whether the drug is a substrate for the common CYP450 subfamilies (FDA Guidance for Industry, 1999, 2006). An understanding of the mechanistic basis of metabolic drug–drug interactions enables the prediction of whether the coadministration of two or more drugs may have clinical consequences affecting safety and efficacy. In practice, an investigational drug under development is coadministered with an approved drug (interacting drug) which utilizes similar CYP pathways. Examples of substrates include (1) midazolam for CYP3A; (2) theophylline for CYP1A2; (3) repaglinide for CYP2C8; (4) warfarin for CYP2C9 (with the evaluation of S-warfarin); (5) omeprazole for CYP2C19; and (6) desipramine for CYP2D6. Additional examples of substrates, along with inhibitors and inducers of specific CYP enzymes, are listed in Table A-2 in Appendix A in the FDA draft guidance (2006). Examples of substrates include, but are not limited to, (1) midazolam, buspirone, felodipine, simvastatin, or lovastatin for CYP3A4; (2) theophylline for CYP1A2; (3) S-warfarin for CYP2C9; and (4) desipramine for CYP2D6.

Since metabolism usually occurs in the liver (some enzymes such as CYP3A4 are also important in gut metabolism), human liver microsomes provide a convenient way to study CYP450 metabolism. Microsomes are a subcellular fraction of tissue obtained by differential high-speed centrifugation.

The key CYP450 enzymes are collected in the microsomal fraction. The CYP450 enzymes retain their activity for many years in microsomes or whole liver stored at low temperature. Hepatic microsomes can be obtained commercially, with or without prior phenotyping, for most important CYP450 enzymes. The cDNAs for the common CYP450s have been cloned, and the recombinant human enzymatic proteins have been expressed in a variety of cells. These recombinant enzymes provide an excellent way to confirm results using microsomes. Pharmacokinetic endpoints recommended for assessment of the substrate are (1) exposure measures such as AUC, C_{max}, time to C_{max} (T_{max}), and others as appropriate; and (2) pharmacokinetic parameters such as clearance, volumes of distribution, and half-lives (FDA Guidance for Industry, 1999). For metabolism induction studies, *in vivo* studies are more relied upon because enzyme induction may not be well predicted from *in vitro* results. Considerations in drug-metabolizing/interaction studies include: (1) acute or chronic use of the substrate and/or interacting drug; (2) safety considerations, including whether a drug is likely to be an NTR (narrow therapeutic range) or non-NTR drug; (3) pharmacokinetic and pharmacodynamic characteristics of the substrate and interacting drugs; and (4) the need to assess induction as well as inhibition. The inhibiting/inducing drugs and the substrates should be dosed so that the exposures of both drugs are relevant to their clinical use.

Transporter-Based Drug–Drug Interactions

Transporter-based interactions have been increasingly documented. Examples include the inhibition or induction of transport proteins, such as P-glycoprotein (P-gp), organic anion transporter (OAT), organic anion transporting polypeptide (OATP), organic cation transporter (OCT), multidrug resistance–associated proteins (MRP), and breast cancer–resistant protein (BCRP). Examples of transporter-based interactions include the interactions between digoxin and quinidine, fexofenadine and ketoconazole (or erythromycin), penicillin and probenecid, and dofetilide and cimetidine. Of the various transporters, P-gp is the most well understood and may be appropriate to evaluate during drug development. Table 12-11 lists some of

TABLE 12-11   **Major Human Transporters and Known Substrates, Inhibitors, and Inducers**

Gene	Aliases	Tissue	Drug Substrate	Inhibitor	Inducer
ABCB1	P-gp, MDR1	Intestine, liver, kidney, brain, placenta, adrenal, testes	Digoxin, fexofenadine, indinavir, vincristine, colchicine, topotecan, paclitaxel	Ritonavir, cyclosporine, verapamil, erythromycin, ketocoanzole, itraconazole, quinidine, elacridar (GF120918) LY335979 valspodar (PSC833)	Rifampin, St John's wort
ABCB4	MDR3	Liver	Digoxin, paclitaxel, vinblastine		
ABCB11	BSEP	Liver	Vinblastine		
ABCC1	MRP1	Intestine, liver, kidney, brain	Adefovir, indinavir		
ABCC2	MRP2, CMOAT	Intestine, liver, kidney, brain	Indinavir, cisplatin	Cyclosporine	
ABCC3	MRP3, CMOAT2	Intestine, liver, kidney, placenta, adrenal	Etoposide, methotrexate, tenoposide		
ABCC4	MRP4				
ABCC5	MRP5				
ABCC6	MRP6	Liver, kidney	Cisplatin, daunorubicin		
ABCG2	BCRP	Intestine, liver, breast, placenta	Daunorubicin, doxorubicin, topotecan, rosuvastatin, sulfasalazine	Elacridar (GFI20918), gefitinib	
SLCOIB1	OATP1B1, OATP-C, OATP2	Liver	Rifampin, rosuvastatin, methotrexate, pravastatin, thyroxine	Cyclosporine, rifampin	
SLCOIB3	OATP1B3, OATP8	Liver	Digoxin, methotrexate, rifampin,		
SLC02B1	SLC21A9, OATP-B	Intestine, liver, kidney, brain	Pravastatin		
SLC1OA1	NTCP	Liver, pancreas	Rosuvastatin		

From FDA Guidance (draft) 2006.

the major human transporters and known substrates, inhibitors, and inducers.

In the simple hepatic clearance model, intrinsic clearance is assumed to be constant within the same subject. This model describes how clearance can change in response to physiologic changes such as blood flow or enzymatic induction. Patient variability and changes in intrinsic clearance may be due to (1) patient factors such as age and genetic polymorphism, (2) enzymatic induction or inhibition due to coadministered drugs, (3) modification of influx and efflux transporters in the liver and the bile canaliculi.

Some hepatic transporters in the liver include P-gp and OATPs (Huang et al, 2009). When a transporter is known to play a major role in translocating drug in and out of cells and organelles within the liver, the simple hepatic clearance model may not adequately describe the pharmacokintics of the drug within the liver. Micro constants may be needed to describe how the drug moves kinetically in and out within a group of cells or compartment. Canalicular transporters are present for many drugs. Biliary excretion should also be incorporated into the model as needed. For this reason, local drug concentration in the liver may be very high, leading to serious liver toxicity. Huang et al (2009) have discussed the importance of drug transporters, drug disposition, and how to study drug interaction in the new drugs.

Knowledge of drug transporters and CYPs can help predict whether many drug interactions have the clinical significance. Pharmacists should realize that the combined effect of efflux and CYP inhibition can cause serious or even fatal adverse reaction due to severalfold increase in AUC or C_{max}. Impairment of bile flow, saturation of conjugation enzymes (phase II) such as glucoronide, and sulfate conjugate formation can lead to adverse toxicity.

CLINICAL EXAMPLE

Digoxin is an MDR1/P-gp substrate.

1. Which of the following sites is important to influence on the plasma levels of digoxin after oral administration?
   a. Hepatocyte (canalicular)
   b. Hepatocyte (sinusoidal)
   c. Intestinal enterocyte
2. Ritonavir and quinidine are examples of P-gp inhibitors. What changes in AUC or C_{max} would you expect for digoxin when coadministered with either one of these two inhibitors?
3. Using your knowledge of drug transporters and their substrate inhibitors, can you determine whether the above change in digoxin plasma level is due to a change in metabolism or distribution?

Solution

1. According to Table 12-11, MDR1 is an efflux transporter for digoxin in the liver (canaliculi) and enterocyte. Digoxin is also a substrate for MDR3, SLCO1B1, and other transporters. MDR1 is inhibited by quinidine and ritonavir.

2. Literature search shows that digoxin transport by P-gp occurs at the liver canaliculi and P-gp will interact with ritonavir or quinidine with coadministration (both are inhibitors of MDR1). Inhibition of efflux will increase the plasma level of digoxin. Other effects may also occur since most transport inhibitors are not 100% specific and may affect metabolism/disposition in other ways.

3. The package insert should be consulted on drug distribution and drug interaction. A pharmacist should realize that although either one of the two inhibitors can increase AUC of digoxin (by 1.5–2 x) in this hypothetical case, in reality, a comprehensive evaluation of pharmacokinetics and pharmacodynamics of the drug doses involved and the medical profile of the patient is needed to determine if an interaction is clinically significant.

FIRST-PASS EFFECTS

For some drugs, the route of administration affects the metabolic rate of the compound. For example, a drug given parenterally, transdermally, or by inhalation may distribute within the body prior to metabolism by the liver. In contrast, drugs given orally are normally absorbed in the duodenal segment of the small intestine and transported via the mesenteric vessels to the hepatic portal vein and then to the liver before entering the systemic circulation. Drugs that are highly metabolized by the liver or by the intestinal mucosal cells demonstrate poor systemic availability when given orally. This rapid metabolism of an orally administered drug before reaching the general circulation is termed *first-pass effect* or *presystemic elimination*.

Evidence of First-Pass Effects

First-pass effects may be suspected when there is relatively low concentrations of parent (or intact) drug in the systemic circulation after oral compared to IV administration. In such a case, the AUC for a drug given orally also is less than the AUC for the same dose of drug given intravenously. From experimental findings in animals, first-pass effects may be assumed if the intact drug appears in a cannulated hepatic portal vein but not in general circulation.

For an orally administered drug that is chemically stable in the gastrointestinal tract and is 100% systemically absorbed ($F = 1$), the area under the plasma drug concentration curve, $\mathrm{AUC}_{0,\,\mathrm{oral}}^{\infty}$, should be the same when the same drug dose is given intravenously, $\mathrm{AUC}_{0,\,\mathrm{IV}}^{\infty}$. Therefore, the absolute bioavailability (F) may reveal evidence of drug being removed by the liver due to first-pass effects as follows:

$$F = \frac{[\mathrm{AUC}]_{0,\,\mathrm{oral}}^{\infty}/D_{0,\,\mathrm{oral}}}{[\mathrm{AUC}]_{0,\,\mathrm{IV}}^{\infty}/D_{0,\,\mathrm{IV}}} \qquad (12.34)$$

For drugs that undergo first-pass effects, $\mathrm{AUC}_{0,\,\mathrm{oral}}^{\infty}$ is smaller than $\mathrm{AUC}_{0,\,\mathrm{IV}}^{\infty}$ and $F < 1$. Drugs such as propranolol, morphine, and nitroglycerin have F values less than 1 because these drugs undergo significant first-pass effects.

Liver Extraction Ratio

Because there are many other reasons for a drug to have a reduced F value, the extent of first-pass effects is not precisely measured from the F value. The liver extraction ratio (ER) provides a direct measurement of drug removal from the liver after oral administration of a drug.

$$\mathrm{ER} = \frac{C_a - C_v}{C_a} \qquad (12.35)$$

where C_a is the drug concentration in the blood entering the liver and C_v is the drug concentration leaving the liver.

Because C_a is usually greater than C_v, ER is usually less than 1. For example, for propranolol, ER or [E] is about 0.7—that is, about 70% of the drug is actually removed by the liver before it is available for general distribution to the body. By contrast, if the drug is injected intravenously, most of the drug would be distributed before reaching the liver, and less of the drug would be metabolized the first time the drug reaches the liver.

The ER may vary from 0 to 1.0. An ER of 0.25 means that 25% of the drug is removed by the liver.

If both the ER for the liver and the blood flow to the liver are known, then hepatic clearance, Cl_h, may be calculated by the following expression:

$$Cl_h = \frac{Q(C_a - C_v)}{C_a} = Q \times \mathrm{ER} \qquad (12.36)$$

where Q is the effective hepatic blood flow.

Relationship between Absolute Bioavailability and Liver Extraction

Liver ER provides a measurement of liver extraction of a drug orally administered. Unfortunately, sampling of drug from the hepatic portal vein and artery is difficult and performed mainly in animals. Animal ER values may be quite different from those in humans. The following relationship between bioavailability and liver extraction enables a rough estimate of the extent of liver extraction:

$$F = 1 - \mathrm{ER} - F'' \qquad (12.37)$$

where F is the fraction of bioavailable drug, ER is the drug fraction extracted by the liver, and F'' is the fraction of drug removed by nonhepatic process prior to reaching the circulation.

If F'' is assumed to be negligible—that is, there is no loss of drug due to chemical degradation, gut metabolism, and incomplete absorption—ER may be estimated from

$$F = 1 - \mathrm{ER} \qquad (12.38)$$

After substitution of Equation 12.34 into Equation 12.38,

$$\mathrm{ER} = 1 - \frac{[\mathrm{AUC}]_{0,\mathrm{oral}}^{\infty}/D_{0,\mathrm{oral}}}{[\mathrm{AUC}]_{0,\mathrm{IV}}^{\infty}/D_{0,\mathrm{IV}}} \qquad (12.39)$$

ER is a rough estimation of liver extraction for a drug. Many other factors may alter this estimation: the size of the dose, the formulation of the drug, and the pathophysiologic condition of the patient all may affect the ER value obtained.

Liver ER provides valuable information in determining the oral dose of a drug when the intravenous dose is known. For example, propranolol requires a much higher oral dose compared to an

IV dose to produce equivalent therapeutic blood levels, because of oral drug extraction by the liver. Because liver extraction is affected by blood flow to the liver, dosing of drug with extensive liver metabolism may produce erratic plasma drug levels. Formulation of this drug into an oral dosage form requires extensive, careful testing.

Estimation of Reduced Bioavailability Due to Liver Metabolism and Variable Blood Flow

Blood flow to the liver plays an important role in the amount of drug metabolized after oral administration. Changes in blood flow to the liver may substantially alter the percentage of drug metabolized and therefore alter the percentage of bioavailable drug. The relationship between blood flow, hepatic clearance, and percent of drug bioavailable is

$$F' = 1 - \frac{Cl_h}{Q} = 1 - \text{ER} \qquad (12.40)$$

where Cl_h is the hepatic clearance of the drug and Q is the effective hepatic blood flow. F' is the bioavailability factor obtained from estimates of liver blood flow and hepatic clearance, ER.

This equation provides a reasonable approach for evaluating the reduced bioavailability due to first-pass effect. The usual effective hepatic blood flow is 1.5 L/min, but it may vary from 1 to 2 L/min depending on diet, food intake, physical activity, or drug intake (Rowland, 1973). For the drug propoxyphene hydrochloride, F' has been calculated from hepatic clearance (990 mL/min) and an assumed liver blood flow of 1.53 L/min:

$$F' = 1 - \frac{0.99}{1.53} = 0.35$$

The results, showing that 35% of the drug is systemically absorbed after liver extraction, are reasonable compared with the experimental values for propranolol.

Presystemic elimination or *first-pass effect* is a very important consideration for drugs that have a high extraction ratio (Table 12-12). Drugs with low extraction ratios, such as theophylline, have very little presystemic elimination, as demonstrated by complete systemic absorption after oral administration.

TABLE 12-12   Hepatic and Renal Extraction Ratios of Representative Drugs

Extraction Ratios		
Low (<0.3)	**Intermediate (0.3–0.7)**	**High (>0.7)**
HEPATIC EXTRACTION		
Amobarbital	Aspirin	Arabinosylcytosine
Antipyrine	Quinidine	Encainide
Chloramphenicol	Desipramine	Isoproterenol
Chlordiazepoxide	Nortriptyline	Meperidine
Diazepam		Morphine
Digitoxin		Nitroglycerin
Erythromycin		Pentazocine
Isoniazid		Propoxyphene
Phenobarbital		Propranolol
Phenylbutazone		Salicylamide
Phenytoin		Tocainide
Procainamide		Verapamil
Salicylic acid		
Theophylline		
Tolbutamide		
Warfarin		

Data from Rowland (1978) and Brouwer et al (1992).

In contrast, drugs with high extraction ratios have poor bioavailability when given orally. Therefore, the oral dose must be higher than the intravenous dose to achieve the same therapeutic response. In some cases, oral administration of a drug with high presystemic elimination, such as nitroglycerin, may be impractical due to very poor oral bioavailability, and thus a sublingual, transdermal, or nasal route of administration may be preferred.

Furthermore, if an oral drug product has slow dissolution characteristics or release rate, then more of the drug will be subject to first-pass effect compared to doses of drug given in a more bioavailable form (such as a solution). In addition, drugs with high presystemic elimination tend to demonstrate more variability in drug bioavailability between and within individuals. Finally, the quantity and quality of the metabolites formed may vary according to the route of drug administration, which may be clinically important if one or more of the metabolites has pharmacologic or toxic activity.

To overcome first-pass effect, the route of administration of the drug may be changed. For example, nitroglycerin may be given sublingually or topically, and xylocaine may be given parenterally to avoid the first-pass effects. Another way to overcome first-pass effects is to either enlarge the dose or change the drug product to a more rapidly absorbable dosage form. In either case, a large amount of drug is presented rapidly to the liver, and some of the drug will reach the general circulation in the intact state.

Although Equation 12.40 seems to provide a convenient way of estimating the effect of liver blood flow on bioavailability, this estimation is actually more complicated. A change in liver blood flow may alter hepatic clearance and F'. A large blood flow may deliver enough drug to the liver to alter the rate of metabolism. In contrast, a small blood flow may decrease the delivery of drug to the liver and become the rate-limiting step for metabolism (see below). The hepatic clearance of a drug is usually calculated from plasma drug data rather than whole-blood data. Significant nonlinearity may be the result of drug equilibration due to partitioning into the red blood cells.

EXAMPLES ▶▶▶

1. A new propranolol 5-mg tablet was developed and tested in volunteers. The bioavailability of propranolol from the tablet was 70%, compared to an oral solution of propranolol, and 21.6%, compared to an intravenous dose of propranolol. Calculate the relative and absolute bioavailability of the propranolol tablet. Comment on the feasibility of further improving the absolute bioavailability of the propranolol tablet.

Solution

The relative bioavailability of propranolol from the tablet compared to the solution is 70% or 0.7. The absolute bioailability, F, of propranolol from the tablet compared to the IV dose is 21.6%, or $F = 0.216$. From the table of ER values (Table 12-13), the ER for propranolol is 0.6 to 0.8. If the product is perfectly formulated, ie, the tablet dissolves completely and all the drug is released from the tablet, the fraction of drug absorbed after deducting for the fraction of drug extracted by the liver is

$$F' = 1 - ER$$
$$F' = 1 - 0.7 \quad \text{(mean ER} = 0.7)$$
$$F' = 0.3$$

Thus, under normal conditions, total systemic absorption of propranolol from an oral tablet would be about 30% ($F = 0.3$). The measurement of relative bioavailability for propranolol is always performed against a reference standard given by the same route of administration and can have a value greater than 100%.

The following shows a method for calculating the absolute bioavailability from the relative bioavailability provided the ER is accurately known. Using the above example,

Absolute availability of the solution $= 1 - ER = 1 - 0.7 = 0.3 = 30\%$

Relative availability of the solution $= 100\%$

Absolute availability of the tablet $= x\%$

Relative availability of the tablet $= 70\%$

$$x = \frac{30 \times 70}{100} = 21\%$$

Therefore, this product has a theoretical absolute bioavailability of 21%. The small difference of calculated and actual (the difference between 21.6% and 21%) absolute bioavailability is due largely to liver extraction fluctuation. All calculations are performed with the assumption of linear pharmacokinetics, which is generally a good approximation. ER may deviate significantly with changes in blood flow or other factors.

TABLE 12-13　Pharmacokinetic Classification of Drugs Eliminated Primarily by Hepatic Metabolism

Drug Class	Extraction Ratio (Approx.)	Percent Bound
Flow Limited		
Lidocaine	0.83	45–80[a]
Propranolol	0.6–0.8	93
Pethidine (meperidine)	0.60–0.95	60
Pentazocine	0.8	—
Propoxyphene	0.95	—
Nortriptyline	0.5	95
Morphine	0.5–0.75	35
Capacity Limited, Binding Sensitive		
Phenytoin	0.03	90
Diazepam	0.03	98
Tolbutamide	0.02	98
Warfarin	0.003	99
Chlorpromazine	0.22	91–99
Clindamycin	0.23	94
Quinidine	0.27	82
Digitoxin	0.005	97
Capacity Limited, Binding Insensitive		
Theophylline	0.09	59
Hexobarbital	0.16	—
Amobarbital	0.03	61
Antipyrine	0.07	10
Chloramphenicol	0.28	60–80
Thiopental	0.28	72
Acetaminophen	0.43	5[a]

[a]Concentration dependent in part.

From Blaschke (1977), with permission.

2. Fluvastatin sodium (Lescol®, Novartis) is a drug used to lower cholesterol. The absolute bioavailability after an oral dose is reported to be 19% to 29%. The drug is rapidly and completely absorbed (manufacturer's product information). What are the reasons for the low oral bioavailability in spite of reportedly good absorption? What is the extraction ratio of fluvastatin? (The absolute bioavailability, F, is 46%, according to values reported in the literature.)

Solution

Assuming the drug to be completely absorbed as reported, using Equation 12.38,

$$ER = 1 - 0.46 = 0.54$$

Thus, 54% of the drug is lost due to first-pass effect because of a relatively large extraction ratio. Since bioavailability is only 19% to 29%, there is probably some nonhepatic loss according to Equation 12.37. Fluvastatin sodium was reported to be extensively metabolized, with some drug excreted in feces.

Relationship between Blood Flow, Intrinsic Clearance, and Hepatic Clearance

Although Equation 12.40 seems to provide a convenient way of estimating the effect of liver blood flow on bioavailability, this estimation is actually more complicated. For example, factors that affect the hepatic clearance of a drug include (1) blood flow to the liver, (2) intrinsic clearance, and (3) the fraction of drug bound to protein.

A change in liver blood flow may alter hepatic clearance and F'. A large blood flow may deliver enough drug to the liver to alter the rate of metabolism. In contrast, a small blood flow may decrease the delivery of drug to the liver and become the rate-limiting step for metabolism. The hepatic clearance of a drug is usually calculated from plasma drug data rather than whole-blood data. Significant nonlinearity may be the result of drug equilibration due to partitioning into the red blood cells.

High-Extraction Ratio Drugs

For some drugs (such as isoproterenol, lidocaine, and nitroglycerin), the extraction ratio is high (>0.7), and the drug is removed by the liver almost as rapidly as the organ is perfused by blood in which the drug is contained. For drugs with very high extraction ratios, the rate of drug metabolism is sensitive to changes in hepatic blood flow. Thus, an increase in blood flow to the liver will increase the rate of drug removal by the organ. Propranolol, a β-adrenergic blocking agent, decreases hepatic blood flow by decreasing cardiac output. In such a case, the drug decreases its own clearance through the liver when given orally. Many drugs that demonstrate first-pass effects are drugs that have high extraction ratios with respect to the liver.

Intrinsic clearance (Cl_{int}) is used to describe the total ability of the liver to metabolize a drug in the absence of flow limitations, reflecting the inherent activities of the mixed-function oxidases and all other enzymes. Intrinsic clearance is a distinct characteristic of a particular drug, and as such, it reflects the inherent ability of the liver to metabolize the drug. Intrinsic clearance may be shown to be analogous to the ratio V_{max}/K_M for a drug that follows Michaelis–Menten kinetics. Hepatic clearance is a concept that characterizes drug elimination based on both blood flow and the intrinsic clearance of the liver, as shown in Equation 12.41.

$$Cl_h = Q \frac{Cl_{int}}{Q + Cl_{int}} \qquad (12.41)$$

Low-Extraction Ratio Drugs

When the blood flow to the liver is constant, hepatic clearance is equal to the product of blood flow (Q) and the extraction ratio (ER) (Equation 12.36). However, the hepatic clearance of a drug is not constant. Hepatic clearance changes with blood flow (Fig. 12-18) and the intrinsic clearance of the drug are described in Equation 12.41. For drugs with low extraction ratios (eg, theophylline, phenylbutazone, and procainamide), the hepatic clearance is less affected by hepatic blood flow. Instead, these drugs are more affected by the intrinsic activity of the mixed-function oxidases. Describing clearance in

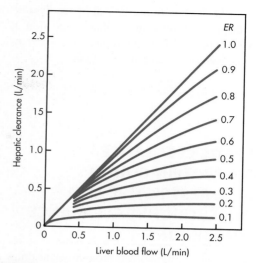

FIGURE 12-18 The relationship between liver blood flow and total hepatic clearance for drugs with varying extraction rates (ER).

terms of all the factors in a physiologic model allows drug clearance to be estimated when physiologic or disease conditions cause changes in blood flow or intrinsic enzyme activity. Smoking, for example, can increase the intrinsic clearance for the metabolism of many drugs.

Changes or alterations in mixed-function oxidase activity or biliary secretion can affect the intrinsic clearance and thus the rate of drug removal by the liver. Drugs that show low extraction ratios and are eliminated primarily by metabolism demonstrate marked variation in overall elimination half-lives within a given population. For example, the elimination half-life of theophylline varies from 3 to 9 hours. This variation in $t_{1/2}$ is thought to be due to genetic differences in intrinsic hepatic enzyme activity. Moreover, the elimination half-lives of these same drugs are also affected by enzyme induction, enzyme inhibition, age of the individual, nutritional, and pathologic factors.

Clearance may also be expressed as the rate of drug removal divided by plasma drug concentration:

$$Cl_h = \frac{\text{rate of drug removed by the liver}}{C_a} \qquad (12.42)$$

Because the rate of drug removal by the liver is usually the rate of drug metabolism, Equation 12.42 may be expressed in terms of hepatic clearance and drug concentration entering the liver (C_a):

$$\text{Rate of liver drug metabolism} = Cl_h C_a \quad (12.43)$$

HEPATIC CLEARANCE OF A PROTEIN-BOUND DRUG: RESTRICTIVE AND NONRESTRICTIVE CLEARANCE FROM BINDING

It is generally assumed that protein-bound drugs are not easily metabolized (*restrictive clearance*), while free (unbound) drugs are subject to metabolism. Protein-bound drugs do not easily diffuse through cell membranes, while free drugs can reach the site of the mixed-function oxidase enzymes easily. Therefore, an increase in the unbound drug concentration in the blood will make more drug available for hepatic extraction. The concept is discussed under restrictive and nonrestrictive clearance (Gillette, 1973) of protein-bound drugs (see Chapter 11).

Most drugs are *restrictively* cleared—for example, diazepam, quinidine, tolbutamide, and warfarin. The clearance of these drugs is proportional to the fraction of unbound drug (f_u). However, some drugs, such as propranolol, morphine, and verapamil, are *nonrestrictively* extracted by the liver regardless of drug bound to protein or free. Kinetically, a drug is nonrestrictively cleared if its hepatic extraction ratio (ER) is greater than the fraction of free drug (f_u), and the rate of drug clearance is unchanged when the drug is displaced from binding. Mechanistically, the protein binding of a drug is a reversible process and for a nonrestrictively bound drug, the free drug gets "stripped" from the protein relatively easily compared to a restrictively bound drug during the process of drug metabolism. The elimination half-life of a nonrestrictively cleared drug is not significantly affected by a change in the degree of protein binding. This is an analogous situation to a protein-bound drug that is actively secreted by the kidney.

For a drug with restrictive clearance, the relationship of blood flow, intrinsic clearance, and protein binding is

$$Cl_h = Q \left(\frac{f_u Cl'_{int}}{Q + f_u Cl'_{int}} \right) \quad (12.44)$$

where f_u is the fraction of drug unbound in the blood and Cl'_{int} is the intrinsic clearance of free drug. Equation 12.44 is derived by substituting $f_u Cl'_{int}$ for Cl_{int} in Equation 12.41.

From Equation 12.44, when Cl'_{int} is very small in comparison to hepatic blood flow (ie, $Q \geq Cl'_{int}$), then Equation 12.45 reduces to Equation 12.46.

$$Cl_h = \frac{Q f_u Cl'_{int}}{Q} \quad (12.45)$$

$$Cl_h = f_u Cl'_{int} \quad (12.46)$$

As shown in Equation 12.46, a change in Cl'_{int} or f_u will cause a proportional change in Cl_h for drugs with protein binding.

In the case where Cl'_{int} for a drug is very large in comparison to flow ($Cl'_{int} \gg Q$), Equation 12.47 reduces to Equation 12.48.

$$Cl_h = \frac{Q f_u Cl'_{int}}{f_u Cl'_{int}} \quad (12.47)$$

$$Cl_h \approx Q \quad (12.48)$$

Thus, for drugs with a very high Cl'_{int}, Cl_h is dependent on hepatic blood flow and independent of protein binding.

For restrictively cleared drugs, change in binding generally alters drug clearance. For a drug with low hepatic extraction ratio and low plasma binding, clearance will increase, but not significantly, when the drug is displaced from binding. For a drug highly bound to plasma proteins (more than 90%), a displacement from these binding sites will significantly increase the free concentration of the drug, and clearance (both hepatic and renal clearance) will increase (see Chapter 11). There are some drugs that are exceptional and show a paradoxical increase in hepatic clearance despite an increase in protein binding. In one case, increased binding to AAG (α acid glycoprotein) was found to concentrate drug in the liver, leading to an increased rate of metabolism because the drug was nonrestrictively cleared in the liver.

Effect of Changing Intrinsic Clearance and/or Blood Flow on Hepatic Extraction and Elimination Half-Life after IV and Oral Dosing

The effects of altered hepatic intrinsic clearance and liver blood flow on the blood level–time curve have been described by Wilkinson and Shand (1975) after both IV and oral dosing. These illustrations show how changes in intrinsic clearance and blood flow affect the elimination half-life, first-pass effects, and bioavailability of the drug as represented by the area under the curve.

Effect of Theoretical Change in Cl_{int} and F on Drug Clearance

The relationship between blood flow (F), intrinsic clearance, and hepatic clearance was simulated with hypothetic examples by Wilkinson and Shand (1975). However, due to the prevalence of transporters, the relationship may only apply unless all model assumptions are met.

For drugs with low ER, the effect of doubling Cl_{int} from 0.167 to 0.334 L/min increases both the extraction ratio (ER) and clearance (Cl) of the drug, leading to a much shorter $t_{1/2}$. The elimination half-life decreases about 50% due to the increase in intrinsic clearance. Simulation shows the change in drug concentrations after oral administration when Cl_{int} doubles. In this case, there is a decrease in both AUC and $t_{1/2}$ (dashed line) due to the increase in clearance of the drug.

For drugs with high ER, the effect of doubling Cl_{int} from 13.7 to 27.0 L/min increases both the extraction ratio and clearance only. The elimination half-life decreases only marginally. After oral administration, when simulated, some decrease in AUC is observed and the $t_{1/2}$ is shortened moderately.

The elimination half-life of a drug with a low extraction ratio is decreased significantly by an increase in hepatic enzyme activity. In contrast, the elimination half-life of a drug with a high extraction ratio is not markedly affected by an increase in hepatic enzyme activity because enzyme activity is already quite high. In both cases, an orally administered drug with a higher extraction ratio results in a greater first-pass effect as shown by an increase in hepatic clearance.

Effect of Changing Blood Flow on Drugs with High or Low Extraction Ratio

Drug clearance and elimination half-life are both affected by changing blood flow to the liver. For drugs with low extraction ($E = 0.1$), a decrease in hepatic blood flow from normal (1.5 L/min) to one-half decreases clearance only slightly, and blood level is slightly higher. In contrast, for a drug with high extraction ratio ($E = 0.9$), decreasing the blood flow to one-half of normal greatly decreases clearance, and the blood level is much higher.

Alterations in hepatic blood flow significantly affect the elimination of drugs with high extraction ratios (eg, propranolol) and have very little effect on the elimination of drugs with low extraction ratios (eg, theophylline). For drugs with low extraction ratios, any concentration of drug in the blood that perfuses the liver is more than the liver can eliminate. Consequently, small changes in hepatic blood flow do not affect the removal rate of such drugs. In contrast, drugs with high extraction ratios are removed from the blood as rapidly as they are presented to the liver. If the blood flow to the liver decreases, then the elimination of these drugs is prolonged. Therefore, drugs with high extraction ratios are considered to be *flow dependent*. A number of drugs have been investigated and classified according to their extraction by the liver.

Effect of Changing Protein Binding on Hepatic Clearance

The effect of protein binding on hepatic clearance is often difficult to quantitate precisely, because it is not always known whether the bound drug is restrictively or nonrestrictively cleared. For example, animal tissue levels of imipramine, a nonrestrictively cleared drug, were shown to change as the degree of plasma protein binding changes (see Chapter 11). As discussed, drug protein binding is not a factor in hepatic clearance for drugs that have high extraction ratios. These drugs are considered to be *flow limited*. In contrast, drugs that have low extraction ratios may be affected by plasma protein binding, depending on the fraction of drug bound. For a drug that has a low extraction ratio and is less than 75% to 80% bound, small changes in protein binding will not produce significant changes in hepatic clearance. These drugs are considered *capacity-limited, binding-insensitive drugs* (Blaschke, 1977) and are listed in Table 12-13. Drugs that are highly bound to plasma protein but with low extraction ratios are considered *capacity limited and binding sensitive*, because a small displacement in the protein binding of these drugs will cause a very large increase in the free drug concentration. These drugs are good examples of restrictively cleared drugs. A large increase in free drug concentration will cause an increase in the rate of drug metabolism, resulting in an overall increase in hepatic clearance. Figure 12-19 illustrates the relationship of protein binding, blood flow, and extraction.

BILIARY EXCRETION OF DRUGS

The biliary system of the liver is an important system for the secretion of bile and the excretion of drugs. Anatomically, the intrahepatic bile ducts join outside the liver to form the common hepatic duct (Fig. 12-20). The bile that enters the gallbladder becomes highly concentrated. The hepatic duct, containing hepatic bile, joins the cystic duct that drains the gallbladder to form the common bile duct. The common bile duct then empties into the duodenum. Bile consists primarily of water, bile salts, bile pigments, electrolytes, and, to a lesser extent, cholesterol and fatty acids. The hepatic cells lining the bile canaliculi are responsible for the production of bile. The production of bile appears to be an active secretion process. Separate active biliary secretion processes have been reported for organic anions, organic cations, and for polar, uncharged molecules.

Drugs that are excreted mainly in the bile have molecular weights in excess of 500. Drugs with molecular weights between 300 and 500 are excreted both in urine and in bile. For these drugs, a decrease in one excretory route results in a compensatory

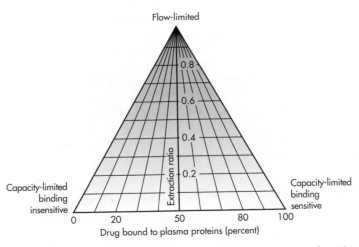

FIGURE 12-19 This diagram illustrates the way in which two pharmacokinetic parameters (hepatic extraction ratio and percent plasma protein binding) are used to assign a drug into one of three classes of hepatic clearance (flow limited; capacity limited, binding sensitive; and capacity limited, binding insensitive). Any drug metabolized by the liver can be plotted on the triangular graph, but the classification is important only for those eliminated primarily by hepatic processes. The closer a drug falls to a corner of the triangle (shaded areas), the more likely it is to have the characteristic changes in disposition in liver disease as described for the three drug classes in the text. (From Blaschke, 1977, with permission.)

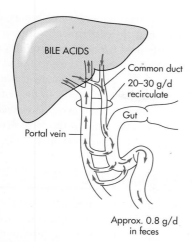

FIGURE 12-20   Enterohepatic recirculation of bile acids and drug. (From Dow, 1963.)

TABLE 12-14   Examples of Drugs Undergoing Enterohepatic Circulation and Biliary Excretion

Enterohepatic Circulation	
Imipramine	
Indomethacin	
Morphine	
Pregnenolone	

Biliary Excretion (intact or as metabolites)	
Cefamandole	Fluvastatin
Cefoperazone	Lovastatin
Chloramphenicol	Moxalactam
Diazepam	Practolol
Digoxin	Spironolactone
Doxorubicin	Testosterone
Doxycycline	Tetracycline
Estradiol	Vincristine

increase in excretion via the other route. Compounds with molecular weights of less than 300 are excreted almost exclusively via the kidneys into urine.

In addition to relatively high molecular weight, drugs excreted into bile usually require a strongly polar group. Many drugs excreted into bile are metabolites, very often glucuronide conjugates. Most metabolites are more polar than the parent drug. In addition, the formation of a glucuronide increases the molecular weight of the compound by nearly 200, as well as increasing the polarity.

Drugs excreted into the bile include the digitalis glycosides, bile salts, cholesterol, steroids, and indomethacin (Table 12-14). Compounds that enhance bile production stimulate the biliary excretion of drugs normally eliminated by this route. Furthermore, phenobarbital, which induces many mixed-function oxidase activities, may stimulate the biliary excretion of drugs by two mechanisms: by an increase in the formation of the glucuronide metabolite and by an increase in bile flow. In contrast, compounds that decrease bile flow or pathophysiologic conditions that cause cholestasis decrease biliary drug excretion. The route of administration may also influence the amount of the drug excreted into bile. For example, drugs given orally may be extracted by the liver into the bile to a greater extent than the same drugs given intravenously.

Estimation of Biliary Clearance

In animals, bile duct cannulation allows both the volume of the bile and the concentration of drug in the bile to be measured directly using a special intubation technique that blocks off a segment of the gut with an inflating balloon. The rate of drug elimination may then be measured by monitoring the amount of drug secreted into the GI perfusate.

Assuming an average bile flow of 0.5 to 0.8 mL/min in humans, biliary clearance can be calculated if the bile concentration, C_{bile}, is known.

$$Cl_{biliary} = \frac{\text{bile flow} \times C_{bile}}{C_p} \qquad (12.49)$$

Alternatively, using the perfusion technique, the amount of drug eliminated in bile is determined from the GI perfusate, and $Cl_{biliary}$ may be calculated without the bile flow rate, as follows:

$$Cl_{biliary} = \frac{\text{amount of drug secreted from bile per minute}}{C_p}$$

$$(12.50)$$

To avoid any complication of unabsorbed drug in the feces, the drug should be given by parenteral administration (eg, IV) during biliary determination experiments. The amount of drug in the GI perfusate recovered periodically may be determined. The extent of biliary elimination of digoxin has been determined in humans using this approach.

Enterohepatic Circulation

A drug or its metabolite is secreted into bile and upon contraction of the gallbladder is excreted into the duodenum via the common bile duct. Subsequently, the drug or its metabolite may be excreted into the feces or the drug may be reabsorbed and become systemically available. The cycle in which the drug is absorbed, excreted into the bile, and reabsorbed is known as *enterohepatic circulation*. Some drugs excreted as a glucuronide conjugate become hydrolyzed in the gut back to the parent drug by the action of a β-glucuronidase enzyme present in the intestinal bacteria. In this case, the parent drug becomes available for reabsorption.

Significance of Biliary Excretion

When a drug appears in the feces after oral administration, it is difficult to determine whether this presence of drug is due to biliary excretion or incomplete absorption. If the drug is given parenterally and then observed in the feces, one can conclude that some of the drug was excreted in the bile. Because drug secretion into bile is an active process, this process can be saturated with high drug concentrations. Moreover, other drugs may compete for the same carrier system.

Enterohepatic circulation after a single dose of drug is not as important as after multiple doses or a very high dose of drug. With a large dose or multiple doses, a larger amount of drug is secreted in the bile, from which drug may then be reabsorbed. This reabsorption process may affect the absorption and elimination rate constants. Furthermore, the biliary secretion process may become saturated, thus altering the plasma level–time curve.

Drugs that undergo enterohepatic circulation sometimes show a small secondary peak in the plasma drug–concentration curve. The first peak occurs as the drug in the GI tract is depleted; a small secondary peak then emerges as biliary-excreted drug is reabsorbed. In experimental studies involving animals, bile duct cannulation provides a means of estimating the amount of drug excreted through the bile. In humans, a less accurate estimation of biliary excretion may be made from the recovery of drug excreted through the feces. However, if the drug was given orally, some of the fecal drug excretion could represent unabsorbed drug.

CLINICAL EXAMPLE

Leflunomide, an immunomodulator for rheumatoid arthritis, is metabolized to a major active metabolite and several minor metabolites. Approximately 48% of the dose is eliminated in the feces due to high biliary excretion. The active metabolite is slowly eliminated from the plasma. In the case of serious adverse toxicity, the manufacturer recommends giving cholestyramine or activated charcoal orally to bind the active metabolite in the GI tract to prevent drug reabsorption and to facilitate drug elimination. The use of cholestyramine or activated charcoal reduces the plasma levels of the active metabolite by approximately 40% in 24 hours and by about 50% in 48 hours.

Frequently Asked Questions

► *Why do we use the term hepatic drug clearance to describe drug metabolism in the liver?*

► *Please explain why many drugs with significant metabolism often have variable bioavailability.*

► *The metabolism of some drugs is affected more than others when there is a change in protein binding. Why?*

► *Give some examples that explain why the metabolic pharmacokinetics of drugs are important in patient care.*

ROLE OF TRANSPORTERS ON HEPATIC CLEARANCE AND BIOAVAILABILITY

In the simple hepatic clearance model, intrinsic clearance is assumed to be constant within the same subject. This model describes how clearance can change in response to physiologic changes such as blood flow or enzymatic induction. Patient variability and changes in intrinsic clearance may be due to (1) patient factors such as age and genetic polymorphism, (2) enzymatic induction or inhibition due to coadministered drugs, and (3) modification of influx and efflux transporters in the liver and the bile canaliculi. When a transporter is known to play a major role in translocating drug in and out of cells and organelles within the liver, the simple hepatic clearance model may not adequately describe the pharmacokinetics of the drug within the liver. Micro constants may be needed to describe how the drug moves kinetically in and out within a group of cells or compartment. Biliary excretion should also be incorporated into the model as needed. Since the development of the hepatic model based on intrinsic clearance, much more information is now known about the interplay between transporters and strategically located CYP isoenzymes in the GI, the hepatocytes in various parts of the liver (see Figs. 12-11 and 12-12). More elaborate models are now available to relate transporters to drug disposition. Huang et al (2009) has discussed the importance of drug transporters, drug disposition, and how to study drug interaction of the new drugs. The interplay between transporters, drug permeability in GI, and hepatic drug extraction are important to the bioavailability and the extent of drug metabolism.

It appears that drugs may be classified in several classes to facilitate prediction of drug disposition. A drug substance is considered to be "highly permeable" when the extent of the absorption (parent drug plus metabolites) in humans is determined to be 90% of an administered dose based on a mass balance determination or in comparison to an intravenous reference dose. Drugs may be classified into four BCS (biopharmaceutical classification system) classes. With respect to oral bioavailability, Wu and Benet (2005) proposed categorizing drugs into the four classes based on solubility and permeability as criteria may provide significant new insights to predicting routes of elimination, effects of efflux, and absorptive transporters on oral absorption, when transporter–enzyme interplay will yield clinically significant effects such as low bioavailability and drug–drug interactions (DDI), the direction and importance of food effects, and transporter effects

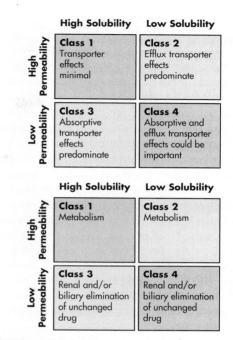

FIGURE 12-21   Classification of Drugs Based on Biopharmaceutics Drug Disposition Classification System (BDDCS). Data from Wu and Benet (2009).

on post-absorption systemic levels following oral and intravenous dosing.

Figure 12-21 provides a good summary of how various physiologic and physiochemical factors influence drug disposition. For example, Class 1 drugs are not so much affected by transporters because absorption is generally good already due to high solubility and permeability. Class 2 drugs are very much affected by efflux transporters because of low solubility and high permiability. The limited amount of drug solubilized and absorbed could efflux back into the GI lumen due to efflux transporters, thus resulting in low plasma level. Further, efflux transporter may pump drug into bile if located in the liver canaliculi.

Frequently Asked Questions

▶ *What are the effects of metabolism on Class 1 and 2 drugs?*

▶ *What are the effects of transporters on Class 3 and 4 drugs?*

CHAPTER SUMMARY

The elimination of most drugs from the body involves the processes of both metabolism (biotransformation) and renal excretion. Drugs that are highly metabolized often demonstrate large intersubject variability in elimination half-lives and are dependent on the intrinsic activity of the biotransformation enzymes. Renal drug excretion is highly dependent on the glomerular filtration rate (GFR) and blood flow to the kidney.

Hepatic clearance is influenced by hepatic blood flow, drug–protein binding, and intrinsic clearance. The liver extraction ratio (ER) provides a direct measurement of drug removal from the liver after oral administration of a drug. Drugs that are metabolized by the liver enzymes follow Michaelis–Menton kinetics. At low drug concentrations the rate of metabolism is first order, whereas at very high drug concentrations, the rate of drug metabolism may approach zero-order pharmacokinetics. Phase 1 reactions are generally oxidation and reduction reactions and involve the mixed function oxidases or cytochrome enzymes. These enzymes may be altered by genetic and environmental factors. Phase 2 reactions are generally conjugation reactions such as the formation of glucuronide and sulfate conjugations. Cytochrome-mediated and acetylation reactions demonstrate polymorphic variability in humans.

First-pass effects or presystemic elimination may occur after oral drug administration in which some of the drugs may be metabolized or not absorbed prior to reaching the general circulation. Alternate routes of drug administration are often used to circumnavigate presystemic elimination. Large-molecular-weight, polar drugs may be eliminated by biliary drug excretion. Enterohepatic drug elimination occurs when the drug is secreted into the GI tract and then reabsorbed.

The role of transporters on hepatic clearance and bioavailability in addition to hepatic drug metabolism are important considerations when considering drug–drug interactions and oral drug absorption.

LEARNING QUESTIONS

1. A drug fitting a one-compartment model was found to be eliminated from the plasma by the following pathways with the corresponding elimination rate constants.
   Metabolism: $k_m = 0.200$ h^{-1}
   Kidney excretion: $k_e = 0.250$ h^{-1}
   Biliary excretion: $k_b = 0.150$ h^{-1}
   a. What is the elimination half-life of this drug?
   b. What would be the half-life of this drug if biliary secretion was completely blocked?
   c. What would be the half-life of this drug if drug excretion through the kidney was completely impaired?
   d. If drug-metabolizing enzymes were induced so that the rate of metabolism of this drug doubled, what would be the new elimination half-life?

2. A new broad-spectrum antibiotic was administered by rapid intravenous injection to a 50-kg woman at a dose of 3 mg/kg. The apparent volume of distribution of this drug was equivalent to 5% of body weight. The elimination half-life for this drug is 2 hours.
   a. If 90% of the unchanged drug was recovered in the urine, what is the renal excretion rate constant?
   b. Which is more important for the elimination of the drugs, renal excretion or biotransformation? Why?

3. Explain briefly:
   a. Why does a drug that has a high extraction ratio (eg, propranolol) demonstrate greater differences between individuals after oral administration than after intravenous administration?

b. Why does a drug with a low hepatic extraction ratio (eg, theophylline) demonstrate greater differences between individuals after hepatic enzyme induction than a drug with a high hepatic extraction ratio?

4. A drug is being screened for antihypertensive activity. After oral administration, the onset time is 0.5 to 1 hour. However, after intravenous administration, the onset time is 6 to 8 hours.

   a. What reasons would you give for the differences in the onset times for oral and intravenous drug administration?

   b. Devise an experiment that would prove the validity of your reasoning.

5. Calculate the hepatic clearance for a drug with an intrinsic clearance of 40 mL/min in a normal adult patient whose hepatic blood flow is 1.5 L/min.

   a. If the patient develops congestive heart failure that reduces hepatic blood flow to 1.0 L/min but does not affect the intrinsic clearance, what is the hepatic drug clearance in this patient?

   b. If the patient is concurrently receiving medication, such as phenobarbital, which increases the Cl_{int} to 90 mL/min but does not alter the hepatic blood flow (1.5 L/min), what is the hepatic clearance for the drug in this patient?

6. Calculate the hepatic clearance for a drug with an intrinsic clearance of 12 L/min in a normal adult patient whose hepatic blood flow is 1.5 L/min. If this same patient develops congestive heart failure that reduces his hepatic blood flow to 1.0 L/min but does not affect intrinsic clearance, what is the hepatic drug clearance in this patient?

   a. Calculate the extraction ratio for the liver in this patient before and after congestive heart failure develops.

   b. From the above information, estimate the fraction of bioavailable drug, assuming the drug is given orally and absorption is complete.

7. Why do elimination half-lives of drugs eliminated primarily by hepatic biotransformation demonstrate greater intersubject variability than those drugs eliminated primarily by glomerular filtration?

8. A new drug demonstrates high presystemic elimination when taken orally. From which of the following drug products would the drug be most bioavailable? Why?

   a. Aqueous solution

   b. Suspension

   c. Capsule (hard gelatin)

   d. Tablet

   e. Sustained release

9. For a drug that demonstrated presystemic elimination, would you expect qualitative and/or quantitative differences in the formation of metabolites from this drug given orally compared to intravenous injection? Why?

10. The bioavailability of propranolol is 26%. Propranolol is 87% bound to plasma proteins and has an elimination half-life of 3.9 hours. The apparent volume of distribution of propranolol is 4.3 L/kg. Less than 0.5% of the unchanged drug is excreted in the urine.

   a. Calculate the hepatic clearance for propranolol in an adult male patient (43 years old, 80 kg).

   b. Assuming the hepatic blood flow is 1500 mL/min, estimate the hepatic extraction ratio for propranolol.

   c. Explain why hepatic clearance is more important than renal clearance for the elimination of propranolol.

   d. What would be the effect of hepatic disease such as cirrhosis on the (1) bioavailability of propranolol and (2) hepatic clearance of propranolol?

   e. Explain how a change in (1) hepatic blood flow, (2) intrinsic clearance, or (3) plasma protein binding would affect hepatic clearance of propranolol.

   f. What is meant by first-pass effects? From the data above, why is propranolol a drug with first-pass effects?

11. The following pharmacokinetic information for erythromycin was reported by Gilman et al (1990, p. 1679):
Bioavailability: 35%
Urinary excretion: 12%
Bound in plasma: 84%
Volume of distribution: 0.78 L/kg

Elimination half-life: 1.6 hours

An adult male patient (41 years old, 81 kg) was prescribed 250 mg of erythromycin base every 6 hours for 10 days. From the given data, calculate the following:

a. Total body clearance

b. Renal clearance

c. Hepatic clearance

12. Why would you expect hepatic clearance of theophylline in identical twins to be less variable compared to hepatic clearance in fraternal twins?

13. Which of the following statements describe(s) correctly the properties of a drug that follows nonlinear or capacity-limited pharmacokinetics?

a. The elimination half-life will remain constant when the dose changes.

b. The area under the plasma curve (AUC) will increase proportionately with an increase in dose.

c. The rate of drug elimination $= C_p \times K_M$.

d. At maximum saturation of the enzyme by the substrate, the reaction velocity is at V_{max}.

e. At very low substrate concentrations, the reaction rate approximates a zero-order rate.

14. The V_{max} for metabolizing a drug is 10 μm/h. The rate of metabolism (v) is 5 μm/h when drug concentration is 4 μm. Which of the following statements is/are true?

a. K_M is 5 μm for this drug.

b. K_M cannot be determined from the information given.

c. K_M is 4 μm for this drug.

15. Which of the following statements is/are true regarding the pharmacokinetics of diazepam (98% protein bound) and propranolol (87% protein bound)?

a. Diazepam has a long elimination half-life due to its lack of metabolism and its extensive plasma protein binding.

b. Propranolol is a drug with high protein binding but unrestricted (unaffected) metabolic clearance.

c. Diazepam exhibits low hepatic extraction.

16. The hepatic intrinsic clearance of two drugs are as follows:

Drug A: 1300 mL/min

Drug B: 26 mL/min

Which drug is likely to show the greatest increase in hepatic clearance when hepatic blood flow is increased from 1 L/min to 1.5 mL/min? Which drug will likely be blood-flow limited?

17. Pravastatin is a statin drug commonly prescribed. The package insert (approved labeling) states that, "The risk of myopathy during treatment with another HMG-CoA reductase inhibitor is increased with concurrent therapy with either erythromycin or cyclosporine." How does cyclosporine change the pharmacokinetics of pravastatin? Is pravastatin uptake involved? Pravastatin is 18% oral bioavailability and 17% urinary excreted.

ANSWERS

Frequently Asked Questions

Why do we use the term hepatic drug clearance to describe drug metabolism in the liver?

- Hepatic drug clearance describes drug metabolism in the liver and accounts for both the effect of blood flow and the intrinsic ability of the liver to metabolize a drug. Hepatic drug clearance is added to renal clearance and other clearances to obtain total (body) clearance, which is important in determining the maintenance dose of a drug. Hepatic drug clearance is often considered nonrenal clearance when it is measured as the difference between total clearance and renal clearance.

Please explain why many drugs with significant metabolism often have variable bioavailability.

- Most orally administered drugs pass through the liver prior to systemic absorption. The rate of blood flow can greatly affect the extent of drug that reaches the systemic circulation. Also, intrinsic metabolism may differ among individuals and may be genetically determined. These factors may cause drug levels to be more erratic for drugs that undergo extensive metabolism compared to drugs that are excreted renally.

The metabolism of some drugs is affected more than others when there is a change in protein binding. Why?

- Protein synthesis may be altered by liver dysfunction. In general, when drug–protein binding is reduced, the free drug may be metabolized more easily. However, some drugs may be metabolized regardless of whether the drug is bound or free (for discussion of nonrestrictive binding, see Chapter 11). In such cases, there is little change in pharmacodynamic activity due to changes in drug–protein binding.

Give some examples that explain why the metabolic pharmacokinetics of drugs are important in patient care.

- Erythromycin, morphine, propranolol, various steroids, and other drugs have large metabolic clearance. In hepatic disease, highly potent drugs that have a narrow therapeutic index should be monitored carefully. Troglitazone (Rezulin), for example, is a drug that can cause severe side effects in patients with liver dysfunction; liver transaminase should be monitored in diabetic patients.

Learning Questions

1. a. $k = k_m + k_e + k_b = 0.20 + 0.25 + 0.15$

$$= 0.60 \text{ h}^{-1}$$

$$t_{1/2} = \frac{0.693}{k} = \frac{0.693}{0.60} = 1.16 \text{ h}$$

b. $k = k_m + k_e = 0.45 \text{ h}^{-1}$

$$t_{1/2} = 1.54 \text{ h}$$

c. $k = 0.35 \text{ h}^{-1}$

$$t_{1/2} = 1.98 \text{ h}$$

d. $k = 0.80 \text{ h}^{-1}$

$$t_{1/2} = 0.87 \text{ h}$$

2. a. $k = 0.347 \text{ h}^{-1}$

$$k_e = (0.9)(0.347) = 0.312 \text{ h}^{-1}$$

b. Renal excretion, 90% of the drug is excreted unchanged.

5. Normal hepatic clearance, Cl_H:

$$Cl_H = Q\left(\frac{Cl_{int}}{Q + Cl_{int}}\right)$$

$$Q = 1.5 \text{ L/min} \quad Cl_{int} = 0.040 \text{ L/min}$$

$$Cl_H = 1.5\left(\frac{0.040}{1.5 + 0.040}\right) = 0.039 \text{ L/min}$$

a. Congestive heart failure:

$$Cl_H = 1.0\left(\frac{0.040}{1.0 + 0.040}\right) = 0.0381 \text{ L/min}$$

b. Enzyme induction:

$$Cl_H = 1.5\left(\frac{0.090}{1.5 + 0.090}\right) = 0.085 \text{ L/min}$$

Note: A change in blood flow, Q, did not markedly affect Cl_H for a drug with low Cl_{int}.

6. Normal hepatic clearance:

$$Cl_H = 1.5\left(\frac{12}{1.5 + 12}\right) = 1.33 \text{ L/min}$$

Congestive heart failure (CHF):

$$Cl_H = 1.0\left(\frac{12}{1.0 + 12}\right) = 0.923 \text{ L/min}$$

a. $Cl_H = Q(\text{ER}) = Q\left(\dfrac{Cl_{int}}{Q + Cl_{int}}\right)$

$$\text{ER} = \frac{Cl_{int}}{Q + Cl_{int}}$$

$$\text{Normal ER} = \frac{12}{1.5 + 12} = 0.89 \text{ L/min}$$

$$\text{CHR ER} = \frac{12}{1.0 + 12} = 0.92 \text{ L/min}$$

b. $F = 1 - \text{ER} = 1 - 0.89$

$$F = 0.11 \, or \, 11\%$$

10. a. Because <0.5% of the unchanged drug is excreted in the urine, hepatic clearance nearly approximates total body clearance.

$$Cl_H \approx Cl_T = kV_D = \left(\frac{0.693}{3.9}\right)(4.3)(80)$$

$$= 61.1 \text{ L/h}$$

b. $Cl_H = Q(ER)$

$$Q = (1.5 \text{ L/min})(60 \text{ min}) = 90 \text{ L/h}$$

$$ER = 61.1/90 = 0.68$$

11. a. $Cl_T = kV_D\left(\dfrac{0.693}{1.6}\right)(0.78)(81) = 27.4 \text{ L/h}$

$$Cl_R = k_e V_D$$

$$k_e = 0.12k = 0.12\left(\frac{0.693}{1.6}\right) = 0.052 \text{ h}^{-1}$$

b. $Cl_R = (0.052)(0.78)(81) = 3.29 \text{ L/h}$

Alternatively,

$$Cl_R = f_e Cl_T$$

$$Cl_R = 0.12 Cl_T = (0.12)(27.4) = 3.29 \text{ L/h}$$

c. $Cl_H = Cl_T - Cl_R = 27.4 - 3.29 = 24.11 \text{ L/h}$

REFERENCES

Alvares AP, Pratt WB: Pathways of drug metabolism. In Pratt WB, Taylor P (eds). *Principles of Drug Action*, 3rd ed. New York, Churchill Livingstone, 1990, Chap 5.

Ariens EJ, Wuis EW: Commentary: Bias in pharmacokinetics and clinical pharmacology. *Clin Pharm Ther* 42:361–363, 1987.

Baily DG, Arnold JMO, Munoz C, Spence JD: Grapefruit juice–felodipine interaction: Mechanism, predictability, and effect of naringin. *Clin Pharm Ther* **53**:637–642, 1993b.

Baily DG, Arnold JMO, Strong HA, Munoz C, Spence JD: Effect of grapefruit juice and naringin on nisoldipine pharmacokinetics. *Clin Pharm Ther* **54**:589–593, 1993a.

Bertilsson L: Geographic/interracial differences in polymorphic drug oxidation. *Clin Pharmacokinet* **29**(4):192–209, 1995.

Blaschke TF: Protein binding and kinetics of drugs in liver diseases. *Clin Pharmacokinet* **2**:32–44, 1977.

Brouwer KL, Dukes GE, Powell JR: Influence of liver function on drug disposition. Applied pharmacokinetics. In Evans WE, Schentag JJ, Jusko WJ, et al (eds). *Principles of Therapeutic Drug Monitoring*. Vancouver, WA, Applied Therapeutics, 1992, Chap 6.

Caldwell J: Conjugation reactions. In Jenner P, Testa B (eds). *Concepts in Drug Metabolism*. New York, Marcel Dekker, 1980, Chap 4.

Campbell TC: Nutrition and drug-metabolizing enzymes. *Clin Pharm Ther* 22:699–706, 1977.

Caraco Y, Sheller J, Wood AJJ: Pharmacogenetic determination of the effects of codeine and prediction of drug interactions. *J Pharmacol Exp Ther* **278**:1165–1174, 1996.

Cer RZ, Mudunuri U, Stephens R, Lebeda F: IC50-to-Ki: A web-based tool for converting IC50 to Ki values for inhibitors of enzyme activity and ligand binding. (Nucleic Acids Research, 2009, Vol. 37, Web Server issue W441–W445 doi:10.1093/nar/gkp253).

Cheng Y, Prusoff WH: Relationship between the inhibition constant (K1) and the concentration of inhibitor which causes 50 per cent inhibition (I50) of an enzymatic reaction. *Biochem Pharmacol* **22**(23):3099–3108, 1973 (http://www.ncbi.nlm.nih.gov/pubmed/8739548).

Cupp MJ, Tracy TS: Cytochrome P-450: New nomenclature and clinical implications. *Am Family Physician* **57**(1):107–116, January 1, 1998 (http://www.aafp.org/afp/980101ap/cupp.html).

Desta Z, Xiaox, Shin JG, et al: Clinical significance of the cytochrome P450 2C19 genetic polymorphism. *Clin Pharmacokinet* **41**(12):913–958, 2002.

Dow P: *Handbook of Physiology*, vol 2, *Circulation*. Washington, DC, American Physiology Society, 1963, p 1406.

Drugs@FDA, http://www.accessdata.fda.gov/scripts/cder/drugsatfda/

Evans DAP: Genetic variations in the acetylation of isoniazid and other drugs. *Ann N Y Acad Sci* **151**:723, 1968.

Evans DAP, Manley KA, McKusik VC: Genetic control of isoniazid metabolism in man. *Br Med J* **2**:485, 1968.

FDA: Drug development and drug interactions: Table of substrates, inhibitors and inducers (http://www.fda.gov/drugs/developmentapprovalprocess/developmentresources/druginteractionslabeling/ucm081177.htm#cypEnzymes). Accessed in 2011.

FDA Guidance for Industry: *In Vivo Drug Metabolism/Drug Interaction Studies–Study Design, Data Analysis, and Recommendations for Dosing and Labeling*, issued 11/24/1999 (www.fda.gov/cder/guidance.htm).

FDA Guidance for Industry: *Drug Interaction Studies: Study design, Data analysis and Implications for Dosing and Labeling* (issued for public comment, 9/11/2006, www.fda.gov/cder/guidance/6695dft.pdf).

Flockhart: Drug interaction table maintained by David Flockhart. Division of Clinical Pharmacology, Indiana University (http://medicine.iupui.edu/flockhart/). Accessed in 2011.

Gilman AG, Rall TW, Nies AS, Taylor (eds): *Goodman and Gilman's The Pharmacological Basis of Therapeutics*, 8th ed. Elmsford, NY, Pergamon Press, 1990.

Gillette JR: Overview of drug-protein binding. *Ann N Y Acad Sci* **226**:6–17, 1973.

Hansch C, Zhang L: Quantitative structure-activity relationships of cytochrome P-450. *Drug Metab Rev* **25**:1–48, 1993.

Huang, S Lesko, L, Temple R: Adverse drug reactions and pharmacokinetic drug interactions. In Waldman SA, Terzic A (eds). *Fundamental Principles: Clinical Pharmacology, Pharmacology and Therapeutics: Principles to Practice*. New York, Elsevier, 2009, Chap 21.

Hucker HB, Kwan KC, Duggan DE: Pharmacokinetics and metabolism of nonsteroidal antiinflammatory agents. In Bridges JW, Chasseaud LF (eds). *Progress in Drug Research*, vol 5. New York, Wiley, 1980, Chap 3.

Hukkinen SK, Varhe A, Olkkola KT, Neuvonen PJ: Plasma concentrations of triazolam are increased by concomitant ingestion of grapefruit juice. *Clin Pharm Ther* **58**:127–131, 1995.

Iwakawa S, Suganuma T, Lee S, et al: Direct determination of diastereomeric carprofen glucuronides in human plasma and urine and preliminary measurements of stereoselective metabolic and renal elimination after oral administration of carprofen in man. *Drug Metab Disp* **17**:414–419, 1989.

Katzung B, Masters S, Trevor A: *Basic & Clinical Pharmacology*, 11th ed. McGraw-Hill, 2009.

Katzung Bertram G. (ed): *Basic & Clinical Pharmacology*, 11th ed. McGraw-Hill, 2009.

Kupferschmidt HH, Ha HR, Ziegler WH, Meier PJ, Krahenbuhl S: Interaction between grapefruit juice and midazolam in humans. *Clin Pharm Ther* **58**:20–28, 1995.

Lai ML, Wang SL, Lai MD, Lin ET, Tse M, Huang JD: Propranolol disposition in Chinese subjects of different CYT2D6 genotypes. *Clin Pharm Ther* **58**:264–268, 1995.

Lindner HH: *Clinical Anatomy*. Norwalk, CT, Appleton & Lange, 1989.

May GD: Genetic differences in drug disposition. *J Clin Pharmacol* **34**:881–897, 1994.

Merkel U, Sigusch H, Hoffmann A: Grapefruit juice inhibits 7-hydroxylation of coumarin in healthy volunteers. *Eur J Clin Pharm* **46**:175–177, 1994.

Nebert DW, Nelson DR, Adesnik M, et al: The P-450 superfamily: Updated listing of all genes and recommended nomenclature for the chromosomal loci. *DNA* **8**:1, 1989.

Negishi M, Tomohide U, Darden TA, Sueyoshi T, Pedersen LG: Structural flexibility and functional versatility of mammalian P-450 enzymes. *FASEB J* **10**:683–689, 1996.

Nelson DR: The cytochrome P450 homepage. *Human Genomics* **4**:59–65, 2009 (http://drnelson.uthsc.edu/cytochromeP450.html).

Parkinson A: Biotransformation of xenobiotics. In Klaassen, CD (ed). *Casarett & Doull's Toxicology*, 5th ed. New York, McGraw-Hill, 1996, Chap 6.

Rahmani R, Zhou XJ: Pharmacokinetics and metabolism of vinca alkaloids. *Cancer Surv* **17**:269–281, 1993.

Rowland M: Effect of some physiologic factors on bioavailability of oral dosage forms. In Swarbrick J (ed). *Current Concepts in the Pharmaceutical Sciences: Dosage Form Design and Bioavailability*. Philadelphia, Lea & Febiger, 1973, Chap 6.

Rowland M: Drug administration and regimens. In Melmon K, Morelli HF (eds). *Clinical Pharmacology*. New York, Macmillan, 1978.

Takao Watanabe, Hiroyuki Kusuhara, Kazuya Maeda, Yoshihisa Shitara, Yuichi Sugiyama: Physiologically based pharmacokinetic modeling to predict transporter-mediated clearance and distribution of pravastatin in humans. *JPET* **328**:652–662, 2009.

Toney GB, Ereshefsky L: Cyclic antidepressants. In Schumacher GE (ed). *Therapeutic Drug Monitoring*. Norwalk, CT, Appleton & Lange, 1995, Chap 13.

Tucker GT: Clinical implications of genetic polymorphism in drug metabolism. *J Pharm Pharmacol* **46**(suppl):417–424, 1994.

Tucker GT, Lennard MS: Enantiomer-specific pharmacokinetics. *Pharmacol Ther* **45**:309–329, 1990.

Wilkinson GR, Guengerich FP, Branch RA: Genetic polymorphism of S-mephenytoin hydroxylation. *Pharmacol Ther* **43**:53–76, 1989.

Wilkinson GR, Shand DG: A physiological approach to hepatic drug clearance. *Clin Pharmacol Ther* **18**:377–390, 1975.

Wolf CR: Distribution and regulation of drug-metabolizing enzymes in mammalian tissues. In Caldwell J, Paulson GD (eds). *Foreign Compound Metabolism*. London, Taylor & Francis, 1984.

Wu CY, Benet LZ: Predicting drug disposition via application of BCS: Transport/absorption/elimination interplay and development of a biopharmaceutics drug disposition classification system. *Pharm Res* **22**:11–23, 2005.

Yee GC, Stanley DL, Pessa LJ, et al: Effect of grapefruit juice on blood cyclosporin concentration. *Lancet* **345**:955–956, 1995.

BIBLIOGRAPHY

Anders MW: *Bioactivation of Foreign Compounds*. New York, Academic Press, 1985.

Balant LP, McAinsh JM: Use of metabolite data in the evaluation of pharmacokinetics and drug action. In Jenner P, Testa B (eds). *Concepts in Drug Metabolism*. New York, Marcel Dekker, 1980, Chap 7.

Benet LZ: Effect of route of administration and distribution on drug action. *J Pharm Biopharm* **6**:559–585, 1978.

Bourne HR, von Zastrow M: Drug receptors and pharmacodynamics. In Katzung BG (ed). *Basic and Clinical Pharmacology*, 9th ed. New York, McGraw-Hill, 2004, Chap 2.

Brosen K: Recent developments in hepatic drug oxidation. *Clin Pharmacokinet* **18**:220, 1990.

Brown C (ed): *Chirality in drug design and synthesis: Racemic Therapeutics–Problems All Along the Line* (EJ Ariens). New York, Academic Press, 1990.

Ducharme MP, Warbasse LH, Edwards DJ: Disposition of intravenous and oral cyclosporine after administration with grapefruit juice. *Clin Pharm Ther* **57:**485–491, 1995.

FDA Guidance for Industry: *Drug Metabolism/Drug Interaction Studies in the Drug Development Process: Studies in vitro,* issued 4/1997.

FDA Drug Development and Drug Interactions Website: www.fda.gov/cder/drug/drugInteractions/default.htm, established May 2006. Drug Development and Drug Interactions www.fda.gov/drugs/developmentapprovalprocess/developmentresources/druginteractionslabeling/ucm080499.htm. Accessed in 2011.

Geroge CF, Shand DG, Renwick AG (eds): *Presystemic Drug Elimination.* Boston, Butterworth, 1982.

Gibaldi M, Perrier D: Route of administration and drug disposition. *Drug Metab Rev* **3:**185–199, 1974.

Gibson GG, Skett P: *Introduction to Drug Metabolism,* 2nd ed. New York, Chapman & Hall, 1994.

Glocklin VC: General considerations for studies of the metabolism of drugs and other chemicals. *Drug Metab Rev* **13:**929–939, 1982.

Gorrod JW, Damani LA: *Biological Oxidation of Nitrogen in Organic Molecules: Chemistry, Toxicology and Pharmacology.* Deerfield Beach, FL, Ellis Horwood, 1985.

Gray H: *Anatomy of the Human Body,* 30th ed. Philadelphia, Lea & Febiger, 1985, p 1495.

Harder S, Baas H, Rietbrock S: Concentration effect relationship of levodopa in patients with Parkinson's disease. *Clin Pharmacokinet* **29:**243–256, 1995.

Hildebrandt A, Estabrook RW: Evidence for the participation of cytochrome b5 in hepatic microsomal mixed-function oxidation reactions. *Arch Biochem Biophys* **143:**66–79, 1971.

Houston JB: Drug metabolite kinetics. *Pharmacol Ther* **15:**521–552, 1982.

Huang SM: New era in drug interaction evaluation: US Food and Drug Administration update on CYP enzymes, transporters, and the guidance process. *J Clin Pharmacol* **48:**662–670, 2008.

Jakoby WB: *Enzymatic Basis of Detoxification.* New York, Academic Press, 1980.

Jenner P, Testa B: *Concepts in Drug Metabolism.* New York, Marcel Dekker, 1980–1981.

Kaplan SA, Jack ML: Physiologic and metabolic variables in bioavailability studies. In Garrett ER, Hirtz JL (eds). *Drug Fate and Metabolism,* vol 3. New York, Marcel Dekker, 1979.

LaDu BL, Mandel HG, Way EL: *Fundamentals of Drug Metabolism and Drug Disposition.* Baltimore, Williams & Wilkins, 1971.

Lanctot KL, Naranjo CA: Comparison of the Bayesian approach and a simple algorithm for assessment of adverse drug events. *Clin Pharm Ther* **58:**692–698, 1995.

Levy RH, Boddy AV: Stereoselectivity in pharmacokinetics: A general theory. *Pharm Res* **8:**551–556, 1991.

Levine WG: Biliary excretion of drugs and other xenobiotics. *Prog Drug Res* **25:**361–420, 1981.

Morris ME, Pang KS: Competition between two enzymes for substrate removal in liver: Modulating effects due to substrate recruitment of hepatocyte activity. *J Pharm Biopharm* **15:**473–496, 1987.

Nies AS, Shand DG, Wilkinson GR: Altered hepatic blood flow and drug disposition. *Clin Pharmacokinet* **1:**135–156, 1976.

Pang KS, Rowland M: Hepatic clearance of drugs, 1. Theoretical considerations of a "well-stirred" model and a "parallel tube" model. Influence of hepatic blood flow, plasma, and blood cell binding and the hepatocellular enzymatic activity on hepatic drug clearance. *J Pharmacokinet Biopharmacol* **5:**625, 1977.

Papadopoulos J, Smithburger PL: Common drug interactions leading to adverse drug event in the intensive care unit: Management and pharmacokinetic considerations, *Crit Care Med* Jun: 35 (suppl 6),126–35, 2010.

Perrier D, Gibaldi M: Clearance and biologic half-life as indices of intrinsic hepatic metabolism. *J Pharmacol Exp Therapeut* **191:**17–24, 1974.

Plaa GL: The enterohepatic circulation. In Gillette JR, Mitchell JR (eds). *Concepts in Biochemical Pharmacology.* New York, Springer-Verlag, 1975, Chap 63.

Pratt WB, Taylor P: *Principles of Drug Action: The Basis of Pharmacology,* 3rd ed. New York, Churchill Livingstone, 1990.

Riddick DS, Ding X, C. Wolf R, Porter TD, Pandey AV, Zhang Q-Y, Gu J, Finn RD, Ronseaux S, McLaughlin LA, Henderson CJ, Zou L, Flück CE: NADPH-Cytochrome P450 Oxidoreductase: Roles in Physiology, Pharmacology, and Toxicology, *Drug Metab Dispos* **41:**12–23, 2013.

Roberts MS, Donaldson JD, Rowland M: Models of hepatic elimination: Comparison of stochastic models to describe residence time distributions and to predict the influence of drug distribution, enzyme heterogeneity, and systemic recycling on hepatic elimination. *J Pharm Biopharm* **16:**41–83, 1988.

Routledge PA, Shand DG: Presystemic drug elimination. *Annu Rev Pharmacol Toxicol* **19:**447–468, 1979.

Semple HA, Tam YK, Coutts RT: A computer simulation of the food effect: Transient changes in hepatic blood flow and Michaelis–Menten parameters as mediators of hepatic first-pass metabolism and bioavailability of propranolol. *Biopharm Drug Disp* **11:**61–76, 1990.

Shand DG, Kornhauser DM, Wilkinson GR: Effects of route administration and blood flow on hepatic drug elimination. *J Pharmacol Exp Therapeut,* **195:**425–432, 1975.

Stoltenborg JK, Puglisi CV, Rubio F, Vane FM: High performance liquid chromatographic determination of stereoselective disposition of carprofen in humans. *J Pharm Sci* **70:**1207–1212, 1981.

Testa B, Jenner B: *Drug Metabolism: Chemical and Biochemical Aspects.* New York, Marcel Dekker, 1976.

Venot A, Walter E, Lecourtier Y, et al: Structural identifiability of "first-pass" models. *J Pharm Biopharm* **15:**179–189, 1987.

Wilkinson GR: Pharmacodynamics of drug disposition: Hemodynamic considerations. *Annu Rev Pharmacol* **15:**11–27, 1975.

Wilkinson GR: Pharmacodynamics in disease states modifying body perfusion. In Benet LZ (ed). *The Effect of Disease States on Drug Pharmacokinetics.* Washington, DC, American Pharmaceutical Association, 1976.

Wilkinson GR, Rawlins MD: *Drug Metabolism and Disposition: Considerations in Clinical Pharmacology.* Boston, MTP Press, 1985.

Williams RT: Hepatic metabolism of drugs. *Gut* **13:**579–585, 1972.

13

Pharmacogenetics and Drug Metabolism

Thomas Abraham and Michael Adams

Chapter Objectives

▶ Define pharmacogenetics and pharmacogenomics.

▶ Define genetic polymorphism and explain the difference between genotype and phenotype.

▶ Explain with relevant examples how genetic variability influences drug response, pharmacokinetics, and dosing regimen design.

▶ Describe the relevance of CYP enzymes and their genetic variability to pharmacokinetics and dosing.

▶ List the major drug transporters and describe how their genetic variability can impact pharmacokinetics.

▶ Discuss the main issues in applying genomic data to patient care, for example, clinical interpretation of data from various laboratories and accuracy of record keeping of large amounts of genomic data.

Variable response to a drug in the general population is thought to follow a normal or Gaussian distribution about a mean or average dose, ED_{50} (Fig. 13-1). Patients who fall within region A of the curve may be described as hyper-responders while those in region B may be characterized as poor or hypo-responders. While pharmacokinetic and pharmacodynamic differences are thought to be primarily responsible for this Gaussian variation in drug response, the extremes in drug response may be due to unique interindividual genetic variability. Modern genetic methods have identified alterations in drug-metabolizing enzymes, drug transporters, and drug receptors that, at least in part, explain many of these extremes in drug response. This has given birth to the field of *pharmacogenetics*, which seeks to characterize inter-individual drug-response variability at the genetic level (Mancinelli et al, 2000). A related term, *pharmacogenomics*, is often used interchangeably but includes the study of the genetic basis of disease and the pharmacological impact of drugs on the disease process (Mancinelli et al, 2000).

Advances in pharmacogenetics have been enabled by high-throughput technology that allows for the screening of tens of thousands of genes rapidly and simultaneously. For example, the DNA chip is a microchip that uses hybridization technology to concurrently detect the presence of tens of thousands of sequences in a small sample. The probes (of known sequence) are spotted onto discreet locations on the chip, so that complementary DNA hybridization from the patient's sample to a probe residing in a defined location indicates the presence of a specific sequence (Mancinelli et al, 2000; Dodgan et al, 2013). Other rapid and low-cost sequencing technologies such as ULCS (ultra-low-cost sequencing) or cyclic array technologies will also permit rapid and high-volume sequencing and/or sequencing of individual genomes. These technologies usually rely on some combination of miniaturization, multiplex or parallel assays, analyte amplification and/or concentration, and detection signal amplification.

Application of pharmacogenetics to pharmacokinetics and pharmacodynamics helps in development of models that may predict an individual's risk to an adverse drug event and therapeutic

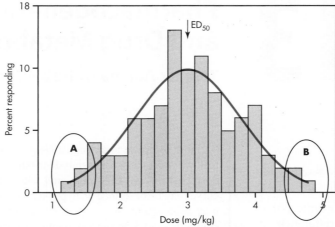

FIGURE 13-1   Simulated Gaussian distribution of population response to a hypothetical drug. The ED_{50} indicates the mean dose producing a therapeutic outcome while regions A and B highlight patients who are hyper- or hyporesponders to the drug effect, respectively.

response (Fernandez-Rozadilla et al, 2013; Meyer et al, 2013). The promise of such modeling efforts is that more individualized dosing regimens may be developed resulting in more "personalized medicine" with fewer adverse events and better therapeutic outcomes (Phillips et al, 2001). This chapter will focus on variations in pharmacokinetic components due to pharmacogenetic factors. Variations in drug response due to genetic variations in the drug's receptor or downstream processes can also be identified using pharmacogenetic principles and screening; however, that is beyond the scope of this chapter.

GENETIC POLYMORPHISMS

Historically, population variability in drug metabolism or therapeutic response was described in terms of the observed phenotype, for example, slow metabolizers or sensitive responders. With our understanding of genetics, we are often able to ascribe specific alterations in gene sequence, or genotype, to explain such observed effects. *Genetic polymorphisms* are variations in gene sequences that occur in at least 1% of the general population, resulting in multiple alleles or variants of a gene sequence. Polymorphisms are distinct from *mutations* that occur in less than 1% of the population. The most commonly occurring

form of genetic variability is the *single nucleotide polymorphism* (SNP, often called "snip"), resulting from a change in a single nucleotide base pair within the gene sequence (Ahles and Engelhardt, 2014). Synonymous SNPs in the coding region of a gene generally result in no change in the amino acid sequence of the eventual protein product. Non-synonymous SNPs in the coding region will result in a change in the amino acid sequence of the protein. In some cases, this alteration may have little effect on the protein's structure and function, for example, if one acidic amino acid is replaced by another. However, non-synonymous SNPs have the potential to drastically alter the function of protein (Ahles and Engelhardt, 2014). An example of such an effect occurs if nucleotide position 2935 of the CYP2D6 gene has a C instead of an A (c.2935A>C). During translation this results in the insertion of a proline instead of histidine at amino acid position 324 generating the CYP2D6*7 allele, with no drug metabolizing activity (The Human Cytochrome P450 Allele Nomenclature Database, 2014). Genetic variants that result from the insertion or deletion of a nucleotide in the coding region are also classified as SNPs. Since the mRNAs from genes are translated to protein in 3-nucleotide codons, such insertions or deletions can have a significant effect on the eventual protein product. An example of such a polymorphism is the CYP2D6*3 allele where a single nucleotide deletion (A_{2637}) results in a frame shift in translation that produces an enzyme with no catalytic activity (The Human Cytochrome P450 Allele Nomenclature Database, 2014). Each variant of a gene is represented by the star designation (*) followed by a number, and each gene could potentially contain multiple variants. A grouping of select variants is called a haplotype and results in unique combinations of polymorphisms with potentially novel phenotypes.

Single nucleotide polymorphisms outside the coding region of the gene can result in altered levels of protein activity as well. Polymorphisms in the promoter sequence of a gene can influence gene transcription rates resulting in greater or lesser amounts of mRNA, and consequently protein expression. Alternatively, SNPs in a splicing control region of the gene can result in the production of a unique protein often missing one or more exons and resulting in a unique (often truncated or inactive) protein. In some cases, multiple copies of a gene on a chromosome can result in increased levels of protein being expressed, and once again the CYP2D6 gene serves as a relevant example. The CYP2D6xN variant (where N = 2–12 copies) results in very high expression of the functional enzyme in patients who are considered ultrarapid metabolizers of certain drugs (The Human Cytochrome P450 Allele Nomenclature Database, 2014; see below). Polymorphic induction of gene expression is distinct from that induced by drugs such as phenytoin, barbiturates, etc. However, it isn't difficult to see that a mixed form of CYP gene expression due to genetics and drug induction could increase metabolic activity to an even greater extent. Deletion or inversion of entire genes on the chromosome would obviously have the opposite effect on enzyme activity and drug metabolism.

Genetic Polymorphism in Drug Metabolism

As discussed in Chapter 12, drug metabolism is responsible for the chemical modification of drugs or other xenobiotics that usually results in increased polarity to enhance elimination from the body. The enzymes that perform drug metabolism are classified as either phase I or phase II enzymes and their relative contributions to drug metabolism are highlighted in Fig. 13-2. Phase I enzymes perform oxidation, reduction, and hydrolysis reactions while phase II enzymes perform conjugation reactions. Polymorphisms have been reported in both phases of drug-metabolizing enzymes and can affect the pharmacokinetic profile of a drug for a given patient. Understanding a patient's genetic determinants of drug metabolism and the consequences of these polymorphisms could be used to design optimum, personalized dosing regimens in the clinic that would avoid adverse reactions or treatment failures due to subtherapeutic doses. While this may appear perfectly logical, the redundancy of drug metabolism and potential contribution from numerous other factors (such as diet, other drugs, age, weight, etc) make it difficult to translate enzyme status data to a clinical decision. For example, warfarin therapy is complicated by a combination of metabolic (CYP2C9 polymorphisms contribute 2%–10%), pharmacodynamic (VKORC1 polymorphisms contribute 10%–25%), and environmental factors (20%–25% contribution). Several algorithms that take into account genetic information have been developed for warfarin dosing and some are available online (Warfarin Dosing, 2009; Pharmacogenetics Knowledge Base, 2014). While these appear to be useful tools to account for genetic differences, the reported effectiveness of achieving an optimal anticoagulant dose of warfarin using algorithms is variable (Caraco et al, 2008; Wang et al, 2012; Kimmel et al, 2013). These confounding results demonstrate the need for more investigation into the factors (including pharmacokinetic and pharmacodynamic factors) that contribute to variable responses, as well as robust clinical investigations to validate these observations. There are 70 drugs that include pharmacogenetic information related to polymorphisms in drug-metabolizing enzymes that contribute to variable drug response (Pharmacogenetics Knowledge Base, 2014). Drugs that are thought to be affected by the polymorphisms, the consequence, and label information are included in Table 13-1 (Evans, 1999; Pharmacogenetics Knowledge Base, 2014). Further examples of polymorphism affecting drugs among different race and special subject groups are shown in Table 13-2.

TABLE 13-1 Clinically Important Genetic Polymorphisms of Drug Metabolism and Transporters That Influence Drug Response

Enzyme	Drug	Drug Effect/Side Effect	FDA Label Information^ (Pharmacogenetics Knowledge Base, 2014)
CYP2C9	Warfarin	Hemorrhage	Actionable
	Tolbutamide	Hypoglycemia	-
	Phenytoin	Phenytoin toxicity	-
	Glipizide	Hypoglycemia	-
	Losartan	Decreased antihypertensive effect	-
CYP2D6	Antiarrhythmics	Proarrhythmic and other toxic effects in poor metabolizers	-
	Antidepressants	Inefficacy in ultrarapid metabolizers	Actionable/Information*
	Antipsychotics	Tardive dyskinesia	Actionable/Information*
	Eliglustat	Inefficacy in ultrarapid metabolizers	Testing recommended
	Opioids	Inefficacy of codeine as analgesic, narcotic side effects, dependence	Actionable
	Pimozide	Toxicity with high dose in poor metabolizers	Testing recommended
	Tetrabenazine	Toxicity with high dose in poor metabolizers or inefficacy in ultrarapid metabolizers	Testing recommended
	Warfarin	Higher risk of hemorrhage	-
	β-Adrenoceptor antagonists	Increased blockade	Actionable/Information*
CYP2C19	Omeprazole	Higher cure rates when given with clarithromycin	Information
	Diazepam	Prolonged sedation	Actionable
	Clopidogrel	Inefficacy in poor metabolizers	Testing recommended
Dihydropyrimidine dehydrogenase	Fluorouracil	Myelotoxicity, neurotoxicity	Actionable
Plasma pseudo-cholinesterase	Succinylcholine	Prolonged apnea	-
N-acetyltransferase	Sulfonamides	Hypersensitivity	-
	Amonafide	Myelotoxicity	-
	Procainamide	Drug-induced lupus erythematosus	-
	Hydralazine	Drug-induced lupus erythematosus	Information
	Isoniazid	Drug-induced lupus erythematosus	Information

(Continued)

TABLE 13-1   **Clinically Important Genetic Polymorphisms of Drug Metabolism and Transporters That Influence Drug Response (Continued)**

Enzyme	Drug	Drug Effect/Side Effect	FDA Label Information^ (Pharmacogenetics Knowledge Base, 2014)
Thiopurine methyltransferase	Mercaptopurine	Myelotoxicity	Testing recommended
	Thioguanine	Myelotoxicity	Actionable
	Azathioprine	Myelotoxicity	Testing recommended
UDP-**G**lucuronosyltransferase	Irinotecan	Diarrhea, Myelotoxicity	Actionable
Multidrug-resistance gene (**MDR1**)	Digoxin	Increased concentrations of digoxin in plasma	-
Organic anion transporter protein (**SLCO1B1**)	Simvastatin	Myopathy	-

^Information: Drug label contains information on gene or protein responsible for drug metabolism but does not include evidence of variations in drug response.

Actionable: Drug label contains information about changes in efficacy, dosage, or toxicity of a drug due to gene variants but does not discuss genetic or other testing.

Testing recommended: Drug label recommends testing or states testing should be performed for specific gene or protein variants prior to use, sometimes in a specific population.

*Depends upon the specific drug agent.

From Evans and Relling (1999)

CYTOCHROME P-450 ISOZYMES

Cytochrome P-450 (CYP450) isozymes are the primary phase I oxidative enzymes that are found in many species with functionality in the metabolism of xenobiotics and endogenous biochemical process. The CYP450s are divided into families identified with numbers (CYP1, CYP2, CYP3, etc) and subfamilies identified with letters (CYP2A, CYP2B, etc) based on amino acid similarities. The major drug-metabolizing CYP450 families are CYP1, CYP2, and CYP3 (see Fig. 13-2) and those will be the focus of this section.

CYP2D6

CYP2D6 is the most highly polymorphic CYP with more than 70 allelic variants reported (The Human Cytochrome P450 Allele Nomenclature Database, 2014). Many of these allelic variants are clinically important because although CYP2D6 only makes up about 5% of hepatic CYP activity, it is responsible for the metabolism of as much as 25% of commonly prescribed drugs (Fig. 13-2). These drugs include

antidepressants, antiarrhythmics, beta-adrenergic antagonists, and opioids, which frequently have narrow therapeutic indices. While we now have more detailed information on the genotypes, the phenotypic differences in CYP2D6 were originally observed with debrisoquine, resulting in the more general descriptions of poor metabolizer (PM), extensive metabolizer (EM), and ultrarapid metabolizer (UM) (Mahgoub et al, 1977; Idle et al, 1978).

It is estimated that approximately 10% of the Caucasian population, 1% of the Asian population, and between 0% and 19% of the African population have a PM phenotype of CYP2D6 (McGraw and Waller, 2012), resulting in increased plasma concentration of the parent drug due to decreased metabolic clearance. In the case of debrisoquine, the increased plasma concentration results in an exaggerated hypotensive response. When a patient with a PM phenotype is administered a tricyclic antidepressant, the increased plasma concentration increases the potential for CNS depression. If metabolism is required for a drug to have activity, the patient with a PM phenotype is more likely to have a treatment failure

TABLE 13-2 Examples of Polymorphisms Affecting Drug Receptors and Enzymes Showing Frequency of Occurrence

Enzyme/Receptor	Frequency of Polymorphism	Drug	Drug Effect/Side Effect
CYP2C9	14%–28% (heterozygotes)	Warfarin	Hemorrhage
		Tolbutamide	Hypoglycemia
	0.2%–1% (homozygotes)	Phenytoin	Phenytoin toxicity
		Glipizide	Hypoglycemia
		Losartan	Decreased antihypertensive effect
CYP2D6	5%–10% (poor metabolizers)	Antiarrhythmics	Proarrhythmic and other toxic effects
			Toxicity in poor metabolizers
	1%–10% (ultrarapid metabolizers)	Antidepressants	Inefficacy in ultrarapid metabolizers
		Antipsychotics	Tardive dyskinesia
		Opioids	Inefficacy of codeine as analgesic, narcotic side effects, dependence
		Warfarin	Higher risk of hemorrhage
		β-Adrenoceptor antagonists	Increased—blockade
CYP2C19	3%–6% (whites)	Omeprazole	Higher cure rates when given with clarithromycin
	8%–23% (Asians)	Diazepam	Prolonged sedation
Dihydropyrimidine dehydrogenase	0.1%	Fluorouracil	Myelotoxicity, Neurotoxicity
Plasma pseudo-cholinesterase	1.5%	Succinylcholine	Prolonged apnea
N-acetyltransferase	40%–70% (whites)	Sulphonamides	Hypersensitivity
	10%–20% (Asians)	Amonafide	Myelotoxicity (rapid acetylators)
		Procainamide, hydralazine, isoniazid	Drug-induced lupus erythematosus
Thiopurine methyltransferase	0.3%	Mercaptopurine, thioguanine, azothioprine	Myelotoxicity
UDP-glucuronosyltransferase	10%–15%	Irinotecan	Diarrhea, myelosuppression
ACE		Enalapril, lisinapril captopril	Renoprotective effect, cardiac indexes, blood pressure
Potassium channels		Quinidine	Drug-induced QT syndrome
HERG		Cisapride	Drug-induced torsade de pointes
KvLQT1		Terfenadine disopyramide	Drug-induced long-QT syndrome
VKORC		Warfarin	Over-anticoagulation
Epidermal growth factor receptor (EGFR)		Gefitinib	Certain polymorphs susceptible
HKCNE2		Meflaquine clarithromycin	Drug-induced arrhythmia

From Meyer (2000) with permission, and from Evans and Relling (1999) as well as Limdi and Veenstra (2010).

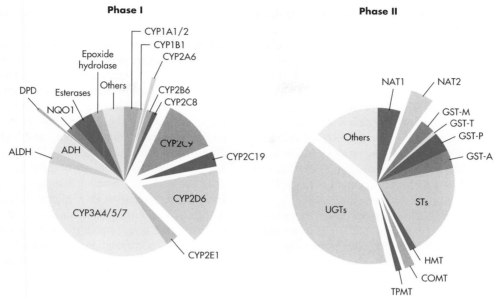

FIGURE 13-2   Drug-metabolizing enzymes that exhibit clinically relevant genetic polymorphisms. Essentially all of the major human enzymes responsible for modification of functional groups (classified as phase I reactions [left]) or conjugation with endogenous substituents (classified as phase II reactions [right]) exhibit common polymorphisms at the genomic level; those enzyme polymorphisms that have already been associated with changes in drug effects are separated from the corresponding pie charts. The percentage of phase I and phase II metabolism of drugs that each enzyme contributes is estimated by the relative size of each section of the corresponding chart. ADH, alcohol dehydrogenase; ALDH, aldehyde dehydrogenase; CYP, cytochrome P-450; DPD, dihydropyrimidine dehydrogenase; NQO1, NADPH, quinone oxidoreductase or DT diaphorase; COMT, catechol O-methyltransferase; GST, glutathione S-transferase; HMT, histamine methyltransferase; NAT, *N*-acetyltransferase; STs, sulfotransferases; TPMT, thiopurine methyltransferase; UGTs, uridine 5′-triphosphate glucuronosyltransferases. (From Evans and Relling, 1999, with permission.)

than an adverse event. This has been reported with the breast cancer agent tamoxifen (Rolla et al, 2012). Tamoxifen has an active metabolite (endoxifen) produced by CYP2D6 that is thought to be responsible for much of its antiestrogenic activities. The patient with the PM phenotype would not metabolize tamoxifen to the active metabolite and, therefore, does not benefit from clinically relevant endoxifen concentrations (Rolla et al, 2012). Genotypically, PM have two null alleles, which do not code for functional CYP2D6 due to a frame shift (CYP2D6*3 and *6), a splicing defect (CYP2D6*4), or a gene deletion (CYP2D6*5).

The UM have very high rates of CYP2D6 enzymatic activity resulting in low plasma concentrations of drugs with consequent lower efficacy. Active drugs like the tricyclic antidepressant amitriptyline may require doses several-fold higher than standard

doses to achieve therapeutic activity when the patient is a UM. On the other hand, drugs that require metabolism to an active metabolite are extremely active, with potentially serious consequences. Codeine is converted to morphine by a CYP2D6 O-demethylation reaction to provide analgesic effects, and morphine-associated toxicity has been reported after codeine administration in patients who are UM (Gasche et al, 2004). The FDA label for codeine-containing products includes a black box warning to highlight the risk of death in children with CYP2D6 UM phenotypes. The UM phenotype is the result of multiple copies (up to 12 copies) of either the wild-type CYP2D6*1 or the *2 gene on a single chromosome resulting in greatly enhanced functional CYP2D6 activity (The Human Cytochrome P450 Allele Nomenclature Database, 2013). The UM phenotype is found in Caucasian populations (1%–10%), but is more common in others such as Saudi Arabians (20%) and Ethiopians (29%) (Samer et al, 2013).

CYP2D6 EM phenotype includes 60%–85% of the Caucasian population and has normal enzymatic activity (CYP2D6*1). In addition to PM, EM, and UM, an intermediate metabolizer (IM) phenotype has also been identified. The IM phenotype is a result of either one null allele or two deficient alleles and is prevalent in up to 50% of Asians, 30% of Africans, and around 10%–15% of Caucasians (Samer et al, 2013). The deficient alleles include CYP2D6*2, *10, and *17, each of which has enzymatic activity that is less than the wild-type enzyme (CYP2D6*1).

Understanding this complex interplay between all the different alleles of CYP2D6 and the many drugs that it metabolizes provides a great opportunity for accurate genotyping to provide for sound clinical decisions to prevent adverse events and prevent therapeutic failures.

CYP1A2

CYP1A2 activity varies widely with genetic polymorphisms contributing to observed differences in levels of gene expression. CYP1A2 is responsible for the metabolism of about 5% of marketed drugs including fluvoxamine, clozapine, olanzapine, and theophylline. Approximately 15% of the Japanese, 5% of the Chinese, and 5% of the Australian populations are classified as CYP1A2 poor metabolizers. The most frequent allelic variant is CYP1A2*1F, which results in an increased expression caused by an SNP in the upstream promoter region. Enhanced enzyme levels are thought to cause faster substrate clearance, which has been associated with treatment failures for clozapine in smokers with the *1F allele (Eap et al, 2004). CYP1A2*1C is also an SNP in the upstream promoter region that results in decreased enzyme expression and has a prevalence up to 25% in Asian populations (McGraw and Waller, 2012).

CYP2C9

CYP2C9 has at least 30 different allelic variants with the two most common being CYP2C9*2 and *3. Both of these variants result in reduced CYP2C9 activity and are carried by about 35% of the Caucasian population. CYP2C9 is a major contributor to the metabolism of the narrow therapeutic index blood thinner warfarin. When a patient has one of these two polymorphisms, the dose of warfarin needed for clinically relevant anticoagulation is generally much less since drug clearance is reduced. If the dose of warfarin is not appropriately lowered, then there is an increased risk of bleeding. There are several other drugs affected by the polymorphisms of CYP2C9, including many nonsteroidal anti-inflammatory drugs, sulfonylureas, angiotensin II receptor antagonists, and phenytoin. For each of these, the CYP2C9*2 and *3 polymorphisms result in higher plasma concentrations but, because of their high therapeutic indices (except phenytoin), do not usually result in adverse effects. In the case of phenytoin, the polymorphisms result in drug accumulation and require dose reduction to prevent toxicity (ie, dizziness, nystagmus, ataxia).

CYP2C19

CYP2C19 is a highly polymorphic drug-metabolizing enzyme with at least 30 variants reported (The Human Cytochrome P450 Allele Nomenclature Database, 2013). Polymorphisms in CYP2C19 result in variable drug response to clopidogrel and several antidepressants. The PM phenotype is often the result of two null alleles, CYP2C19*2, and *3. Both alleles produce truncated, nonfunctional CYP2C19 through the introduction of a stop codon. The stop codon in the CYP2C19*2 allele is the result of a splicing defect that introduces a frame shift while in the CYP2C19*3 allele, an SNP introduces the early stop codon (de Morais et al, 1994). The allelic frequency of CYP2C19*2 has been shown to be 15% in Africans, 29%–35% in Asians, 12%–15% in Caucasians, and 61% in Oceanians. CYP2C19*3 is mainly found in Asians (5%–9%) with very low frequency in Caucasians (0.5%) (Samer et al, 2013).

The CYP2C19 PM phenotype results in a lack of efficacy for the antiplatelet prodrug clopidogrel. For activation, clopidogrel requires a two-step metabolism by several different CYP450 with CYP2C19 being a significant contributor. Studies have demonstrated, and the FDA has added to the label, that deficiencies in CYP2C19 activity may result in the increased risk of adverse cardiovascular outcomes because the PM does not activate clopidogrel sufficiently (Scott et al, 2011). With omeprazole the opposite occurs since metabolism inactivates the drug. The PM phenotype results in higher plasma concentrations, larger AUC values, and greater efficacy in lowering gastric pH than extensive metabolizers with CYP2C19*1 alleles (Ogawaa and Echizen, 2010). The higher plasma concentration of omeprazole is particularly useful in the multiple-drug treatment of *Helicobacter pylori*. In the PM patients treated with omeprazole, the *H. pylori* eradication rate is higher when they have one or more of the null alleles (Shi and Klotz, 2008).

The CYP2C19*17 allele results in a gain of function and, therefore, has more metabolic capacity than the wild-type enzyme, CYP2C19*1, because of an SNP in the upstream noncoding region that induces transcription (Sim et al, 2006). Patients that have this UM phenotype are either heterozygous or homozygous for CYP2C19*17. Carriers of this allele are associated with higher risk for bleeding due to the increased metabolism of clopidogrel to the active metabolite (Sibbing et al, 2010). These examples demonstrate that both loss and gain of function alleles can have significant effects on patient outcomes depending upon the blood levels and activity of the parent drug and the metabolite.

CYP3A4

CYP3A4 is the most abundant CYP450 in the liver and metabolizes over 50% of the clinically used drugs (Fig. 13-2). In addition, the liver expression of CYP3A4 is variable between individuals. To date, over 20 allelic variants of CYP3A4 have been identified (The Human Cytochrome P450 Allele Nomenclature Database, 2013). Despite the large number of variants, there is limited data demonstrating any clinical significance for CYP3A4 substrates. Some of the variability may be caused by allelic variants that influence the upstream noncoding region of the gene, specifically in CYP3A4*1B allele, which may influence gene expression, although the exact transcription factor binding site has not been identified (Sata et al, 2000). The CYP3A4*2 allele has a non-synonymous SNP that is found in about 2.7% of the Caucasian population and has some decreased clearance for the calcium channel blocker nifedipine

but not for testosterone 6β-hydroxylation (Sata et al, 2000). The effects of the polymorphisms in CYP3A4 are still under investigation but currently there are no null phenotypes.

Other Phase I Enzymes

While the CYP450s are the most abundant and extensively studied phase I drug-metabolizing enzymes, others have polymorphisms that have an effect on the clearance (or activation) of drugs and, therefore, affect the clinical outcomes of patients secondary to, at least partially, changes in pharmacokinetics.

Plasma pseudocholinesterase or serum butyrylcholinesterase

Plasma pseudocholinesterase is responsible for the inactivation through ester hydrolysis of the neuromuscular blockers succinylcholine and mivacurium. While mivacurium is no longer marketed in the US market, succinylcholine is used to provide skeletal muscle relaxation or paralysis for surgery or mechanical ventilation. There are at least 65 allelic variants of pseudocholinesterase that have been identified in approximately 1.5% of the population that result in various levels of pseudocholinesterase deficiencies (Soliday et al, 2010). These allelic variants include non-synonymous point mutations or frame shift mutations that result in a PM phenotype for succinylcholine. Patients with slowed metabolism of succinylcholine have elevated blood levels, prolonged duration of action, and prolonged apnea compared to patients with fully functional pseudocholinesterase.

Dihydropyrimidine dehydrogenase (DPD)

DPD is the first reduction and rate-limited step in breakdown of the pyrimidine nucleic acids and their analogs. Polymorphisms in DPD result in a loss of enzymatic activity leading to the accumulation of the chemotherapeutic agent 5-flourouracil (5-FU), which leads to significant toxicity including leukopenia, thrombocytopenia, and stomatitis. It is estimated that approximately 3%–5% of population has low or deficient DPD activity (Lu et al, 1993; Etienne et al, 1994). There are three alleles, each with low frequency, that appear to account for the majority of the deficient DPD activity observed and more than 20%

of the serious toxicity observed with 5-FU administration. DPYD*2A is the most common allelic variant, although the exact frequency is not clear. This variant results in a nonfunctional enzyme due to a point mutation that creates an exon skipping splice variant. DPYD*13 and c.2846A>T variants are non-synonymous SNPs that decrease the activity of the DPD produced. There are many other allelic variants that have been identified to date but have only been found in very small numbers or have unknown clinical consequences.

PHASE II ENZYMES

As discussed in the previous chapter (drug metabolism), phase II drug-metabolizing enzymes are commonly referred to as transferases and perform conjugation reactions that add a biochemical compound to a xenobiotic to facilitate its elimination. Just like the phase I reactions, there are genetic variations in the several phase II enzymes that influence the pharmacokinetics of drugs.

Thiopurine S-methyltransferase

Thiopurine drugs including 6-mercaptopurine (MP) and azathioprine are used for their anticancer and immunosuppressive properties but can have significant adverse effects including myelosuppression. The phase II metabolizing enzyme thiopurine S-methyltransferase (TPMT) is involved in the degradation of thiopurine drugs and TPMT polymorphisms account for about one-third of the variable responses to MP and azathioprine (Colombel et al, 2000; Ansari et al, 2002). While TPMT alone only explains one-third of the variability, other factors are known to contribute, which highlights the challenge and multifactorial nature of personalized medicine to account for intraindividual differences. At least twenty-eight allelic variants in the coding and splicing region of TPMT have been identified with most of the null phenotypes being associated with TPMT*2, TPMT*3A, and TPMT*3B alleles resulting in non-synonymous mutations that lead to the production of an unstable enzyme and reduced activity overall. The loss of TPMT function is present in about 5% of the Caucasian population and results in

accumulation of MP leading to an increased risk for adverse effects like leukopenia (Ameyaw et al, 1999; Schaeffeler et al, 2008). Although not well understood, variations in the promoter region for TPMT can also account for some of the observed differences in expression and susceptibility for adverse effects. The remaining variability may be accounted for with numerous other factors including some genetic and some environmental.

Uridine Diphosphate (UDP)-glucuronosyltransferase

UDP-glucuronosyltransferase (UGT) is a super-family of phase II drug-metabolizing enzymes that produce glucuronidation metabolites through conjugation reactions (see Chapter 12). Like the CYP450s, the UGTs are divided into families identified with numbers (UGT1, UGT2, etc) and subfamilies identified with letters (UGT1A, UGT2B, etc) based on amino acid similarities. Drug metabolism is catalyzed almost exclusively by UGT1 and UGT2 (Meech et al, 2012). At least 200 alleles for UGT1 and UGT2 gene families have been reported causing changes in enzymatic activity or expression levels that may contribute to individual variations in drug response (UGT Alleles Nomenclature Home Page, June 2005). One of the most frequently studied genetic variations in Caucasians is the UGT1A1*28 allele (32%) (Stingl et al, 2014) due to changes in the promoter region that decrease the expression of UGT1A1 (Beutler et al, 1998). The UGT1A1*6 allele is found most frequently in the Asian population (18%) and contains a non-synonymous SNP in the coding region that results in decreased UGT1A1 activity (Stingl et al, 2014).

The potential effect of variable activity of UGT is dependent on the relationship between parent drug and metabolite. While most UGT metabolites are inactive, there are examples of activation including morphine metabolism to the active 6-glucuronide metabolite and various carboxylic acids metabolism to reactive, potentially toxic, acylglucuronides (Stingl et al, 2014). The potential effects of these changes have been reported for over 22 different drugs with various changes to pharmacokinetic profiles including AUC and clearance (Stingl et al, 2014).

A summary of the pharmacogenetics for all 22 drugs is beyond the scope of this chapter, but one example of a drug that includes FDA labeling related to UGT polymorphisms, irinotecan, will be briefly discussed.

Irinotecan is a prodrug topisomerase-1 inhibitor that is approved to treat metastatic colon or rectal cancer. The active metabolite of irinotecan, SN-38, is produced by ester hydrolysis and is primarily cleared through biliary excretion after inactivation by UGT (Rothenberg, 1998). The accumulation of SN-38 is associated with dose- and treatment-limiting adverse effects including bone marrow toxicity and diarrhea. The FDA-approved label for irinotecan recommends a dosage reduction in patients that are homozygous for UGT1A1*28 due to an increased risk of neutropenia (Food and Drug Administration, 2014). In Asian populations, the UGT1A1*6 allele is associated with increased irinotecan toxicity and decreased clearance compared to the UGT1A1*1 (wild-type) allele (Han et al, 2009). Other UGT alleles including UGT1A7*3 and UGT1A9*22 may contribute to irinotecan toxicity by metabolizing SN-38 but the consequences of these variations are not so clear.

N-Acetyltransferase

N-acetyltransferase (NAT) was identified as a polymorphic enzyme through phenotypic observations of fast or slow acetylators of the anti-tuberculosis drug, isoniazid (Evans and White, 1964). There are two different human genes, NAT1 and NAT2, that code for functional NAT activity. While both NAT1 and NAT2 are polymorphic, the fast and slow acetylator phenotype is associated with the NAT2 gene. The slow acetylator phenotype is found in about 50% of Caucasians, 90% of Arabs, and 10% of Japanese populations (Green et al, 2000). Several NAT2 alleles, *5, *6, *7, *10, *14, and *17, are either null genes or encode of defective enzymes that contribute to the slow phenotype (Pharmacogenetics Knowledge Base, 2014). Patients that are slow metabolizers of isoniazid exhibit increased blood levels of the drug, which results in an increased incidence of neurotoxicity (Pharmacogenetics Knowledge Base, 2014). The metabolism of both procainamide and hydralazine is also dependent upon the activity of NAT2 such that

slow metabolizers are associated with an increased risk of lupus erythematosus (Chen et al, 2007). With fast metabolizers, there can also be an increased toxicity of the topoisomerase II inhibitor, amonafide, which is associated with a higher incidence of myelosuppression (Innocenti et al, 2001).

TRANSPORTERS

Several membrane transporter proteins are involved in drug absorption from the intestinal tract and distribution through the body. An increased appreciation of the influence of these transporters on the uptake and efflux of drugs into or out of tissues has enhanced interest in the pharmacogenetics of these transporters. It is likely that significant issues in oral drug bioavailability and variable pharmacokinetics result from genetic polymorphisms in transporters. Unlike many of the drug-metabolizing enzymes discussed above, our current understanding of transporter pharmacogenetics is not as well developed and the consequences of the SNPs are not so clear.

MDR1 (P-Glycoprotein)

The MDR1 or ABCB1 gene codes for the efflux protein P-glycoprotein (P-gp) that is frequently associated with drug resistance to antineoplastic agents including vincristine and doxorubicin. In cancers that express PGP, the drug is transported out of the cells, keeping the drug concentrations inside the target cell low. In addition to this resistance function, expression of PGP also contributes to the efflux of some drugs from various tissues that affect the pharmacokinetics of these compounds. There are many PGP substrates and inhibitors as outlined in Chapter 11. At least 66 SNPs in the ABCB1 gene have been reported, and the three most studied SNPs include two synonymous and one non-synonymous variants (Brambila-Tapia, 2013). The synonymous SNPs are reported to result in decreased expression of PGP due to decreased mRNA expression, unstable mRNA, or alterations in protein folding (Sissung et al, 2012). The effects of these SNPs on drug serum levels have been examined in multiple studies with substrates including digoxin and docetaxel. The reported results on the pharmacokinetic profile of these two drugs have been inconsistent with studies showing increased blood levels or no change compared to the wild-type gene (Sissung et al, 2012). These results highlight the dependency on the individual substrate, the complexity, and the effect of specific tissue transporter expression, which contributes to the pharmacokinetic profile of each drug. Additionally, there are also known inhibitors to PGP that complicate the prediction of the pharmacokinetic profile in patients that are administered multiple drugs.

ABC Transporters

The multidrug resistance-associated proteins (MRPs) are members of the ATP-binding cassette (ABC) superfamily with six members currently, of which MRP1 (ABCC1), MRP2 (ABCC2), and MRP3 (ABCC3) are commonly known to effect drug disposition. Like MDR, these transporters can also be expressed in cancer cells, which confer resistance to the chemotherapeutic agent tamoxifen. It appears that polymorphisms in this family are rare and occur at different frequencies among different populations. Despite numerous studies, the functional importance of these polymorphisms remains unclear (Sissung et al, 2012). Future studies with specific substrates and polymorphisms may ultimately provide additional information on the variable responses or adverse effects of drugs.

Solute Carrier Transporters

Another important class of drug transporters is the solute carriers (SLCs) such as the organic anion transporter protein (OATP) and organic cation transporter (OCT). These transporters are located throughout the body and have various roles in the transport of many different drugs. OATP1B1 (coded by the SLCO1B1 gene) is a hepatic influx transporter with at least 40 non-synonymous SNPs identified that result in either an altered expression or activity of OATP1B1 (Sissung et al, 2012). While the clinical consequences of all of these SNPs are unknown, one SNP (c.521T>C) has been associated with an increased risk of simvastatin-induced myopathy (Ramesy et al, 2014). This non-synonymous SNP is associated with a lower plasma clearance of simvastatin and is found in the SLCLO1B1*5, *15, and *17 alleles (Ramesy et al, 2014). These alleles are present in most populations with a frequency between 5% and 20% and warrant the avoidance of high-dose simvastatin (>40 mg) or treatment with another statin to decrease the risk of simvastatin-induced myopathies (Sissung et al, 2012).

CHAPTER SUMMARY

The overarching theme for the effects of polymorphisms in drug-metabolizing enzymes and transporters is that they have the potential to modify the pharmacokinetic profile by influencing drug clearance or activation, secondary to metabolism. While the pharmacogenetics of these pharmacokinetic determinants can account for some of this variability, it is not able to explain all therapeutic or adverse event variations. So currently the FDA only recommends pharmacogenetic testing, due to pharmacokinetic factors, in a limited number of drug therapy regimens (see Table 13-1). One instance where genetic testing is strongly suggested (based on pharmacokinetic parameters) is in the use of tetrabenazine for the treatment of Huntington's disease chorea, where daily dosing is guided by CYP2D6 phenotypes to prevent adverse events and achieve therapeutic efficacy. A second instance is genotyping for polymorphisms in CYP2C19, which is responsible for the bioactivation of clopidogrel, an antiplatelet agent. In either case the clinician's decision to order a genetic test prior to drug therapy may be predicated on multiple factors such as whether there are alternative drug choices; whether the test results can be obtained in an appropriate time frame; and whether the insurance or patient is willing to pay for the test. In the two examples above, a genetic test may be ordered prior to tetrabenazine (since good alternatives are not available), while prasugrel or ticagrelor may be selected instead of clopidogrel as they are not affected by

CYP2C19 variants. Genetic polymorphisms that affect pharmacodynamic interactions also contribute to the variability of drug response, and genetic testing is required in multiple instances where such variations alter the response to drug therapy, for example, imitanib for c-KIT-positive tumors. Additionally, there are many other factors including concomitant medications that may act as metabolism inducers or inhibitors, disease states, and age that cannot be accounted for by genetics alone. It is these observations that temper the excitement of personalized medicine in preventing all adverse effects and therapeutic failures.

GLOSSARY

Allele: An alternative form of a gene at a given locus.

Minor allele: A less common allele at a polymorphic locus.

Biological marker (biomarker): A characteristic that is objectively measured and evaluated as an indicator of normal biologic processes, pathogenic processes, or pharmacologic responses to a therapeutic intervention.

Genetic polymorphism: Minor allele frequency of ≥1% in the population.

Genome: The complete DNA sequence of an organism.

Genotype: The alleles at a specific locus an individual carries.

Haplotype: A group of alleles from two or more loci on a chromosome, inherited as a unit.

Pharmacogenetic test: An assay intended to determine interindividual variations in DNA sequence related to drug absorption and disposition (pharmacokinetics) or drug action (pharmacodynamics), including polymorphic variation in the genes that encode the functions of transporters, metabolizing enzymes, receptors, and other proteins.

Pharmacogenetics: A study of genetic causes of individual variations in drug response. In this chapter, the term "pharmacogenetics" is interchangeable with "pharmacogenomics."

Pharmacogenomic test: An assay intended to study interindividual variations in whole-genome or candidate gene, single-nucleotide polymorphism (SNP) maps, haplotype markers, or alterations in gene expression or inactivation that may be correlated with pharmacological function and therapeutic response. In some cases, the *pattern or profile of change* is the relevant biomarker, rather than changes in individual markers.

Pharmacogenomics: Genome-wide analysis of the genetic determinants of drug efficacy and toxicity. Pharmacogenetics focuses on a single gene while pharmacogenomics studies multiple genes.

Phenotype: Observable expression of a particular gene or genes.

Promoter: A segment of DNA sequence that controls initiation of transcription of the gene and is usually located upstream of the gene.

Single-nucleotide polymorphism: A DNA sequence variation occurring when a single nucleotide—A, T, C, or G—in the gene (or other shared sequence) is altered.

ABBREVIATIONS

ABC transporters: ATP-binding cassette transporters

CYP: Cytochrome P450

EM: Extensive metabolizer

IM: Intermediate metabolizer

NAT: *N*-acetyltransferase

OATP: Organic anion transporter protein

OCT: Organic cation transporter

P-gp: P-glycoprotein, MDR1, ABCB1

PGt: Pharmacogenetics

PM: Poor metabolizer

SLC: Solute carrier transporter

SNP: Single-nucleotide polymorphism

UM: Ultrarapid metabolizer

Frequently Asked Questions

▶ *What are the differences between pharmacogenetics and pharmacogenomics? How are PGx and PGt used to improve healthcare?*

▶ *What is the difference between a mutation, polymorphism, SNP, and haplotype? Why are these distinctions important for individualizing drug therapy?*

▶ *What types of genes are important to drug therapy? How would variability in these genes impact drug therapy?*

▶ *How common and clinically relevant are metabolic polymorphisms?*

▶ *How can genetic information be used to improve drug therapy for individuals and/or groups of patients?*

REFERENCES

Ahles A, Engelhardt S: Polymorphic variants of adrenoceptors: Pharmacology, physiology, and role in diseases. *Pharmacol Rev* **66**:598, 2014.

Ameyaw MM, Collie-Duguid ES, Powrie RH, Ofori-Adjei D, Mcleod HL: Thiopurine methyltransferase alleles in British and Ghanaian populations. *Hum Mol Genet* **8**:367, 1999.

Ansari A, Hassan C, Duley J, et al: Thipurine methyltransferase activity and the use of azathioprine in inflammatory bowel disease. *Aliment Pharmacol Ther* **16**:1743, 2002.

Beutler E, Gelbart T, Demina A: Racial variability in the UDP-glucuronosyltransferase 1 (UGT1A1) promoter: A balanced polymorphism for regulation of bilirubin metabolism? *Proc Natl Acad Sci USA* **95**:8170, 1998.

Brambila-Tapia AJL: MDR1 (ABCB1) polymorphisms: Functional effects and clinical implications. *Revista de Investigacion Clinica* **65**:445, 2013.

Caraco Y, Blotnick, S, Muszkat M: CYP2C9 genotype-guided warfarin prescribing enhances the efficacy and safety of anticoagulation: A prospective randomized controlled study. *Clin Pharmacol Ther* **83**:460, 2008.

Chen M, Xiz B, Chen B, et al: N-acetyltransferase 2 slow acetylator genotype associated with adverse effects of sulphasalazine in the treatment of inflammatory bowel disease. *Can J Gastroenterol* **21**:155, 2007.

Colombel JF, Ferrari N, Debuysere H, et al: Genotypic analysis of thiopurine S-methyltransferase in patients with Crohn's disease and severe myelosuppression during azathioprine therapy. *Gastroenterology* **118**:1025, 2000.

de Morais SM, Wilkinson GR, Blaisdell J, Nakamura K, Meyer UA, Goldstein JA: The major genetic defect responsible for the polymorphism of S-mephenytoin metabolism in humans. *J Biol Chem* **269**:15419, 1994.

Dodgan TM, Hochfeld WE, Fickl H, et al: Introduction of the AmpliChip CYP450 test to a South African cohort: a platform comparative prospective cohort study. *BMC Med Genetics* **14**:20, 2013.

Eap CB, Bender S, Jaquenoud Sirot E, et al: Nonresponse to clozapine and ultrarapid CYP1A2 activity: Clinical data and analysis of *CYP1A2* gene. *J Clin Psychopharmacol* **24**:214, 2004.

Etienne MC, Lagrange JL, Dassonville O, et al: Population study of dihydropyrimidine dehydrogenase in cancer-patients. *J Clin Oncol* **12**:2248, 1994.

Evans DAP, White TA: Human acetylation polymorphism. *J Lab Clin Med* **63**:394, 1964.

Evans WE, Relling MV: Pharmacogenomics: Translating functional genomics into rational therapeutics. *Science* **286**:487, 1999.

Fernandez-Rozadilla C, Cazier JB, Moreno V, et al: Pharmacogenomics in colorectal cancer: A genome-wide association study to predict toxicity after 5-fluorouracil or FOLFOX administration. *Pharmacogen J* **13**:209, 2013.

Food and Drug Administration: Drugs at FDA. http://www.accessdata.fda.gov/scripts/cder/drugsatfda/. Silver Spring, MD, 2014.

Gasche Y, Daali R, Fathi M, et al: Codeine intoxication associated with ultrarapid CYP2D6 metabolism. *N Engl J Med* **351**:2827, 2004.

Green J, Banks E, Berrington A, Darby S, Deo H, Newton R: N-acetyltransferase 2 and bladder cancer: An overview and consideration of the evidence for gene-environment interaction. *Br J Cancer* **83**:412, 2000.

Han JY, Lim HS, Park YH, Lee SY, Lee JS: Integrated pharmacogenetic prediction of irinotecan pharmacokinetics and toxicity in patients with advanced non-small cell lung cancer. *Lung Cancer* **63**:115, 2009.

Idle JR, Mahgoub A, Lancaster R, Smith RL: Hypotensive response to debrisoquine and hydroxylation phenotype. *Life Sci* **11**:979, 1978.

Innocenti F, Iyer L, Ratain MJ: Pharmacogenetics of anticancer agents: Lessons from amonafide and irinotecan. *Drug Metab Dispos* **26**:596, 2001.

Kimmel SE, French B, Kasner SE, et al: A pharmacogenetic versus a clinical algorithm for warfarin dosing. *N Engl J Med* **369**:2283, 2013.

Limdi NA, Veenstra DL: Expectations, validity, and reality in pharmacogenetics. *J Clin Epidemiol* **63**(9):960, 2010.

Lu ZH, Zhang RW, Diasio RB: Dihydropyrimidine dehydrogenase-activity in human peripheral-blood mononuclear-cells and liver-population characteristics, newly identified deficient patients, and clinical implication in 5-fluorouracil chemotherapy. *Cancer Res* **53:**5433, 1993.

Mahgoub A, Idle JR, Dring LG, Lancaster R, Smith RL: Polymorphic hydroxylation of debrisoquine in man. *Lancet* **ii:**584, 1977.

Mancinelli L, Cronin M, Sadee W: Pharmacogenomics: The promise of personalized medicine. *AAPS PharmSci* **2**(1):29, 2000.

McGraw J, Waller D: Cytochrome P450 variations in different ethnic populations. *Expert Opin Drug Metab Toxicol* **8:**371, 2012.

Meech R, Miners JO, Lewis BC, Mackenzie PI: The glycosidation of xenobiotics and endogenous compounds: Versatility and redundancy in the UDP glycosyltransferase superfamily. *Pharmacol Ther* **134:**200, 2012.

Meyer UA: Pharmacogenetics and adverse drug reactions. *Lancet* **356:**1667–1171, 2000.

Meyer UA, Zanger UM, Schwab M: Omics and drug response. *Ann Rev Pharm Tox* **53:**475, 2013.

Ogawaa R, Echizen H: Drug-drug interaction profiles of proton pump inhibitors. *Clin Pharmacokinet* **49:**509, 2010.

Pharmacogenetics Knowledge Base, PharmGKB. http://www.pharmgkb.org/. Palo Alto, California, 2014.

Phillips KA, Veenstra DL, Ores E, et al: Potential role of pharmacogenetics in reducing adverse drug reactions-A systematic review. *JAMA* **286:**2270, 2001.

Ramesy LB, Johnson SG, Caudle KE, et al: The Clinical Pharmacogenetics Implementation Consortium guideline for SLCO1B1 and simvastatin-induced myopathy: 2014 update. *Clin Pharmacol Ther* **96:**423, 2014.

Rothenberg ML: Efficacy and toxicity of irinotecan in patients with colorectal cancer. *Semin Oncol* **25:**39, 1998.

Rolla R, Vidali M, Meola S, et al: Side effects associated with ultrarapid cytochrome P450 2D6 genotype among women with early stage breast cancer treated with tamoxifen. *Clin Lab* **58:**1211, 2012.

Samer CF, Ing Lorenzini K, Rollason V, Daali Y, Desmeules JA: Applications of CYP450 testing in the clinical setting. *Mol Diagn Ther* **17:**165, 2013.

Sata F, Sapone A, Elizondo G, et al: CYP3A4 allelic variants with amino acid substitutions in exons 7 and 12: Evidence for an allelic variant with altered catalytic activity. *Clin Pharmacol Ther* **67:**45, 2000.

Schaeffeler E, Zanger UM, Eichelbaum M, Asante-Poku S, Shin JG, Schwab M: Highly multiplexed genotyping of thiopurine S-methyltransferase variants using MALD-TOF mass spectrometry: Reliable genotyping in different ethnic groups. *Clin Chem* **54:**1637, 2008.

Scott SA, Sangkuhl K, Gardner EE, et al: Clinical Pharmacogenetics implementation consortium guidelines for cytochrome P450-2C19 (CYP2C19) genotype and clopidogrel therapy. *Clin Pharmacol Ther* **90:**328, 2011.

Shi S, Klotz U: Proton pump inhibitors: An update of their clinical use and pharmacokinetics. *Eur J Clin Pharmacol* **64:**935, 2008.

Sibbing D, Koch W, Gebhard D, et al: Cytochrome 2C19*17 allelic variant, platelet aggregation, bleeding events and stent thrombosis in clopidogrel-treated patients with coronary stent placement. *Circulation* **121:**512, 2010.

Sim SC, Risinger, C, Dahl ML, et al: A common novel CYP2C19 gene variant causes ultrarapid drug metabolism relevant for the drug response to proton pump inhibitors and antidepressants. *Clin Pharmacol Ther* **79:**103, 2006.

Sissung TM, Troutman SM, Campbell TJ, et al: Transporter pharmacogenetics: Transporter polymorphisms affect normal physiology, diseases, and pharmacotherapy. *Discov Med* **13:**19, 2012.

Soliday FK, Conley YP, Henker R: Pseudocholinesterase deficiency: A comprehensive review of genetic, acquired, and drug influences. *AANA J* **78:**313, 2010.

Stingl JC, Bartels H, Viviani R, Lehmann ML, Brockmoller J: Relevance of UDP-glucuronosyltransferase polymorphisms for drug dosing: A quantitative systematic review. *Pharmacol Ther* **141:**92, 2014.

The Human Cytochrome P450 Allele Nomenclature Database. http://www.cypalleles.ki.se/. Eds. Ingelman-Sundberg M, Daly AK, and Nebert DW. Stockholm, Sweden, 2014.

UGT Alleles Nomenclature Home Page. UGT Nomenclature Commitee. http://www.ugtalleles.ulaval.ca. Quebec, Canada, June 2005.

Wang M, Lang X, Cui S, et al: Clinical application of pharmacogenetic-based warfarin-dosing algorithm in patients of Han nationality after rheumatic valve replacement: A randomized and controlled trial. *Int J Med Sci* **9:**472, 2012.

Warfarin Dosing. http://www.warfarindosing.org/Source/Home.aspx. St. Louis, MO 2014.

14

Physiologic Factors Related to Drug Absorption

Phillip M. Gerk, Andrew B. C. Yu, and Leon Shargel

Chapter Objectives

▶ Define passive and active drug absorption.

▶ Explain how Fick's law of diffusion relates to passive drug absorption.

▶ Calculate the percent of drug nonionized and ionized for a weak acid or weak-base drug using the Henderson–Hasselbalch equation, and explain how this may affect drug absorption.

▶ Define transcellular and paracellular drug absorption and explain using drug examples.

▶ Describe the anatomy and physiology of the GI tract and explain how stomach emptying time and GI transit time can alter the rate and extent of drug absorption.

▶ Explain the effect of food on gastrointestinal physiology and systemic drug absorption.

▶ Describe the various transporters and how they influence the pharmacokinetics of drug disposition in the GI tract.

DRUG ABSORPTION AND DESIGN OF A DRUG PRODUCT

Major considerations in the design of a drug product include the therapeutic objective, the application site, and systemic drug absorption from the application site. If the drug is intended for systemic activity, the drug should ideally be completely and consistently absorbed from the application site. In contrast, if the drug is intended for local activity, then systemic absorption from the application should be minimal to prevent systemic drug exposure and possible systemic side effects. For extended-release drug products, the drug product should remain at or near the application site and then slowly release the drug for the desired period of time. The systemic absorption of a drug is dependent on (1) the physicochemical properties of the drug, (2) the nature of the drug product, and (3) the anatomy and physiology of the drug absorption site.

In order to develop a drug product that elicits the desired therapeutic objective, the pharmaceutical scientist must have a thorough understanding of the biopharmaceutic properties of the drug and drug product and the physiologic and pathologic factors affecting drug absorption from the application site. A general description of drug absorption, distribution, and elimination is shown in Fig. 14-1. Pharmacists must also understand the relationship of drug dosage to therapeutic efficacy and adverse reactions and the potential for drug–drug and drug–nutrient interactions. This chapter will focus on the anatomic and physiologic considerations for the systemic absorption of a drug, whereas Chapters 15 to 18 will focus on the biopharmaceutic aspects of the drug and drug-product design including considerations in manufacturing and performance tests. Since the major route of drug administration is the oral route, major emphasis in the chapter will be on gastrointestinal drug absorption.

▶ Explain the pH-partition
hypothesis and how
gastrointestinal pH and the pK$_a$
of a drug may influence systemic
drug absorption. Describe how
drug absorption may be affected
by a disease that causes changes
in intestinal blood flow and/or
motility.

▶ List the major factors that
affect drug absorption from
oral and nonoral routes of drug
administration.

▶ Describe various methods
that may be used to study
oral drug absorption from the
gastrointestinal transit.

ROUTE OF DRUG ADMINISTRATION

Drugs may be given by parenteral, enteral, inhalation, intranasal, transdermal (percutaneous), or intranasal route for systemic absorption. Each route of drug administration has certain advantages and disadvantages. Some characteristics of the more common routes of drug administration are listed in Table 14-1. The systemic availability and onset of drug action are affected by blood flow at the administration site, the physicochemical characteristics of the drug and the drug product, and any pathophysiologic condition at the absorption site. After a drug is systemically absorbed, drug distribution and clearance follow normal physiological conditions of the body. Drug distribution and clearance are not usually altered by the drug formulation but may be altered by pathology, genetic polymorphism, and drug–drug interactions, as discussed in other chapters.

Many drugs are not administered orally because of insufficient systemic absorption from the GI tract. The diminished oral drug absorption may be due to drug instability in the gastrointestinal tract, drug degradation by the digestive enzymes in the intestine, high hepatic clearance (first-pass effect), and efflux transporters such as P-glycoprotein resulting in poor and/or erratic systemic drug availability. Some orally administered drugs, such as cholestyramine and others (Table 14-2), are not intended for systemic absorption but may be given orally for local activity in the gastrointestinal tract. However, some oral drugs such as mesalamine and balsalazide that are intended for local activity in the GI tract may also have a significant amount of systemic drug absorption. Small, highly lipid-soluble drugs such as nitroglycerin and fentanyl that are subject to high first-pass effects if swallowed but may be given by buccal or sublingual routes to bypass degradation in the GI tract and/or first-pass effects. Insulin is an example of protein peptide drug generally not given orally due to degradation and inadequate absorption in the GI tract.

Biotechnology-derived drugs (see Chapter 20) are usually given by the parenteral route because they are too labile in the GI tract to be administered orally. For example, erythropoietin and human growth hormone (somatrophin) are administered intramuscularly, and insulin is given subcutaneously or intramuscularly. Subcutaneous injection results in relatively slow absorption from the site of administration compared to intravenous injection, which provides immediate delivery to the plasma. Pathophysiologic conditions such as burns will increase the permeability of drugs across the skin compared with normal intact skin. Currently, pharmaceutical research is being directed to devise approaches for the oral absorption of various protein drugs such as insulin (Dhawan et al, 2009). Recently, inhaled insulin was approved for use by the FDA

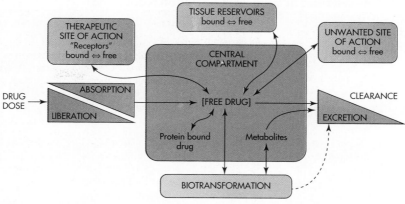

FIGURE 14-1   The interrelationship of the absorption, distribution, binding, metabolism, and excretion of a drug and its concentration at its sites of action. (From Buxton and Benet, 2011.)

TABLE 14-1   Common Routes of Drug Administration

Route	Bioavailability	Advantages	Disadvantages
Parenteral Routes			
Intravenous bolus (IV)	Complete (100%) systemic drug absorption. Rate of bioavailability considered instantaneous.	Drug is given for immediate effect.	Increased chance for adverse reaction. Possible anaphylaxis.
Intravenous infusion (IV inf)	Complete (100%) systemic drug absorption. Rate of drug absorption controlled by infusion rate.	Plasma drug levels more precisely controlled. May inject large fluid volumes. May use drugs with poor lipid solubility and/or irritating drugs.	Requires skill in insertion of infusion set. Tissue damage at site of injection (infiltration, necrosis, or sterile abscess).
Subcutaneous injection (SC)	Prompt from aqueous solution. Slow absorption from repository formulations.	Generally, used for insulin injection.	Rate of drug absorption depends on blood flow and injection volume. Insulin formulaton can vary from short to intermediate and long acting.
Intradermal injection	Drug injected into surface area (dermal) of skin.	Often used for allergy and other diagnostic tests, such as tuberculosis.	Some discomfort at site of injection.
Intramuscular injection (IM)	Rapid from aqueous solution. Slow absorption from nonaqueous (oil) solutions.	Easier to inject than intravenous injection. Larger volumes may be used compared to subcutaneous solutions.	Irritating drugs may be very painful. Different rates of absorption depending on muscle group injected and blood flow.
Intra-arterial injection	100% of solution is absorbed.	Used in chemotherapy to target drug to organ.	Drug may also distribute to other tissues and organs in the body.
Intrathecal Injection	100% of solution is absorbed.	Drug is directly injected into cerebrospinal fluid (CSF) for uptake into brain.	

(Continued)

TABLE 14-1   Common Routes of Drug Administration (Continued)

Route	Bioavailability	Advantages	Disadvantages
Intraperitoneal injection	In laboratory animals, (eg, rat) drug absorption resembles oral absorption.	Used more in small laboratory animals. Less common injection in humans. Used for renally impaired patients on peritoneal dialysis who develop peritonitis.	Drug absorption via mesenteric veins to liver, may have some hepatic clearance prior to systemic absorption.
Enteral Routes			
Buccal or sublingual (SL)	Rapid absorption from lipidsoluble drugs.	No "first-pass" effects. Buccal route may be formulated for local prolonged action. Eg, adhere to the buccal mucosa with some antifungal. Buccal is different from sublingual which is usually placed "under tongue."	Some drugs may be swallowed. Not for most drugs or drugs with high doses.
Oral (PO)	Absorption may vary. Generally, slower absorption rate compared to IV bolus or IM injection.	Safest and easiest route of drug administration. May use immediate-release and modified-release drug products.	Some drugs may have erratic absorption, be unstable in the gastointestinal tract, or be metabolized by liver prior to systemic absorption.
Enteral Routes			
Rectal (PR)	Absorption may vary from suppository. More reliable absorption from enema (solution).	Useful when patient cannot swallow medication. Used for local and systemic effects.	Absorption may be erratic. Suppository may migrate to different position. Some patient discomfort.
Other Routes			
Transdermal	Slow absorption, rate may vary. Increased absorption with occlusive dressing.	Transdermal delivery system (patch) is easy to use. Used for lipid-soluble drugs with low dose and low MW (molecular weight).	Some irritation by patch or drug. Permeability of skin variable with condition, anatomic site, age, and gender. Type of cream or ointment base affects drug release and absorption.
Inhalation and intranasal	Rapid absorption. Total dose absorbed is variable.	May be used for local or systemic effects.	Particle size of drug determines anatomic placement in respiratory tract. May stimulate cough reflex. Some drug may be swallowed.

but the product was fairly quickly discontinued by the manufacturer because of poor patient and physician acceptance of this new route of administration. Biotechnology-derived drugs are discussed more fully in Chapter 20.

When a drug is administered by an extravascular route of administration (eg, oral, topical, intranasal, inhalation, rectal), the drug must first be absorbed into the systemic circulation and then diffuse or be transported to the site of action before eliciting biological and therapeutic activity. The general principles and kinetics of absorption from these extravascular sites follow the same principles as oral dosing, although the physiology of the site of administration differs.

TABLE 14-2   Drugs Given Orally for Local Drug Activity in the Gastrointestinal Tract

Drug	Example	Comment
Cholestyramine	Questran	Cholestyramine resin is the chloride salt of a basic anion exchange resin, a cholesterol-lowering agent. Cholestyramine resin is hydrophilic, but insoluble in water and not absorbed from the digestive tract.
Balsalazide disodium	Colazal	Balsalazide disodium is a prodrug that is enzymatically cleaved in the colon to produce mesalamine, an anti-inflammatory drug. Balsalazide disodium is intended for local action in the treatment of mildly to moderately active ulcerative colitis. Balsalazide disodium and its metabolites are absorbed from the lower intestinal tract and colon.
Mesalamine[a] delayed-release tablet	Asacol HD tablet	Asacol HD delayed-release tablets have an outer protective coat and an inner coat which dissolves at pH 7 or greater, releasing mesalamine in the terminal ileum for topical antiinflammatory action in the colon.
Mesalamine controlled-release capsule	Pentasa capsule	Pentasa capsule is an ethylcellulose-coated, controlled-release capsule formulation of mesalamine designed to release therapeutic quantities of mesalamine throughout the gastrointestinal tract.

[a]Mesalamine (also referred to as 5-aminosalicylic acid or 5-ASA). Although mesalamine is indicated for local anti-inflammatory activity in the lower GI tract, mesalamine is systemically absorbed from the GI tract.

NATURE OF CELL MEMBRANES

Many drugs administered by extravascular routes are intended for local effect. Other drugs are designed to be absorbed from the site of administration into the systemic circulation. For systemic drug absorption, the drug may cross cellular membranes. After oral administration, drug molecules must cross the intestinal epithelium by going either through or between the epithelial cells to reach the systemic circulation. The permeability of a drug at the absorption site into the systemic circulation is intimately related to the molecular structure and properties of the drug and to the physical and biochemical properties of the cell membranes. Once in the plasma, the drug may act directly or have to cross biological membranes to reach the site of action. Therefore, biological membranes potentially pose a significant barrier to drug delivery.

Transcellular absorption is the process of drug movement across a cell. Some polar molecules may not be able to traverse the cell membrane but, instead, go through gaps or *tight junctions* between cells, a process known as *paracellular drug diffusion*. Figure 14-2 shows the difference between the two processes. Some drugs are probably absorbed by a mixed mechanism involving one or more processes.

Membranes are major structures in cells, surrounding the entire cell (plasma membrane) and acting as a boundary between the cell and the interstitial fluid. In addition, membranes enclose most of the cell organelles (eg, the mitochondrion membrane). Functionally, cell membranes are semipermeable partitions that act as selective barriers to the passage of molecules. Water, some selected small molecules, and lipid-soluble molecules pass through such membranes, whereas highly charged molecules and large molecules, such as proteins and protein-bound drugs, do not.

The transmembrane movement of drugs is influenced by the composition and structure of the plasma membranes. Cell membranes are generally thin, approximately 70–100 Å in thickness. Cell membranes are composed primarily of phospholipids in the form of a bilayer interdispersed with carbohydrates and protein groups. There are several theories as to the structure of the cell membrane. The *lipid bilayer* or *unit membrane theory,* originally proposed by Davson and Danielli (1952), considers the plasma membrane to be composed of two layers of phospholipid between two surface layers of proteins, with the hydrophilic "head" groups of the phospholipids facing the protein layers and the hydrophobic "tail" groups of the phospholipids

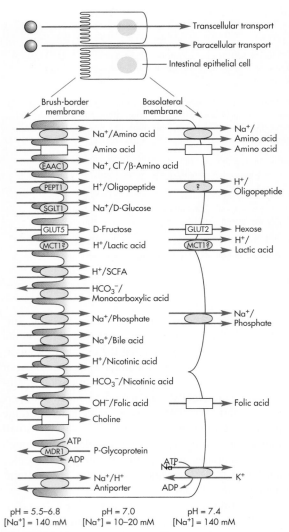

pH = 5.5–6.8   pH = 7.0   pH = 7.4
[Na⁺] = 140 mM   [Na⁺] = 10–20 mM [Na⁺] = 140 mM

FIGURE 14-2 Summary of intestinal epithelial transporters. Transporters shown by square and oval shapes demonstrate active and facilitated transporters, respectively. Names of cloned transporters are shown with square or oval shapes. In the case of active transporters, arrows in the same direction represent symport of substance and the driving force. Arrows going in the reverse direction mean the antiport. (From Tsuji and Tamai, 1996, with permission.) Note that BCRP and MRP2 are positioned similarly to MDR1 (P-glycoprotein).

structure does not account for the diffusion of water, small-molecular-weight molecules such as urea, and certain charged ions.

The *fluid mosaic model*, proposed by Singer and Nicolson (1972), explains the transcellular diffusion of polar molecules (Lodish, 1979). According to this model, the cell membrane consists of globular proteins embedded in a dynamic fluid, lipid bilayer matrix (Fig. 14-3). These proteins provide a pathway for the selective transfer of certain polar molecules and charged ions through the lipid barrier. As shown in Fig. 14-3, transmembrane proteins are interdispersed throughout the membrane. Two types of pores of about 10 nm and 50–70 nm were inferred to be present in membranes based on capillary membrane transport studies (Pratt and Taylor, 1990). These small pores provide a channel through which water, ions, and dissolved solutes such as urea may move across the membrane.

Membrane proteins embedded in the bilayer serve special purposes. These membrane proteins function as structural anchors, receptors, ion channels, or transporters to transduce electrical or chemical signaling pathways that facilitate or prevent selective actions. In contrast to simple bilayer structure, membranes are highly ordered and compartmented (Brunton, 2011). Indeed many early experiments on drug absorption or permeability using isolated gut studies were proven not valid because the membrane proteins and electrical properties of the membrane were compromised in many epithelial cell membranes, including those of the gastrointestinal tract.

PASSAGE OF DRUGS ACROSS CELL MEMBRANES

Passive Diffusion

Theoretically, a lipophilic drug may pass through the cell or go around it. If the drug has a low molecular weight and is lipophilic, the lipid cell membrane is not a barrier to drug diffusion and absorption. *Passive diffusion* is the process by which molecules spontaneously diffuse from a region of higher concentration to a region of lower concentration. This process is *passive* because no external energy is

aligned in the interior. The lipid bilayer theory explains the observation that lipid-soluble drugs tend to penetrate cell membranes more easily than polar molecules. However, the bilayer cell membrane

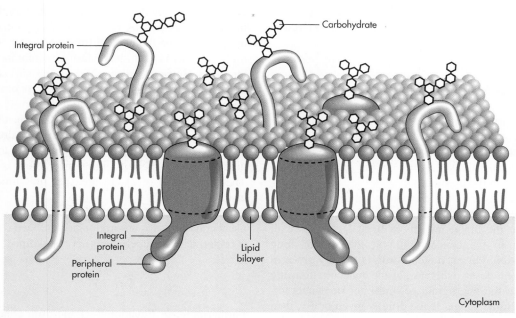

FIGURE 14-3   Model of the plasma membrane including proteins and carbohydrates as well as lipids. Integral proteins are embedded in the lipid bilayer; peripheral proteins are merely associated with the membrane surface. The carbohydrate consists of monosaccharides, or simple sugars, strung together in chains attached to proteins (forming glycoproteins) or to lipids (forming glycolipids). The asymmetry of the membrane is manifested in several ways. Carbohydrates are always on the exterior surface and peripheral proteins are almost always on the cytoplasmic, or inner, surface. The two lipid monolayers include different proportions of the various kinds of lipid molecules. Most important, each species of integral protein has a definite orientation, which is the same for every molecule of that species. (©George V. Kelvin.)

expended. In Fig. 14-4, drug molecules move forward and back across a membrane. If the two sides have the same drug concentration, forward-moving drug molecules are balanced by molecules moving back, resulting in no net transfer of drug. When one side is higher in drug concentration at any given time, the number of forward-moving drug molecules will be higher than the number of backward-moving molecules; the net result will be a transfer of molecules to the alternate side downstream from the concentration gradient, as indicated in the figure by the big arrow. The rate of transfer is called *flux*, and is represented by a vector to show its direction in space. The tendency of molecules to move in all directions is natural, because molecules possess kinetic energy and constantly collide with one another in space. Only left and right molecule movements are shown in Fig. 14-4, because movement of molecules in other directions will not result in concentration changes because of the limitation of the container wall.

Passive diffusion is the major absorption process for most drugs. The driving force for passive diffusion is higher drug concentrations, typically on the mucosal side compared to the blood as in the case of oral drug absorption. According to *Fick's law of diffusion*,

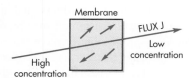

FIGURE 14-4   Passive diffusion of molecules. Molecules in solution diffuse randomly in all directions. As molecules diffuse from left to right and vice versa (small arrows), a net diffusion from the high-concentration side to the low-concentration side results. This results in a net flux (*J*) to the right side. Flux is measured in mass per unit time (eg, ng/min).

drug molecules diffuse from a region of high drug concentration to a region of low drug concentration.

$$\frac{dQ}{dt} = \frac{DAK}{h}(C_{GI} - C_p) \qquad (14.1)$$

where dQ/dt = rate of diffusion, D = diffusion coefficient, A = surface area of membrane, K = lipid–water partition coefficient of drug in the biologic membrane that controls drug permeation, h = membrane thickness, and $C_{GI} - C_p$ = difference between the concentrations of drug in the gastrointestinal tract and in the plasma.

Because the drug distributes rapidly into a large volume after entering the blood, the concentration of drug in the blood initially will be quite low with respect to the concentration at the site of drug absorption. For example, a drug is usually given in milligram doses, whereas plasma concentrations are often in the microgram-per-milliliter or nanogram-per-milliliter range. If the drug is given orally, then $C_{GI} \gg C_p$ and a large concentration gradient is maintained until most of the drug is absorbed, thus driving drug molecules into the plasma from the gastrointestinal tract.

Given Fick's law of diffusion, several other factors can be seen to influence the rate of passive diffusion of drugs. For example, the degree of lipid solubility of the drug influences the rate of drug absorption. The partition coefficient, K, represents the lipid–water partitioning of a drug across the hypothetical membrane in the mucosa. Drugs that are more lipid soluble have a larger value of K. The surface area, A, of the membrane also influences the rate of absorption. Drugs may be absorbed from most areas of the gastrointestinal tract. However, the duodenal area of the small intestine shows the most rapid drug absorption, due to such anatomic features as villi and microvilli, which provide a large surface area. These villi are less abundant in other areas of the gastrointestinal tract.

The thickness of the hypothetical model membrane, h, is a constant for any particular absorption site. Drugs usually diffuse very rapidly through capillary plasma membranes in the vascular compartments, in contrast to diffusion through plasma membranes of capillaries in the brain. In the brain, the capillaries are densely lined with glial cells, so a drug diffuses slowly into the brain as if a thick lipid membrane exists. The term *blood–brain barrier* is used to describe the poor diffusion of water-soluble molecules across capillary plasma membranes into the brain. However, in certain disease states such as meningitis these membranes may be disrupted or become more permeable to drug diffusion.

The diffusion coefficient, D, is a constant for each drug and is defined as the amount of a drug that diffuses across a membrane of a given unit area per unit time when the concentration gradient is unity. The dimensions of D are area per unit time—for example, cm^2/sec.

Because D, A, K, and h are constants under usual conditions for absorption, a combined constant P or permeability coefficient may be defined.

$$P = \frac{DAK}{h} \qquad (14.2)$$

Furthermore, in Equation 14.1 the drug concentration in the plasma, C_p, is extremely small compared to the drug concentration in the gastrointestinal tract, C_{GI}. If C_p is negligible and P is substituted into Equation 14.1, the following relationship for Fick's law is obtained:

$$\frac{dQ}{dt} = P(C_{GI}) \qquad (14.3)$$

Equation 14.3 is an expression for a first-order process. In practice, the extravascular absorption of most drugs tends to be a first-order absorption process. Moreover, because of the large concentration gradient between C_{GI} and C_p, the rate of drug absorption is usually more rapid than the rate of drug elimination.

Many drugs have both lipophilic and hydrophilic chemical substituents. Those drugs that are more lipid soluble tend to traverse cell membranes more easily than less lipid-soluble or more water-soluble molecules. For drugs that act as weak electrolytes, such as weak acids and bases, the extent of ionization influences the drug's diffusional permeability. The ionized species of the drug contains a charge and is more water soluble than the nonionized species of the drug, which is more lipid soluble. The extent of ionization of a weak electrolyte will depend on both the pK$_a$ of the drug and the pH of the medium in which the drug is dissolved. *Henderson and Hasselbalch* used the following expressions pertaining to weak acids and weak bases to describe the relationship between pK$_a$ and pH:

For weak acids,

$$\text{Ratio} = \frac{[\text{Salt}]}{[\text{Acid}]} = \frac{[\text{A}^-]}{[\text{HA}]} = 10^{(\text{pH}-\text{pK}_a)} \quad (14.4)$$

For weak bases,

$$\text{Ratio} = \frac{[\text{Base}]}{[\text{Salt}]} = \frac{[\text{RNH}_2]}{[\text{RNH}_3^+]} = 10^{(\text{pH}-\text{pK}_a)} \quad (14.5)$$

With Equations 14.4 and 14.5, the proportion of free acid or free base existing as the nonionized species may be determined at any given pH, assuming the pK$_a$ for the drug is known. For example, at a plasma pH of 7.4, salicylic acid (pK$_a$ = 3.0) exists mostly in its ionized or water-soluble form, as shown below:

$$\text{Ratio} = \frac{[\text{Salt}]}{[\text{Acid}]} = 10^{(7.4-3.0)}$$

$$\log\frac{[\text{Salt}]}{[\text{Acid}]} = 7.4 - 3.0 = 4.4$$

$$\frac{[\text{Salt}]}{[\text{Acid}]} = 2.51 \times 10^4$$

In a simple system, the total drug concentration on either side of a membrane should be the same at equilibrium, assuming Fick's law of diffusion is the only distribution factor involved. For diffusible drugs, such as nonelectrolyte drugs or drugs that do not ionize, the drug concentrations on either side of the membrane are the same at equilibrium. However, for electrolyte drugs or drugs that ionize, the total drug concentrations on either side of the membrane are not equal at equilibrium if the pH of the medium differs on respective sides of the membrane. For example, consider the concentration of salicylic acid (pK$_a$ = 3.0) in the stomach (pH 1.2) as opposed to its concentration in the plasma (pH 7.4) (Fig. 14-5). According to the Henderson–Hasselbalch equation (Equation 14.4) for weak acids, at pH 7.4 and at pH 1.2, salicylic acid exists in the ratios that follow.

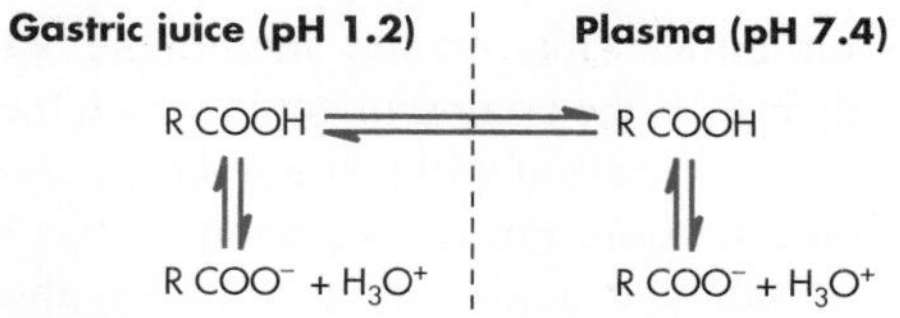

Gastric juice (pH 1.2)   **Plasma (pH 7.4)**

R COOH ⇌ R COOH

R COO$^-$ + H$_3$O$^+$ R COO$^-$ + H$_3$O$^+$

FIGURE 14-5   Model for the distribution of an orally administered weak electrolyte drug such as salicylic acid.

In the plasma, at pH 7.4

$$\text{Ratio} = \frac{(\text{RCOO}^-)}{(\text{RCOOH})} = 2.51 \times 10^4$$

In gastric juice, at pH 1.2

$$\text{Ratio} = \frac{(\text{RCOO}^-)}{(\text{RCOOH})} = 10^{(1.2-3.0)} = 1.58 \times 10^{-2}$$

The total drug concentration on either side of the membrane is determined as shown in Table 14-3.

Thus, the pH affects distribution of salicylic acid (RCOOH) and its salt (RCOO$^-$) across cell membranes. It is assumed that the acid, RCOOH, is freely permeable and the salt, RCOO$^-$, is not permeable across the cell membrane. In this example the total concentration of salicylic acid at equilibrium is approximately 25,000 times greater in the plasma than in the stomach (see Table 14-3). These calculations can also be applied to weak bases, using Equation 14.5.

According to the *pH-partition hypothesis*, if the pH on one side of a cell membrane differs from the pH on the other side of the membrane, then (1) the drug (weak acid or base) will ionize to different degrees on respective sides of the membrane; (2) the total drug concentrations (ionized plus nonionized

TABLE 14-3   Relative Concentrations of Salicylic Acid as Affected by pH

Drug	Gastric Juice (pH 1.2)	Plasma (pH 7.4)
RCOOH	1.0000	1
RCOO-	0.0158	25,100
Total drug concentration	1.0158	25,101

drug) on either side of the membrane will be unequal; and (3) the compartment in which the drug is more highly ionized will contain the greater total drug concentration. For these reasons, a weak acid (such as salicylic acid) will be rapidly absorbed from the stomach (pH 1.2), whereas a weak base (such as quinidine) will be poorly absorbed from the stomach.

Another factor that can influence drug concentrations on either side of a membrane is a particular *affinity* of the drug for a tissue component, which prevents the drug from moving freely back across the cell membrane. For example, a drug such as dicumarol binds to plasma protein, and digoxin binds to tissue protein. In each case, the protein-bound drug does not move freely across the cell membrane. Drugs such as chlordane are very lipid soluble and will partition into adipose (fat) tissue. In addition, a drug such as tetracycline might form a complex with calcium in the bones and teeth. Finally, a drug may concentrate in a tissue due to a specific uptake or active transport process. Such processes have been demonstrated for iodide in thyroid tissue, potassium in the intracellular water, and certain catecholamines into adrenergic storage sites. Such drugs may have a higher total drug concentration on the side where binding occurs, yet the free drug concentration that diffuses across cell membranes will be the same on both sides of the membrane.

Instead of diffusing into the cell, drugs can also diffuse into the spaces around the cell as an absorption mechanism. In *paracellular drug absorption,* drug molecules smaller than 500 MW diffuse through the tight junctions, or spaces between intestinal epithelial cells. Generally, paracellular drug absorption is very slow, being limited by tight junctions between cells. For example, if mannitol is dosed orally, it would be absorbed minimally and only through this route; mannitol has very, very low oral bioavailability.

Carrier-Mediated Transport

Enterocytes are simple columnar epithelial cells that line the intestinal walls in the small intestine and colon. They express various drug transporters, are connected by tight junctions, and often play an important role in determining the rate and extent of drug absorption. Uptake transporters move drug molecules into the blood and increase plasma drug concentration, whereas efflux transporters move drug molecules back into the gut lumen and reduce systemic drug absorption. These cells also express some drug-metabolizing enzymes, and can contribute to presystemic drug metabolism (Doherty, 2002).

Theoretically, a lipophilic drug may either pass through the cell or go around it. If the drug has a low molecular weight and is lipophilic, the lipid cell membrane is not a barrier to drug diffusion and absorption. In the intestine, drugs and other molecules can go through the intestinal epithelial cells by either diffusion or a carrier-mediated mechanism. Numerous specialized carrier-mediated transport systems are present in the body, especially in the intestine for the absorption of ions and nutrients required by the body.

Active Transport

Active transport is a carrier-mediated transmembrane process that plays an important role in the gastrointestinal absorption and in renal and biliary secretion of many drugs and metabolites. A few lipid-insoluble drugs that resemble natural physiologic metabolites (such as 5-fluorouracil) are absorbed from the gastrointestinal tract by this process. Active transport is characterized by the ability to transport drug against a concentration gradient—that is, from regions of low drug concentrations to regions of high drug concentrations. Therefore, this is an energy-consuming system. In addition, active transport is a specialized process requiring a carrier that binds the drug to form a carrier–drug complex that shuttles the drug across the membrane and then dissociates the drug on the other side of the membrane (Fig. 14-6).

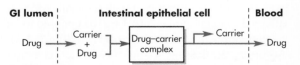

FIGURE 14-6   Hypothetical carrier-mediated transport process.

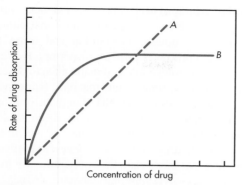

FIGURE 14-7 Comparison of the rates of drug absorption of a drug absorbed by passive diffusion (line *A*) and a drug absorbed by a carrier-mediated system (line *B*).

The carrier molecule may be highly selective for the drug molecule. If the drug structurally resembles a natural substrate that is actively transported, then it is likely to be actively transported by the same carrier mechanism. Therefore, drugs of similar structure may compete for sites of adsorption on the carrier. Furthermore, because only a fixed number of carrier molecules are available, all the binding sites on the carrier may become saturated if the drug concentration gets very high. A comparison between the rate of drug absorption and the concentration of drug at the absorption site is shown in Fig. 14-7. Notice that for a drug absorbed by passive diffusion, the rate of absorption increases in a linear relationship to drug concentration (first-order rate). In contrast, for drugs that are absorbed by a carrier-mediated process, the

rate of drug absorption increases with drug concentration until the carrier molecules are completely saturated. At higher drug concentrations, the rate of drug absorption remains constant, or zero order.

Several transport proteins are expressed in the intestinal epithelial cells (Suzuki and Sugiyama et al, 2000; Takano et al, 2006) (Fig. 14-8). Although some transporters facilitate absorption, other transporters such as P-gp may effectively inhibit drug absorption. P-gp (also known as MDR1), an energy-dependent, membrane-bound protein, is an *efflux transporter* that mediates the secretion of compounds from inside the cell back out into the intestinal lumen, thereby limiting overall absorption (see Chapter 13). Thus, drug absorption may be reduced or increased by the presence or absence of efflux proteins. The role of efflux proteins is generally believed to be a defense mechanism for the body to excrete and reduce drug accumulation.

P-gp is expressed also in other tissues such as the blood–brain barrier, liver, and kidney, where it limits drug penetration into the brain, mediates biliary drug secretion, and mediates renal tubular drug secretion, respectively. Efflux pumps are present throughout the body and are involved in transport of a diverse group of hydrophobic drugs, natural products, and peptides. Many drugs and chemotherapeutic agents, such as cyclosporin A, verapamil, terfenadine, fexofenadine, and most HIV-1 protease inhibitors, are substrates of P-gp (see Chapter 13). In addition, individual genetic differences in intestinal absorption may be the result of genetic differences in P-gp and other transporters.

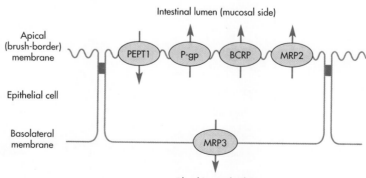

FIGURE 14-8 Localization of efflux transporters and PEPT1 in intestinal epithelial cell. (From Takano et al, 2006, with permission.)

Facilitated Diffusion

Facilitated diffusion is also a carrier-mediated transport system, differing from active transport in that the drug moves along a concentration gradient (ie, moves from a region of high drug concentration to a region of low drug concentration). Therefore, this system does not require energy input. However, because this system is carrier mediated, it is saturable and structurally selective for the drug and shows competition kinetics for drugs of similar structure. In terms of drug absorption, facilitated diffusion seems to play a very minor role.

Transporters and Carrier-Mediated Intestinal Absorption

Various carrier-mediated systems (transporters) are present at the intestinal brush border and basolateral membrane for the absorption of specific ions and nutrients essential for the body (Tsuji and Tamai, 1996). Both influx and efflux transporters are present in the brush border and basolateral membrane that will increase drug absorption (influx transporter) or decrease drug absorption (efflux transporter).

Uptake transporters. For convenience, influx transporters were referred to as those that enhance absorption as uptake transporters and those that cause drug outflow as efflux transporters. However, this concept is too simple and inadequate to describe the roles of many transporters that have bidirectional efflux and other functions related to their location in the membrane. Recent progress has been made in understanding the genetic role of membrane transporters in drug safety and efficacy. In particular, more than 400 membrane transporters in two major superfamilies—ATP-binding cassette (ABC) and solute carrier (SLC)—have been annotated in the human genome. Many of these transporters have been cloned, characterized, and localized in the human body including the GI tract. The subject was reviewed recently by The International Transporter Consortium (ITC) (Giacomini, 2010).

Many drugs are absorbed by carrier systems because of the structural similarity to natural substrates or simply because they encounter the transporters located in specific part of the GI tract (Table 14-4). The small intestine expresses a variety of uptake

TABLE 14-4   Intestine Transporters and Examples of Drugs Transported

Transporter	Examples	
Amino acid transporter	Gabapentin	D-Cycloserine
	Methyldopa	Baclofen
	L-dopa	
Oligopeptide transporter	Cefadroxil	Cephradine
	Cefixime	Ceftibuten
	Cephalexin	Captopril
	Lisinopril	Thrombin inhibitor
Phosphate transporter	Fostomycin	Foscarnet
Bile acid transporter	S3744	
Glucose transporter	p-Nitrophenyl-β-d-glucopyranoside	
P-glycoprotein efflux	Etoposide	Vinblastine
	Cyclosporin A	
Monocarboxylic acid transporter	Salicylic acid	Benzoic acid
	Pravastatin	

Data from Tsuji and Tamai (1996).

transporters (see Fig. 14-2) for amino acids, peptides, hexoses, organic anions, organic cations, nucleosides, and other nutrients (Tsuji and Tamai, 1996; Giacomini, 2010). Among these uptake (absorptive) transporters are the intestinal oligopeptide transporter, or di-/tripeptide transporter, PepT1 has potential for enhancing intestinal absorption of peptide drugs. The expression and function of PepT1 (gene symbol *SLC15A1*) are now well analyzed for this application. Proteins given orally are digested in the gastrointestinal tract to produce a variety of short-chain peptides; these di- and tripeptides could be taken up by enterocytes and the proton/peptide cotransporter (PepT1) localized on the brush-border membrane. These uptake transporters are located at the brush border as well as in the basolateral membrane to allow efficient absorption of essential nutrients into the body. Uptake transporters such as those for hexoses and amino acids also favor absorption (see arrows as shown in Fig. 14-7).

Efflux transporters. Many of the efflux transporters in the GI tract are membrane proteins located strategically in membranes to protect the body from influx of undesirable compounds. A common example is MDR1 or P-gp (alias), which has the gene symbol *ABCB1*. P-gp is an example of the ABC subfamily. MDR1 is one of the many proteins known as *multidrug-resistance associated protein*. It is important in pumping drugs out of cells and causing treatment resistance in some cell lines (see Chapter 13).

P-gp has been identified in the intestine and reduces apparent intestinal epithelial cell permeability from lumen to blood for various lipophilic or cytotoxic drugs. P-gp is highly expressed on the apical surface of superficial columnar epithelial cells of the ileum and colon, and expression decreases proximally into the jejunum, duodenum, and stomach. Takano et al (2006) reported that P-gp is present in various human tissues and ranked as follows: (1) adrenal medulla (relative level to that in KB-3-1 cells, > 500-fold); (2) adrenal (160-fold); (3) kidney medulla (75-fold); (4) kidney (50-fold); (5) colon (31-fold); (6) liver (25-fold); (7) lung, jejunum, and rectum (20-fold); (8) brain (12-fold); (9) prostate (8-fold); and so on, including skin, esophagus, stomach, ovary, muscle, heart, and kidney cortex. The widespread presence of P-gp in the body appears to be related to its defensive role in effluxing drugs and other xenobiotics out of different cells and vital body organs. This transporter is sometimes called an efflux transporter while others are better described as "influx" proteins. P-gp has the remarkable ability to efflux drug out of many types of cells including endothelial lumens of capillaries. The expression of P-gp is often triggered in many cancer cells making them drug resistant due to drug efflux.

For many GI transporters, the transport of a drug is often bidirectional (Fig. 14-9), and whether the transporter causes drug absorption or exsorption depends on which direction the flux dominates with regard to a particular drug at a given site. An example of how P-gp affects drug absorption can be seen with the drug digoxin. P-gp is present in the liver and the GI tract. In Caco-2 cells and other model systems, P-gp is known to efflux drug out of the enterocyte. Digoxin was previously known to have erratic/incomplete absorption or bioavailability problems. While reported bioavailability issues were attributed to formulation or other factors, it is also now known that knocking out the P-gp gene in mice increases bioavailability of the drug. In addition, human P-gp genetic polymorphisms occur. Hoffmeyer et al (2000) demonstrated that a polymorphism in exon 26 (C3435T) resulted in reduced intestinal P-gp, leading to increased oral bioavailability of digoxin in the subject involved. However, direct determination of P-gp substrate *in vivo* is not always readily possible. Most early determinations are done using *in vitro* cell assay methods, or *in vivo* studies involving a cloned animal with the gene knocked out such as the P-gp, a KO (knock-out) mouse, for example, P-gp (−/−), which is the most sensitive method to identify P-gp substrates.

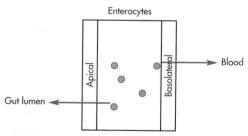

FIGURE 14-9 Diagram showing possible directional movement of a substrate drug by a transporter.

Changes in the expression of P-gp may be triggered by diseases or other drugs, contributing to variability in P-gp activity and variable plasma drug concentrations after a given dose is administered. Results from *in vitro* and preclinical (animal) studies may need to be verified with by clinical drug–drug interaction studies to establish the role of P-gp in the oral bioavailability of a drug.

The breast cancer resistance protein (BCRP; gene symbol *ABCG2*) is like P-gp in that it is also found in many important fluid barrier layers, including the intestine, liver, kidney, and brain. BCRP also transports many drugs out of cells, working (like P-gp) to keep various compounds out of the body (by decreasing their absorption) or helping to eliminate them. Drugs transported by BCRP include many anticancer drugs (methotrexate, irinotecan, mitoxantrone), statins (rosuvastatin), as well as nitrofurantoin and various sulfated metabolites of drugs and endogenous compounds. The FDA requires all investigational new drugs to be tested for their potential activity as substrates of both P-gp and BCRP, and also recommends determining if they are inhibitors (Huang and Zhang, 2012).

Frequently Asked Questions
▶ *What is the effect of intestinal P-gp on the blood level of the substrate drug digoxin when a substrate inhibitor (ketoconazole) is present?*

▶ *According to the diagram in Fig. 14-9, in which direction is P-gp pumping the drug? Is P-gp acting as an efflux transporter in this diagram?*

▶ *Why is it too simple to classify transporters based on an "absorption" and "exsorption" concept?*

▶ *Would a drug transport process involving ABC transporter be considered a passive or active transport process?*

▶ *How does a transporter influence the level of drug within the cell?*

P-gp affects the bioavailability of many substrate drugs listed in Table 14-5. P-gp inhibitors should be carefully evaluated before coadministration with a P-gp substrate drug. Other transporters are also present in the intestines (Tsuji and Tamai, 1996). For example, many oral cephalosporins are absorbed through amino acid transporters. Cefazolin, a parenteral-only cephalosporin, is not available orally because it cannot be absorbed to a significant degree through this mechanism.

Frequently Asked Questions
▶ *The bioavailability of an antitumor drug is provided in the package insert. Why is it important to know whether the drug is an efflux transporter substrate or not?*

▶ *Can the expression of efflux transporter in a cell change as the disease progresses?*

▶ *Why is blockade of efflux transporter efflux of a drug, its glucuronide, or sulfate metabolite into the bile clinically important?*

Clinical Examples of Transporter Impact

Multidrug resistance (MDR) to cancer cells has been linked to efflux transporter proteins such as P-gp that can efflux or pump out chemotherapeutic agents from the cells (Sauna et al, 2001). Paclitaxel (Taxol) is an example of coordinated metabolism, efflux, and triggering of hormone nuclear receptor to induce efflux protein (Fig. 14-10). P-gp (see MDR1 in Fig. 14-2) is responsible for 85% of paclitaxel excretion back into the GI tract (Synold et al, 2001). Paclitaxel activates the pregnane X receptor (also known as PXR, or alternatively as steroid X receptor [SXR]), which in turn induces MDR1 transcription and P-gp expression, resulting in even further excretion of paclitaxel into the intestinal fluid. Paclitaxel also induces CYP3A4 and CYP2C8 transcription, resulting in increased paclitaxel metabolism. Thus, in response to a xenobiotic challenge, PXR can induce both a first line of defense (intestinal excretion) and a backup system (hepatic drug inactivation) that limits exposure to potentially toxic compounds. In contrast to paclitaxel, docetaxel is a closely related antineoplastic agent that does not activate PXR but has a much better absorption profile.

Mutations of other transporters, particularly those involved in reuptake of serotonin, dopamine, and gamma-aminobutyric acid (GABA), are presently being studied with regard to clinically relevant changes in drug response. Pharmacogenetic variability in these transporters is an important consideration

TABLE 14-5   Reported Substrates of P-gp—A Member of ATP-Binding Cassette (ABC) Transporters

Acebutolol, acetaminophen, actinomycin d, h-acetyldigoxin, amitriptyline, amprenavir, apafant, asimadoline, atenolol, atorvastatin, azidopine, azidoprocainamide methoiodide, azithromycin

Benzo(a)pyrene, betamethasone, bisantrene, bromocriptine, bunitrolol, calcein-AM

Camptothecin, carbamazepine, carvedilol, celiprolol, cepharanthin, cerivastatin, chloroquine, chlorpromazine, chlorothiazide, Clarithromycin, colchicine, corticosterone, cortisol, cyclosporin A

Daunorubicin (daunomycin), debrisoquine, desoxycorticoster one, dexamethasone, digitoxin,

Digoxin, diltiazem, dipyridamole, docetaxel, dolastatin 10, domperidone, doxorubicin (adriamycin)

Eletriptan, emetine, endosulFan, erythromycin, estradiol, estradiol-17h-d-glucuronide, etoposide (VP-16)

Fexofenadine, gf120918, grepafloxacin

Hoechst 33342, hydroxyrubicin, imatinib, indinavir, ivermectin

Levofloxacin, loperamide, losartan, lovastatin

Methadone, methotrexate, methylprednisolone, metoprolol, mitoxantrone, monensin

Morphine, $_{99m}$tc-sestamibi

N-desmethyltamoxifen, nadolol, nelfinavir, nicardipine, nifedipine, nitrendipine, norverapamil

Olanzapine, omeprazole

PSC-833 (valspodar), perphenazine, prazosin, prednisone, pristinamycin IA, puromycin

Quetiapine, quinidine, quinine

Ranitidine, reserpine

Rhodamine 123, risperidone, ritonavir, roxithromycin

Saquinavir, sirolimus, sparfloxacin, sumatriptan,

Tacrolimus, talinolol, tamoxifen, Taxol (paclitaxel), telithromycin, terfenadine, timolol, toremifene

Tributylmethylammonium, trimethoprim

Valinomycin, vecuronium, verapamil, vinblastine

Vincristine, vindoline, vinorelbine

Adapted from Takano et al (2006), with permission.

in patient dosing. When therapeutic failures occur, the following questions should be asked: (1) Is the drug a substrate for P-gp and/or CYP3A4? (2) Is the drug being coadministered with anything that inhibits P-gp and/or CYP3A4? For example, grapefruit juice and many drugs can affect drug metabolism and oral absorption.

Vesicular Transport

Vesicular transport is the process of engulfing particles or dissolved materials by the cell. Pinocytosis and phagocytosis are forms of vesicular transport that differ by the type of material ingested. *Pinocytosis* refers to the engulfment of small solutes or fluid, whereas *phagocytosis* refers to the engulfment of larger particles or macromolecules, generally by macrophages. *Endocytosis* and *exocytosis* are the processes of moving specific macromolecules into and out of a cell, respectively.

During pinocytosis, phagocytosis, or transcytosis, the cell membrane invaginates to surround the material and then engulfs the material, incorporating it inside the cell (Fig. 14-11). Subsequently, the cell membrane containing the material forms a vesicle or vacuole within the cell. *Transcytosis* is the process by which various macromolecules are transported across the interior of a cell. In transcytosis, the vesicle fuses with the plasma membrane to release the encapsulated material to another side of the cell. Vesicles are employed to intake the macromolecules on one side of the cell, draw them across the cell, and eject them on the other side. Transcytosis (sometimes referred to as vesicular transport) is the proposed process for the absorption of orally

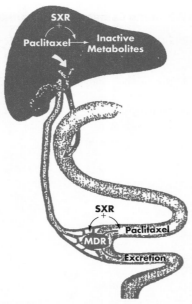

FIGURE 14-10 Mechanism of coordinated efflux and metabolism of paclitaxel by PXR (SXR). (From Synold et al, 2001, with permission.)

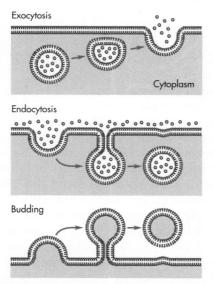

FIGURE 14-11 Diagram showing exocytosis and endocytosis. (From Alberts et al, 1989, with permission.)

administered Sabin polio vaccine and various large proteins.

Pinocytosis is a cellular process that permits the active transport of fluid from outside the cell through the membrane surrounding the cell into the inside of the cell. In pinocytosis, tiny incuppings called caveolae (little caves) in the surface of the cell close and then pinch off to form pinosomes, little fluid-filled bubbles, that are free within the cytoplasm of the cell.

An example of *exocytosis* is the transport of a protein such as insulin from insulin-producing cells of the pancreas into the extracellular space. The insulin molecules are first packaged into intracellular vesicles, which then fuse with the plasma membrane to release the insulin outside the cell.

Pore (Convective) Transport

Very small molecules (such as urea, water, and sugars) are able to cross cell membranes rapidly, as if the membrane contained channels or pores. Although such pores have never been directly observed by microscopy, the model of drug permeation through aqueous pores is used to explain renal excretion of drugs and the uptake of drugs into the liver.

A certain type of protein called a *transport protein* may form an open channel across the lipid membrane of the cell (see Fig. 14-2). Small molecules including drugs move through the channel by diffusion more rapidly than at other parts of the membrane.

Ion-Pair Formation

Strong electrolyte drugs are highly ionized or charged molecules, such as quaternary nitrogen compounds with extreme pK_a values. Strong electrolyte drugs maintain their charge at all physiologic pH values and penetrate membranes poorly. When the ionized drug is linked with an oppositely charged ion, an *ion pair* is formed in which the overall charge of the pair is neutral. This neutral drug complex diffuses more easily across the membrane. For example, the formation of ion pairs to facilitate drug absorption has been demonstrated for propranolol, a basic drug that forms an ion pair with oleic acid, and quinine, which forms ion pairs with hexylsalicylate (Nienbert, 1989).

An interesting application of ion pairs is the complexation of amphotericin B and DSPG (distearoylphosphatidylglycerol) in some amphotericin B/liposome products. Ion pairing may transiently alter distribution, reduce high plasma free drug concentration, and reduce renal toxicity.

DRUG INTERACTIONS IN THE GASTROINTESTINAL TRACT

Many agents (drug or chemical substances) may have dual roles as substrate and/or inhibitor between CYP3A4 and P-glycoprotein, P-gp. Simultaneous administration of these agents results in an increase in the oral drug bioavailability of one or both of the drugs. Various drug–drug and drug–nutrient interactions involving oral bioavailability have been reported in human subjects (Thummel and Wilkinson, 1998; Di Marco et al, 2002; von Richter et al, 2004).

Many commonly used medications (eg, dextromethorphan hydrobromide) and certain food groups (eg, grapefruit juice) are substrates both for the efflux transporter, P-gp, and for the CYP3A enzymes involved in biotransformation of drugs (see Chapter 12). Grapefruit juice also affects drug transport in the intestinal wall. Certain components of grapefruit juice (such as naringin and bergamottin) are responsible for the inhibition of P-gp and CYP3A. Di Marco et al (2002) demonstrated the inhibitory effect of grapefruit and Seville orange juice on the pharmacokinetics of dextromethorphan. Using dextromethorphan as the substrate, these investigators showed that grapefruit juice inhibits both CYP3A activity as well as P-gp resulting in an increased bioavailability of dextromethorphan. Grapefruit juice has been shown to increase the oral bioavailability of many drugs, such as cyclosporine or saquinavir, by inhibiting intestinal metabolism.

Esomeprazole (Nexium) and omeprazole (Prilosec) are proton pump inhibitors that inhibit gastric acid secretion, resulting an increased stomach pH. Esomeprazole and omeprazole may interfere with the absorption of drugs where gastric pH is an important determinant of bioavailability (eg, ketoconazole, iron salts, and digoxin). Both esomeprazole and omeprazole are extensively metabolized in the liver by CYP2C19 and CYP3A4. The prodrug clopidogrel (Plavix) inhibits platelet aggregation entirely due to an active metabolite. Coadministration of clopidogrel with omeprazole, an inhibitor of CYP2C19, reduces the pharmacological activity of clopidogrel if given either concomitantly or 12 hours apart.

The dual effect of a CYP isoenzyme and a transporter on drug absorption is not always easy to determine or predict based on pharmacokinetic studies alone. A well-studied example is the drug digoxin. Digoxin is minimally metabolized (CYP3A4), orally absorbed (Suzuki and Sugiyama, 2000), and a substrate for P-gp based on:

1. Human polymorphism single-nucleotide polymorphism (SNP) in exon 26 (C3435T) results in a reduced intestinal expression level of P-gp, along with increased oral bioavailability of digoxin.
2. Ketoconazole increases the oral bioavailability and shortens mean absorption time from 1.1 to 0.3 hour. Ketoconazole is a substrate and inhibitor of P-gp; P-gp can subsequently influence bioavailability. The influence of P-gp is not always easily detected unless studies are designed to investigate its presence.

For this analysis, a drug is given orally and intravenously before and after administration of an inhibitor drug. The AUC of the drug is calculated for each case. For example, ketoconazole causes an increase in the oral bioavailability of the immunosuppressant tacrolimus from 0.14 to 0.30, without affecting hepatic bioavailability (0.96–0.97) (Suzuki and Sugiyama, 2000). Since hepatic bioavailability is similar, the increase in bioavailability from 0.14 to 0.30 is the result of ketoconazole suppression on P-gp.

Mouly and Paine (2003) reported P-gp expression determined by Western blotting along the entire length of the human small intestine. They found that relative P-gp levels increased progressively from the proximal to the distal region. von Richter et al (2004) measured P-gp as well as CYP3A4 in paired human small intestine and liver specimens obtained from 15 patients. They reported that much higher levels of both P-gp (about seven times) and CYP3A4 (about three times) were found in the intestine than in the liver, suggesting the critical participation of intestinal P-gp in limiting oral drug bioavailability.

The concept of drug–drug interactions has received increased attention in recent years, as they may be responsible for many drug therapy-induced medical problems (Johnson et al, 1999).

Frequently Asked Questions

▶ *Animal studies are not definitive when extrapo-lated to humans. Why are animal studies or in vitro transport studies in human cells often performed to decide whether a drug is a P-gp substrate?*

▶ *How would you demonstrate that digoxin metabo-lism is solely due to hepatic extraction and not due to intestinal extraction since both CYP3A4 and P-gp are present in the intestine in larger amounts?*

ORAL DRUG ABSORPTION

The oral route of administration is the most common and popular route of drug dosing. The oral dosage form must be designed to account for extreme pH ranges, the presence or absence of food, degradative enzymes, varying drug permeability in the different regions of the intestine, and motility of the gastrointestinal tract. In this chapter we will discuss intestinal variables that affect absorption; dosage-form considerations are discussed in Chapters 15–18.

Anatomic and Physiologic Considerations

The normal physiologic processes of the alimentary canal may be affected by diet, contents of the gastrointestinal (GI) tract, hormones, the visceral nervous system, disease, and drugs. Thus, drugs given by the enteral route for systemic absorption may be affected by the anatomy, physiologic functions, and contents of the alimentary tract. Moreover, the physical, chemical, and pharmacologic properties of the drug and the formulation of the drug product will also affect systemic drug absorption from the alimentary canal.

The *enteral system* consists of the alimentary canal from the mouth to the anus (Fig. 14-12). The major physiologic processes that occur in the GI system are secretion, digestion, and absorption. Secretion includes the transport of fluid, electrolytes, peptides, and proteins into the lumen of the alimentary canal. Enzymes in saliva and pancreatic secretions are also

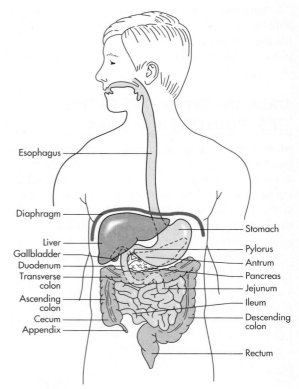

FIGURE 14-12   Gastrointestinal tract.

involved in the digestion of carbohydrates and proteins. Other secretions, such as mucus, protect the linings of the lumen of the GI tract. Digestion is the breakdown of food constituents into smaller structures in preparation for absorption. Food constituents are mostly absorbed in the proximal area (duodenum) of the small intestine. The process of absorption is the entry of constituents from the lumen of the gut into the body. Absorption may be considered the net result of both lumen-to-blood and blood-to-lumen transport movements.

Drugs administered orally pass through various parts of the enteral canal, including the oral cavity, esophagus, and various parts of the gastrointestinal tract. Residues eventually exit the body through the anus. The total transit time, including gastric emptying, small intestinal transit, and colonic transit, ranges from 0.4 to 5 days (Kirwan and Smith, 1974). The small intestine, particularly the duodenum area, is the most important site for drug absorption. Small intestine transit time (SITT) ranges from 3 to 4 hours for most healthy subjects. If absorption is not completed by the time a drug leaves the small intestine, absorption may be erratic or incomplete.

The small intestine is normally filled with digestive juices and liquids, keeping the lumen contents fluid. In contrast, the fluid in the colon is reabsorbed, and the lumenal content in the colon is either semisolid or solid, making further drug dissolution and absorption erratic and difficult. The lack of the solubilizing effect of the chyme and digestive fluid contributes to a less favorable environment for drug absorption.

Oral Cavity

Saliva is the main secretion of the oral cavity, and it has a pH of about 7. Saliva contains ptyalin (salivary amylase), which digests starches. Mucin, a glycoprotein that lubricates food, is also secreted and may interact with drugs. About 1500 mL of saliva is secreted per day.

The oral cavity can be used for the buccal absorption of lipid-soluble drugs such as fentanyl citrate (Actiq®) and nitroglycerin, also formulated for sublingual routes. Recently, orally disintegrating tablets, ODTs, have become available. These ODTs, such as aripiprazole (Abilify Discmelt®), rapidly disintegrate in the oral cavity in the presence of saliva. The resulting fragments, which are suspended in the saliva, are swallowed and the drug is then absorbed from the gastrointestinal tract. A major advantage for ODTs is that the drug may be taken without water. In the case of the antipsychotic drug, aripiprazole, a nurse may give the drug in the form of an ODT (Abilify Discmelt) to a schizophrenic patient. The nurse can easily ascertain that the drug was taken and swallowed.

Esophagus

The esophagus connects the pharynx and the cardiac orifice of the stomach. The pH of the fluids in the esophagus is between 5 and 6. The lower part of the esophagus ends with the esophageal sphincter, which prevents acid reflux from the stomach. Tablets or capsules may lodge in this area, causing local irritation. Very little drug dissolution occurs in the esophagus.

Stomach

The stomach is innervated by the vagus nerve. However, local nerve plexus, hormones, mechanoreceptors sensitive to the stretch of the GI wall, and chemoreceptors control the regulation of gastric secretions, including acid and stomach emptying. The fasting pH of the stomach is about 2–6. In the presence of food, the stomach pH is about 1.5–2, due to hydrochloric acid secreted by parietal cells. Stomach acid secretion is stimulated by gastrin and histamine. Gastrin is released from G cells, mainly in the antral mucosa and also in the duodenum. Gastrin release is regulated by stomach distention (swelling) and the presence of peptides and amino acids. A substance known as intrinsic factor enhances vitamin B-12 (cyanocobalamin) absorption. Various gastric enzymes, such as pepsin, which initiates protein digestion, are secreted into the gastric lumen to initiate digestion.

Basic drugs are solubilized rapidly in the presence of stomach acid. Mixing is intense and pressurized in the antral part of the stomach, a process of breaking down large food particles described as *antral milling*. Food and liquid are emptied by opening the pyloric sphincter into the duodenum. Stomach emptying is influenced by the food content and osmolality. Fatty acids and mono- and diglycerides delay gastric emptying (Hunt and Knox, 1968). High-density foods generally are emptied from the stomach more slowly. The relation of gastric emptying time to drug absorption is discussed more fully in the next section.

Stomach pH may be increased due to the presence of food and certain drugs such as omeprazole, a proton pump inhibitor used in gastroesophageal reflux disease (GERD). Increased stomach pH may cause a drug interaction with enteric-coated drug products (eg, diclofenac enteric-coated tablets, Voltaren). Such drug products require acid pH in the stomach to delay drug release from the dosage form until it reaches the higher pH of the intestine. If the stomach pH is too high, the enteric-coated drug product may release the drug in the stomach, thus causing irritation to the stomach.

A few fat-soluble, acid-stable drugs may be absorbed from the stomach by passive diffusion. Ethanol is completely miscible with water, easily crosses cell membranes, and is efficiently absorbed from the stomach. Ethanol is more rapidly absorbed from the stomach in the fasting state compared to the fed state (Levitt et al, 1997).

Duodenum

A common duct from both the pancreas and the gallbladder enters into the duodenum. The duodenal pH is about 6–6.5, because of the presence of bicarbonate that neutralizes the acidic chyme emptied from the stomach. The pH is optimum for enzymatic digestion of protein and peptide-containing food. Pancreatic juice containing enzymes is secreted into the duodenum from the bile duct. Trypsin, chymotrypsin, and carboxypeptidase are involved in the hydrolysis of proteins into amino acids. Amylase is involved in the digestion of carbohydrates. Pancreatic lipase secretion hydrolyzes fats into fatty acid. The complex fluid medium in the duodenum helps dissolve many drugs with limited aqueous solubility.

The duodenum is the major site for passive drug absorption due to both its anatomy, which creates a high surface area, and high blood flow. The duodenum is a site where many ester prodrugs are hydrolyzed during absorption. Proteolytic enzymes in the duodenum degrade many protein drugs preventing adequate absorption of the intact protein drug.

Jejunum

The jejunum is the middle portion of the small intestine, between the duodenum and the ileum. Digestion of protein and carbohydrates continues after addition of pancreatic juice and bile in the duodenum. This portion of the small intestine generally has fewer contractions than the duodenum and is preferred for *in vivo* drug absorption studies.

Ileum

The ileum is the terminal part of the small intestine. This site also has fewer contractions than the duodenum and may be blocked off by catheters with an inflatable balloon and perfused for drug absorption studies. The pH is about 7, with the distal part as high as 8. Due to the presence of bicarbonate secretion, acid drugs will dissolve in the ileum. Bile secretion helps dissolve fats and hydrophobic drugs. The ileocecal valve separates the small intestine from the colon.

Colon

The colon lacks villi and has limited drug absorption due to lack of large surface area, blood flow, and the more viscous and semisolid nature of the lumen contents. The colon is lined with mucin that functions as lubricant and protectant. The pH in this region is 5.5–7 (Shareef et al, 2003). A few drugs, such as theophylline and metoprolol, are absorbed in this region. Drugs that are absorbed well in this region are good candidates for an oral sustained-release dosage form. The colon contains both aerobic and anaerobic microorganisms that may metabolize some drugs. For example, L-dopa and lactulose are metabolized by enteric bacteria. Crohn's disease affects the colon and thickens the bowel wall. The microflora also become more anaerobic. Absorption of clindamycin and propranolol is increased, whereas other drugs have reduced absorption with this disease (Rubinstein et al, 1988). A few delayed-release drug products such as mesalamine (Asacol tablets, Pentasa capsules) have a pH-sensitive coating that dissolves in the higher pH of the lower bowel, releasing the mesalamine to act locally in Crohn's disease. Balsalazide disodium capsules (Colazal), also used in Crohn's disease, is a prodrug containing an azo group that is cleaved by anaerobic bacteria in the lower bowel to produce mesalamine (5-aminosalicylic acid or 5-ASA), an anti-inflammatory drug.

Rectum

The rectum is about 15 cm long, ending at the anus. In the absence of fecal material, the rectum has a small amount of fluid (approximately 2 mL) with a pH of about 7. The rectum is perfused by the superior, middle, and inferior hemorrhoidal veins. The inferior hemorrhoidal vein (closest to the anal sphincter) and the middle hemorrhoidal vein feed into the vena cava and back to the heart, thus bypassing the liver and avoiding hepatic first-pass effect. The superior hemorrhoidal vein joins the mesenteric circulation, which feeds into the hepatic portal vein and then to the liver.

The small amount of fluid present in the rectum has virtually no buffer capacity; as a consequence, the dissolving drug(s) or even excipients can have a determining effect on the existing pH in the anorectal area. Drug absorption after rectal administration may be variable, depending on the placement of the suppository or drug solution within the rectum. A portion of the drug dose may be absorbed via the lower hemorrhoidal veins, from which the drug feeds directly into the systemic circulation; some drugs may be absorbed via the superior hemorrhoidal vein, which feeds into the mesenteric veins to the hepatic portal vein to the liver, and be metabolized before systemic absorption. Thus some of the variability in drug absorption following rectal administration may occur due to variation in the site of absorption within the rectum.

Factors Affecting Drug Absorption in the Gastrointestinal Tract

Drugs may be absorbed by passive diffusion from all parts of the alimentary canal including sublingual, buccal, GI, and rectal absorption. For most drugs, the optimum site for drug absorption after oral administration is the upper portion of the small intestine or duodenum region. The unique anatomy of the duodenum provides an immense surface area for the drug to diffuse passively (Fig. 14-13). The large surface area of the duodenum is due to the presence of valve-like folds in the mucous membrane on which are small projections known as *villi*. These villi contain even smaller projections known as *microvilli*, forming a brush border. In addition, the duodenal region is highly perfused with a network of capillaries, which

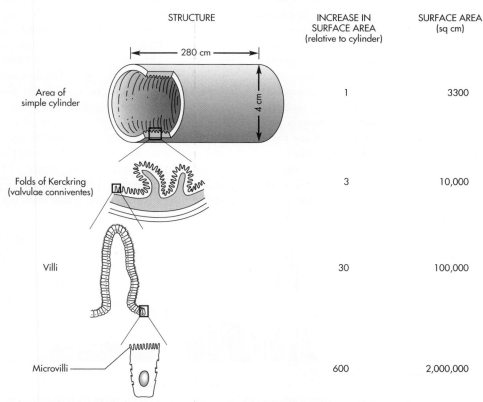

STRUCTURE	INCREASE IN SURFACE AREA (relative to cylinder)	SURFACE AREA (sq cm)
Area of simple cylinder	1	3300
Folds of Kerckring (valvulae conniventes)	3	10,000
Villi	30	100,000
Microvilli	600	2,000,000

FIGURE 14-13 Three mechanisms for increasing surface area of the small intestine. The increase in surface area is due to folds of Kerkring, villi, and microvilli. (From Wilson, 1962, with permission.)

helps maintain a concentration gradient from the intestinal lumen and plasma circulation.

Gastrointestinal Motility

Once a drug is given orally, the exact location and/or environment of the drug product within the GI tract is difficult to discern. GI motility tends to move the drug through the alimentary canal, so the drug may not stay at the absorption site. For drugs given orally, an anatomic absorption window may exist within the GI tract in which the drug is efficiently absorbed. Drugs contained in a nonbiodegradable controlled-release dosage form should be completely released into this absorption window to be absorbed before the movement of the dosage form into the large bowel.

The transit time of the drug in the GI tract depends on the physicochemical and pharmacologic properties of the drug, the type of dosage form, and various physiologic factors. Movement of the drug within the GI tract depends on whether the alimentary canal contains recently ingested food (digestive or fed state) or is in the fasted or interdigestive state (Fig. 14-14). During the fasted or interdigestive state, alternating cycles of activity known as the *migrating motor complex* (MMC) act as a propulsive movement that empties the upper GI tract to the cecum. Initially, the alimentary canal is quiescent. Then, irregular contractions followed by regular contractions with high amplitude (housekeeper waves) push any residual contents distally or farther down the alimentary canal. In the fed state, the migrating motor complex is replaced by irregular contractions, which have the effect of mixing intestinal contents and advancing the intestinal stream toward the colon in short segments

(Table 14-6). The pylorus and ileocecal valves prevent regurgitation or movement of food from the distal to the proximal direction.

Gastric Emptying Time

Anatomically, a swallowed drug rapidly reaches the stomach. Eventually, the stomach empties its contents into the small intestine. Because the duodenum has the greatest capacity for the absorption of drugs from the GI tract, a delay in the gastric emptying time for the drug to reach the duodenum will slow the rate and possibly the extent of drug absorption, thereby prolonging the onset time for the drug. Some drugs, such as penicillin, are unstable in acid and decompose if stomach emptying is delayed. Other drugs, such as aspirin, may irritate the gastric mucosa during prolonged contact.

A number of factors affect gastric emptying time. Some factors that tend to delay gastric emptying include consumption of meals high in fat, cold beverages, and anticholinergic drugs (Burks et al, 1985; Rubinstein et al, 1988). Liquids and small particles less than 1 mm are generally not retained in the stomach. These small particles are believed to be emptied due to a slightly higher basal pressure in the stomach over the duodenum. Different constituents of a meal empty from the stomach at different rates. Feldman et al (1984) observed that 10 oz of liquid soft drink, scrambled egg (digestible solid), and a radio-opaque marker (undigestible solid) were 50% emptied from the stomach in 30 minutes, 154 minutes, and 3–4 hours, respectively. Thus, liquids are generally emptied faster than digested solids from the stomach (Fig. 14-15).

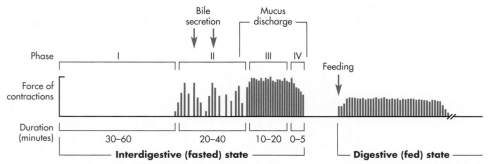

FIGURE 14-14   A pictorial representation of the typical motility patterns in the interdigestive (fasted) and digestive (fed) state. (From Rubinstein et al, 1988, with permission.)

TABLE 14-6   Characteristics of the Motility Patterns in the Fasted Dog

Phase	Duration	Characteristics
Fasted State		
I	30–60 min	Quiescence.
II	20–40 min	• Irregular contractions • Medium amplitude but can be as high as phase III • Bile secretion begins • Onset of gastric discharge of administered fluid of small volume usually occurs before that of particle discharge • Onset of particle and mucus discharge may occur during the latter part of phase II
III	5–15 min	• Regular contractions (4–5 contractions/min) with high amplitude • Mucus discharge continues • Particle discharge continues
IV	0–5 min	• Irregular contractions • Medium descending amplitude • Sometimes absent
Fed State		
One phase only	As long as food is present in the stomach	• Regular, frequent contractions. • Amplitude is lower than phase III • 4–5 contractions/min

From Rubinstein et al (1988), with permission.

Large particles, including tablets and capsules, are delayed from emptying for 3–6 hours by the presence of food in the stomach. Indigestible solids empty very slowly, probably during the interdigestive phase, a phase in which food is not present and the stomach is less motile but periodically empties its content due to housekeeper wave contraction (Fig. 14-16).

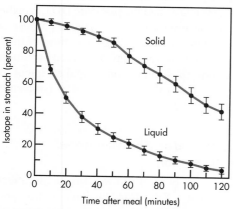

FIGURE 14-15   Gastric emptying of a group of normal subjects using the dual-isotope method. The mean and 1 SE of the fraction of isotope remaining in the stomach are depicted at various time intervals after ingestion of the meal. Note the exponential nature of liquid emptying and the linear process of solid emptying. (From Minami and McCallum, 1984, with permission.)

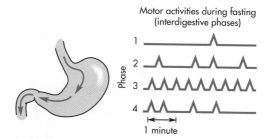

FIGURE 14-16   Motor activity responsible for gastric emptying of indigestible solids. Migrating myoelectric complex (MMC), usually initiated at proximal stomach or lower esophageal sphincter, and contractions during phase 3 sweep indigestible solids through open pylorus. (From Minami and McCallum, 1984, with permission.)

Intestinal Motility

Normal peristaltic movements mix the contents of the duodenum, bringing the drug particles into intimate contact with the intestinal mucosal cells. The drug must have a sufficient time (*residence time*) at the absorption site for optimum absorption. In the case of high motility in the intestinal tract, as in diarrhea, the drug has a very brief residence time and less opportunity for adequate absorption.

The average normal SITT was about 7 hours as measured in early studies using indirect methods based on the detection of hydrogen after an oral dose of lactulose (fermentation of lactulose by colon bacteria yields hydrogen in the breath). Newer studies using gamma scintigraphy have shown SITT to be about 3–4 hours. Thus a drug may take about 4–8 hours to pass through the stomach and small intestine during the fasting state. During the fed state, SITT may take 8–12 hours. For modified-release or controlled-dosage forms, which slowly release the drug over an extended period of time, the dosage form must stay within a certain segment of the intestinal tract so that the drug contents are released and absorbed before loss of the dosage form in the feces. Intestinal transit is discussed further in relation to the design of sustained-release products in Chapter 19.

In one study reported by Shareef et al (2003), utilizing a radio-opaque marker, mean mouth-to-anus transit time was 53.3 hours. The mean colon transit time was 35 hours, with 11.3 hours for the right (ascending transverse portion), 11.4 hours for the left (descending and portion of the transverse), and 12.4 hours for the recto sigmoid colon. Dietary fiber has the greatest effect on colonic transit. Dietary fiber increases fecal weight, partly by retaining water and partly by increasing bacterial mass (Shareef et al, 2003).

Perfusion of the Gastrointestinal Tract

The blood flow to the GI tract is important in carrying absorbed drug to the systemic circulation. A large network of capillaries and lymphatic vessels perfuse the duodenal region and peritoneum. The splanchnic circulation receives about 28% of the cardiac output and is increased after meals. This high degree of perfusion helps to maintain a concentration gradient favoring absorption. Once the drug is absorbed from the small intestine, it enters via the mesenteric vessels to the hepatic-portal vein and goes to the liver prior to reaching the systemic circulation. Any decrease in mesenteric blood flow, as in the case of congestive heart failure, will decrease the rate of drug removal from the intestinal tract, thereby reducing the rate of drug bioavailability (Benet et al, 1976).

Absorption through the Lymphatic System

The role of the lymphatic circulation in drug absorption is well established. Lipophilic drugs may be absorbed through the lacteal or lymphatic vessels under the microvilli. Absorption of drugs through the lymphatic system bypasses the liver and avoids the first-pass effect due to liver metabolism, because the lymphatic vessels drain into the vena cava rather than the hepatic-portal vein. The lymphatics are important in the absorption of dietary lipids and may be partially responsible for the absorption of some lipophilic drugs. Many poorly water-soluble drugs are soluble in oil and lipids, which may dissolve in chylomicrons and be absorbed systemically via the lymphatic system. Bleomycin or aclarubicin were prepared in chylomicrons to improve oral absorption through the lymphatic system (Yoshikawa et al, 1983, 1989). Other drugs that can be significantly absorbed through the lymphatic system include halofantrine, certain testosterone derivatives, temarotene, ontazolast, vitamin D-3, and the pesticide DDT. Notably, as the trend in drug development is to produce more highly potent lipophilic drugs, targeting of the lymphatic system is receiving increased attention. In such efforts, the formulation of lipid excipients plays a very dramatic role in the success of lymphatic targeting (Yanez et al, 2011).

Effect of Food on Gastrointestinal Drug Absorption

The presence of food in the GI tract can affect the bioavailability of the drug from an oral drug product (Table 14-7). Digested foods contain amino acids, fatty acids, and many nutrients that may affect intestinal pH and solubility of drugs. The effects of food are not always predictable and can have clinically significant consequences. Some effects of food on

TABLE 14-7   The Affect of Food on the Bioavailability of Selected Drugs

Drug	Food Affect
Decreased bioavailability with food	
Doxycycline Hyclate Delayed-Release Tablets	The mean Cmax and $AUC_{0-\infty}$ of doxycycline are 24% and 13% lower, respectively, following single dose administration with a high-fat meal (including milk) compared to fasted conditions.
Atorvastatin calcium tablets	Food decreases the rate and extent of drug absorption by approximately 25% and 9%, respectively, as assessed by Cmax and AUC.
Clopidogrel bisulfate tablets	Clopidogrel is a prodrug and is metabolized to a pharmacologically active metabolite and inactive metabolites. The active metabolite AUC_{0-24} was unchanged in the presence of food, while there was a 57% decrease in active metabolite Cmax
Naproxen delayed-release tablets	Naproxen delayed-release tablets are enteric coated tablets with a pH-sensitive coating. The presence of food prolonged the time the tablets remained in the stomach. Tmax is delayed but peak naproxen levels, Cmax was not affected.
Alendronate sodium tablets	Bioavailability was decreased by approximately 40% when 10 mg alendronate was administered either 0.5 or 1 hour before a standardized breakfast. Alendronate must be taken at least one-half hour before the first food, beverage, or medication of the day with plain water only. Other beverages (including mineral water), food, and some medications are likely to reduce drug absorption.
Tamsulosin HCl capsules	Taking tamsulosin capsules under fasted conditions results in a 30% increase in bioavailability (AUC) and 40% to 70% increase in peak concentrations (C_{max}) compared to fed conditions.
Increased bioavailability with food	
Oxycodone HCl CR tablets	Food has no significant effect on the extent of absorption of oxycodone from OxyContin. However, the peak plasma concentration of oxycodone increased by 25% when a OxyContin 160 mg tablet was administered with a high-fat meal.
Metaxalone Tablets	A high-fat meal increased Cmax by 177.5% and increased AUC (AUC_{0-t}, AUC_∞) by 123.5% and 115.4%, respectively. T_{max} was delayed (4.3 h versus 3.3 h) and terminal $t_{1/2}$ was decreased (2.4 h versus 9.0 h).
Spironolactone tablets	Food increased the bioavailability of unmetabolized spironolactone by almost 100%. The clinical importance of this finding is not known
Food has very little affect on bioavailability	
Gabapentin capsules	Food has only a slight effect on the rate and extent of absorption of gabapentin (14% increase in AUC and C_{max}).
Tramadol HCl tablets	Oral administration of Tramadol hydrochloride tablets with food does not significantly affect its rate or extent of absorption.
Digoxin tablets	When digoxin tablets are taken after meals, the rate of absorption is slowed, but the total amount of digoxin absorbed is usually unchanged. When taken with meals high in bran fiber, however, the amount absorbed from an oral dose may be reduced.
Bupropion HCl ER tablets	Food did not affect the C_{max} or AUC of bupropion.
Methylphenidate HCl ER tablets (Concerta®)	In patients, there were no differences in either the pharmacokinetics or the pharmacodynamic performance of Concerta® when administered after a high fat breakfast. There is no evidence of dose dumping in the presence or absence of food.
Fluoxetine HCl capsules	Food does not appear to affect the 846 systemic bioavailability of fluoxetine, although it may delay its absorption by 1 to 2 hours, which is probably not clinically significant.
Dutasteride soft gelatin capsules	Food reduces the Cmax by 10% to 15%. This reduction is of no clinical significance.

Food can affect bioavailability of the drug by affecting the rate and/or extent of drug absorption. In some cases, food may delay the Tmax for enteric coated drugs due to a delay in stomach emptying time. For each drug, the clinical importance of the change in bioavailability due to food must be assessed.

the bioavailability of a drug from a drug product include (US Food and Drug Administration, Guidance for Industry, December 2002):

- Delay in gastric emptying
- Stimulation of bile flow
- A change in the pH of the GI tract
- An increase in splanchnic blood flow
- A change in luminal metabolism of the drug substance
- Physical or chemical interaction of the meal with the drug product or drug substance

Food effects on bioavailability are generally greatest when the drug product is administered shortly after a meal is ingested. The nutrient and caloric contents of the meal, the meal volume, and the meal temperature can cause physiologic changes in the GI tract in a way that affects drug product transit time, luminal dissolution, drug permeability, and systemic availability. In general, meals that are high in total calories and fat content are more likely to affect GI physiology and thereby result in a larger effect on the bioavailability of a drug substance or drug product. The FDA recommends the use of high-calorie and high-fat meals to study the effect of food on the bioavailability and bioequivalence of drug products (FDA Guidance for Industry, 2002; see also Chapter 16).

The absorption of some antibiotics, such as penicillin and tetracycline and certain hydrophilic drugs, is decreased with food, whereas other drugs, particularly lipid-soluble drugs such as griseofulvin, metaxalone, and metazalone, are better absorbed when given with food containing a high-fat content (Fig. 14-17). The presence of food in the GI lumen stimulates the flow of bile. Bile contains bile acids, which are surfactants involved in the digestion and solubilization of fats, and also increases the solubility of fat-soluble drugs through micelle formation. For some basic drugs (eg, cinnarizine) with limited aqueous solubility, the presence of food in the stomach stimulates hydrochloric acid secretion, which lowers the pH, causing more rapid dissolution of the drug and better absorption. Absorption of this basic drug is reduced when gastric acid secretion is reduced (Ogata et al, 1986).

Most drugs should be taken with a full glass (approximately 8 fluid oz or 250 mL) of water to

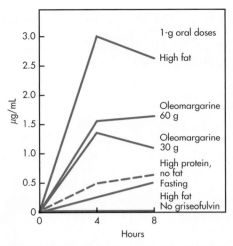

FIGURE 14-17   A comparison of the effects of different types of food intake on the serum griseofulvin levels following a 1.0-g oral dose. (From Crounse, 1961, with permission.)

ensure that drugs will wash down the esophagus and be more available for absorption. Generally, the bioavailability of drugs is better in patients in the fasted state and with a large volume of water (Fig. 14-18). The solubility of many drugs is limited, and sufficient fluid is necessary for dissolution of the drug. Some patients may be on several drugs that are dosed frequently for months. These patients are often nauseous and are reluctant to take a lot of fluid. For example, HIV patients with active viral counts may be on an AZT or DDI combination with one or more of the protease inhibitors, Invirase (Hoffmann-La Roche), Crixivan (Merck), or Norvir (Abbott). These HIV treatments appear to be better than any previous treatments but depend on patient compliance in taking up to 12–15 pills daily for weeks. Any complications affecting drug absorption can influence the outcome of these therapies. With antibiotics, unabsorbed drug may influence the GI flora. For drugs that cause GI disturbances, residual drug dose in the GI tract can potentially aggravate the incidence of diarrhea.

Some drugs, such as erythromycin, iron salts, aspirin, and nonsteroidal anti-inflammatory agents (NSAIDs), are irritating to the GI mucosa and are given with food to reduce this irritation. For these drugs, the rate of absorption may be reduced in the

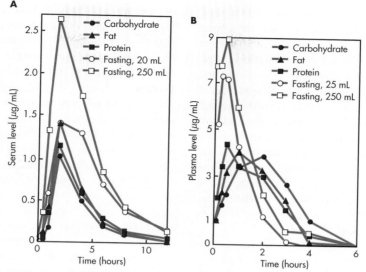

FIGURE 14-18   Effect of water volume and meal on the bioavailability of erythromycin and aspirin (ASA). (**A**) From Welling PG, et al: Bioavailability of erythromycin state: influence of food and fluid volume. *J Pharm Sci* **67**(6):764–766, June 1978, with permission. (**B**) From Koch PA, et al: Influence of food and fluid ingestion on aspirin bioavailability. *J Pharm Sci* **67**(11):1533–1535, November 1978, with permission.

presence of food, but the extent of absorption may be the same and the efficacy of the drug is retained.

The GI transit time for enteric-coated and non-disintegrating drug products may also be affected by the presence of food. Enteric-coated tablets may stay in the stomach for a longer period of time because food delays stomach emptying. Thus, the enteric-coated tablet does not reach the duodenum rapidly, delaying drug release and systemic drug absorption. The presence of food may delay stomach emptying of enteric-coated tablets or nondisintegrating dosage forms for several hours. In contrast, since enteric-coated beads or microparticles disperse in the stomach, stomach emptying of the particles is less affected by food, and these preparations demonstrate more consistent drug absorption from the duodenum. Fine granules (smaller than 1–2 mm in size) and tablets that disintegrate are not significantly delayed from emptying from the stomach in the presence of food.

Food can also affect the integrity of the dosage form, causing an alteration in the release rate of the drug. For example, theophylline bioavailability from Theo-24 controlled-release tablets is much more

rapid when given to a subject in the fed rather than fasted state because of dosage form failures, known as *dose-dumping* (Fig.14-19).

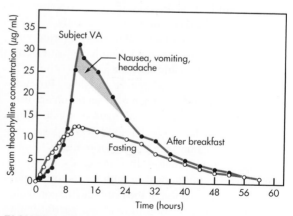

FIGURE 14-19   Theophylline serum concentrations in an individual subject after a single 1500-mg dose of Theo-24 taken during fasting and after breakfast. The shaded area indicates the period during which this patient experienced nausea, repeated vomiting, or severe throbbing headache. The pattern of drug release during the food regimen is consistent with "dose-dumping." (From Hendeles et al, 1985, with permission.)

Food may enhance the absorption of a drug beyond 2 hours after meals. For example, the timing of a fatty meal on the absorption of cefpodoxime proxetil was studied in 20 healthy adults (Borin et al, 1995). The area under the plasma concentration–time curve and peak drug concentration was significantly higher after administration of cefpodoxime proxetil tablets with a meal and 2 hours after a meal relative to dosing under fasted conditions or 1 hour before a meal. The time to peak concentration was not affected by food, which suggests that food increased the extent but not the rate of drug absorption. These results indicate that absorption of cefpodoxime proxetil is enhanced with food or if the drug is taken closely after a heavy meal.

Timing of drug administration in relation to meals is often important. Pharmacists regularly advise patients to take a medication either 1 hour before or 2 hours after meals to avoid any delay in drug absorption.

Alendronate sodium (Fosamax®) is a bisphosphonate that acts as a specific inhibitor of osteoclast-mediated bone resorption used to prevent osteoporosis. Bisphosphonates are very soluble in water and their systemic oral absorption is greatly reduced in the presence of food. The approved labeling for alendronate sodium states that (Fosamax) "must be taken at least one-half hour before the first food, beverage, or medication of the day with plain water only."

Since fatty foods may delay stomach emptying time beyond 2 hours, patients who have just eaten a heavy, fatty meal should take these drugs 3 hours or more after the meal, whenever possible. Products that are used to curb stomach acid secretion are usually taken before meals, in anticipation of acid secretion stimulated by food. Famotidine (Pepcid) and cimetidine (Tagamet) are taken before meals to curb excessive acid production. In some cases, drugs are taken directly after a meal or with meals to increase the systemic absorption of the drug (eg, itraconazole, metaxalone) or with food to decrease gastric irritation of the drug (eg, ibuprofen). Many lipophilic drugs have increased bioavailability with food possibly due to formation of micelles in the GI tract and some lymphatic absorption.

Fluid volume tends to distend the stomach and speed up stomach emptying; however, a large volume of nutrients with high caloric content supersedes that faster rate and delays stomach emptying time. Reduction in drug absorption may be caused by several other factors. For example, tetracycline hydrochloride absorption is reduced by milk and food that contains calcium, due to tetracycline chelation. However, significant reduction in absorption may simply be the result of reduced dissolution due to increased pH. Coadministration of sodium bicarbonate raises the stomach pH and reduces tetracycline dissolution and absorption (Barr et al, 1971).

Ticlopidine (Ticlid®) is an antiplatelet agent that is commonly used to prevent thromboembolic disorders. Ticlopidine has enhanced absorption after a meal. The absorption of ticlopidine was compared in subjects who received either an antacid or food or were in a control group (fasting). Subjects who received ticlopidine 30 minutes after a fatty meal had an average increase of 20% in plasma concentrations over fasting subjects, whereas antacid reduced ticlopidine plasma concentrations by approximately the same amount. There was a higher incidence of gastrointestinal complaint in the fasting group. Many other drugs have reduced gastrointestinal side effects when taken with food. The decreased gastrointestinal side effects associated with food consumption may greatly improve tolerance and compliance in patients.

Double-Peak Phenomenon

Some drugs, such as ranitidine, cimetidine, and dipyridamole, after oral administration produce a blood concentration curve consisting of two peaks (Fig. 14-20). This double-peak phenomenon is generally observed after the administration of a single dose to fasted patients. The rationale for the double-peak phenomenon has been attributed to variability in stomach emptying, variable intestinal motility, presence of food, enterohepatic recycling, or failure of a tablet dosage form.

The double-peak phenomenon observed for cimetidine (Oberle and Amidon, 1987) may be due to variability in stomach emptying and intestinal flow rates during the entire absorption process after a single dose. For many drugs, very little absorption occurs in the stomach. For a drug with high water solubility, dissolution of the drug occurs in the stomach, and partial emptying of the drug into the duodenum will

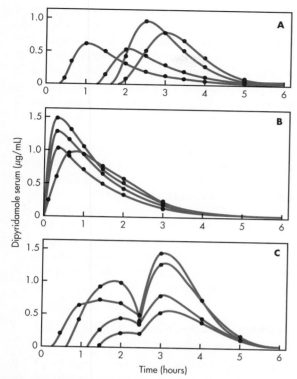

FIGURE 14-20 Serum concentrations of dipyridamole in three groups of four volunteers each. **(A)** After taking 25 mg as tablet intact. **(B)** As crushed tablet. **(C)** As tablet intact 2 hours before lunch. (From Mellinger TJ, Bohorfoush JG: Blood levels of dipyridamole (Persantin) in humans. *Arch Int Pharmacodynam Ther* **163**:471–480, 1966, with permission.)

result in the first absorption peak. A delay in stomach emptying results in a second absorption peak as the remainder of the dose is emptied into the duodenum.

In contrast, ranitidine (Miller, 1984) produces a double peak after both oral or parenteral (IV bolus) administration. Ranitidine is apparently concentrated in the bile within the gallbladder from the general circulation after IV administration. When stimulated by food, the gallbladder contracts and bile-containing drug is released into the small intestine. The drug is then reabsorbed and recycled (enterohepatic recycling).

Tablet integrity may also be a factor in the production of a double-peak phenomenon. Mellinger and Bohorfoush (1966) compared a whole tablet or a crushed tablet of dipyridamole in volunteers and showed that a tablet that does not disintegrate or incompletely disintegrates may have delayed gastric emptying, resulting in a second absorption peak.

ORAL DRUG ABSORPTION DURING DRUG PRODUCT DEVELOPMENT

Prediction of Oral Drug Absorption

During the screening of new chemical entities for possible therapeutic efficacy, some drugs might not be discovered due to lack of systemic absorption after oral administration. Lipinski et al (2001) reviewed the chemical structure of many orally administered drugs and published the Rule of Five. During drug screening, "Rule of Five" predicts that poor drug absorption or permeation is more likely when there are more than five H-bond (hydrogen-bond) donors. For 10 H-bond acceptors, the molecular weight (MWT) is greater than 500, and the calculated log P (Clog P) is greater than 5 (or Mlog $P > 4.15$). The rule is based on molecular computation and simulation and the effect of hydrophobicity, hydrogen bond, molecular size, and other relevant factors in assessing absorption using computational methods. The method is not applicable to drugs whose absorption involves transporters. These rules were developed to avoid types of chemical structures during early drug development that are unlikely to have adequate bioavailability. These rules have been modified by others (Takano et al, 2006). Rules for drug molecules that would improve the chance for oral absorption would include:

- Molecular weight ≤500 Da
- Not more than five *H-bond* donors (*nitrogen* or *oxygen atoms* with one or more *hydrogen atoms*) (O–H or N–H group)
- Not more than 10 *H-bond* acceptors (*nitrogen* or *oxygen atoms*)
- An octanol–water partition coefficient, log $P \leq 5.0$

These rules only help predict adequate drug absorption and do not predict adequate pharmacodynamic activity. Moreover, some chemical structures do not follow the above rules, but may have good therapeutic properties.

Burton et al (2002) reviewed the difficulty in predicting drug absorption based only on physicochemical activity of drug molecules and discussed other factors that can affect oral drug absorption. Burton et al state that drug absorption is a complex process dependent upon drug properties such as solubility and permeability, formulation factors, and physiological variables, including regional permeability differences, pH, mucosal enzymology, and intestinal motility, among others. These investigators point out that intestinal drug absorption, permeability, fraction absorbed, and, in some cases, even bioavailability are not equivalent properties and cannot be used interchangeably. Often these properties are influenced by the nature of the drug product and physical and chemical characteristics of the drug.

Software programs, such as GastroPlus™, have recently been developed to predict oral drug absorption, pharmacokinetics, and pharmacodynamic drugs in human and preclinical species. Simulation programs may use physicochemical data, such as molecular weight, pK_a, solubility at various pH, log P/log D, type of dosage form, *in vitro* inputs such as dissolution, permeability/Caco-2, CYP metabolism (gut/liver), transporter rates, and *in vivo* inputs such as drug clearance and volume of distribution.

METHODS FOR STUDYING FACTORS THAT AFFECT DRUG ABSORPTION

Gamma Scintigraphy to Study Site of Drug Release

Gamma scintigraphy is a technique commonly used to track drug dosage form movement from one region to another within the GI tract after oral administration. Gamma scintigraphy also has many research applications and is widely used for formulation studies, such as the mechanism of drug release from a hydrophilic matrix tablet (Abrahamsson et al, 1998). Generally a nonabsorbable radionuclide that emits gamma rays is included as marker in the formulation. In some studies, two radiolabels may be used for simultaneous detection of liquid and solid phases. One approach is to use labeled technetium (Tc[99m]) in a capsule matrix to study how a drug is absorbed. The image of the capsule breaking up in the stomach or the GI tract is monitored using a gamma camera. Simultaneously, blood levels or urinary excretion of the drug may be measured. This study can be used to correlate residence time of the drug in a given region after capsule breakup to drug absorption. The same technique is used to study drug absorption mechanisms in different regions of the GI tract before a drug is formulated for extended release.

Gamma scintigraphy has been used to study the effect of transit time on the absorption of theophylline (Sournac et al, 1988). *In vitro* drug release characteristics were correlated with total gastrointestinal transit time. The results showed a significant correlation between the *in vitro* release of theophylline and the percent of the total amount of theophylline absorbed *in vivo*. This study illustrates the importance of gamma scintigraphy for the development of specialized drug dosage forms.

Markers to Study Effect of Gastric and GI Transit Time on Absorption

Many useful agents are available that may be used as tools to study absorption and understand the mechanism of the absorptive process. For example, mannitol has a concentration-dependent effect on small intestinal transit. Adkin et al (1995) showed that small concentrations of mannitol included in a pharmaceutical formulation could lead to reduced uptake of many drugs absorbed exclusively from the small intestine. No significant differences between the gastric emptying times of the four solutions of different concentrations tested were observed.

Similarly, Hebden et al (1999) demonstrated that codeine slowed GI transit, decreased stool water content, and diminished drug absorption when compared to controls. The results indicated that stool water content may be an important determinant in colonic drug absorption. In contrast, the sugar lactulose accelerated GI transit, increased stool water content, and enhanced drug absorption from the distal gut. Quinine absorption was greater when given with lactulose compared to no lactulose.

Riley et al (1992) studied the effects of gastric emptying and GI transit on the absorption of several drug solutions (furosemide, atenolol, hydrochlorothiazide, and salicylic acid) in healthy subjects. These drugs may potentially be absorbed differently at various sites in the GI system. Subjects were given 20 mg oral metoclopramide or 60 mg oral codeine phosphate to slow gastric emptying. The study showed that gastric emptying time affects the absorption of salicylic acid, but not that of furosemide, hydrochlorothiazide, or atenolol. *In vivo* experiments are needed to determine the effect of changing transit time on drug absorption.

Remote Drug Delivery Capsules (RDDCs)

Drug absorption *in vivo* may be studied either directly by an intubation technique that directly takes samples from the GI tract or remotely with a special device, such as the Heidelberg capsule. The *Heidelberg capsule* (Barrie, 1999) is a device used to determine the pH of the stomach. The capsule contains a pH sensor and a miniature radio transmitter (invented by H. G. Noeller and used at Heidelberg University in Germany decades ago). The capsule is about 2 cm × 0.8 cm and can transmit data to outside after the device is swallowed and tethered to the stomach. Other, newer telemetric methods may be used to take pictures of various regions of the GI tract.

An interesting *remote drug delivery capsule* (RDDC) with electronic controls for noninvasive regional drug absorption study was reported by Parr et al (1999). This device was used to study absorption of ranitidine hydrochloride solution in 12 healthy male volunteers. Mean gastric emptying of the RDDC was 1.50 hours, and total small intestine transit was 4.79 hours. The capsule was retrieved from the feces at 30.25 hours. The onset of ranitidine serum levels depended on the time of capsule activation and the site of drug release.

Osmotic Pump Systems

The osmotic pump system is a drug product that contains a small hole from which dissolved drug is released (pumped out) at a rate determined by the rate of entrance of water from the GI tract across a semipermeable membrane due to osmotic pressure (see Chapter 18). The drug is either mixed with an osmotic agent or located in a reservoir. Osmotic pump systems may be used to study drug absorption

in different parts of the GI tract because the rate of drug release is constant (zero order) and generally not altered by the environment of the gastrointestinal tract. The constant rate of drug release provides relatively constant blood concentrations.

In Vivo *GI Perfusion Studies*

In the past, segments of guinea pig or rat ileums were cut and used to study drug absorption; however, we now know that many of the isolated preparations were not viable shortly after removal, making the absorption data collected either invalid or difficult to evaluate. In addition, the differences among species make it difficult to extrapolate animal data to humans.

GI perfusion is an *in vivo* method used to study absorption and permeability of a drug in various segments of the GI tract. A tube is inserted from the mouth or anus and placed in a specific section of the GI tract. A drug solution is infused from the tube at a fixed rate, resulting in drug perfusion of the desired GI region. The jejunal site is peristaltically less active than the duodenum, making it easier to intubate, and therefore, it is often chosen for perfusion studies. Perfusion studies in other sites such as the duodenum, ileum, and even the colon have also been performed by gastroenterologists and pharmaceutical scientists.

Lennernas et al (1992, 1995) have applied perfusion techniques in humans to study permeability in the small intestine and the rectum. These methods yield direct absorption information in various segments of the GI tract. The regional jejunal perfusion method was reported to have great potential for mechanistic evaluations of drug absorption.

Buch and Barr (1998) evaluated propranolol HCl in the proximal and distal intestine in humans ($n = 7$ subjects) using direct intubation. Propranolol HCl is a beta blocker that has high inter- and intrasubject variability in absorption and metabolism. These investigators showed that propranolol was better absorbed from a solution in the distal region of the intestine. This study is difficult to relate to the propranolol extended-release oral products for which differences in drug release rates and GI transit time may also influence inter- and intrasubject variability in bioavailability.

More recently, balloon-isolated jejunal drug administration has been used to determine the absorption characteristics of (-)epicatechin, vitamin E, and vitamin E acetate (Actis-Goretta et al, 2013). The current efforts to determine intestinal regional drug absorption have been recently reviewed, and data generated from these studies will be useful to refine models for predicting drug absorption (Lennernas, 2014).

Intestinal Permeability to Drugs

Drugs that are completely absorbed ($F > 90\%$) after oral administration generally demonstrate high permeability in *in vitro* models. Previously, poor drug absorption was mostly attributed to poor dissolution, slow diffusion, degradation, or poor intestinal permeation. Modern technology has shown that poor or variable oral drug bioavailability among individuals is also the result of individual genetic differences in intestinal absorption (see Chapter 13). Interindividual differences in membrane proteins, ion channels, uptake transporters, and efflux pumps (such as P-glycoprotein, P-gp) that mediate directional transport of drugs and their metabolites across biological membranes can change the extent of drug absorption, or even transport to the site of action elsewhere in the body. It is now clear that the behavior of drugs in the body is the result of an intricate interplay between these receptors, drug transporters, and the drug-metabolizing systems. This insight provides another explanation for erratic drug absorption beyond poor formulation and first-pass metabolism.

Alternative methods to study intestinal drug permeability include *in vivo* or *in situ* intestinal perfusion in a suitable animal model (eg, rats), and/or *in vitro* permeability methods using excised intestinal tissues, or monolayers of suitable epithelial cells such as Caco-2 cells. In addition, the physicochemical characterization of a drug substance (eg, oil–water partition coefficient) provides useful information to predict a drug's permeability.

Caco-2 Cells for In Vitro Permeability Studies

Although *in vivo* studies yield much definitive information about drug permeability in humans, they are tedious and costly to perform. The *Caco-2* cell line is a human colon adenocarcinoma cell line that differentiates in culture and resembles the epithelial lining of the human small intestine. The permeability of the cellular monolayer may vary with the stage of cell growth and the cultivation method used. However, using monolayers of Caco-2 cells under controlled conditions, the permeability of a drug may be determined. Caco-2 cells can also be used to study interactions of drugs with the transporter P-gp discussed below.

Drug permeability using the Caco-2 cell line has been suggested as an *in vitro* method for passively transported drugs. In some cases, the drug permeability may appear to be low due to efflux of drugs via membrane transporters such as P-gp. Permeability studies using the Caco-2 cell line have been suggested as a method for classifying the permeability of a drug according to the Biopharmaceutics Classification System, BCS (Tolle-Sander and Polli, 2002; US Food and Drug Administration, Guidance 2003, August 2002; Sun and Pang, 2007). The main purpose of the BCS is to identify a drug as having high or low permeability as a predictor of systemic drug absorption from the GI tract (see Chapter 16).

Drug Transporters

Many methods are available to study the actions of drug transporters in the GI tract. In addition to Caco-2 cells, there are several commercially available expression systems to study various transporters, including those required by the FDA in drug development. These systems include transporters recombinantly expressed in insect, frog, or mammalian cells. Also, the plasma membranes of some of these expression systems can also be isolated, providing membrane vesicle preparations that are devoid of drug-metabolizing activity.

Determinations of Artificial Membrane Permeability

To accelerate early determinations of factors involved in drug absorption, permeability and solubility of a novel drug candidate are determined early in the drug development process. Permeability of drug candidates may be determined using high-throughput screening techniques, such as the parallel artificial membrane permeability assay (PAMPA). In this technique, artificial lipid membranes are supported on a filter between two fluid compartments, one of which contains the drug candidate. The rate of appearance into the opposite compartment is then measured to determine the permeability of the compound. Several models and variations of this approach are available, and investigators should pay attention particularly to the lipid composition of the artificial membranes as well as other experimental details. Notably, the PAMPA can only predict simple diffusional permeability, which does not involve uptake or efflux transporters (Avdeef et al, 2007).

EFFECT OF DISEASE STATES ON DRUG ABSORPTION

Drug absorption may be affected by any disease that causes changes in (1) intestinal blood flow, (2) gastrointestinal motility, (3) changes in stomach emptying time, (4) gastric pH that affects drug solubility, (5) intestinal pH that affects the extent of ionization, (6) the permeability of the gut wall, (7) bile secretion, (8) digestive enzyme secretion, or (9) alteration of normal GI flora. Some factors may dominate, while other factors sometimes cancel the effects of one another. Pharmacokinetic studies comparing subjects with and without the disease are generally necessary to establish the effect of the disease on drug absorption. Patients in an advanced stage of *Parkinson's disease* may have difficulty swallowing and greatly diminished gastrointestinal motility.

Patients on tricyclic antidepressants (imiprimine, amitriptyline, and nortriptyline) and antipsychotic drugs (phenothiazines) with anticholinergic side effects may have reduced gastrointestinal motility or even intestinal obstructions. Delays in drug absorption, especially with slow-release products, have occurred.

Achlorhydric patients may not have adequate production of acids in the stomach; stomach HCl is essential for solubilizing insoluble free bases. Many weak-base drugs that cannot form soluble salts will remain undissolved in the stomach when there is no hydrochloric acid present and are therefore unabsorbed. Salt forms of these drugs cannot be prepared

because the free base readily precipitates out due to the weak basicity.

Dapsone, itraconazole, and ketoconazole may also be less well absorbed in the presence of achlorhydria. In patients with acid reflux disorders, proton pump inhibitors, such as omeprazole, render the stomach achlorhydric, which may also affect drug absorption. Coadministering orange juice, colas, or other acidic beverages can facilitate the absorption of some medications requiring an acidic environment.

HIV–AIDS patients are prone to a number of gastrointestinal (GI) disturbances, such as decreased gastric transit time, diarrhea, and achlorhydria. Rapid gastric transit time and diarrhea can alter the absorption of orally administered drugs. Achlorhydria may or may not decrease absorption, depending on the acidity needed for absorption of a specific drug. Indinavir, for example, requires a normal acidic environment for absorption. The therapeutic window of indinavir is extremely narrow, so optimal serum concentrations are critical for this drug to be efficacious.

Congestive heart failure (CHF) *patients* with persistent edema have reduced splanchnic blood flow and develop edema in the bowel wall. In addition, intestinal motility is slowed. The reduced blood flow to the intestine and reduced intestinal motility results in a decrease in drug absorption. For example, furosemide (Lasix), a commonly used loop diuretic, has erratic and reduced oral absorption in patients with CHF and a delay in the onset of action.

As discussed above, *Crohn's disease* is an inflammatory disease of the distal small intestine and colon. The disease is accompanied by regions of thickening of the bowel wall, overgrowth of anaerobic bacteria, and sometimes obstruction and deterioration of the bowel. The effect on drug absorption is unpredictable, although impaired absorption may potentially occur because of reduced surface area and thicker gut wall for diffusion. For example, higher plasma propranolol concentration has been observed in patients with Crohn's disease after oral administration of propranolol. Serum α-1-acid glycoprotein levels are increased in Crohn's disease patients and may affect the protein binding and distribution of propranolol in the body and result in higher plasma concentrations.

Celiac disease is an inflammatory disease affecting mostly the proximal small intestine. Celiac disease is caused by sensitization to gluten, a viscous protein found in cereals and grains. Patients with celiac disease generally have an increased rate of stomach emptying and increased permeability of the small intestine. Cephalexin absorption appears to be increased in celiac disease, although it is not possible to make general predictions about these patients. Other intestinal conditions that may potentially affect drug absorption include corrective surgery involving peptic ulcer, antrectomy with gastroduodenostomy, and selective vagotomy.

Recently, hypoxemia and hypovolemia have been shown to have adverse effects on the intestinal microvilli (Harrois et al, 2013). Since the microvilli are important for many aspects of drug absorption, patients with significant blood loss, hypoxemia, or intestinal ischemia may be reasonably expected to have altered drug oral absorption. Caregivers may need to consider non-enteral routes of drug administration.

Drugs That Affect Absorption of Other Drugs

Anticholinergic drugs in general may reduce stomach acid secretion. Propantheline bromide is an anticholinergic drug that may also slow stomach emptying and motility of the small intestine. Tricyclic antidepressants and phenothiazines also have anticholinergic side effects that may cause slower peristalsis in the GI tract. Slower stomach emptying may cause delay in drug absorption.

Metoclopramide is a drug that stimulates stomach contraction, relaxes the pyloric sphincter, and, in general, increases intestinal peristalsis, which may reduce the effective time for the absorption of some drugs and thereby decrease the peak drug concentration and the time to reach peak drug concentration. For example, digoxin absorption from a tablet is reduced by metoclopramide but increased by an anticholinergic drug, such as propantheline bromide. Allowing more time in the stomach for the tablet to dissolve generally helps with the dissolution and absorption of a poorly soluble drug, but would not be helpful for a drug that is not soluble in stomach acid.

Antacids should not be given with cimetidine, because antacids may reduce drug absorption.

Antacids containing aluminum, calcium, or magnesium may complex with drugs such as tetracycline, ciprofloxacin, and indinavir, resulting in a decrease in drug absorption. To avoid this interaction, antacids should be taken 2 hours before or 6 hours after drug administration.

Proton pump inhibitors such as omeprazole (Prilosec®), lansoprazole (Prevacid®), pantoprazole (Protonix®), and others decrease gastric acid production, thereby raising gastric pH. These drugs may interfere with drugs for which gastric pH affects bioavailability (eg, ketoconazole, iron salts, ampicillin esters, and digoxin) and enteric-coated drug products (eg, aspirin, diclofenac) in which the pH-dependent enteric coating may dissolve in the higher gastric pH and release drug prematurely ("dose-dumping").

Cholestyramine is a nonabsorbable ion-exchange resin for the treatment of hyperlipidemia. Cholestyramine binds warfarin, thyroxine, and loperamide, similar to activated charcoal, thereby reducing absorption of these drugs.

Nutrients That Interfere with Drug Absorption

Many nutrients substantially interfere with the absorption or metabolism of drugs in the body (Anderson, 1988; Kirk, 1995). The effect of food on bioavailability was discussed earlier. Oral drug–nutrient interactions are often drug specific and can result in either an increase or a decrease in drug absorption.

Absorption of calcium in the duodenum is an active process facilitated by vitamin D, with calcium absorption as much as four times more than that in vitamin D deficiency states. It is believed that a calcium-binding protein, which increases after vitamin D administration, binds calcium in the intestinal cell and transfers it out of the base of the cell to the blood circulation.

Grapefruit juice often increases bioavailability, as observed by an increase in plasma levels of many drugs that are substrates for cytochrome P-450 (CYP) 3A4 (see Chapter 12). Grapefruit juice contains various flavonoids such as naringin and furanocoumarins such as bergamottin, which inhibit certain cytochrome P-450 enzymes involved in drug metabolism (especially CYP3A4). In this case, the observed increase in the plasma drug–blood levels is due to decreased presystemic elimination in the GI tract and/or liver. Indirectly, the amount of drug absorbed systemically from the drug product is increased. Grapefruit juice can also block drug efflux by inhibiting P-gp for some drugs.

MISCELLANEOUS ROUTES OF DRUG ADMINISTRATION

For systemic drug absorption, the oral route is the easiest, safest, and most popular route of drug administration. Alternate routes of drug administration have been used successfully to improve systemic drug absorption or to localize drug effects in order to minimize systemic drug exposure and adverse events. Furthermore, enteral drug administration (through nasogastric tubes and the like) may be necessary in patients incapable of swallowing medications but requiring chronic dosing. In such cases, oral liquid (solutions, suspensions, or emulsions) may be administered; some of these may require extemporaneous compounding. Increasingly popular nonparenteral alternatives to oral drug delivery for systemic drug absorption include nasal, inhalation, and transdermal drug delivery. Nasal, inhalation, and topical drug delivery may also be used for local drug action (Mathias et al, 2010).

Nasal Drug Delivery

Nasal drug delivery may be used for either local or systemic effects. Because the nasal region is richly supplied with blood vessels, nasal administration is also useful for systemic drug delivery. However, the total surface area in the nasal cavity is relatively small, retention time in the nasal cavity is generally short, and some drug may be swallowed. The swallowed fraction of the dose would have all the disadvantages of oral route, including low oral bioavailability and undesirable taste, as seen with sumatriptan nasal spray (Imitrex). These factors may limit the nose's capacity for systemic delivery of drugs requiring large doses. Surfactants are often used to increase systemic penetration, although the effect of chronic drug exposure on the integrity of

nasal membranes must also be considered. In general, a drug must be sufficiently lipophilic to cross the membranes of the nasal epithelium in order to be absorbed. Small molecules with balanced lipophilic and hydrophilic properties tend to be absorbed more easily. This observation poses a challenge for nasal delivery of larger molecules such as proteins and peptides, which would benefit from delivery routes that avoid the degradative environment of the intestine. Dosage forms intended for nasal drug delivery include nasal drops, nasal sprays, aerosols, and nebulizers (Su and Campanale, 1985).

Depending on the metabolic absorption, and chemical profile of the drug, some drugs are rapidly absorbed through the nasal membrane and can deliver rapid therapeutic effect. Various hormones and insulin have been tested for intranasal delivery. In some cases the objective is to improve availability, and in other cases it is to reduce side effects. Vasopressin and oxytocin are older examples of drugs marketed as intranasal products. In addition, many opioids are known to be rapidly absorbed from the nasal passages and can deliver systemic levels of the drug almost as rapidly as an intravenous injection (Dale et al, 2002). A common problem with nasal drug delivery is the challenge of developing a formulation with nonirritating ingredients. Many surfactants that facilitate absorption tend to be moderately or very irritating to the nasal mucosa.

Intranasal corticosteroids for treatment of allergic and perennial rhinitis have become more popular since intranasal delivery is believed to reduce the total dose of corticosteroid required. A lower dose also leads to minimization of side effects such as growth suppression. This logic has led to many second-generation corticosteroids such as beclomethasone dipropionate, budesonide, flunisolide, fluticasone propionate, mometasone furoate, and triamcinolone acetonide that are being considered or developed for intranasal delivery (Szefler, 2002). However, the potential for growth suppression in children varies. In one study, beclomethasone dipropionate reduced growth in children, but mometasone furoate nasal spray used for 1 year showed no signs of growth suppression. Overall, the second-generation corticosteroids are given by nasal delivery to cause minimal systemic side effects (Szefler, 2002).

Inhalation Drug Delivery

Inhalation drug delivery may also be used for local or systemic drug effects. The lung has a potential absorption surface of some 70 m², a much larger surface than the small intestine or nasal passages. When a substance is inhaled, it is exposed to membranes of the mouth or nose, pharynx, trachea, bronchi, bronchioles, alveolar sacs, and alveoli. The lungs and their associated airways are designed to remove foreign matter from the highly absorptive peripheral lung surfaces via mucociliary clearance. However, if compounds such as aerosolized drug can reach the peripheral region of the lung, absorption can be very efficient.

Particle (droplet) size and velocity of application control the extent to which inhaled substances penetrate into airway spaces. Optimum size for deep airway penetration of drug particles is 3–5 μm. Large particles tend to deposit in upper airways, whereas very small molecules (<3 μm) are exhaled before absorption can occur. Most inhalation devices deliver approximately 10% of the administered dose to the lower respiratory tract. A number of devices such as spacers (to reduce turbulence and improve deep inhalation) have been developed to increase lung delivery. An *in vitro* device useful to measure the particle size emitted from an aerosol or a mechanically produced fine mist is the cascade impacter.

Recently, recombinant human insulin for inhalation (Exubera®) was approved by the FDA, demonstrating the viability of this delivery route even for large biological drugs. Insulin inhalation was withdrawn from the US market in 2007 due to lack of consumer demand for the product.

Topical and Transdermal Drug Delivery

Topical drug delivery is generally used for local drug effects at the site of application. Dosing is dependent upon the concentration of the drug in the topical product (eg, cream, ointment) and the total surface area applied. Drug may be applied as an ointment or cream to the skin or various mucous membranes such as intravaginally. Even though the objective is to obtain a local drug effect, some of the drug may be absorbed systemically.

Transdermal products are generally used for systemic drug absorption. For transdermal drug delivery the drug is incorporated into a transdermal therapeutic system or patch, but it may be incorporated into an ointment as well (see Chapter 15). The advantages of transdermal delivery include continuous release of drug over a period of time, low presystemic clearance, and good patient compliance.

Other routes of drug administration are discussed elsewhere and in Chapter 15.

Frequently Asked Questions

▶ *What is an "absorption window"?*

▶ *Why are some drugs orally absorbed better with food, whereas the oral absorption of other drugs are slowed or decreased by food?*

▶ *What type of food is expected to have the greatest effect on gastrointestinal pH and gastrointestinal transit time?*

▶ *Are drugs that are administered as an oral solution completely absorbed from the gastrointestinal tract?*

▶ *What factors influence drug absorption?*

CHAPTER SUMMARY

Oral systemic drug absorption is a complex process dependent upon many biopharmaceutic factors including (1) the physicochemical properties of the drug, (2) the nature of the drug product, (3) the anatomy and physiology of the drug absorption site, and (4) the type and amount of food or other drugs present in the gut. Most drugs are passively absorbed as described by Fick's law of diffusion according to the *pH-partition hypothesis*, which may be a first-order process depending on permeability and how much drug is dissolved at the absorption site. Orally administered drugs may not be absorbed all along the gastrointestinal tract. The duodenum affords the optimum area for absorption due to the high surface area and blood flow. Several substrate-specific transporters may be the dominant factor responsible for bioavailability of some drugs. These drugs are absorbed by active transport, which is a carrier-mediated process that requires energy and transports the drug against a concentration gradient. Active drug absorption may be saturable depending on the carrier protein involved and is often site specific. Influx and efflux transporters in the gastrointestinal tract influence systemic drug absorption. A well-known class of transporters in the GI tract is known as the ABC family. MDR1 (alias P-gp) is an example. P-gp reduces drug absorption by effluxing the drug out of the enterocytes and back into the gut lumen. When the absorption process becomes saturated, the rate of drug absorption no longer follows a first-order process. Many efflux transporters in the GI and other parts of the body are now recognized, and their presence and quantity are genetically expressed and may be activated by certain diseases, such as cancer. P-glycoprotein is a common efflux transporter in the GI tract, which may be inhibited by coadministered drugs and nutrients leading to enhanced systemic absorption. In addition to normal gastrointestinal and physiologic factors such as stomach emptying time, small intestine transit time, local pH, content of the GI tract, presystemic metabolism,

and drug dosage form factors jointly influence systemic drug absorption.

Biopharmaceutic factors such as drug aqueous solubility, permeability of cell membranes, the degree of ionization, molecular size, particle size, and nature of the dosage form will also affect systemic drug absorption. The prediction of drug absorption based on physicochemical activity of drug molecules and other factors have been attempted during drug screening and discovery. Often these properties are influenced by biopharmaceutic factors such as formulation, physiological variables, pH, intestinal regional permeability differences, lumenal contents, transporters, and intestinal motility. Drug absorption is greatly dependent on routes of administration. Parenteral, inhalation, transdermal, and intranasal routes all present physiologic and biopharmaceutic issues that must be understood in order to develop an optimum formulation that is consistently absorbed systemically. Various methods are used to study drug absorption depended on the route involved. Gamma scintigraphy and marker methods are used to study stomach emptying time and GI transit time. GI perfusion methods are used to determine the influence of transporters and the effect of presystemic clearance and regional drug absorption.

LEARNING QUESTIONS

1. A recent bioavailability study in adult human volunteers demonstrated that after the administration of a single enteric-coated aspirin granule product given with a meal, the plasma drug levels resembled the kinetics of a sustained-release drug product. In contrast, when the product was given to fasted subjects, the plasma drug levels resembled the kinetics of an immediate-release drug product. Give a plausible explanation for this observation.

2. The aqueous solubility of a weak-base drug is poor. In an intubation (intestinal perfusion) study, the drug was not absorbed beyond the jejunum. Which of the following would be the correct strategy to improve drug absorption from the intestinal tract?

   a. Give the drug as a suspension and recommend that the suspension be taken on an empty stomach.
   b. Give the drug as a hydrochloride salt.
   c. Give the drug with milk.
   d. Give the drug as a suppository.

3. What is the primary reason that protein drugs such as insulin are not given orally for systemic absorption?

4. Which of the following statements is true regarding an acidic drug with a pK_a of 4?

   a. The drug is more soluble in the stomach when food is present.
   b. The drug is more soluble in the duodenum than in the stomach.
   c. The drug is more soluble when dissociated.

5. Which region of the gastrointestinal tract is most populated by bacteria? What types of drugs might affect the gastrointestinal flora?

6. Discuss methods by which the first-pass effect (presystemic absorption) may be circumvented.

7. Misoprostol (Cytotec, GD Searle) is a synthetic prostaglandin E1 analog. According to the manufacturer, the following information was obtained when misoprostol was taken with an antacid or high-fat breakfast:

Condition	C_{max} (pg/mL)	$AUC_{0-24\ hour}$ (pg·h/mL)	t_{max} (minutes)
Fasting	811 ± 317^a	417 ± 135	14 ± 8
With antacid	689 ± 315	349 ± 108^b	20 ± 14
With high-fat breakfast	303 ± 176^b	373 ± 111	64 ± 79^b

[a]Results are expressed as the mean ± SD (standard deviation).
[b]Comparisons with fasting results statistically significant, $p < 0.05$.

What is the effect of antacid and high-fat breakfast on the bioavailability of misoprostol? Comment on how these factors affect the rate and extent of systemic drug absorption.

8. Explain why the following occur.
   a. Drug *A* is given by IV bolus injection and the onset of the pharmacodynamic effect is immediate. When Drug *A* is given orally in the same dose, the onset of the pharmacodynamic effect is delayed and the intensity of the pharmacodynamic effect is less than the drug given by IV bolus injection.
   b. Drug *B* is given by IV bolus injection and the onset of the pharmacodynamic effect is delayed. When Drug *B* is given orally in the same dose to fasted subjects, the onset of the pharmacodynamic effect is shorter and the pharmacodynamic effect is more intense after IV bolus injection.

ANSWERS TO QUESTIONS

Frequently Asked Questions

What is an "absorption window"?

- An *absorption window* refers to the segment of the gastrointestinal tract from which the drug is well absorbed and beyond which the drug is either poorly absorbed or not absorbed at all. After oral administration, most drugs are well absorbed in the duodenum and to a lesser extent in the jejunum. A small amount of drug absorption may occur from the ileum.

Why are some drugs absorbed better with food whereas the oral absorption of other drugs is slowed or decreased by food?

- Food, particularly food with a high fat content, stimulates the production of bile, which is released into the duodenum. The bile helps to solubilize a lipid-soluble drug, thereby increasing drug absorption. Fatty food also slows gastrointestinal motility, resulting in a longer *residence time* for the drug to be absorbed from the small intestine.

Are drugs that are administered as an oral solution completely absorbed from the gastrointestinal tract?

- After oral administration, the drug in solution may precipitate in the gastrointestinal tract. The precipitated drug needs to redissolve before it can be absorbed. Some drug solutions are prepared with a co-solvent, such as alcohol or glycerin, and form coarse crystals on precipitation that dissolve slowly, whereas other drugs precipitate into fine crystals that redissolve rapidly. The type of precipitate is influenced by the solvent, by the degree of agitation, and by the physical environment. *In vitro* mixing and dilution of the drug solution in artificial gastric juice, artificial intestinal juice, or other pH buffers may predict the type of drug precipitate that is formed.

  In addition, drugs dissolved in a highly viscous solution (eg, simple syrup) may have slower absorption because of the viscosity of the solution. Furthermore, drugs that are readily absorbed across the gastrointestinal membrane may not be completely bioavailable (ie, 100% systemic absorption) due to *first-pass effects* (discussed in Chapter 12). Finally, drugs that are absorbed by saturable mechanisms may have concentrations exceeding the capacity of the intestine to absorb all the drug within the absorption window.

What factors contribute to a delay in drug absorption?

- The major biologic factor that delays gastrointestinal drug absorption is a delay in gastric emptying time. Any factor that delays stomach emptying time, such as fatty food, will delay the drug entering into the duodenum from the stomach and, thereby, delay drug absorption.

Learning Questions

1. In the presence of food, undissolved aspirin granules larger than 1 mm are retained up to several hours longer in the stomach. In the absence of food, aspirin granules are emptied from the stomach within 1–2 hours. When the aspirin granules empty into the duodenum slowly, drug absorption will be as slow as with a sustained-release drug product. Enteric-coated aspirin granules taken with an evening meal may provide relief of pain for arthritic patients late into the night.

2. The answer is **b**. A basic drug formulated as a suspension will depend on stomach acid for dissolution as the basic drug forms a hydrochloric acid (HCl) salt. If the drug is poorly soluble, adding milk may neutralize some acid so that the drug may not be completely dissolved. Making an HCl salt rather than a suspension of the base ensures that the drug is soluble without being dependent on stomach HCl for dissolution.

3. Protein drugs are generally digested by proteolytic enzymes present in the GI tract and, therefore, are not adequately absorbed by the oral route. Protein drugs are most commonly given parenterally. Other routes of administration, such as intranasal and rectal administration, have had some success or are under current investigation for the systemic absorption of protein drugs.

4. The answer is **c**. Raising the pH of an acid drug above its pK_a will increase the dissociation of the drug, thereby increasing its aqueous solubility.

5. The large intestine is most heavily populated by bacteria, yeasts, and other microflora. Some drugs that are not well absorbed in the small intestine are metabolized by the microflora to products that are absorbed in the large bowel. For example, drugs with an azo link (eg, sulfasalazine) are cleaved by bacteria in the bowel and the cleaved products (eg, 5-aminosalicylic acid and sulfapyridine) are absorbed. Other drugs, such as antibiotics (eg, tetracyclines), may destroy the bacteria in the large intestine, resulting in an overgrowth of yeast (eg, *Candida albicans*) and leading to a yeast infection. Destruction of the microflora in the lower bowel can also lead to cramps and diarrhea.

6. First-pass effects are discussed more fully in Chapter 12. Alternative routes of drug administration such as buccal, inhalation, sublingual, intranasal, and parenteral will bypass the first-pass effects observed after oral drug administration.

7. Although antacid statistically decreased the extent of systemic drug absorption ($p < .05$) as shown by an $AUC_{0-4\,h}$ of 349 ± 108 pg·h/mL, compared to the control (fasting) $AUC_{0-4\,h}$ value of 417 ± 135 pg·h/mL, the effect of antacid is not clinically significant. A high-fat diet decreased the rate of systemic drug absorption, as shown by a longer t_{max} value (64 minutes) and lower C_{max} value (303 pg/mL).

REFERENCES

Abrahamsson B, Alpsten M, Bake B, et al: Drug absorption from nifedipine hydrophilic matrix extended release (ER) tablet—Comparison with an osmotic pump tablet and effect of food. *J Controlled Release* (Netherlands) **52**:301–310, 1998.

Adkin DA, Davis SS, Sparrow RA, et al: Effect of different concentrations of mannitol in solution on small intestinal transit: Implications for drug absorption. *Pharm Res* **12**:393–396, 1995.

Actis-Goretta L, Lévèques A, Giuffrida F, et al: Elucidation of (-)-epicatechin metabolites after ingestion of chocolate by healthy humans. *Free Radic Biol Med* **53**:787–795.

Alberts B, Bray D, Lewis J, et al: *Molecular Biology of the Cell.* New York, Garland, 1994.

Anderson KE: Influences of diet and nutrition on clinical pharmacokinetics. *Clin Pharm* **14**:325–346, 1988.

Barr WH, Adir J, Garrettson L: Decrease in tetracycline absorption in man by sodium bicarbonate. *Clin Pharmacol Ther* **12**:779–784, 1971.

Avdeef A, Bendels S, Di L, et al: PAMPA—critical factors for better predictions of absorption. *J Pharm Sci* **96**:2893–2909.

Barrie S: Heidelberg pH capsule gastric analysis. In Pizzorno JE, Murray MT (eds). *Textbook of Natural Medicine*, 2nd ed. London, Churchill Livingstone, 1999, Chap 16.

Benet LZ, Greither A, Meister W: Gastrointestinal absorption of drugs in patients with cardiac failure. In Benet LZ (ed). *The Effect of Disease States on Drug Pharmacokinetics.* Washington, DC, American Pharmaceutical Association, 1976, Chap 3.

Borin MT, Driver MR, Forbes KK: Effect of timing of food on absorption of cefpodoxime proxetil. *J Clin Pharmacol* **35**(5):505–509, 1995.

Brunton L, Chabner B, Knollman B: Goodman & Gilman's The Pharmacological Basis of Therapeutics, 12th Edition. New York, McGraw-Hill, 2011.

Buch A, Barr WH: Absorption of propranolol in humans following oral, jejuna and ileal administration. *Pharm Res* **15**(6):953–957, 1998.

Burks TF, Galligan JJ, Porreca F, Barber WD: Regulation of gastric emptying. *Fed Proc* **44**:2897–2901, 1985.

Burton PS, Goodwin JT, Vidimar TJ. Amore BM: Predicting drug absorption: How nature made it a difficult problem, *J Pharmacol Exp Ther* **303**(3):889–895, 2002.

Buxton IAO, Benet LZ: Pharmacokinetics: Dynamics of drug absorption, distribution, metabolism, and elimination. In *Goodman & Gilman's Pharmacological Basis of Therapeutics.* New York, McGraw-Hill, 2011, Chap 2.

Crounse RG: Human pharmacology of griseofulvin: The effect of fat intake on gastrointestinal absorption. *J Invest Dermatol* **37**:529–533, 1961.

Dale O, Hoffer C, Sheffels P, Kharasch ED: Disposition of nasal, intravenous, and oral methadone in healthy volunteers. *Clin Pharmacol Therapeut* **72**:536–545, 2002.

Davson H, Danielli JF: *The Permeability of Natural Membranes.* Cambridge, UK, Cambridge University Press, 1952.

Dhawan S, Chopra S, Kapil R, Kapoor D: Novel approaches for oral insulin delivery *Pharm Tech* **33** (7), 2009. (http://pharmtech .findpharma.com/pharmtech/Formulation+Article/Novel -Approaches-for-Oral-Insulin-Delivery/ArticleStandard/Article /detail/609407).

Di Marco MP, Edwards DJ, Irving IW, Murray P, Ducharme WP: The effect of grapefruit juice and Seville orange juice on the pharmacokinetics of dextromethorphan: The role of gut CYP3A and P-glycoprotein. *Life Sci* **71**:1149–1160, 2002.

Doherty MM, Charman WN: The mucosa of the small intestine: How clinically relevant as an organ of drug metabolism? *Clin Pharmacokinet* **41**(4):235–253, 2002.

FDA Guidance for Industry: Food-Effect Bioavailability and Fed Bioequivalence Studies, 2002.

Feldman M, Smith HJ, Simon TR: Gastric emptying of solid radio-opaque markers: Studies in healthy and diabetic patients. *Gastroenterology* **87**:895–902, 1984.

GastroPlus™, Simulations Plus, Inc (www.simulations-plus.com /Products.aspx?grpID=3&cID=16&pID=11).

Giacomini KM: The International Transporter Consortium Membrane transporters in drug development. *Nat Rev Drug Discov* **9**:216–236, 2010.

Harrois A, Baudry N, Huet O, et al: Synergistic deleterious effect of hypoxemia and hypovolemia on microcirculation in intestinal villi. *Crit Care Med* **41**(11):e376–84, 2013.

Hebden JM, et al: Stool water content and colonic drug absorption: contrasting effects of lactulose and codeine. *Pharm Res* **16**: 1254–1259, 1999.

Hendeles L, Weinberger M, Milavetz G, et al: Food induced dumping from "once-a-day" theophylline product as cause of theophylline toxicity. *Chest* **87**:758–785, 1985.

Hoffmeyer S, Burke O, von Richter O: Functional polymorphism of the human multidrung-resitance gene: Multiple sequence variations and correlation of one allele with P-glycoprotein expression and activity in vivo. *Proc Natl Acad Sci USA* **97**(7): 3473–8, 2000.

Huan SM, Zhang L: Drug Interaction Studies. http://www.fda.gov /downloads/drugs/guidancecomplianceregulatoryinformation /guidances/ucm292362.pdf. Accessed [2/23/2012]

Hunt JN, Knox M: Regulation of gastric emptying. In Code CF (ed). *Handbook of Physiology. Section 6: Alimentary Canal.* Washington, DC, American Physiological Society, 1968, pp 1917–1935.

Johnson MD, Newkirk G, White JR Jr: Clinically significant drug interactions. *Postgrad Med* **105**(2):193–5, 200, 205-6 passim, 1999.

Kirk JK: Significant drug-nutrient interactions. *Am Fam Physician* **51**:1175–1182, 1185, 1995.

Kirwan WO, Smith AN: Gastrointestinal transit estimated by an isotope capsule. *Scand J Gastroenterol* **9**:763–766, 1974.

Lennernas H, Ahrenstedt O, Hallgren R, et al: Regional jejunal perfusion, a new in vivo approach to study oral drug absorption in man. *Pharm Res* **9**:1243–1251, 1992.

Lennernas H, Falgerholm U, Raab Y, et al: Regional rectal perfusion: New in vivo approach to study rectal drug absorption in man. *Pharm Res* **12**:426–432, 1995.

Lennernas H: Human in vivo regional intestinal permeability: Importance for pharmaceutical drug development. *Mol Pharm* **11**:12–23, 2014.

Levitt DL, Li R, Demaster EG, Elson M, Furne J, Levitt DG: Use of measurements of ethanol absorption from stomach and intestine to assess human ethanol metabolism. *Am J Physiol Gastrointest Liver Physiol* **273**:G951–G957, 1997 (http://ajpgi .physiology.org/cgi/content/full/273/4/G951).

Lipinski CA, Lombardo F, Dominy BW, Feeney PJ: Experimental and computational approaches to estimate solubility and permeability in drug discovery and development settings. *Adv Drug Del Rev* **46**(1–3):3–26, 2001.

Lodish HF, Rothman JE: The assembly of cell membranes. *Sci Am* **240**:48–63, 1979.

Mathias NR, Hussain MA: Non-invasive systemic drug delivery: Developability considerations for alternate routes of administration. *J Pharm Sci* **9**:1–20, 2010.

Mellinger TJ, Bohorfoush JG: Blood levels of dipyridamole (Persantin) in humans. *Arch Int Pharmacodynam Ther* **163**:465–480, 1966.

Miller R: Pharmacokinetics and bioavailability of ranitidine in humans. *J Pharm Sci* **73**:1376–1379, 1984.

Minami H, McCallum RW: The physiology and pathophysiology of gastric emptying in humans. *Gastroenterology* **86**:1592–1610, 1984.

Mouly S, Paine MF: P-glycoprotein increases from proximal to distal regions of human small intestine. *Pharm Res* **20**(10):1595–1599, 2003.

Nienbert R: Ion pair transport across membranes. *Pharm Res* **6**:743–747, 1989.

Oberle RL, Amidon GL: The influence of variable gastric emptying and intestinal transit rates on the plasma level curve of cimetidine: An explanation for the double-peak phenomenon. *J Pharmacokinet Biopharmacol* **15**:529–544, 1987.

Ogata H, Aoyagi N, Kaniwa N, et al: Gastric acidity dependent bioavailability of cinnarizine from two commercial capsules in healthy volunteers. *Int J Pharm* **29**:113–120, 1986.

Parr AF, Sandefer EP, Wissel P, et al: Evaluation of the feasibility and use of a prototype remote drug delivery capsule (RDDC) for noninvasive regional drug absorption studies in the GI tract of man and beagle dog. *Pharm Res* **16**:266–271, 1999.

Pratt P, Taylor P (eds): *Principles of Drug Action: The Basis of Pharmacology*, 3rd ed. New York, Churchill Livingstone, 1990, p 241.

Riley SA, Sutcliffe F, Kim M, et al: Influence of gastrointestinal transit on drug absorption in healthy volunteers. *Br J Clin Pharm* **34**:32–39, 1992.

Rubinstein A, Li VHK, Robinson JR: Gastrointestinal–physiological variables affecting performance of oral sustained release dosage forms. In Yacobi A, Halperin-Walega E (eds). *Oral Sustained Release Formulations: Design and Evaluation*. New York, Pergamon, 1988, Chap 6.

Sauna ZE, Smith MM, Muller M, Kerr KM, Ambudkar SV: The mechanism of action of multidrug resitance linked P-glycoprotein. *J Bioener Biomembr* **33**:481–491, 2001.

Shareef MA, Ahuja A, Ahmad FJ, Raghava S: Colonic drug delivery: An updated review. *AAPS PharmSci* **5**:161–186, 2003.

Singer SJ, Nicolson GL: The fluid mosaic model of the structure of cell membranes. *Science* **175**:720–731, 1972.

Sournac S, Maublant JC, Aiache JM, et al: Scintigraphic study of the gastrointestinal transit and correlations with the drug absorption kinetics of a sustained release theophylline tablet. Part 1. Administration in fasting state. *J Controll Release* **7**:139–146, 1988.

Su KSE, Campanale KM: Nasal drug delivery systems requirements, development and evaluations. In Chien YW (ed). *Transnasal Systemic Medications*. Amsterdam, Elsevier Scientific, 1985, pp 139–159.

Sun H, Pang KS: Permeability, transport, and metabolism of solutes in Caco-2 cell monolayers: A theoretical study *Drug Metab Disp*, **36**(1):102–123, 2007.

Suzuki H, Sugiyama Y: Role of metabolic enzymes and efflux transporters in the absorption of drugs from the small intestine. *Eur J Pharm Sci* **12**:3–12, 2000.

Synold TW, Dussault I, Forman BM: The orphan nuclear receptor SXR coordinately regulates drug metabolism and efflux. *Nature Med* **7**(5):584–590, 2001.

Szefler SJ: Pharmacokinetics of intranasal corticosteroids. *J Allergy Clin Immunol* **108**:S26–S31, 2002.

Takano M, Yumoto R, Murakami T: Expression and function of efflux drug transporters in the intestine. *Pharmacol Therapeut* **109**:137–161, 2006.

Thummel K, Wilkinson GR: In vitro and in vivo drug interactions involving human CYP3A. *Annu Rev Pharmacol Toxicol* **38**:389–430, 1998.

Tolle-Sander S, Polli JE: Method considerations for Caco-2 permeability assessment in the biopharmaceutics classification system. *Pharmacopoeial Forum* **28**:164–172, 2002.

Tsuji A, Tamai I: Carrier-mediated intestinal transport of drugs. *Pharm Res* **13**(7):963–977, 1996.

US Food and Drug Administration: *FDA Guidance for Industry: Waiver of In Vivo Bioavailability and Bioequivalence Studies for Immediate-Release Solid Oral Dosage Forms Based on a Biopharmaceutics Classification System*, August 2002.

US Food and Drug Administration: *FDA Guidance for Industry: Food-Effect Bioavailability and Fed Bioequivalence Studies*, December 2002.

von Richter O, Burk O, Fromm MF, Thon KP, Eichelbaum M, Kivisto KT: Cytochrome P450 3A4 and P-glycoprotein expression in human small intestinal enterocytes and hepatocytes: A comparative analysis in paired tissue specimens. *Clin Pharmacol Ther* **75**:172–183, 2004.

Welling PG: Drug bioavailability and its clinical significance. In Bridges KW, Chasseaud LF (eds). *Progress in Drug Metabolism*, Vol 4. London, Wiley, 1980, Chap 3.

Wilson TH: *Intestinal Absorption*. Philadelphia, Saunders, 1962.

Yoshikawa H, Muranishi S, Sugihira N, Seaki H: Mechanism of transfer of bleomycin into lymphatics by bifunctional delivery system via lumen of small intestine. *Chem Pharm Bull* **31**:1726–1732, 1983.

Yoshikawa H, Nakao Y, Takada K, et al: Targeted and sustained delivery of aclarubicin to lymphatics by lactic acid oligomer microsphere in rat. *Chem Pharm Bull* **37**:802–804, 1989.

BIBLIOGRAPHY

Berge S, Bighley L, Monkhouse D: Pharmaceutical salts. *J Pharm Sci* **66**:1–19, 1977.

Blanchard J: Gastrointestinal absorption, II. Formulation factors affecting bioavailability. *Am J Pharm* **150**:132–151, 1978.

Davenport HW: *Physiology of the Digestive Tract*, 5th ed. Chicago, Year Book Medical, 1982.

Evans DF, Pye G, Bramley R, et al: Measurement of gastrointestinal pH profiles in normal ambulant human subjects. *Gut* **29**:1035–1041, 1988.

Eye IS: A review of the physiology of the gastrointestinal tract in relation to radiation doses from radioactive materials. *Health Phys* **12**:131–161, 1966.

Houston JB, Wood SG: Gastrointestinal absorption of drugs and other xenobiotics. In Bridges JW, Chasseaud LF (eds). *Progress in Drug Metabolism*, Vol 4. London, Wiley, 1980, Chap 2.

Leesman GD, Sinko PJ, Amidon GL: Stimulation of oral drug absorption: Gastric emptying and gastrointestinal motility. In Welling PW, Tse FLS (eds). *Pharmacokinetics: Regulatory, Industry, Academic Perspectives*. New York, Marcel Dekker, 1988, Chap 6.

Mackowiak PA: The normal microbial flora. *N Engl J Med* **307**:83–93, 1982.

Martonosi AN (ed): *Membranes and Transport*, Vol 1. New York, Plenum, 1982.

McElnay JC: Buccal absorption of drugs. In Swarbick J, Boylan JC (eds). *Encyclopedia of Pharmaceutical Technology*, Vol 2. New York, Marcel Dekker, 1990, pp 189–211.

Palin K: Lipids and oral drug delivery. *Pharm Int* 272–275, November 1985.

Palin K, Whalley D, Wilson C, et al: Determination of gastric-emptying profiles in the rat: Influence of oil structure and volume. *Int J Pharm* **12**:315–322, 1982.

Pisal DS, Koslowski MP, Balu-Iyer SV: Delivery of therapeutic proteins. *J Pharm Sci* **99**(5):2557–2575, 2010.

Welling PG: Interactions affecting drug absorption. *Clin Pharmacokinet* **9**:404–434, 1984.

Welling PG: Dosage route, bioavailability and clinical efficacy. In Welling PW, Tse FLS (eds). *Pharmacokinetics: Regulatory, Industry, Academic Perspectives*. New York, Marcel Dekker, 1988, Chap 3.

Welling PG: Absorption of drugs. In Swarbrick J, Boylan JC (eds). *Encyclopedia of Pharmaceutical Technology*. New York, Marcel Dekker, 2002, pp 8–22.

Wilson TH: *Intestinal Absorption*. Philadelphia, Saunders, 1962.

15

Biopharmaceutic Considerations in Drug Product Design and *In Vitro* Drug Product Performance

Sandra Suarez, Patrick J. Marroum, and Minerva Hughes

Chapter Objectives

▶ Describe the biopharmaceutic factors affecting drug design.

▶ Define the term "rate-limiting step" and discuss how the rate-limiting step relates to the bioavailability of a drug.

▶ Differentiate between the terms solubility and dissolution.

▶ Differentiate between the concept of drug absorption and bioavailability.

▶ Describe the various *in vitro* and *in vivo* tests commonly used to evaluate drug products.

▶ Describe the statistical methods for comparing two dissolution profiles for similarity.

▶ List the USP dissolution apparatus and provide examples of drug products for which the dissolution apparatus might be appropriate.

▶ Define sink conditions and explain why dissolution medium must maintain sink conditions.

▶ Define *in vitro–in vivo* correlation (IVIVC) and explain why a Level A correlation is the most important correlation for IVIVC.

Biopharmaceutics is the study of the physicochemical properties of the drug and the drug product, *in vitro*, as it relates to the bioavailability of the drug, *in vivo*, and its desired therapeutic effect. Biopharmaceutics thus links the physical and chemical properties of the drug and the drug product to their clinical performance, *in vivo*. Consequently, a primary concern in biopharmaceutics is the bioavailability of drugs. *Bioavailability* refers to the measurement of the rate and extent of active drug that becomes available at the site of action. For the majority of orally administered drugs, the site of action is within the systemic circulation and the drug must be absorbed to achieve a pharmacological response. Oral drug absorption involves at least three distinct steps: drug release or dissolution from the drug product in the body's fluids, permeation of the drug across the gastrointestinal (GI) linings into the systemic circulation, and drug disposition during GI transit (eg, GI stability, motility, metabolism, etc). Additional drug disposition may occur in the systemic circulation and thus reduce the concentration of drug available to the target tissues. However, because the systemic blood circulation ultimately delivers therapeutically active drug to the tissues and to the drug's site of action, changes in oral bioavailability affect changes in the pharmacodynamics and toxicity of a drug.

A drug product may also be designed to deliver the drug directly to the site of action before reaching the systemic circulation, which is often termed *locally acting* drug. Some examples of products in this class include ophthalmic, pulmonary, and nasal drug products. Similar to systemic bioavailability, local drug bioavailability is strongly influenced by physicochemical properties of the drug and drug product, the rate and extent of drug release from the drug product, and permeation at the target site (eg, skin physiology compared with that in the cornea). Regardless of the intended site of drug action, biopharmaceutics aims to balance the amount and extent of drug delivered from the drug product to achieve optimal therapeutic efficacy and safety for the patient.

▶ Define clinically relevant drug product specifications and describe the methods to establish them.

▶ Explain the biopharmaceutic classification system and how solubility, dissolution, and permeation apply to BCS classification.

▶ Provide a description of some common oral drug products and explain how biopharmaceutic principles may be used to formulate a product that will extend the duration of activity of the active drug.

BIOPHARMACEUTIC FACTORS AND RATIONALE FOR DRUG PRODUCT DESIGN

In broad terms, the factors affecting drug bioavailability may be related to the formulation of the drug product or the biological constraints of the patient.

Drugs are not usually given as pure chemical drug substances, but are formulated into finished dosage forms (ie, drug products). These drug products include the active drug substance combined with selected additional ingredients (*excipients*) that make up the dosage form. Although excipients are considered inert with respect to pharmacodynamic activity, excipients are important in the manufacture of the drug product and provide functionality to the drug product with respect to drug release and dissolution (see also Chapter 18).

Some common drug products include liquids, tablets, capsules, injectables, suppositories, transdermal systems, and topical creams and ointments. These finished dosage forms or drug products are then given to patients to achieve a specific therapeutic objective. The design of the dosage form, the formulation of the drug product, and the manufacturing process require a thorough understanding of the biopharmaceutic principles of drug delivery. Considerations in the design of a drug product to deliver the active drug with the desired bioavailability characteristics and therapeutic objectives include (1) the physicochemical properties of the drug molecule, (2) the finished dosage form (eg, tablet, capsule, etc), (3) the nature of the excipients in the drug product, (4) the method of manufacturing, and (5) the route of drug administration.

Biopharmaceutics allows for the rational design of drug products and is based on:

- The physical and chemical properties of the drug substance
- The route of drug administration, including the anatomic and physiologic nature of the application site (eg, oral, topical, injectable, implant, transdermal patch, etc)
- Desired pharmacodynamic effect (eg, immediate or prolonged activity)
- Toxicologic properties of the drug
- Safety of excipients
- Effect of excipients and dosage form on drug product performance
- Manufacturing processes

As mentioned above, some drugs are intended for topical or local therapeutic action at the site of administration. Drugs intended for local activity are designed to have a direct pharmacodynamic action without affecting other body organs, and systemic drug absorption is often undesirable. Locally acting drugs may be administered orally (eg, local GI effect) or applied topically to the skin, nose, eye, mucous membranes, buccal cavity, throat, or rectum. A drug intended for local activity may also be given intravaginally, into the urethral tract, or intranasally; inhaled into the lungs; and applied into the ear or on the eye. Examples of drugs used for local action include anti-infectives, antifungals, local anesthetics, antacids, astringents, vasoconstrictors, antihistamines, bronchodilators, and corticosteroids. Though systemic absorption is undesired, it may occur with locally acting drugs and modifying the drug product design may help to mitigate systemic effects.

Each route of drug administration presents special biopharmaceutic considerations in drug product design. For example, the design of a vaginal tablet formulation for the treatment of a fungal infection must use ingredients compatible with vaginal anatomy and physiology. An eye medication requires special considerations for formulation pH, isotonicity, sterility, the need to minimize local irritation to the cornea, potential for drug loss from draining by tears, and residual systemic drug absorption. For a drug administered by an extravascular route (eg, intramuscular injection), local irritation, drug dissolution at the application site, and drug absorption from the intramuscular site are some of the factors that must be considered. Systemic absorption after extravascular administration is influenced by the anatomic and physiologic properties of the site and the physicochemical properties of the drug and the drug product. On the other hand, if the drug is given by an intravascular route (eg, IV administration), systemic drug absorption is considered complete or 100% bioavailable, because the drug is placed directly into the general circulation. However, drug disposition can be altered by modifying the composition of the drug product (eg, addition on mannitol may change the renal clearance of the drug).

A drug product may also be designed as a combination drug/device product to allow the drug formulation to be used in conjunction with a specialized medical device or packaging component. For example, a drug solution or suspension may be formulated to work with a nebulizer or metered-dose inhaler for administration into the lungs. Both the physical characteristics of the nebulizer and the formulation of the drug product can influence the droplet particle size and its distribution, the spray pattern, and plume geometry of the emitted dose, which may affect its *in vivo* performance. Also, drug-polymer coating may be applied to a cardiac stent for local delivery of antiproliferative drugs directly to diseased tissue during percutaneous coronary intervention to treat a blocked artery.

By choosing the route of drug administration carefully and properly designing the drug product, the bioavailability of the active drug can be varied from rapid and complete absorption to a slow, sustained rate of absorption or even virtually no absorption, depending on the therapeutic objective. Once the drug is systemically absorbed, normal physiologic processes for drug distribution and elimination occur. These intrinsic factors may also be influenced by the specific formulation of the drug (eg, encapsulated drug in liposome or microspheres may change the drug distribution and systemic clearance). The rate of drug release from the product and the rate and extent of drug absorption are important in determining the onset, intensity, and duration of drug action.

Biopharmaceutic considerations often determine the ultimate dose and dosage form of a drug product. For example, the dosage form for a locally acting drug such as a topical drug product (eg, ointment) is often expressed in concentration or as a percentage of the active drug in the formulation (eg, 0.5% hydrocortisone ointment). The amount of drug applied is not specified because the concentration of the drug at the active site relates to the pharmacodynamic action. However, biopharmaceutic studies must be performed to ensure that the drug product does not irritate, cause an allergic response, or allow significant systemic drug absorption. In contrast, the dosage form for a systemically acting drug is expressed in terms of mass, such as milligrams or grams. In this case, the dose is based on the amount of drug that is absorbed systemically and dissolved in an apparent volume of distribution to produce a desired drug concentration at the target site. The therapeutic dose may also be adjusted based on the weight or surface area of the patient, to account for the differences in the apparent volume of distribution, which is expressed as mass per unit of body weight (mg/kg) or mass per unit of body surface area (mg/m^2). For many commercial drug

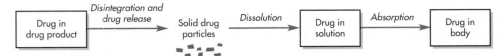

FIGURE 15-1   Rate processes of drug bioavailability.

products, the dose is determined based on average body weights and may be available in several dose strengths, such as 10-mg, 5-mg, and 2.5-mg tablets, to accommodate differences in body weight and possibly to titrate the dose in the patient.

> **Frequently Asked Questions**
> ▶ *How do excipients improve the manufacturing of an oral drug product?*
>
> ▶ *If excipients do not have pharmacodynamic activity, how do excipients affect the performance of the drug product?*

RATE-LIMITING STEPS IN DRUG ABSORPTION

Systemic drug absorption from a drug product consists of a succession of rate processes (Fig. 15-1). For solid oral, immediate-release drug products (eg, tablets, capsules), the rate processes include (1) disintegration of the drug product and subsequent release of the drug, (2) dissolution of the drug in an aqueous environment, and (3) absorption across cell membranes into the systemic circulation. In the process of drug disintegration, dissolution, and absorption, the rate at which drug reaches the circulatory system is determined by the slowest step in the sequence. The slowest step in a series of kinetic processes is called the *rate-limiting step*. For drugs that have very poor aqueous solubility, the rate at which the drug dissolves (*dissolution*) is often the slowest step and therefore exerts a rate-limiting effect on drug bioavailability. In contrast, for a drug that has a high aqueous solubility, the dissolution rate is rapid, and the rate at which the drug crosses or permeates cell membranes is the slowest or rate-limiting step. In general, for drug products that slowly release the drug from the formulation such as extended- or controlled-release formulations or for drug products

where dissolution of the drug is the rate-limiting step in the appearance in the systemic circulation, with a discriminating dissolution method, the probability of establishing a predictive *in vitro–in vivo* correlation (IVIVC) is higher.

Disintegration

For immediate-release, solid oral dosage forms, the drug product must disintegrate into small particles and release the drug. To monitor uniform tablet disintegration, the *United States Pharmacopeia* (USP) has established an official disintegration test (Fig. 15-2). Solid drug products exempted from disintegration tests include troches, tablets that are intended to be chewed, and drug products intended for sustained release or prolonged or repeat action as well as liquid-filled soft gelatin capsules.

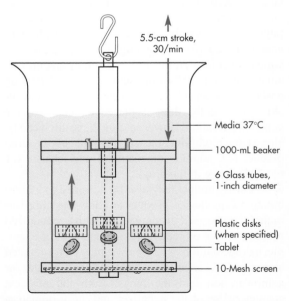

FIGURE 15-2   USP disintegration testing apparatus. (Hanson and Gray, 2004, with permission.)

The process of disintegration does not imply complete dissolution of the tablet and/or the drug. Complete disintegration is defined by the USP-NF (National Formulary) as "that state in which any residues of the tablet, except fragments of insoluble coating, remaining on the screen of the test apparatus in the soft mass have no palpably firm core." The official apparatus for the disintegration test and procedure is described in the USP-NF. Separate specifications are given for drug products that are designed not to disintegrate. These products include troches, chewable tablets, and modified-release (MR) drug products.

Although disintegration tests allow for measurement of the formation of fragments, granules, or aggregates from solid dosage forms, no information is obtained from these tests on the rate of dissolution of the active drug. However, there has been some interest in using only the disintegration test and no dissolution test for drug products that meet the Biopharmaceutical Classification System (BCS) for highly soluble and highly permeable drugs (Chapter 16). In general, the disintegration test serves as a component in the overall quality control of tablet manufacture. Disintegration testing can be used in lieu of dissolution testing, provided the following ICH Q6A guidelines are met: (1) The product under consideration is rapidly dissolving (dissolution >80% in 15 minutes at pH 1.2, 4.0, and 6.8); (2) the drug product contains drugs that are highly soluble throughout the physiological range (dose/solubility volume <250 mL from pH 1.2 to 6.8); and (3) a relationship to dissolution has been established or when disintegration is shown to be more discriminating than dissolution and dissolution characteristics do not change on stability.

Dissolution and Solubility

Dissolution is the process by which a solid drug substance becomes dissolved in a solvent over time. *Solubility* is the mass of solute that dissolves in a specific mass or volume of solvent at a given temperature (eg, 1 g of NaCl dissolves in 2.786 mL of water at 25°C). Solubility by definition is an *equilibrium* property, whereas dissolution is a *dynamic* property. In biologic systems, drug dissolution in an aqueous medium is an important prior condition for predicting systemic drug absorption. The rate at which drugs with poor aqueous solubility dissolve from an intact or disintegrated solid dosage form in the gastrointestinal tract often controls the rate of systemic absorption of the drug. Thus, dissolution tests may be used to predict bioavailability and may be used to discriminate formulation factors that affect drug bioavailability. As per 21 CFR (Code of Federal Regulations), dissolution testing is required for US Food and Drug Administration (FDA)-approved solid oral drug products.

Noyes and Whitney (1897) and other investigators studied the rate of dissolution of solid drugs. According to their observations, the steps in dissolution include the process of drug dissolution at the surface of the solid particle, thus forming a saturated solution around the particle. The dissolved drug in the saturated solution, known as the *stagnant layer*, diffuses to the bulk of the solvent from regions of high drug concentration to regions of low drug concentration (Fig. 15-3).

The overall rate of drug dissolution may be described by the *Noyes–Whitney equation* (Equation 15.1):

$$\frac{dC}{dt} = \frac{DA}{h}(C_s - C)$$ (15.1)

where dC/dt = rate of drug dissolution at time t, D = diffusion rate constant, A = surface area of the particle, C_s = concentration of drug (equal to solubility of drug) in the stagnant layer, C = concentration of drug in the bulk solvent, and h = thickness of the stagnant layer.

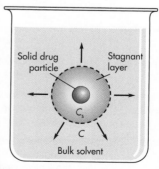

FIGURE 15-3   Dissolution of a solid drug particle in a solvent. (C_s = concentration of drug in the stagnant layer, C = concentration of drug in the bulk solvent.)

The rate of dissolution, dC/dt, is the rate of drug dissolved per time expressed as concentration change in the dissolution fluid.

The Noyes–Whitney equation shows that dissolution in a flask may be influenced by the physicochemical characteristics of the drug, the formulation, and the solvent. The dissolution of drug in the body, particularly in the gastrointestinal tract, is considered to be dissolving in an aqueous environment. Permeation of drug across the gut wall (a model lipid membrane) is affected by the ability of the drug to diffuse (D) and to partition between the lipid membranes. A favorable partition coefficient ($K_{oil/water}$) will facilitate drug absorption (see Chapter 14).

In addition to these factors, the temperature of the medium and the agitation rate also affect the rate of drug dissolution. *In vivo*, body temperature is maintained at a constant 37°C, and the agitation (primarily peristaltic movements in the gastrointestinal tract) is reasonably constant. In contrast, *in vitro* studies of dissolution kinetics require maintenance of constant temperature and agitation. Temperature is generally kept at 37°C, and the agitation or stirring rate is held to a specified agitation rate such as 75 rpm (revolutions per minute). An increase in temperature will increase the kinetic energy of the molecules and increase the diffusion constant, D. Moreover, an increase in agitation of the solvent medium will reduce the thickness, h, of the stagnant layer, allowing for more rapid drug dissolution.

Factors that affect drug dissolution of a solid oral dosage form include (1) the physical and chemical nature of the active drug substance, (2) the nature of the excipients, (3) the method of manufacture, and (4) the dissolution test conditions.

Frequently Asked Questions

▶ *What is meant by the rate-limiting step in drug bioavailability from a solid oral drug product?*

▶ *What is the usual rate-limiting step for a poorly soluble and highly permeable drug (BCS 2)?*

▶ *How could the manufacturing process affect drug product performance?*

PHYSICOCHEMICAL PROPERTIES OF THE DRUG

In addition to their effect on dissolution kinetics, the physical and chemical properties of the drug substance as well as the excipients are important considerations in the design of a drug product (Table 15-1).

TABLE 15-1   Physicochemical Properties for Consideration in Drug Product Design

pK_a and pH profile	Necessary for optimum stability and solubility of the final product.
Particle size	May affect the particle surface of the drug and therefore the dissolution rate of the product.
Polymorphism	The ability of a drug to exist in various crystal forms may change the solubility of the drug. Also, the stability of each form is important, because polymorphs may convert from one form to another.
Hygroscopicity	Moisture absorption may affect the physical structure as well as stability of the product.
Partition coefficient	May give some indication of the relative affinity of the drug for oil and water. A drug that has high affinity for oil may have poor release and dissolution from the drug product.
Excipient interaction	The compatibility of the excipients with the drug and sometimes trace elements in excipients may affect the stability of the product. It is important to have specifications of all raw materials.
pH stability profile	The stability of solutions is often affected by the pH of the vehicle; furthermore, because the pH in the stomach and gut is different, knowledge of the stability profile would help avoid or prevent degradation of the product during storage or after administration.
Impurity profile	The presence of impurities may depend upon the synthetic route for the active drug and subsequent purification. Impurities need to be "qualified" or tested for safety. Changes in the synthetic method may change the impurity profile.
Chirality	The presence of chirality may show that the isomers have differences in pharmacodynamic activity.

For example, intravenous solutions are difficult to prepare with drugs that have poor aqueous solubility. Drugs that are physically or chemically unstable may require special excipients, coatings, or manufacturing processes to protect the drug from degradation. Drugs with a potent pharmacodynamic response, such as estrogens and other hormones, penicillin antibiotics, cancer chemotherapeutic agents, and others, may cause adverse reactions to personnel who are exposed to these drugs during manufacture and also present a problem for manufacturing.

Solubility, pH, and Drug Absorption

The *solubility–pH profile* is a plot of the solubility of the drug at various physiologic pH values. In designing oral dosage forms, the formulator must consider that the natural pH environment of the gastrointestinal tract varies from acidic in the stomach to slightly alkaline in the small intestine. A basic drug is more soluble in an acidic medium, forming a soluble salt. Conversely, an acid drug is more soluble in the intestine, forming a soluble salt in the more alkaline pH environment found there. The solubility–pH profile gives a rough estimation of the completeness of dissolution for a dose of a drug in the stomach or in the small intestine.

Solubility may be improved with the addition of an acidic or basic excipient. Solubilization of aspirin, for example, may be increased by the addition of an alkaline buffer. In the formulation of controlled-release drugs, buffering agents may be added to slow or modify the release rate of a fast-dissolving drug. Typically, the controlled-release drug product of this type is a nondisintegrating. The buffering agent is released slowly rather than rapidly, so that the drug does not dissolve immediately in the surrounding gastrointestinal fluid.

In addition to considering the potential for *in situ* salt formation at different pH values for ionizable drug substances, direct salt formation of the drug is a common approach for tailoring the dissolution rate, and consequently, drug absorption for many ionizable drugs. Salt formation may change the drug's physicochemical properties in many aspects, including its solubility, chemical stability, polymorphism, and manufacturability, all of which must be considered by the formulator during development. Also, the potential for converting from the salt form to the unionized drug form during drug product manufacturing must be considered for optimal drug product design.

Stability, pH, and Drug Absorption

The *stability–pH profile* is a plot of the reaction rate constant for drug degradation versus pH. If drug decomposition occurs by acid or base catalysis, some prediction of degradation of the drug in the gastrointestinal tract may be made. For example, erythromycin has a pH-dependent stability profile. In acidic medium, as in the stomach, erythromycin decomposition occurs rapidly, whereas in neutral or alkaline pH, the drug is relatively stable. Consequently, erythromycin tablets are coated with an acid-resistant film, which is referred to as enteric coating, to protect against acid degradation in the stomach. The knowledge of erythromycin stability subsequently led to the preparation of a less water-soluble erythromycin salt that is more stable in the stomach. The dissolution rate of erythromycin drug substance powder, without excipients, varied from 100% dissolved in 1 hour for the water-soluble version to less than 40% dissolved in 1 hour for the less water-soluble version. The slow-dissolving erythromycin drug substance also resulted in slow-dissolving drug products formulated with the modified drug. Thus, in the erythromycin case, the dissolution rate of the powdered drug substance was a very useful *in vitro* tool for predicting bioavailability problems of the resulting erythromycin product in the body.

Particle Size and Drug Absorption

Dissolution kinetics is also affected by particle size. As previously described in the Noyes–Whitney dissolution model, the dissolution rate is proportional to the surface area of the drug. Dissolution takes place at the surface of the solute (drug), and thus, the greater the surface area, the better the water saturation, and the more rapid the rate of drug dissolution. The effective surface area of a drug is increased enormously by a reduction in the particle size (ie, more particles for a given volume). The geometric shape of the particle also affects the surface area, and, during dissolution, the surface is constantly changing. For dissolution calculations using the various models, however, the solute particle is usually assumed to have retained its geometric shape.

Particle size and particle size distribution studies are important for drugs that have low water solubility, particularly class II drugs according to the Biopharmaceutical Classification System (BCS) (see Chapter 16) where dissolution is often rate limiting for absorption. Consequently, there are many drugs that are very active when administered intravenously but are not very effective when given orally because of poor oral absorption owing to the drug's poor aqueous solubility. Griseofulvin, nitrofurantoin, and many steroids are drugs with low aqueous solubility; reduction of the particle size by milling to a micronized form has improved the oral absorption of these drugs. A disintegrant may also be added to the formulation to ensure rapid disintegration of the tablet and release of the particles. The addition of surface-active agents may increase wetting as well as solubility of these drugs.

Sometimes micronization and varying the choice of excipient are not sufficient to overcome solubility-related bioavailability problems. In these cases, so-called *nanosizing*, or producing even smaller drug substance particles, may be beneficial. As compared with micronization, nanosized particles may be formulated for injection drug products (eg, nano-suspension) in addition to traditional oral dosage forms.

It is possible that nanosized drug particles may not dissolve readily after IV administration and end up sequestered by the *reticuloendothelial system* (RES). However, the nanoparticles will eventually dissolve, permeate into the cytoplasm, and contribute to overall systemic drug exposure in a pseudo extended-release pharmacokinetic profile.

Polymorphism, Solvates, and Drug Absorption

Polymorphism refers to the arrangement of a drug substance in various crystal forms or polymorphs. In recent years, the term polymorph has been used frequently to describe polymorphs, solvates, amorphous forms, and desolvated solvates. *Amorphous forms* are

noncrystalline forms, *solvates* are forms that contain a solvent (solvate) or water (hydrate), and *desolvated* solvates are forms that are made by removing the solvent from the solvate. Many drugs exist in an *anhydrous* state (no water of hydration) or in a hydrous state.

Polymorphs have the same chemical structure but different physical properties, such as different solubility, hygroscopicity, density, hardness, and compression characteristics. Some polymorphic crystals have much lower aqueous solubility than the amorphous forms, causing a product to be incompletely absorbed.

Chloramphenicol, for example, has several crystal forms, and when given orally as a suspension, the drug concentration in the body was found to be dependent on the percent of β-polymorph in the suspension. The β form is more soluble and better absorbed (Fig. 15-4). In general, the crystal form that has the lowest free energy is the most stable polymorph. A drug that exists as an amorphous form (noncrystalline form) generally dissolves more rapidly than the same drug in a more structurally rigid crystalline form. Some polymorphs are *metastable* and may convert to a more stable form over time. A change in crystal form may cause problems in manufacturing the product. For example, a change

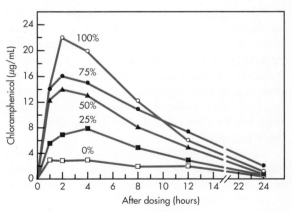

FIGURE 15-4 Comparison of mean blood serum levels obtained with chloramphenicol palmitate suspensions containing varying ratios of α- and β-polymorphs, following single oral dose equivalent to 1.5 g chloramphenicol. Percentage polymorph β in the suspension. (From Aguiar et al, 1967, with permission.)

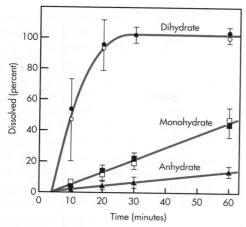

FIGURE 15-5 Dissolution behavior of erythromycin dihydrate, monohydrate, and anhydrate in phosphate buffer (pH 7.5) at 37°C. (From Allen et al, 1978, with permission.)

absorption from the absorption site, increase drug bioavailability, etc. Some of the excipients used in the manufacture of solid and liquid drug products are listed in Tables 15-2 and 15-3.

Excipients in the drug product may also affect the dissolution kinetics of the drug, either by altering the medium in which the drug is dissolving or by reacting with the drug itself. Some of the more common manufacturing problems that affect dissolution are listed in Table 15-4. Other excipients include suspending agents that increase the viscosity of the drug vehicle and thereby diminish the rate of drug dissolution from suspensions. Tablet lubricants, such as magnesium stearate, may repel water and reduce dissolution when used in large quantities. Coatings, particularly shellac, will crosslink upon aging and decrease the dissolution rate.

in the crystal structure of the drug may cause cracking in a tablet or even prevent a granulation from being compressed into a tablet. Re-formulation of a product may be necessary if a new crystal form of a drug is used.

Some drugs interact with solvent during the manufacturing process to form a crystal called a *solvate*. Water may form special crystals with drugs called *hydrates*; for example, erythromycin hydrates have quite different solubility compared to the anhydrous form of the drug (Fig. 15-5). Ampicillin trihydrate, on the other hand, was reported to be less absorbed than the anhydrous form of ampicillin because of faster dissolution of the latter.

FORMULATION FACTORS AFFECTING DRUG PRODUCT PERFORMANCE

Excipients are added to a formulation to provide certain functional properties to the drug and dosage form; excipients also affect drug product performance, *in vivo* (Amidon et al, 2007; Chapter 18). Some of these functional properties of the excipients are used to improve the manufacturability of the dosage form, stabilize the drug against degradation, decrease gastric irritation, control the rate of drug

TABLE 15-2   Common Excipients Used in Solid Drug Products

Excipient	Property in Dosage Form
Lactose	Diluent
Dibasic calcium phosphate	Diluent
Starch	Disintegrant, diluent
Microcrystalline cellulose	Disintegrant, diluent
Magnesium stearate	Lubricant
Stearic acid	Lubricant
Hydrogenated vegetable oil	Lubricant
Talc	Lubricant
Sucrose (solution)	Granulating agent
Polyvinyl pyrrolidone (solution)	Granulating agent
Hydroxypropylmethyl-cellulose	Tablet-coating agent
Titinium dioxide	Combined with dye as colored coating
Methylcellulose	Coating or granulating agent
Cellulose acetate phthalate	Enteric-coating agent

TABLE 15-3 Common Excipients Used in Oral Liquid Drug Products

Excipient	Property in Dosage Form
Sodium carboxy-methyl cellulose	Suspending agent
Tragacanth	Suspending agent
Sodium alginate	Suspending agent
Xanthan gum	Thixotropic suspending agent
Veegum	Thixotropic suspending agent
Sorbitol	Sweetener
Alcohol	Solubilizing agent, preservative
Propylene glycol	Solubilizing agent
Methyl, propylparaben	Preservative
Sucrose	Sweetener
Polysorbates	Surfactant
Sesame oil	For emulsion vehicle
Corn oil	For emulsion vehicle

Surfactants, on the other hand, may affect drug dissolution in an unpredictable fashion. Low concentrations of surfactants decrease the surface tension and increase the rate of drug dissolution, whereas higher surfactant concentrations tend to form micelles with the drug and thus decrease the dissolution rate. Large drug particles have a smaller surface area and dissolve more slowly than smaller particles. Poor disintegration of a compressed tablet may be due to high compression of tablets without sufficient disintegrant.

Some excipients, such as sodium bicarbonate, may change the pH of the medium surrounding the active drug substance. Aspirin, a weak acid when formulated with sodium bicarbonate, will form a water-soluble salt in an alkaline medium, in which the drug rapidly dissolves. The term for this process is *dissolution in a reactive medium*. The solid drug dissolves rapidly in the reactive solvent surrounding the solid particle. However, as the dissolved drug molecules diffuse outward into the bulk solvent, the drug may precipitate out of solution with a very fine particle size. These small particles have enormous collective surface area, dispersing and redissolving readily for more rapid absorption upon contact with the mucosal surface.

Excipients in a formulation may interact directly with the drug to form a water-soluble or water-insoluble complex. For example, if tetracycline is formulated with calcium carbonate, an insoluble complex

TABLE 15-4 Effect of Excipients on the Pharmacokinetic Parameters of Oral Drug Products[a]

Excipients	Example	k_a	t_{max}	AUC
Disintegrants	Avicel, Explotab	↑	↓	↑/–
Lubricants	Talc, hydrogenated vegetable oil	↓	↑	↓/–
Coating agent	Hydroxypropylmethyl cellulose	–	–	–
Enteric coat	Cellulose acetate phthalate	↓	↑	↓/–
Sustained-release agents	Methylcellulose, ethylcellulose	↓	↑	↓/–
Sustained-release agents (waxy agents)	Castorwax, Carbowax	↓	↑	↓/–
Sustained-release agents (gum/viscous)	Veegum, Keltrol	↓	↑	↓/–

[a]This may be concentration and drug dependent. ↑ = Increase, ↓ = decrease, – = no effect, k_a = absorption rate constant, t_{max} = time for peak drug concentration in plasma, AUC = area under the plasma drug concentration–time curve.

of calcium tetracycline is formed that has a slow rate of dissolution and poor absorption.

Excipients may be added intentionally to the formulation to enhance the rate and extent of drug absorption or to delay or slow the rate of drug absorption (see Table 15-4). For example, excipients that increase the aqueous solubility of the drug generally increase the rate of dissolution and drug absorption. Excipients may increase the retention time of the drug in the gastrointestinal tract and therefore increase the total amount of drug absorbed. Excipients may also act as carriers to increase drug diffusion across the intestinal wall. In contrast, certain excipients may create a barrier between the drug and body fluids that retard drug dissolution and thus reduce the rate or extent of drug absorption.

Common excipients found in oral drug products are listed in Tables 15-2 and 15-3. Excipients should be pharmacodynamically inert. However, excipients may change the functionality (performance) of the drug substance and the bioavailability of the drug from the dosage form. For solid oral dosage forms such as compressed tablets, excipients may include (1) a diluent (eg, lactose), (2) a disintegrant (eg, starch), (3) a lubricant (eg, magnesium stearate), and (4) other components such as binding and stabilizing agents. If used improperly in a formulation, the rate and extent of drug absorption may be affected. For example, Fig. 15-6 shows that an excessive quantity of magnesium stearate (a hydrophobic lubricant) in

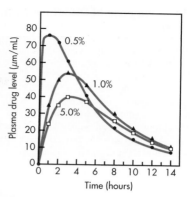

FIGURE 15-7   Effect of lubricant on drug absorption. Percentage of magnesium stearate in formulation. Incomplete drug absorption occurs for formulation with 5% magnesium stearate.

the formulation may retard drug dissolution and slow the rate of drug absorption. The total amount of drug absorbed may also be reduced (Fig. 15-7). To prevent this problem, the lubricant level should be decreased or a different lubricant selected. Sometimes, increasing the amount of disintegrant may overcome the retarding effect of lubricants on dissolution. However, with some poorly soluble drugs an increase in disintegrant level has little or no effect on drug dissolution because the fine drug particles are not wetted. The influence of some common ingredients on drug absorption parameters is summarized in Table 15-4. These are general trends for typical preparations.

DRUG PRODUCT PERFORMANCE, *IN VITRO*: DISSOLUTION AND DRUG RELEASE TESTING

Dissolution and drug release tests are *in vitro* tests that measure the rate and extent of dissolution or release of the drug substance from a drug product, usually in an aqueous medium under specified conditions. *In vitro* dissolution testing provides useful information throughout the drug development process (Table 15-5).

The dissolution test is an important quality control procedure used to confirm batch-to-batch reproducibility and to show typical variability in composition

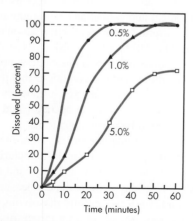

FIGURE 15-6   Effect of lubricant on drug dissolution. Percentage of magnesium stearate in formulation.

TABLE 15-5 Purpose of Dissolution and Drug Release Tests

Formulation development and selection
Confirmation of batch-to-batch reproducibility
Establish drug product stability
Demonstrate that the product performs consistently throughout its use period or shelflife
Establish *in vivo–in vitro* correlations (IVIVC)
Evaluate the biopharmaceutic implications of a product change, rather than to require a bioequivalence study (SUPAC—scale-up and postapproval changes)

and manufacturing parameters. Dissolution and drug release tests are also used as a measure of drug product performance, *in vitro* when linked to product performance *in vivo*. The dissolution test should reflect relevant changes in the drug product formulation or changes in the manufacturing process that might affect drug release characteristics and consequently *in vivo* performance. Ideally, the dissolution method used for a particular drug product *in vitro* should mimic the release characteristics of the drug product *in vivo* and should potentially be able to differentiate among formulations with different release characteristics.

In vitro drug dissolution studies are often used for monitoring drug product stability and manufacturing process control. In this case, the dissolution test provides evidence that the product will perform consistently throughout its use period or shelf life.

The dissolution test is not only useful for the quality control of finished product, but can provide valuable information during formulation development (ie, salt form selection, excipient selection, etc). A suitable dissolution method may uncover a formulation problem with the drug product that could result in a bioavailability problem.

Each dissolution method is specific for the drug product and its formulation. When developing optimal dissolution parameters, a variety of conditions (ie, apparatus, media pH, etc) should be explored. The ultimate goal is to identify a dissolution test that is capable of distinguishing between acceptable and unacceptable drug formulations as observed by different drug dissolution rates under the same experimental conditions. Overall, a suitable dissolution test

should be able to reflect changes in the formulation, manufacturing process, and physical and chemical characteristics of the drug, such as particle size, polymorphs, and surface area (Gray et al, 2001).

The dissolution test is typically a requirement for routine batch testing and qualification of certain scale-up and postapproval changes (SUPAC) for many marketed drug products (see Chapter 18). After a change is made to a formulation, the manufacturer needs to assess the potential effect of the change on the drug's bioavailability. If the changes are deemed minor, the impact on its *in vivo* performance can be assessed by comparing the pre- and postchange product dissolution profile using the approved dissolution method or under different pH conditions. If differences exist between the dissolution profiles, an *in vivo* bioequivalence study may be performed to determine whether the observed difference *in vitro* translates into different pharmacokinetics *in vivo*, which could affect the safety and efficacy profile of the drug product. Major postapproval manufacturing changes require a bioequivalence study to support approval of the change, but this bioequivalence study may be waived in the presence of an acceptable *in vitro–in vivo* correlation (see Chapter 16).

Development and Validation of Dissolution and Drug Release Tests

The USP dissolution test is an *in vitro* performance test applicable to many dosage forms such as tablets, capsules, transdermals, suppositories, suspensions, etc. The development and validation of dissolution tests is discussed in several USP general information chapters (eg, USP <711>, USP <1092>, USP <724>). The dissolution procedure requires a dissolution apparatus, dissolution medium, and test conditions that provide a method that is *discriminating* yet sufficiently rugged and reproducible for day-to-day operation and capable of being transferred between laboratories.

The choice of apparatus and dissolution medium is based on the physicochemical characteristics of the drug (including solubility, stability) and the type of formulation (such as immediate release, enteric coated, extended release, rapidly dissolving, etc).

The development of an appropriate dissolution test requires the investigator to explore different

TABLE 15-6   Conditions That May Affect Drug Dissolution and Release

Drug substance
    Particle size
    Polymorph
    Surface area
    Chemical stability in dissolution media
Formulation of drug product
    Excipients (lubricants, suspending agents, etc)
Medium
    Volume
    pH
    Molarity
    Co-solvents, added enzymes/surfactants
Temperature of medium
Apparatus
Hydrodynamics
    Agitation rate
    Shape of dissolution vessel
    Placement of tablet in vessel
    Sinkers (for floating products and products that stick to side of vessel)

agitation rates, different media (including volume and pH of medium), and different kinds of dissolution apparatus (Table 15-6). For solid oral dosage forms, USP Apparatus 1 and Apparatus 2 are used most frequently. The dissolution test conditions should be able to discriminate a change in formulation that might affect drug product performance. In addition, the dissolution test should be sufficiently rugged and reproducible for day-to-day operation and capable of being transferred between laboratories. The current USP-NF lists officially recognized dissolution apparatus (Table 15-7). Once a suitable dissolution test is obtained, acceptable dissolution criteria (specifications) are developed for the drug product. For example, Philip and Daly (1983) devised a method using pH 6.6 phosphate buffer as the dissolution medium instead of 0.1 N HCl to avoid instability of the antibiotic drug erythromycin. Using the USP paddle method at 50 rpm and a temperature of 22°C, the dissolution of the various erythromycin tablets was shown to vary with the source of the bulk active drug (Table 15-8 and Fig. 15-8).

Visual observations of the dissolution and disintegration behavior of the drug product are important and should be recorded. Dissolution and disintegration patterns can indicate manufacturing variables. These observations are particularly useful during

TABLE 15-7   USP-NF and Non-USP-NF Dissolution Apparatus

Apparatus[a]	Name	Agitation Method	Drug Product
Apparatus 1	Rotating basket	Rotating stirrer	Tablets, capsules
Apparatus 2	Paddle	Rotating stirrer	Tablets, capsules, modified drug products, suspensions
Apparatus 3	Reciprocating cylinder	Reciprocation	Extended-release drug products
Apparatus 4	Flow cell	Fluid movement	Drug products containing low water-soluble drugs
Apparatus 5	Paddle over disk	Rotating stirrer	Transdermal drug products
Apparatus 6	Cylinder	Rotating stirrer	Transdermal drug products
Apparatus 7	Reciprocating disk	Reciprocation	Extended-release drug products
Rotating bottle	(Non-USP-NF)		Extended-release drug products (beads)
Diffusion cell (Franz)	(Non-USP-NF)		Ointments, creams, transdermal drug products

[a]USP-NF dissolution apparatus and non-USP-NF dissolution apparatus.

TABLE 15-8   Dissolution of Erythromycin Stearate Bulk Drug and Corresponding Tablets

Curve No.	Bulk Drug	500-mg Tablet	250-mg Tablet
	Percent Dissolution after 1.0 h		
4	49	44	
6	72	70	
7	75	70	
–	78	–	80
8	82	75	
9	92	85	

From Philip and Daly (1983), with permission.

dissolution method development and formulation optimization.

The size and shape of the dissolution vessel may affect the rate and extent of dissolution. For example, dissolution vessels range in size from several milliliters to several liters. The shape may be round-bottomed or flat, so the tablet might lie in a different

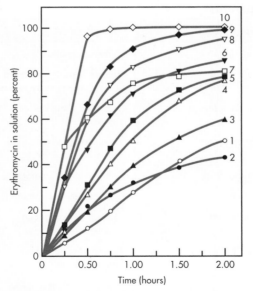

FIGURE 15-8   Dissolution profile of various lots of erythromycin stearate as a function of time (0.05 M, pH 6.6 phosphate buffer). (From Philip and Daly, 1983, with permission.)

position in different experiments. The usual medium volume is 500–1000 mL. Drugs that are poorly water soluble may require use of a very large-capacity vessel (up to 2000 mL) to observe significant dissolution. In some cases, a surfactant (eg, sodium lauryl sulfate, Triton X-100, etc) may be added to the dissolution medium for water-insoluble drugs. *Sink conditions* is a term referring to an excess volume of medium (at least 3×) that allows the solid drug to dissolve continuously. If the drug solution becomes saturated, no further net drug dissolution will take place. According to the USP-NF, "the quantity of medium used should not be less than 3 times that needed to form a saturated solution of the drug substance."

The amount of agitation and the nature of the stirrer affect hydrodynamics of the system, thereby affecting the dissolution rate. Stirring rates must be controlled, and criteria differ among drug products. Low stirring rates (50–75 rpm) are more discriminating of formulation factors affecting dissolution than higher stirring rates. However, a higher dissolution rate may be needed for some special formulations in order to obtain reproducible dissolution rates. Suspensions that contain viscous or thickening agents may settle into a diffusion-controlled "cone-shape" region in the flask when stirring rate is too slow. The temperature of the dissolution medium must be controlled, and variations in temperature must be avoided. Most dissolution tests are performed at 37°C. However, for transdermal drug products, the recommended temperature is 32°C.

The nature of the dissolution medium will also affect the dissolution test. The solubility of the drug must be considered, as well as the total amount of drug in the dosage form. The dissolution medium should not be saturated by the drug (ie, sink conditions are maintained). Usually, a volume of medium larger than the amount of solvent needed to completely dissolve the drug is used in the dissolution test. Which medium is best is determined through careful investigative studies. The dissolution medium in many USP dissolution tests is deaerated water or, if substantiated by the solubility characteristics of the drug or formulation, a buffered aqueous solution (typically pH 4–8) or dilute HCl may be used. The significance of deaeration of the medium should be determined. Various investigators have used 0.1 N HCl, phosphate buffer, simulated gastric fluid, water, and simulated intestinal fluid, depending on the nature of the drug product and the location in the gastrointestinal tract where the drug is expected to dissolve.

The design of the dissolution apparatus, along with the other factors previously described, has a marked effect on the outcome of the dissolution test. No single apparatus and test can be used for all drug products. Each drug product must be considered individually with the dissolution test (method and limit(s)) that best correlates to *in vivo* bioavailability to the extent feasible.

Usually, the dissolution test will state that a certain percentage of the labeled amount of drug product must dissolve within a specified period of time. In practice, the absolute amount of drug in the drug product may vary from tablet to tablet. Therefore, a prescribed number of tablets from each lot are usually considered to get a representative dissolution rate for the product.

Frequently Asked Questions

▶ *Drug absorption involves at least three distinct steps: dissolution, permeation, and disposition during transit in GI (an additional step of drug disposition in the body is involved as well for bioavailability). How are these processes validated* in vitro *when the* in vivo *requirement for drug bioavailability is waived?*

▶ *What are the risk mitigating steps taken above if some manufacturing processes cannot be validated* in vitro?

▶ *Why is it important to maintain sink conditions?*

COMPENDIAL METHODS OF DISSOLUTION

The USP-NF describes the official dissolution apparatus and includes information for performing dissolution tests on a variety of drug products including tablets, capsules, and other special products such as transdermal preparations. The selection of a particular dissolution method for a drug may be specified in

the USP-NF monograph for a particular drug product or may be recommended by the FDA.[1] The USP-NF sets standards for dissolution and drug release tests of most drug products listed in USP monographs. Alternative dissolution methods, particularly the use of comparative dissolution rate profiles under various conditions, are often used during drug development to better understand the relationship of the formulation components and manufacturing process on drug release.

The USP dissolution apparatus and the type of drug products that is often used with the apparatus are listed in Table 15-7. For USP Apparatus 1 (basket) and 2 (paddle), low rotational speeds affect the reproducibility of the hydrodynamics, whereas at high rotational speeds, turbulence may occur. Dissolution profiles that show the drug dissolving too slowly or too rapidly may justify increasing or decreasing the rotational speed (Gray et al, 2001). The choice of apparatus for solid oral dosage forms is often Apparatus 1 (rotating basket) or Apparatus 2 (paddle) due to the ease of use, availability of the apparatus, and availability of automated methods.

Apparatus 1: Rotating Basket

The rotating basket apparatus (Apparatus 1) consists of a cylindrical basket held by a motor shaft. The basket holds the sample and rotates in a round flask containing the dissolution medium. The entire flask is immersed in a constant-temperature bath set at 37°C. Agitation is provided by rotating the basket. The rotating speed and the position of the basket must meet specific requirements set forth in the current USP. The most common rotating speed for the basket method is 100–150 rpm. A disadvantage of the rotating basket is that the formulation may clog to the 40-mesh screen.

Apparatus 2: Paddle Method

The paddle apparatus (Apparatus 2) consists of a special, coated paddle that minimizes turbulence due to stirring (Fig. 15-9). The paddle is attached vertically

---

[1]The FDA provides recommendations for many drug products on its website, www.accessdata.fda.gov/scripts/cder/dissolution/index.cfm.

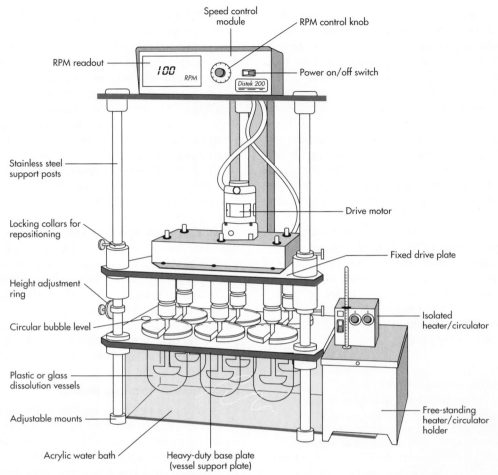

FIGURE 15-9 Typical setup for performing the USP dissolution test with the Distek 2000. The system is equipped with a height adjustment ring for easy adjustment of paddle height. (Drawing courtesy of Distek Inc, Somerset, NJ.)

to a variable-speed motor that rotates at a controlled speed. The tablet or capsule is placed into the round-bottom dissolution flask, which minimizes turbulence of the dissolution medium. The apparatus is housed in a constant-temperature water bath maintained at 37°C, similar to the rotating-basket method. The position and alignment of the paddle are specified in the USP. The paddle method is very sensitive to tilting. Improper alignment may drastically affect the dissolution results with some drug products. The most common operating speeds for Apparatus 2 are 50 or 75 rpm for solid oral dosage forms and 25 rpm for oral suspensions. Apparatus 2 is generally preferred for

tablets. A *sinker*, such as a few turns of platinum wire, may be used to prevent a capsule or tablet from floating. A sinker may also be used for film-coated tablets that stick to the vessel walls or to help position the tablet or capsule under the paddle (Gray et al, 2001). The sinker should not alter the dissolution characteristics of the dosage form.

Apparatus 3: Reciprocating Cylinder

The reciprocating cylinder apparatus (Apparatus 3) consists of a set of cylindrical, flat-bottomed glass vessels equipped with reciprocating cylinders for dissolution testing of extended-release products, particularly bead-type modified-release dosage forms. Reciprocating agitation moves the dosage form up and down in the media. The agitation rate is generally 5–30 dpm (dips per minute). The reciprocating cylinder can be programmed for dissolution in various media for various times. The media can be changed easily. This apparatus may be used during drug product development to attempt to mirror pH changes and transit times in the GI tract such as starting at pH 1 and then pH 4.5 and then at pH 6.8.

Apparatus 4: Flow-through-Cell

The flow-through-cell apparatus (Apparatus 4) consists of a reservoir for the dissolution medium and a pump that forces dissolution medium through the cell holding the test sample. The media may be a non-recirculating, continuous flow solution, or recirculating solution. The flow rate is critical. Flow rate ranges from 4 to 32 mL/min. Apparatus 4 may be used for modified-release dosage forms that contain active ingredients having very limited solubility. The high volume provides "infinite" sink conditions.

There are many variations of this method. Essentially, the sample is held in a fixed position while the dissolution medium is pumped through the sample holder, thus dissolving the drug. Laminar flow of the medium is achieved by using a pulseless pump. Peristaltic or centrifugal pumps are not recommended. The flow rate is usually maintained between 10 and 100 mL/min. The dissolution medium may be fresh or recirculated. In the case of fresh medium, the dissolution rate at any moment may be obtained, whereas in the official paddle or basket method, cumulative dissolution rates are monitored. A major advantage of the flow-through method is the easy maintenance of a sink condition for dissolution. A large volume of dissolution medium may also be used, and the mode of operation is easily adapted to automated equipment.

Apparatus 5: Paddle-over-Disk

The USP-NF also lists a paddle-over-disk method for testing the release of drugs from transdermal products. The apparatus (Apparatus 5) uses the paddle and vessel assembly from Apparatus 2 with the addition of a stainless steel disk assembly designed for holding the transdermal system at the bottom of the vessel. The entire preparation is placed in a dissolution flask filled with specified medium maintained at 32°C. The paddle is placed directly over the disk assembly. Samples are drawn midway between the surface of the dissolution medium and the top of the paddle blade at specified times. Matrix transdermal patches can be cut to size of the disk assembly.

Apparatus 6: Cylinder

The cylinder method (Apparatus 6) for testing transdermal preparation is modified from the basket method (Apparatus 1). In place of the basket, a stainless steel cylinder is used to hold the sample. The sample is mounted onto cuprophan (an inert porous cellulosic material) and the entire system adheres to the cylinder. Testing is maintained at 32°C. Apparatus 6 may be used for reservoir transdermal patches that cannot be cut smaller. Samples are drawn midway between the surface of the dissolution medium and the top of the rotating cylinder for analysis.

Apparatus 7: Reciprocating Disk

The reciprocating disk method for testing transdermal products uses a motor drive assembly (Apparatus 7) that reciprocates vertically. The samples are placed on disk-shaped holders using cuprophan supports. The test is also carried out at 32°C, and reciprocating frequency is about 30 cycles per minute.

ALTERNATIVE METHODS OF DISSOLUTION TESTING

Rotating Bottle Method

The rotating bottle method was suggested in NF-XIII (National Formulary) but has become less popular since. The rotating bottle method was used mainly for controlled-release beads. For this purpose the dissolution medium may be easily changed, such as from artificial gastric juice to artificial intestinal juice. The equipment consists of a rotating rack that holds the sample drug products in bottles. The bottles are capped tightly and rotated in a 37°C temperature bath. At various times, the samples are removed from the bottle, decanted through a 40-mesh screen, and the residues are assayed. An equal volume of fresh medium is added to the remaining drug residues within the bottles and the dissolution test is continued. A dissolution test with pH 1.2 medium for 1 hour, pH 2.5 medium for the next 1 hour, followed by pH 4.5 medium for 1.5 hours, pH 7.0 medium for 1.5 hours, and pH 7.5 medium for 2 hours was recommended to simulate the condition of the gastrointestinal tract. The main disadvantage is that this procedure is manual and tedious.

Intrinsic Dissolution Method

Most methods for dissolution deal with a finished drug product. Sometimes a new drug or substance may be tested for dissolution without the effect of excipients or the fabrication effect of processing. The dissolution of a drug powder by maintaining a constant surface area is called *intrinsic dissolution*. Intrinsic dissolution is usually expressed as mg/cm²/min. In one method, the basket method is adapted to test dissolution of powder by placing the powder in a disk attached with a clipper to the bottom of the basket.

Peristalsis Method

The peristalsis method attempts to simulate the hydrodynamic conditions of the gastrointestinal tract in an *in vitro* dissolution device. The apparatus consists of a rigid plastic cylindrical tubing fitted with a septum and rubber stoppers at both ends. The dissolution chamber consists of a space between the septum and the lower stopper. The apparatus is placed in a beaker containing the dissolution medium. The dissolution medium is pumped with peristaltic action through the dosage form.

Diffusion Cells

Static and flow-through diffusion cells are commercially available to characterize *in vitro* drug release and drug permeation kinetics from topically applied dosage form (eg, ointment, cream) or transdermal drug product. The *Franz diffusion cell* is a static diffusion system that is used for characterizing drug permeation through a skin model (Fig. 15-10).

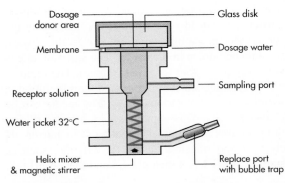

FIGURE 15-10   The Franz diffusion cell. (Courtesy of Hanson Research Corporation [www.hansonresearch.com /vert_diffusion_cell.htm], with permission.)

The source of skin may be human cadaver skin or animal skin (eg, hairless mouse skin). Anatomically, each skin site (eg, abdomen, arm) has different drug permeation qualities. The skin is mounted on the Franz diffusion cell system. The drug product (eg, ointment) is placed on the skin surface and the drug permeates across the skin into a receptor fluid compartment that may be sampled at various times. The Franz diffusion cell system is useful for comparing *in vitro* drug release profiles and skin permeation characteristics to aid in selecting an appropriate formulation that has optimum drug delivery.

Dissolution Testing of Enteric-Coated Products

USP-NF lists two methods (Method A and Method B) for testing enteric-coated products. The latest revision of the USP-NF should be consulted for complete details of the methods.

Both methods require that the dissolution test be performed in the apparatus specified in the drug monograph (usually Apparatus 2 or Apparatus 1). The product is first studied with 0.1 N HCl for 2 hours and then the medium is changed to pH 6.8 buffer medium. The buffer stage generally runs for 45 minutes or for the time specified in the monograph. The objective is that no significant dissolution occurs in the acid phase (less than 10% for any sample unit), and a specified percentage of drug is released in the buffer phase. Dissolution acceptance criteria are defined in the individual drug monographs for commercial products. Appropriate criteria will need to be established for novel drugs formulated as enteric-coated drug products.

Dissolution Approaches for Novel/Special Dosage Forms

New or specialized dosage forms are being developed for improving patient compliance, to enhance therapeutic response and for marketing exclusivity. Some of these dosage forms include osmotic capsules, orally disintegrating tablets, medicated chewing gums, soft gelatin capsules containing drug dissolved in oil, nanomaterial, liposomal drug products, implants, intrauterine devices, and drug-eluting stents. While conventional apparatus may be used to evaluate the dissolution kinetics of nonconventional dosage forms, specialized or modified systems may be needed for others. For example, medicated chewing gum and extended-release parenteral products may need a specialized dissolution apparatus or a modified dissolution apparatus (Siewart et al, 2003).

USP Performance Verification Test and Mechanical Calibration

Dissolution is a complex system that mainly consists of three components: (1) the analyst, (2) the dissolution apparatus, and (3) the analytical procedure/instrument. In order for the dissolution test to be performed properly, and give meaningful results, these three components must interact together optimally, or the results can be misleading. The USP general chapter for dissolution includes *performance verification test* (PVT), to assure the suitability of Apparatus 1 and 2 when used for testing drug products. PVT requires chemical calibration with calibrator tablets that may be obtained from USP-NF. The calibration tablets, either prednisone tablets for dissolution tests requiring disintegrating tablets or salicylic acid as a standard for nondisintegrating tablets, are used to qualify USP dissolution Apparatus 1 and Apparatus 2. PVT is also useful to compare performance of different dissolution apparatus used in different laboratories.

Mechanical calibration is a critical component of the qualification of the dissolution apparatus. The FDA has introduced a mechanical calibration approach that considers mechanical specifications of the instrument design and its manufacture (FDA Guidance for Industry, January 2010). Instead of using a calibrator tablet, a pharmaceutical manufacturer can use an appropriately rigorous method of mechanical calibration for dissolution Apparatus 1 and 2.

> **Frequently Asked Questions**
> ▶ *Which dissolution apparatus are most often used for tablets and capsules?*
> ▶ *What is meant by "sink" conditions?*
> ▶ *How is the discriminating ability of the method assessed?*
> ▶ *Can the discriminating ability of the dissolution method be improved by tightening the dissolution acceptance criteria?*

Discriminating Dissolution Test

The value of *in vitro* dissolution testing is its ability to characterize drug products and assist in decision making including (1) ensuring quality control through a linkage to batches used in pivotal clinical studies; (2) information on batch-to-batch consistency; and (3) guide in formulation development. Dissolution testing is the only product test that truly measures the effect of formulation and physical properties of the active pharmaceutical ingredient (API) on the rate of drug solubilization. In addition, under certain circumstances (eg, presence of an adequate IVIVC) *in vitro* dissolution testing can serve as a surrogate for bioequivalence studies to assess the impact of some pre- and postapproval changes. The dissolution testing procedure should be discriminating to ensure its value.

A discriminating method is the one that is appropriately sensitive to manufacturing changes. A discriminating method is able to differentiate drug products manufactured under target conditions versus drug products that are intentionally manufactured with meaningful variations (ie, ±10%–20% change) to the specification ranges of the most relevant material attributes and manufacturing variables (eg, drug substance particle size, polymorphism, compression force, tablet hardness, etc). The choice of experimental design to evaluate the most relevant variables will depend on the design of the dosage form, the manufacturing process, and intrinsic properties of the API (Brown et al, 2004).

Developing a discriminating method is crucial when setting drug product specifications (eg, dissolution acceptance criterion) because the value of this specification depends on the discriminating ability of the method. If the method is over-discriminating, batches with adequate performance will be rejected creating a burden for the pharmaceutical companies. If it is under-discriminating, batches with an inadequate performance will be accepted, which may put the patient to risk. However, unless an *in vitro–in vivo* relationship (IVIVR) or correlation (IVIVC) has been established between dissolution and *in vivo* data (eg, plasma concentrations), the biorelevancy of the method (ability of the method to reject for batches with inadequate *in vivo* performance) cannot be determined.

Ideally, dissolution (or release) method and acceptance criterion should be further evaluated using *in vivo* bioavailability or bioequivalence studies with product variants manufactured during the course of pharmaceutical development, including batches used in clinical trials. A dissolution method and acceptance criterion should be modified if they are found to be over-discriminating or under-discriminating when compared with the results of *in vivo* studies.

One should note that the discriminating ability is determined not only by the dissolution method settings but also by the selected specification-sampling time point and specification value. Figure 15-11 illustrates the importance of selecting the right specification-sampling time point and specification value to establish a discriminating method. Batches A through C are commercial batches. The fast release batch corresponds to a pivotal Phase 3 clinical batch. What can we say about the discriminating ability of the dissolution method? The method seems sensitive to particle size changes; however, because batch A failed similarity testing (eg, f_2 statistical testing), then the dissolution acceptance criterion should be selected in a way that rejects this batch, increasing in this way the method's discriminating ability. Selecting a criterion of $Q = 80\%$ at 30 minutes fulfills this purpose. Note that setting a dissolution acceptance criterion

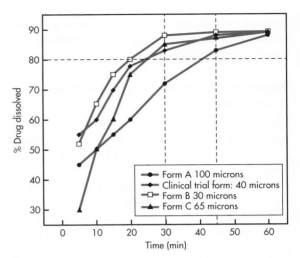

FIGURE 15-11   Effect of particle size and drug release rate—Importance of selecting the right specification-sampling time point and specification value to establish a discriminating dissolution method.

to $Q = 80\%$ at 45 minutes may not be appropriate because it would be accepting a batch that does not have the same performance as that for the clinical batch. Selecting the wrong acceptance criterion (eg, overly permissive criterion), despite the method's intrinsic discriminating ability, renders the method not discriminating.

DISSOLUTION PROFILE COMPARISONS

Dissolution profile comparisons are used to assess the similarity of the dissolution characteristics of two formulation or different strengths of the same formulation to decide whether *in vivo* bioavailability/bioequivalence studies are needed. The SUPAC-IR and SUPAC-MR (FDA guidances for immediate-release and modified-release oral formulations, respectively) provide recommendations to firms who intend, during the postapproval period, to change (a) the components or compositions; (b) the site of manufacture; (c) the scale-up/scale-down of manufacture; and/or (d) the manufacturing (process and equipment) of the drug product. For each type of change, these guidances list documentation (eg, dissolution testing, bioequivalence, etc) that should be normally provided to support the change depending on the level of complexity of the proposed change (Levels 1, 2, and 3). Note that the principles listed in these guidances can also be applicable for manufacturing changes occurring during product development.

For minor changes and some major changes (eg, manufacturing site change for an immediate-release formulation) for which *in vivo* bioequivalence is not warranted, dissolution profile comparisons either in the proposed media or in multimedia can be submitted to support the change.

Dissolution profiles may be considered similar by virtue of overall profile similarity and/or similarity at every dissolution sample time point. The FDA guidance on dissolution testing (FDA Guidance for Industry, 1997a) describes three statistical methods for the evaluation of similarity: (1) model-independent approach using a similarity factor; (2) model-independent multivariate confidence region procedure; and (3) model-dependent approach. The first approach is described below. Refer to the dissolution testing guidance for details on the other two approaches.

A model-independent approach uses a difference factor (f_1) and a similarity factor (f_2) to compare dissolution profiles. The difference factor (f_1) calculates the percent (%) difference between the two curves at each time point and is a measurement of the relative error between the two curves.

$$f_1 = \left[\left(\sum_{t=1}^{n} |R_t - T_t| \right) \Big/ \left(\sum_{t=1}^{n} R_t \right) \right] \times 100$$

where n is the number of time points, R is the dissolution value of the reference batch at time t, and T is the dissolution value of the test batch at time t.

The *similarity factor* (f_2) is a logarithmic reciprocal square root transformation of the sum of squared error and is a measurement of the similarity in the percent (%) dissolution between the two curves.

$$f_2 = 50 \times \log \left[\left(1 + (1/n) \sum_{t=1}^{n} (R_t - T_t)^2 \right)^{-0.5} \times 100 \right]$$

where n is the number of time points, R is the dissolution value of the reference (prechange) batch at time t, and T is the dissolution value of the test (postchange) batch at time t.

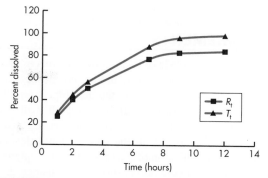

FIGURE 15-12   Dissolution of test and reference ER tablets. R_t = reference and T_t = text.

The similarity factor (f_2) is determined by comparing the dissolution profiles of 6–12 units each of the test and reference products (Fig. 15-12). Using the mean dissolution values from both profiles at each time interval, the similarity factor (f_2) is calculated. For this calculation, three to four or more dissolution time points should be available. The dissolution measurements of the test and reference batches should be performed under exactly the same conditions, and only one measurement should be considered after 85% dissolution of both products. The dissolution time points for both profiles should be the same (eg, 15, 30, 45, and 60 minutes). f_2 values greater than 50 mean that there is less than 10% difference between the two dissolution profiles. f_2 values greater than 50 (50–100) ensure sameness or equivalence of the two curves and, thus, of the performance of the test (postchange) and reference (prechange) products. Note that to allow use of mean data, the percent coefficient of variation at the earlier time points (eg, 15 minutes) should not be more than 20%, and at other time points should not be more than 10%. If these criteria are not met, then other approaches such as multivariate approaches (refer to the dissolution guidance for details on these approaches) should be used to determine similarity. In addition, dissolution profile comparisons are not applicable from statistical perspective when the release characteristics are very fast achieving greater than 85% in 15 minutes.

MEETING DISSOLUTION REQUIREMENTS

According to the Code of Federal Regulations (CFR), a drug product application should include the specifications necessary to ensure the identity, strength, quality, purity, potency, and bioavailability of the drug product, including, and acceptance criteria relating to, dissolution rate in the case of solid dosage forms. For the selection of the dissolution acceptance criteria, the following points should be considered:

1. The dissolution profile data from the pivotal clinical batches and primary (registration) stability batches should be used for the setting of the dissolution acceptance criteria of your product (ie, specification-sampling time point and specification value). A significant trend in the change in dissolution profile during stability should be justified with dissolution profile comparisons and *in vivo* data in those instances where the similarity testing fails.

2. Specifications should be established based on average *in vitro* dissolution data for each lot under study, equivalent to USP Stage 2 testing ($n = 12$).

3. For immediate-release formulations, the last time point should be the time point where at least 80% of drug has been released. If the maximum amount released is less than 80%, the last time point should be the time when the plateau of the release profile has been reached. Percent release of less than 80% should be justified with data (eg, sink conditions information).

4. For extended-release formulations, a minimum of three time points is recommended to set the specifications. These time points should cover the early, middle, and late stages of the release profile. The last time point should be the time point where at least 80% of drug has been released. If the maximum amount released is less than 80%, the last time point should be the time when the plateau of the release profile has been reached.

5. The dissolution acceptance criterion should be set in a way to ensure consistent performance from lot to lot, and this criterion should not allow the release of any lots with dissolution profiles outside those that were studied clinically.

The term Q means the amount of drug dissolved within a given time period established in the drug product specification table and is expressed as a percentage of label content. For example, a value of $Q = 80\%$ at 30 minutes means that the mean percent dissolved of 12 units individually tested is at least 80% at the selected time point of 30 minutes. Note that when implementing dissolution as a quality control tool for batch release and stability analysis, the testing should follow the recommendations listed in the USP method <711> for immediate-release dosage forms and <724> for modified-release dosage forms. For example, for Stage 1, which considers the testing of 6 units, each unit must meet the criterion of not less than 85% at 30 minutes for a drug product whose acceptance criterion was set to $Q = 80\%$ at 30 minutes. Testing should continue through the three stages (S_1, S_2, S_3) unless the results conform at either Stage 1 or Stage 2 (Table 15-9).

TABLE 15-9 Theophylline Extended-Release Capsules, USP

Test 1	
Time (h)	**Amount Dissolved**
1	Between 10% and 30%
2	Between 30% and 55%
4	Between 55% and 80%
8	Not less than 80%
Test 2	
Time (h)	**Amount Dissolved**
1	Between 3% and 15%
2	Between 20% and 40%
4	Between 50% and 75%
6	Between 65% and 100%
8	Not less than 80%

Both of these theophylline ER capsule products are for products labeled for dosing every 12 h. These products are bioequivalent *in vivo* and are approved by FDA as therapeutic equivalents.

The USP-NF monographs may have multiple dissolution tests for generic drug products that are approved by the FDA as therapeutic equivalents. Although both the brand and approved generic drug products are bioequivalent, their *in vitro* dissolution profiles may be different. Ideally, both methods should have very similar discriminating ability; however, this can only be determined when an IVIVR or an IVIVC has been established for the drug products rending the method not only discriminating but also predictive of *in vivo* performance.

PROBLEMS OF VARIABLE CONTROL IN DISSOLUTION TESTING

As described above, various equipment and operating variables are associated with dissolution testing. Understating the effects of operating conditions, the hydrodynamics and the geometric variables on the velocity distribution in the dissolution system are critical to enhance the reliability of dissolution testing and to avoid product recalls.

Dissolution testing is a complex process involving various steps such as solid–liquid mass transfer, particle erosion, possible particle disintegration, particle suspension, and particle–liquid interactions. However, this process is further complicated by other factors such as shear stress distribution as a function of tablet location within the apparatus, and the location of the tablet upon its release inside the apparatus.

Depending on the particular dosage form involved, the variables may or may not exert a pronounced effect on the rate of dissolution of the drug or drug product. Variations may occur with the same type of equipment and procedure. The centering and alignment of the paddle is critical in the paddle method. Turbulence can create increased agitation, resulting in a higher dissolution rate. Wobbling and tilting due to worn equipment should be avoided. The basket method is less sensitive to the tilting effect. However, the basket method is more sensitive to clogging due to gummy materials. Pieces of small particles can also clog up the basket screen and create a local nonsink condition for dissolution. Furthermore, dissolved gas in the medium may form air bubbles on the surface of the dosage form unit and can affect dissolution in both the basket and paddle methods.

Several published articles are available describing high variability in dissolution results, due to hydrodynamic effects, unpredictability, and randomness of observed results even for dissolution apparatus calibrator tablets (Bocanegra et al, 1990; Gray and Hubert, 1994; Achanta et al, 1995; Qureshi and McGilveray, 1999). Small variations in the location of the tablet on the vessel bottom caused by the randomness of the tablet descent through the liquid are likely to result in significantly different velocities and velocity gradients near the tablet (Armenante and Muzzio, 2005). Experiments were conducted using USP paddle apparatus by placing (aligned to the walls) a metal strip (1.7 mm thick × 6.4 mm wide) to evaluate the effect of variable mixing/stirring and flow pattern in a drug dissolution vessel. The majority of products evaluated gave significantly higher dissolution results with vessels containing metal strip than without. The extent of increased dissolution with the metal strip varied from products indicating that, employing the current apparatuses, products may provide lower-than-anticipated results that may not be reflective of the product drug release characteristics (Qureshi and Shabnam, 2001).

PERFORMANCE OF DRUG PRODUCTS: *IN VITRO–IN VIVO* CORRELATION

For controlled-release or extended-release formulation, since dissolution or release of the drug from the formulation is the rate-limiting step in the appearance of the drug into the systemic circulation, it is possible to establish a relationship between the release of the drug *in vitro* and its release *in vivo* or its absorption into the systemic circulation. If such correlation exists, then one is able to predict the plasma concentration time profile of a drug from its *in vitro* dissolution. Usually such a correlation is developed with two or more formulations with different release characteristics. It is recommended that a correlation be established with three or more formulations. However, if the dissolution of the drug is independent of the dissolution conditions (such as apparatus agitation rate, pH, etc), then it is possible to establish such a correlation with only one formulation. The establishment of a predictive IVIVC not only provides you with a better understanding of the release properties of the drug product but also enables one to decrease the number of *in vivo* studies needed to approve and maintain a drug product on the market resulting in an economic benefit as well as a decreased regulatory burden. It also enables one to set clinically meaningful dissolution specifications based on the predicted plasma concentration time profile.

A meaningful and predictive IVIVC is a correlation that is able to predict the C_{max} and AUC within 20% (FDA guidance for industry, 1997b). There are two ways in evaluating the predictability of the correlation: (1) Internal predictability refers to the ability to predict the pharmacokinetic profile of the formulations that were used to develop the correlation; (2) external predictability refers to the ability to detect the profile of a lot or formulation that was not used to develop the IVIVC. In the United States and in Europe, a bioequivalence study can be waived based on the IVIVC if the predicted mean AUC and C_{max} of the test and reference do not differ from each other by more than 20% (US IVIVC guidance for industry; EMA, August 2012).

Categories of *In Vitro–In Vivo* Correlations
Level A Correlation

Level A correlation is the highest level of correlation and represents a point-to-point (1:1) relationship between an *in vitro* dissolution and the *in vivo* input rate of the drug from the dosage form. Level A correlation compares the percent (%) drug released versus percent (%) drug absorbed. Generally, the percentage of drug absorbed may be calculated by the Wagner–Nelson or Loo–Riegelman procedures (see Chapter 8) or by direct mathematical deconvolution, a process of mathematical resolution of blood level into an input (absorption) and an output (disposition) component (Fig. 15-13).

The major advantage of a Level A correlation is that a point-to-point correlation is developed. All *in vitro* dissolution data and all *in vivo* plasma drug concentration–time profile data are used. Once a Level A correlation is established, an *in vitro* dissolution profile can serve as a surrogate for *in vivo* performance. A change in manufacturing site, method of manufacture, raw material supplies, minor

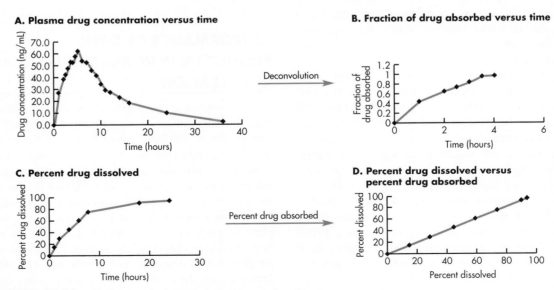

FIGURE 15-13   Deconvolution of plasma drug concentration–time curve.

formulation modification, and even product strength using the same formulation can be justified without the need for additional human studies. Level A correlation enables the *in vitro* dissolution test to become meaningful and clinically relevant quality control test that can predict *in vivo* drug product performance.

Level B Correlation

Level B correlation utilizes the principle of statistical moment (see Chapter 25) in which the mean *in vitro* dissolution time is compared to either the mean residence time (MRT)[2] or the mean *in vivo* dissolution time (MDT). Level B correlation uses all of the *in vitro* and *in vivo* data, but is not a point-to-point correlation. Different profiles can give the same parameter values. The Level B correlation alone cannot justify formulation modification, manufacturing site change, excipient source change, batch-to-batch quality, etc.

Level C Correlation

A Level C correlation is not a point-to-point correlation. A Level C correlation establishes a single-point relationship between a dissolution parameter such as percent dissolved at a given time and a pharmacokinetic parameter of interest such as AUC and C_{max}. Level C correlation is useful for formulation selection and development but has limited application. *Multiple Level C correlation* relates one or several pharmacokinetic parameters of interest to the amount of drug dissolved at several time points of the dissolution profile. In general, if one is able to develop a multiple Level C correlation, then it may be feasible to develop a Level A correlation. Several examples of Level C correlation are given below.

Dissolution rate versus absorption rate. If dissolution of the drug is rate limiting, a faster dissolution rate may result in a faster rate of appearance of the drug in the plasma. It may be possible to establish a correlation between rate of dissolution and rate of absorption of the drug.

The absorption rate is usually more difficult to determine than peak absorption time. Therefore, the absorption time may be used in correlating dissolution data to absorption data. In the analysis of *in vitro–in vivo* drug correlation, rapid drug dissolution may be distinguished from the slower drug absorption by observation of the absorption time for the preparation. The absorption time refers to the time for a constant amount of drug to be absorbed. In one study involving three sustained-release aspirin products (Levy et al, 1965), the dissolution times for the preparations were linearly correlated to the absorption times (Fig. 15-14). The results from this study demonstrated that aspirin was rapidly absorbed and was very much dependent on the dissolution rate for absorption.

Percent of drug dissolved versus percent of drug absorbed. If a drug is absorbed completely after dissolution, a linear correlation may be obtained by comparing the percentage of drug absorbed to the percentage of drug dissolved. In choosing the dissolution method, one must consider the appropriate dissolution medium and use a slow dissolution stirring rate so that *in vivo* dissolution is approximated.

Aspirin is absorbed rapidly, and a slight change in formulation may be reflected in a change in the

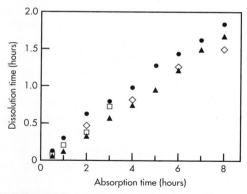

FIGURE 15-14   An example of correlation between time required for a given amount of drug to be absorbed and time required for the same amount of drug to be dissolved *in vitro* for three sustained-release aspirin products. (From Wood, 1966, with permission.)

---

[2]MRT is the mean (average) time that the drug molecules stay in the body, whereas the MDT is the mean time for drug dissolution.

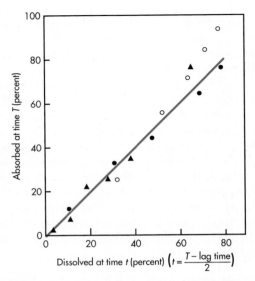

FIGURE 15-15   An example of continuous *in vivo–in vitro* correlation of aspirin. (From Levy et al, 1965, with permission.)

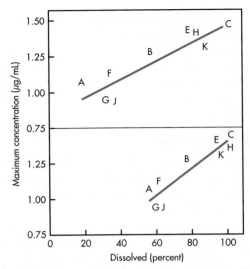

FIGURE 15-16   *In vitro–in vivo* correlation between C_{max} and percent drug dissolved. A, 30 min (slope = 0.06, r = 0.902, $p < 0.001$). B, 60 min (slope = 0.10, r = 0.940, $p < 0.001$). (Letters on graph indicate different products.) (From Shah et al, 1983, with permission.)

amount and rate of drug absorption during the period of observation (see Figs. 15-14 and 15-15). If the drug is absorbed slowly, which occurs when absorption is the rate-limiting step, a difference in dissolution rate of the product may not be observed. In this case, the drug would be absorbed very slowly independent of the dissolution rate.

Maximum plasma concentrations versus percent of drug dissolved *in vitro*. When different drug formulations are studied for dissolution, a poorly formulated drug may not be completely dissolved and released, resulting in lower plasma drug concentrations. The percentage of drug released at any time interval will be greater for the more bioavailable drug product. When such drug products are studied *in vivo*, the peak drug serum concentration will be higher for the drug product that shows the highest percent of drug dissolved. An example of *in vitro–in vivo* correlation for 100-mg phenytoin sodium capsules is shown in Fig. 15-16. Several products were tested (Shah et al, 1983). A linear correlation was observed between the maximum drug concentration in the body and the percent of drug dissolved *in vitro*.

The dissolution study on the phenytoin sodium products (Shah et al, 1983) showed that the fastest dissolution rate was product C, for which about 100% of the labeled contents dissolved in the test (Fig. 15-17). Interestingly, these products also show the shortest time to reach peak concentration (t_{max}). The t_{max} is dependent on the absorption rate constant.

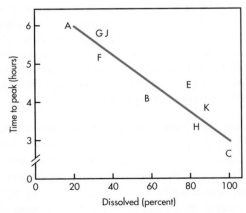

FIGURE 15-17   *In vitro–in vivo* correlation between t_{max} and percent drug dissolved in 30 minutes by basket method. Letters on graph indicate different products. (From Shah et al, 1983, with permission.)

In this case, the fastest absorption would also result in the shortest t_{max}.

Serum drug concentration versus percent of drug dissolved.

In a study on aspirin absorption, the serum concentration of aspirin was correlated to the percent of drug dissolved using an *in vitro* dissolution method (Wood, 1966). The dissolution medium was simulated gastric juice. Because aspirin is rapidly absorbed from the stomach, the dissolution of the drug is the rate-limiting step, and various formulations with different dissolution rates will cause differences in the serum concentration of aspirin by minutes (Fig. 15-18).

Biopharmaceutic Drug Classification System

The biopharmaceutic drug classification system, BCS, discussed more fully in Chapter 16, is a predictive approach to relate certain physicochemical characteristics of a drug substance and drug product to *in vivo* bioavailability. The BCS is not a direct *in vitro*–*in vivo* correlation. For example, the drug substance from an immediate-release (IR) oral drug product would tend to be rapidly and mostly absorbed if the drug substance and drug product meet the criteria for BCS Class I drugs. A BCS Class I drug product contains a highly soluble drug substance that is highly permeable and from which the drug rapidly dissolves from the drug product over the physiologic pH range of 1–7.4. Highly permeable drugs are drugs whose absolute bioavailability is greater than 90%. It is to be noted that the BCS only applies to oral immediate-release formulations and cannot be applied to modified-release formulations or for buccally absorbed drug products (FDA Guidance for Industry, August 2000).

APPROACHES TO ESTABLISH CLINICALLY RELEVANT DRUG PRODUCT SPECIFICATIONS

Establishing the appropriate product specifications is critical in assuring that the manufacture of the dosage form is consistent and successful throughout the product's life cycle. Product specifications are typically considered as those limits that define adequate quality and that support the *in vitro* determinations of identity, purity, potency, and strength of the drug product. On the other hand, clinically relevant specifications are those specifications that, in addition, take into consideration the clinical impact assuring consistent safety and efficacy profile. In this case, the choice of acceptance criteria is no longer made based on the *in vitro* results but on predetermined clinical acceptable outcomes. Understanding the relationship between the *in vitro* measures and the clinical outcomes may provide flexibility in setting specifications.

How are clinically relevant specifications set? The ideal approach would be to adopt the *quality by design* (QbD) approach in the drug development process. This approach should include the understanding of the *critical quality attributes* (CQA) and interactions and the impact that these may have on the *quality target product profile* (QTPP). Under the QbD paradigm it is assumed that all the batches manufactured within the *design space* (DS) have the same *in vivo* performance, in such a way that once the DS is verified, no studies are needed for movements within the DS. The key question arises as: How do we achieve the goal of demonstrating that all the batches within

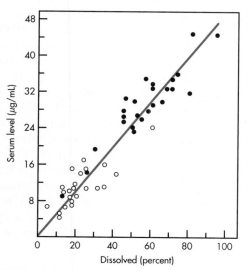

FIGURE 15-18 Example of *in vivo–in vitro* two-point correlation between 10-minute serum level and percent dissolved at 1.2 minutes (○) and the 20-minute serum level and percent dissolved at 4.2 minutes (●). (From Wood, 1966, with permission.)

the DS have the same *in vivo* performance? In answering this question the use of biopharmaceutic tools such as dissolution and BA/BE studies become relevant because it would be rather impractical to determine the clinical relevance of movements within the DS through clinical efficacy and safety trials.

As such, one approach to establishing clinically relevant drug product specifications may be to manufacture several product variants with different dissolution characteristics resulting in markedly different plasma concentration versus time profiles. In so doing, one can also (a) assess the impact of changes in various product attributes or process parameters on *in vitro* dissolution and *in vivo* performance, (b) explore relationship between *in vitro* dissolution and *in vivo* bioavailability, and (c) determine relative bioavailability or bioequivalence among product variants, using clinical trial material as a reference. Consequently, this approach not only facilitates the identification of the *critical material attributes* (CMA) and *critical process parameters* (CPP) but also facilitates establishing clinically relevant drug product specifications. This understanding helps in defining and verifying the DS limits, which links the important *in vitro* performance of the drug product to the desired clinical performance.

Due to the critical role that dissolution plays in defining the bioavailability of the drug, *in vitro* dissolution, if identified as a CQA, can serve as a relevant predictor of the *in vivo* performance of the drug product. In this case, clinically meaningful dissolution method and specifications will minimize the variability to the patient and therefore will optimize drug therapy.

There are several general approaches that can be used for determining clinically relevant dissolution specifications, depending on whether *in vivo* data (ie, systemic exposure) are available (Suarez-Sharp, 2011a, 2011b, 2012).

Approach A: Data linking *in vitro* and *in vivo* performance are NOT available.

In this approach, although there is PK and efficacy and safety data for the relevant phases of product development, no relationship has been established linking variations on the CMAs, and CPPs, and dissolution on clinical performance. Therefore, drug product specifications (ie, dissolution acceptance criterion) are established

based on the mean dissolution values of batches tested in pivotal clinical trials. Any major changes implemented to a pivotal clinical trial formulation need to be supported by additional BA/BE studies since dissolution can only support the implementation of minor changes.

It is widely accepted that minor changes can be evaluated by dissolution profile comparisons and they would have no or minimal effect on the bioavailability and consequently the safety and efficacy profile; however, there may be the case when certain minor apparent changes may have an *in vivo* impact and the assessment of the impact on clinical performance depends on the discriminating ability of the method (ie, established using data from DOE studies). These limitations make this approach less desirable.

Approach B: Data linking *in vitro* and *in vivo* performance ARE available.

In this case, studies have been carried out to determine whether changing the CMAs or CPPs have an effect on dissolution and systemic exposure. The *in vitro–in vivo* assessment (IVIVA) process often involves the following steps: (a) Prepare product variants using critical formulation and/or manufacturing variables to study their *in vitro* dissolution characteristics, (b) develop a discriminating dissolution method, (c) conduct *in vivo* pharmacokinetic study(ies) in appropriate groups of human subjects to test these product variants along with a reference standard (ie, the formulation used in pivotal Phase 3 clinical trials), (d) identify the products exhibiting the fastest and slowest dissolution characteristics, and (e) evaluate relative bioavailability and/or bioequivalence of the product variants and determine if an IVIVC or an IVIVR (eg, established by determining whether the drug product variants with extreme dissolution profiles are bioequivalent) can be established for the drug products under study. In general, data analysis from these approaches will result in one of the following outcomes:

Sub-Approach B1: An IVIVR Has Been Established. In those cases where an IVIVC has been attempted but cannot be established, an IVIVR should be investigated as this would provide some leeway and support for further drug product formulation refinement. While an IVIVR is not as robust as an IVIVC, it can be an important tool in the QbD approach to formulation development and justification. For example, verification of the DS and the clinical relevancy of the specifications for material attributes and process parameters can still be determined in the absence of an IVIVC; however, clinical relevancy can only be assured for those changes whose dissolution profiles fall within the extremes of dissolution profiles for batches that were bioequivalent to the clinical trial formulation.

Figure 15-19 illustrates the advantage of this approach over approach A. This figure shows the relationship between drug substance particle size, dissolution, and BE. Under approach A with batch D failing similarity testing (ie, f_2 testing) and in the absence of BA/BE data, the appropriate specification was set at $Q = 80\%$ at 15 minutes in order to reject batch D. However, for this particle case there was actually a BE study showing that all the batches considered were BE to the clinical batch. Under these conditions, one can then set an acceptance criterion that does not reject this batch, which in this case is

$Q = 80\%$ at 20 minutes. Setting a wider dissolution acceptance criterion based on *in vivo* data allows for the setting of wider particle size specifications determined in this particular case, on the slowest releasing batch that is BE to the clinical batch.

A small variation to this approach as described above would be to use data from an *in vivo* BA/BE study where at least two formulation variants have been evaluated and determine whether the dissolution method and acceptance criterion are able to reject for batches that are not bioequivalent. As explained above, when this happens the method and acceptance criteria may be considered clinically relevant.

Sub-Approach B2: An IVIVC Has Been Established. This is the most desirable approach for setting clinically relevant product specifications, including dissolution acceptance criteria. It may be challenging to develop an IVIVC for IR products as compared to extended-release dosage forms. Since the mechanisms for release of drug from IR dosage forms is simpler than that for modified-release dosage forms, one might expect that an IVIVC would be easier to develop with IR formulations. However, mainly Level C correlation for IR products have been successful and useful in guiding

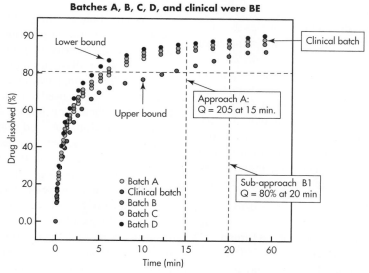

FIGURE 15-19   Setting clinically relevant dissolution acceptance criterion. The advantage of approach A versus sub-approach B1.

drug product development and the identification of critical process parameters and material attributes affecting product performance such as dissolution (see IVIVC section on how to set appropriate dissolution specifications for these dosage forms using an IVIVC).

A properly validated IVIVC enhances drug product understanding and provides justification of manufacturing changes during drug product development. It enhances the significance of the *in vitro* testing leading to drug product specifications' (eg, dissolution acceptance criteria) setting based on targeted clinically relevant plasma concentrations. In addition, it allows for the prediction of the clinical impact of movements within the DS without the need for additional *in vivo* studies.

Failure of Correlation of *In Vitro* Dissolution to *In Vivo* Absorption

A robust IVIVC should demonstrate its ability to predict the *in vivo* performance of a drug product from its *in vitro* dissolution characteristics over the range of *in vitro* release rates evaluated during the construction and validation of the correlation. Well-defined IVIVCs have been reported for modified-release drug products (see Chapter 19) but have been more difficult to predict for IR drug products. The success for establishing a robust IVIVC depends on several factors including (1) the selection of a discriminating dissolution method that mimics the drug product's *in vivo* performance; (2) the number of formulations used in the construction of the correlation; (3) inclusion of formulation with significant different release characteristics as demonstrated by dissolution similarity test; (4) design of the *in vivo* BA/BE study (eg, fast vs. feed conditions); (5) modeling approach (mechanistic vs. not mechanistic), etc. The following is a list of the most common reasons (besides not meeting the validation requirements) for a lack of successful IVIVCs (Suarez-Sharp, 2012):

1. Failing to meet the criteria for *in vitro* and *in vivo* experimentation in terms of the number of *in vitro* release characteristics of the formulations used in the construction of the IVIVC. Differences in *in vitro* release rate may be verified by conducting a similarity test. A failed similarity test is an indication of a significant difference in the *in vitro* release rate.

2. Lack of a rank order correlation.

3. Gut wall metabolism that can affect the bioavailability of the drug.

4. Instability of the drug in the GI tract.

5. The IVIVC should be developed in the fasted state and only in fed conditions when the drug is not tolerated.

6. The use of mean-based deconvolution instead of individual-based deconvolution in the case of a two-stage approach correlation.

7. The IVIVC was over-parameterized and not fully mechanistic.

8. Complex absorption processes were not captured by the model.

9. The use of different scaling factors for the formulations.

10. When it comes to the applicability of the IVIVC (eg, postapproval changes, support of wider dissolution acceptance criteria), similarity test (eg, f_2 testing) is often used instead of IVIVC predictions. It should be noted that IVIVC supersedes similarly testing in such a way that when an IVIVC is approved, the data that should be included to support the change should be the difference in predicted means for C_{max} and AUC.

As noted above, the problem of no correlation between systemic exposure and dissolution may be due to the complexity of drug absorption and the weakness of the dissolution method. The use of the so-called "physiologically relevant *in vitro* release approaches" can be used to understand the effects of formulation factors on release (dispersion, dissolution, drug precipitation, and stability), and the interactions between active pharmaceutical ingredients, dosage form, excipients, and the *in vivo* environment. These "physiologically relevant dissolution approaches" may increase the likelihood for the development of successful IVIVCs.

"Physiologically relevant approaches" can range from using physiologically relevant media in standard dissolution apparatus as stated in the guidance for industry documents (FDA Guidance for Industry,

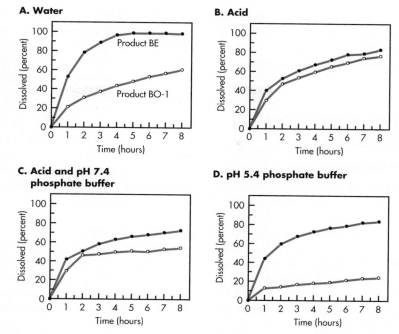

FIGURE 15-20 Dissolution profile of two quinidine gluconate sustained-release products in different dissolution media. Each data point is the mean of 12 tablets. f(● = product BE, ○ = product BO-1.) (Data from Prasad et al, 1983.)

1997a) to more complicated media to mimic *in vivo* conditions such as food effects and alcohol dose dumping (Klein, 2010). Note, however, that successful IVIVCs have been possible when simple dissolution methods are used (Suarez-Sharp, 2012).

An excellent example of the importance of dissolution design is shown in Fig. 15-20. Dissolution tests using four different dissolution media were performed for two quinidine gluconate sustained-release tablets (Prasad et al, 1983). Brand BE was known to be bioavailable, whereas product BO-1 was known to be incompletely absorbed. It is interesting to see that using acid medium as well as acid followed by pH 7.4 buffer did not distinguish the two products well, whereas using water or pH 5.4 buffer as dissolution medium clearly distinguished the "good" product from the one that was not completely available. In this case, the use of an acid medium is consistent with the physiologic condition in the stomach, but this procedure would be misleading as a quality control tool. It is important that any new

dissolution test be carefully researched before being adopted as a method for predicting drug absorption.

DRUG PRODUCT STABILITY

The long-term stability of any drug product is a critical attribute of overall product quality, given that it defines the time period for which product quality, safety, and effectiveness are assured. Product stability is usually determined by testing a variety of stability indicating attributes such as drug potency, impurities, dissolution, and other relevant physicochemical measures of performance as necessary.

Stability studies are generally performed under well-controlled storage and testing conditions and provide evidence on how the quality of a drug product varies with time under the influence of a variety of environmental factors such as temperature, humidity, oxygen, and light. The time period during which a drug product is expected to remain within the established product quality specification under the labeled storage conditions is generally termed "*shelf-life*"; however, this term is often used interchangeably with expiration period, expiry date, or expiration date.

CONSIDERATIONS IN THE DESIGN OF A DRUG PRODUCT

Biopharmaceutic Considerations

As mentioned above, biopharmaceutics is the study of the manufacturing factors and physicochemical properties influencing the rate and extent of drug absorption from the site of administration of a drug and the use of this information to (1) anticipate potential clinical problems arising from poor absorption of a candidate drug and (2) optimize bioavailability of newly developed compounds. Some of the major biopharmaceutic considerations in the design of a drug product are given in Table 15-10.

The essential elements of the biopharmaceutical considerations in drug product design include (Kaplan, 1972) (1) studies done to decide the physicochemical nature of the drug to be used, for example, salt and particle size; (2) the timing of these studies in relation to the preclinical studies with the drug; (3) the determination of the solubility and dissolution characteristics; (4) the evaluation of drug absorption and physiological disposition studies; and (4) the design and evaluation of the final drug formulation.

TABLE 15-10   Dissolution Acceptance

Stage	Number Tested	Acceptance Criteria
S_1	6	Each unit is not less than $Q + 5\%$
S_2	6	Average of 12 units ($S_1 + S_2$) is equal to or greater than Q, and no unit is less than $Q - 15\%$
S_3	12	Average of 24 units ($S_1 + S_2 + S_3$) is equal to or greater than Q, not more than 2 units are less than $Q - 15\%$, and no unit is less than $Q - 25\%$

Adapted with permission from *United States Pharmacopeia*, 2004.

The drug product must effectively deliver the active drug at an appropriate rate and amount to the target receptor site so that the intended therapeutic effect is achieved. To achieve this goal, the drug must traverse the required biological membrane barriers, escape widespread distribution to unwanted areas, endure metabolic attack, and cause an alteration of cellular function. The finished dosage form should not produce any additional side effects or discomfort due to the drug and/or excipients. Ideally, all excipients in the drug product should be pharmacologically inactive ingredients alone or in combination in the final dosage form.

The finished drug product is a compromise of various factors, including therapeutic objectives, pharmacokinetics, physical and chemical properties, manufacturing, cost, and patient acceptance. Most important, the finished drug product should meet the therapeutic objective by delivering the drug with maximum bioavailability and minimum adverse effects.

Pharmacodynamic Considerations

Pharmacodynamics is the study of the effect of a drug in the body and its mechanism of action. Therapeutic considerations include the desired pharmacodynamic and pharmacologic properties of the drug, including the desired therapeutic response and the type and frequency of adverse reactions to the drug. The therapeutic objective influences the design of the drug product, route of drug administration, dose, dosage regimen, and manufacturing process. An oral drug used to treat an acute illness is generally formulated to release the drug rapidly, allowing for quick absorption and rapid onset. If more rapid drug absorption is desired (or if oral absorption is not feasible for chemical, metabolic, or tolerability reasons), then an injectable drug formulation might be formulated. In the case of nitroglycerin, which is highly metabolized if swallowed, a sublingual tablet formulation allows for rapid absorption of the drug from the buccal area of the mouth for the treatment of angina pectoris.

In order to reduce unwanted systemic side effects, locally acting drugs such as inhaled drugs have been developed. The advantage of inhaled therapy for local action is that it is possible to deliver the drug directly into the lungs, reducing the amount needed to reach a therapeutic effect at the site of action and thereby reducing systemic side effects resulting in an improved benefit:risk ratio.

For the treatment of certain diseases, such as hypertension, chronic pain, etc, an extended- or controlled-release dosage form is preferred. The extended-release dosage form releases the drug slowly, thereby controlling the rate of drug absorption and allowing for more constant plasma drug concentrations. In some cases, an immediate-drug-release component is included in the extended-release dosage form to allow for both rapid onset followed by a slower sustained release of the drug, for example, zolpidem tartrate extended-release tablets (Ambien® CR tablets). Controlled-release and modified-release dosage forms are discussed in Chapter 19.

Drug Substance Considerations

The physicochemical properties of the drug substance (see Table 15-1) are major factors that are controlled or modified by the formulator. Important physicochemical properties include solubility, stability, chirality, polymorphs, solvate, hydrate, salt form, ionizable behavior, and impurity profile. These physicochemical properties influence the type of dosage form, the formulation, and the manufacturing process. Physical properties of the drug—such as intrinsic dissolution rate, particle size, and crystalline form—are influenced by methods of processing and manufacturing. If the drug has low aqueous solubility and an intravenous injection is desired, a soluble salt of the drug may be prepared. Chemical instability or chemical interactions with certain excipients will also affect the type of drug product and its method of fabrication. There are many creative approaches to improve the product; only a few are discussed in this chapter.

Pharmacokinetics of the Drug

Drug development is a laborious process that can be roughly grouped into the following five stages: (1) disease target identification, (2) target validation, (3) high-throughput identification of drug leads, (4) lead optimization, and (5) preclinical and clinical evaluation. Stages 3–5 mainly involve the characterization

of the pharmacokinetic properties, namely absorption, distribution, metabolism, and excretion (ADME), of the molecules being investigated as potential drug candidates. The data obtained from these studies allow the development of a dose(s) and dosage regimen that are age appropriate including avoidance of drug–drug interactions, food effect interactions, and achieving an appropriate drug release rate that will maintain a desired drug level in the body. Clinical failures of about 50% of the Investigational New Drug (IND) filings are attributed to their inadequate ADME attributes. It is, therefore, not surprising that the pharmaceutical industry is searching for ever more effective means to minimize this problem.

Building mathematical models (known as in silico screens) to reliably predict ADME attributes solely from molecular structure is at the heart of this effort in reducing costs as well as development cycle times (Gombar et al, 2003). Also, the integration of PK and PD allows for the characterization of the onset, intensity, and duration of the pharmacological effect of a drug and its interaction to the mechanism of action. In understanding the interrelationship of these two disciplines, light can be shed on situations where one or the other needs to be optimized in drug development. As such PK/PD modeling and simulation provides quantitative assessment of dose/exposure-response relationships with extensive applications at the early and late-stage drug development as well as during decision making.

Until recently, it is well known that there is a great degree of individual variation, called polymorphism in the genes coding for drug-metabolizing enzymes. The degree of polymorphism can significantly affect the drug metabolism and, therefore, the pharmacokinetics and the clinical outcome of the drug. Thus, variations in oxidation of some drugs have been attributed to genetic differences in certain CYP enzymes. Genetic polymorphisms of CYP2D6 and CYP2C19 enzymes are well characterized, and human populations of "extensive metabolizers" and "poor metabolizers" have been identified. Applying pharmacogenomics (eg, genomic biomarkers) into the drug development and clinical trial evaluation allows for the selection of an optimal group of patients to be enrolled into trials and reduce the number of adverse events. This will lead to more successful clinical trials and decrease the time to market for compounds.

Bioavailability of the Drug

Bioavailability is a pharmacokinetic term that describes the rate and extent to which the active drug ingredient is absorbed from a drug product and becomes available at the site of drug action. As such, bioavailability is concerned with how quickly (eg, when rapid onset of action is needed) and how much of a drug (since this represent the "effective dose") appears in the blood after a specific dose is administered. Given that the pharmacologic response is generally related to the concentration of drug at its site of action, the availability of a drug from a dosage form is a critical element of a drug product's clinical efficacy. However, most bioavailability studies involve the determination of drug concentration mainly in the plasma since it is rather difficult to measure the concentration at the site of action.

Before a systemically acting drug reaches the systemic circulation, the drug must be absorbed; however, before the drug is absorbed, the drug product must disintegrate and the drug substance must be dissolved and transferred across the gastrointestinal tract membrane into the systemic circulation. Therefore, any factors affecting these three processes such as psychochemical properties of the drug, formulation and manufacturing variables, physiological factors, drug–drug interactions, and food effect interactions will also affect bioavailability.

The stability of the drug in the gastrointestinal tract, including the stomach and intestine, is another consideration. Some drugs, such as penicillin G, are unstable in the acidic medium of the stomach. The addition of buffering in the formulation or the use of an enteric coating on the dosage form will protect the drug from degradation at a low pH.

Some drugs have poor bioavailability because of first-pass effects (presystemic elimination). If oral drug bioavailability is poor due to metabolism by enzymes in the gastrointestinal tract or in the liver, then a higher dose may be needed, as in the case of propranolol, or an alternative route of drug administration, as in the case of nitroglycerin. Incompletely absorbed drugs and drugs with highly variable bioavailability have a risk that, under unusual conditions (eg, change in diet or disease condition, drug–drug interaction), excessive drug bioavailability can occur leading to more intense pharmacodynamic activity and possible adverse events. If the drug is not absorbed after the oral route or a higher dose causes toxicity, then the drug must be given by an alternative route of administration, and a different dosage form such as a parenteral drug product might be needed.

Dose Considerations

Some patients experience unique differences from the regular adult population in pharmacokinetic parameters due to differences in metabolic background, renal clearance, weight, volume of distribution, age, and disease stage (eg, liver impairment, renal impairment) and, consequently, require individualized dosing. Therefore, the drug product must usually be available in several dose strengths to allow for individualized dosing and possibly dose titration. Some tablets are also scored for breaking, to potentially allow (as supported by appropriate data) the administration of fractional tablet doses.

The absence of an available pediatric dosage form for some medications increases the potential for dosing errors and may produce serious complications in this patient population. Congress enacted the *Pediatric Research Equity Act* (PREA) and other laws requiring drug companies to study their products in children under certain circumstances. When pediatric studies are necessary, they must be conducted with the same drug and for the same use for which they were approved in adults. Thus, specific dosing guidelines and useful dosage forms for pediatric patients are being developed in order to optimize therapeutic efficacy and limit, or prevent serious adverse side effects.

In the presence of renal or liver impairment, the drug metabolism or excretion process may be altered requiring smaller dose. For example, in case of renal insufficiency, phenobarbitone, which is mainly excreted by the kidneys, should be given in smaller dose, and in case of patients with liver impairment, morphine should be given in smaller dose.

The size and the shape of a solid oral drug product are designed for easy swallowing. The total size of a drug product is determined by the dose of the drug and any additional excipients needed to manufacture the desired dosage form. For oral dosage forms, if the recommended dose is large (1 g or more), then the patient may have difficulty in swallowing the drug product. For example, many patients may find a capsule-shaped tablet (caplet) easier to swallow than a large round tablet. Large or oddly shaped tablets, which may become lodged in the esophageal sphincter during swallowing, are generally not manufactured. Some esophageal injuries due to irritating drug lodged in the esophagus have been reported with potassium chloride tablets and other drugs. Older patients may have more difficulties in swallowing large tablets and capsules. Most of these swallowing difficulties may be overcome by taking the product with a large amount of fluid.

Dosing Frequency

Both the dose and the dosing frequency including the total daily dose should be considered when developing a therapeutic dosage regimen for a patient (see Chapter 22). The dose is the amount of drug taken at any one time. This can be expressed as the weight of drug (eg, 100 mg), volume of drug solution (eg, 5 mL, 5 drops), or some other quantity (eg, 2 puffs). The dosage regimen is the frequency at which the drug doses are given. Examples include two puffs twice a day, one capsule two times a day, etc. The total daily dose is calculated from the dose and the number of times per day the dose is taken.

The dosing frequency is in part determined by the clearance of the drug and the target plasma drug concentration. When the dosing frequency or interval is less than the half-life, $(t_{1/2})$, greater accumulation occurs, that is, steady-state levels are higher and there is less fluctuation. If the dosing interval is much greater than the half-life of the drug, then minimum concentration, $C_{p\ min}$, approaches zero. Under these conditions, no accumulation will occur and the plasma concentration–time profile will be the result of administration of a series of single doses.

As such if the drug has a short elimination half-life or rapid clearance from the body, the drug must be given more frequently or given in an extended-release drug product. Simplifying the medication dosing frequency could improve compliance markedly (Jin et al, 2008). Thus to minimize fluctuating plasma drug concentrations and improve patient compliance, an extended-release drug product may be preferred.

Patient Considerations

The drug product and therapeutic regimen must be acceptable to the patient. Poor patient compliance may result from poor product attributes, such as difficulty in swallowing, disagreeable odor, bitter medicine taste, or two frequent and/or unusual dosage requirements.

In recent years, creative packaging has allowed the patient to remove one tablet each day from a specially designed package so that the daily doses are not missed. Orally disintegrating tablets and chewable tablets allow the patient to typically take the medication without water. These innovations improve compliance. Of course, pharmacodynamic factors, such as side effects of the drug or an allergic reaction, also influence patient compliance.

Transmucosal (nasal) administration of antiepileptic drugs may be more convenient, easier to use, just as safe, and is more socially acceptable than rectal administration.

Route of Drug Administration

The route of drug administration (see Chapter 14) affects the rate and extent (bioavailability) of the drug, thereby affecting the onset, duration, and intensity of the pharmacologic effect (efficacy and safety). For intravenous (IV) delivery, the total dose of drug reaches the systemic circulation. However, drug delivery by other routes may result in only partial absorption, resulting in lower bioavailability. For example, following oral administration, a drug dissolves in the GI and then gets absorbed through the epithelial cells of the intestinal mucosa; however, this process may be affected by factors such as presence of food. In the design of a drug dosage form, the pharmaceutical manufacturer must consider (1) the intended route of administration; (2) the size of the dose;

(3) the anatomic and physiologic characteristics of the administration site, such as membrane permeability and blood flow; (4) the physicochemical properties of the site, such as pH, osmotic pressure, and presence of physiologic fluids; and (5) the interaction of the drug and dosage form at the administration site, including alteration of the administration site due to the drug and/or dosage form.

Although the pharmacodynamic activity of the drug at the receptor site is similar with different routes of administration, severe differences in the intensity of the pharmacodynamic response and the occurrence of adverse events may be observed. For example, isoproterenol has a thousandfold difference in activity when given orally or by IV injection. Figure 15-21 shows the change in heart rate due to isoproterenol with different routes of administration. Studies have shown that isoproterenol is metabolized in the gut and during passage through the liver (presystemic elimination or first-pass effects). The rate and types of metabolite formed are different depending on the routes of administration.

The use of novel drug delivery methods could enhance the efficacy and reduce the toxicity of antiepileptic drugs (AEDs). As such, slow-release oral forms of medication or depot drugs such as skin patches might improve compliance and, therefore, seizure control. In emergency situations, administration via rectal, nasal, or buccal mucosa can deliver the drug more quickly than can oral administration (Fisher and Ho, 2002).

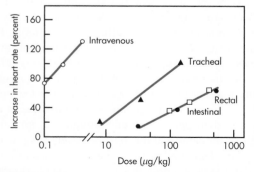

FIGURE 15-21   Dose–response curve to isoproterenol by various routes in dogs. (From Gillette and Mitchell, 1975, with permission.)

DRUG PRODUCT CONSIDERATIONS

Pharmaceutical development companies are looking at new approaches to deliver drugs safely and improve efficacy and patient compliance. Noninvasive systemic drug delivery such as oral, inhalation, intranasal, transdermal, etc are much more preferred compared to invasive drug delivery such as intramuscular, intravenous, and subcutaneous (Mathias and Hussain, 2010). Although the oral route of drug administration is preferred and is the most popular route of drug administration, alternate noninvasive systemic drug delivery is being considered for biotechnology-derived drugs (proteins), ease of self-administration (orally disintegrating tablets), or prolonged drug delivery (transdermal patch). The discussion below briefly describes some of the more popular drug products.

Oral Drug Products

Oral administration of drug products is the most common, convenient, and economic route. The major advantages of oral drug products are the convenience of administration, safety, and the elimination of discomforts involved with injections. The hazard of rapid intravenous administration causing toxic high concentration of drug in the blood is avoided. The main disadvantages of oral drug products are the potential issues of reduced, erratic, or incomplete bioavailability due to solubility, permeability, and/or stability problems. Unabsorbed drug may also alter the contents and microbiologic flora of the gastrointestinal tract. Some orally administered drugs may irritate the gastrointestinal linings causing nausea or gastrointestinal discomfort. Bioavailability may be altered by drug and food interactions and any pathology of the GI tract such as ulcerative colitis (see Chapter 14). The oral route is nevertheless problematic because of the unpredictable nature of gastrointestinal drug absorption due to factors such as the presence of food that may alter the gastrointestinal tract pH, gastric motility, and emptying time, as well as the rate and extent of drug absorption.

Highly ionized drug molecules are not absorbed easily. The ganglion-blocking drugs hexamethonium, pentolinium, and bretylium are ionized at intestinal pH. Therefore, they are not sufficiently absorbed orally to be effective systemically. Neomycin, gentamicin, and cefamandole are not well absorbed orally. Drugs with large molecular weights may not be well absorbed when given orally. The antibiotics neomycin and vancomycin are not absorbed after oral administration and are used for local antibacterial effect in the gastrointestinal tract. Some large molecules are absorbed when administered in solution with a surface-active agent. For example, cyclosporine has been given orally with good absorption when formulated with a surfactant in oil. A possible role of the oil is to stimulate the flow of lymph as well as to delay retention of the drug. Oily vehicles have been used to lengthen the gastrointestinal transit time of oral preparations.

Delivering proteins and peptides by the oral route has been a big challenge, given the lack of stability such as enzymatic degradation in the digestive system prior to absorption. Considerable progress has been made over past few years in developing innovative technologies for promoting absorption across GI and numbers of these approaches are demonstrating potential in clinical studies. In developing oral protein delivery systems with high bioavailability, three practical approaches might be most helpful (Morishita and Peppas, 2006): (1) modification of the physicochemical properties of macromolecules; (2) addition of novel function to macromolecules; or (3) use of improved delivery carriers. Chemical modification and use of mucoadhesive polymeric system for site-specific drug delivery seem to be promising candidates for protein and peptide drug delivery (Shaji and Patole, 2008). Also, nanoparticles with peptidic ligands are especially worthy of notice because they can be used for specific targeting in the gastrointestinal tract.

Absorption of Lipid-Soluble Drugs

Lipid solubility of drugs is a major factor affecting the extent of drug distribution, particularly to the brain, where the blood–brain barrier restricts the penetration of polar and ionized molecules. Inconsistently, drugs that are highly hydrophobic are also poorly absorbed, because they are poorly soluble in aqueous fluid and, therefore, cannot get to the surface of cells. For a drug to be readily absorbed, it must be mainly

hydrophobic, but have some solubility in aqueous solutions. This is one reason why many successfully developed drugs are weak acids or weak bases to begin with.

The most significant issue to consider when formulating poorly water-soluble drugs is the risk of precipitation in the lumen of the gastrointestinal tract. The *lipid formulation classification system* (LFCS) provides a simple framework that can be used, in combination with appropriate *in vitro* tests, to predict how the fate of a drug is likely to be affected by formulation, and to optimize the choice of lipid formulation for a particular drug (Puoton, 2006). Poorly water-soluble drug candidates present considerable formulation challenges. These drugs can be successfully formulated for oral administration. Some options available involve either reduction of particle size (of crystalline drug) or formulation of the drug in solution, as an amorphous system or lipid formulation (Puoton, 2006).

Lipophilic drugs are more soluble in lipids or oily vehicles. Lipid-soluble drugs given with fatty excipients mix with digested fatty acids, which are emulsified by bile in the small intestine. The emulsified drug is then absorbed through the GI mucosa or through the lymphatic system. A normal digestive function of the small intestine is the digestion and absorption of fats such as triglycerides. These fats are first hydrolyzed into monoglycerides and fatty acids by pancreatic lipase. The fatty acids then react with carrier lipoproteins to form chylomicrons, which are absorbed through the lymph. The chylomicrons eventually release the fatty acids, and any lipophilic drugs incorporated in the oil phase. Fat substances trigger receptors in the stomach to delay stomach emptying and reduce GI transit rates. Prolonged transit time allows more contact time for increased drug absorption.

When griseofulvin or phenytoin was given orally in corn oil suspensions, an increase in drug absorption was demonstrated (Bates and Equeira, 1975). The increase in absorption was attributed to the formation of mixed micelles with bile secretions, which aid drug dissolution. Hydrophobic drugs such as griseofulvin and metaxalone have greater bioavailability when given with a high-fat meal. A meal high in lipids will delay stomach emptying depending on the volume and nature of the oil. For example, the bioavailability of a water-insoluble antimalarial drug was increased in dogs when oleic acid was incorporated as part of a vehicle into a soft gelatin capsule (Stella et al, 1978). Calcium carbonate, a source of calcium for the body, was only about 30% available in a solid dosage form, but was almost 60% bioavailable when dispersed in a special vehicle as a soft gelatin capsule (Fordtran et al, 1986). Bleomycin, an anticancer drug (MW 1500), is poorly absorbed orally and therefore was formulated for absorption through the lymphatic system. The lymphotropic carrier was dextran sulfate. Bleomycin was linked by ionic bonds to the carrier to form a complex. The carrier dextran (MW 500,000) was too large to be absorbed through the membrane and pass into the lymphatic vessels (Yoshikawa et al, 1989).

Gastrointestinal Side Effects

Many orally administered drugs such as aspirin are irritating to the stomach. These drugs may cause nausea or stomach pain due to local irritation when taken on an empty stomach. In some cases, food or antacids may be given together with the drug to reduce stomach irritation. Alternatively, the drug may be enteric coated to reduce gastric irritation. Buffered aspirin tablets, enteric-coated aspirin tablets, and rapidly dissolving effervescent tablets and granules are available to minimize local gastric irritation. However, enteric coating may sometimes delay or reduce the amount of drug absorbed. Furthermore, enteric coating may not abolish gastric irritation completely, because the drug may occasionally be regurgitated back to the stomach after the coating dissolves in the intestine. Enteric-coated tablets may be greatly affected by the presence of food in the stomach. The drug may not be released from the stomach for several hours when stomach emptying is delayed by food.

Buffering material or antacid ingredients have also been used with aspirin to reduce stomach irritation. When a large amount of antacid or buffering material is included in the formulation, dissolution of aspirin may occur quickly, leading to reduced irritation to the stomach. However, many buffered aspirin formulations do not contain sufficient buffering material to make a difference in dissolution in the stomach.

It has been shown that acute aspirin-induced damage to the gastric mucosa can be reduced by chemically associating aspiring with the phospholipid, phosphatidylcholine (PC) and that the mechanism of mucosal protection provided by this compound is not related to any alteration in the ability of aspirin to inhibit mucosal COX activity (Bhupinderjit et al, 1999). Also, certain drugs have been formulated into soft gelatin capsules to improve drug bioavailability and reduce gastrointestinal side effects. If the drug is formulated in the soft gelatin capsule as a solution, the drug may disperse and dissolve more rapidly, leaving less residual drug in the gut and causing less irritation. This approach may be useful for a drug that causes local irritation but will be ineffective if the drug is inherently ulcerogenic. Indomethacin, for example, may cause ulceration in animals even when administered parenterally.

There are many options available to the formulator to improve the tolerance of the drug and minimize gastric irritation. The nature of excipients and the physical state of the drugs are important and must be carefully assessed before a drug product is formulated. Some excipients may improve the solubility of the drug and facilitate absorption, whereas others may physically adsorb the drug to reduce irritation. Often, a great number of formulations must be considered before an acceptable one is chosen.

Immediate-Release and Modified-Release Drug Products

The USP differentiates between an immediate-release (IR) drug product and a modified-release (MR) drug product. For the IR drug product, no deliberate effort has been made to modify the drug release rate. IR drug products disintegrate rapidly after administration. IR dosage forms release the active drug(s) within short time (eg, 80% of drug after 60 min). Applying particular formulation and process technologies, even faster drug release can be achieved. The basic approach used in development of tablets is the use of superdisintegrants like cross-linked crospovidone, sodium starch glycolate, carboxymethylcellulose, etc. These superdisintegrants provide instantaneous disintegration of tablets following oral administration.

For MR drug products, the pattern of drug release from the dosage form has been deliberately changed from that of a conventional (immediate-release) form of the drug. Types of MR drug products include delayed release (eg, enteric coated) and extended release (ER). ER formulations are designed to reduce dosing frequency for drugs with a short elimination half-life and duration of effect. These forms reduce the fluctuation in plasma drug concentration, providing a more uniform therapeutic effect while minimizing adverse effects. Absorption rate is slowed by different methods including coating drug particles with wax or other water-insoluble material, by embedding the drug in a matrix that releases it slowly during transit through the GI tract, or by complexing the drug with ion-exchange resins.

An ER oral dosage form should meet the following characteristics: (1) The BA profile established for the drug product rules out the occurrence of any dose dumping; (2) the drug product's steady-state performance is comparable (eg, degree of fluctuation is similar or lower) to a currently marketed noncontrolled release or controlled-release drug product that contains the same active drug ingredient or therapeutic moiety and that is subject to an approved full NDA; (3) the drug product's formulation provides consistent pharmacokinetic performance between individual dosage units; and (4) the drug product has a less frequent dosing interval compared to a currently marketed noncontrolled release drug product. Chapter 19 discusses MR drug products in more detail.

Buccal and Sublingual Tablets

A drug that diffuses and penetrates rapidly across mucosal membranes may be placed under the tongue and be rapidly absorbed. A tablet designed for release under the tongue is called a *sublingual tablet*. Nitroglycerin, isoproterenol, erythrityl tetranitrate, and isosorbide dinitrate are common examples. A tablet designed for release and absorption of the drug in the buccal (cheek) pouch is called a *buccal tablet*. The buccal cavity is the space between the mandibular arch and the oral mucosa, an area well supplied with blood vessels for efficient drug absorption.

Oral transmucosal absorption is generally rapid because of the rich vascular supply to the mucosa and the lack of a stratum corneum epidermis. This minimal barrier to drug transport results in a rapid rise in blood concentrations. Sublingual and buccal medications are compounded in the form of small, quick-dissolving tablets, sprays, lozenges, or liquid suspensions. A buccal tablet may be designed to release drug slowly for a prolonged effect. This form of drug product administration is very effective as it avoids first-pass metabolism by the liver before general distribution. Consequently, for a drug with significant first-pass effect, buccal/sublingual absorption may provide better bioavailability than oral administration and rapid unset of action as it may be absorbed in the blood stream in minutes.

For example, Sorbitrate sublingual tablet, Sorbitrate chewable tablet, and Sorbitrate oral tablet (Zeneca) are three different dosage forms of isosorbide dinitrate for the relief and prevention of angina pectoris. The sublingual tablet is a lactose formulation that dissolves rapidly under the tongue and is then absorbed. The chewable tablet is chewed, and some drug is absorbed in the buccal cavity; the oral tablet is simply a conventional product for GI absorption. The chewable tablet contains flavor, confectioner's sugar, and mannitol, which are absent in both the oral and sublingual tablets. The sublingual tablet contains lactose and starch for rapid dissolution. The onset of sublingual nitroglycerin is rapid, much faster than when nitroglycerin is taken orally or absorbed through the skin. The duration of action, however, is shorter than with the other two routes. Some peptide drugs have been reported to be absorbed by the buccal route, which provides a route of administration without the drug being destroyed by enzymes in the GI tract.

A newer approach to drug absorption from the oral cavity has been the development of a translingual nitroglycerin spray (Nitrolinqual Pumpspray). The spray, containing 0.4 mg per metered dose, is given by spraying one or two metered doses onto the oral mucosa at the onset of an acute angina attack.

Fentanyl citrate is a potent, lipid-soluble opioid agonist that crosses mucosal membranes rapidly. Fentanyl has been formulated as a transdermal drug product (Durapress®) and as an oral lozenge on a handle (Actiq®) containing fentanyl citrate for oral transmucosal delivery. According to the manufacturer, fentanyl bioavailability from Actiq is about 50%, representing a combination of rapid absorption across the oral mucosa and slower absorption through swallowing and transport across the gastrointestinal mucosa.

Colonic Drug Delivery

Drugs that are destroyed following oral administration by the acidic environment of the stomach or metabolized by enzymes may only be slightly affected in the colon. Oral drug products for colonic drug delivery have been studied not only for the delivery of drugs for the treatment of local diseases associated with the lower bowel and colon (eg, Crohn's disease) but also for their potential for the delivery of proteins and therapeutic peptides (eg, insulin) for systemic absorption (Chourasia and Jain, 2003; Shareef, et. al, 2003). Targeting drug delivery to the colon has several therapeutic advantages. Crohn's disease or chronic inflammatory colitis may be more effectively treated by direct drug delivery to the colon. For example, mesalamine (5-aminosalicylic acid, Asacol®) is available in a delayed-release tablet coated with an acrylic-based resin that delays the release of the drug until it reaches the distal ileum and beyond. Other approaches include prodrugs (sulfasalazine and balsalazine) to deliver 5-aminosalicylic acid (5-ASA) for localized chemotherapy of inflammatory bowel disease (IBD). Drugs containing an azo bond (balsalazide) and azo cross-linked polymers used as a coating are degraded by anaerobic microbes in the lower bowel.

Protein drugs are generally unstable in the acidic environment of the stomach and are also degraded by proteolytic enzymes present in the stomach and small intestine. Researchers are investigating the oral delivery of protein and peptide drugs by protecting them against enzymatic degradation for later release in the colon.

Drug delivery to the colon is highly influenced by several factors including high bacterial level, the physiology of the colonic environment, level of fluid, and transit time. Thus availability of most drugs to the absorptive membrane is low because of the high water absorption capacity of the colon, the colonic contents are considerably viscous, and their mixing is not efficient. The human colon has over 500 distinct species of bacteria as resident flora. Within the cecum and colon, anaerobic species dominate and bacterial counts of 10^{12}/mL have been reported. Among the reactions carried out by these gut flora are azoreduction and enzymatic cleavage, that is, glycosides. These metabolic processes may be responsible for the metabolism of many drugs and may also be applied to colon-targeted delivery of peptide-based macromolecules such as insulin by oral administration (Philip and Philip, 2010).

Drugs such as the beta-blockers, oxprenolol and metoprolol, and isosorbide-5-mononitrate, nonsteroidal anti-inflammatory drugs (NSAIDs), steroids, peptides, and vaccines are well absorbed in the colon, similar to absorption in the small intestine. Thus, these drugs are suitable candidates for colonic delivery. The NSAID naproxen has been formed into a prodrug naproxen–dextran that survives intestinal enzyme and intestinal absorption. The prodrug reaches the colon, where it is enzymatically decomposed into naproxen and dextran (Harboe et al, 1989).

Rectal and Vaginal Drug Delivery

Products for rectal or vaginal drug delivery may be administered in either solid or liquid dosage forms. Rectal drug administration can be used for either local or systemic drug delivery. Rectal drug delivery for systemic absorption is preferred for drugs that cannot be tolerated orally (eg, when a drug causes nausea) or in situations where the drug cannot be given orally (eg, during an epileptic attack). Rectal route offers potential advantages for drug delivery such as rapid absorption of many low-molecular-weight drugs, partial avoidance of first-pass metabolism, potential for absorption into the lymphatic system, retention of large volumes, rate-controlled drug delivery, and absorption enhancement (Lakshmi et al, 2012). However, this route also has some disadvantages as many drugs are poorly or erratically absorbed across the rectal mucosa, dissolution problems, and drug metabolism in microorganisms among other factors. Thus to overcome these, various absorption-enhancing adjuvants, surfactants, mixed micelle, and cyclodextrins have been investigated.

The rate of absorption from this route can be affected by several factors including formulation, concentration of drug, pH of the rectal content, presence of stools, volume of fluid, etc. A sustained-release preparation may be prepared for rectal administration. The rate of release of the drug from this preparation is dependent on the nature of the base composition and on the solubility of the drug involved.

Release of drug from a suppository depends on the composition of the suppository base. A water-soluble base, such as polyethylene glycol and glycerin, generally dissolves and releases the drug; on the other hand, an oleaginous base with a low melting point may melt at body temperature and release the drug. Some suppositories contain an emulsifying agent that keeps the fatty oil emulsified and the drug dissolved in it.

Vaginal drug delivery offers a valuable route for drug delivery through the use of specifically designed carrier systems for both local and systemic applications. A range of drug delivery platforms suitable for intravaginal administration have been developed such as intravaginal rings, vaginal tablets, creams, hydrogels, suppositories, and particulate systems.

For example, progesterone vaginal suppositories have been evaluated for the treatment of premenstrual symptoms of anxiety and irritability. Antifungal agents are often formulated into suppositories for treating vaginal infections. Fluconazole, a triazole antifungal agent, has been formulated to treat vulvovaginal candidiasis. The result of oral doses is comparable to that of a clotrimazole vaginal suppository. Many vaginal preparations are used for the delivery of antifungal agents.

The rate and extent of drug absorption after intravaginal administration may vary depending on formulation factors, age of the patient, vaginal physiology, and menstrual cycle. As such exhaustive efforts have been made recently to evaluate the vagina as a potential route for the delivery of molecules, such as proteins, peptides, small interfering RNAs, oligonucleotides, antigens, vaccines, and hormones. However, successful delivery of drugs through the vagina remains a challenge, primarily due to the poor absorption across the vaginal epithelium, cultural sensitivity, hygiene, personal, gender specificity, local irritation, and other factors that need to be addressed during the design of a vaginal formulation (Ashok et al, 2012).

Parenteral Drug Products

The parenteral route of administration refers to all forms of drugs administered via a syringe, needle, or catheter into body tissues or fluids such as intravenous, intra-arterial, intraosseous, intramuscular, subcutaneous, and intrathecal routes.

In general, intravenous (IV) bolus administration of a drug provides the most rapid onset of drug action. After IV bolus injection, the drug is distributed via the circulation to all parts of the body within a few minutes. After intramuscular (IM) injection, drug is absorbed from the injection site into the bloodstream (Fig. 15-22). Plasma drug input after oral and IM administration involves an absorption phase in which the drug concentration rises slowly to a peak and then declines according to the elimination half-life of the drug. (Note that the systemic elimination of all products is essentially similar; only the rate and extent of absorption may be modified by formulation.) The plasma drug level peaks instantaneously after an IV bolus injection, so a peak is usually not visible. After 3 hours, however, the plasma level of the drug after intravenous administration has declined

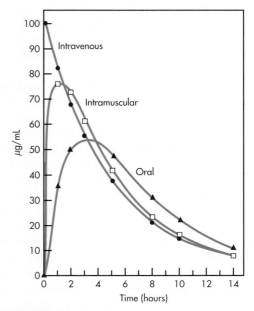

FIGURE 15-22   Plasma concentration of a drug after the same dose is administered by three different routes.

to a lower level than after the oral and intramuscular administration. In this example (see Fig. 15-22), the areas under the plasma curves are all approximately equal, indicating that the oral and intramuscular preparations are both well formulated and 100% available. Frequently, because of incomplete absorption or metabolism, oral preparations may have a lower area under the curve.

Drug absorption after an intramuscular injection may be faster or slower than after oral drug administration. Intramuscular preparations are generally injected into a muscle mass such as in the buttocks (gluteus muscle) or in the deltoid muscle. Drug absorption occurs as the drug diffuses from the muscle into the surrounding tissue fluid and then into the blood. Different muscle tissues have different blood flow. For example, blood flow to the deltoid muscle is higher than blood flow to the gluteus muscle. Intramuscular injections may be formulated to have a faster or slower drug release by changing the vehicle of the injection preparation. Aqueous solutions release drug more rapidly, and the drug is more rapidly absorbed from the injection site, whereas a viscous, oily, or suspension vehicle may result in a slow drug release and consequently slow and sustained drug absorption. Viscous vehicles generally slow down drug diffusion and distribution. A drug in an oily vehicle must partition into an aqueous phase before systemic absorption. A drug that is very soluble in oil and relatively insoluble in water may have a relatively long and sustained release from the absorption site because of slow partitioning.

Modified-release parenteral dosage forms have been developed in which the drug is entrapped or encapsulated into inert polymeric or lipophilic matrices that slowly release the drug *in vivo* over a week or up to several years (Patil and Burgess, 2010). The polymers or lipophilic carriers used to deliver the drugs in MR parenterals are either biodegradable *in vivo* or are nonbiodegradable. Nonerodible, nonbiodegradable systems are removed at the end of therapy. Drugs, including peptides and proteins, have also been formulated as emulsions, suspensions, liposomes, and nanoparticles for parenteral injection. A change in a parenteral drug product from a solution to an emulsion, liposome, etc will alter the drug's distribution and pharmacokinetic profile.

CLINICAL EXAMPLE

Hyperlipidemia is the medical term for high levels of cholesterol and triglycerides in the blood. Individuals with hyperlipidemia are predisposed to clogged blood vessels, or atherosclerosis, which puts them at a high risk for heart disease and stroke. Fenofibrate is the dimethyl ester prodrug of fenofibric acid, a lipid-modulating agent commonly used to treat hyperlipidemia. Fenofibrate is practically insoluble in water and it has the lowest and most variable bioavailability within the class of lipid-modulating fibrates (Najib, 2002). The drug is marketed in capsule or tablet dosage forms, and dissolution is most likely the rate-limiting step for oral absorption. Consequently, drug product design focused heavily on biopharmaceutic principles to improve the reliability and predictability of drug absorption from the initial 100-mg capsule formulation, previously marketed under the trade name Lipidil®. The bioavailability of the original 100-mg capsule formulation was first enhanced through micronization, or particle size reduction. Based on relative bioavailability studies, a 100-mg fenofibrate original capsule is bioequivalent to a 67-mg micronized fenofibrate capsule, Tricor® (fenofibrate capsules, micronized).

However, despite improved oral bioavailability, the Tricor micronized fenofibrate capsule formulation still demonstrated increased drug exposure when taken with food, up to 35%. Further particle size reduction through NanoCrystal® colloidal dispersion technology, and optimizing tableting excipients, led to a new reduced dose tablet that could be administered without regards to food, Tricor fenofibrate tablet. A 145-mg nanosized Tricor fenofibrate tablet is bioequivalent to the 200-mg micronized Tricor fenofibrate capsule (Tricor Package Insert, 2004).

A second formulation of fenofibric acid, the choline salt, was tailored based on the different physicochemical properties between the salt and free acid, and effects of modified-release excipients, to address the food effect and drug solubility challenges, Trilipix® fenofibric acid delayed-release capsules. Compared with fenofibrate, the choline salt form is freely water soluble and readily absorbed. Thus, through biopharmaceutic design considerations, researchers were able to develop a 135-mg fenofibric acid salt product with equivalent exposures to the 200-mg Tricor micronized capsule product that could be taken without regard to food (Trilipix Package Insert, 2008).

Nasal Drug Products

The nasal route of administration has been used for the delivery of drug products for both topical and systemic actions. A variety of different drug products such as antihistamines, corticosteroids, anticholinergics, and vasoconstrictors are currently being marketed for the local treatment of congestion, rhinitis, sinusitis, and related allergic or chronic conditions. Recently, increasing investigations of the nasal route have focused especially on nasal application for systemic drug delivery. The intranasal delivery of drugs for systemic action is aimed at optimizing drug bioavailability, given its large surface area, porous endothelial membrane, high total blood flow, and the avoidance of first-pass metabolism. Thus, peptides such as calcitonin and pituitary hormones have been successfully delivered through the nasal route. Intranasal delivery is also currently being marketed for treatments for migraine, smoking cessation, acute pain relief, osteoporosis, and vitamin B_{12} deficiency. In addition, MedImmune Inc. and Wyeth marketed the first intranasal vaccine in the United States: FluMist®.

Recently, the nasal route of administration has gained increasing consideration for obtaining systemic absorption or brain uptake of drugs. The delivery of drugs to the CNS from the nasal route may occur via olfactory neuroepithelium. Drug delivery through nasal route into CNS has been reported for Alzheimer's disease, brain tumors, epilepsy, pain, and sleep disorders (Pavan et al, 2008).

There are various factors that affect the systemic bioavailability of drugs that are administered through the nasal route (Kumari et al, 2013). These factors can be classified as follows:

1. Physiochemical properties of the drugs: lipophilic–hydrophilic balance, chemical form, polymorphism, enzymatic degradation in nasal cavity, molecular size, solubility, and dissolution rate
2. Delivery effect: formulation (concentration, pH, osmolarity), droplet/particle size distribution, viscosity
3. Nasal effect: mucociliary clearance, cold, rhinitis, membrane permeability, environmental pH, the anatomical and physiological

Nasal devices have progressively evolved from the pipettes and the droppers through to spraying devices such as squeeze bottles, toward, a nasal gel pump, pressurized metered dose inhalers (MDIs), and dry-powder inhalers (Djupesland, 2013). Drug development in the near future should not only rely on innovative new compounds and sophisticated formulations but also rely on the efficiency, safety, and comfort of the dispensing systems. The ideal nasal drug delivery system should have optimum performance (accurate and reproducible dose, narrow droplet/particle size distribution, in particular) and support patient compliance, thus contributing to the reduction in global health expenditure.

Certain studies should be performed to characterize the performance properties of the nasal drug product and to provide support in defining the optimal labeling statements regarding use. Delivery systems for nasal administration can vary in both design and mode of operation, and these characteristics may be unique to a particular drug product. Regardless of the design, the most crucial attributes are the reproducibility of the dose, the spray plume, and the particle/droplet size distribution, since these parameters can affect the delivery of the drug substance to the intended biological target. Studies to define these characteristics will help facilitate correct use and maintenance of the drug product and contribute to patient compliance. For the most part, these should be one-time studies, preferably performed on multiple batches (eg, two or three) of drug product representative of the product intended for distribution (FDA Guidance for Industry, 2002).

The concept of classical bioequivalence and bioavailability may not be applicable for all nasal drug products specially those for local action. In addition, the doses administered are typically so small that blood or serum concentrations may not be detectable by routine analytical procedures. Therefore, for locally acting drug product, major manufacturing changes may require the need for clinical trials.

Inhalation Drug Products

Localized drug delivery to the lungs is an important and effective therapeutic method for treating a variety of pulmonary disorders including asthma, bronchitis, and cystic fibrosis. The advantages of inhalation therapy for the treatment of lung disorders are the following: (1) Relatively small doses are needed for effective therapy, reducing exposure of drug to the systemic circulation, and potentially minimizes adverse effects; (2) wide surface area for absorption and relatively low metabolic activity of the lungs; (3) the lungs provide substantially greater bioavailability for macromolecules than any other port of entry to the systemic circulation.

The therapeutic effect for locally acting inhaled drugs and the duration of this effect are determined mainly by the dose deposited at the site of action and its pulmonary clearance. In turn, drug distribution and deposition along the respiratory tract (RT) depend on several factors such as (1) characteristics of the inhaled formulation (particle size distribution, shape, electrical charge, density, and hygroscopicity) and (2) breathing patterns such as frequency, depth, and flow rate. An ideal inhalation aerosol for local delivery may be one with a relatively slow rate of pulmonary absorption and clearance. It has been shown that increasing the lipophilicity (Derendorf et al, 2006) and optimization of particle size (MMAD <5 μm) (Labiris and Dolovich, 2003; Gonda 1987) and release rate (Gonda, 1987; Suarez et al, 1998), it is possible to increase the lung residence time of the drug. Currently, there are more than 65 different inhaled products of more than 20 active ingredients marketed to treat respiratory diseases (Labiris and Dolovich, 2003). Inhaled glucocorticoids (eg, fluticasone propionate, budesonide, triamcinolone acetonide, mometasone furoate, etc) are some drugs usually prescribed for the treatment of local pulmonary diseases. The modification of the physicochemical (eg, side chains added to the D-ring of the structure to slow the dissolution of the drug in the aqueous bronchial fluid) and biopharmaceutical properties (eg, low oral bioavailability) of these drugs made possible to increase its targeting (high benefit:risk ratio) to the site of action, the lungs.

Inhalation therapy for local action is generated by different devices that aim to deliver the drug to the lower airways. Inhalation devices can be classified into three different categories: MDIs, dry-powder inhalers (eg, Aerolizer®, Diskus®, Flexaler®, Turbohaler®, etc), and nebulizer inhalers. Some examples of inhalation and intranasal products are shown in Table 15-11. The recent development of new inhalation devices makes it

TABLE 15-11   Failure of *In Vitro–In Vivo* Correlation (IVIVC)

Biorelevant dissolution method needed

Immediate-release drug product containing a rapidly dissolving and rapidly absorbed drug (BCS1)

Dissolution media may not reflect physiological conditions in the GI tract

    GI transit time

    pH in different regions of GI tract

    Contents of GI tract

    Fed or fasted state

    Normal digestive enzymes

    Flora of GI tract

Other factors affecting systemic drug absorption

    In vitro dissolution is a closed system, whereas *in vivo* drug absorption is an open system

    Pre-systemic drug elimination (first-pass effects)

    Enterohepatic circulation

possible to deliver larger drug doses (milligram compared with microgram dosing) to the airways and achieve greater deposition efficiency than the older devices (>50% lung deposition vs. ≤20% with older devices) (Dolovich, 1999).

The development of drugs for pulmonary drug delivery has focused mainly on the optimization of particle or device technologies to improve the aerosol generation and pulmonary deposition of inhaled drugs. Although substantial progress has been made in these areas, no significant advances have been made that would lead pulmonary drug delivery beyond the treatment of some respiratory diseases. One main reason for this stagnation is the poor knowledge about (1) details on the fate of inhaled drug or carrier particles after deposition in the lungs; (2) how much drug (total amount) reaches the lungs and validated method to demonstrate this; and (3) differential assessment on the region of drug deposition (eg, central portion vs. periphery lung deposition). Inhalation products are complex drug–device combination products, bearing quite distinctive performance characteristics and patient instructions for use and handling. Thus, bioavailability/bioequivalence studies alone may not be sufficient for documentation of the locally acting drug products (FDA Guidance for Industry, 1989a; FDA, 2013), following major manufacturing changes or for approval of generics because for delivery to the target sites these drugs do not depend upon systemic circulation. Following administration of the locally acting drug product, drug moieties detected in the systemic circulation (i) appear subsequent to its delivery to and absorption from the local site, and (ii) contain drug absorbed from multiple sites. Despite these arguments, some experts (Adams et al, 2010; O'Connor et al, 2011) believe that pharmacokinetic studies might be able to provide some key information (how much drug is deposited, where is it deposited, how long does it stay in the lung) needed for demonstration of bioequivalence of inhalation drugs for local action.

The role of aerosol therapy is emerging beyond the initial focus. This expansion has been driven by the Montreal protocol and the need to eliminate chlorofluorocarbons (CFCs) from traditional metered-dose inhalers, by the need for delivery devices and formulations that can efficiently and reproducibly target the systemic circulation for the delivery of proteins and peptides, and by developments in medicine that have made it possible to consider curing lung diseases with aerosolized gene therapy and preventing epidemics of influenza and measles with aerosolized vaccines. The rate of absorption from the periphery of the lung has been shown to be twice as fast as that taking place from the central portions, owing to the variable thickness of the epithelial cells versus alveolar cells (Brown and Schanker, 1983). Therefore, to achieve maximum bioavailability of drugs aimed for systemic delivery, attention should be paid on delivering the drug to the periphery of the lungs.

The continued expansion of the role of aerosol therapy will probably depend on several factors such as the demonstration of the safety of this route of administration for drugs that have their targets outside the lung and are administered long term (eg, insulin aerosol) (Laube, 2005).

Transdermal Drug Products

Transdermal drug products, sometimes referred to as transdermal delivery systems or "patches,"[3] are placed on the skin to deliver drug into the patient's systemic

circulation for systemic activity. Scopolamine® (Transderm Scop) delivers drug through the skin of the ear for relief of motion sickness. Transdermal administration may release the drug over an extended period of several hours or days (eg, estrogen replacement therapy) without the discomforts of gastrointestinal side effects or first-pass effects. Many transdermal products deliver drug at a constant rate to the body, similar to a zero-order infusion process. As a result, a stable, plateau level of the drug may be maintained. Many therapeutic categories of drugs are now available as transdermal products (Table 15-12).

Transdermal products vary in design (Gonzalez and Cleary, 2010). In general, the patch contains several parts: (1) a backing or support layer; (2) a drug layer (reservoir containing the dose); (3) a release-controlling layer (usually a semipermeable film), (4) a pressure-sensitive adhesive (PSA); and (5) a protective strip, which must be removed prior to application (see Chapter 19, Fig. 19-14). The release-controlling membrane may be a polymeric

TABLE 15-12 Biopharmaceutic Considerations in Drug Product Design

Pharmacodynamic considerations
Therapeutic objective
Toxic effects
Adverse reactions
Drug considerations
Chemical and physical properties of drug
Drug product considerations
Pharmacokinetics of drug
Bioavailability of drug
Route of drug administration
Desired drug dosage form
Desired dose of drug
Patient considerations
Compliance and acceptability of drug product
Cost
Manufacturing considerations
Cost
Availability of raw materials
Stability
Quality control
Method of manufacturing
Patents

---

[3]Several "patches" are available for local activity on the skin. Examples include lidocaine patch for local anesthetic activity due to pain from shingles and diclofenac sodium patch, a topical nonsteroidal anti-inflammatory drug (NSAID).

film such as ethylvinyl copolymer, which controls the release rate of the dose and its duration of action. The PSA layer is important for maintaining uninterrupted skin contact for drug diffusion through the skin. In some cases, the drug is blended directly into an adhesive, such as acrylate or silicone; performing the dual functions of release control and adhesion, this product is known as "drug in adhesive." In other products, the drug dose may be placed in a separate insoluble matrix layer, which helps control the release rate. This is generally known as a "matrix patch," and provides a little more control of the release rate as compared to the simple "reservoir" type of patch. Multilayers of drugs may be involved in other transdermal products using a "laminate" design. In many cases, drug permeation through the skin is the slowest step in the transdermal delivery of drug into the body. See Chapter 19 for a discussion of modified-release drug products.

Absorption Enhancers

A variety of excipients known as *absorption enhancers* or *permeation enhancers* have been incorporated into the drug product to promote systemic drug absorption from the application site. For oral drug products that contain poorly absorbed hydrophobic drugs, surfactants have been added to the formulation to help solubilize the drug by making the drug more miscible in water. The stratum corneum is the major barrier to systemic drug absorption from transdermal drug products. The addition of excipients or the use of physical approaches has been used to enhance drug permeation from transdermal products. For example, Estraderm®, a estradiol transdermal system, contains ethanol, which promotes drug delivery through the stratum corneum of the skin. The use of ultrasound (phonophoresis or sonophoresis) has been used by physical therapists to enhance percutaneous absorption of hydrocortisone ointments and creams from intact skin. Iontophoresis is a technique using a small electric charge to deliver drug containing an ionic charge through the stratum corneum. Most of these absorption enhancement approaches attempt to disrupt the cellular barriers to drug transport and allow the drug to permeate better.

Scale-Up and Postapproval Changes (SUPAC)

Any change in a drug product after it has been approved for marketing by the FDA is known as a *postapproval change*. Postapproval changes may include formulation (component and composition), equipment, manufacturing process, site, and scale-up in a drug product after it has been approved for marketing by the FDA (FDA Guidance for Industry, November 1999). A major concern of industry and the FDA is that if a pharmaceutical manufacturer makes any such, whether these changes will affect the identity, strength, purity, quality, bioavailability safety, or efficacy of the approved drug product. In addition, any changes in raw material (ie, material used for preparing active pharmaceutical ingredient), excipients, or packaging (including container closure system) should also be shown not to affect the quality of the drug product. There are three levels of manufacturing changes.

Level 1 changes are defined as changes that are unlikely to have any detectable impact on formulation quality and performance and are usually reported in the annual report.

Level 2 changes could have a significant impact in formation quality and performance and are usually reported in a change being affected supplement. Level 2 changes usually require dissolution profile comparisons in multiple media.

Level 3 changes are likely to have a significant impact on quality and performance and are usually reported in a prior approval supplement. Level 3 changes usually require the conduct of a bioequivalence study unless a predictive IVIVC is present.

Frequently Asked Questions

▶ *What physical or chemical properties of a drug substance are important in designing a drug for (a) oral administration or (b) parenteral administration?*

▶ *For a lipid-soluble drug that has very poor aqueous solubility, what strategies could be used to make this drug more bioavailable after oral administration?*

▶ *For a weak ester drug that is unstable in highly acidic or alkaline solutions, what strategies could be used to make this drug more bioavailable after oral administration?*

CHAPTER SUMMARY

Biopharmaceutics is the study of the physicochemical properties of the drug and the drug product and links these properties to drug product quality and drug product performance. Biopharmaceutics has a crucial role in establishing a link between the *in vivo* product performance such as bioavailability, onset of action, safety, and efficacy to the drug product critical process parameters and material attributes. Both *in vitro* (eg, dissolution) and *in vivo* methods (bioavailability) are applied to evaluate drug product quality and drug product performance. Thus, the selection of a suitable salt form of the drug that has improved stability, aqueous solubility, and bioavailability is based on the drug's physicochemical properties. Polymorphism refers to the arrangement of a drug substance in various crystalline forms. The selection of a suitable crystal, solvate, or hydrates may be crucial to improve the solubility and dissolution of a drug, and therefore its bioavailability. The particle size distribution of the drug is an important property for insoluble, hydrophobic drugs. Decreasing the particle size for some low-solubility drugs may result in improved bioavailability. Systemic drug absorption from a drug product consists of a succession of rate processes including (1) disintegration of the drug product and subsequent release of the drug, (2) dissolution of the drug in an aqueous environment, and (3) absorption of the drug across cell membranes into the systemic circulation. The slowest step in a series of kinetic processes is called the rate-limiting step. Dissolution is a dynamic process by which a solid drug substance becomes dissolved in a dissolution medium. Developing a discriminating dissolution method and setting the appropriate product specifications is critical in assuring that the manufacture of the dosage form is consistent and successful throughout the product's life cycle. Clinically relevant specifications are those specifications that, in addition, take into consideration the clinical impact assuring consistent safety and efficacy profile. In this case, clinically meaningful dissolution method and specifications will minimize the variability to the patient and, therefore, will optimize drug therapy. Due to the critical role that dissolution plays in defining the bioavailability of the drug, *in vitro* dissolution, if identified as CQA, can serve as a relevant predictor of the *in vivo* performance of the drug product.

An *in vitro–in vivo* correlation (IVIVC) establishes a relationship between a biological property of the drug (such as pharmacodynamic effect or plasma drug concentration) and a physicochemical property of the drug product containing the drug substance, such as dissolution rate. A properly validated IVIVC enhances drug product understanding and provides justification of manufacturing changes during drug product development. It enhances the significance of the *in vitro* testing leading to drug product specifications' (eg, dissolution acceptance criteria) setting based on targeted clinically relevant plasma concentrations. In addition, it allows for the prediction of the clinical impact of movements within the design space without the need for additional *in vivo* studies.

The use of biopharmaceutic tools such as dissolution and BA/BE studies become very relevant in setting clinically relevant drug product specifications because it would be rather impractical to determine the clinical relevance of movements within the design space through clinical efficacy and safety trials.

LEARNING QUESTIONS

1. What are the two rate-limiting steps possible in the oral absorption of a solid drug product? Which one would apply to a soluble drug? Which one could be altered by the pharmacist? Give examples.

2. What is the physiologic transport mechanism for the absorption of most drugs from the gastrointestinal tract? What area of the gastrointestinal tract is most favorable for the absorption of drugs? Why?

3. Explain why the absorption rate of a soluble drug tends to be greater than the elimination rate of the drug.

4. What type of oral dosage form generally yields the greatest amount of systemically available drug in the least amount of time? (Assume that the drug can be prepared in any form.) Why?

5. What effect does the oral administration of an anticholinergic drug, such as atropine sulfate, have on the bioavailability of aspirin from an enteric-coated tablet? (*Hint:* Atropine sulfate decreases gastrointestinal absorption.)

6. Drug formulations of erythromycin, including its esters and salts, have significant differences in bioavailability. Erythromycin is unstable in an acidic medium. Suggest a method for preventing a potential bioavailability problem for this drug.

7. Why can two generic drug products have different dissolution profiles *in vitro* and still be bioequivalent *in vivo*?

ANSWERS

Frequently Asked Questions

What physical or chemical properties of a drug substance are important in designing a drug for (a) oral administration or (b) parenteral administration?

- For optimal drug absorption after oral administration, the drug should be water soluble and highly permeable so that it can be absorbed throughout the gastrointestinal tract. Ideally, the drug should not change into a polymorphic form that could affect its solubility. The drug should be stable in both gastric and intestinal pH and preferably should not be hygroscopic.

   For parenteral administration, the drug should be water soluble and stable in solution, preferably at autoclave temperature. The drug should be non-hydroscopic and preferably should not change into another polymorphic form.

For a lipid-soluble drug that has very poor aqueous solubility, what strategies could be used to make this drug more bioavailable after oral administration?

- A lipid-soluble drug may be prepared in an oil-in-water (o/w) emulsion or dissolved in a nonaqueous solution in a soft gelatin capsule. A co-solvent may improve the solubility and dissolution of the drug.

For a weak ester drug that is unstable in highly acidic or alkaline solutions, what strategies could be used to make this drug more bioavailable after oral administration?

- The rate of hydrolysis (decomposition) of the ester drug may be reduced by formulating the drug in a co-solvent solution. A reduction in the percent of the aqueous vehicle will decrease the rate of hydrolysis. In addition, the drug should be formulated at the pH in which the drug is most stable.

Learning Questions

1. The rate-limiting steps in the oral absorption of a solid drug product are the rate of drug dissolution within the gastrointestinal tract and the rate of permeation of the drug molecules across the intestinal mucosal cells. Generally, disintegration of the drug product is rapid and not rate limiting. Water-soluble drugs dissolve rapidly in the aqueous environment of the gastrointestinal tract, so the permeation of the intestinal mucosal cells may be the rate-limiting step. The drug absorption rate may be altered by a variety of methods, all of which depend on knowledge of the biopharmaceutic properties of the drug and the drug product and on the physiology of the gastrointestinal tract. Drug examples are described in detail in this chapter and in Chapter 14.

2. Most drugs are absorbed by passive diffusion. The duodenum area provides a large surface area and blood supply that maintains a large drug concentration gradient favorable for drug absorption from the duodenum into the systemic circulation.

3. If the initial drug absorption rate, dD_A/dt, was slower than the drug elimination rate, dD_E/dt, then therapeutic drug concentrations in the body would not be achieved. It should be noted that the rate of absorption is generally first order, $dD_A/dt = D_0 k_a$, where D_0 is the drug dose, which is great initially. Even if $k_a < k$, the initial drug absorption rate may be greater than the drug elimination rate. After the drug is absorbed from the absorption site, $dD_A/dt \le dD_E/dt$.

4. A drug prepared as an oral aqueous drug solution is generally the most bioavailable. However, the same drug prepared as a well-designed immediate-release tablet or capsule may have similar bioavailability. In the case of an oral drug solution, there is no dissolution step; the drug molecules come into contact with intestinal membrane, and the drug is rapidly absorbed. As a result of first-pass effects (discussed in Chapter 12), a drug given in an oral drug solution may not be 100% bioavailable. If the drug solution is formulated with a high solute concentration—such as sorbitol solution, which yields a high osmotic pressure—gastric motility may be slowed, thus slowing the rate of drug absorption.

5. Anticholinergic drugs prolong gastric emptying, which will delay the absorption of an enteric-coated drug product.

6. Erythromycin may be formulated as enteric-coated granules to protect the drug from degradation at the stomach pH. Enteric-coated granules are less affected by gastric emptying and food (which delays gastric emptying) compared to enteric-coated tablets.

REFERENCES

Abbvie Incorporated. 2012 Trilipix (Fenofibric Acid) Delayed-Release Capsules, 45 mg and 135 mg Package Insert. North Chicago, Ill., USA. Original market approval in 2008.

Abbvie Incorporated. 2013 Tricor (Fenofibrate) Tablets, 48 mg and 145 mg Package Insert. North Chicago, Ill., USA. Original market approval in 2004.

Achanta AS, Gray VA, Cecil TL, et al: Evaluation of the performance of prednisone and salicylic acid calibrators. *Drug Develop Ind Pharm* **21**:1171–1182, 1995.

Adams W, et al: Demonstrating bioequivalence of locally acting orally inhaled drug products (OIPs): Workshop Summary Report. *J Aerol Med* **23**(1):1–29, 2010.

Aguiar AJ, Krc J, Kinkel AW, Samyn JC: Effect of polymorphism on the absorption of chloramphenical from chloramphenical palmitate. *J Pharm Sci* **56**:847–853, 1967.

Allen PV, Rahn PD, Sarapu AC, Vandewielen AJ: Physical characteristic of erythromycin anhydrate, and dihydrate crystalline solids. *J Pharm Sci* **67**:1087–1093, 1978.

Amidon GE, Peck GE, Block LH, et al: Proposed new USP general information chapter, Excipient performance <1059>. *Pharmacopeial Forum* **33**(6):1311–1323, 2007.

Armenante P, Muzzio F: Inherent Method Variability in Dissolution Testing: The Effect of Hydrodynamics in the USP II Apparatus. A Technical Report Submitted to the Food

and Drug Administration, 2005. http://www.fda.gov/ohrms
/dockets/ac/05/briefing/2005-4187B1_01_04-Effect-
Hydrodynamics.pdf.

Ashok V, Kumar MR, Murali D, Chatterjee A: A review of vaginal route as a systemic drug delivery. *Critical Rev in Pharm Sci* 1(1):1–19, 2012.

Bates TR, Equeira JA: Bioavailability of micronized grieseofulvin from corn oil in water emulsion, aqueous suspension and commercial dosage form in humans. *J Pharm Sci* **64**:793–797, 1975.

Bhupinderjit SA, et al: Phospholipid association reduces the gastric mucosal toxicity of aspirin in human subjects. *Am J Gastroent* **94**(7):1817–1822, 1999.

Bocanegra LB, Morris GJ, Jurewicz JT, et al: Fluid and particle laser Doppler velocity measurements and mass transfer predictions for USP paddle method dissolution apparatus. *Drug Dev Ind Pharm* **16**:1441–1462, 1990.

Brown CK, Chokshi HP, Nickerson B, et al: Acceptable analytical practices for dissolution testing of poorly soluble compounds. *Pharm Tech* **28**(12):56, 2004.

Brown R, Schanker L: Absorption of aerosolized drugs from the rat lung. *Drug Metab Dispos* **11**:355–360, 1983.

Chourasia MK, Jain SK: Pharmaceutical approaches to colon targeted drug delivery systems. *J Pharm Pharm Sci* **6**(1): 33–66, January–April 2003.

Derendorf H, Nave R, Drollmann A, et al: Relevance of pharmacokinetics and pharmacodynamics of inhaled corticosteroids to asthma. *ERJ* **28**(5):1042–1050, 2006.

Djupesland PG: Nasal drug delivery devices: characteristics and performance in a clinical perspective—A review. *Drug Deliv Transl Res* **3**(1):42–62, 2013.

Dolovich M: New propellant-free technologies under investigation. *J Aerosol Med* **12**(1):s9–s17, 1999.

EMA: Guideline on quality of oral modified release product (draft), August 2012.

FDA Guidance for Industry: *In-vitro Bioequivalence Studies of Metaproterenol Sulfate and Albuterol Inhalation Aerosols (Metered Dose Inhalers)*, Division of Bioequivalence, Food and Drug Administration, Rockville, Maryland, 1989.

FDA Guidance for Industry:[4] *Dissolution Testing of Immediate Release Solid Oral Dosage Forms*, FDA, 1997a.

FDA Guidance for Industry: *Extended Release Oral Dosage Forms: Development, Evaluation, and Application of In Vitro/In Vivo Correlations*, FDA, 1997b.

FDA Guidance for Industry: *Changes to an Approved NDA or ANDA*, November 1999.

FDA Guidance for Industry: *Waiver of In Vivo Bioavailability and Bioequivalence Studies for Immediate-Release Solid Oral Dosage Forms Based on a Biopharmaceutics Classification System*, August 2000.

FDA Guidance for Industry: *Nasal Spray and Inhalation Solution, Suspension, and Spray Drug Products—Chemistry, Manufacturing, and Controls Documentation*, 2002.

FDA Guidance for Industry: *The Use of Mechanical Calibration of Dissolution Apparatus 1 and 2: Current Good Manufacturing Practice (CGMP)*, January 2010.

FDA: Draft guidance for industry on fluticasone propionate; salmeterol xinafoate, 2013.

Fisher RS, Ho J: Potential new methods for antiepileptic drug delivery. *CNS Drugs* **16**(9):579–593, 2002.

Fordtran J, Patrawala M, Chakrabarti S: Influence of vehicle composition on *in vivo* absorption of calcium from soft elastic gelatin capsule. *Pharm Res* **3**(suppl):645, 1986.

Gillette JR, Mitchell JR: Routes of drug administration and response. In *Concepts in Biochemical Pharmacology*. Berlin, Springer-Verlag, 1975, Chap 64.

Gonda I: Drugs administered directly into the respiratory tract: Modeling of the duration of effective drug levels. *J Pharm Sci* **77**:340–346, 1987.

Gombar VK, Silver IS, Zhao Z: Role of ADME characteristics in drug discovery and their in silico evaluation: In silico screening of chemicals for their metabolic stability. *Curr Top Med Chem* **3**(11):1205–1225, 2003.

Gonzalez MA, Cleary GW: Transdermal dosage forms. In Shargel L, Kanfer I (eds). *Generic Drug Product Development–Specialty Dosage Forms*. New York, Informa Healthcare, 2010, Chap 8.

Gray VA, Brown CK, Dressman JB, Leeson J: A new general chapter on dissolution. *Pharm Forum* **27**:3432–3439, 2001.

Gray VA, Hubert BB: Calibration of dissolution apparatuses 1 and 2. What to do when equipment fails. *Pharmacop Forum* **20**:8571–8573, 1994.

Hanson R, Gray V: *Handbook of Dissolution Testing*, 3rd ed. Hockessin, DE, Dissolution Technologies, Inc., 2004, Chap 1.

Harboe E, Larsen C, Johansen A, Olesen HP: Macromolecular prodrugs. XV. Colon-targeted delivery–bioavailability of naproxen from orally administered dextran-naproxen ester prodrugs varying in molecular size in the pig. *Pharm Res* **6**(11): 919–923, 1989.

Jin J, Sklar, GE, Sen Oh VM, et al: Factors affecting therapeutic compliance: A review from the patient's perspective. *Ther Clin Risk Manag* **4**(1):269–286, 2008.

Kaplan SA: Biopharmaceutical considerations in drug formulation design and evaluation. *Drug Metab Rev* **1**:15–34, 1972.

Klein S: The use of biorelevant dissolution media to forecast the *in vivo* performance of a drug. *AAPS J* **12**(3):397–406, 2010.

Kumari N, Kalyanwat R, Singh VK. Complete review on nasal drug delivery systems. *Int J Med Pharm Res* **1**(2):235–249, 2013.

Labiris NR, Dolovich MB: Pulmonary drug delivery. Part I: Physiological factors affecting therapeutic effectiveness of aerosolized medications. *Br J Clin Pharmacol* **56**(6):588–599, 2003.

Lakshmi PJ, Deepthi B, Rama RN: Rectal drug delivery: A promising route for enhancing drug absorption. *Asian J Res Pharm Sci* **2**(4):143–149, 2012.

Laube B: The expanding role of aerosols in systemic drug delivery, therapy, and vaccination. *Resp Care* **50**(9):1161–1176, 2005.

---

[4]FDA Guidance for Industry may be obtained on the Internet at www.fda.gov/cder/guidance/index.htm.

Levy G, Leonards J, Procknal JA: Development of *in vitro* tests which correlate quantitatively with dissolution rate-limited drug absorption in man. *J Pharm Sci* **54:**1719, 1965.

Mathias NR, Hussain MA: Non-invasive systemic drug delivery: Developability considerations for alternate routes of administration, *J Pharm Sci* **99**(1):1–20, 2010.

Morishita M, Peppas N: Is the oral route possible for peptide and protein drug delivery? *Drug Discovery Today* **11**(19–20): 905–910, 2006.

Najib J: Fenofibrate in the treatment of dyslipidemia: A review of the data as they relate to the new suprabioavailable tablet formulation. *Clin Ther* **24**(12):2022, 2002.

Noyes AA, Whitney WR: The rate of solution of solid substances in their own solutions. *J Am Chem Soc* **19:**930–934, 1897.

O'Connor D, et al: Role of pharmacokinetics in establishing bioequivalence for orally inhaled drug products: Workshop Summary Report. *J Aerol Med* **24**(3):119–135, 2011.

Patil SD, Burgess DJ: Pharmaceutical development of modified release parenteral dosage forms using bioequivalence (BE), quality by design (QBD) and in vito in vivo correlation (IVIVC) principles. In Shargel, L, Kanfer I (eds). *Generic Drug Product Development–Specialty Dosage Forms.* New York, Informa Healthcare, 2010, Chap 9.

Pavan B, Dalpiaz A, Ciliberti N, et al: Progress in drug delivery to the central nervous system by the prodrug approach. *Molecules* **13:**1035–1065, 2008.

Philip J, Daly RE: Test for selection of erythromycin stearate bulk drug for tablet preparation. *J Pharm Sci* **72:**979–980, 1983.

Philip AK, Philip B: Colon targeted drug delivery systems: A review on primary and novel approaches. *OMJ* **25:**70–78, 2010.

Puoton CW: Formulation of poorly water-soluble drugs for oral administration: Physicochemical and physiological issues and the lipid formulation classification system. *Eur J Pharm Sci* **29**(3–4):27, 2006.

Prasad V, Shah V, Knight P, et al: Importance of media selection in establishment of *in vitro–in vivo* relationship for quinidine gluconate. *Int J Pharm* **13:**1–7, 1983.

Qureshi SA, McGilveray IJ. Typical variability in drug dissolution testing: Study with USP and FDA calibrator tablets and a marketed drug (Glibenclamide) product. *Eur J Pharm Sci* **7:**249, 1999.

Qureshi SA, Shabnam J: Cause of high variability in drug dissolution testing and its impact on setting tolerances. *Eur J Pharm Sci* **12:**271–276, 2001.

Shah VP, Prasad VK, Alston T, et al: Phenytoin I: *In vitro* correlation for 100 mg phenytoin sodium capsules. *J Pharm Sci* **72:**306–308, 1983.

Shaji J, Patole V: Protein and peptide drug delivery: Oral approaches. *Indian J Pharm Sci* **70**(3):269–277, 2008.

Shareef MA, Ahuja A, Ahmad FJ, Raghava S: Colonic drug delivery: An updated review. *AAPS Pharm Sci* **54:**161–186, 2003.

Siewart M, Dressman J, Brown CK, Shah VP: FIP/AAPS Guidelines to dissolution/in vitro release testing of novel/special dosage forms. *AAPS Pharm Sci Tech* **4**(1):1–10, 2003.

Stella V, Haslam J, Yata N, et al: Enhancement of bioavailability of a hydrophobic amine antimalarial by formulation with oleic acid in a soft gelatin capsule. *J Pharm Sci* **67:**1375–1377, 1978.

Suarez S, et al. Effect of dose and release rate on pulmonary targeting of glucocorticoids using liposomes as a model dosage form. *Pharm Res* **15:**461–463, 1998.

Suarez-Sharp S: Models to Establish Clinically Relevant Drug Product Specifications. AAPS Annual Meeting and Exposition, Baltimore, MD, 2011a. http://www.fda.gov/downloads/AboutFDA/CentersOffices/OfficeofMedicalProductsandTobacco/CDER/UCM301057.pdf.

Suarez-Sharp S: Establishing Clinically Relevant Drug Product Specifications: FDA Perspective. AAPS Annual Meeting and Exposition, Chicago, IL, 2011b. http://www.fda.gov/downloads/AboutFDA/CentersOffices/OfficeofMedicalProductsandTobacco/CDER/UCM341185.pdf.

Suarez-Sharp S: FDA's Experience on IVIVC- New Drugs. PQRI Workshop on Application of IVIVC in Formulation Development. Bethesda, MD, 2012. http://www.pqri.org/workshops/ivivc/suarez.pdf.

Wood JH: *In vitro* evaluation of physiological availability of compressed tablets. *Pharm Acta Helv* **42:**129, 1966.

Yoshikawa H, Nakao Y, Takada K, et al: Targeted and sustained delivery of aclarubicin to lymphatics by lactic acid oligomer microsphere in rat. *Chem Pharm Bull* **37:**802–804, 1989.

BIBLIOGRAPHY

Aguiar AJ: Physical properties and pharmaceutical manipulations influencing drug absorption. In Forth IW, Rummel W (eds). *Pharmacology of Intestinal Absorption: Gastrointestinal Absorption of Drugs,* Vol 1. New York, Pergamon, 1975, Chap 6.

Amidon GL, Lennernas H, Shah VP, Crison JR: A theoretical basis for a biopharmaceutic drug classification: The correlation of *in vitro* drug product dissolution and *in vivo* bioavailability. *Pharm Res* **12**:413–420, 1995.

Barr WH: The use of physical and animal models to assess bioavailability. *Pharmacology* **8**:88–101, 1972.

Berge S, Bighley L, Monkhouse D: Pharmaceutical salts. *J Pharm Sci* **66**:1–19, 1977.

Blanchard J: Gastrointestinal absorption, II. Formulation factors affecting bioavailability. *Am J Pharm* **150**:132–151, 1978.

Blanchard J, Sawchuk RJ, Brodie BB: *Principles and Perspectives in Drug Bioavailability*. New York, Karger, 1979.

Burks TF, Galligan JJ, Porreca F, Barber WD: Regulation of gastric emptying. *Fed Proc* **44**:2897–2901, 1985.

Cabana BE, O'Neil R: FDA's report on drug dissolution. *Pharm Forum* **6**:71–75, 1980.

Cadwalder DE: *Biopharmaceutics and Drug Interactions*. Nutley, NJ, Roche Laboratories, 1971.

Christensen J: The physiology of gastrointestinal transit. *Med Clin N Am* **58**:1165–1180, 1974.

Dakkuri A, Shah AC: Dissolution methodology: An overview. *Pharm Technol* **6**:28–32, 1982.

Dressman JB, Amidon GL, Reppas C, Shah VP: Dissolution testing as a prognostic tool for oral drug absorption: Immediate release dosage forms. *Pharm Res* **15**:11–22, 1998.

Eye IS: A review of the physiology of the gastrointestinal tract in relation to radiation doses from radioactive materials. *Health Phys* **12**:131–161, 1966.

Gilbaldi M: *Biopharmaceutics and Clinical Pharmacokinetics*. Philadelphia, Lea & Febiger, 1977.

Hansen WA: *Handbook of Dissolution Testing*. Springfield, OR, Pharmaceutical Technology Publications, 1982.

Hardwidge E, Sarapu A, Laughlin W: Comparison of operating characteristics of different dissolution test systems. *J Pharm Sci* **6**:1732–1735, 1978.

Houston JB, Wood SG: Gastrointestinal absorption of drugs and other xenobiotics. In Bridges JW, Chasseaud LF (eds). *Progress in Drug Metabolism,* Vol 4. London, Wiley, 1980, Chap 2.

Jollow DJ, Brodie BB: Mechanisms of drug absorption and drug solution. *Pharmacology* **8**:21–32, 1972.

LaDu BN, Mandel HG, Way EL: *Fundamentals of Drug Metabolism and Drug Disposition*. Baltimore, Williams & Wilkins, 1971.

Leesman GD, Sinko PJ, Amidon GL: Simulation of oral drug absorption: Gastric emptying and gastrointestinal motility. In Welling PW, Tse FLS (eds). *Pharmacokinetics: Regulatory, Industry, Academic Perspectives*. New York, Marcel Dekker, 1988, Chap 6.

Leeson LJ, Carstensen JT: Industrial pharmaceutical technology. In Leeson L, Carstensen JT (eds). *Dissolution Technology*. Washington, DC, Academy of Pharmaceutical Sciences, 1974.

Levine RR: Factors affecting gastrointestinal absorption of drugs. *Dig Dis* **15**:171–188, 1970.

McElnay JC: Buccal absorption of drugs. In Swarbrick J, Boylan JC (eds). *Encyclopedia of Pharmaceutical Technology,* Vol 2. New York, Marcel Dekker, 1990, pp 189–211.

Mojaverian P, Vlasses PH, Kellner PE, Rocci ML Jr: Effects of gender, posture and age on gastric residence of an indigestible solid: Pharmaceutical considerations. *Pharm Res* **5**:639–644, 1988.

Neinbert R: Ion pair transport across membranes. *Pharm Res* **6**:743–747, 1989.

Niazi S: *Textbook of Biopharmaceutics and Clinical Pharmacokinetics*. New York, Appleton, 1979.

Notari RE: *Biopharmaceutics and Pharmacokinetics: An Introduction*. New York, Marcel Dekker, 1975.

Palin K: Lipids and oral drug delivery. *Pharm Int* **11**:272–279, November 1985.

Palin K, Whalley D, Wilson C, et al: Determination of gastric-emptying profiles in the rat: Influence of oil structure and volume. *Int J Pharm* **12**:315–322, 1982.

Parrott EL: *Pharmaceutical Technology*. Minneapolis, Burgess, 1970.

Pernarowski M: Dissolution methodology. In Leeson L, Carstensen JT (eds). *Dissolution Technology*. Washington, DC, Academy of Pharmaceutical Sciences, 1975, p 58.

Pharmacopeial Forum: FDA report on drug dissolution. *Pharm Forum* **6**:71–75, 1980.

Prasad VK, Shah VP, Hunt J, et al: Evaluation of basket and paddle dissolution methods using different performance standards. *J Pharm Sci* **72**:42–44, 1983.

Robinson JR: *Sustained and Controlled Release Drug Delivery Systems*. New York, Marcel Dekker, 1978.

Robinson JR, Eriken SP: Theoretical formulation of sustained release dosage forms. *J Pharm Sci* **55**:1254, 1966.

Rubinstein A, Li VHK, Robinson JR: Gastrointestinal–physiological variables affecting performance of oral sustained release dosage forms. In Yacobi A, Halperin-Walega E (eds). *Oral Sustained Release Formulations: Design and Evaluation*. New York, Pergamon, 1988, Chap 6.

Schwarz-Mann WH, Bonn R: Principles of transdermal nitroglycerin administration. *Eur Heart J* **10**(suppl A):26–29, 1989.

Shaw JE, Chandrasekaran K: Controlled topical delivery of drugs for system in action. *Drug Metab Rev* **8**:223–233, 1978.

Siewart M, Dressman J, Brown CK, Shah VP: *FIP/AAPS Guidelines to dissolution/in vitro release testing of novel/special dosage forms. AAPS Pharm Sci Tech* **4**(1):1–10, 2003.

Swarbrick J: *In vitro* models of drug dissolution. In Swarbrick J (ed). *Current Concepts in the Pharmaceutical Sciences: Biopharmaceutics*. Philadelphia, Lea & Febiger, 1970.

Wagner JG: *Biopharmaceutics and Relevant Pharmacokinetics.* Hamilton, IL, Drug Intelligence Publications, 1971.

Welling PG: Dosage route, bioavailability and clinical efficacy. In Welling PW, Tse FLS (eds). *Pharmacokinetics: Regulatory, Industry, Academic Perspectives.* New York, Marcel Dekker, 1988, Chap 3.

Wurster DE, Taylor PW: Dissolution rates. *J Pharm Sci* **54:** 169–175, 1965.

Yoshikawa H, Muranishi S, Sugihira N, Seaki H: Mechanism of transfer of bleomycin into lymphatics by bifunctional delivery system via lumen of small intestine. *Chem Pharm Bull* **31:**1726–1732, 1983.

York P: Solid state properties of powders in the formulation and processing of solid dosage form. *Int J Pharm* **14:**1–28, 1983.

Zaffaroni A: Therapeutic systems: The key to rational drug therapy. *Drug Metab Rev* **8:**191–222, 1978.

16

Drug Product Performance, *In Vivo*: Bioavailability and Bioequivalence

Barbara Davit, Dale Conner, and Leon Shargel

Chapter Objectives

▶ Define bioavailability, bioequivalence, and drug product performance.

▶ Explain why certain drugs and drug products have low bioavailability.

▶ Explain why first-pass effect as well as chemical instability of a drug can result in low relative bioavailability.

▶ Distinguish between bioavailability and bioequivalence.

▶ Explain why relative bioavailability may have values greater than 100%.

▶ Explain why bioequivalence may be considered as a measure of drug product performance.

▶ Describe various methods for measuring bioavailability and the advantages and disadvantages of each.

▶ Describe the statistical criteria for bioequivalence and 90% confidence intervals.

DRUG PRODUCT PERFORMANCE

Drug product performance,[1] *in vivo,* may be defined as the release of the drug substance from the drug product leading to bioavailability of the drug substance. The assessment of drug product performance is important since bioavailability is related both to the pharmacodynamic response and to adverse events. Thus, performance tests relate the quality of a drug product to clinical safety and efficacy. Bioavailability studies are drug product performance studies used to define the effect of changes in the physicochemical properties of the drug substance, the formulation of the drug, and the manufacture process of the drug product (dosage form). Drug product performance studies are used in the development of new and generic drug products.

Bioavailability is one aspect of drug product quality that links the *in vivo* performance of a new drug product to the original formulation that was used in clinical safety and efficacy studies. Bioequivalence studies are drug product performance tests that compare the bioavailability of the same active pharmaceutical ingredient from one drug product (test) to a second drug product (reference). Bioavailability and bioequivalence can be considered as measures of the drug product performance *in vivo*.

Bioequivalence Studies in New Drug Development (NDA)

During drug development, bioequivalence studies are used to compare (a) early and late clinical trial formulations; (b) formulations used in clinical trials and stability studies, if different; (c) clinical trial formulations and to-be-marketed drug products, if different; and (d) product strength equivalence, as appropriate. Bioequivalence study designs are used to support new formulations of previously approved products, such as a new fixed-dose combination version of two products approved for coadministration, or modified-release versions of immediate-release products. Postapproval, *in vivo*

---

[1]A glossary of important terms appears at the end of this chapter.

▶ Explain the conditions under which a generic drug product manufacturer may request a waiver (biowaiver) for performing an *in vivo* bioequivalence study.

▶ Define therapeutic equivalence and explain why bioequivalence is only one component of the regulatory requirements for therapeutic equivalence.

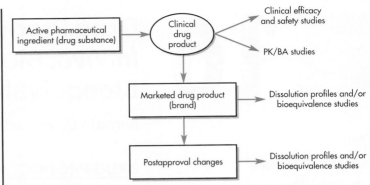

FIGURE 16-1 Drug product performance and new drug product development for NDAs. Drug product performance may be determined *in vivo* by bioequivalence studies or *in vitro* by comparative drug dissolution studies. BA = bioavailability.

bioequivalence studies may be needed to support regulatory approval of major changes in formulation, manufacturing, or site, in comparison to reference formulation (usually the prechange formulation) (Fig. 16-1).

The initial safety and clinical efficacy studies during new drug development may use a simple formulation such as a hard gelatin capsule containing only the active ingredient diluted with lactose. If the new drug demonstrates appropriate human efficacy and safety, a to-be-marketed drug product (eg, compressed tablet) may be developed. Since the initial safety and efficacy studies were performed using a different formulation (ie, hard gelatin capsule), the pharmaceutical manufacturer must demonstrate that the to-be-marketed drug product demonstrates equivalent drug product performance to the original formulation (Fig. 16-1). Equivalent drug product performance is generally demonstrated by an *in vivo* bioequivalence study in normal healthy volunteers. Under certain conditions, equivalent drug product performance may be demonstrated *in vitro* using comparative dissolution profiles (see Chapter 15).

As stated above, the marketed drug product that is approved by the US Food and Drug Administration (FDA) may not be the same formulation that was used in the original safety and clinical efficacy studies. After the drug product is approved by the FDA and marketed, the manufacturer may perform changes to the formulation. These changes to the marketed drug product are known as postapproval changes (see also Chapter 17). These postapproval changes, often termed SUPAC (scale-up and postapproval change based on several FDA guidance documents), could include a change in the supplier of the active ingredient, a change in the formulation, a change in the manufacturing process, and/or a

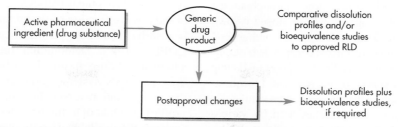

FIGURE 16-2   Drug product performance and generic drug product development. Drug product performance may be determined *in vivo* by bioequivalence studies or *in vitro* by comparative drug/release dissolution studies.

change in the manufacturing site. In each case, the manufacturer must demonstrate that drug product performance did not change and is the same for the drug product manufactured before and after the SUPAC change. As shown in Fig. 16-1, drug product performance may be determined by *in vivo* bioequivalence studies or by *in vitro* comparative drug release or dissolution profiles.

Bioequivalence Studies in Generic Drug Development (ANDA)

Comparative drug product performance studies are important in the development of generic drug products (Fig. 16-2). A generic drug product is a multisource drug product[2] that has been approved by the FDA as a therapeutic equivalent to the reference listed drug product[3] (usually the brand or innovator drug product) and has proven equivalent drug product performance. Clinical safety and efficacy studies are not generally performed on generic drug products. Since the formulation and method of manufacture of a drug product can affect the bioavailability and stability of the drug, the generic drug manufacturer must demonstrate that the generic drug product is pharmaceutically equivalent, bioequivalent, and therapeutically equivalent to the comparator brand-name drug product. Drug product performance comparison for oral generic drug products is usually measured by

[2]Multisource drug products are drug products that contain the same active drug substance in the same dosage form and are marketed by more than one pharmaceutical manufacturer.

[3]Reference listed drugs corresponding to proposed generic versions are listed by the US-FDA in its publication *Approved Drug Products with Therapeutic Equivalence Evaluations* (*Orange Book*).

in vivo bioequivalence studies in normal healthy adult subjects under fasted and fed conditions. Drug product performance comparisons *in vitro* may also include comparative drug dissolution/release profiles. Similar to the brand-name drug product manufacturer, the generic drug manufacturer may make changes after FDA approval in the formulation, in the source of the active pharmaceutical ingredient, manufacturing process, or other changes. For any postapproval change, the manufacturer must demonstrate that the change did not alter the performance of the drug product.

PURPOSE OF BIOAVAILABILITY AND BIOEQUIVALENCE STUDIES

Bioavailability and bioequivalence studies are important in the process of approving pharmaceutical products for marketing. *Bioavailability* is defined as the rate and extent to which the active ingredient or active moiety is absorbed from a drug product and becomes available at the site of action (US-FDA, CDER, 2014a). Bioavailability data provide an estimate of the fraction of drug absorbed from the formulation, and provide information about the pharmacokinetics of the drug. *Relative bioavailability* studies compare two drug product formulations. A bioequivalence study is a specialized type of relative bioavailability study. *Bioequivalence* is defined as the absence of a significant difference in the rate and extent to which the active ingredient or active moiety becomes available at the site of drug action when administered at the same molar dose under similar conditions in an appropriately designed study.

Bioavailability and bioequivalence data play pivotal roles in regulatory submissions for marketing approval of new and generic drugs throughout the world. Each regulatory agency has developed its own unique system of guidelines advising new and generic drug applicants on how to conduct acceptable bioavailability and bioequivalence studies to support marketing approval. A recent survey of international bioequivalence guidelines showed that there are more similarities than differences among approaches used by various international jurisdictions (Davit et al, 2013). In this chapter, discussion of the relationship between bioavailability, bioequivalence, and drug approval requirements will focus on the perspective of the FDA. Where appropriate, the reader will be directed to references covering international jurisdictions for further reading.

In summary, clinical studies are used to determine the safety and efficacy of drug products. Bioavailability studies are drug product performance studies used to define the effect of changes in the physicochemical properties of the drug substance, the formulation of the drug, and manufacture process of the drug product (dosage form). Bioequivalence studies are used to compare the bioavailability of the same drug (same salt or ester) from various drug products. Bioavailability and bioequivalence can be considered as performance measures of the drug product *in vivo*. If the drug products are pharmaceutically equivalent, bioequivalent, and therapeutically equivalent (as defined by the regulatory agency such as the FDA), then the clinical efficacy and the safety profile of these drug products are assumed to be similar and may be substituted for each other.

Frequently Asked Questions

▶ *Why are bioequivalence studies considered as drug product performance studies?*

▶ *What are the differences between a safety/efficacy study and an in vivo bioequivalence study? How do the study objectives differ?*

▶ *What's the difference between drug product performance and bioequivalence?*

RELATIVE AND ABSOLUTE AVAILABILITY

Regulatory agencies such as the FDA require submission of bioavailability data in applications to market new drug products (US-FDA, CDER, 2014b).

A drug product's bioavailability provides an estimate of the relative fraction of the administered dose that is absorbed into the systemic circulation (US-FDA, CDER, 2014c). Determining the fraction (*f*) of administered dose absorbed involves comparing the drug product's systemic exposure (represented by the concentration-versus-time or pharmacokinetic profile) with that of a suitable reference product. For systemically available drug products, bioavailability is most often assessed by determining the area under the drug plasma concentration-versus-time profile (AUC). The AUC is considered the most reliable measure of a drug's bioavailability, as it is directly proportional to the total amount of unchanged drug that reaches the systemic circulation (Le, 2014). Figure 16-3 shows how the drug concentration-versus-time profile is used to identify the pharmacokinetic parameters that form the basis of bioavailability and bioequivalence comparisons.

Absolute Bioavailability

Absolute bioavailability compares the bioavailability of the active drug in the systemic circulation following extravascular administration with the bioavailability of the same drug following intravenous administration (Fig. 16-4). Intravenous drug administration is considered 100% absorbed. The route of extravascular administration can be inhaled, intramuscular, oral, rectal, subcutaneous, sublingual, topical, transdermal, etc. The absolute bioavailability is the dose-corrected AUC of the extravascularly administered drug product divided by the AUC of the drug product given intravenously. Thus, for an oral formulation, the absolute bioavailability is calculated as follows:

$$F_{abs} = \frac{AUC_{po} \cdot D_{iv}}{AUC_{iv} \cdot D_{po}}$$

where
F_{abs} is the fraction of the dose absorbed, expressed as a percentage;
AUC_{po} is the AUC following oral administration;
D_{iv} is the dose administered intravenously;
AUC_{iv} is the AUC following intravenous administration; and
D_{po} is the dose administered orally.

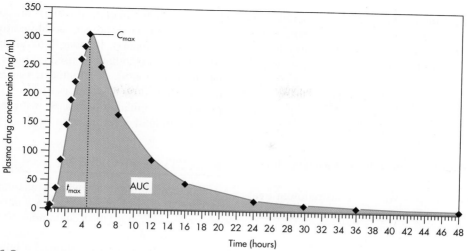

FIGURE 16-3 Plasma drug concentration–time curve after oral drug administration.

Absolute availability, F_{abs}, may be expressed as a fraction or as a percent by multiplying $F_{abs} \times 100$. A drug given by the intravenous route will have an absolute bioavailability of 100% ($f = 1$). A drug given by an extravascular route may have an $F_{abs} = 0$ (no systemic absorption) and $F_{abs} = 1.0$ (100% systemic absorption).

Relative Bioavailability

Another type of comparative bioavailability assessment is provided by a relative bioavailability study. In a relative bioavailability study, the systemic exposure of a drug in a designated formulation (generally referred to as treatment A or reference formulation) is compared with that of the same drug administered

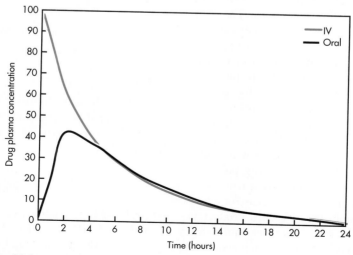

FIGURE 16-4 Relationship between plasma drug concentration-versus-time profiles for an intravenously administered formulation versus an orally administered formulation. In an absolute bioavailability study, the systemic exposure profile of a drug administered by the oral route (black curve) is compared with that of the drug administered by the intravenous route (green curve).

in a reference formulation (generally referred to as treatment B or test formulation). In a relative bioavailability study, the AUCs of the two formulations are compared as follows:

$$F_{rel} = 100 \cdot \frac{AUC_A \cdot D_B}{AUC_B \cdot D_A}$$

where

F_{rel} is the relative bioavailability of treatment (formulation) A, expressed as a percentage;

AUC_A is the AUC following administration of treatment (formulation) A;

D_A is the dose of formulation A;

AUC_B is the AUC of formulation B; and

D_B is the dose of formulation B.

Relative bioavailability studies are frequently included in regulatory submissions. For example, the FDA recommends that new drug developers routinely use an oral solution as the reference for a new oral formulation, for the purpose of assessing how formulation impacts bioavailability. Other types of relative bioavailability studies used in drug development include studies to characterize food effects and drug–drug interactions. In a *food-effect* bioavailability study, oral bioavailability of the drug product given with food (usually a high-fat, high-calorie meal) is compared to oral bioavailability of the drug product given under fasting conditions. The drug product given under fasting conditions is treated as the reference treatment. The goal of a *drug–drug interaction* study is to determine whether there is an increase or decrease in bioavailability in the presence of the interacting drug. As such, the general drug–drug interaction study design compares drug relative bioavailability with and without (reference treatment) the interacting drug. Relative bioavailability studies are used in developing new formulations of existing immediate-release drug products, such as new modified-release versions or new fixed-dose combination formulations. In the case of a new modified-release version, the reference product is the approved immediate-release product. In the case of a new fixed-dose combination, the reference product can be the single-entity drug products administered either separately (ie, three treatments for a fixed-dose combination doublet) or concurrently according to an approved combination regimen (ie, two treatments). Relative bioavailability study designs are also commonly used for bridging formulations during drug development, for example, to evaluate how drug systemic availability from a new premarket formulation compares with that from an existing premarket formulation.

PRACTICE PROBLEM

The bioavailability of a new investigational drug was studied in 12 volunteers. Each volunteer received either a single oral tablet containing 200 mg of the drug, 5 mL of a pure aqueous solution containing 200 mg of the drug, or a single IV bolus injection containing 50 mg of the drug. Plasma samples were obtained periodically up to 48 hours after the dose and assayed for drug concentration. The average AUC values (0–48 hours) are given in the table below. From these data, calculate (a) the relative bioavailability of the drug from the tablet compared to the oral solution and (b) the absolute bioavailability of the drug from the tablet.

Drug Product	Dose (mg)	AUC ($\mu g \cdot h/mL$)	Standard Deviation
Oral tablet	200	89.5	19.7
Oral solution	200	86.1	18.1
IV bolus injection	50	37.8	5.7

Solution

The relative bioavailability of the drug from the tablet is estimated in the equation below. No adjustment for the dose is necessary since the nominal doses are the same.

$$\text{Relative bioavailability} = \frac{89.5}{86.1} = 1.04 \quad \text{or} \quad 104\%$$

The relative bioavailability of the drug from the tablet is 1.04, or 104%, compared to the solution. In this study, the difference in drug bioavailability between tablet and solution would need to be analyzed statistically to determine whether the difference in drug bioavailability is statistically significant. It is possible for the relative bioavailability to be greater than 100%. In this case, the tablet formulation may have some property or excipient that increases bioavailability.

The absolute drug bioavailability from the tablet is calculated and adjusted for the dose.

$$F = \text{absolute bioavailability} = \frac{89.5/200}{37.5/50}$$

$$= 0.592 \quad \text{or} \quad 59.2\%$$

Because F, the fraction of dose absorbed from the tablet, is less than 1, the drug from the oral tablet is not completely absorbed systemically, as a result of either poor oral absorption of the drug itself, formulation effects that reduce oral bioavailability, or metabolism by first-pass effect (presystemic elimination). The relative bioavailability of the drug from the tablet is approximately 100% when compared to the oral solution.

The comparison between oral solution (little to no formulation effect) and IV administration gives information on the absorption of the drug itself when formulation effects are virtually nonexistent. With this knowledge, one can interpret the absolute bioavailability from the tablet and know if there is an effect of that formulation to change bioavailability or relative bioavailability is the same whether the tablet formulation wasn't even there.

Results from bioequivalence studies may show that the relative bioavailability of the test oral product is greater than, equal to, or less than 100% compared to the reference oral drug product. However, the results from these bioequivalence studies should not be misinterpreted to imply that the absolute bioavailability of the drug from the oral drug products is also 100% unless the oral formulation was compared to an intravenous injection (completely bioavailable) of the drug.

METHODS FOR ASSESSING BIOAVAILABILITY AND BIOEQUIVALENCE

Direct and indirect methods may be used to assess drug bioavailability. Bioequivalence of a drug product is demonstrated by the rate and extent of drug absorption, as determined by comparison of measured parameters. The FDA's regulations (US-FDA, CDER, 2014a) list the following approaches to determining bioequivalence, in descending order of accuracy, sensitivity, and reproducibility:

- *In vivo* measurement of active moiety or moieties in biological fluid (ie, a pharmacokinetic study)
- *In vivo* pharmacodynamic (PD) comparison
- *In vivo* limited clinical comparison
- *In vitro* comparison
- Any other approach deemed acceptable (by the FDA)

For drug products that are not intended to be absorbed into the bloodstream, bioavailability may be assessed by measurements intended to reflect the rate and extent to which the active ingredient or active moiety becomes available at the site of action. The design of the bioavailability study depends on the objectives of the study, the ability to analyze the drug (and metabolites) in biological fluids, the pharmacodynamics of the drug substance, the route of drug administration, and the nature of the drug product. For all systemically active drugs, with a few exceptions, bioequivalence should be demonstrated by an *in vivo* study based on pharmacokinetic (PK) endpoints, as this is the most sensitive, accurate, and reproducible approach. The other approaches—PD, clinical, or *in vitro*—may be more appropriate for locally acting drugs that are not systemically absorbed, such as those administered topically or those that act locally within the gastrointestinal (GI) tract. These latter BE approaches are considered on a case-by-case basis (Table 16-1). Detailed examples to illustrate when PD, clinical, or *in vitro* approaches are most suitable for establishing BE are presented below.

IN VIVO MEASUREMENT OF ACTIVE MOIETY OR MOIETIES IN BIOLOGICAL FLUIDS

Plasma Drug Concentration

Measurement of drug concentrations in blood, plasma, or serum after drug administration is the most direct and objective way to determine systemic drug bioavailability. By appropriate blood sampling,

TABLE 16-1   Methods for Assessing Bioavailability and Bioequivalence

***In vivo* measurement of active moiety or moieties in biological fluids**

Plasma drug concentration
Time for peak plasma (blood) concentration (t_{max})
Peak plasma drug concentration (C_{max})
Area under the plasma drug concentration–time curve (AUC)

Urinary drug excretion
Cumulative amount of drug excreted in the urine (D_u)
Rate of drug excretion in the urine (dD_u/dt)
Time for maximum urinary excretion (t)

***In vivo* pharmacodynamic (PD) comparison**
Maximum pharmacodynamic effect (E_{max})
Time for maximum pharmacodynamic effect
Area under the pharmacodynamic effect–time curve
Onset time for pharmacodynamic effect

Clinical endpoint study
Limited, comparative, parallel clinical study using predetermined clinical endpoint(s) and performed in patients

***In vitro* studies**
Comparative drug dissolution, f_2 similarity factor
In vitro binding studies
Examples: Cholestyramine resin—*In vitro* equilibrium and kinetic binding studies

Any other approach deemed acceptable (by the FDA)

an accurate description of the plasma drug concentration–time profile of the therapeutically active drug substance(s) can be obtained using a validated drug assay.

***t*_{max}:** The *time of peak plasma concentration*, t_{max}, corresponds to the time required to reach maximum drug concentration after drug administration. At t_{max}, peak drug absorption occurs and the rate of drug absorption exactly equals the rate of drug elimination (Fig. 16-3). Drug absorption still continues after t_{max} is reached, but at a slower rate. When comparing drug products, t_{max} can be used as an approximate indication of drug absorption rate. The value for t_{max} will become smaller (indicating less time required to reach peak plasma concentration) as the absorption rate for the drug becomes more rapid. Units for t_{max} are units of time (eg, hours, minutes).

For many systemically absorbed drugs, small differences in t_{max} may have little clinical effect on overall drug product performance. However, for some drugs, such as delayed action drug products, large differences in t_{max} may have clinical impact.

***C*_{max}:** The *peak plasma drug concentration*, C_{max}, represents the maximum plasma drug concentration obtained after oral administration of drug. For many drugs, a relationship is found between the pharmacodynamic drug effect and the plasma drug concentration. C_{max} provides indications that the drug is sufficiently systemically absorbed to provide a therapeutic response. In addition, C_{max} provides warning of possibly toxic levels of drug. The units of C_{max} are concentration units (eg, mg/mL, ng/mL). Although not a unit for rate, C_{max} is often used in bioequivalence studies as a surrogate measure for the rate of drug bioavailability. So, the expectation is that as the rate of drug absorption goes up, the peak or C_{max} will also be larger. If the rate of drug absorption goes down, then the peak or C_{max} is smaller.

AUC: The *area under the plasma level–time curve*, AUC, is a measurement of the *extent* of drug bioavailability (see Fig. 16-3). The AUC reflects the total amount of active drug that reaches the systemic circulation. The AUC is the area under the drug plasma level–time curve from $t = 0$ to $t = \infty$, and is equal to the amount of unchanged drug reaching the general circulation divided by the clearance.

$$[AUC]_0^\infty = \int_0^\infty C_p dt \qquad (16.1)$$

$$[AUC]_0^\infty = \frac{FD_0}{\text{clearance}} = \frac{FD_0}{kV_D} \qquad (16.2)$$

where F = fraction of dose absorbed, D_0 = dose, k = elimination rate constant, and V_D = volume of distribution. The AUC is independent of the route of administration and processes of drug elimination as long as the elimination processes do not change. The AUC can be determined by a numerical integration procedure, such as the trapezoidal rule method. The units for AUC are concentration × time (eg, $\mu g \cdot h/mL$).

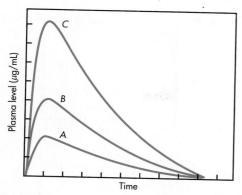

FIGURE 16-5   Plasma level–time curve following administration of single doses of (**A**) 250 mg, (**B**) 500 mg, and (**C**) 1000 mg of drug.

For many drugs, the AUC is directly proportional to dose. For example, if a single dose of a drug is increased from 250 to 1000 mg, the AUC will also show a fourfold increase (Figs. 16-5 and 16-6).

In some cases, the AUC is not directly proportional to the administered dose for all dosage levels. For example, as the dosage of drug is increased, one of the pathways for drug elimination may become saturated (Fig. 16-7). Drug elimination includes the processes of metabolism and excretion. Drug metabolism is an enzyme-dependent process. For drugs such as salicylate and phenytoin, continued increase of the dose causes saturation of one of the enzyme pathways for drug metabolism and consequent prolongation of the elimination half-life. The AUC thus increases disproportionally to the increase in dose, because a smaller amount of drug is being eliminated (ie, more drug is retained).

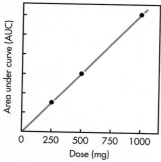

FIGURE 16-6   Linear relationship between AUC and dose (data from Fig. 16-5).

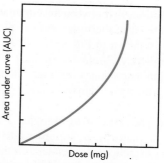

FIGURE 16-7   Relationship between AUC and dose when metabolism (elimination) is saturable.

When the AUC is not directly proportional to the dose, bioavailability of the drug is difficult to evaluate because drug kinetics may be dose dependent. Conversely, absorption may also become saturated resulting in lower-than-expected changes in AUC.

Urinary Drug Excretion Data

Urinary drug excretion data is an indirect method for estimating bioavailability. The drug must be excreted in significant quantities as unchanged drug in the urine. In addition, timely urine samples must be collected and the total amount of urinary drug excretion must be obtained (see Chapter 3).

D_u^∞: The *cumulative amount of drug excreted in the urine*, D_u^∞, is related directly to the total amount of drug absorbed. Experimentally, urine samples are collected periodically after administration of a drug product. Each urine specimen is analyzed for free drug using a specific assay. A graph is constructed that relates the cumulative drug excreted to the collection-time interval (Fig. 16-8).

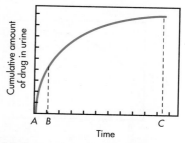

FIGURE 16-8   Corresponding plots relating the plasma level–time curve and the cumulative urinary drug excretion.

The relationship between the cumulative amount of drug excreted in the urine and the plasma level–time curve is shown in Fig. 16-8. When the drug is almost completely eliminated (point C), the plasma concentration approaches zero and the maximum amount of drug excreted in the urine, D_u^∞, is obtained.

dD_u/dt: The *rate of drug excretion*. Because most drugs are eliminated by a first-order rate process, the rate of drug excretion is dependent on the first-order elimination rate constant, k, and the concentration of drug in the plasma, C_p. In Fig. 16-9, the *maximum rate of drug excretion*, $(dD_u/dt)_{max}$, is at point B, whereas the minimum rate of drug excretion is at points A and C. Thus, a graph comparing the rate of drug excretion with respect to time should be similar in shape to the plasma level–time curve for that drug (Fig. 16-10).

t^∞: The *total time for the drug to be excreted*. In Figs. 16-9 and 16-10, the slope of the curve segment A–B is related to the rate of drug absorption, whereas point C is related to the total time required after drug administration for the drug to be absorbed and completely excreted, $t = \infty$. The t^∞ is a useful parameter in bioequivalence studies that compare several drug products.

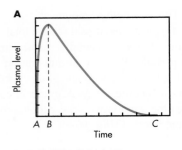
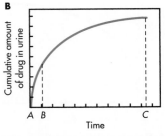

FIGURE 16-9   Corresponding plots relating the plasma level–time curve and the cumulative urinary drug excretion.

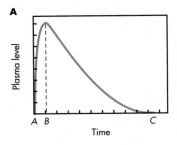
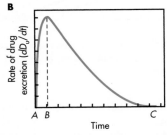

FIGURE 16-10   Corresponding plots relating the plasma level–time curve and the rate of urinary drug excretion.

BIOEQUIVALENCE STUDIES BASED ON PHARMACODYNAMIC ENDPOINTS—*IN VIVO* PHARMACODYNAMIC (PD) COMPARISON

In some cases, the quantitative measurement of a drug in plasma is not available or *in vitro* approaches are not applicable. The following criteria for a PD endpoint study are important:

- A dose–response relationship is demonstrated.
- The PD effect of the selected dose should be at the rising phase of the dose–response curve, as shown in Fig. 16-11.
- Sufficient measurements should be taken to assure an appropriate PD response profile.
- All PD measurement assays should be validated for specificity, accuracy, sensitivity, and precision.

For locally acting, nonsystemically absorbed drug products, such as topical corticosteroids, plasma drug concentrations may not reflect the bioavailability of the drug at the site of action. An acute

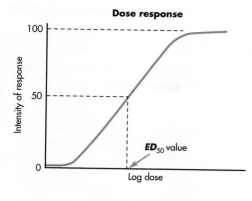

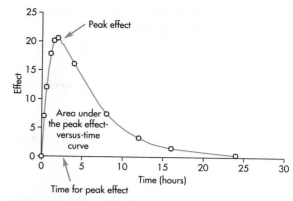

FIGURE 16-12   Acute pharmacodynamic effect–time curve. It shows an acute pharmacologic effect that is measured periodically after a single oral dose. The effect curve is similar to Fig. 16-3.

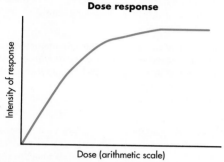

FIGURE 16-11   Dose–response curves. Dose–response curves for dose versus response graphed on a log or arithmetic scale.

pharmacodynamic effect,[4] such as an effect on forced expiratory volume, FEV_1 (inhaled bronchodilators), or skin blanching (topical corticosteroids) can be used as an index of drug bioavailability. In this case, the acute pharmacodynamic effect is measured over a period of time after administration of the drug product. Measurements of the pharmacodynamic effect should be made with sufficient frequency to permit a reasonable estimate for a time period at least three times the half-life of the drug (Gardner, 1977). This approach may be particularly applicable to dosage forms that are not intended to deliver the active moiety to the bloodstream for systemic distribution (Zou and Yu, 2014).

The use of an acute pharmacodynamic effect to determine bioavailability generally requires demonstration of a dose–response curve (Fig. 16-11 and Chapter 21). Bioavailability is determined by characterization of the dose–response curve. For bioequivalence determination, pharmacodynamic parameters including the total area under the acute pharmacodynamic effect–time curve, peak pharmacodynamic effect, and time for peak pharmacodynamic effect are obtained from the pharmacodynamic effect–time curve (Fig. 16-12). The onset time and duration of the pharmacokinetic effect may also be included in the analysis of the data. The use of pharmacodynamic endpoints for the determination of bioavailability and bioequivalence is much more variable than the measurement of plasma or urine drug concentrations. Some examples of drug products for which bioequivalence PD endpoints are recommended are listed on Table 16-2.

BIOEQUIVALENCE STUDIES BASED ON CLINICAL ENDPOINTS— CLINICAL ENDPOINT STUDY

The clinical endpoint study is the least accurate, least sensitive to bioavailability differences, and most variable. A predetermined clinical endpoint is used to evaluate comparative clinical effect in the

---

[4]A pharmacodynamic endpoint is an acute pharmacologic effect that is directly related to the drug's activity that can be measured quantitatively.

TABLE 16-2   Examples of Drug Products for Which FDA Recommends That Bioequivalence Studies Use Pharmacodynamic Endpoints

Drug Product	Indication	Mechanism of Action	Endpoint
Acarbose tablet (if no Q1/Q2 sameness between test and reference)	Treatment of type 2 diabetes	Inhibition of intestinal α-glucosidase, thereby decreasing absorption of starch and oligosaccharides	Reduction in blood glucose concentrations
Lanthanum carbonate tablet	Reduction of serum phosphate levels in patients with end-stage renal disease	Inhibits phosphate absorption by forming highly insoluble lanthanum phosphate complexes in GI tract	Reduction in urinary phosphate excretion
Orlistat capsules	Treatment of obesity	Inhibition of intestinal lipase, thereby reducing absorption of free fatty acids and monoacylglycerols	Amount of fat excreted in feces over 24 hours at steady state
Fluticasone propionate cream	Relief of skin itching and inflammation	The application of corticosteroids causes blanching in the microvasculature of the skin (not the mechanism of action, but quantitatively measurable)	Skin chromameter measurements through at least 24 hours after application
Albuterol sulfate metered dose inhaler	Relaxes smooth muscle of airways, thus protecting against bronchoconstrictor challenges	A beta$_2$-adrenergic agonist	• Either a bronchoprovocation or bronchodilatation assay is suitable • For bronchoprovocation, measure the concentration or dose of methacholine required to decrease FEV_1 by 20% • For bronchodilatation, measure the $AUEC_{0-4\,hr}$ $AUEC_{0-6\,hr}$ and maximum FEV_1 through 6 hours post-dose
Fluticasone propionate/salmeterol xinafoate inhalation power	Treatment of asthma and chronic obstructive pulmonary disease (COPD)	• Fluticasone is an anti-inflammatory corticosteroid • Salmeterol is a beta$_2$-adreneric agonist	Measure area under the FEV_1-time curve at designated intervals on first day and last day of 4-week daily treatment period
Low-molecular-weight heparins for IV administration	Anticoagulant	Inactivation of Factor Xa and Factor IIa in coagulation cascade	• To assure pharmaceutical equivalence of two formulations, measure anti-Xa and anti-IIa activities • Demonstration of *in vivo* bioequivalence is waived because product is a true solution

Adapted from Zou and Yu (2014).

TABLE 16-3   Examples of Drug Products for Which FDA Recommends Bioequivalence Studies with Clinical Endpoints

Product	Study Patients	Study Duration	Endpoint(s)
Calcipotriene cream	Plaque psoriasis	56 days	Proportions of subjects in the PP population with treatment success on PGA and clinical success of PASI
Imiquimod cream	Actinic keratosis	14 weeks	Proportion of subjects in the PP population with treatment success (100% clearance of all AK lesions)
Ketoconazole shampoo	Dandruff	28 days	Proportion of subjects with treatment success or cure, defined as a score of 0 or 1 on the Global Evaluation Scale (erythema rating)
Miconazole nitrate vaginal cream	Vulvovaginal candidiasis	21–30 days	Proportion of patients with therapeutic cure, defined as both mycological and clinical cure, at the test-of-cure visit
Nitazoxanide tablets	Diarrhea caused by Giardia lamblia	10 days	Proportion of patients with a "well" clinical response, defined as either (1) no symptoms, no watery stool, and no more than 2 soft stools with no hematochezia within the past 24 hours or (2) no symptoms and no unformed stools within the past 48 hours
Sucralfate tablets	Active duodenal ulcer disease; patients must be *Helicobacter pylori* negative or continue to have the presence of an ulcer after appropriate *H. pylori* treatment	8 weeks	Proportion of patients with ulcer healing at week 8 by endoscopic examination; if more than one ulcer is observed at enrollment, both must demonstrate healing at week 8 for success ("cure")

chosen patient population. Highly variable clinical responses require the use of a large number of patient study subjects, which increases study costs and requires a longer time to complete compared to the other approaches for determination of bioequivalence. A placebo arm is usually included to demonstrate that the study is sufficiently sensitive to identify the clinical effect in the patient population enrolled in the study. The FDA considers this approach only when analytical methods and pharmacodynamic methods are not available to permit use of one of the approaches described above. The clinical study is usually a limited, comparative, parallel clinical study using predetermined clinical endpoint(s).

Clinical endpoint BE studies are recommended for those products that have negligible systemic uptake, for which there is no identified PD measure, and for which the site of action is local. Comparative clinical studies have been used to establish bioequivalence for topical antifungal drug products (eg, ketoconazole) and for topical acne preparations. For dosage forms intended to deliver the active moiety to the bloodstream for systemic distribution, this approach may be considered acceptable only when analytical methods cannot be developed to permit use of one of the other approaches. Some examples of drug products where a clinical endpoint bioequivalence study is recommended (Davit and Conner, 2015) are listed in Table 16-3.

IN VITRO STUDIES

Comparative drug release/dissolution studies under certain conditions may give an indication of drug bioavailability and bioequivalence. Ideally, the *in vitro* drug dissolution rate should correlate with *in vivo* drug bioavailability (see Chapter 15 on *in vivo–in vitro* correlation, IVIVC). The test and reference products for which *in vitro* release rates form the basis of the bioequivalence usually demonstrate Q1/Q2 sameness (qualitatively same inactive ingredients in the quantitative same amounts). Comparative dissolution studies are often performed on several test formulations of the same drug during drug development. Comparative dissolution profiles may be considered similar if the similarity factor (f_2) is greater than 50 (see Chapter 15). For drugs whose dissolution rate is related to the rate of systemic absorption, the test formulation that demonstrates the most rapid rate of drug dissolution *in vitro* will generally have the most rapid rate of drug bioavailability *in vivo*. Under certain conditions, comparative dissolution profiles of higher and lower dose strengths of a solid oral drug product such as an immediate-release tablet are used to obtain a waiver (biowaiver) of performing additional *in vivo* bioequivalence studies (see section on biowaivers).

OTHER APPROACHES DEEMED ACCEPTABLE (BY THE FDA)

The FDA may also use *in vitro* approaches other than comparative dissolution for establishing bioequivalence. The use of *in vitro* biomarkers and *in vitro* binding studies has been proposed to establish bioequivalence. For example, cholestyramine resin is a basic quaternary ammonium anion-exchange resin that is hydrophilic, insoluble in water, and not absorbed in the gastrointestinal tract. The bioequivalence of cholestyramine resin is performed by equilibrium and kinetic binding studies of the resin to bile acid salts (US-FDA, CDER, 2012a). For calcium acetate tablets, which exert the therapeutic response by binding phosphate in the GI tract, the FDA recommends a relatively simple *in vitro* binding assay based on the test/reference binding ratio over a range of phosphate concentrations. Since this test is thought to be highly reproducible, the BE acceptance criterion is that the test/reference binding ratio should fall within limits of 0.9–1.1 (US-FDA, CDER, 2011a). The FDA accepts various other *in vitro* approaches for BE assessment of proposed generic locally acting drug products. For the acyclovir topical ointment,

recommended BE approaches consist of comparative *in vitro* release testing and physicochemical characterization (US-FDA, CDER, 2012b).

BIOEQUIVALENCE STUDIES BASED ON MULTIPLE ENDPOINTS

The FDA may recommend two or more bioequivalence studies, each based on a different approach, for some drug products with complex delivery systems or mechanisms of action. Some examples of drug products that FDA requires multiple bioequivalence studies (Davit and Conner, 2015) are listed in Table 16-4.

BIOEQUIVALENCE STUDIES

Differences in the predicted clinical response or an adverse event may be due to differences in the pharmacokinetic and/or pharmacodynamic behavior of the drug among individuals or to differences in the bioavailability of the drug from the drug product. Bioequivalent drug products that have the same systemic drug bioavailability will have the same predictable drug response. However, variable clinical responses among individuals that are unrelated to bioavailability may also be due to differences in the pharmacodynamics of the drug. Differences in pharmacodynamics, that is, the relationship between the drug and the receptor site, may be due to differences in receptor sensitivity to the drug (see Chapter 21). Various factors affecting pharmacodynamic drug behavior may include age, drug tolerance, drug interactions, and unknown pathophysiologic factors.

Bases for Determining Bioequivalence

Bioequivalence is established if the *in vivo* bioavailability of a test drug product (usually the generic product) does not differ significantly (ie, statistically not significant) from that of the *reference listed drug* (usually the brand-name product approved through the NDA route) in the product's rate and extent of drug absorption. Bioequivalence is determined by comparison of measured parameters (eg, concentration of the active drug ingredient in the blood, urinary

TABLE 16-4   Drug Products for Which FDA Recommends Multiple Bioequivalence Approaches

Product	Indicated to Treat	Approach	Endpoint
Diclofenac gel	Osteoarthritis of the knee	Clinical	Pain score change from baseline
		In vivo PK	AUC, C_{max}
Nitazoxanide oral	Diarrhea caused by *Giardia lamblia*	Clinical	Proportion of patients with a "well" clinical response
		In vivo PK	AUC, C_{max}
Fluticasone propionate nasal suspension	Allergic rhinitis	Clinical	Total nasal symptom score (TNSS) change from baseline
		In vivo PK	AUC, C_{max}
		In vitro	Comparison of device performance with regard to the amount of drug per actuation, droplet size distribution, and plume shape
Mesalamine DR and ER oral formulations	Ulcerative colitis	*In vivo* PK	AUC, pAUC, C_{max}
		In vitro	Comparison of dissolution profiles in several different media of varying pH values
Mesalamine rectal enema	Distal ulcerative colitis, proctitis, and proctosigmoiditis	*In vivo* PK	AUC, C_{max}
		In vitro	Dissolution profiles at pH 4.5, 6.8, 7.2 (Apparatus 2), 900 mL, 35, 50 rpm
Mesalamine suppository	Ulcerative proctitis	*In vivo* PK	AUC, C_{max}
		In vitro	Comparison of physicochemical properties
Risperidone long-acting injectable	Bipolar I disorder and schizophrenia	Steady-state PK in patients	AUC_τ, $(C_{max})_{SS}$
		In vitro	Comparison of the time for 50% of drug to be released at two bracketing sampling times
Lansoprazole DR capsule	Gastroesophageal reflux disease	*In vivo* PK	AUC, C_{max}
		In vitro	Comparison of sedimentation volume, granule dispersion, recovery, and acid resistance, after dispersing into apple juice and dispensing into nasogastric tubes
Dexamethasone/ Tobramycin Ophthalmic Suspension	Prophylaxis against inflammation and infection during cataract surgery	*In vivo* PK	AUC, C_{max}, in aqueous humor of cataract surgery patients
		In vitro	Microbial kill rates against specified microorganisms

excretion rates, or pharmacodynamic effects), when administered at the same molar dose of the active moiety under similar experimental conditions, either single dose or multiple dose.

In a few cases, a drug product that differs from the reference listed drug in its rate of absorption, but not in its extent of absorption, may be considered bioequivalent if the difference in the rate of absorption is intentional and appropriately reflected in the labeling and/or the rate of absorption is not detrimental to the safety and effectiveness of the drug product.

DESIGN AND EVALUATION OF BIOEQUIVALENCE STUDIES

Objective

All scientific studies should have clearly stated objectives. The main objective for a bioequivalence study is that the drug bioavailability from test and reference products is not statistically different when administered to patients or subjects at the same molar dose from pharmaceutically equivalent drug products through the same route of administration under similar experimental conditions.

Study Considerations

The basic design for a bioequivalence study is determined by (1) the scientific questions and objectives to be answered, (2) the nature of the reference material and the dosage form to be tested, (3) the availability of analytical methods, (4) the pharmacokinetics and pharmacodynamics of the drug substance, (5) the route of drug administration, and (6) benefit–risk and ethical considerations with regard to testing in humans.

Since bioequivalence studies are performed to compare the bioavailability of the test or generic drug product to the reference or brand-name product, the statistical techniques should be of sufficient sensitivity to detect differences in rate and extent of absorption that are not attributable to subject variability. Once bioequivalence is established, it is likely that both the generic and brand-name dosage forms will produce the same therapeutic effect. The FDA publishes guidances for bioequivalence studies (US-FDA, CDER, 2010a). Sponsors may also request a meeting with the FDA to review the study design for a specific drug product. Pharmacokinetic

parameters, pharmacodynamic parameters, clinical observations, and/or *in vitro* studies may be used to determine drug bioavailability from a drug product.

The design and evaluation of well-controlled bioequivalence studies require cooperative input from pharmacokineticists, statisticians, clinicians, bioanalytical chemists, and others. For some generic drugs, the FDA offers general guidelines for conducting these studies. For example, *Statistical Procedures for Bioequivalence Studies Using a Standard Two-Treatment Crossover Design* is available from the FDA (US-FDA, CDER, 2000a); the publication addresses three specific aspects, including (1) logarithmic transformation of pharmacokinetic data, (2) sequence effect, and (3) outlier consideration. However, even with the availability of such guidelines, the principal investigator should prepare a detailed protocol for the study. Some of the elements of a protocol for an *in vivo* bioavailability study are listed in Table 16-5.

For bioequivalence studies, the test and reference drug formulations must contain the same drug in the same dose strength and in similar dosage forms (eg, immediate release or controlled release), and must be given by the same route of administration. Before beginning the study, the *Institutional Review Board* (IRB) of the clinical facility in which the study is to be performed must approve the study. The IRB is composed of both professional and lay persons with diverse backgrounds who have clinical experience and expertise as well as sensitivity to ethical issues and community attitudes. The IRB is responsible for all ethical issues including safeguarding the rights and welfare of human subjects.

The basic guiding principle in performing studies is *do not do unnecessary human research*. Generally, the study is performed in normal, healthy male and female volunteers who have given informed consent to be in the study. Critically ill patients are not included in an *in vivo* bioavailability study unless the attending physician determines that there is a potential benefit to the patient. The number of subjects in the study will depend on the expected intersubject and intrasubject variability. Patient selection is made according to certain established criteria for inclusion in, or exclusion from, the study. For example, the study might exclude any volunteers who have known allergies to the drug, are overweight, or have taken any medication within a specified period (often 1 week) prior to the study.

TABLE 16-5   Elements of a Bioavailability Study Protocol

I. Title
    A. Principal investigator (study director)
    B. Project/protocol number and date
II. Study objective
III. Study design
    A. Design
    B. Drug products
        1. Test product(s)
        2. Reference product
    C. Dosage regimen
    D. Sample collection schedule
    E. Housing/confinement
    F. Fasting/meals schedule
    G. Analytical methods
IV. Study population
    A. Subjects
    B. Subject selection
        1. Medical history
        2. Physical examination
        3. Laboratory tests
    C. Inclusion/exclusion criteria
        1. Inclusion criteria
        2. Exclusion criteria
    D. Restrictions/prohibitions
V. Clinical procedures
    A. Dosage and drug administration
    B. Biological sampling schedule and handling procedures
    C. Activity of subjects
VI. Ethical considerations
    A. Basic principles
    B. Institutional review board
    C. Informed consent
    D. Indications for subject withdrawal
    E. Adverse reactions and emergency procedures
VII. Facilities
VIII. Data analysis
    A. Analytical validation procedure
    B. Statistical treatment of data
IX. Drug accountability
X. Appendix

Moderate smokers may be included in these studies. The subjects generally fast for 10–12 hours (overnight) prior to drug administration and may continue to fast for a 2- to 4-hour period after dosing.

Reference Listed Drug (RLD)

For bioequivalence studies of generic products, one formulation of the drug is chosen as a reference standard against which all other formulations of the drug are compared. The FDA designates a single reference listed drug[5] as the standard drug product to which all generic versions must be shown to be bioequivalent. The FDA hopes to avoid possible significant variations among generic drugs and their brand-name counterparts. Such variations could result if generic drugs were compared to different reference listed drugs.

The reference drug product should be administered by the same route as the comparison formulations unless an alternative route or additional route is needed to answer specific pharmacokinetic questions. For example, if an active drug is poorly bioavailable after oral administration, the drug may be compared to an oral solution or an intravenous injection. For bioequivalence studies on a proposed generic drug product, the reference standard is the *reference listed drug* (RLD), which is listed in the FDA's *Approved Drug Products with Therapeutic Equivalence Evaluations*—the Orange Book (US-FDA, CDER, 2014d), and the proposed generic drug product is often referred to as the "test" drug product. The RLD is generally a formulation currently marketed with a fully approved NDA for which there are valid scientific safety and efficacy data. The RLD is usually the innovator's or original manufacturer's brand-name product and is administered according to the dosage recommendations in the labeling.

Before beginning an *in vivo* bioequivalence study, the total content of the active drug substance in the test product (generally the generic product) must be within 5% of that of the reference product. Moreover, *in vitro* comparative dissolution or drug-release studies under various specified conditions are usually performed for both test and reference products before performing the *in vivo* bioequivalence study.

Regulatory Recommendations for Optimizing Bioavailability Study Design

The FDA lists a number of recommendations to consider in designing clinical relative bioavailability studies in drug development. These recommendations include the following:

- Use of a randomized crossover design whenever possible

---

[5]The reference listed drug (RLD) is listed in the Orange Book, *Approved Drug Products with Therapeutic Equivalence Evaluations.* http://www.accessdata.fda.gov/scripts/cder/ob/default.cfm.

- Enrolling both male and female subjects whenever possible
- Administering single doses rather than multiple doses, as single-dose studies are more sensitive, although multiple-dose studies may be more suitable in some cases
- Conducting the studies under fasting and fed conditions[6]
- Measuring the parent drug rather than metabolites, unless the parent cannot be reliably measured. Presystemically formed metabolites that contribute meaningfully to safety and efficacy should also be measured

In addition, the FDA recommends that C_{max} and t_{max} be measured to compare peak exposure and rate of absorption, and that AUC_{0-t} (AUC to the last measurable drug concentration) and $AUC_{0-\infty}$ (AUC extrapolated to infinity) be measured to compare total exposure or extent of drug absorption. Drug exposure parameters should be log-transformed before statistical comparisons. Further detail about the statistical tests will be provided later in the discussion on bioequivalence study designs.

Frequently Asked Questions

▶ *What are the study protocol considerations for conducting a bioequivalence study?*

▶ *What is the reference listed drug (RLD), and how is the RLD selected?*

▶ *How is a bioavailability study of a new molecular entity conducted?*

▶ *Why does the value for relative bioavailability sometimes exceed 1.0, whereas the value for absolute bioavailability cannot exceed 1.0?[7]*

---

[6]In a food-effect bioavailability study, the reference treatment is the oral formulation of the drug product given on an empty stomach, which is compared with the same oral formulation given with food, usually a high-fat, high-calorie meal.

[7]F will appear to exceed 1.0, if the absolute bioavailability is near 100% and variability yields a result slightly higher than 1.0.

Factors Influencing Bioavailability and Impact on Drug Development

Various factors influence bioavailability (Table 16-6). Some of these factors are listed below with implications for formulation development and optimization of dosing regimens.

Physicochemical properties of the drug and formulation. Formulations can be designed to improve the bioavailability of poorly soluble drugs, extend the absorption phase by slowing the rate of release of drugs (controlled-release formulations), or prevent dissolution in the gastric lumen for drugs that are destroyed by gastric acidity (enteric-coated formulations) (see also Chapter 15).

An example of how formulation design can improve bioavailability is shown by comparing the immunosuppressant drug cyclosporine systemic exposures provided by the Neoral® microemulsion formulation to those provided by the Sandimmune® formulation. The Neoral label states that, in a relative bioavailability study in renal transplant, rheumatoid arthritis, and psoriasis patients, the mean cyclosporine AUC was 20%–50% greater, and the mean cyclosporine C_{max} was 40%–106% greater, compared to following administration with Sandimmune. In addition, the dose-normalized AUC in liver transplant patients administered Neoral for 28 days was 50% greater and C_{max} was 90% greater than in those patients administered Sandimmune.

Drug stability and pH effects. Acid-labile drugs potentially have low bioavailability, as they are subject to acid-induced degradation in the low pH conditions of the stomach. For such drugs to achieve therapeutic plasma concentrations, it is necessary to deliver them by formulations that protect against acid-induced degradation, such as buffered products or enteric-coated products. Enteric-coated formulations are used to deliver acid-labile drugs such as didanosine (Damle et al, 2002), a purine nucleoside analog indicted to treat HIV disease, and omeprazole and lansoprazole (Horn and Howden, 2005), which are proton pump inhibitors indicated to treat acid reflux.

Presystemic and first-pass metabolism. The effects of presystemic metabolism on oral bioavailability is (Jagdale et al, 2009) illustrated by propranolol, a

TABLE 16-6   Factors Influencing Bioavailability and Impacting Drug Development

- Physicochemical properties of the drug and formulation
  - The active drug ingredient has low solubility in water (eg, less than 5 mg/mL)
  - The dissolution rate of the product is slow (eg, <50% in 30 min when tested with a general method specified by the FDA)
  - The particle size and surface area of the active drug ingredient is critical in determining its bioavailability
  - Certain structural forms of the active drug ingredient (eg, polymorphic forms, solvates, complexes, and crystal modifications) dissolve poorly, thus affecting bioavailability
- Drug product
  - Drug products that have a high ratio of excipients to active ingredients (eg, >5:1)
  - Specific inactive ingredients (eg, hydrophilic or hydrophobic excipients and lubricants) either may be required for absorption of the active drug or may interfere with such absorption
- Drug stability
  - The drug (and drug product) has poor stability leading to short shelf life
  - The active drug ingredient or therapeutic moiety is unstable in specific portions of the GI tract and requires special coatings or formulations (eg, buffers, enteric coatings, etc) to ensure adequate absorption
- pH effects (eg, pH within the gastrointestinal lumen)
- Surface of dosage form and time available for absorption
- Presystemic metabolism, including hepatic first-pass effect
- Food effects, for orally administered formulations
- The active drug ingredient or its precursor is absorbed mostly in a particular segment of the GI tract or is absorbed from a localized site
- Drug–drug interactions
- Efflux transporters (such as P-glycoprotein)
- The drug product is subject to dose-dependent kinetics in or near the therapeutic range, and the rate and extent of absorption are important in establishing bioequivalence
- Age
- Disease state

nonselective beta adrenergic receptor blocking agent used as an antihypertensive, antianginal, and antiarrhythmic, presystemic metabolism. Propranolol is almost completely absorbed after oral administration, but due to extensive first-pass metabolism in the liver, only about 25% of the parent drug reaches the systemic circulation.

Prodrugs that undergo rapid presystemic metabolism can be used to improve bioavailability, as illustrated by valacyclovir, a prodrug of the nucleoside analog antiviral compound acyclovir. Valacyclovir undergoes rapid presystemic conversion to acyclovir. Both valacyclovir and acyclovir are effective in treating herpes infections. However, because acyclovir bioavailability is greatly enhanced when delivered by its prodrug valacyclovir, for treating herpes zoster, it is only necessary to administer Valtrex® (valacyclovir) tablets administered once daily, compared to 5 times daily for Zovirax® (acyclovir) capsules.

Food effects. Food can either decrease drug bioavailability or increase bioavailability, or have no effect on bioavailability (Davit and Conner, 2008; Dehaven and Conner, 2014). Food can influence bioavailability in a number of ways, such as affecting gastrointestinal pH, gastric emptying, intestinal transit, splanchnic blood flow, and first-pass metabolism. Food can also affect bioavailability by physical or chemical interactions. Most food effects on drug bioavailability are not considered clinically significant, and, consequentially, most drug products are labeled to be administered without regard to meals. If the food effects on drug bioavailability are clinically significant, then the drug product labeling will provide instructions about how to achieve the optimal dosing regimen—either to take the drug only on an empty stomach, or only with food, depending on the nature of the bioavailability effect and clinical consequences.

An example of food reducing bioavailability and the implications for drug product labeling is illustrated by didanosine, discussed earlier. As food prolongs gastric emptying, this increases the length of time that the acid-labile didanosine will be in contact with a low pH environment. The Videx® EC label states that food reduced the didanosine C_{max} by 46% and its AUC by 19%. Consequently, the Videx EC label recommends that didanosine should be taken on an empty stomach in order to avoid the possibility of exposing a patient to subtherapeutic plasma levels.

Food-induced increases in drug bioavailability can be either desirable or undesirable. The food effect on isotretinoin (indicated to treat severe recalcitrant nodular acne) bioavailability is used to optimize the dosing regimen. The Accutane® label states that for isotretinoin capsules, both the C_{max} and AUC were more than doubled when the drug product was taken with a meal compared with fasted conditions. Consequently, the label recommends that isotretinoin capsules should always be taken with food. By contrast, in some cases, food-induced increases in oral bioavailability may be associated with safety concerns. This situation is illustrated by the drug efavirenz, a non-nucleoside reverse transcriptase inhibitor indicated to treat HIV disease. The Sustiva® label describes how coadministration of a high-fat, high-calorie meal increased the efavirenz AUC and C_{max} by 22% and 39%, respectively, and coadministration of a lower-fat, lower-calorie meal increased the efavirenz AUC and C_{max} by 17% and 51%, respectively. Due to concern that exposure to higher efavirenz systemic bioavailability could result in increased serious adverse events, the Sustiva® label recommends that efavirenz capsules and tablets be taken on an empty stomach, preferably at bedtime.

Effects of drug–drug interactions. Changes in drug bioavailability due to drug–drug interactions can occur via a variety of mechanisms, such as inhibition of metabolizing enzymes, induction of metabolizing enzymes, inhibitor of transporters, and induction of transporters. The FDA recommends that interactions between an investigational new drug and other drugs be defined during drug development (US-FDA, CDER, 2012c). Two examples of drug–drug interactions, one of enzyme inhibition and the second of enzyme induction, will show how the ability of coadministered drugs to alter systemic bioavailability impacts both recommendations for optimal dosing regimens and development of new formulations to maximize bioavailability.

An example of a drug–drug interaction that increases bioavailability is provided by ritonavir (an HIV protease inhibitor indicated for treating HIV disease), which is a potent inhibitor of cytochrome P450 3A (CYP3A). As such, ritonavir coadministration increases systemic bioavailability of drugs that are metabolized by CYP3A. For drugs such as sedative hypnotics, antiarrhythmic, and ergot alkaloid preparations, large increases in systemic bioavailability caused by ritonavir coadministration can result in potentially serious and/or life-threatening adverse events; thus, ritonavir coadministration with these drugs is contraindicated. For other coadministered CYP3A substrate drugs for which ritonavir increases bioavailability, such as antidepressants, clarithromycin, immunomodulators, rifabutin, and trazadone, the Norvir® labeling recommends either dose-adjustment or additional monitoring of the coadministered drug to maintain systemic bioavailability levels associated with safety and efficacy.

Because ritonavir can significantly increase the bioavailability of CYP3A substrates, it has been developed as a "booster" to improve systemic exposure of HIV therapies that are CYP3A substrates and that have low oral bioavailability due to extensive hepatic clearance (de Mendoza et al, 2006). Notably, ritonavir is formulated together with the HIV-1 protease inhibitor lopinavir in the fixed-dose combination product Kaletra®. Ritonavir in the Kaletra formulation inhibits the CYP3A-mediated metabolism of lopinavir, thereby increasing lopinavir systemic bioavailability to levels that achieve antiviral activity.

Enzyme inducers coadministered with drugs can potentially lower systemic bioavailability to subtherapeutic levels. An example is the antibacterial drug rifampin (used in treatment of tuberculosis), which is a potent inducer of cytochrome P-450 enzymes. Coadministration of rifampin with drugs metabolized by metabolic pathways induced by rifampin can result in lower bioavailability due to acceleration of metabolism. The Rifadin® label states that, to maintain optimum therapeutic bioavailability, dosages of drugs metabolized by these enzymes may require dose adjustment when starting or stopping concomitantly administered rifampin. Some examples of these drugs for which rifampin lowers systemic bioavailability to the extent that dose adjustment is needed include anticonvulsants, antiarrhythmics, beta-blockers, calcium channel blockers, fluoroquinolones, oral hypoglycemic agents, transplant drugs, and tricyclic antidepressants. For some drugs, such as oral contraceptives, coadministration with rifampin is contraindicated due to concerns that rifampin coadministration can lower oral contraceptive systemic bioavailability to sub-therapeutic levels.

Efflux transporters. The cardiac glycoside digoxin is a substrate for P-glycoprotein, at the level of intestinal absorption, renal tubular secretion, and biliary-intestinal secretion (Hughes and Crowe, 2010). Therefore, drugs that induce or inhibit P-glycoprotein have the potential to alter digoxin bioavailability. Examples of such drugs include amiodarone, propafenone, quinidine, and verapamil. As digoxin is a narrow therapeutic index drug, small changes in bioavailability can potentially result in serious adverse events due to loss of efficacy (bioavailability is lower than the therapeutic range) or life-threatening toxicity (bioavailability exceeds the therapeutic range). Digoxin oral solution USP labeling instructs the practitioner to measure serum digoxin concentrations before initiating concomitant drugs, reduce the digoxin dose once concomitant therapy is initiated, and continue to monitor digoxin serum concentrations.

Age. The systemic bioavailability of a drug is controlled by its absorption, distribution, metabolism, and elimination (ADME). In pediatric patients, growth and developmental changes in factors influencing ADME lead to drug bioavailability that can differ from that of adult patients (US-FDA, CDER, 2014e).

The FDA recommends that sponsors developing pediatric formulations conduct pharmacokinetic studies in the pediatric population to determine how the dosing regimen should be adjusted to achieve the same systemic exposure that is safe and effective in adults (Chapter 23).

Systemic bioavailability of drugs can change with aging (Klotz, 2009). Impairments in the functional reserve of multiple organs can occur with advancing age, and such impairments might affect drug metabolism and pharmacokinetics. Advancing age is associated with changes such as decreases in liver mass and perfusion, changes in body composition, and decreases in renal function. Many of these changes result in increased drug bioavailability. As a result, it is recommended that clinicians carefully monitor dosing regimens and drug action in geriatric patients.

Disease state. The bioavailability of drugs eliminated primarily through renal excretory mechanisms is likely to increase in patients with impaired renal function (Chapter 24). The FDA recommends that, where appropriate, drug pharmacokinetics be characterized in patients with varying degrees of renal impairment. The results of such studies are used to determine how doses can be adjusted in patients with renal impairment in order to achieve the same systemic drug bioavailability as in patients with normal renal function (US-FDA, CDER, 2010b). Similarly, it may be advisable to conduct pharmacokinetic studies of drugs that are primarily cleared by the liver in patients with varying degrees of hepatic impairment (US-FDA, CDER, 2003a). The results of pharmacokinetic studies in hepatic-impaired patients can be useful in determining whether dose adjustments are required in such patients to achieve the same systemic drug bioavailability as in patients with normal liver function.

The systemic bioavailability of a drug in patients can differ from that in healthy normal subjects. Ordinarily, sponsors conduct single- and multiple-dose pharmacokinetic studies in both healthy normal subjects and the target patient population in early stage development, to characterize similarities and differences in drug systemic bioavailability.

Analytical Methods

Analytical methods used in an *in vivo* bioavailability, bioequivalence, or pharmacodynamic studies must be validated for accuracy and sufficient sensitivity. The actual concentration of the active drug ingredient or therapeutic moiety, or its active metabolite(s), must be measured with appropriate precision in body fluids or excretory products. For bioavailability and bioequivalence studies, both the parent drug and its major active metabolites are generally measured. For bioequivalence studies, the parent drug is measured. Measurement of the active metabolite is important for very high-hepatic clearance (first-pass metabolism) drugs when the parent drug concentrations are too low to be reliable.

The analytical method for measurement of the drug must be validated for accuracy, precision, sensitivity, specificity, and robustness. The use of more than one analytical method during a bioequivalence study may not be valid, because different methods may yield different values. Data should be presented in both tabulated and graphic form for evaluation. The plasma drug concentration–time curve for each drug product and each subject should be available.

STUDY DESIGNS

For many drug products, the FDA, Division of Bioequivalence, Office of Generic Drugs, provides guidance for the performance of *in vitro* dissolution and *in vivo* bioequivalence studies (US-FDA, CDER, 2010a). Generally, two bioequivalence studies are required for solid oral dosage forms, including (1) a fasting study and (2) a food intervention study. For extended-release capsules containing beads (pellets) that might be poured on a semisolid food such as applesauce, an additional "sprinkle" bioequivalence study is recommended. Other study designs such as parallel design, replicate design, and multiple-dose (steady-state) bioequivalence studies have been proposed by the FDA. Proper study design and statistical evaluation are important considerations for the determination of bioequivalence. Some of the designs listed above are summarized here.

Fasting Study

Bioequivalence studies are usually evaluated by a single-dose, two-period, two-treatment, two-sequence, open-label, randomized crossover design comparing equal doses of the test and reference products in fasted, adult, healthy subjects. This study is requested for all immediate-release and modified-release oral dosage forms. Both male and female subjects may be used in the study. Blood sampling is performed just before (zero time) the dose and at appropriate intervals after the dose to obtain an adequate description of the plasma drug concentration–time profile. The subjects should be in the fasting state (overnight fast of at least 10 hours) before drug administration and should continue to fast for up to 4 hours after dosing. No other medication is normally given to the subject for at least 1 week prior to the study. In some cases, a parallel design may be more appropriate for certain drug products, containing a drug with a very long elimination half-life. A replicate design may be used for a drug product containing a drug that has high intrasubject variability.

Food Intervention Study

Coadministration of food with an oral drug product may affect the bioavailability of the drug. Food intervention or food effect studies are generally conducted using meal conditions that are expected to provide the greatest effects on GI physiology so that systemic drug availability is maximally affected. Food effects on bioavailability are generally greatest when the drug product is administered shortly after a meal is ingested. The nutrient and caloric contents of the meal, the meal volume, and the meal temperature can cause physiological changes in the GI tract in a way that affects drug product transit time, luminal dissolution, drug permeability, and systemic availability.

Meals that are high in total calories and fat content are more likely to affect the GI physiology and thereby result in a larger effect on the bioavailability of a drug substance or drug product (US-FDA, CDER, 2003b). In addition, the high fat meal can have a significant effect on certain modified-release drug products causing them to dose dump. The test meal is a high-fat (approximately 50% of total caloric content of the meal) and high-calorie (approximately 800–1000 calories) meal. A typical test meal is two eggs fried in butter, two strips of bacon, two slices of toast with butter, 4 oz of brown potatoes, and 8 oz of milk. This test meal derives approximately 150, 250, and 500–600 calories from protein, carbohydrate, and fat, respectively (www.fda.gov/cder/guidance/4613dft.pdf).

For bioequivalence studies for generic drugs, drug bioavailability from both the test and reference products should be affected similarly by food. The usual study design uses a single-dose, randomized, two-treatment, two-period, crossover study comparing equal doses of the test and reference products. Following an overnight fast of at least 10 hours, subjects are given the recommended meal 30 minutes before dosing. The meal is consumed over 30 minutes, with administration of the drug product immediately after the meal. The drug product is given with 240 mL (8 fluid oz) of water. No food is allowed for at least 4 hours postdose. This study is requested for all modified-release dosage forms and may be requested for immediate-release dosage forms if the bioavailability of the active drug ingredient is known to be affected by food (eg, ibuprofen, naproxen). According to the labeling for certain extended-release capsules that contain coated beads, the capsule contents can be sprinkled over soft foods such as applesauce. This is taken by the fasted subject and the bioavailability of the drug is then measured for the NDA. For generic drug products in Abbreviated New Drug Applications (ANDAs), this study is performed as a bioequivalence study to demonstrate that both products, sprinkled on food, will have equivalent bioavailability. Bioavailability studies might also examine the effects of other foods and special vehicles such as apple juice.

CROSSOVER STUDY DESIGNS

Subjects who meet the inclusion and exclusion study criteria and have given informed consent are selected at random. A complete crossover design is usually employed, in which each subject receives the test drug product and the reference product. Examples of *Latin-square crossover designs* for a bioequivalence study in human volunteers, comparing three different drug formulations (A, B, C) or four different

drug formulations (A, B, C, D), are described in Tables 16-7 and 16-8. The Latin-square design plans the clinical trial so that each subject receives each drug product only once, with adequate time between medications for the elimination of the drug from the body. In this design, each subject is his own control, and subject-to-subject variation is reduced. Moreover, variations due to sequence, period, and treatment (formulation) are reduced, so that all patients do not receive the same drug product on the same day and in the same order. The order in which the drug treatments are given should not stay the same in order to prevent any bias in the data due to a residual effect from the previous treatment. Possible carryover effects from any particular drug product are minimized by changing the sequence or order in which the drug products are given to the subject. Thus, drug product B may be followed by drug product A, D, or C (Table 16-8). After each subject receives a drug product, blood samples are collected at appropriate time intervals so that a valid blood drug level–time curve is obtained. The time intervals should be spaced so that the peak blood concentration, the total area under the curve, and the absorption and elimination phases of the curve may be well described.

Period refers to the time period in which a study is performed. A two-period study is a study that is performed on two different days (time periods) separated by a *washout period* during which most of the drug is eliminated from the body—generally about

TABLE 16-7   Latin-Square Crossover Design for a Bioequivalence Study of Three Drug Products in Six Human Volunteers

Subject	Drug Product		
	Study Period 1	Study Period 2	Study Period 3
1	A	B	C
2	B	C	A
3	C	A	B
4	A	C	B
5	C	B	A
6	B	A	C

TABLE 16-8 Latin-Square Crossover Design for a Bioequivalency Study of 4 Drug Products in 16 Human Volunteers

	Drug Product			
Subject	Study Period 1	Study Period 2	Study Period 3	Study Period 4
1	A	B	C	D
2	B	C	D	A
3	C	D	A	B
4	D	A	B	C
5	A	B	D	C
6	B	D	C	A
7	D	C	A	B
8	C	A	B	D
9	A	C	B	D
10	C	B	D	A
11	B	D	A	C
12	D	A	C	B
13	A	C	D	B
14	C	D	B	A
15	D	B	A	C
16	B	A	C	D

10 elimination half-lives. A *sequence* refers to the number of different orders in the treatment groups in a study. For example, a two-sequence, two-period study would be designed as follows:

	Period 1	Period 2
Sequence 1	T	R
Sequence 2	R	T

where R = reference and T = treatment.

Replicated Crossover Study Designs

The standard bioequivalence criterion using the two-way crossover design does not give an estimate of within-subject (intrasubject) variability. By giving the same drug product twice to the same subject, the replicate design provides a measure for within-subject variability. Replicate design studies may be used for highly variable drugs and for narrow therapeutic index drugs. In the case of highly variable drugs (%CV greater than 30), a large number of subjects (>80) would be needed to demonstrate bioequivalence using the standard two-way crossover design. Drugs with high within-subject variability generally have a wide therapeutic window and despite high variability, these products have been demonstrated to be both safe and effective. Replicate designs for highly variable drugs/products require a smaller number of subjects and, therefore, do not unnecessarily expose a large number of healthy subjects to a drug when this large number of subjects is not needed for assurance of bioequivalence (Haidar et al, 2008).

Replicated crossover designs are used for the determination of individual bioequivalence, to estimate within-subject variance for both the test and reference drug products, and to provide an estimate of the subject-by-formulation interaction variance. A four-period, two-sequence, two-formulation design is shown below:

	Period 1	Period 2	Period 3	Period 4
Sequence 1	T	R	T	R
Sequence 2	R	T	R	T

where R = reference and T = treatment.

In this design, the same reference and the same test are each given twice to the same subject. Other sequences are possible. In this design, reference-to-reference and test-to-test comparisons may also be made.

Narrow Therapeutic Index Drugs

Narrow therapeutic index (NTI) drugs, also referred to as critical dose drugs, are drugs in which small changes in dose or concentration may lead to serious therapeutic failures or serious adverse drug reactions in patients. Narrow therapeutic index drugs consistently display the following characteristics: (a) Subtherapeutic concentrations may lead to serious therapeutic failure;

(b) there is little separation between therapeutic and toxic doses (or the associated plasma concentrations); (c) they are subject to therapeutic monitoring based on pharmacokinetic or pharmacodynamic measures; (d) they possess low-to-moderate within-subject variability (<30%); and (e) in clinical practice, doses are generally adjusted in very small increments (<20%). The FDA currently recommends that bioequivalence studies of narrow therapeutic index drugs should employ a four-way, fully replicated, crossover study design. The replicated study design permits comparison of both test and reference means and test and reference within-subject variability (Davit et al, 2013).

An additional test recommended in bioequivalence studies of generic narrow therapeutic index drugs is a test for within-subject variability. The test determines whether within-subject variability of the test narrow therapeutic index drug does not differ significantly from that of the reference by evaluating the test/reference ratio of the within-subject standard deviation. The FDA currently recommends that all bioequivalence studies on narrow therapeutic index drugs must pass both the reference-scaled approach and the unscaled average bioequivalence limits of 80.00%–125.00%.

Reference Scaled Average Bioequivalence

Recently a three-sequence, three-period, two-treatment partially replicated crossover design for bioequivalence studies of highly variable drugs has been recommended by the FDA (Haidar et al, 2008). The partially replicated design allows the estimation of the within-subject variance and subject-by-formulation interaction for the reference product. The time for completion of this study is shorter than the fully replicated four-way crossover design.

This design is usually used for highly variable drugs with within-subject variability ≥30%. Large numbers of subjects may be needed in bioequivalence studies of highly variable drugs; the FDA implemented the reference-scaled average bioequivalence approach to ease regulatory burden and reduce unnecessary human testing. Using this approach, the implied BE limits can widen to be larger than 80%–125% for drugs that are highly

variable, provided that certain constraints are applied to this approach in order to maintain an acceptable type I error rate and satisfy any public health concerns (Davit et al, 2012).

	Period 1	Period 2	Period 3
Sequence 1	T	R	R
Sequence 2	R	T	R
Sequence 3	R	R	T

Under this design, if the test product has lower variability than the reference product, the study will need a smaller number of subjects to pass the bioequivalence criteria. Scaled average bioequivalence is evaluated for both AUC and C_{max}.

Parallel Study Designs

A nonreplicate, parallel design is used for drug products that contain drugs that have a long elimination half-life or drug products such as depot injections in which the drug is slowly released over weeks or months. In this design, two separate groups of volunteers are used. One group will be given the test product and the other group will be given the reference product. It is important to balance the demographics of both groups of volunteers. Blood sample collection time should be adequate to ensure completion of gastrointestinal transit (approximately 2–3 days) of the drug product and absorption of the drug substance. C_{max} and a suitably truncated AUC, generally to 72 hours after dose administration, can be used to characterize peak and total drug exposure, respectively. For drugs that demonstrate low intrasubject variability in distribution and clearance, an AUC truncated at 72 hours (AUC_0^{72} hours) can be used in place of AUC_0^t or AUC_0^∞. This design is not recommended for drugs that have high intrasubject variability in distribution and clearance.

Multiple-Dose (Steady-State) Study Design

A bioequivalence study may be performed using a multiple-dose study design. Multiple doses of the same drug are given consecutively to reach steady-state plasma drug levels. The multiple-dose study is designed as a steady-state, randomized, two-treatment, two-way, crossover study comparing equal doses of the test and reference products in healthy adult subjects. Each subject receives either the test or the reference product separated by a "washout" period, which is the time needed for the drug to be completely eliminated from the body.

To ascertain that the subjects are at steady state, three consecutive trough concentrations (C_{min}) are determined. The last morning dose is given to the subject after an overnight fast, with continual fasting for at least 2 hours following dose administration. Blood sampling is then performed over one dosing interval. The area under the curve during a dosing interval at steady state should be the same as the area under the curve extrapolated to infinite time after a single dose.

Pharmacokinetic analyses for multiple-dose studies include calculation of the following parameters for each subject:

AUC_{0-tau}—Area under the curve during a dosing interval

t_{max}—Time to C_{max} during a dosing interval
C_{max}—Maximum drug concentration during dosing interval
C_{min}—Drug concentration at the end of a dosing interval
C_{av}—The average drug concentration during a dosing interval
Degree of fluctuation $= (C_{max} - C_{min})/C_{max}$
Swing $= (C_{max} - C_{min})/C_{min}$

The data are analyzed statistically using analysis of variance (ANOVA) on the log-transformed AUC and C_{max}. To establish bioequivalence, both AUC and C_{max} for the test (generic) product should be within 80%–125% of the reference product using a 90% confidence interval. Estimation of the absorption rate constant during multiple dosing is difficult, because the residual drug from the previous dose superimposes on the dose that follows. However, the data obtained in multiple doses are useful in calculating a steady-state plasma level.

The extent of bioavailability, measured by assuming the $[AUC]_0^\infty$, is dependent on clearance:

$$[AUC]_0^\infty = \frac{FD_0}{Cl_T}$$

Determination of bioavailability using multiple doses reveals changes that are normally not detected in a single-dose study. For example, nonlinear pharmacokinetics may occur after multiple drug doses due to the higher plasma drug concentrations saturating an enzyme system involved in absorption or elimination of the drug. Nonlinear pharmacokinetics after multiple-dose studies may be observed by rising C_{min} drug concentrations and AUC_t after each dosing interval. With some drugs, a drug-induced malabsorption syndrome can also alter the percentage of drug absorbed. In this case, drug bioavailability may decrease after repeated doses if the fraction of the dose absorbed (F) decreases or if the total body clearance (kV_D) increases. It should be noted that nonlinear PK can also be observed by high single doses of the drug.

There are several disadvantages of using the multiple-dose crossover method for the determination of bioequivalence. (1) The study takes more time to perform, because steady-state conditions must be reached. A longer time for completion of a study leads to greater clinical costs and the possibility of a subject dropping out and not completing the study. (2) More plasma samples must be obtained from the subject to ascertain that steady state has been reached and to describe the plasma level–time curve accurately. (3) Because C_{av}^∞ depends primarily on the dose of the drug and the time interval between doses, the extent of drug systemically available is more important than the rate of drug availability. Small differences in the rate of drug absorption may not be observed with steady-state study comparisons

Clinical Endpoint Bioequivalence Study

Study design for a clinical endpoint study generally consists of a randomized, double-blind, placebo-controlled, parallel-designed study comparing test product, reference product, and placebo product in patients. A placebo arm is usually included to demonstrate that the treatments are active (above the no-effect part of the effect versus dose curve, see Fig. 16-11) and the study is sufficiently sensitive to identify the clinical effect in the patient population enrolled in the study. In some cases, the use of a placebo may not be included for safety reasons.

The primary analysis for bioequivalence is determined by evaluating the difference between the proportion of patients in the test and reference treatment groups who are considered a "therapeutic cure" at the end of study. The superiority of the test and reference products against the placebo is also tested using the same dichotomous endpoint of "therapeutic cure."

Determination of Bioequivalence of Drug Products in Patients Maintained on a Therapeutic Drug Regimen

A bioequivalence study may be performed in patients already maintained on the reference (brand-name) drug. Due to safety concerns, certain drugs such as clozapine, a dibenzodiazepine derivative with potent antipsychotic properties, should not be given to normal healthy subjects (US-FDA, CDER, 2011b). Instead, bioequivalence studies on clozapine should be performed in patients who have been stabilized on the highest strength (eg, 100 mg) using a multiple-dose bioequivalence study design. Patients on these or other drugs such as antipsychotics (US-FDA, CDER, 2013a) or cancer chemotherapeutic drugs (Kaur et al, 2013) would be at risk if a washout

period is used between drug treatments. Therefore, the patient is maintained on his or her previous dose of medication or an equal dose of the test product, and blood sampling is performed during a dosage interval (Fig. 16-13, reference product A). Once blood sampling is accomplished, the patient takes equal oral doses of the other drug product (test or reference) and the previous drug product is discontinued. Drug dosing with each drug product continues until attainment of steady state. When steady state is reached, the plasma level–time curve for a dosage interval with the second drug product is described (Fig. 16-13, drug product B). Using the same plasma measures as before, the bioequivalence or lack of bioequivalence may be determined. The patient then continues with his or her therapy with the original drug product.

Products are given in random order: A then B, B then A. Failure to do this might lead to a sequence effect. The reference product that is tested is provided by the investigator from a known lot (not the patient's own prescription).

Since the patients are being treated with the reference (brand) product A, the drug concentrations are at steady state prior to the start of the study and the accumulation phase is not observed. The test

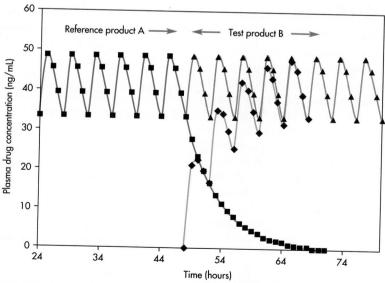

FIGURE 16-13 Multiple-dose bioequivalence study in patients. Bioequivalence is determined by comparison of the steady-state plasma drug-versus-time profile after administration of the reference drug product A to the steady-state plasma drug–time profile after administration of the test drug product B.

drug product B is started and the reference drug product A is stopped. The total plasma drug concentrations are maintained. Bioequivalence is determined by comparison of the steady-state plasma drug-versus-time profile after administration of the reference drug product A to the steady-state plasma drug–time profile after administration of the test drug product B.

If the blood level–time curve of the second drug product is bioequivalent, as shown by AUC_t and C_{max}, to that of the reference drug product, the second product is considered to be bioequivalent. If the second drug has less bioavailability (assuming that only the extent of drug absorption is less than that of the reference drug), the resulting C_{av}^{∞} will be smaller than that obtained with the first drug. C_{av}^{∞} is not actually used as a direct measurement. Usually, the drug manufacturer will perform dissolution and content uniformity tests before performing a bioequivalence study. These *in vitro* dissolution tests will help ensure that the C_{av}^{∞} obtained from each drug product *in vivo* will not be largely different from each other. In contrast, if the extent of drug availability is greater in the second drug product, the C_{av}^{∞} will be higher.

CLINICAL EXAMPLE

Levothyroxine Sodium Oral Tablets

A multiple dose relative bioavailability study[8] of two synthetic branded levothyroxine sodium oral tablets, product A and product B, were evaluated in 20 euthyroid patients. The investigation was designed as a two-way crossover study in which the patients who had been diagnosed as hypothyroid by their primary-care physician were given a single 100-μg daily dose of either product A or product B levothyroxine sodium tablets for 50 days and then switched over immediately to the other treatment for 50 days. Predose blood samples were taken on days 1, 25, 48, 49, and 50 of each phase, and, on day 50, a complete blood sampling was performed. The serum from

---

[8]For the FDA-recommended bioequivalence study for levothyroxine sodium tablets, see FDA Guidance for Industry: Levothyroxine Sodium Tablets—In Vivo Pharmacokinetic and Bioavailability Studies, and In Vitro Dissolution Testing, December 2000.

each blood sample was analyzed for total and free thyroxine (T4), total and free triiodothyronine (T3), the major metabolite of T4, and thyrotropin (TSH).

a. Why were hypothyroid patients used in this study?

b. Why were the subjects dosed for 50 days with each thyroid product?

c. Why were blood samples obtained on days 48, 49, and 50?

d. Why was T3 measured?

e. Why was TSH measured?

Solution

a. Normal healthy euthyroid subjects would be at risk if they were to take levothyroxine sodium for an extended period of time.

b. The long (50-day) daily dosing for each product was required to obtain steady-state drug levels because of the long elimination half-life of levothyroxine.

c. Serum from blood samples was taken on days 48, 49, and 50 to obtain three consecutive C_{min} drug levels.

d. T3 is the active metabolite of T4.

e. The serum TSH concentration is inversely proportional to the free serum T4 concentrations and gives an indication of the pharmacodynamic activity of the active drug.

CLINICAL EXAMPLE

Mercaptopurine (Purinethol) Oral Tablets

Mercaptopurine (Purinethol) is a cytotoxic drug used to treat cancer and is available in a 50-mg oral tablet. The FDA recommends bioequivalence steady-state studies (US-FDA, CDER, 2011c) in patients receiving therapeutic oral doses (usually 100–200 mg/d in the average adult) or maintenance daily doses (usually 50–100 mg/d in the average adult).

Patients should be on a stable regimen using the same dosage unit (multiples of the same 50-mg strength). Plasma drug concentration–time profiles are obtained in these patients at steady state with the brand product. The proposed generic drug product is then given to these patients at the same dosage regimen until steady state is reached. Plasma drug concentration–time profiles are obtained for the generic drug product; then the patients return to the original brand medication.

Frequently Asked Questions

▶ *What do sequence, washout period, and period mean in a crossover bioavailability study?*

▶ *Why does the FDA request a food intervention (food-effect) study for new and generic drug products before granting approval?*

▶ *What type of bioequivalence studies are requested for drugs that are not systemically absorbed or for those drugs in which the C_{max} and AUC cannot be measured in the plasma?*

▶ *How do inter- and intrasubject variability affect the statistical demonstration of bioequivalence for a drug product?*

PHARMACOKINETIC EVALUATION OF THE DATA

For single-dose studies, including a fasting study or a food intervention study, the pharmacokinetic analyses include calculation for each subject of the area under the curve to the last quantifiable concentration (AUC_0^t) and to infinity (AUC_0^∞), t_{max}, and C_{max}. Additionally, the elimination rate constant, k, the elimination half-life, $t_{1/2}$, and other parameters may be estimated. For multiple-dose studies, pharmacokinetic analysis includes calculation for each subject of the steady-state area under the curve, (AUC_∞^t), t_{max}, C_{min}, C_{max}, and the percent fluctuation [$100 \times (C_{max} - C_{min})/C_{min}$]. Proper statistical evaluation should be performed on the estimated pharmacokinetic parameters.

Statistical Evaluation of the Data

Bioequivalence is generally determined using a comparison of population averages of a bioequivalence metric, such as AUC and C_{max}. This approach, termed *average bioequivalence*, involves the calculation of a 90% confidence interval for the ratio of averages (population geometric means) of the bioequivalence

metrics for the test and reference drug products (US-FDA, CDER, 2000a).

Many statistical approaches (parametric tests) assume that the data are distributed according to a normal distribution or "bell-shaped curve" (see Appendix A). The pharmacokinetic parameters such as C_{max} and AUC may not be normally distributed, and the true distribution is difficult to ascertain because of the small number of subjects used in a bioequivalence study. The distribution of data that have been transformed to log values resembles more closely a normal distribution compared to the distribution of non-log-transformed data.

Two One-Sided Tests Procedure

The two one-sided tests procedure is also referred to as the *confidence interval approach* (Schuirmann, 1987). This statistical method is used to demonstrate if the bioavailability of the drug from the test formulation is too low or high in comparison to that of the reference product. The objective of the approach is to determine if there are large differences (ie, greater than 20%) between the mean parameters.

The 90% confidence limits are estimated for the sample means. The interval estimate is based on Student's t distribution of the data. In this test, presently required by the FDA, a 90% confidence interval about the ratio of means of the two drug products must be within ±20% for measurement of the rate and extent of drug bioavailability. For most drugs, up to a 20% difference in AUC or C_{max} between two formulations would have no clinical significance. The lower 90% confidence interval for the ratio of means cannot be less than 0.80, and the upper 90% confidence interval for the ratio of the means cannot be greater than 1.20. When log-transformed data are used, the 90% confidence interval is set at 80%–125%. These confidence limits have also been termed the *bioequivalence interval* (Midha et al, 1993). The 90% confidence interval is a function of sample size and study variability, including inter- and intrasubject variability.

For a single-dose, fasting or food intervention bioequivalence study, an ANOVA is usually performed on the log-transformed AUC and C_{max} values. There should be no statistical differences between the mean AUC and C_{max} parameters for the test (generic) and reference drug products. In addition, the 90%

TABLE 16-9   Statistical Analysis for Average Bioequivalence

- Based on log-transformed data
- Point estimates of the mean ratios
  Test/reference for AUC and C_{max} are between 80% and 125%
- AUC and C_{max}
  90% confidence intervals (CI) must fit between 80% and 125%
- Bioequivalence criteria
  Two one-sided tests procedure
  - Test (T) is not significantly less than reference
  - Reference (R) is not significantly less than test
  - Significant difference is 20% ($\alpha = 0.05$ significance level)
    T/R = 80/100 = 80%
    R/T = 80% (all data expressed as T/R, so this becomes 100/80 = 125%)
- The statistical model typically includes factors accounting for the following sources of variation: sequence, subjects nested in sequences, period, and treatment

From US-FDA, CDER (2000).

confidence intervals about the ratio of the means for AUC and C_{max} values of the test drug product should not be less than 0.80 (80%) nor greater than 1.25 (125%) of that of the reference product based on log-transformed data. Table 16-9 summarizes the statistical analysis for average bioequivalence. Presently, the FDA accepts only average bioequivalence estimates used to establish bioequivalence of generic drug products.

Analysis of Variance

An analysis of variance (see ANOVA) is a statistical procedure (see Appendix A) used to test the data for differences within and between treatment and control groups. A bioequivalent product should produce no significant difference in all pharmacokinetic parameters tested. The parameters tested statistically usually include AUC_0^t, AUC_0^∞, and C_{max} obtained for each treatment or dosage form. Other metrics of bioavailability have also been used to compare the bioequivalence of two or more formulations. The ANOVA may evaluate variability in subjects, treatment groups, study period, formulation, and other variables, depending on the study design. If the variability in the data is large, the difference in means for

each pharmacokinetic parameter, such as AUC, may be masked, and the investigator might erroneously conclude that the two drug products are bioequivalent.

A statistical difference between the pharmacokinetic parameters obtained from two or more drug products is considered statistically significant if there is a probability of less than 1 in 20 times or 0.05 probability ($p \leq .05$) that these results would have happened on the basis of chance alone. The probability, p, is used to indicate the level of statistical significance. If $p < .05$, the differences between the two drug products are not considered statistically significant.

To reduce the possibility of failing to detect small differences between the test products, a *power test* is performed to calculate the probability that the conclusion of the ANOVA is valid. The power of the test will depend on the sample size, variability of the data, and desired level of significance. Usually, the power is set at 0.80 with a $\beta = 0.2$ and a level of significance of 0.05. The higher the power, the test is more sensitive and the greater the probability that the conclusion of the ANOVA is valid.

THE PARTIAL AUC IN BIOEQUIVALENCE ANALYSIS

Several new drug delivery systems have a complex approach to drug release (eg, combinations of zero-order and first-order release) that produces an unusually shaped plasma drug concentration-versus-time profile. The shape of this plasma drug concentration-versus-time profile is related to the pharmacodynamics of the drug.

To evaluate a generic dosage form of these new drug delivery systems, the FDA recommends including the partial AUC (pAUC) as a pivotal BE metric. The pAUC is defined as the area under the plasma concentration-versus-time profile over two specified time points. The choice of sampling time points for calculating the pAUC is based on the pharmacokinetic/pharmacodynamic or efficacy/safety data for the drug under examination.

The FDA currently expects the pAUC to be analyzed statistically when determining bioequivalence of multiphasic modified-release (MR) formulations designed to achieve a rapid therapeutic response followed by a sustained response. Such products are

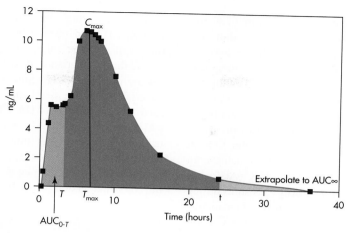

FIGURE 16-14   Partial AUC analysis in a bioequivalence study. The partial AUC (pAUC) refers to the AUC between two specified, clinically relevant, time points on the drug plasma concentration-versus-time profile. The sampling time *T* should be selected based on the pharmacokinetic and pharmacodynamic properties of the active ingredient.

generally formulated with both an immediate-release component and a delayed- or extended-release component. Figure 16-14 illustrates how a pAUC analysis, based on two partial AUCs, is applied. The two partial AUCs consist of an early pAUC measure AUC_{0-T} to compare test and reference exposure responsible for early onset of response, and a late pAUC measure AUC_{T-t} to compare test and reference exposure responsible for sustained response. The early AUC_{0-T} is measured beginning at sampling time 0 to a truncation time T. The late AUC_{T-t} is measured from the truncation time T to the last sampling point with measurable drug concentration. These two metrics replace AUC_{0-t} in bioequivalence evaluation. The bioequivalence determination is based on comparison of test and reference C_{max}, $AUC_{0-\infty}$, AUC_{0-T}, and AUC_{T-t}.

The partial AUC (pAUC) refers to the AUC between two specified, clinically relevant, time points on the drug plasma concentration-versus-time profile. The sampling time T should be selected based on the pharmacokinetic and pharmacodynamic properties of the active ingredient.

Examples of Partial AUC Analyses

The first product to which this approach was applied was the zolpidem extended-release formulation. The reference for this product, Ambien CR®, exhibits

biphasic absorption characteristics, which result in rapid initial absorption from the gastrointestinal tract similar to zolpidem tartrate immediate release, and then provide extended plasma concentrations beyond 3 hours of administration. As a result, patients receiving Ambien CR experience both rapid onset of sleep and maintenance of sleep. To ensure that a test zolpidem tartrate extended-release tablet provides the same pharmacodynamic response (timing of sleep onset and maintenance) when switched with the reference product, the FDA expects that, in a bioequivalence study comparing the two, the parameters $AUC_{0-1.5h}$, $AUC_{1.5h-t}$, $AUC_{0-\infty}$, and C_{max} will all pass bioequivalence limits of 80.00%–125.00% (US-FDA, CDER, 2011d). The sampling time for the early and late pAUCs for the zolpidem extended-release tablet were selected based on zolpidem pharmacokinetic–pharmacodynamic relationships.

The FDA recently posted a draft guidance for industry recommending the application of three pAUC metrics, for bioequivalence studies of generic versions of the methylphenidate multiphasic MR tablet (US-FDA, CDER, 2014f). The reference listed drug for this product is Concerta®, indicated for the treatment of attention deficit hyperactivity disorder. The product is labeled to be administered once in the morning, before the start of the school day, for pediatric patients. The three pAUC metrics are proposed to ensure that when patients for whom Concerta treatment is indicated switch formulations, they will experience equivalent therapeutic responses over the course of the day. Thus, for an acceptable bioequivalence study, the 90% confidence intervals of the geometric mean test/reference ratios C_{max}, AUC_{0-T_1}, $AUC_{T_1-T_2}$, $AUC_{T_2-T_3}$, and AUC_∞ should fall within the limits of 80.00%–125.00%. The sampling time T_1 for the first pAUC (AUC_{0-T_1}) is based on the time at which 90%–95% of subjects are likely to achieve an early onset of response. The middle pAUC ($AUC_{T_1-T_2}$) comparison is to ensure similar drug exposures during the remaining school hours (for pediatric patients) after early onset of exposure. The late pAUC comparison ($AUC_{T_2-T_3}$) is to ensure equivalent methylphenidate exposures during the latter part of the dosing interval, corresponding to the duration of the sustained response.

The pAUC is also used as a BE metric in studies comparing test and reference versions of mesalamine orally administered MR formulations (Table 16-10). Mesalamine is indicated to treat inflammatory diseases of the colon and rectum, and is thought to act locally rather than systemically. Table 16-10 summarizes the mesalamine RLD oral MR formulations, associated indications, and Pauc metrics used in BE studies against each of these RLDs. Mesalamine is well absorbed, most likely throughout the small and large intestines, with the result that it is possible to measure plasma concentrations and determine PK profiles following oral administration (US-FDA, CDER, 2013b). However, because the site of mesalamine action is the colon and rectum, the FDA concluded that comparisons of AUC and C_{max} alone in BE studies would not distinguish between products with materially different mesalamine release profiles at the sites of drug action (US-FDA, CDER, 2010c). Thus, the pAUC is used to analyze systemic mesalamine concentrations over specified time intervals to determine whether mesalamine from test and reference products is available at the same rate and to the same extent at the colon and rectum (Davit and Conner, 2015).

BIOEQUIVALENCE EXAMPLES

A simulated example of the results for a single-dose, fasting study is shown in Table 16-11 and in Fig. 16-15. As shown by the ANOVA, no statistical differences for the pharmacokinetic parameters, AUC_0^t, AUC_0^∞, and C_{max}, were observed between the test product and the brand-name product. The 90% confidence limits for the mean pharmacokinetic parameters of the test product were within 0.80–1.25 (80%–125%) of the reference product means based on log transformation of the data. The power test for the AUC measures was above 99%, showing good precision of the data. The power test for the C_{max} values was 87.9%, showing that this parameter was more variable.

Table 16-12 shows the results for a hypothetical bioavailability study in which three different tablet

TABLE 16-10   Bioequivalence Metrics for *In Vivo* Studies of Mesalamine Modified-Release Oral Dosage Forms

Formulation	Reference	Bioequivalence Metrics
Mesalamine delayed-release capsule	Delzicol®	For both fasting and fed studies: C_{max}, $AUC_{8-48\,h}$, AUC_{0-t}
Mesalamine delayed-release tablet	Asacol®	
Mesalamine delayed-release tablet	Asacol HD®	
Mesalamine delayed-release tablet	Lialda®	
Mesalamine extended-release capsule	Pentasa®	For fasting study: C_{max}, $AUC_{0-3\,h}$, $AUC_{3\,h-t}$, AUC_{0-t} For fed study: C_{max} and AUC_{0-t} are pivotal; $AUC_{0-3\,h}$ and AUC_{0-t} are supportive
Mesalamine extended-release capsule	Apriso®	

TABLE 16-11   **Bioavailability Comparison of a Generic (Test) and Brand-Name (Reference) Drug Products (Log-Normal Transformed Data)**

Variable	Units	Geometric Mean		% Ratio	90% Confidence Interval (Lower Limit, Upper Limit)	p Values for Product Effects	Power of ANOVA	ANOVA %CV
		Test	Reference					
C_{max}	ng/mL	344.79	356.81	96.6	(89.5, 112)	0.3586	0.8791	17.90%
	ng·h/mL	2659.12	2674.92	99.4	(95.1, 104)	0.8172	1.0000	12.60%
AUC_∞		2708.63	2718.52	99.6	(95.4, 103)	0.8865	1.0000	12.20%
t_{max}	h	4.29	4.24	101				
K_{elim}	1/h	0.0961	0.0980	98.1				
$t_{1/2}$	h	8.47	8.33	101.7				

The results were obtained from a two-way, crossover, single-dose study in 36 fasted, healthy, adult male and female volunteers. No statistical differences were observed for the mean values between test and reference products.

formulations were compared to a solution of the drug given in the same dose. As shown in the table, the bioavailability from all three tablet formulations was greater than 80% of that of the solution. According to the ANOVA, the mean AUC values were not statistically different from one another, nor different from that of the solution. However, the 90% confidence interval for the AUC showed that for tablet A, the bioavailability was less than 80% (ie, 74%), compared to the solution at the low-range estimate, and would not be considered bioequivalent based on the AUC.

For illustrative purposes, consider a drug that has been prepared at the same dosage level in three

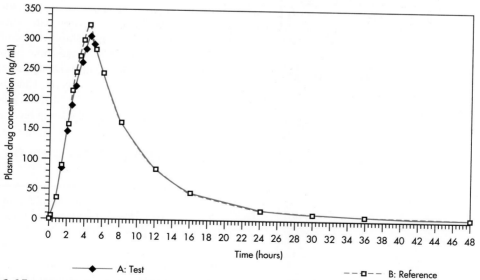

FIGURE 16-15   Bioequivalence of test and reference drug products: mean plasma drug concentrations.

TABLE 16-12   **Summary of the Results of a Bioavailability Study**[a]

Dosage Form	C_{max} (μg/mL)	t_{max} (h)	AUC_{0-24} (μg h/mL)	F[b]	90% Confidence Interval for AUC
Solution	16.1 ± 2.5	1.5 ± 0.85	1835 ± 235		
Tablet A	10.5 ± 3.2[c]	2.5 ± 1.0[c]	1523 ± 381	81	74%–90%
Tablet B	13.7 ± 4.1	2.1 ± 0.98	1707 ± 317	93	88%–98%
Tablet C	14.8 ± 3.6	1.8 ± 0.95	1762 ± 295	96	91%–103%

[a]The bioavailability of a drug from four different formulations was studied in 24 healthy, adult male subjects using a four-way Latin-square crossover design. The results represent the mean ± standard deviation.

[b]Oral bioavailability relative to the solution.

[c]$p \leq .05$.

formulations, A, B, and C. These formulations are given to a group of volunteers using a three-way, randomized crossover design. In this experimental design, all subjects receive each formulation once. From each subject, plasma drug level and urinary drug excretion data are obtained. With these data we can observe the relationship between plasma and urinary excretion parameters and drug bioavailability (Fig. 16-16). The rate of drug absorption from formulation A is more rapid than that from formulation B, because the t_{max} for formulation A is shorter. Because the AUC for formulation A is identical to the AUC for formulation B, the extent of bioavailability from both of these formulations is the same. Note, however, the C_{max} for A is higher than that for B, because the rate of drug absorption is more rapid.

The C_{max} is generally higher when the extent of drug bioavailability is greater. The rate of drug absorption from formulation C is the same as that from formulation A, but the extent of drug available is less. The C_{max} for formulation C is less than that for formulation A. The decrease in C_{max} for formulation C is proportional to the decrease in AUC in comparison to the drug plasma level data for formulation A. The corresponding urinary excretion data confirm these observations. These relationships are summarized in Table 16-13. The table illustrates how bioavailability parameters for plasma and urine change when only the extent and rate of bioavailability are changed, respectively. Formulation changes in a drug product may affect both the rate and extent of drug bioavailability.

STUDY SUBMISSION AND DRUG REVIEW PROCESS

The contents of New Drug Applications (NDAs) and Abbreviated New Drug Applications (ANDAs) are similar in terms of the quality of manufacture (Table 16-14). The submission for an NDA must contain safety and efficacy studies as provided by animal toxicology studies, clinical efficacy studies, and pharmacokinetic/bioavailability studies. For the

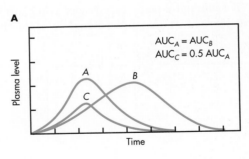

A

AUC$_A$ = AUC$_B$
AUC$_C$ = 0.5 AUC$_A$

Plasma level — Time

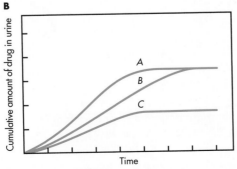

B

Cumulative amount of drug in urine — Time

FIGURE 16-16   Corresponding plots relating plasma concentration and urinary excretion data.

TABLE 16-13   Relationship of Plasma Level and Urinary Excretion Parameters to Drug Bioavailability

Extent of Drug Bioavailability Decreases		Rate of Drug Bioavailability Decreases	
Parameter	**Change**	**Parameter**	**Change**
Plasma data			
t_{max}	Same	t_{max}	Increase
C_{max}	Decrease	C_{max}	Decrease
AUC	Decrease	AUC	Same
Urine data			
t^{∞}	Same	t^{∞}	Increase
$[dD_u/dt]_{max}{}^{a}$	Decrease	$[dD_u/dt]_{max}{}^{a}$	Decrease
D_u^{∞}	Decrease	D_u^{∞}	Same

^{a}Maximum rate of urinary drug excretion.

generic drug manufacturer, the bioequivalence study is the pivotal study in the ANDA that replaces the animal, clinical, and pharmacokinetic studies.

An outline for the submission of a completed bioavailability to the FDA is shown in Table 16-15. The investigator should be sure that the study has been properly designed, the objectives are clearly defined, and the method of analysis has been validated (ie, shown to measure precisely and accurately the plasma drug concentration). The results are analyzed both statistically and pharmacokinetically.

TABLE 16-14   NDA Versus ANDA Review Process

Brand-Name Drug NDA Requirements	Generic Drug ANDA Requirements
1. Chemistry	1. Chemistry
2. Manufacturing	2. Manufacturing
3. Controls	3. Controls
4. Labeling	4. Labeling
5. Testing	5. Testing
6. Animal studies	6. Bioequivalence
7. Clinical studies	
8. Bioavailability	

Source: Center for Drug Evaluation & Research, US Food & Drug Administration, http://www.fda.gov.

These results, along with case reports and various data supporting the validity of the analytical method, are included in the submission. The FDA reviews the study in detail according to the outline presented in Table 16-16. If necessary, an FDA investigator may inspect both the clinical and analytical facilities used in the study and audit the raw data used in support of the bioavailability study. For ANDA applications, the FDA Office of Generic Drugs reviews the entire ANDA as shown in Fig. 16-17. If the application is incomplete, the FDA will not review the submission and the sponsor will receive a *Refusal to File* letter.

Frequently Asked Questions

▶ *What is the most appropriate bioequivalence design for a solid oral drug product containing a drug for systemic absorption?*

▶ *What are some of the problems associated with clinical endpoint bioequivalence studies?*

WAIVERS OF *IN VIVO* BIOEQUIVALENCE STUDIES (BIOWAIVERS)

In some cases, *in vitro* dissolution testing may be used in lieu of *in vivo* bioequivalence studies. When the drug product is in the same dosage form but in different strengths and is proportionally similar in active and

TABLE 16-15 Proposed Format and Contents of an *In Vivo* Bioequivalence Study Submission and Accompanying *In Vitro* Data

Title page
Study title
Name of sponsor
Name and address of clinical laboratory
Name of principal investigator(s)
Name of clinical investigator
Name of analytical laboratory
Dates of clinical study (start, completion)
Signature of principal investigator (and date)
Signature of clinical investigator (and date)

Table of contents
I. Study Résumé
Product information
Summary of bioequivalence study
Summary of bioequivalence data
Plasma
Urinary excretion
Figure of mean plasma concentration–time profile
Figure of mean cumulative urinary excretion
Figure of mean urinary excretion rates

II. Protocol and Approvals
Protocol
Letter of acceptance of protocol from FDA
Informed consent form
Letter of approval of Institutional Review Board
List of members of Institutional Review Board

III. Clinical Study
Summary of the study
Details of the study
Demographic characteristics of the subjects
Subject assignment in the study
Mean physical characteristics of subjects arranged by sequence
Details of clinical activity
Deviations from protocol
Vital signs of subjects
Adverse reactions report

IV. Assay Methodology and Validation
Assay method description
Validation procedure
Summary of validation
Data on linearity of standard samples
Data on interday precision and accuracy
Data on intraday precision and accuracy
Figure for standard curve(s) for low/high ranges
Chromatograms of standard and quality control samples
Sample calculation

V. Pharmacokinetic Parameters and Tests
Definition and calculations
Statistical tests
Drug levels at each sampling time and pharmacokinetic parameters
Figure of mean plasma concentration–time profile
Figures of individual subject plasma concentration–time profiles
Figure of mean cumulative urinary excretion
Figures of individual subject cumulative urinary excretion
Figure of mean urinary excretion rates
Fgures of individual subject urinary excretion rates
Tables of individual subject data arranged by drug, drug/period, drug/sequence

VI. Statistical Analyses
Statistical considerations
Summary of statistical significance
Summary of statistical parameters
Analysis of variance, least squares estimates, and least squares means
Asessment of sequence, period, and treatment effects
90% confidence intervals for the difference between test and reference products for the log-normal transformed parameters of AUC_{0-t}, $AUC_{0-\infty}$, and C_{max} should be within 80% and 125%

VII. Appendices
Randomization schedule
Sample identification codes
Analytical raw data
Chromatograms of at least 20% of subjects
Medical record and clinical reports
Clinical facilities description
Analytical facilities description
Curricula vitae of the investigators

VIII. *In Vitro* Testing
Dissolution testing
Dissolution assay methodology
Content uniformity testing
Potency determination

IX. Batch Size and Formulation
Batch record
Quantitative formulation

Modified from Dighe and Adams (1991), with permission.

TABLE 16-16   General Elements of a Biopharmaceutics Review

Introduction	Summary and analysis of data
Study design	Comments
Study objective(s)	Deficiencies
Assay description and validation	Recommendation

inactive ingredients, an *in vivo* bioequivalence study of one or more of the lower strengths can be waived based on the dissolution tests and an *in vivo* bioequivalence

study on the highest strength. Ideally, if there is a strong correlation between dissolution of the drug and the bioavailability of the drug, then the comparative dissolution tests comparing the test product to the reference product should be sufficient to demonstrate bioequivalence. For most drug products, especially immediate-release tablets and capsules, no strong correlation exists, and the FDA requires an *in vivo* bioequivalence study. For oral solid dosage forms, an *in vivo* bioequivalence study may be required to support at least one dose strength of the product. Usually, an *in vivo* bioequivalence study is required for the highest dose strength. If the lower-dose-strength test product is

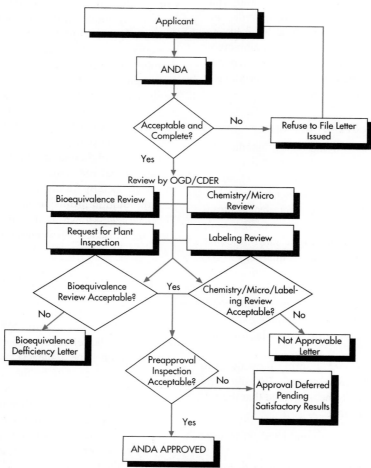

FIGURE 16-17   Generic drug review process. (*Source*: Office of Generic Drugs, Center for Drug Evaluation & Research, US Food & Drug Administration.)

substantially similar in active and inactive ingredients, then only a comparative *in vitro* dissolution between the test and brand-name formulations may be used.

For example, an immediate-release (IR) tablet is available in 200-mg, 100-mg, and 50-mg strengths. The 100- and 50-mg-strength tablets are made the same way as the highest-strength tablet. A human bioequivalence study is performed on the highest or 200-mg strength. Comparative *in vitro* dissolution studies are performed on the 100-mg and 50-mg dose strengths. If these drug products have no known bioavailability problems, are well absorbed systemically, are well correlated with *in vitro* dissolution, and have a large margin of safety, then arguments for not performing an *in vivo* bioavailability study may be valid. Methods for correlation of *in vitro* dissolution of the drug with *in vivo* drug bioavailability are discussed in Chapters 15 and 19. The manufacturer does not need to perform additional *in vivo* bioequivalence studies on the lower-strength products if the products meet all *in vitro* criteria.

Regulatory Perspective for Biowaiver

The FDA permits the waiving of BE studies for products for which BE is self-evident. This includes solutions for parenteral, oral, or local use. There are generally additional criteria to be met before a biowaiver can be granted. Test and reference solutions intended for parenteral use should have the same active and inactive ingredients in the same amounts. The FDA generally refers to this as qualitative (Q1) and quantitative (Q2) sameness. Generic drug product solutions that are intended for oral or topical use can have different excipients than their corresponding RLD products, but should not contain excipients that could potentially cause differences in drug substance absorption.

The FDA will consider granting biowaivers to non-biostudy strengths of a generic IR solid oral dosage form drug product line, provided that the following three criteria are met:

- An acceptable BE study is conducted on at least one strength.
- The strength(s) for which the biowaiver is sought should be proportionally similar to the strength on which BE was demonstrated.

- Acceptable *in vitro* dissolution should be demonstrated for the strength(s) for which the biowaiver is sought.

The FDA does not grant biowaivers for generic modified-release products, but may deem non-biostudy strength(s) BE to the corresponding biostudy strength(s) subject to certain criteria. This policy applies to all MR dosage forms, including but not limited to delayed-release tablets and capsules, extended-release tablets, transdermal products, and long-acting injectables (Davit et al, 2013).

Dissolution Profile Comparisons

Comparative dissolution profiles are used as (1) the basis for formulation development of bioequivalent drug products and proceeding to the pivotal *in vivo* bioequivalence study (Chapter 15); (2) comparative dissolution profiles are used for demonstrating the equivalence of a change in the formulation of a drug product after the drug product has been approved for marketing (see SUPAC in Chapter 17); and (3) the basis of a biowaiver of a lower-strength drug product that is dose proportional in active and inactive ingredients to the higher-strength drug product.

A model-independent mathematical method was developed by Moore and Flanner (1996) to compare dissolution profiles using two factors, f_1 and f_2. The factor f_2, known as the *similarity factor*, measures the closeness between the two profiles:

$$f_2 = 50 \times \log\left[\left(1 + \frac{1}{n}\sum_{t=1}^{n}(R_1 - T_1)^2\right)^{-0.5} \times 100\right]$$

where n is the number of time points, R_1 is the dissolution value of the reference product at time t, and T_1 is the dissolution value of the test product batch at time t.

The reference may be the original drug product before a formulation change (prechange) and the test may be the drug product after the formulation was changed (postchange). Alternatively, the reference may be the higher-strength drug product and the test may be the lower-strength drug product. The f_2 comparison is the focus of several FDA guidances and is of regulatory interest in knowing the similarity of the two dissolution curves. When the two profiles are identical, $f_2 = 100$. An average difference of 10% at all measured time points results in an f_2 value of 50 (Shah et al, 1998). The FDA has set a public standard for f_2 value between 50 and 100 to indicate similarity between two dissolution profiles (US-FDA, CDER, 1997).

In some cases, two generic drug products may have dissimilar dissolution profiles and still be bioequivalent *in vivo*. For example, Polli et al (1997) have shown that slow-, medium-, and fast-dissolving formulations of metoprolol tartrate tablets were bioequivalent. Furthermore, bioequivalent modified-release drug products may have different drug release mechanisms and therefore different dissolution profiles. For example, for theophylline extended-release capsules, the *United States Pharmacopeia* (USP) lists 10 individual drug release tests for products labeled for dosing every 12 hours. However, only generic drug products that are FDA approved as bioequivalent drug products and listed in the current edition of the Orange Book may be substituted for each other.

Frequently Asked Questions

▶ *Why are preclinical animal toxicology studies and clinical efficacy drug studies in human subjects not required by the FDA to approve a generic drug product as a therapeutic equivalent to the brand-name drug product?*

▶ *Are bioequivalence studies needed for each dose strength of an oral drug product? For example, an oral drug product is commercially available in 200-mg, 100-mg, and 50-mg dose strengths.*

THE BIOPHARMACEUTICS CLASSIFICATION SYSTEM (BCS)

The BCS is a scientific framework for classifying drug substances based on their aqueous solubility and intestinal permeability. When combined with the dissolution of the drug product, the BCS takes into account three major factors that govern the rate and extent of drug absorption from IR solid oral dosage forms. These factors are dissolution, solubility, and intestinal permeability.

According to the BCS, drug substances are classified as follows:

- Class 1: high solubility–high permeability
- Class 2: low solubility–high permeability
- Class 3: high solubility–low permeability
- Class 4: low solubility–low permeability

A theoretical basis for correlating *in vitro* drug dissolution with *in vivo* bioavailability was developed by Amidon et al (1995). This approach is based on the aqueous solubility of the drug and the permeation of the drug through the gastrointestinal tract. The classification system is based on Fick's first law applied to a membrane:

$$J_w = P_w C_w$$

where J_w is the drug flux (mass/area/time) through the intestinal wall at any position and time, P_w is the permeability of the membrane, and C_w is the drug concentration at the intestinal membrane surface.

This approach assumes that no other components in the formulation affect the membrane permeability and/or intestinal transport. Using this approach, Amidon et al (1995) studied the solubility and permeability characteristics of various representative drugs and obtained a biopharmaceutic drug classification for predicting the *in vitro* drug dissolution of IR solid oral drug products with *in vivo* absorption.

The FDA may waive the requirement for performing an *in vivo* bioavailability or bioequivalence study for certain IR solid oral drug products that meet very specific criteria, namely, the permeability, solubility, and dissolution of the drug. These characteristics include the *in vitro* dissolution of the drug product in various media, drug permeability information, and assuming ideal behavior of the drug product, drug dissolution, and absorption in the GI tract. For regulatory purposes, drugs are classified according to the BCS in accordance with the solubility, permeability, and dissolution characteristics of the drug (US-FDA, CDER, 2000b).

Solubility

An objective of the BCS approach is to determine the equilibrium solubility of a drug under approximate physiologic conditions. For this purpose, determination of pH–solubility profiles over a pH range of 1–8 is suggested. The solubility class is determined by calculating what volume of an aqueous medium is sufficient to dissolve the highest anticipated dose strength. A drug substance is considered highly soluble when the highest dose strength is soluble in 250 mL or less of aqueous medium over the pH range 1–8. The volume estimate of 250 mL is derived from typical bioequivalence study protocols that prescribe administration of a drug product to fasting human volunteers with a glass (8 oz) of water.

Permeability

Studies of the extent of absorption in humans, or intestinal permeability methods, can be used to determine the permeability class membership of a drug. To be classified as highly permeable, a test drug should have an extent of absorption >90% in humans. Supportive information on permeability characteristics of the drug substance should also be derived from its physical–chemical properties (eg, octanol: water partition coefficient).

Some methods to determine the permeability of a drug from the gastrointestinal tract include (1) *in vivo* intestinal perfusion studies in humans; (2) *in vivo* or *in situ* intestinal perfusion studies in animals; (3) *in vitro* permeation experiments using excised human or animal intestinal tissues; and (4) *in vitro* permeation experiments across a monolayer of cultured human intestinal cells. When using these methods, the experimental permeability data should correlate with the known extent-of-absorption data in humans.

After oral drug administration, *in vivo* permeability can be affected by the effects of efflux and absorptive transporters in the gastrointestinal tract, by food, and possibly by the various excipients present in the formulation.

Dissolution

The dissolution class is based on the *in vitro* dissolution rate of an IR drug product under specified test conditions and is intended to indicate rapid *in vivo* dissolution in relation to the average rate of gastric emptying in humans under fasting conditions. An IR

drug product is considered rapidly dissolving when not less than 85% of the label amount of drug substance dissolves within 30 minutes using USP Apparatus I (see Chapter 14) at 100 rpm or Apparatus II at 50 rpm in a volume of 900 mL or less in each of the following media: (1) acidic media such as 0.1 N HCl or simulated gastric fluid USP without enzymes, (2) a pH 4.5 buffer, and (3) a pH 6.8 buffer or simulated intestinal fluid USP without enzymes.

The FDA is in the process of revising the BCS guidance to permit biowaivers for generic formulations of Class 3 drugs (Mehta, 2014). Table 16-17 summarizes the recently proposed FDA criteria to be met for BCS biowaivers.

Biopharmaceutics Drug Disposition Classification System

The major aspects of BCS are the consideration of solubility and permeation. According to BCS, permeability *in vivo* is considered high when the active drug is systemically absorbed ≥90%. Wu and Benet (2005) and Benet et al (2008) have proposed modification of the BCS system known as the *Biopharmaceutics Drug Disposition Classification System* (BDDCS), which takes into account drug metabolism (hepatic clearance) and transporters in the gastrointestinal tract for drugs that are orally administered. For BCS 1 drugs (ie, high solubility and high permeability), transporter effects will be minimal. However, BCS 2 drugs (low solubility and high permeability), transporter effects are more important. These investigators suggest that the BCS should be modified on the basis of the extent of drug metabolism, overall drug disposition, including routes of drug elimination and the effects of efflux, and absorptive transporters on oral drug absorption.

Drug Products for Which Bioavailability or Bioequivalence May Be Self-Evident

The best measure of a drug product's performance is to determine the *in vivo* bioavailability of the drug. For some well-characterized drug products and for certain drug products in which bioavailability is self-evident (eg, sterile solutions for injection), *in vivo* bioavailability studies may be

TABLE 16-17   Criteria Proposed by FDA for Consideration of BCS-Based Biowaivers of Immediate-Release Generic Drug Products

BCS Class 1			
Highly Soluble	**Oral Bioavailability**	**Dissolution**	**Criteria on Excipients**
Highest strength, over range of pH 1.0–6.8	≥85%	• ≥85% in 30 minutes at pH 1.0, 4.5, 6.8 ("rapidly dissolving") • Volume = 500 mL • Paddles at 50 rpm, or basket at 100 rpm	• Test and reference should be pharmaceutical equivalents • Test and reference should not differ in amounts of excipients known to affect bioavailability

BCS Class 3			
Highly Soluble	**Oral Bioavailability**	**Dissolution**	**Criteria on Excipients**
Highest strength, over range of pH 1.0–6.8	<85%	• ≥85% in 15 minutes at pH 1.0, 4.5, 6.8 ("very rapidly dissolving") • Volume = 500 mL • Paddles at 50 rpm, or basket at 100 rpm	• Test and reference should be pharmaceutical equivalents • Test and reference formulations should be Q1 and Q2 the same

unnecessary or unimportant to the achievement of the product's intended purposes. The FDA will waive the requirement for submission of *in vivo* evidence demonstrating the bioavailability of the drug product if the product meets one of the following criteria (US-FDA, CDER, 2014a). However, there may be specific requirements for certain drug products, and the appropriate FDA division should be consulted.

1. The drug product (a) is a solution intended solely for intravenous administration and (b) contains an active drug ingredient or therapeutic moiety combined with the same solvent and in the same concentration as in an intravenous solution that is the subject of an approved, full NDA.

2. The drug product is a topically applied preparation (eg, a cream, ointment, or gel intended for local therapeutic effect). The FDA has released guidances for the performance of bioequivalence studies on topical corticosteroids and antifungal agents. The FDA is also considering performing dermatopharmacokinetic (DPK) studies on other topical drug products. In addition, *in vitro* drug release and diffusion studies may be required.

3. The drug product is in an oral dosage form that is not intended to be absorbed (eg, an antacid or a radiopaque medium). Specific *in vitro* bioequivalence studies may be required by the FDA. For example, the bioequivalence of cholestyramine resin is demonstrated *in vitro* by the binding of bile acids to the resin.

4. The drug product meets both of the following conditions:
   a. It is administered by inhalation as a gas or vapor (eg, as a medicinal or as an inhalation anesthetic).
   b. It contains an active drug ingredient or therapeutic moiety in the same dosage form as a drug product that is the subject of an approved, full NDA.

5. The drug product meets all of the following conditions:
   a. It is an oral solution, elixir, syrup, tincture, or similar other solubilized form.
   b. It contains an active drug ingredient or therapeutic moiety in the same concentration as a drug product that is the subject of an approved, full NDA.
   c. It contains no inactive ingredient that is known to significantly affect absorption of the active drug ingredient or therapeutic moiety.

GENERIC BIOLOGICS (BIOSIMILAR DRUG PRODUCTS)

Biologics, or biotechnology-derived drugs, in contrast to drugs that are chemically synthesized, are derived from living sources such as humans, animals, or microorganisms. Many biologics are complex mixtures that are not easily identified or characterized and are manufactured using biotechnology or are purified from natural sources. Other biological drugs, such as insulin and growth hormone, are proteins derived by biotechnology and have been well characterized. Advances in analytical sciences (both physicochemical and biological) enable some protein products to be characterized extensively in terms of their physicochemical and biological properties. These analytical procedures have improved the ability to identify and characterize not only the desired product but also product-related substances and product- and process-related impurities. Advances in manufacturing science and production methods may enhance the likelihood that a product will be highly similar to another product by better targeting the original product's physicochemical and functional properties.

The assessment of biosimilarity between a proposed biosimilar product and its reference product involves the robust characterization of the proposed biosimilar product, including comparative physicochemical and functional studies. The FDA recommends the following factors that must be considered in assessing whether products are highly similar (US-FDA, CDER, 2014g).

- *Expression system*: Therapeutic protein products can be produced by microbial cells (prokaryotic, eukaryotic), cell lines of human or animal origin (eg, mammalian, avian, insect), or tissues derived from animals or plants. It is expected that the expression construct for a proposed biosimilar product will encode the same primary amino acid sequence as its reference product.
- *Manufacturing process*: A comprehensive understanding of all steps in the manufacturing process for the proposed biosimilar product should be established during product development.
- *Assessment of physicochemical properties*: Physicochemical assessment of the proposed biosimilar product and the reference product should consider all relevant characteristics of the protein product (eg, the primary, secondary, tertiary, and quaternary structure, post-translational modifications, and functional activity[ies]). The objective of this assessment is to maximize the potential for detecting differences in quality attributes between the proposed biosimilar product and the reference product.
- *Functional activities*: Functional assays serve multiple purposes in the characterization of protein products. These tests act to complement physicochemical analyses and are a quality measure of the function of the protein product.
- *Receptor binding and immunochemical properties*: When binding or immunochemical properties are part of the activity attributed to the protein product, analytical tests should be performed to characterize the product in terms of these specific properties.
- *Impurities*: The applicant should characterize, identify, and quantify impurities (product and process related) in the proposed biosimilar product and the reference product.
- *Reference product and reference standards*: A thorough physicochemical and biological assessment of the reference product should provide a base of information from which to develop the proposed biosimilar product and justify reliance on certain existing scientific knowledge about the reference product.
- *Finished drug product*: Product characterization studies should be performed on the most downstream intermediate best suited for the analytical procedures used.
- *Stability*: An appropriate physicochemical and functional comparison of the stability of the proposed biosimilar product with that of the reference product should be initiated including accelerated and stress stability studies, or forced degradation studies.

The foundation for an assessment of biosimilarity between a proposed biosimilar product and its reference product involves the robust characterization of the proposed biosimilar product, including comparative physicochemical and functional studies.

Biosimilarity Versus Interchangeability

The Patient Protection and Affordable Care Act of 2010 contains provisions that establish an abbreviated regulatory approval pathway for generic versions of biological medicines (ie, biosimilars). The new legislation establishes two distinct categories of biosimilar products: (1) biological products that are "biosimilar" to a reference biological product, and (2) biological products that are "interchangeable" with the reference product.

Biosimilar biological drug products are biological products that are highly similar to the reference product notwithstanding minor differences in clinically inactive components. In addition, there are no clinically meaningful differences between the biological product and the reference product in terms of the safety, purity, and potency of the product.

Interchangeable biological drug products are biological products that are interchangeable with a reference biological product if (1) it meets the criteria for being biosimilar to the reference product, (2) it can be expected to produce the same clinical result as the reference product in any given patient, and (3) the risk in terms of safety or diminished efficacy in alternating or switching between use of the biological and reference product is not greater than the risk of using the reference product without such alteration or switch.

FDA determination of biosimilar drug products is based on the totality of the evidence provided by a sponsor to support a demonstration of biosimilarity. The FDA recommends that sponsors use a stepwise approach in their development of biosimilar products. FDA regulatory approval of a biosimilar drug product is based on a stepwise approach includes a comparison of the proposed product and the reference product including:

- Analytical studies that demonstrate that the biological product is highly similar to the reference product notwithstanding minor differences in clinically inactive components
- Animal studies (including the assessment of toxicity)
- Clinical study or studies (including the assessment of immunogenicity and pharmacokinetics or pharmacodynamics) that are sufficient to demonstrate safety, purity, and potency

Biosimilars and interchangeable biotechnology-derived drugs will be considered on a case-by-case basis. After FDA approval, the manufacturer must provide robust postmarketing safety monitoring as an important component in ensuring the safety and effectiveness of biological products,

FDA Guidance Documents

The legislation makes clear that the FDA will play a central role in defining the specific criteria needed to demonstrate biosimilarity for a given class of biological. In deference to the FDA's expertise in this area, the legislation specifically states that the FDA can issue guidance documents with respect to the approval of a biosimilar product. The guidance can be general or specific in nature, and the public must be provided with an opportunity to comment.

Advocates for the manufacture of generic biologics argue that bioequivalent biotechnology-derived drug products can be made on a case-by-case basis. Those opposed to the development of generic biologics or biosimilar drug products have claimed that generic manufacturers do not have the ability to fully characterize the active ingredient(s), that immunogenicity-related impurities may be present in the product, and that the manufacture of a biologic drug product is process dependent. Several biosimilar drug products have been approved in Europe. Currently, there are several applications for biosimilar drug products under review by the FDA. In the United States, FDA regulatory approval is based on a stepwise approach that includes a comparison of the proposed product and the reference product with respect to structure, function, animal toxicity, human pharmacokinetics (PK) and pharmacodynamics (PD), clinical immunogenicity, and clinical safety and effectiveness.

CLINICAL SIGNIFICANCE OF BIOEQUIVALENCE STUDIES

Bioequivalence of different formulations of the same drug substance involves equivalence with respect to the rate and extent of systemic drug absorption. Clinical interpretation is important in evaluating the results of a bioequivalence study. A small difference between drug products, even if statistically significant, may produce very little difference in therapeutic response. Generally, two formulations whose rate and extent of absorption differ by 20% or less are considered bioequivalent. The Report by the Bioequivalence Task Force (1988) considered that differences of less than 20% in AUC and C_{max} between drug products are "unlikely to be clinically significant in patients." The Task Force further stated that "clinical studies of effectiveness have difficulty detecting differences in doses of even 50%–100%." Therefore, normal variation is observed in medical practice and plasma drug levels may vary among individuals greater than 20%.

According to Westlake (1973), a small, statistically significant difference in drug bioavailability from two or more dosage forms may be detected if the study is well controlled and the number of subjects is sufficiently large. When the therapeutic objectives of the drug are considered, an equivalent clinical response should be obtained from the comparison dosage forms if the plasma drug concentrations remain above the minimum effective concentration (MEC) for an appropriate interval and do not reach the minimum toxic concentration (MTC). Therefore, the investigator must consider whether any statistical difference in bioavailability would alter clinical efficiency.

Special populations, such as the elderly or patients on drug therapy, are generally not used for bioequivalence studies. Normal, healthy volunteers are preferred for bioequivalence studies, because these subjects are less at risk and may more easily endure the discomforts of the study, such as blood sampling. Furthermore, the objective of these studies is to evaluate the bioavailability of the drug from the dosage form, and use of healthy subjects should minimize both inter- and intrasubject variability. It is theoretically possible that the excipients in one of the dosage forms tested may pose a problem in a patient who uses the generic dosage form.

For the manufacture of a dosage form, specifications are set to provide uniformity of dosage forms. With proper specifications, quality control procedures should minimize product-to-product variability by different manufacturers and lot-to-lot variability with a single manufacturer (see Chapter 18).

EXAMPLE ▶▶▶

IMPACT OF EFFLUX TRANSPORTERS ON BIOEQUIVALENCE STUDY

Digoxin is a drug that may be absorbed differently in individuals that expressed the efflux gene MDR1.

Questions
- What would be the impact of such an individual recruited into a bioavailability study?
- Would a protocol with the usual crossover design be able to adequately evaluate the bioequivalence of a generic digoxin product with a reference? Explain why or why not.

Solution
Bioequivalence studies for generic drug products compare the bioavailability of the drug from the test (generic) product to the bioavailability of the drug from the reference (brand) product. The study design is a two-way, crossover design in which each subject takes each drug product. The study design usually includes males and females with different ethnic backgrounds. In addition, some studies include both smokers and nonsmokers. Although there may be large intersubject variability due to gender, environmental, and genetic factors, the crossover design minimizes intrasubject variability by comparing the bioavailability of test and reference products in the same individual. Thus each individual subject should have similar drug absorption characteristics after taking the test or reference drug products.[9]

SPECIAL CONCERNS IN BIOAVAILABILITY AND BIOEQUIVALENCE STUDIES

The general bioequivalence study designs and evaluation, such as the comparison of AUC, C_{max}, and t_{max}, may be used for systemically absorbed

---

[9]For a few drug products, a high intrasubject variability (>30% CV) may be observed for which the bioavailability response changes for the same drug product each time the drug is dosed in the same subject.

TABLE 16-18   Issues in Establishing in Bioavailability and Bioequivalence

Drugs with high intrasubject variability

Drugs with long elimination half-life

Biotransformation of drugs

   Stereoselective drug metabolism

   Drugs with active metabolites

   Drugs with polymorphic metabolism

Nonbioavailable drugs (drugs intended for local effect)

   Antacids

   Local anesthetics

   Anti-infectives

   Anti-inflammatory steroids

Dosage forms for nonoral administration

   Transdermal

   Inhalation

   Ophthalmic

   Intranasal

Bioavailable drugs that should not produce peak drug levels

   Potassium supplements

Endogenous drug levels

   Hormone replacement therapy

Biotechnology-derived drugs

   Erythropoietin interferon

   Protease inhibitors

Complex drug substances

   Conjugated estrogens

drugs and conventional oral dosage forms. However, for certain drugs and dosage forms, systemic bioavailability and bioequivalence are difficult to ascertain (Table 16-18). Drugs and drug products (eg, cyclosporine, chlorpromazine, verapamil, isosorbide dinitrate, sulindac) are considered to be highly variable if the intrasubject variability in bioavailability parameters is greater than 30% by analysis of variance coefficient of variation (Shah et al, 1996). The number of subjects required to demonstrate bioequivalence for these drug products may be excessive, requiring more than 60 subjects to meet current FDA bioequivalence criteria. The intrasubject variability may be due to the drug itself or to the drug formulation or to both. The FDA has held public forums to determine whether the current bioequivalence guidelines need to be changed for these highly variable drugs (Davit et al, 2012).

For drugs with very long elimination half-lives or a complex elimination phase, a complete plasma drug concentration–time curve (ie, three elimination half-lives or an AUC representing 90% of the total AUC) may be difficult to obtain for a bioequivalence study using a crossover design. For these drugs, a truncated (shortened) plasma drug concentration–time curve (0–72 hours) may be more practical. The use of a truncated plasma drug concentration–time curve allows for the measurement of peak absorption and decreases the time and cost for performing the bioequivalence study.

Many drugs are stereoisomers, and each isomer may give a different pharmacodynamic response and may have a different rate of biotransformation. The bioavailability of the individual isomers may be difficult to measure because of problems in analysis. Some drugs have active metabolites, which should be quantitated as well as the parent drug. Drugs such as thioridazine and selegilene have two active metabolites. The question for such drugs is whether bioequivalence should be proven by matching the bioavailability of both metabolites and the parent drug. Assuming both biotransformation pathways follow first-order reaction kinetics, then the metabolites should be in constant ratio to the parent drug. Genetic variation in metabolism may present a bioequivalence problem. For example, the acetylation of procainamide to *N*-acetylprocainamide demonstrates genetic polymorphism, with two groups of subjects consisting of rapid acetylators and slow acetylators. To decrease intersubject variability, a bioequivalence study may be performed on only one phenotype, such as the rapid acetylators.

Some drugs (eg, benzocaine, hydrocortisone, anti-infectives, antacids) are intended for local effect and formulated as topical ointments, oral suspensions, or

TABLE 16-19   Possible Surrogate Markers for Bioequivalence Studies

Drug Product	Drug	Possible Surrogate Marker for Bioequivalence
Metered-dose inhaler	Albuterol	Forced expiratory volume (FEV_1)
Topical steroid	Hydrocortisone	Skin blanching
Anion-exchange resin	Cholestyramine	Binding to bile acids
Antacid	Magnesium and aluminum hydroxide gel	Neutralization of acid
Topical antifungal	Ketoconazole	Drug uptake into stratum corneum

rectal suppositories. These drugs should not have significant systemic bioavailability from the site of administration. The bioequivalence determination for drugs that are not absorbed systemically from the site of application can be difficult to assess. For these nonsystemic-absorbable drugs, a "surrogate" marker is needed for bioequivalence determination (Table 16-19). For example, the acid-neutralizing capacity of an oral antacid and the binding of bile acids to cholestyramine resin have been used as surrogate markers in lieu of *in vivo* bioequivalence studies.

Various drug delivery systems and newer dosage forms are designed to deliver the drug by a nonoral route, which may produce only partial systemic bioavailability. For the treatment of asthma, inhalation of the drug (eg, albuterol, beclomethasone dipropionate) has been used to maximize drug in the respiratory passages and to decrease systemic side effects. Drugs such as nitroglycerin given transdermally may differ in release rates, in the amount of drug in the transdermal delivery system, and in the surface area of the skin to which the transdermal delivery system is applied. Thus, the determination of bioequivalence among different manufacturers of transdermal delivery systems for the same active drug is difficult. Dermatopharmacokinetic studies investigate drug uptake into skin layers after topical drug administration. The drug is applied topically, the skin is peeled at various time periods after the dose, using transparent tape, and the drug concentrations in the skin are measured.

Drugs such as potassium supplements are given orally and may not produce the usual bioavailability parameters of AUC, C_{max}, and t_{max}. For these drugs,

more indirect methods must be used to ascertain bioequivalence. For example, urinary potassium excretion parameters are more appropriate for the measurement of bioavailability of potassium supplements. However, for certain hormonal replacement drugs (eg, levothyroxine), the steady-state hormone concentration in hypothyroid individuals, the thyroidal-stimulating hormone level, and pharmacodynamic endpoints may also be appropriate to measure.

GENERIC SUBSTITUTION

Drug product selection and generic drug product substitution are major responsibilities for physicians, pharmacists, and others who prescribe, dispense, or purchase drugs. To facilitate such decisions, the FDA publishes annually, in print and on the Internet, *Approved Drug Products with Therapeutic Equivalence Evaluations*, also known as the Orange Book (www.fda.gov/cder/ob/default.htm). The Orange Book identifies drug products approved on the basis of safety and effectiveness by the FDA and contains therapeutic equivalence evaluations for approved multisource prescription drug products. These evaluations serve as public information and advice to state health agencies, prescribers, and pharmacists to promote public education in the area of drug product selection and to foster containment of healthcare costs.

To contain drug costs, most states have adopted generic substitution laws to allow pharmacists to dispense a generic drug product for a brand-name drug product that has been prescribed. Some states have adopted a *positive formulary*, which lists therapeutically equivalent or interchangeable drug products that pharmacists may dispense. Other states use a *negative formulary*, which lists drug products that are not therapeutically equivalent, and/or the interchange of which is prohibited. If the drug is not in the negative formulary, the unlisted generic drug products are assumed to be therapeutically equivalent and may be interchanged.

Approved Drug Products with Therapeutic Equivalence Evaluations (Orange Book)

The Orange Book contains therapeutic equivalence evaluations for approved drug products made by various manufacturers. These marketed drug products

are evaluated according to specific criteria. The evaluation codes used for these drugs are listed in Table 16-20. The drug products are divided into two major categories: "A" codes apply to drug products considered to be therapeutically equivalent to other pharmaceutically equivalent products, and "B" codes apply to drug products that the FDA, at this time, does not consider to be therapeutically equivalent to other pharmaceutically equivalent products. A list of therapeutic-equivalence-related terms and their definitions is also given in the monograph. According to the FDA, evaluations do not mandate that drugs be purchased, prescribed, or dispensed, but provide public information and advice. The FDA evaluation of the drug products should be used as a guide only,

TABLE 16-20   Therapeutic Equivalence Evaluation Codes

A Codes	
Drug products considered to be therapeutically equivalent to other pharmaceutically equivalent products	
AA	Products in conventional dosage forms not presenting bioequivalence problems
AB	Products meeting bioequivalence requirements
AN	Solutions and powders for aerosolization
AO	Injectable oil solutions
AP	Injectable aqueous solutions
AT	Topical products
B Codes	
Drug products that the FDA does not consider to be therapeutically equivalent to other pharmaceutically equivalent products	
B*	Drug products requiring further FDA investigation and review to determine therapeutic equivalence
BC	Extended-release tablets, extended-release capsules, and extended-release injectables
BD	Active ingredients and dosage forms with documented bioequivalence problems
BE	Delayed-release oral dosage forms
BN	Products in aerosol–nebulizer drug delivery systems
BP	Active ingredients and dosage forms with potential bioequivalence problems
BR	Suppositories or enemas for systemic use
BS	Products having drug standard deficiencies
BT	Topical products with bioequivalence issues
BX	Insufficient data

Adopted from *Approved Drug Products with Therapeutic Equivalence Evaluations (Orange Book)* (www.fda.cder/ob/default.htm), 2003.

with the practitioner exercising professional care and judgment.

The concept of therapeutic equivalence as used to develop the Orange Book applies only to drug products containing the same active ingredient(s) and does not encompass a comparison of different therapeutic agents used for the same condition (eg, propoxyphene hydrochloride versus pentazocine hydrochloride for the treatment of pain). Any drug product in the Orange Book that is repackaged and/or distributed by other than the application holder is considered to be therapeutically equivalent to the application holder's drug product even if the application holder's drug product is single source or coded as nonequivalent (eg, BN). Also, distributors or repackagers of an application holder's drug product are considered to have the same code as the application holder. Therapeutic equivalence determinations are not made for unapproved, off-label indications. With this limitation, however, the FDA believes that products classified as therapeutically equivalent can be substituted with the full expectation that the substituted product will produce the same clinical effect and safety profile as the prescribed product (www.fda.gov/cder/ob/default.htm).

Professional care and judgment should be exercised in using the Orange Book. Evaluations of therapeutic equivalence for prescription drugs are based on scientific and medical evaluations by the FDA. Products evaluated as therapeutically equivalent can be expected, in the judgment of the FDA, to have equivalent clinical effect and no difference in their potential for adverse effects when used under the conditions of their labeling. However, these products may differ in other characteristics such as shape, scoring configuration, release mechanisms, packaging, excipients (including colors, flavors, preservatives), expiration date/time, and, in some instances, labeling. If products with such differences are substituted for each other, there is a potential for patient confusion due to differences in color or shape of tablets, inability to provide a given dose using a partial tablet if the proper scoring configuration is not available, or decreased patient acceptance of certain products because of flavor. There may also be better stability of one product over another under adverse storage conditions or allergic reactions in rare cases due to a coloring or a preservative ingredient, as well as differences in cost to the patient.

FDA evaluation of therapeutic equivalence in no way relieves practitioners of their professional responsibilities in prescribing and dispensing such products with due care and with appropriate information to individual patients. In those circumstances where the characteristics of a specific product, other than its active ingredient, are important in the therapy of a particular patient, the physician's specification of that product is appropriate. Pharmacists must also be familiar with the expiration dates/times and labeling directions for storage of the different products, particularly for reconstituted products, to assure that patients are properly advised when one product is substituted for another.

EXAMPLE ▶ ▶ ▶

INTERPRETATION OF THERAPEUTIC EVALUATION CODE FOR NIFEDIPINE EXTENDED-RELEASE TABLETS

The FDA has approved a few drug products containing the same active drug from different pharmaceutical manufacturers, each of which has provided a separate New Drug Application (NDA) for its own product. Since no information is available to demonstrate whether the two NDA-approved drug products are bioequivalent, each branded drug product becomes a separate reference listed drug (Table 16-21). Generic drug manufacturers must demonstrate to which RLD product is bioequivalent.

In Table 16-21, AB1 products are bioequivalent to each other and can be substituted. AB2 products are bioequivalent to each other and can be substituted. However, an AB1 product cannot be substituted for an AB2 product.

TABLE 16-21   Nifedipine Extended-Release Oral Tablet

TE Code	RLD	Active Ingredient	Dosage Form; Route	Strength	Proprietary Name	Applicant
AB1	Yes	Nifedipine tablet	Extended release; oral	90 mg	**Adalat CC**	Bayer Healthcare
AB1	No	Nifedipine tablet	Extended release; oral	90 mg	Nifedipine	Actavis
AB1	No	Nifedipine tablet	Extended release; oral	90 mg	Nifedipine	Valeant Intl
AB2	Yes	Nifedipine tablet	Extended release; oral	90 mg	**Procardia XL**	Pfizer
AB2	No	Nifedipine tablet	Extended release; oral	90 mg	Nifedipine	Mylan
AB2	No	Nifedipine tablet	Extended release; oral	90 mg	Nifedipine	Osmotica Pharm

TE = therapeutic equivalent.

Source: *Approved Drug Products with Therapeutic Equivalence Evaluations (Orange Book)*, [www.accessdata.fda.gov/scripts/cder/ob/default.cfm].

GLOSSARY[10]

Abbreviated New Drug Application (ANDA): Drug manufacturers must file an ANDA for approval to market a generic drug product. The generic manufacturer is not required to perform clinical efficacy studies or nonclinical toxicology studies for the ANDA.

Bioavailability: Bioavailability means the rate and extent to which the active ingredient or active moiety is absorbed from a drug product and becomes available at the site of action. For drug products that are not intended to be absorbed into the bloodstream, bioavailability may be assessed by measurements intended to reflect the rate and extent to which the active ingredient or active moiety becomes available at the site of action.

Bioequivalence requirement: A requirement imposed by the FDA for *in vitro* and/or *in vivo* testing of specified drug products, which must be satisfied as a condition for marketing.

[10]The definitions are from *Approved Drug Products with Therapeutic Equivalence Evaluations* (*Orange Book*). [www.fda.gov/Drugs/InformationOnDrugs/ucm129662.htm], *Code of Federal Regulations*, 21 CFR 320, and other sources.

Bioequivalent drug products: This term describes pharmaceutical equivalent or pharmaceutical alternative products that display comparable bioavailability when studied under similar experimental conditions. For systemically absorbed drugs, the test (generic) and reference listed drug (brand name) shall be considered bioequivalent if (1) the rate and extent of absorption of the test drug do not show a significant difference from the rate and extent of absorption of the reference drug when administered at the same molar dose of the therapeutic ingredient under similar experimental conditions in either a single dose or multiple doses or (2) the extent of absorption of the test drug does not show a significant difference from the extent of absorption of the reference drug when administered at the same molar dose of the therapeutic ingredient under similar experimental conditions in either a single dose or multiple doses and the difference from the reference drug in the rate of absorption of the drug is intentional, is reflected in its proposed labeling, is not essential to the attainment of effective body drug concentrations on chronic use, and is considered medically insignificant for the drug.

When the above methods are not applicable (eg, for drug products that are not intended to be absorbed into the bloodstream), other *in vivo* or *in vitro* test methods to demonstrate bioequivalence may be appropriate. Bioequivalence may sometimes be demonstrated using an *in vitro* bioequivalence standard, especially when such an *in vitro* test has been correlated with human *in vivo* bioavailability data. In other situations, bioequivalence may sometimes be demonstrated through comparative clinical trials or pharmacodynamic studies.

Bioequivalent drug products may contain different inactive ingredients, provided the manufacturer identifies the differences and provides information that the differences do not affect the safety or efficacy of the product.

Biosimilar or biosimilarity: The biological product is highly similar to the reference product notwithstanding minor differences in clinically inactive components, and there are no clinically meaningful differences between the biological product and the reference product in terms of the safety, purity, and potency of the product.

Brand name: The trade name of the drug. This name is privately owned by the manufacturer or distributor and is used to distinguish the specific drug product from competitor's products (eg, Tylenol, McNeil Laboratories).

Chemical name: The name used by organic chemists to indicate the chemical structure of the drug (eg, *N*-acetyl-*p*-aminophenol).

Drug product: The finished dosage form (eg, tablet, capsule, or solution) that contains the active drug ingredient, generally, but not necessarily, in association with inactive ingredients.

Drug product performance: Drug product performance, *in vivo*, may be defined as the release of the drug substance from the drug product, leading to bioavailability of the drug substance and leading to a pharmacodynamic response. Bioequivalence studies are drug product performance tests.

Drug product selection: The process of choosing or selecting the drug product in a specified dosage form.

Drug substance: A drug substance is the active pharmaceutical ingredient (API) or component in the drug product that furnishes the pharmacodynamic activity.

Equivalence: Relationship in terms of bioavailability, therapeutic response, or a set of established standards of one drug product to another.

Generic name: The established, nonproprietary, or common name of the active drug in a drug product (eg, acetaminophen).

Generic substitution: The process of dispensing a different brand or an unbranded drug product in place of the prescribed drug product. The substituted drug product contains the same active ingredient or therapeutic moiety as the same salt or ester in the same dosage form but is made by a different manufacturer. For example, a prescription for Motrin brand of ibuprofen might be dispensed by the pharmacist as Advil brand of ibuprofen or as a nonbranded generic ibuprofen if generic substitution is permitted and desired by the physician.

Pharmaceutical alternatives: Drug products that contain the same therapeutic moiety but as different salts, esters, or complexes. For example, tetracycline phosphate and tetracycline hydrochloride equivalent to 250-mg tetracycline base are considered pharmaceutical alternatives. Different dosage forms and strengths within a product line by a single manufacturer are pharmaceutical alternatives (eg, an extended-release dosage form and a standard immediate-release dosage form of the same active ingredient). The FDA currently considers a tablet and capsule containing the same active ingredient in the same dosage strength as pharmaceutical alternatives.

Pharmaceutical equivalents: Drug products in identical dosage forms that contain the same active ingredient(s), that is, the same salt or ester, are of the same dosage form, use the same route of administration, and are identical in strength or concentration (eg, chlordiazepoxide hydrochloride, 5-mg capsules). Pharmaceutically equivalent drug products are formulated to contain the same amount of active ingredient in the same dosage form and to meet the same or compendial or other applicable standards (ie, strength, quality, purity, and identity), but they may differ in characteristics such as shape, scoring configuration, release mechanisms, packaging, excipients (including colors, flavors, preservatives), expiration time, and, within certain limits, labeling. When applicable, pharmaceutical equivalents must meet the same content uniformity, disintegration times, and/or dissolution rates. Modified-release dosage forms that require a reservoir or overage or certain dosage forms such as prefilled syringes in which residual volume may vary must deliver identical amounts of active drug ingredient over an identical dosing period.

Pharmaceutical substitution: The process of dispensing a pharmaceutical alternative for the prescribed drug product. For example, ampicillin suspension is dispensed in place of ampicillin capsules, or tetracycline hydrochloride is dispensed in place of tetracycline phosphate. Pharmaceutical substitution generally requires the physician's approval.

Reference listed drug: The reference listed drug (RLD) is identified by the FDA as the drug product on which an applicant relies when seeking approval of an ANDA. The RLD is generally the brand-name drug that has a full NDA. The FDA designates a single RLD as the standard to which all generic versions must be shown to be bioequivalent. The FDA hopes to avoid possible significant variations among generic drugs and their brand-name counterparts. Such variations could result if generic drugs were compared to different RLDs.

Therapeutic alternatives: Drug products containing different active ingredients that are indicated for the same therapeutic or clinical objectives. Active ingredients in therapeutic alternatives are from the same pharmacologic class and are expected to have the same therapeutic effect when administered to patients for such condition of use. For example, ibuprofen is given instead of aspirin; cimetidine may be given instead of ranitidine.

Therapeutic equivalents: Drug products are considered to be therapeutic equivalents only if they are pharmaceutical equivalents and if they can be expected to have the same clinical effect and safety profile when administered to patients under the conditions specified in the labeling. The FDA classifies as therapeutically equivalent those products that meet the following general criteria: (1) they are approved as safe and effective; (2) they are pharmaceutical equivalents in that they (a) contain identical amounts of the same active drug ingredient in the same dosage form and route of administration, and (b) meet compendial or other applicable standards of strength, quality, purity, and identity; (3) they are bioequivalent in that (a) they do not present a known or potential bioequivalence problem, and they meet an acceptable *in vitro* standard, or (b) if they do present such a known or potential problem, they are shown to meet an appropriate bioequivalence standard; (4) they are adequately labeled; and (5) they are manufactured in compliance with Current Good Manufacturing Practice regulations. The FDA believes that products classified as therapeutically equivalent can be substituted with the full expectation that the substituted product will produce the same clinical effect and safety profile as the prescribed product.

Therapeutic substitution: The process of dispensing a therapeutic alternative in place of the prescribed drug product. For example, amoxicillin is dispensed instead of ampicillin or ibuprofen is dispensed instead of naproxen. Therapeutic substitution can also occur when one NDA-approved drug is substituted for the same drug that has been approved by a different NDA, for example, the substitution of Nicoderm (nicotine transdermal system) for Nicotrol (nicotine transdermal system).

Frequently Asked Questions

▶ *Can pharmaceutic equivalent drug products that are not bioequivalent have similar clinical efficacy?*

▶ *What is the difference between generic substitution and therapeutic substitution?*

CHAPTER SUMMARY

Drug product performance may be defined as the release of the drug substance from the drug product leading to bioavailability of the drug substance. Bioequivalence is a measure of comparative drug product performance and relates the quality of a drug product to clinical safety and efficacy. The absolute availability of drug is the systemic availability of a drug after extravascular administration (eg, oral, rectal, transdermal, subcutaneous) compared to IV dosing, whereas relative bioavailability compares the bioavailability of a drug from two or more drug products. The most direct method to assess drug bioavailability is to determine the rate and extent of systemic drug absorption by measurement of the active drug concentrations in plasma. The main pharmacokinetic parameters, C_{max} and AUC, are used to determine bioequivalence. However, other pharmacokinetic parameters such as t_{max} and elimination $t_{1/2}$ should also be assessed. The most common statistical design for bioequivalence studies is the two-way, crossover design in normal healthy volunteers. Bioequivalence is generally determined if the 90% confidence intervals for C_{max} and AUC fall within 80%–125% of the reference listed drug based on log transformation of the data. Food intervention or food effect studies are generally conducted using meal conditions that are expected to provide the greatest effects on GI physiology so that systemic drug availability is maximally affected. The Biopharmaceutics Classification System (BCS) is based on the solubility, permeability, and dissolution characteristics of the drug. However, systemic drug bioavailability may also be affected by transporters in the GI tract, hepatic clearance, GI transit and motility, and the contents of the GI tract.

Drug product selection and generic substitution are important responsibilities of the pharmacist. A listing of approved drug products of generic drug products that may be safely substituted is available in *Approved Drug Products with Therapeutic Equivalence Evaluations* (Orange Book).

LEARNING QUESTIONS

1. An antibiotic was formulated into two different oral dosage forms, A and B. Biopharmaceutic studies revealed different antibiotic blood level curves for each drug product (Fig. 16-18).

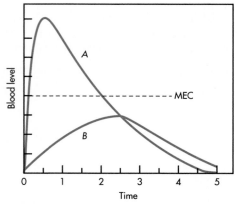

FIGURE 16-18 Blood level curves for two different oral dosage forms of a hypothetical antibiotic.

Each drug product was given in the same dose as the other. Explain how the various possible formulation factors could have caused the differences in blood levels. Give examples where possible. How would the corresponding urinary drug excretion curves relate to the plasma level–time curves?

2. Assume that you have just made a new formulation of acetaminophen. Design a protocol to compare your drug product against the acetaminophen drug products on the market. What criteria would you use for proof of bioequivalence for your new formulation? How would you determine if the acetaminophen was completely (100%) systemically absorbed?

3. The data in Table 16-22 represent the average findings in antibiotic plasma samples taken from 10 humans (average weight 70 kg), tabulated in a 4-way crossover design.

TABLE 16-22   Comparison of Plasma Concentrations of Antibiotic, as Related to Dosage Form and Time

Time after Dose (h)	Plasma Concentration (μg/mL)			
	IV Solution (2 mg/kg)	Oral Solution (10 mg/kg)	Oral Tablet (10 mg/kg)	Oral Capsule (10 mg/kg)
0.5	5.94	23.4	13.2	18.7
1.0	5.30	26.6	18.0	21.3
1.5	4.72	25.2	19.0	20.1
2.0	4.21	22.8	18.3	18.2
3.0	3.34	18.2	15.4	14.6
4.0	2.66	14.5	12.5	11.6
6.0	1.68	9.14	7.92	7.31
8.0	1.06	5.77	5.00	4.61
10.0	0.67	3.64	3.16	2.91
12.0	0.42	2.30	1.99	1.83
$\mathrm{AUC}\left(\dfrac{\mu g}{mL} \times h\right)$	29.0	145.0	116.0	116.0

a. Which of the four drug products in Table 16-22 would be preferred as a reference standard for the determination of relative bioavailability? Why?

b. From which oral drug product is the drug absorbed more rapidly?

c. What is the absolute bioavailability of the drug from the oral solution?

d. What is the relative bioavailability of the drug from the oral tablet compared to the reference standard?

e. From the data in Table 16-15, determine:
  (i) Apparent V_D
  (ii) Elimination $t_{1/2}$
  (iii) First-order elimination rate constant k
  (iv) Total body clearance

f. From the data above, graph the cumulative urinary excretion curves that would correspond to the plasma concentration–time curves.

4. Aphrodisia is a new drug manufactured by the Venus Drug Company. When tested in humans, the pharmacokinetics of the drug assumes a one-compartment open model with first-order absorption and first-order elimination:

$$D_{GI} \xrightarrow{k_a} D_B V_D \xrightarrow{k}$$

The drug was given in a single oral dose of 250 mg to a group of college students 21–29 years of age. Mean body weight was 60 kg. Samples of blood were obtained at various time intervals after the administration of the drug, and the plasma fractions were analyzed for active drug. The data are summarized in Table 16-23.

a. The minimum effective concentration of Aphrodisia in plasma is 2.3 μg/mL. What is the onset time of this drug?

b. The minimum effective concentration of Aphrodisia in plasma is 2.3 μg/mL. What is the duration of activity of this drug?

c. What is the elimination half-life of Aphrodisia in college students?

d. What is the time for peak drug concentration (t_{max}) of Aphrodisia?

e. What is the peak drug concentration (C_{max})?

TABLE 16-23 Data Summary of Active Drug Concentration in Plasma Fractions

Time (h)	C_p (μg/mL)	Time (h)	C_p (μg/mL)
0	0	12	3.02
1	1.88	18	1.86
2	3.05	24	1.12
3	3.74	36	0.40
5	4.21	48	0.14
7	4.08	60	0.05
9	3.70	72	0.02

   f. Assuming that the drug is 100% systemically available (ie, fraction of drug absorbed equals unity), what is the AUC for Aphrodisia?

5. You wish to do a bioequivalence study on three different formulations of the same active drug. Lay out a Latin-square design for the proper sequencing of these drug products in six normal, healthy volunteers. What is the main reason for using a crossover design in a bioequivalence study? What is meant by a "random" population?

6. Four different drug products containing the same antibiotic were given to 12 volunteer adult males (age 19–28 years, average weight 73 kg) in a 4-way crossover design. The volunteers fasted for 12 hours prior to taking the drug product. Urine samples were collected up to 72 hours after the administration of the drug to obtain the maximum urinary drug excretion, D_u^∞. The data are presented in Table 16-24.

TABLE 16-24 Urinary Drug Excretion Data Summary

Drug Product	Dose (mg/kg)	Cumulative Urinary Drug Excretion 0–72 h
IV solution	0.2	20
Oral solution	4	380
Oral tablet	4	340
Oral capsule	4	360

   a. What is the absolute bioavailability of the drug from the tablet?

   b. What is the relative bioavailability of the capsule compared to the oral solution?

7. According to the prescribing information for cimetidine (Tagamet®), following IV or IM administration, 75% of the drug is recovered from the urine after 24 hours as the parent compound. Following a single oral dose, 48% of the drug is recovered from the urine after 24 hours as the parent compound. From this information, determine what fraction of the drug is absorbed systemically from an oral dose after 24 hours.

8. Define *bioequivalence requirement*. Why does the FDA require a bioequivalence requirement for the manufacture of a generic drug product?

9. Why can we use the time for peak drug concentration (t_{max}) in a bioequivalence study for an estimate of the rate of drug absorption, rather than calculating the k_a?

10. Ten male volunteers (18–26 years of age) weighing an average of 73 kg were given either 4 tablets each containing 250 mg of drug (drug product A) or 1 tablet containing 1000 mg of drug (drug product B). Blood levels of the drug were obtained and the data are summarized in Table 16-25.

   a. State a possible reason for the difference in the time for peak drug concentration ($t_{max,A}$) after drug product A compared to the $t_{max,B}$ after drug product B. (Assume that all the tablets were made from the same formulation—ie, the drug is in the same particle size, same salt form, same excipients, and same ratio of excipients to active drug.)

   b. Draw a graph relating the cumulative amount of drug excreted in urine of patients given drug product A compared to the cumulative drug excreted in urine after drug product B. Label axes.

   c. In a second study using the same 10 male volunteers, a 125-mg dose of the drug was given by IV bolus and the AUC was computed as 20 μg·h/mL. Calculate the fraction of drug systemically absorbed from drug product B (1×1000-mg) tablet using the data in Table 16-25.

TABLE 16-25   Blood Level Data Summary for Two Drug Products

| | | Drug Product | | |
Kinetic Variable	Unit	A, 4 × 250-mg Tablet	B, 1000-mg Tablet	Statistic
Time for peak drug concentration (range)	h	1.3 (0.7–1.5)	1.8 (1.5–2.2)	$p < .05$
Peak concentration (range)	μg/mL	53 (46–58)	47 (42–51)	$p < .05$
AUC (range)	μg·h/mL	118 (98–125)	103 (90–120)	NS
$t_{1/2}$	h	3.2 (2.5–3.8)	3.8 (2.9–4.3)	NS

11. After performing a bioequivalence test comparing a generic drug product to a brand-name drug product, it was observed that the generic drug product had greater bioavailability than the brand-name drug product.
    a. Would you approve marketing the generic drug product, claiming it was superior to the brand-name drug product?
    b. Would you expect identical pharmacodynamic responses to both drug products?
    c. What therapeutic problem might arise in using the generic drug product that might not occur when using the brand-name drug product?

12. The following study is from Welling et al (1982):
    Tolazamide Formulations: Four tolazamide tablet formulations were selected for this study. The tablet formulations were labeled A, B, C, and D. Disintegration and dissolution tests were performed by standard USP-23 procedures.
    Subjects: Twenty healthy adult male volunteers between the ages of 18 and 38 years (mean, 26 years) and weighing between 61.4 and 95.5 kg (mean, 74.5 kg) were selected for the study. The subjects were randomly assigned to four groups of five each. The 4 treatments were administered according to 4 × 4 Latin-square design. Each treatment was separated by 1-week intervals. All subjects fasted overnight before receiving the tolazamide tablet the following morning. The tablet was given with

180 mL of water. Food intake was allowed at 5 hours postdose. Blood samples (10 mL) were taken just before the dose and periodically after dosing. The serum fraction was separated from the blood and analyzed for tolazamide by high-pressure liquid chromatography.
Data Analysis: Serum data were analyzed by a digital computer program using a regression analysis and by the percent of drug unabsorbed by the method of Wagner and Nelson (1963). AUC was determined by the trapezoidal rule and an analysis of variance was determined by Tukey's method.
    a. Why was a Latin-square crossover design used in this study?
    b. Why were the subjects fasted before being given the tolazamide tablets?
    c. Why did the authors use the Wagner–Nelson method rather than the Loo–Riegelman method for measuring the amount of drug absorbed?
    d. From the data in Table 16-26 only, from which tablet formulation would you expect the highest bioavailability? Why?
    e. From the data in Table 16-26, did the disintegration times correlate with the dissolution times? Why?
    f. Do the data in Table 16-27 appear to correlate with the data in Table 16-26? Why?
    g. Draw the expected cumulative urinary excretion–time curve for formulations A and B. Label axes and identify each curve.

TABLE 16-26   Disintegration Times and Dissolution Rates of Tolazamide Tablets[a]

Tablet	Mean Disintegration Time[b] min (Range)	Percent Dissolved in 30 min[c] (Range)
A	3.8 (3.0–4.0)	103.9 (100.5–106.3)
B	2.2 (1.8–2.5)	10.9 (9.3–13.5)
C	2.3 (2.0–2.5)	31.6 (26.4–37.2)
D	26.5 (22.5–30.5)	29.7 (20.8–38.4)

[a]N = 6.

[b]By the method of USP-23.

[c]Dissolution rates in pH 7.6 buffer.

From Welling et al (1982), with permission.

h. Assuming formulation A is the reference formulation, what is the relative bioavailability of formulation D?

i. Using the data in Table 16-27 for formulation A, calculate the elimination half-life ($t_{1/2}$) for tolazamide.

13. If *in vitro* drug dissolution and/or release studies for an oral solid dosage form (eg, tablet) does not correlate with the bioavailability of the drug *in vivo*, why should the pharmaceutical manufacturer continue to perform *in vitro* release studies for each production batch of the solid dosage form?

TABLE 16-27   Mean Tolazamide Concentrations[a] in Serum

Time (h)	Treatment (μg/mL)				Statistic[b]
	A	**B**	**C**	**D**	
0	10.8 ± 7.4	1.3 ± 1.4	1.8 ± 1.9	3.5 ± 2.6	$\overline{\text{ADCB}}$
1	20.5 ± 7.3	2.8 ± 2.8	5.4 ± 4.8	13.5 ± 6.6	$\overline{\text{ADCB}}$
3	23.9 ± 5.3	4.4 ± 4.3	9.8 ± 5.6	20.0 ± 6.4	$\overline{\text{ADCB}}$
4	25.4 ± 5.2	5.7 ± 4.1	13.6 ± 5.3	22.0 ± 5.4	$\overline{\text{ADCB}}$
5	24.1 ± 6.3	6.6 ± 4.0	15.1 ± 4.7	22.6 ± 5.0	$\overline{\text{ADCB}}$
6	19.9 ± 5.9	6.8 ± 3.4	14.3 ± 3.9	19.7 ± 4.7	$\overline{\text{ADCB}}$
8	15.2 ± 5.5	6.6 ± 3.2	12.8 ± 4.1	14.6 ± 4.2	$\overline{\text{ADCB}}$
12	8.8 ± 4.8	5.5 ± 3.2	9.1 ± 4.0	8.5 ± 4.1	$\overline{\text{CADB}}$
16	5.6 ± 3.8	4.6 ± 3.3	6.4 ± 3.9	5.4 ± 3.1	$\overline{\text{CADB}}$
24	2.7 ± 2.4	3.1 ± 2.6	3.1 ± 3.3	2.4 ± 1.8	$\overline{\text{CBAD}}$
C_{max}, μg/mL[c]	27.8 ± 5.3	7.7 ± 4.1	16.4 ± 4.4	24.0 ± 4.5	$\overline{\text{ADCB}}$
t_{max}, h[d]	3.3 ± 0.9	7.0 ± 2.2	5.4 ± 2.0	4.0 ± 0.9	$\text{BC}\overline{\text{DA}}$
AUC_{0-24}, μg h/mL[e]	260 ± 81	112 ± 63	193 ± 70	231 ± 67	$\overline{\text{ADCB}}$

[a]Concentrations ± 1 SD, n = 20.

[b]For explanation see text.

[c]Maximum concentration of tolazamide in serum.

[d]Time of maximum concentration.

[e]Area under the 0–24-h serum tolazamide concentration curve calculated by trapezoidal rule.

From Welling et al (1982), with permission.

14. Is it possible for two pharmaceutically equivalent solid dosage forms containing different inactive ingredients (ie, excipients) to demonstrate bioequivalence *in vivo* even though these drug products demonstrate differences in drug dissolution tests *in vitro*?

15. For bioequivalence studies, t_{max}, C_{max}, and AUC, along with an appropriate statistical analysis, are the parameters generally used to demonstrate the bioequivalence of two similar drug products containing the same active drug.
    a. Why are the parameters t_{max}, C_{max}, and AUC acceptable for proving that two drug products are bioequivalent?
    b. Are pharmacokinetic models needed in the evaluation of bioequivalence?
    c. Is it necessary to use a pharmacokinetic model to completely describe the plasma drug concentration–time curve for the determination of t_{max}, C_{max}, and AUC?
    d. Why are log-transformed data used for the statistical evaluation of bioequivalence?
    e. What is an add-on study?

ANSWERS

Frequently Asked Questions

Why are preclinical animal toxicology studies and clinical efficacy drug studies in human subjects not required by the FDA to approve a generic drug product as a therapeutic equivalent to the brand-name drug product?

- Preclinical animal toxicology and clinical efficacy studies were performed on the marketed *brand* drug product as part of the New Drug Application (NDA) prior to FDA approval. These studies do not have to be repeated for the *generic* bioequivalent drug product. The manufacturer of the generic drug product must submit an Abbreviated New Drug Application (ANDA) to the FDA, demonstrating that the generic drug product is a therapeutic equivalent (see definitions in Chapter 15) to the brand drug product.

What do sequence, washout period, and period mean in a crossover bioavailability study?

- The *sequence* is the order in which the drug products (ie, treatments) are given (eg, brand product followed by generic product or vice versa). Sequence is important to prevent any bias due to the order of the treatments in the study. The term *washout* refers to the time for total elimination of the dose. The time for washout is determined by the elimination half-life of the drug. *Period* refers to the drug-dosing day on which the drug is given to the subjects. For example, for Period 1, half the subjects receive treatment A, brand product, and the other half of the subjects receive treatment B, generic product.

Why does the FDA require a food intervention (food-effect) study for generic drug products before granting approval?

- Manufacturers are required to perform a food-intervention bioavailability study on all drugs whose bioavailability is known to be affected by food. In addition, a food-intervention bioavailability study is required on all modified-release products since (1) the modified-release formulation (eg, enteric coating, sustained-release coating) may be affected by the presence of food and (2) modified-release products have a greater potential to be affected by food due to their longer residence time in the gastrointestinal tract and changes in gastrointestinal motility.

What type of bioequivalence studies are required for drugs that are not systemically absorbed or for those drugs in which the C_{max} and AUC cannot be measured in the plasma?

- If the drug is not absorbed systemically from the drug product, a surrogate marker must be used as a measure of bioequivalence. This surrogate marker may be a pharmacodynamic effect or, as in the case of cholestyramine resin, the binding capacity for bile acids *in vitro*.

Learning Questions

3. **a.** Oral solution: The drug is in the most bio-available form.

   b. Oral solution: Same reason as above.

   c. Absolute bioavailability

$$= \frac{[AUC]_{soln}/dose_{soln}}{[AUC]_{IV}/dose_{IV}}$$

$$= \frac{145/10}{29/2} = 1.0$$

   d. Relative bioavailability

$$= \frac{[AUC]_{tab}/dose_{tab}}{[AUC]_{soln}/dose_{soln}}$$

$$= \frac{116/10}{145/10} = 0.80$$

   e. (1) $C_p^0 = 6.67 \ \mu g/mL$
   (by extrapolation of IV curve)

$$V_D = \frac{2000 \ \mu g/kg}{6.67 \ \mu g/mL} = 300 \text{ mL/kg}$$

   (2) $t_{1/2} = 3.01$ h
   (3) $k = 0.23$ h^{-1}
   (4) $Cl_T = kV_D = 69$ m/kg·h

4. Plot the data on both rectangular and semi-log graph paper. The following answers were obtained from estimates from the plotted plasma level–time curves. More exact answers may be obtained mathematically by substitution into the proper formulas.

   a. 1.37 hours
   b. 13.6 hours

   c. 8.75 hours
   d. 5 hours
   e. 4.21 $\mu g/mL$
   f. 77.98 μg h/mL

5. Drug Product

Subject	Period 1	Period 2	Week 3
1	A	B	C
2	B	C	A
3	C	A	B
4	A	C	B
5	C	B	A
6	B	A	C

6. **a.** Absolute bioavailability

$$= \frac{D_{u,PO}^{\infty}/dose_{PO}}{D_{u,IV}^{\infty}/dose_{IV}} = \frac{340/4}{20/0.2}$$

$$= 0.85 \text{ or } 85\%$$

   b. Relative bioavailability

$$= \frac{D_{ucap}^{\infty}/dose_{cap}}{D_{usoln}^{\infty}/dose_{sol}} = \frac{360/4}{380/4}$$

$$= 0.947 \text{ or } 94.7\%$$

7. The fraction of drug absorbed systemically is the absolute bioavailability.

   Fraction of drug absorbed

$$= \frac{\% \text{ of dose excreted after PO}}{\% \text{ of dose excreted after IV}}$$

$$= \frac{48\%}{75\%} = 0.64$$

REFERENCES

Amidon, GL, Lennernas H, Shah VP, Crison JR: A theoretical basis for a biopharmaceutic drug classification: The correlation of *in vitro* drug product dissolution and *in vivo* bioavailability. *Pharm Res* **12**:413, 1995.

Benet LZ, Amidon, GL, Barends DM, et al: The use of BDDCS in classifying the permeability of marketed drugs. *Pharm Res* **52**:483, 2008.

Damle BD, Kaul S, Behr D, Knupp C: Bioequivalence of two formulations of didanosine, encapsulated enteric-coated beads and buffered tablets, in healthy volunteers and HIV-infected subjects. *J Clin Pharmacol* **42**:791, 2002.

Davit B, Braddy A, Conner D, Yu X: International guidelines for bioequivalence of systemically-available orally-administered generic drug products: a survey of similarities and differences. *AAPSJ* **15**:974, 2013.

Davit BM, Chen ML, Conner DP, et al: Implementation of a reference-scaled average bioequivalence approach for highly variable generic drug products by the US Food and Drug Administration. *AAPSJ* **14**:915, 2012.

Davit BM, Conner DP: Food effects on drug bioavailability: implications for new and generic drug development. In Yu L, Krishna R (eds). *Biopharmaceutics Applications in Drug Development.* New York, Springer, 2008, p 317.

Davit BM, Conner DP: United States of America. In Kanfer I, Shargel L (eds). *Generic Drug Product Development—International Regulatory Requirements for Bioequivalence.* Boca Raton, CRC Press, 2015, in press (with permission).

de Mendoza C, Valer L, Ribera E, et al: Performance of six different ritonavir-boosted protease inhibitor-based regimens in heavily antiretroviral-experienced HIV-infected patients. *HIV Clin Trials* **7**:163, 2006.

Dehaven WI, Conner DP: The effects of food on drug bioavailability and bioequivalence. In Li BV, Yu LX (eds). *FDA Bioequivalence Standards.* New York, Springer, 2014, p 95.

Gardner S: Bioequivalence requirements and *in vivo* bioavailability procedures. *Fed Reg* **42**:1651, 1977.

Haidar SH, Davit BM, Chen ML, et al: Bioequivalence approaches for highly variable drugs and drug products. *Pharm Res* **25**: 237, 2008.

Horn JR, Howden CW: Review article: similarities and differences among delayed-release proton pump inhibitor formulations. *Aliment Pharmacol Ther* **22**(S3):20, 2005.

Hughes J, Crowe A: Inhibition of P-glycoprotein-mediated efflux of digoxin and its metabolites by macrolide antibiotics. *J Pharmacol Sci* **113**:315, 2010.

Jagdale SC, Agavekar AJ, Pandya SV, Kuchekar BS, Chabukswar AR: Formulation and evaluation of a gastroretentive drug delivery system of propranolol hydrochloride. *AAPS PharmSciTech* **10**:1071, 2009.

Kaur P, Chaurasia CS, Davit BM, Conner DP: Bioequivalence study designs for generic solid oral anticancer drug products: Scientific and regulatory considerations. *J Clin Pharmacol* **53**:1252, 2013.

Klotz U: Pharmacokinetics and drug metabolism in the elderly. *Drug Metab Rev* **41**:67, 2009.

Le J: Drug Bioavailability, The Merck Manual Professional Edition. http://merckmanuals.com/professional/clinical_pharmacology /pharmacokinetics/drug_bioavailability.html. Kenilworth, NJ, 2014.

Mehta M: The criteria for BCS-based biowaiver and the regulatory experience gathered in the US. Open Forum presentation, American Association of Pharmaceutical Sciences Annual Meeting, San Diego, CA, 2014.

Midha KA, Ormsby ED, Hubbard JW, et al: Logarithmic transformation in bioequivalence: Application with two formulations of perphenazine. *J Pharm Sci* **82**:138, 1993.

Moore JW, Flanner HH: Mathematical comparison of curves with an emphasis on *in vitro* dissolution profiles. *Pharm Tech* **20**:64, 1996.

Polli JE, Rekhi GS, Augsburger LL, Shah VP: Methods to compare dissolution profiles and a rationale for wide dissolution specifications for metoprolol tartrate tablets. *J Pharm Sci* **86**:690, 1997.

Report by the Bioequivalence Task Force 1988 on Recommendations from the Bioequivalence Hearings Conducted by the Food and Drug Administration, Sept 29–Oct 1, 1986. Rockville, MD, 1988.

Shah VP, Tsong Y, Sathe P: In vitro dissolution profile comparison—Statistics and analysis of the similarity factor, f_2. *Pharm Res* **15**:896, 1998.

Shah PV, Yacobi A, Barr WH, et al: Evaluation of orally administered highly variable drugs and drug formulations. *Pharm Res* **13**:1590, 1996.

Schuirmann DJ: A comparison of the two one-sided tests procedure and the power approach for assessing the equivalence of average bioavailability. *J Pharmacokinet Biopharm* **15**:657, 1987.

US-FDA, CDER: Guidance for Industry, Dissolution Testing of Immediate-Release Solid Oral Dosage Forms. http://www.fda.gov /downloads/Drugs/GuidanceComplianceRegulatoryInformation /Guidances/UCM070237.pdf. Silver Spring, MD, 1997.

US-FDA, CDER: Guidance for Industry, Statistical Approaches to Establishing Bioequivalence. http://www.fda.gov/downloads /GuidanceComlianceRegulatoryInformation/Guidances /UCM070244.pdf. Silver Spring, MD, 2000a.

US-FDA, CDER: Guidance for Industry, Waiver of In Vivo Bioavailability and Bioequivalence Studies for Immediate-Release Solid Oral Dosage Forms Based on A Biopharmaceutics Classification System. http://www.fda.gov/downloads /Drugs/GuidanceComplianceRegulatoryInfomration/Guidances /UCM070246.pdf. Silver Spring, MD, 2000b.

US-FDA, CDER: Guidance for Industry, Pharmacokinetics in Patients with Impaired Hepatic Function: Study Design, Data Analysis, and Impact on Dosing and Labeling. http://www.fda.gov /downloads/Drugs/GuidanceComplianceRegulatoryInformation /Guidances/UCM072123.pdf. Silver Spring, MD, 2003a.

US-FDA, CDER: Guidance for Industry, Food-Effect Bioavailability Studies and Fed Bioequivalence Studies. http://www.fda.gov /downloads/Drugs/GuidanceComplianceRegulatoryInformation /Guidances/UCM070241.pdf. Silver Spring, MD, 2003b.

US-FDA, CDER: Guidance for Industry, Bioequivalence Recommendations for Specific Products. http://www.fda.gov /downloads/GuidanceComplianceRegulatoryInformatoin /Guidances/UCM072872.pdf Silver Spring, MD, 2010a.

US-FDA, CDER: Guidance for Industry Pharmacokinetics in Patients with Impaired Renal Function—Study Design, Data Analysis, and Impact on Dosing and Labelling. http://www.fda.gov/downloads /Drugs/GuidanceComplianceRegulatoryInformation/Guidances /UCM204959.pdf. Silver Spring, MD, 2014.

US-FDA, CDER: Response to Warner Chilcott Company LLC petition part approval and denial. http://www.regulations .Gov/#!documentDetail;D=FDA-2010-P-0111-0011. Silver Spring, MD, 2010c.

US-FDA, CDER: Draft Bioequivalence Recommendations for Cholestyramine Oral Powder. US-FDA, CDER: Draft Bioequivalence Recommendations for Calcium Acetate Tablets. http://www.fda .gov/downloads/GuidanceComplianceRegulatoryInformation /Guidances/UCM148185.pdf. Silver Spring, MD, 2011a.

US-FDA, CDER: Draft Bioequivalence Recommendations for Clozapine Tablets. http://www.fda.gov/downloads/Drugs /GuidanceComplianceRegulatoryInformation/Guidances /UCM249219.pdf. Silver Spring, MD, 2011b.

US-FDA, CDER: Draft Bioequivalence Recommendations for Mercaptopurine Tablets. http://www.fda.gov/downloads/Drugs /GuidanceComplianceRegulatoryInformation/Guidances /ucm088658.pdf. Silver Spring, MD, 2011c.

US-FDA, CDER: Bioequivalence Recommendations for Zolpidem Extended-Release Tablets. http://www.fda.gov/downloads/Drugs /GuidanceComplianceRegulatoryInformation/Guidances /UCM175029.pdf. Silver Spring, MD, 2011d.

http://www.fda.gov/downloads/Drugs/ComplianceGuidanceRegulatoryInformation/Guidances/UCM273910.pdf. Silver Spring, MD, 2012a.

US-FDA, CDER: Draft Bioequivalence Recommendations for Acyclovir Topical Ointment. http://www.fda.gov/downloads /GuidanceComplianceRegulatoryInformation/Guidances /UCM296733.pdf. Silver Spring, MD, 2012b.

US-FDA, CDER: Guidance for Industry Drug-Drug Interaction Studies—Study Design, Data Analysis, Implications for Dosing, and Labeling Recommendations. http://www.fda.gov/downloads /Drugs/GuidanceComplianceRegulatoryInformation /Guidances/UCM292362.pdf. Silver Spring, MD, 2012c.

US-FDA, CDER: Draft Bioequivalence Recommendations for Risperidone Intramuscular Injection. http://www.fda.gov/downloads /Drugs/GuidanceComplianceRegulatoryInformation/Guidances /UCM201272.pdf. Sliver Spring, MD 2013a.

US-FDA, CDER: Drugs@FDA, Delzicol® Approval Summary. http:// www.accessdata.fda.gov/drugsatfda_docs/nda/2013/204412 _delzicol_toc.cfm. Silver Spring, MD, 2013b.

US-FDA, CDER: CFR Code of Federal Regulations Title 21 Part 320 Bioavailability Bioequivalence Requirements. http://www .accessdata.fda.gov/scripts/cdrh/cfdocs/cfcfr/CFRSearch.cfm ?CFRPart=320&showFR=1&subpartNode=21:5.0.1.1.8.1. Silver Spring, MD 2014a.

US-FDA, CDER: CFR Code of Federal Regulations Title 21 Part 314 Applications for FDA Approval to Market a New Drug. http://www.accessdata.fda.gov/scripts/cdrh/cfdocs/cfcfr /cfrsearch.cfm?cfrpart=314. Silver Spring, MD, 2014b.

US-FDA, CDER: Draft Guidance for Industry Bioavailability and Bioequivalence Studies Submitted in NDAs or INDs— General Considerations. http://www.fda.gov/downloads/Drugs /GuidanceComplianceRegulatoryInformation/Guidances /UCM389370.pdf. Silver Spring, MD, 2014c.

US-FDA, CDER: Orange Book: *Approved Drug Products with Therapeutic Equivalence Evaluations*. http://www.accessdata .fda.gov/scripts/cder/ob/default.cfm. Silver Spring, MD, 2014d.

US-FDA, CDER: Guidance for Industry General Considerations for Pediatric Pharmacokinetic Studies for Drugs and Biological Products. U.S. Food and Drug Administration Drugs Guidance. http://www.fda.gov/downloads/Drugs/GuidanceCompliance-RegulatoryInformation/Guidances/UCM425885.pdf. Silver Spring, MD, 2014e.

US-FDA, CDER: Draft Bioequivalence Recommendations for Methylphenidate Extended-Release Tablets. http://www.fda .gov/downloads/Drugs/GuidanceComplianceRegulatoryInformation/Guidances/UCM320007.pdf. Silver Spring, MD, 2014f.

US-FDA, CDER. Guidance for Industry, Clinical Pharmacology Data to Support a Finding of Biosimilarity to a Reference Product. http://www.fda.gov/downloads/drugs/guidancecompliance-regulatoryinformation/guidances/ucm397017.pdf. Silver Spring, MD, 2014g.

Wagner JG, Nelson E: Per cent absorbed time plots derived from blood level and/or urinary excretion data. *J Pharm Sci* **52**:610, 1963.

Welling PG, Patel RB, Patel UR, et al: Bioavailability of tolazamide from tablets: Comparison of *in vitro* and *in vivo* results. *J. Pharm. Sci* **71**:1259, 1982.

Westlake WJ: Use of statistical methods in evaluation of *in vivo* performance of dosage forms. *J Pharm Sci* **61**:1340, 1973.

Wu CY, Benet LZ: Predicting drug disposition via application of BCS: Transport/absorption/elimination interplay and development of a biopharmaceutics drug disposition classification system. *Pharm Res* **22**:11, 2005.

Zou P, Yu LX: Pharmacodynamic endpoint bioequivalence studies. In LX Yu, Li BV (eds). *FDA Bioequivalence Standards*. New York, Springer, 2014, p 217.

17

Biopharmaceutical Aspects of the Active Pharmaceutical Ingredient and Pharmaceutical Equivalence

Changquan Calvin Sun, Leon Shargel, and Andrew BC Yu

Chapter Objectives

▶ Define active pharmaceutical ingredient[1] (API) and drug product (finished dosage form).

▶ Define pharmaceutical equivalence (PE) and therapeutic equivalence (TE).

▶ Describe the physical and biopharmaceutical properties of API important in the design and performance of drug products.

▶ Discuss why physical and biopharmaceutical properties of the API and the drug product are interrelated and important in drug product design and performance.

▶ Describe the main methods used to test (PE) of the active ingredient (API) or the dosage form (drug product).

▶ Explain the relationship of PE, bioequivalence (BE), and therapeutic equivalence (TE).

▶ Explain whether a generic drug product that is not an exact PE can be TE.

INTRODUCTION

In order to bring a new drug to the market, a company must submit a new drug application (NDA) to the FDA for review and approval. Regulatory approval is based on evidence that establishes the safety and efficacy of the new drug product through one or more clinical trials (FDA, cited June 5, 2014). The development of a new drug, from discovery to entering the market, is a lengthy and expensive process. These clinical studies are typically performed by a large pharmaceutical company known as the innovator company. The innovator company patents the new drug and gives it a brand name. The brand drug product is available from only one manufacturer until patent expiration. These drug products are also known as single-source drugs, which are marketed at a high price, a practice that allows the company to recover the costs in development and to make a profit. The patents are critical for encouraging innovation that is needed for developing new drugs to effectively treat diseases. Once the patent expires, other companies can make and market the generic versions of the brand drug product after gaining approval for marketing by a regulatory agency through an Abbreviated New Drug Application (ANDA) process, which presents a substantially lower barrier than the NDA process (Fig. 17-1). At that point, the drug becomes a multisource drug, provided the generic drug products contain the same active pharmaceutical ingredient (API) in the same dosage form and given by the same route of administration (Chapter 16). Through market competition, the price of a multisource drug is significantly lower than the single-source brand drug. It was estimated that the substitution of for brand-name drugs by generics saved buyers $8–10 billion dollars

---

[1]The active pharmaceutical ingredient (API) is also referred to as the drug substance. Both drug substance and API will be used interchangeably in this chapter.

▶ Explain why a generic drug product with identical PE may not lead to equivalent pharmacokinetic and pharmacodynamic performance.

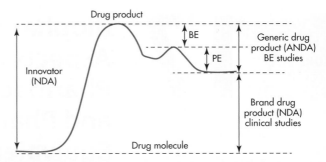

FIGURE 17-1   An illustration of the different barriers that must be overcome to gain the approval of a new drug product through either New Drug Application (NDA) or Abbreviated New Drug Application (ANDA) approval processes. BE = bioequivalence, PE = pharmaceutical equivalence.

in the US in 1994 (Cook et al, 1998). This number is undoubtedly much higher today. This makes the drug more readily affordable to the general public. The competition of generic drug products reduces global healthcare costs and motivates brand name companies to sustain their business through more innovations. Generic drug products are especially important for countries where innovator drug products are not available. Therefore, a balance must be reached to both encourage innovation by brand name companies and curb costs in drug purchasing through generic drugs competition.

The safety and efficacy of a generic drug product is established by demonstrating that the generic drug product is a *therapeutic equivalent* (TE) to the branded or innovator drug product (see Chapter 16). Under the current ANDA process for approval of generic drug products, TE of a generic drug product is assumed if the following conditions are met:

- They are approved as safe and effective.
- They are pharmaceutical equivalents.
- They are bioequivalent in that (a) they do not present a known or potential bioequivalence problem, and they meet an acceptable *in vitro* standard, or (b) if they do present such a known or potential problem, they are shown to meet an appropriate bioequivalence standard.
- They are adequately labeled.
- They are manufactured in compliance with Current Good Manufacturing Practice regulations.

Among the list of criteria, the requirements of pharmaceutically equivalent (PE) and bioequivalent (BE) to the innovator drug product are most crucial for a generic drug product to be considered as being therapeutically equivalent (TE) to the innovator drug product (Fig. 17-2) (FDA Guidance for Industry, 2003). The substitution of innovator drug products with TE generic drug products by a

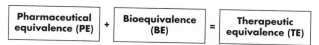

FIGURE 17-2   The relationship between pharmaceutical equivalence, bioequivalence, and therapeutic equivalence in the current regulatory framework.

pharmacist is allowed without the permission of the prescriber. The FDA believes that products classified as therapeutically equivalent can be substituted with the full expectation that the substituted product will produce the same clinical effect and safety profile as the prescribed product.

Although the cost-saving advantage of generic substitution is obvious, the absence of direct clinical studies in patients leads to a lingering concern about efficacy of generic drug products. Patients often ask, "Are they [generic drugs] really as safe and efficacious as the innovator drug products?" To answer this question, the concepts of PE and BE must be carefully examined.[2,3]

> **Frequently Asked Questions**
> ▶ *If two APIs are pharmaceutical equivalents, can we assume that these two APIs are also identical?*
> ▶ *Can drug products that are not pharmaceutical equivalents be bioequivalent in patients?*

Pharmaceutical Equivalents

For generic drug products to be pharmaceutical equivalents, they must be identical dosage forms that contain identical amounts of the chemically identical API. Pharmaceutical equivalents deliver identical amounts of the API over the identical dosing period. They must meet the identical compendial or other applicable standards on potency, content uniformity, disintegration times, and dissolution rates where

applicable (CFR Part 320, 2013). However, in the cases of modified-release dosage forms, such as a transdermal drug delivery product, which require a reservoir or overage, and prefilled syringes, which require residual volume, drug content may vary as long as the delivered amount of drug is identical to the innovator drug product. Different salt forms or prodrugs of the same API do not qualify as being identical under this definition by the FDA. Therefore, strict criteria on API in a drug product must be met in order to be qualified as a pharmaceutical equivalent.

Pharmaceutically equivalent drug products may contain different inactive ingredients, or excipients, for example, colorant, flavor, and preservative. They may contain different amounts of impurities within an allowable range. This flexibility in compositions of the drug product sometimes, though rarely, leads to undesirable consequences on the therapeutic performance as we will discuss later. In addition, pharmaceutically equivalent drug products may differ in characteristics such as shape, release mechanism, scoring (for tablets), packaging, and even labeling to some extent.

Strictly speaking, only identical drug products are truly bioequivalent and therapeutically equivalent. However, for practical reasons, two drug products are generally viewed as bioequivalent (BE), under the current FDA policies, when they do not significantly differ in the rate and extent of the API (or its active moiety) reaching the site of drug action when administered at the same molar dose and under similar conditions in an appropriately designed study (see Chapter 16). If the rate of a product is purposely modified, such as certain extended-release dosage forms, but the change in rate does not significantly affect the extent of availability of the API to the site of drug action (ie, not medically significant for the drug to work), they may still be considered as bioequivalent, provided such change is reflected in the labeling and it does not affect the effective drug concentration in body on chronic use. Some of the issues concerning pharmaceutical equivalence are listed in Table 17-1.

---

[2]As noted in Chapter 16, the currently marketed brand drug product may not have the identical formulation as the original formulation used in the safety and efficacy studies in patients. Brand and generic manufacturers may make changes in the formulation after approval. Both brand and generic manufactures may use BE studies to demonstrate that the change in formulation or manufacturing process did not change the BE of the product.

[3]Definitions appear both in Chapter 16 and at the end of this chapter.

TABLE 17-1 Issues in Establishing Pharmaceutical Equivalence of the API and Drug Product

Active Pharmaceutical Ingredient (API)	Comments
Particle size	Particle size differences can lead to differences in dissolution rates and differences in bulk density. In solution, the API is PE. However, particle size is important in suspensions and can cause a problem in dissolution. In suspensions, PE can be problematic.
Polymorph	Different crystalline forms and also amorphous API may have different dissolution rates. However, in solution the API is PE. In the case of an IV solution made with an API containing a polymorphic form impurity, after initial solubilization, the API may precipitate out during its product cycle. Long-term stability of this solution may be a problem.
Hydrate/Anhydrous	Although differences in the water of hydration, in solution the API is PE. There may be dissolution rate different between different hydrates and anhydrous forms of the API. Different water contents in hydrates and anhydrous forms affect API potency.
Impurities	PE may be synthesized using different synthetic pathways, leading to differences in impurities. Different purification methods can also lead to residual solvents and different impurities that need to be qualified depending on whether these are above or below threshold level.
Stability	Crystal defects as a result of different methods of synthesis and purification may affect the shelf life of the drug substance. Amorphous forms often degrade more rapidly for many APIs. Thus, stability is a PE issue, which may lead to a change in efficacy of the API due to more rapid decomposition.
Racemic/Chirality	Racemic APIs may be PE if the ratio of isomers is the same in both products. However, omeprazole (Prilosec) may not be considered as a PE to esomeprazole (Nexium), the S-isomer of omeprazole, since different isomers may have different pharmacodynamic activity.
Biotechnology-derived drugs	Biotechnology-derived products include proteins and peptides that need to be both pharmaceutical equivalent to the innovator drug and have equivalent pharmacodynamic activity. Additionally, differences in impurities may lead to immunogenicity problems (see Chapter 20).

Dosage Form (Drug Product)	Comments
Drug product delivery system	Transdermal systems and oral ER drug products may have different drug delivery systems but are considered PE to their respective brand drug product provided they meet the additional requirements for therapeutic equivalence.
Size, shape, and other physical attributes of generic tablets and capsules	Differences in physical characteristics (eg, size and shape of the tablet or capsule) are not strictly a PE issue but may affect patient compliance and acceptability of medication regimens, could lead to medication errors, and could have different GI transit times.
Excipients	Generic and brand drug products may have different excipients and still be considered PE provided they meet the requirements for therapeutic equivalence.
Sterile solutions	The ingredients in many sterile drug solutions (eg, ophthalmic solutions) must be the same, both qualitative and quantitative.
Overage	Overage is generally disallowed unless justified by data. Transdermal products using a reservoir system may have an overage to maintain the desired bioavailability.
Liposomes and emulsions	Liposomes and emulsions are dispersed systems with two or more liquid phases, generally composed of lipid and aqueous phases. PE is difficult to establish for these drug products. For example, there may be differences in drug concentration in the lipid phase and in the aqueous phase.

(Continued)

TABLE 17-1   Issues in Establishing Pharmaceutical Equivalence of the API and Drug Product (Continued)

Active Pharmaceutical Ingredient (API)	Comments
Inhalation products	Different designs in inhalation devices may deliver drugs with different particle size, plume geometry, etc, which may produce different clinical efficacy. Certain inhalation products may be considered PE provided they meet the requirements for therapeutic equivalence.
Manufacturing process	The manufacturing process can affect drug product performance. For example, an increase in compaction may produce a harder tablet that disintegrates more slowly, thereby releasing the drug more slowly (see also Chapter 18).

PHARMACEUTICAL ALTERNATIVES

Drug products that contain the same therapeutic moiety or its precursor but differ in dosage form, API amount, or chemical structure (different salt forms, prodrugs, complexes, etc) are considered "pharmaceutical alternatives" by the FDA as long as they meet applicable standards. Therefore, if the API is identical, an 80-mg drug tablet is a pharmaceutical alternative to a 100-mg drug product. Tablet products containing different chemical form of an API, for example, a prodrug or a different salt, are pharmaceutical alternatives regardless whether or not the molar dose is the same. In addition, the route of administration should be the same for two products to qualify as pharmaceutical alternatives. For example, an IV injectible drug product cannot be a pharmaceutical alternative to an oral tablet. Pharmaceutical alternatives may or may not be bioequivalent or therapeutically equivalent with the innovator drug product. In addition, capsule and tablets containing the same API, for example, quinidine sulfate 200-mg tablets versus quinidine sulfate 200-mg capsules are considered as pharmaceutical alternatives even if the products are bioequivalent.

Stability-Related Therapeutic Nonequivalence

Generic IV drug products are bioequivalent if they are pharmaceutically equivalent because their bioavailability is 100% by the nature of their route of administration. However, different drug products may have different stability, which can significantly impact therapeutic performance of a drug product that is otherwise pharmaceutically equivalent to the innovator products. Cefuroxime is an antimicrobial prophylaxis that is used as a single-dose IV injection in patients undergoing coronary artery bypass grafting surgery in the operating room immediately before the induction of general anesthesia. When a brand name drug product was used, a single dose of 3 g of cefuroxime generally achieves and maintains serum levels sufficient to prevent infections during the surgery. Occasionally, a 0.75 g dose is administered 12 hours after the surgery to prevent infections. However, when a generic cefuroxime was used to substitute the brand drug for cost saving, an increased frequency of post-surgical infections occurred (Fujimura et al, 2011). Some patients had to be admitted to the surgical intensive care unit. When the brand name drug product was again used, new cases of severe postoperative infection stopped. When the generic drug product was reintroduced, higher incidence of postoperative infections again occurred. Subsequent investigation confirmed that, although both drug products are chemically identical, the generic product hydrolyzed very quickly to render it less effective by the time it is administered (Fujimura et al, 2011). Although reasons that caused the poor stability in the generic product were not given, it is likely that the differences in formulation and/or manufacturing process are responsible.

Excipients and Impurities-Related Therapeutic Nonequivalence

Drugs are rarely administered alone. Various excipients, such as binder, solubilizer, stabilizer, preservatives, lubricant, diluents, and colorants, are added to make the final drug product. Sometimes, impurities and contaminants are present in the drug product. Unfortunately, the focus of quality control has been traditionally placed on the analysis of drug in the product. The recent safety problem with heparin due to the contamination by over-sulfated chondroitin sulfate, an impurity that is structurally similar to heparin, is a wakeup call to the scientific community that impurities must also be considered to ensure therapeutic equivalence or the sameness between two products (Dodd and Besag, 2009; Vesga et al, 2010). Similarly, although less dramatically, impurities contained in drugs and excipients, degradation during manufacturing and storage, interaction between drug and excipients may also have a negative impact on the safety and efficacy of a drug product. They should be considered when evaluating whether or not a generic drug product is therapeutically equivalent to the innovator drug product. In addition, some adverse reactions may not be evident in a single-dose BE study but may show up during chronic use of the drug. Hence, impurities in the drug and excipients must be controlled to avoid unintended problems in safety and efficacy of generic drug products. It should also be pointed out that the absence of some critical functional excipients or the inappropriate amounts of them in a drug product may lead to poor efficacy even if the drug itself is of high quality (Zuluaga et al, 2010).

The potential problems mentioned above are true for both innovator and generic drug products. However, the innovator drug product has proven its safety and effectiveness through a well-controlled clinical study. Unless there are major changes in the formulation, quality of drug and excipients, or manufacturing process, the potential problems related to excipients and impurities are usually not a concern on the clinical performance of innovator drug products.

PRACTICE PROBLEM

A generic manufacturer wants to make an amoxicillin suspension, 250 mg/5 mL with identical excipients as in the brand product. The generic manufacturer purchased the API from a drug supplier who imported various grades of amoxicillin trihydrate from different countries. The supplier reported that the amoxicillin trihydrate drug substance is a pharmaceutic equivalent (PE) to the innovator' API. A consultant stated further that the proposed product has the same chemical formula, antibacterial activity, potency, and excipients as in the innovator's drug product. The generic drug product will be marketed in a similar package. A bioequivalence study was performed comparing the proposed generic drug product to the brand drug product. The rate and extent of the generic product was found to be within the required BE requirements (see Chapter 16). After submission to the FDA, the product was rejected by the FDA's Office of Generic Drugs. Based on your understanding of the PE definition, what could be the possible reasons for the FDA not approving this product? (Hint: Consult Table 17-1 about the potential issues with PE, TE, and BE.)

Solution

Per the definition of PE below, four attributes are possible sources of failure in PE. The Code of Federal Regulations (CFR) also defines some product performance criteria, which must be met. PE should NOT be defined subjectively. For clarity, it is useful to group the potential issues under those terms in this chapter with PE heading. Other product design factors are discussed in Chapter 15.

Pharmaceutical equivalents (PE) are drug products in identical dosage forms that contain identical amounts of the identical active drug ingredient and meet the identical compendial or other applicable standard of identity, strength, quality, and purity, including potency and, where applicable, content uniformity, disintegration times, and/or dissolution rates.

Possible sources of pharmaceutical inequivalence:

1. Stability is affected by various factors such as residual solvent, reagents, and by-products (impurities) that are the results of different methods of chemical synthesis and purification.

2. Drug substance suppliers may use different starting materials (SM) during synthesis. The starting materials may also have different impurities, depending on the method of crystallization method used for purification. Generally, impurity profiles are synthetic route dependent, and may not always be detected using the same analytical method as the innovator.

3. The stability may not be detected with the BA/BE test. However, the FDA requires clinical samples to be retained, and it is possible that the retained samples may fail stability specification later. In addition, content uniformity may be a quality issue for failure under PE defined.

   Comment 1: The CFR states that the purity and identity criteria must be met. Although the CFR does not directly refer to the impurity profile and all the detail drug substance properties, the comprehensive statements clearly state that the drug substance, which ends up in the drug product, must perform as intended.

   Comment 2: A change in particle size, or crystallinity, during product manufacturing can result in batch-to-batch or within-batch variability failure. When this occurs, even an objective BE study will not preclude regulatory rejection or product failure. Another important issue is the *content uniformity* in the context of the drug substance and the product in a multi-drug source environment. The statistical nature of this is the recognition of an adequate design for sampling, and the relevance of quality-by-design (QbD) (see Chapter 18), which when properly implemented, minimizes the need for more testing of factors that affect PE.

4. Low level of an unsuspicious trace solvent may change the crystal form, solid state stability of a drug substance.

5. By-products in a drug substance from starting materials may cause PE issues that affect quality. In some cases toxicity or even carcinogenicity issues must be considered when different drug sources are used. It is important to note that as progress occurs, more efficient synthetic methods may be discovered for generic drugs. The synthetic process may be quite different even though a higher yield may be achieved, the impurity profile should be also acceptable. Compendial standards such as the European Pharmacopeia or USP-NF are helpful, but additional evaluation may be needed. Some of this information may be in the DMF (drug master file, or also referred to as master file) provided by the drug substance supplier.

6. Chirality is important as the same chemical formula may be structurally different resulting in different solubility and/or activity. Note the reference to "identical active drug ingredients" in the definition. Therefore, *d*-thyroxine and *l*-thyroxine will not be considered as PE.

Polymorphic Form-Related Therapeutic Nonequivalence

For poorly soluble drugs, a change in polymorph form may impact bioavailability. In the FDA's definition of pharmaceutical equivalence, polymorph is not considered. Hence, two products are still considered pharmaceutically equivalent even when different polymorph is used. For patent reasons, some generic manufacturers seek approval of new products that contain a different polymorph than the brand name product. In that case, the potential phase change during manufacture and storage will need to be carefully evaluated and controlled. The potential impact due to polymorph form difference can be masked by appropriate formulation design. In some cases, even difference in drug crystal morphology may lead to different bioavailability (Modi et al, 2013). These factors should be evaluated in the design of generic drug product to ensure bioequivalence and therapeutic equivalence.

Particle Size-Related Therapeutic Nonequivalence

For low-dose tablet products, content uniformity is a challenge. Even for the brand name product, unintended particle size variations have an impact on content uniformity in tablet products, especially those manufactured using the direct compression process (Rohrs et al, 2006). It is possible that the batch of generic tablets used for BE study meets the content uniformity requirement and demonstrates BE with the brand name product. However, some subsequent batches of the generic tablets fail to meet the content uniformity requirement and clinical outcomes unexpectedly vary. This problem is also faced by the brand name drug manufacturers. It can be minimized if stringent quality control is implemented, which is usually the case by the innovator drug companies but not always so by all generic drug manufacturers. In that case, the uncontrolled generic substitution may occasionally cause unintended problems in therapeutic performance that negate any cost saving by the generic substitution to the tax payers. Besides the potential content uniformity issue, variations in particle size can also potentially impact bioavailability of poorly soluble drugs because smaller drug particles correspond to larger surface area for dissolution and potentially much higher bioavailability (Jounela et al, 1975). Consequently, the safety and effectiveness of a solid dosage form drug product may be affected by variations in particle size of the drug. Therefore, inadequate particle size control may lead to non-bioequivalence and poor consistency in clinical performance.

Bioequivalence of Drugs with Multiple Indications

Another interesting point to consider is the validity of extrapolation TE in one indication of a drug to another indication. A generic drug product might have been clinically shown to be therapeutically equivalent to a brand name product in one indication. In that case, can we conclude that the generic drug product is therapeutically equivalent for all other indications of the drug? The demonstration of TE in one population of patients plus the BE in healthy volunteers is certainly a very strong evidence suggesting TE in other indications. However, a definitive answer can only be attained through a clinical study for each indication because different characteristics of the drug may be critical for successful clinical outcomes in different patient populations. For example, a drug may dissolve quickly and get absorbed completely in one patient population with a normal pH environment in their GI tract. Hence, variation in particle size and formulation does not affect bioavailability. However, the bioavailability of the same two drug products in the same cancer patients may be very different because of the much slower dissolution of the drug in their GI tract, which has a higher pH.

FORMULATION AND MANUFACTURING PROCESS CHANGES

Even for innovator drug products, the marketed product may not have been used in the original clinical trials that establish its efficacy and safety. In addition, changes to the formulation, suppliers of excipients, manufacturing process, or manufacturing site may be necessary in order to smoothly manufacture the drug product at large scale after the approval. The FDA requires the manufacturer to demonstrate that drug product performance is not affected by these scale-up and postapproval changes (SUPAC) (FDA, 1995, 1997). It sometimes happens that changes in the formulation and manufacturing process for a brand name drug product are more than allowed by SUPAC. If so, a BE study is required. Compared to the materials that require SUPAC, the differences between a generic drug product and the products used in the clinical trials are likely much more due to different formulations and different manufacturing processes. Hence, the requirement of a BE study for generic products is perhaps a minimum by comparison.

SIZE, SHAPE, AND OTHER PHYSICAL ATTRIBUTES OF GENERIC TABLETS AND CAPSULES

Although a generic drug product, such as a tablet or capsule, is a pharmaceutical equivalent and bioequivalent to the brand drug product, generic drug manufacturers should consider physical attributes of these products to ensure therapeutic equivalence (FDA Guidance for Industry, December 2003). There has been an increasing concern that differences in physical characteristics (eg, size and shape of the tablet or capsule) may affect patient compliance and acceptability of medication regimens or could lead to medication errors. For example, difficulty in swallowing tablets or capsules can be a problem for many individuals and may lead to a variety of adverse events and patient noncompliance with treatment regimens. In addition to possible swallowing difficulty, larger tablets and capsules have been shown to prolong esophageal transit time. This can lead to disintegration of the product in the esophagus and/or cause injury to the esophagus, resulting in pain and localized esophagitis and the potential for serious sequelae including ulceration. Studies in humans have also suggested that oval tablets may be easier to swallow and have faster esophageal transit times than round tablets of the same weight. The weight of the tablet or capsule also may affect transit time, with heavier tablets or capsules having faster transit times compared to similarly sized, lighter tablets or capsules. Surface area, disintegration time, and propensity for swelling when swallowed are additional parameters that can influence esophageal transit time and have the potential to affect the performance of the drug product for its intended use. Consequently, these physical attributes should also be considered for generic drug products intended to be swallowed intact.

> **Frequently Asked Question**
>
> ▶ *How would the shape or size of an oral drug product affect compliance in an elderly patient?*

CHANGES TO AN APPROVED NDA OR ANDA

After the approval of a new drug product or generic drug product, the manufacturer may make a change to the marketed product (FDA Guidance for Industry, April 2004). These changes may include changes in the API, changes in the manufacturing process, change in the formulation, scale-up or an increase in the batch size of the drug product, change in the manufacturing site, and change in the container closure system. In many cases, the manufacturer may make multiple changes to the drug product. For any of these changes, it is important to assess whether the change has a potential to have an adverse effect on the identity, strength, quality, purity, or potency of a drug product as these factors may relate to the safety or effectiveness of the drug product (Table 17-2). The FDA must be notified whenever a manufacturer makes a change to an approved product. The reporting requirement for a change is listed in Table 17-2. The manufacturer

TABLE 17-2. Changes to an Approved NDA or ANDA

Change	Definition	FDA Reporting Requirement	Example
Major change	A change that has a substantial potential to have an adverse effect on the identity, strength, quality, purity, or potency of a drug product as these factors may relate to the safety or effectiveness of the drug product	*Prior Approval Supplement*—requires the submission of a supplement and approval by the FDA prior to distribution of the drug product	A move to a different manufacturing site for the manufacturer of an ER capsule
Moderate change	A change that has a moderate potential to have an adverse effect on the identity, strength, quality, purity, or potency of the drug product as these factors may relate to the safety or effectiveness of the drug product	(1) *Supplement—Changes Being Effected in 30 Days*—requires the submission of a supplement to FDA at least 30 days before the distribution of the drug product made using the change (2) *Supplement—Changes Being Effected*—moderate changes for which distribution can occur when FDA receives the supplement	A change in the manufacturing process for an IR tablet
Minor change	A change that has minimal potential to have an adverse effect on the identity, strength, quality, purity, or potency of the drug product as these factors may relate to the safety or effectiveness of the drug product	*Annual report*—The applicant must describe minor changes in its next annual report	A change in an existing code imprint for a dosage form. For example, changing from a numeric to alphanumeric code

Source: FDA Guidance for Industry (April 2004). The essence of this guidance has been incorporated into 21 CFR 340.70.

must assess the effects of the change before distributing a drug product made with a manufacturing change.

How Prevalent Is the Therapeutic Nonequivalence of a Generic Product?

The assumption of therapeutic equivalence by a generic drug product that meets BE requirement is rarely challenged. For the benefit of all, it is important to ask the following questions: "How often is a generic product not therapeutically equivalent to a brand product?" and "If they occur frequently, why the TE failures are rarely observed?" Insights useful to answering these questions may be gained from analyzing one example of nontherapeutic equivalent vancomycin. A generic injectible vancomycin failed to treat a liver transplant patient against infection. However, switching to the innovator product led to speedy recovery by the patient (Rodriguez et al, 2009). Had this case been non-life-threatening, the different bactericidal activities between the generic and innovator products may have been ignored. A patient that requires longer treatment may be simply attributed to differential individual response to a therapy. The physician may simply switch to a different kind of antibiotics. On the other hand, a death of the patient, in this case caused by ineffective drug therapy, may be simply attributed to the severity of the disease where a death is not an unexpected outcome (Rodriguez et al, 2009). Either scenario will conceal the problem in the antibiotic failure. In another example, several generic oxacillin products do not show similar potency as that of the innovator product, hence, not bioequivalent. Those products that do meet BE requirement, however, lack therapeutic equivalence in an animal model

(Rodriguez et al, 2010). In this case, the brand name oxacillin product was withdrawn from the countries by its original manufacturer because of a lack of profit due to the intense competition from generic products. This left the patients in the entire region who require oxacillin therapy to face a highly dangerous consequence in their health. Patients with life-threatening infections might die due to ineffective drug therapy unnoticed by the physician. Unfortunately, such dismaying situation is also found in other drugs, such as gentamicin (Zuluaga et al, 2010), cefuroxime (Mastoraki et al, 2008), metronidazole (Agudelo and Vesga 2012), vancomycin (Vesga et al, 2010). For drugs with narrow therapeutical indices, such as some antiepileptic drugs, therapeutic nonequivalence have also been reported (Crawford et al, 2006). For antibiotic drugs, the use of substandard drug products may have contributed to the drug resistance. Other concerns on therapeutic nonequivalence of generic products have been discussed (Dettelbach, 1986; Lamy 1986). In any case, the assumption of therapeutic equivalence by a bioequivalent generic product requires more careful examination. The occurrence of therapeutic nonequivalence of generic products may be much higher than what most people believe.

THE FUTURE OF PHARMACEUTICAL EQUIVALENCE AND THERAPEUTIC EQUIVALENCE

In light of the emerging evidences pointing out the potential difference in therapeutic nonequivalence of generic drug products, suggestions have been made to require clinical evaluations on clinical efficacy of generic products with randomized double-blind comparative study for each major indication (Fujimura et al, 2011). Such a requirement, although scientifically rigorous, effectively stifles the competition that is critical for bringing down the cost of prescription drugs. In absence of a predictive *in vitro* analytical method or a valid animal model, a sensible approach to this problem is to allow restricted substitution to the prescribed drugs, say no more than 50%, while closely monitoring the therapeutic performance by medical doctors and regulatory authority. Full substitution by a given generic product is allowed when confidence on its clinical efficacy and safety is established. This approach does not affect the approval process and the entry of generic drug products to the market. However, it does slightly reduce the rate that generic products completely take over the market, thus reducing the chance of therapeutic failure, before their clinical safety and efficacy is firmly established. This approach avoids the catastrophic failures of substandard drug products while still taking advantage of the generic competition.

A reason to the documented failures in therapeutic equivalence of generic products may be attributed to the empirical nature of drug product development. In absence of a clear understanding in the relationship among structure, property, and performance (Sun, 2009), each product by a different manufacture can be potentially very different. Therefore, a successful BE study may not assure the therapeutic equivalence. Having recognized the challenge, the way forward would be for the scientific community, pharmaceutical companies, drug regulatory agencies (DRAs) worldwide to work together to advance the science that enables the design of high-quality and stable drug products in a consistent way. In the short term, DRAs can appropriately tighten the BE requirement, at least for types of products with known TE problems, to minimize the occurrence of drug therapy failure due to substandard generic drug products. In his 1986 editorial, Dr. Dettelbach stated, "However, until we institute a system of evaluating generic drugs in patients, in whom therapeutic and pharmacodynamics differences can be of critical importance, we may be playing a dangerous game" (Dettelbach, 1986). After so many years, his statement still remains largely true.

BIOSIMILAR DRUG PRODUCTS

The Biologics Price Competition and Innovation Act of 2009 (BPCI Act) amended the Public Health Service Act (PHS Act) and other statutes to create an abbreviated licensure pathway in section 351(k) of the PHS Act for biological products shown to be biosimilar to, or interchangeable with, an FDA-licensed biological reference product. Biological products can present challenges given the scientific and technical complexities that are associated with the larger and typically more complex structure of biological products and the processes by which such products are manufactured. Most biological products are produced in a living system such as a microorganism, or plant or animal cells, whereas small-molecule drugs are typically manufactured through chemical synthesis (FDA Guidance for Industry, 2012a, 2012b).

Biosimilar or biosimilarity means that the biological product is highly similar to the reference product notwithstanding minor differences in clinically inactive components, and there are no clinically meaningful differences between the biological product and the reference product in terms of the safety, purity, and potency of the product.

Interchangeable biosimilar drug products include the following:

- The biological product is biosimilar to the reference product.
- It can be expected to produce the same clinical result as the reference product in any given patient.
- For a product administered more than once, the safety and reduced efficacy risks of alternating or switching are not greater than with repeated use of the reference product.

Due to the complexity of these products, the FDA intends to consider the totality of the evidence provided by a sponsor to support a demonstration of biosimilarity. The FDA recommends that sponsors use a stepwise approach in their development of biosimilar products. Evidence demonstrating biosimilarity can include a comparison of the proposed product and the reference product with respect to structure, function, animal toxicity, human pharmacokinetics (PK) and pharmacodynamics (PD), clinical immunogenicity, and clinical safety and effectiveness. In addition, the FDA will consider the biosimilar development program, including the manufacturing process.

§320.1 Definitions (2014 Code of Federal Regulation, Title 21)

(a) *Bioavailability* means the rate and extent to which the active ingredient or active moiety is absorbed from a drug product and becomes available at the site of action. For drug products that are not intended to be absorbed into the bloodstream, bioavailability may be assessed by measurements intended to reflect the rate and extent to which the active ingredient or active moiety becomes available at the site of action.

(b) *Drug product* means a finished dosage form, for example, tablet, capsule, or solution, that contains the active drug ingredient, generally, but not necessarily, in association with inactive ingredients.

(c) *Pharmaceutical equivalents* mean drug products in identical dosage forms that contain identical amounts of the identical active drug ingredient, that is, the same salt or ester of the same therapeutic moiety, or, in the case of modified-release dosage forms that require a reservoir or overage or such forms as prefilled syringes where residual volume may vary, that deliver identical amounts of the active drug ingredient over the identical dosing period; do not necessarily contain the same inactive ingredients; and meet the identical compendial or other applicable standard of identity, strength, quality, and purity, including potency and, where applicable, content uniformity, disintegration times, and/or dissolution rates.

(d) *Pharmaceutical alternatives* mean drug products that contain the identical therapeutic moiety, or its precursor, but not necessarily in the same amount or dosage form or as the same salt or ester. Each such drug product individually meets either the identical or its own respective compendial or other applicable standard of identity, strength, quality, and purity, including potency and, where applicable, content uniformity, disintegration times and/or dissolution rates.

(e) *Bioequivalence* means the absence of a significant difference in the rate and extent to which the active ingredient or active moiety in pharmaceutical equivalents or pharmaceutical alternatives becomes available at the site of drug action when administered at the same molar dose under similar conditions in an appropriately designed study. Where there is an intentional difference in rate (eg, in certain extended-release dosage forms), certain pharmaceutical equivalents or alternatives may be considered bioequivalent if there is no significant difference in the extent to which the active ingredient or moiety from each product becomes available at the site of drug action. This applies only if the difference in the rate at which the active ingredient or moiety becomes available at the site of drug action is intentional and is reflected in the proposed labeling, is not essential to the attainment of effective body drug concentrations on chronic use, and is considered medically insignificant for the drug.

(f) *Bioequivalence requirement* means a requirement imposed by the Food and Drug Administration for *in vitro* and/or *in vivo* testing of specified drug products, which must be satisfied as a condition of marketing.

(g) *Same drug product formulation* means the formulation of the drug product submitted for approval and any formulations that have minor differences in composition or method of manufacture from the formulation submitted for approval, but are similar enough to be relevant to the agency's determination of bioequivalence.

[42 FR 1634, Jan. 7, 1977, as amended at 42 FR 1648, Jan. 7, 1977; 57 FR 17997, Apr. 28, 1992; 67 FR 77672, Dec. 19, 2002; 74 FR 2861, Jan. 16, 2009]. Explanations of related terms are found in the preface in the Orange book.

HISTORICAL PERSPECTIVE

In the last decade, many FDA guidances were developed to guide the control and manufacturing of API that impact PE issues. Many of the guidances were withdrawn with the adoption of the ICH quality guidances by the EU, Japan, and the United States (Step 4, announced in CFR 2008). The quality (Q) guidance for API (referred to as drug substance in ICH) is well discussed in the preamble for Q3A, which fully discuss API issues in the developed world: impurities, by-products, enantiomers, crystallinity, and other quality attributes. The issue of degradation impurities that may still form due to processing in the formulated product is discussed in Q3B (drug product guidance). A series of Q guidances (ich.org) are easily available. As the QbD and progress evolve, the present regulations of drug source supply will be updated accordingly. Revision of compendial and compliance policy notification as well as CFRs announcement should be frequently consulted. For example: Compliance Policy Guide Sec. 420.300

Changes in Compendial Specifications and New Drug Application Supplements; Withdrawal of Guidance. https://www.federalregister.gov/articles/2012/08/30/2012-21415/compliance-policy-guide-sec-420300-changes-in-compendial-specifications-and-new-drug-application.

A Notice by the Food and Drug Administration was posted on August 30, 2012.

A pharmacist should recognize that even a compendial grade drug source, manufactured by a new process may potentially form new degradation impurities that may not be controlled under the drug substance guidance. Therefore, in the new ICH guidance (ICH Q3A, 2006), it advises in the preamble that regardless of new or old molecules, any impurities above defined thresholds must be identified; additionally, total impurities must be reported. If impurities are relatively high with respect to dose, they must be qualified (ie, determined by toxicity studies to be within safe level). Consequently, most generic manufacturers tend to use historically known manufacturing methods without introducing new or unknown impurities.

CHAPTER SUMMARY

Pharmaceutical equivalence (PE), along with bioequivalence, is important for establishing therapeutic equivalence (TE) of generic drug products. PE is also important for postapproval changes in both brand and generic drug products. The determination of PE depends upon the physical and chemical properties of the active pharmaceutical ingredient (API), as well as the design and manufacture of the finished dosage form (drug product). For the API, different synthetic pathways and purification steps can lead to physical and chemical differences in the API, including particle size, degree of hydration, crystalline form, impurities, and stability. The drug product can differ in characteristics such as shape, scoring configuration, release mechanisms, packaging, and excipients (including colors, flavors, and preservatives). PE is more difficult to establish for complex APIs, complex drug products, or multiple APIs within the drug product (eg, combination drug product). Biotechnology-derived drugs, such as proteins and polypeptides, that are proposed for biosimilar drug products have additional issues with respect to structure, function, animal toxicity, human pharmacokinetics (PK) and pharmacodynamics (PD), clinical immunogenicity, and clinical safety and effectiveness.

LEARNING QUESTIONS

1. The reference listed drug marketed by a brand drug company has a patent on the crystalline form of the API. A generic drug manufacturer wants to make a therapeutic equivalent of the brand drug product using an amorphous form of the API. Will the generic manufacturer be able to meet the requirements for pharmaceutical equivalence and therapeutic equivalence with the amorphous form of the API?

2. Why is it more difficult to determine PE for biosimilars, such as erythropoietin injection (Procrit) compared to small molecules, such as atorvastatin calcium tablets (Lipitor)?

3. Explain why a generic drug products can be a pharmaceutical equivalent but not identical to the brand drug product.

4. For a generic drug product to be "pharmaceutical equivalent" to the innovator drug (or reference drug product), which of the following is true? Explain your answer.
   a. API in the generic product must be identical to the API in the reference drug product.
   b. It is desirable but not necessary for API to be identical in the generic and reference drug products.
   c. Many APIs used in generic products are referenced by drug master files and meet compendial standards. For these APIs, does it mean generic products are always pharmaceutically equivalent to the brand name drug?

5. Under what circumstances is particle size distribution of API critical for the product performance?

6. Can a generic drug product containing a different polymorph of an API be pharmaceutically equivalent to an innovator drug product? How about if a different salt or cocrystal is used in the generic drug product?

7. The drug miconazole may contain benzyl chloride-related impurity/imtermediate that may be potentially genotoxic as reported in the literature. This API is supplied by various suppliers with DMFs available. How would a generic manufacturer planning to market a miconazole vaginal cream ensure that the API purchased is safe? Does supplier-designated "EP or USP-NF" grade necessarily ensure that PE is met?

ANSWERS

Frequently Asked Questions

If two active pharmaceutical ingredients are pharmaceutical equivalents, can we assume that these two APIs are also identical?

- No. The API can differ in particle size, crystal structure, hydrate, impurities, and/or stability (see Table 17-1.)

Can drug products that are not pharmaceutical equivalents be bioequivalent in patients?

- Yes. Capsules and tablets containing the same API can be bioequivalent. However, in the United States, capsules and tablets are pharmaceutical alternatives. Extended-release tablets or capsules that have different drug release processes can be bioequivalent *in vivo*. Tablets containing either the API or a salt of the API can be bioequivalent when absorption is not dissolution limited.

How would the shape or size of an oral drug product affect compliance in an elderly patient?

- Certain shape, size, or color may discourage the patient from swallowing the tablet. For many patients, tablets containing a 1000 mg of active drug can be difficult to swallow.

Why do drug manufacturers make changes to an approved drug product that is currently on the market?

- There are many reasons that a manufacturer makes a change in the formulation. For example, changed physical properties of API, due to the use of a more economical API synthesis process, necessitate a change in the formulation to assure the same performance of drug product. A manufacturer may want to enlarge the units manufactured (scale-up), use new manufacturing equipment, and/or change the manufacturing site.

Should a bioequivalence study be performed every time a drug manufacturer makes a change in the formulation of the drug product?

- If the change in formulation is minor, such as removal of the color, and the manufacturer can show the likelihood that the change would not affect the bioequivalence of the formulation after the minor change, no bioequivalence study would be needed.

Where can we find a list of US products with therapeutic equivalence and a discussion of evaluation criteria?

- The publication *Approved Drug Products with Therapeutic Equivalence Evaluations* (the List, commonly known as the Orange Book. http://www.fda.gov/Drugs/DevelopmentApprovalProcess/ucm079068.htm). A discussion of PE, TE, and other terms are found in the preface.

REFERENCES

Agudelo M, Vesga O: Therapeutic equivalence requires pharmaceutical, pharmacokinetic, and pharmacodynamic identities: True bioequivalence of a generic product of intravenous metronidazole. *Antimicrob Agents Chemother* 56(5):2659–2665, 2012.

CFR Part 320: Bioavailability and Bioequivalence Requirements. Title 21—Food and Drugs, Chapter I: Food and Drug Administration, Department of Health and Human Services, Subchapter D—Drugs for Human Use, 2013. [Cited June 29, 2014] Available from http://www.accessdata.fda.gov/scripts/cdrh/cfdocs/cfcfr/cfrsearch.cfm?cfrpart=320.

Cook A, Acton JP, Schwartz E: How Increased Competition from Generic Drugs Has Affected Prices and Returns in the

Pharmaceutical Industry. Congressional Budget Office, Washington, DC, 1998 (http://www.cbo.gov/ftpdocs/6xx/doc655/pharm.pdf1-75).

Crawford P, et al: Are there potential problems with generic substitution of antiepileptic drugs? A review of issues. *Seizure* 15(3):165–176, 2006.

Dettelbach HR: A time to speak out on bioequivalence and therapeutic equivalence. *J Clin Pharmacol* 26(5):307–308, 1986.

Dodd S, Besag FMC: Editorial [Lessons from contaminated heparin]. *Curr Drug Saf* 4(1):1–1, 2009.

FDA: Immediate Release Solid Oral Dosage Forms Scale-Up and Postapproval Changes: Chemistry, Manufacturing, and Controls, In Vitro Dissolution Testing, and In Vivo Bioequivalence Documentation. FDA, US Department of Health and Human Services, Center for Drug Evaluation and Research, Editor, 1995.

FDA: SUPAC-MR: Modified Release Solid Oral Dosage Forms Scale-Up and Postapproval Changes: Chemistry, Manufacturing, and Controls; In Vitro Dissolution Testing and In Vivo Bioequivalence Documentation. FDA, US Department of Health and Human Services, Center for Drug Evaluation and Research, Editor, 1997.

FDA: How Drugs are Developed and Approved. [Cited June 5, 2014] Available from http://www.fda.gov/Drugs/DevelopmentApprovalProcess/HowDrugsareDevelopedandApproved/default.htm.

FDA Guidance for Industry: Bioavailability and Bioequivalence Studies for Orally Administered Drug Products—General Considerations. FDA, US Department of Health and Human Services, Center for Drug Evaluation and Research, Editor, 2003.

FDA Guidance for Industry: Changes to an Approved NDA or ANDA, April 2004.

FDA Guidance for Industry: Biosimilars: Questions and Answers Regarding Implementation of the Biologics Price Competition and Innovation Act of 2009, Draft Guidance, February 2012a.

FDA Guidance for Industry: Scientific Considerations in Demonstrating Biosimilarity to a Reference Product, Draft Guidance, February 2012b.

FDA Guidance for Industry: Size, Shape, and Other Physical Attributes of Generic Tablets and Capsules, (Draft) December 2013.

Fujimura S, et al: Antibacterial effects of brand-name teicoplanin and generic products against clinical isolates of methicillin-resistant *Staphylococcus aureus*. *J Infect Chemother* 17(1):30–33, 2011.

ICH Guidance, Q3A, www.ICH.org. ICH Harmonised Tripartite Guideline—Impurities In New Drug Substances, Q3A(R2), Current Step 4 Version Dated October 25, 2006.

Jounela AJ, Pentikäinen PJ, Sothmann A: Effect of particle size on the bioavailability of digoxin. *Eur J Clin Pharmacol* 8(5):365–370, 1975.

Lamy PP: Generic equivalents: Issues and concerns. *J Clin Pharmacol* 26(5):309–316, 1986.

Mastoraki E, et al: Incidence of postoperative infections in patients undergoing coronary artery bypass grafting surgery receiving antimicrobial prophylaxis with original and generic cefuroxime. *J Infect* 56(1):35–39, 2008.

Modi S.R., et al: Impact of crystal habit on biopharmaceutical performance of celecoxib. *Cryst. Growth Des* 13:2824–2832, 2013.

Rodriguez CA, et al: Potential therapeutic failure of generic vancomycin in a liver transplant patient with MRSA peritonitis and bacteremia. *J Infect* 59(4):277–280, 2009.

Rodriguez C, et al: In vitro and in vivo comparison of the anti-staphylococcal efficacy of generic products and the innovator of oxacillin. *BMC Infect Dis* 10(1):153, 2010.

Rohrs BR, et al: Particle size limits to meet USP content uniformity criteria for tablets and capsules. *J Pharm Sci* 95(5):1049–1059, 2006.

Sun CC: Materials science tetrahedron—A useful tool for pharmaceutical research and development. *J Pharm Sci* 98:1671–1687, 2009.

Vesga O, et al: Generic vancomycin products fail in vivo despite being pharmaceutical equivalents of the innovator. *Antimicrob Agents Chemother* 54(8):3271–3279, 2010.

Wittkowsky AK: Generic warfarin: Implications for patient care. *Pharmacotherapy* 17(4):640–643, 1997.

Zuluaga AF, et al: Determination of therapeutic equivalence of generic products of gentamicin in the neutropenic mouse thigh infection model. *PLoS ONE* 5(5):e10744, 2010.

18

Impact of Biopharmaceutics on Drug Product Quality and Clinical Efficacy

Leon Shargel and Andrew Yu

Chapter Objectives

▶ Describe the types of safety and efficacy risks that may occur after taking a drug product and various means for preventing these risks.

▶ Differentiate between drug product quality and drug product performance.

▶ Differentiate between quality control and quality assurance.

▶ Explain how quality by design (QbD) ensures the development and manufacture of a drug product that will deliver consistent performance.

▶ Define quality target product profile (QTPP) and explain how QTPP is different than conventional quality product criteria.

▶ Identify various formulation and manufacturing process factors that affect product quality and performance and the concept of QTPP.

▶ Describe the quality principles underlying basis for the development, manufacture, and quality assurance of the drug product throughout its life cycle in QbD.

RISKS FROM MEDICINES

Side effects from the use of drugs are the major cause of drug-related injuries, adverse events, and deaths. The FDA (FDA, CDER, 2005, 2007) has summarized various types of safety and efficacy risks from medicines (Fig. 18-1). Side effects are observed in clinical trials or postmarketing surveillance and result in listing of adverse events in the drug's labeling. Some side effects are avoidable, and others are unavoidable. Avoidable side effects may include known drug–drug or drug–food interactions, contraindications, improper compliance, etc. In many cases, drug therapy requires an individualized drug treatment plan and careful patient monitoring. Known side effects occur with the best medical practice and even when the drug is used appropriately. Examples include nausea from antibiotics or bone marrow suppression from chemotherapy. Medication errors include wrong drug, wrong dose, or incorrect drug administration. Some side effects are unavoidable. These uncertainties include unexpected adverse events, side effects due to long-term therapy, and unstudied uses and unstudied populations. For example, a rare adverse event occurring in fewer than 1 in 10,000 persons would not be identified in normal premarket testing. Chapters 13, 21, and 22 discuss how pharmacogenetics, pharmacokinetics, pharmacodynamics, and clinical considerations may improve drug efficacy and safety in many instances. *Drug product quality* is another important consideration. Quality is recognized and defined in ICH (International Conference on Harmonisation,[1] which provides for international standards of new drug product quality; see below) as the suitability of either a drug substance (Chapter 17) or drug product for its intended use. This term includes such attributes as the identity, strength, and purity. Drug product quality defects are an important source of risk that affects drug product performance and can affect patient safety and therapeutic efficacy. Product quality includes strength and purity

---

[1]International Conference on Harmonisation—Quality, http://www.fda.gov/Drugs/GuidanceComplianceRegulatoryInformation/Guidances/ucm065005.htm.

- ▶ Describe how product specifications relate to drug product quality and the relevance to quality assurance of the drug product through QbD.

- ▶ Describe a practical strategy to track risks in a drug product development by drawing a scientific roadmap for validating the overall process of material acquiring, manufacturing, and distributional steps involved in a drug product appropriately labeled for medical use.

- ▶ Define critical quality attributes and how these attributes relate to clinical safety and efficacy.

- ▶ Explain how postapproval changes in a drug product may affect drug quality and performance.

- ▶ List the major reasons that a drug product might be recalled due to quality defects.

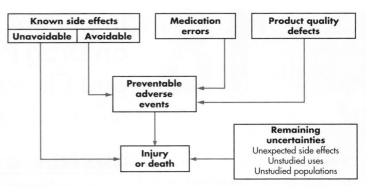

FIGURE 18-1   Sources of risk from drug products (CDER report, FDA).

of the drug substance, the manufacturing process of the drug product, and the monitoring of the manufacturing operations.[2] This chapter will focus on drug product quality and risks of product quality defects that affect drug product performance. To minimize product quality defects, regulatory agencies such as the FDA must consider risk-based regulatory decisions supporting the drug approval process. These decisions depend on the scientific understanding of how formulation and manufacturing process factors affect product quality and performance and are the underlying basis for the development, manufacture, and quality assurance of the drug product throughout its life cycle.[3]

RISK ASSESSMENT

Risk assessment is a valuable science-based process used in quality risk management that can aid in identifying which material attributes and process parameters potentially have an effect on product critical quality attributes (CQAs). Risk assessment is typically performed early in the pharmaceutical development process and is repeated as more information becomes available and greater knowledge is obtained. Risk assessment tools can be used to identify and rank parameters (eg, process, equipment, input materials) with potential to have an impact on product quality, based on prior knowledge and initial experimental data. Once the significant parameters are identified, they can be further studied to achieve a higher level of process understanding.

---

[2]Pharmaceutical manufacturers are required to follow current Good Manufacturing Practices (cGMP) to ensure that the drug products are made consistently with high quality.

[3]A glossary of terms appears at the end of the chapter.

TABLE 18-1   Drug Product Quality and Performance Attributes

Product quality

    Chemistry, manufacturing, and controls (CMC)

    Microbiology

    Information that pertains to the identity, strength, quality, purity, and potency of the drug product

    Validation of manufacturing process and identification of critical quality attributes

Product performance

    In vivo

        Bioavailability and bioequivalence

    In vitro

        Drug release/dissolution

DRUG PRODUCT QUALITY AND DRUG PRODUCT PERFORMANCE

Drug product quality relates to the biopharmaceutic and physicochemical properties of the drug substance and the drug product to the *in vivo* performance of the drug. The performance of each drug product must be consistent and predictable to assure both clinical efficacy and safety. Drug product attributes and performance are critical factors that influence product quality (Table 18-1). Each component of the drug product and the method of manufacture contribute to quality. Quality must be built into the product during research, development, and production. Quality is maintained by implementing systems and procedures that are followed during the development and manufacture of the drug product.

For convenience, drug product quality is listed in Table 18-2 separately from drug product performance. However, drug product quality must be maintained since drug product quality impacts directly on drug product performance.

PHARMACEUTICAL DEVELOPMENT

The pharmaceutical development process must design a quality drug product (QbD, quality by design) using a manufacturing process that provides consistent drug product performance and achieves the desired therapeutic objective. The product development program is based on a sound understanding of the mechanistic activity of the drug substance and its optimal delivery to achieve the desired therapeutic outcome. The integration of biopharmaceutics and QbD optimizes drug product development and performance, which has been described by a biopharmaceutics risk assessment roadmap (Fig. 18-2) (Selen et al, 2014).

This manufacturing process is carefully designed using scientific principles throughout and integrating assurance of product quality into the design of the manufacturing process (quality assurance). Information gained from pharmaceutical development studies and from the manufacturing process provides scientific understanding to support the establishment of the design space (see below), specifications, and manufacturing controls that ensure that each batch of the drug product will be produced with the same quality and performance. The information from pharmaceutical development studies is also the basis for quality risk management. Changes in formulation and manufacturing processes during development and life cycle management after market approval provide additional knowledge and further support the manufacture of the drug product. Every step that affects drug manufacture must also be tested to demonstrate that the desired physical and functional outcomes are achieved (process validation). Once the manufacturing process has been validated, every single lot produced by this method must meet the desired specifications (quality control).

Frequently Asked Questions

▶ *Explain how to "build in" drug quality to ensure that "the performance of a drug product will be predictable to assure clinical efficacy and safety."*

▶ *What do you use as a reference in evaluating performance of a new product in a quality system?*

Quality Risks in Drug Products

Various risks related to drug product quality and performance can impact patient medication. Most serious side effects of drugs are recognized and are described in the approved product label to prevent serious injury. Quality risks are occasionally very serious.

TABLE 18-2   Approaches to Pharmaceutical Development

Aspect	Minimal Approaches	Enhanced, Quality-by-Design Approaches
Overall pharmaceutical development	• Mainly empirical • Developmental research often conducted one variable at a time	• Systematic, relating mechanistic understanding of material attributes and process parameters to drug product CQAs • Multivariate experiments to understand product and process • Establishment of design space • Process analytical technology (PAT) tools utilized
Manufacturing process	• Fixed • Validation primarily based on initial full-scale batches • Focus on optimization and reproducibility	• Adjustable within design space • Life cycle approach to validation and, ideally, continuous process verification • Focus on control strategy and robustness • Use of statistical process control methods
Process controls	• In-process tests primarily for go/no-go decisions • Off-line analysis	• PAT tools utilized with appropriate feed forward and feedback controls • Process operations tracked and trended to support continual improvement efforts postapproval
Product specifications	• Primary means of control • Based on batch data available at the time of registration	• Part of the overall quality control strategy • Based on desired product performance with relevant supportive data
Control strategy	• Drug product quality controlled primarily by intermediates (in-process materials) and end-product testing	• Drug product quality ensured by risk-based control strategy for well-understood product and process • Quality controls shifted upstream, with the possibility of real-time release testing or reduced end-product testing
Life cycle management	• Reactive (ie, problem-solving and corrective action)	• Preventive action • Continual improvement facilitated

From FDA Guidance for Industry: Q8(R2) Pharmaceutical Development, November 2009.

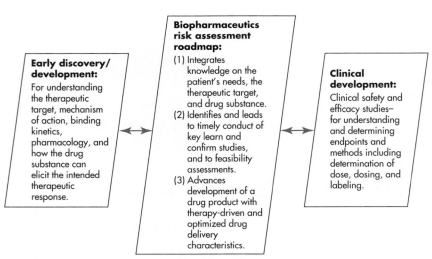

FIGURE 18-2   Biopharmaceutics risk assessment roadmap as a connecting and translational tool for improving and enhancing product quality. (From Selen et al, 2014.)

Mostly, quality risks compromise the intended effect of medicine or produce unintended adverse reactions. Recently, a biopharmaceutics risk assessment roadmap (BioRAM) has been developed for optimizing clinical drug product performance (Selen et al, 2009, 2014). BioRAM uses biopharmaceutic tools to identify and address potential challenges to optimize the drug product for patient benefit (Fig. 18-3). As stated by Selen et al (2014), "Understanding the mode of action of a drug substance and its optimal delivery for generating the desired therapeutic effect is the central tenet of BioRAM. Based on mechanistic knowledge gained about the drug substance and how it elicits the intended response, BioRAM can help to select the optimal drug."

Quality risks may be tracked by following all operation steps involved from drug product development throughout the manufacturing process, distribution, and patient utilization of the drug product. Key operations in manufacturing and pharmaceutical development are listed in Table 18-2. These operations and quality controls are found in the many FDA references essential for proper operation of those steps (http://www.fda.gov/Drugs/GuidanceComplianceRegulatoryInformation/Guidances/ucm065005.htm).

Quality documents are important to ensure FDA compliance, which inspects manufacturing facilities and its operation. The development pharmaceutics

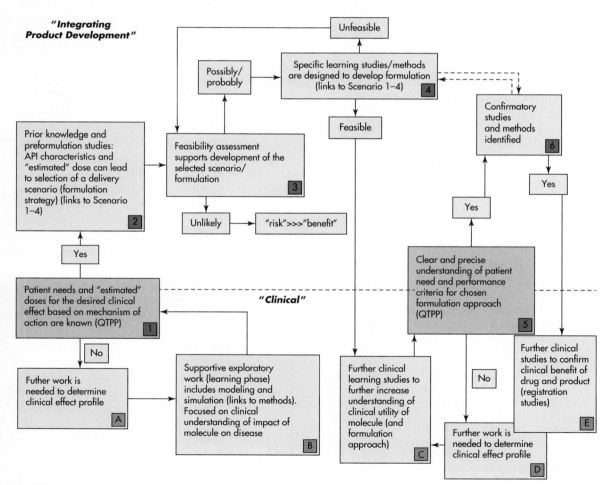

FIGURE 18-3   The biopharmaceutics risk assessment roadmap (BioRAM). (From Selen et al, 2014.)

section can uncover product risks that are often an extension of poor formulation or poor product design. Modern design concepts involve identifying risk sources (variate) that take into account the frequency of occurrence and components (unit process) of the overall operation. The overall process involves many materials and operations. Hence a QbD approach is often multivariate by necessity. An understanding of risk involves some probability and statistics. QbD is very much rooted in statistics. However, an understanding of the basic material science and interplay of functional components should always override the tools and mathematics that are used to implement them. These tools should be viewed as an aid to discover or add more choice to manufacturing through QbD. The risks from drug product quality are sometimes described as *product drug quality defects*. Some of the quality elements important during product development are listed in Table 18-3.

TABLE 18-3   Quality Elements of Pharmaceutical Development and Quality by Design

- Define quality target product quality profile (QTPP).
- Design and develop formulations and manufacturing processes to ensure predefined product quality.
- Identify critical quality attributes (CQA), process parameters, and sources of variability that are critical to quality from the perspective of patients, and then translate them into the attributes that the drug product should possess.
- Perform a risk assessment: linking material attributes and process parameters to drug product CQAs.
- Identify *a design space* for critical processing variables and formulation variables that impact *in vivo* product performance.
- Establish how the critical process parameters can be varied to consistently produce a drug product with the desired characteristics.
- Establish the relationships between formulation and manufacturing process variables (including drug substance and excipient attributes and process parameters); identify desired product characteristics and sources of variability.
- Implement a flexible and robust manufacturing process that can adapt and produce a consistent product over time.
- Develop *process analytical technology* (PAT) to integrate systems during drug product manufacture that provides continuous real-time quality assurance.
- Control manufacturing processes to produce consistent quality over time.
- Apply product life cycle management and continual improvement.

EXAMPLE OF QUALITY RISK

Imported drugs—Quality of the active pharmaceutical ingredient (API) from various sources is regulated by different countries. These regulations involve common risks that are quite critical. It is important that the API or product is properly reviewed to meet either component or FDA criteria.

Development pharmaceutics involves selecting appropriate excipients, the API source, and the fabricating development concept to the drug product (eg, oral tablet, eye product, transdermal patch, etc).

Drug development risks are numerous and vary with the product type. A risk in QbD may be easily overlooked with an inadequate quality strategy. For example, a tablet may be friable and soft due to poor formulation or the tablet blend may be excessively compressed. Too often, inadequate understanding of excipient functions or inclusion of suitable binders (eg, or starch, macrocrystalline cellulose) results in an incorrect QbD strategy, that is, testing friability and hardness at different hardness at inappropriate levels instead of using a suitable binder or increasing the proportion of excipients. The proper inclusion of suitable ingredients may result in a product that is so robust that hardness has little or no effect on disintegration while still maintaining friability. A well-designed QbD study on such a product would do away with need extensive testing.

Method of preparation risks—Preparation broadly describes synthesis, manufacturing, and packaging steps. API risks have been discussed in the previous chapter. API material properties include particle size, crystal forms, and compression characteristics. However, these properties may be reduced by the impact resulting from a poor API that has residual solvents (eg, chloroform, toluene), or solvents that may be classified as carcinogenic. With the adoption of recent FDA quality guidances, residual solvents are generally well controlled with generally recognized standards with FDA-approved products.

Control of starting materials in API synthesis—Sources of impurities such as heavy metals, solvents, and impurities are risks that may impact quality in subsequent steps in unknown ways. For example, metallic impurities, even not harmful, may have an impact on stability of some products, and low level may alter the appearance of a product even not harmful. Related impurities to an API may sometimes have pharmacologic properties of their own. In general, the history or processes that precede starting materials is not documented. Starting materials may not be regulatory controlled or inspected. It is of particularly importance to maintain a good quality practice by the vendor or supplier even though the starting materials are not strictly regulated. A chemical may be produced for chemical or industrial purpose. For example, urea is produced as fertilizer rather than for drug or excipient use.

Control tests on the finished product are quality tests that are specified, including stability, dissolution, and other special product tests. It is important to consider whether the tests will have impact on the performance of the product. Most of the issues raised by this question are addressed in the relevance of the product attributes to clinical performance. Figures 18-2 and 18-3 address these issues. Recently, the concept of product life cycle, learn and confirm using QbD versus the convention concept of "set the specification and maintain" is being debated and will impact on quite new and a both benefit and risk.

Frequently Asked Questions

▶ *Can a QbD strategy for testing hardness and disintegration replace the need for a full dissolution profile testing of all batches?*

▶ *Can a dissolution test of a tablet at the beginning and the end period of stability cycle replace dissolution testing every 3 or 6 months during the stability cycle?*

▶ *Is sterility testing of an injection product at the initial and the end of production batch adequate to justify the stability of a new product?*

Quality (by) Design (QbD)

A major principle that drives manufacturing process development is QbD. *Quality by design* is a systematic, scientific, risk-based, holistic, and proactive approach to pharmaceutical development that begins

with predefined objectives and emphasizes the understanding of product and processes and process control. Product and process performance characteristics are scientifically designed to meet specific objectives (Yu, 2008). To achieve QbD objectives, product and process characteristics important to desired performance must be derived from a combination of prior knowledge and experimental assessment during product development. Quality cannot be tested in drug products. Quality should be built in the design and confirmed by testing. With a greater understanding of the drug product and its manufacturing process, regulatory agencies are working with pharmaceutical manufacturers to use systematic approaches to drug product development that will achieve product quality and the desired drug product performance (FDA Guidance for Industry, 2009). The elements of QbD are listed in Table 18-3.

Quality target product profile (QTPP) is a prospective summary of the quality characteristics of a drug product that ideally will be achieved to ensure the desired quality, taking into account safety and efficacy of the drug product. As part of the quality system, the concept QTPP was introduced in QbD. QTPP summarizes all the important product attributes that are targeted and designed by the manufacturer during design and manufacturing. QTPP helps to maintain the quality throughout the life cycle of the product.

The following steps are informative in understanding various aspects of the overall scheme and its relevance:

1. Quality target product profile (QTPP)-driven specifications
2. BioRAM (see Fig. 18-3)
3. Advancing and leveraging science and technology including mechanistic understanding, *in silico* tools, statistical evaluations
4. Knowledge sharing and collaborations based on multidimensional collaborations and shared database

By the use of an integrated approach to QbD using biopharmaceutic principles, drug products can be manufactured with the assurance that product quality and performance will be maintained throughout its life cycle.

Critical Manufacturing Attributes (CMAs) and Critical Process Parameters (CPPs)

In process development, the most important processes and component properties should be identified in the manufacturing process. A CQA is a physical, chemical, biological, or microbiological property or characteristic that needs to be controlled (directly or indirectly) to ensure product quality. The pharmaceutical manufacturer should identify critical manufacturing attributes (CMAs), critical process parameters (CPPs), and sources of variability that ensure the quality of the finished dosage form. The CQAs should be based on clinical relevance. Thus, the manufacturer of the drug product designs and develops the formulations and manufacturing processes to ensure a predefined quality.

Design Space

The interaction between critical processes and materials should also be studied to optimize manufacturing processes. A *design space* is defined for critical processing variables and formulation variables that impact *in vivo* product performance. There may be several variables that affect the product variability *in vitro*. It is important to identify which of these variables are actually relevant to drug product performance *in vivo*. ICH defines design space in Q8 as follows:

- The multidimensional combination and interaction of input variables (eg, material attributes) and process parameters that have been demonstrated to provide assurance of quality.
- Working within the design space is not considered a change. Movement out of the design space is considered to be a change and would normally initiate a regulatory postapproval change process.
- Design space is proposed by the applicant and is subject to regulatory assessment and approval.

Design space is the geometrical region suitable for quality manufacturing when two or more process/material variables are plotted in a two-dimensional or higher-dimensional space to show the combined effects of the relevant processing variables during manufacturing. Some of these processing variables may or may not be critical to drug product performance. Thus, the manufacturer knows which process variable is critical and must have stricter control.

Process Analytical Technology (PAT)

Like design space, *process analytical technology* (PAT) also uses critical processes and materials to improve the quality of the product, but in PAT the emphasis is on monitoring these variables in a timely manner. PAT is intended to support innovation and efficiency in pharmaceutical development, manufacturing, and quality assurance (FDA Guidance for Industry, September 2004). Conventional pharmaceutical manufacturing is generally accomplished using batch processing with laboratory testing conducted on samples collected during the manufacturing process and after the drug product is made (finished dosage form). These laboratory tests are used to evaluate quality of the drug product (see quality control and quality assurance below). Newer methods based on science and engineering principles now exist for improving pharmaceutical development, manufacturing, and quality assurance starting earlier in the development timeline through innovation in product and process development, analysis, and control.

PAT uses an integrated systems approach to regulating pharmaceutical product quality. PAT assesses mitigating risks related to poor product and process quality, and then monitors and controls them. PAT is characterized by the following:

- Product quality and performance are ensured through the design of effective and efficient manufacturing processes.
- Product and process specifications are based on a mechanistic understanding of how formulation and process factors affect product performance.
- Continuous real-time quality assurance.
- Relevant regulatory policies and procedures are tailored to accommodate the most current level of scientific knowledge.
- Risk-based regulatory approaches recognize:
  - The scientific understanding of how formulation and manufacturing process factors affect product quality and performance.
  - The capability of process control strategies to prevent or mitigate the risk of producing a poor quality product.

PAT enhances manufacturing efficiencies by improving the manufacturing process, through scientific innovation and with better communication between manufacturers and the regulatory agencies. PAT may be considered a part of the overall QbD such that quality is built into the product during manufacture. An increased emphasis on building quality into drug products allows more focus to be placed on relevant multifactorial relationships among material, manufacturing process, environmental variables, and their effects on quality. This enhanced focus provides a basis for identifying and understanding relationships among various critical formulation and process factors and for developing effective risk mitigation strategies (eg, product specifications, process controls, training). The data and information to help understand these relationships can be leveraged through preformulation programs, development and scale-up studies, as well as from improved analysis of manufacturing data collected over the life of a product.

EXCIPIENT EFFECT ON DRUG PRODUCT PERFORMANCE

Drug products are finished dosage forms that contain the API along with suitable diluents and/or excipients. Excipients are generally considered inert in that they have no pharmacodynamic activity of their own. However, excipients have different functional purposes and influence the performance of the drug product (Amidon et al, 2007; Shargel, 2010). Compressed tablets may consist of the active ingredient, a diluent (filler), a binder, buffering agents, a disintegrating agent, and one or more lubricant. Approved FD&C and D&C dyes or lakes (dyes adsorbed onto insoluble aluminum hydroxide), flavors, and sweetening agents may also be present. These excipients provide various functional purposes such as improving compression, improving powder flow, stability of the active ingredient, and other properties (Table 18-4). For example, diluents such as lactose, starch, dibasic calcium phosphate, and microcrystalline cellulose are added where the quantity of active ingredient is small and/or difficult to compress.

The physical and chemical properties of the excipients, the physical and chemical properties of the API, and the manufacturing process all play a role in the performance of the finished dosage form. Each excipient must be evaluated to maintain consistent performance of the drug product throughout the product's life cycle.

TABLE 18-4   Common Excipients for Solid Oral Dosage Forms

Excipient	Function in Compressed Tablet	Possible Effect on Drug Product Performance
Microcrystalline cellulose, lactose, calcium carbonate	Diluent	Very low-dose drug (eg, 5 mg) may have high ratio of excipients to active drug leading to a problem of homogeneous blending and possible interaction of drug with excipients.
Copovidone, starch, methylcellulose	Binder	Binders give adhesiveness to the powder blend and can affect tablet hardness. Harder tablets tend to disintegrate more slowly.
Magnesium stearate	Lubricant	Lubricants are hydrophobic; over-lubrication can slow dissolution of API.
Starch	Disintegrant	Disintegrant allows for more rapid fragmentation of tablet *in vivo*, reducing disintegration time and allowing for more rapid dissolution.
FD&C colors and lakes	Color	
Various	Coating	Coatings may have very little effect (film coat) or have rate-controlling effect on drug release and dissolution (eg, enteric coat).

PRACTICAL FOCUS

BSE in Gelatin

Gelatin and other excipients may be produced from ruminant sources such as bones and hides obtained from cattle. In the early 1990s, the FDA became concerned about transmissible spongiform encephalopathies (TSEs) in animals and Creutzfeldt–Jakob disease in humans. In 1993, the FDA recommended against the use of materials from cattle that had resided in, or originated from, countries in which *bovine spongiform encephalopathy* (BSE, or "mad cow disease") had occurred. The FDA organized a Transmissible Spongiform Encephalopathies Advisory Committee to help assess the safety of imported and domestic gelatin and gelatin by-products in FDA-regulated products with regard to the risk posed by BSE. The FDA published a guidance to industry concerning the sourcing and processing of gelatin used in pharmaceutical products to ensure the safety of gelatin as it relates to the potential risk posed by BSE (http://www.fda.gov/opacom/morechoices/industry/guidance/gelguide.htm). In some cases, such as the magnesium stearates, a vegetative source may be used to avoid the BSE/TSE concern.

Gelatin Capsules Stability

Soft and hard gelatin capsules show a decrease in the dissolution rate as they age in simulated gastric fluid (SGF) with and without pepsin or in simulated intestinal fluid (SIF) without pancreatin. This has been attributed to pellicle formation. When the dissolution of aged or slower-releasing capsules was carried out in the presence of an enzyme (pepsin in SGF or pancreatin in SIF), a significant increase in dissolution was observed. In this setting, multiple dissolution media may be necessary to assess product quality adequately.

Excipient Effects

Excipients can sometimes affect the rate and extent of drug absorption. In general, using excipients that are currently in FDA-approved immediate-release solid oral dosage forms within a suitable range will not affect the rate or extent of absorption of a highly soluble and highly permeable drug substance that is formulated in a rapidly dissolving immediate-release product.

Excessive use of lubricant should be avoided. When new excipients or atypically large amounts of commonly used excipients are included in an immediate-release solid dosage form, additional information documenting the absence of an impact on bioavailability of the drug may be requested by the FDA. Such information can be provided with a relative bioavailability study using a simple aqueous solution as the reference product. Large quantities of certain excipients, such as surfactants (eg, polysorbate 80) and sweeteners (eg, mannitol or sorbitol), may be problematic.

> **Frequently Asked Questions**
>
> ▶ How does a change in drug product quality change drug product performance?
>
> ▶ What is the difference between critical manufacturing attribute (CMA), critical product attribute (CPA), and critical quality attribute (CQA)?
>
> ▶ How can a pharmaceutical manufacturer ensure that a drug product has the same drug product performance before and after a change in the supplier of the active pharmaceutical ingredient or a change in the supplier of an excipient?

QUALITY CONTROL AND QUALITY ASSURANCE

An independent *quality assurance* (QA) unit is a vital part of drug development and manufacture. QA is responsible for ensuring that all the appropriate procedures have been followed and documented. QA provides a high probability that each dose or package of a drug product will have predictable characteristics and perform according to its labeled use. The *quality control* (QC) unit is responsible for the in-process tests beginning from receipt of raw materials, throughout production, finished product, packaging, and distribution.

Principles of quality assurance include the following: (1) Quality, safety, and effectiveness must be designed and built into the product; (2) quality cannot be inspected or tested into the finished product; and (3) each step of the manufacturing process must be controlled to maximize the probability that the finished product meets all quality and design specifications.

QA/QC has the responsibility and authority to approve or reject all components, drug product containers, closures, in-process materials, packaging material, labeling, and drug products, and the authority to review production records to ensure that no errors have occurred or, if errors have occurred, that they have been fully investigated. QA/QC is responsible for approving or rejecting drug products manufactured, processed, packed, or held under contract by another company.

PRACTICAL FOCUS

Tablet compression may affect drug product performance of either immediate-release or extended-release drug products even between products containing the same active drug. Metoprolol is a beta 1-selective (cardioselective) adrenoceptor blocking agent that is available as an immediate-release tablet (metoprolol tartrate tablets, USP—Lopressor®) and an extended-release tablet (metoprolol succinate extended-release tablets—Toprol-XL®). Metoprolol is a highly soluble and highly permeable drug that meets the Biopharmaceutics Classification System, BCS 1 (Chapter 16). Metoprolol is rapidly and completely absorbed from the immediate-release tablet.

Compression makes the powder blend more compact and affects tablet hardness, especially when inadequate amount of binder is added. Excessive compression may cause the tablet to disintegrate more slowly, resulting in a slower rate of dissolution and systemic drug absorption. Adequate use of binder and lubricant during product design obviates the need to use excessive force during compression/compaction.

The metoprolol succinate extended-release tablet (Toprol-XL) is a multiple-unit system containing metoprolol succinate in a multitude of controlled-release pellets. Each pellet acts as a separate drug delivery unit and is designed to deliver metoprolol continuously over the dosage interval (Toprol-XL approved label). The controlled-release pellets are mixed with excipients and compressed into tablets. If the tablet is compressed too strongly, the high compression will not only increase tablet hardness but can also deform the controlled-release pellets. The deformed pellets lose their controlled-release characteristics and the active drug, metoprolol, dissolves more quickly resulting in a faster-than-desired rate of systemic drug absorption. Inadequate amount of lubricant or glidant can also aggravate or damage pellets during compression.

Good Manufacturing Practices

Good Manufacturing Practices (GMPs) are FDA regulations that describe the methods, equipment, facilities, and controls required for producing human and veterinary products. GMPs define a quality system that manufacturers use to build quality into their products. For example, approved drug products developed and produced according to GMPs are considered safe, properly identified, of the correct strength, pure, and of high quality. The US regulations are called *current* Good Manufacturing Practices (cGMPs), to emphasize that the expectations are dynamic. These regulations are minimum requirements that may be exceeded by the manufacturer. GMPs help prevent inadvertent use or release of unacceptable drug products into manufacturing and distribution. GMP requirements include well-trained personnel and management, buildings and facilities, and written and approved Standard Operating Procedures (SOPs), as listed in Table 18-5.

Guidances for Industry

The FDA publishes guidances for the industry to provide recommendations to pharmaceutical manufacturers for the development and manufacture of drug substances and drug products (http://www.fda.gov /drugs/guidancecomplianceregulatoryinformation /guidances/ucm121568.htm). The International Conference on Harmonization of Technical Requirements for Registration of Pharmaceuticals for Human Use (ICH) is composed of the regulatory authorities of Europe, Japan, and the United States, and experts from the pharmaceutical industry. The ICH is interested in the global development and availability of new medicines while maintaining safeguards on quality, safety and efficacy, and regulatory obligations to protect public health (www.ich.org).*

TABLE 18-5   Current Good Manufacturing Practice for Finished Pharmaceuticals

Subpart A—General Provisions
  Scope, definitions

Subpart B—Organization and Personnel
  Responsibilities of quality control unit, personnel qualifications, personnel responsibilities, consultants

Subpart C—Buildings and Facilities
  Design and construction features, lighting, ventilation, air filtration, air heating and cooling, plumbing, sewage and refuse, washing and toilet facilities, sanitation, maintenance

Subpart D—Equipment
  Equipment design, size, and location, equipment construction, equipment cleaning and maintenance, automatic, mechanical, and electronic equipment, filters

Subpart E—Control of Components and Drug Product Containers and Closures
  General requirements, receipt and storage of untested components, drug product containers and closures; testing and approval or rejection of components, drug product containers and closures; use of approved components, drug product containers and closures; retesting of approved components, drug product containers and closures, rejected components, drug product containers and closures, drug product containers and closures

Subpart F—Production and Process Controls
  Written procedures; deviations, change of components, calculation of yield, equipment identification, sampling and testing of in-process materials and drug products, time limitations on production, control of microbiological contamination, reprocessing

Subpart G—Packaging and Labeling Controls
  Materials examination and usage criteria, labeling issuance, packaging and labeling operations, tamper-resistant packaging requirements for over-the-counter human drug products, drug product inspection, expiration dating

Subpart H—Holding and Distribution
  Warehousing procedures, distribution procedures

Subpart I—Laboratory Controls
  General requirements, testing and release for distribution, stability testing, special testing requirements, reserve samples, laboratory animals, penicillin contamination

Subpart J—Records and Reports
  General requirements; equipment cleaning and use log; component, drug product, container, closure, and labeling records; master production and control records, batch production and control records, production record review, laboratory records, distribution, complaint files

Subpart K—Returned and Salvaged Drug Products
  Returned drug products, drug product salvaging

From: US Code of Federal Regulations.

Quality Standards

Public standards are necessary to ensure that drug substances and drug products have consistent and reproducible quality. The *United States Pharmacopeia National Formulary* (USP-NF, www.usp.org) is legally recognized by the US Food, Drug and Cosmetic Act and sets public standards for drug products and drug substances. The USP-NF contains monographs for drug substances and drug products that include standards for strength, quality, and purity. In addition, the USP-NF contains general chapters that describe specific procedures that support the monographs. The tests in the monographs may provide *acceptance criteria*, that is, numerical limits, ranges, or other criteria for the test for the drug substance or drug product. An *impurity* is defined as any component of the drug substance that is not the entity defined as the drug substance. Drugs with a USP or NF designation that do not conform to the USP monograph may be considered adulterated. *Specifications* are the standards a drug product must meet to ensure conformance to predetermined criteria for consistent and reproducible quality and performance.

International Conference on Harmonization (ICH) has published several guidances to regulate drug substance and drug product manufacturing. The main approach is to promote "better understanding of manufacturing processes with quality (by) design." QbD improves the quality of the product and makes it easier for regulatory agencies to evaluate postapproval changes of a drug product. ICH guideline Q8 describes pharmaceutical development and ICH guidance Q10 discusses pharmaceutical quality systems. Earlier guidances such as ICH Q6A provide more specific details on setting acceptance criteria and test specification for new drug substances and new drug products. The ICH guidance Q6A has been recommended for adoption in the United States, the European Union, and Japan. These regulations will be applied to new drug substances and drug products.

RISK MANAGEMENT

Regulatory and Scientific Considerations

The FDA develops rational, science-based regulatory requirements for drug substances and finished drug products. The FDA establishes quality standards and acceptance criteria for each component used in the manufacture of a drug product. Each component must meet an appropriate quality and performance objective.

Drug Manufacturing Requirements

Assurance of product quality is derived from careful attention to a number of factors, including selection of quality parts and materials, adequate product and process design, control of the process, and in-process and end-product testing. Because of the complexity of today's medical products, routine end-product testing alone often is not sufficient to ensure product quality. The *chemistry, manufacturing, and controls* (CMC) section of a drug application describes the composition, manufacture, and specifications of the drug substance and drug product (Table 18-6).

Process Validation

Process validation is the process for establishing documented evidence to provide a high degree of assurance that a specific process will consistently

TABLE 18-6   Guidelines for the Format and Content of the Chemistry, Manufacturing, and Controls Section of an Application

I. Drug Substance
  A. Description, including physical and chemical characteristics and stability
    1. Name(s)
    2. Structural formula
    3. Physical and chemical characteristics
    4. Elucidation of structure
    5. Stability
  B. Manufacturer(s)
  C. Method(s) of manufacturer and packaging
    1. Process controls
    2. Container-closure system
  D. Specifications and analytical methods for the drug substance
  E. Solid-state drug substance forms and their relationship to bioavailability

II. Drug Product
  A. Components
  B. Composition
  C. Specifications and analytical methods for inactive components
  D. Manufacturer(s)
  E. Method(s) of manufacture and packaging
    1. Process controls
    2. Container closure system

III. Methods validation package

IV. Environmental assessment

FDA Guidance (1999).

produce a product meeting its predetermined specifications and quality characteristics. Process validation is a key element in ensuring that these quality assurance goals are met. Proof of validation is obtained through collection and evaluation of data, preferably beginning at the process development phase and continuing through the production phase.

The product's end use should be a determining factor in the development of product (and component) characteristics and specifications. All pertinent aspects of the product that may affect safety and effectiveness should be considered. These aspects include performance, reliability, and stability. Acceptable ranges or limits should be established for each characteristic to set up allowable variations.

Specifications are the quality standards (ie, tests, analytical procedures, and acceptance criteria) that confirm the quality of drug substances, drug products, intermediates, raw material reagents, components, in-process material, container closure systems, and other materials used in the production of the drug substance or drug product. The standards or specifications that are critical to product quality are considered CMAs or CPPs.

Through careful design and validation of both the process and process controls, a manufacturer can establish with a high degree of confidence that all manufactured units from successive lots will be acceptable. Successfully validating a process may reduce the dependence on intensive in-process and finished product testing. In most cases, end-product testing plays a major role in ensuring that quality assurance goals are met; that is, validation and end-product testing are not mutually exclusive.

Drug Recalls and Withdrawals

The FDA coordinates drug recall information and prepares health hazard evaluations to determine the risk to public health from products being recalled. The FDA classifies recall actions in accordance to the level of risk. The FDA and the manufacturer develop recall strategies based on the potential health hazard and other factors, including distribution patterns and market availability. The FDA also determines the need for public warnings and assists the recalling firm with public notification. Table 18-7 lists some of the major reasons for drug recalls.

SCALE-UP AND POSTAPPROVAL CHANGES (SUPAC)

A *postapproval change* is any change in a drug product after it has been approved for marketing by the FDA. Postapproval manufacturing changes may adversely impact drug product quality. Since safety and efficacy are established using clinical batches, the same level of quality must be ensured in the finished drug product released to the public. A change to a marketed drug product can be initiated for a number of reasons, including a revised market forecast, change in an API source, change in excipients,

TABLE 18-7   Major Reasons for Drug Recalls

Failed USP dissolution test requirements

Microbial contamination of nonsterile products

Lack of efficacy

Impurities/degradation products

Lack of assurance of sterility

Lack of product stability—Stability data failing to support expiration date

Cross-contamination with other products

Deviations from good manufacturing practices

Failure or inability to validate manufacturing processes

Failure or inability to validate drug analysis methods

Subpotency or superpotency

Labeling mix-ups including

- Labeling: Label error on declared strength
- Labeling: Correctly labeled product in incorrect carton or package

Misbranded: Promotional literature with unapproved therapeutic claims

Marketed without a new or generic approval

Adapted from Center for Drug Evaluation and Research, CDER 2007 Update and other sources.

optimization of the manufacturing process, and upgrade of the packaging system. A change within a given parameter can have varied effect depending on the type of product. For example, a change in the container closure/system of a solid oral dosage form may have little impact on an oral tablet dosage form unless the primary packaging component is critical to the shelf life of the finished product.

If a pharmaceutical manufacturer makes any change in the drug formulation, scales up the formulation to a larger batch size, or changes the process, equipment, or manufacturing site, the manufacturer should consider whether any of these changes will affect the identity, strength, purity, quality, safety, and efficacy of the approved drug product. Moreover, any changes in the raw material (ie, active pharmaceutical ingredient), excipients (including a change in grade or supplier), or packaging (including container closure system) should also be shown not to affect the quality of the drug product. The manufacturer should assess the effect of the change on the identity, strength (eg, assay, content uniformity), quality (eg, physical, chemical, and biological properties), purity (eg, impurities and degradation products), or potency (eg, biological activity, bioavailability, bioequivalence) of a product as they may relate to the safety or effectiveness of the product.

The FDA has published several SUPAC guidances, including *Changes to an Approved NDA or ANDA* for the pharmaceutical industry. These guidances address the following issues:

- Components and composition of the drug product
- Manufacturing site change
- Scale-up of drug product
- Manufacturing equipment
- Manufacturing process
- Packaging
- Active pharmaceutical ingredient

These documents describe (1) the level of change, (2) recommended CMC tests for each level of change, (3) *in vitro* dissolution tests and/or bioequivalence tests for each level of change, and (4) documentation that should support the change. The level of change is classified as to the likelihood that a change in the drug product as listed above might affect the quality of the drug product. The levels of change as described by the FDA are listed in Table 18-8.

As noted in Table 18-8, a Level 1 change, which could be a small change in the excipient amount (eg, starch, lactose), would be unlikely to alter the quality or performance of the drug product, whereas a Level 3 change, which may be a qualitative or

quantitative change in the excipients beyond an allowable range, particularly for drug products containing a narrow therapeutic window, might require an *in vivo* bioequivalence study to demonstrate that drug quality and performance were not altered by the change.

The SUPAC guidance is an early guidance that assesses changes in manufacturing and its effect on product quality. The basic concepts continue to be a useful guide, and in many respects, QbD extends its scope. With adequate QbD study, some changes in manufacturing may require only an annual report instead of a prior approval supplements for regulatory purposes. The ultimate question to ask is: Will the product quality be assured to be equivalent or better and meet with prior information described in the application with QbD data?

Assessment of the Effects of the Change

Assessment of the effect of a change should include a determination that the drug substance intermediates, drug substance, in-process materials, and/or drug product affected by the change conform to the approved specifications. *Acceptance criteria* are numerical limits, ranges, or other criteria for the tests described. *Conformance* to a specification means that the material, when tested according to the analytical procedures listed in the specification, will meet the listed acceptance criteria. Additional testing may be needed to confirm that the material affected by manufacturing changes continues to meet its specification. The assessment may include, as appropriate, evaluation of any changes in the chemical, physical, microbiological, biological, bioavailability, and/or stability profiles. This additional assessment may involve testing of the postchange drug product itself or, if appropriate, the component directly affected by the change. The type of additional testing depends on the type of manufacturing change, the type of drug substance and/or drug product, and the effect of the change on the quality of the product. Examples of additional tests include:

- Evaluation of changes in the impurity or degradant profile
- Toxicology tests to qualify a new impurity or degradant or to qualify an impurity that is above a previously qualified level
- Evaluation of the hardness or friability of a tablet

TABLE 18-8   FDA Definitions of Level of Changes That May Affect the Quality of an Approved Drug Product

Change Level	Definition of Level
Level 1	Changes that are unlikely to have any detectable impact on the formulation quality and performance.
Level 2	Changes that could have a significant impact on formulation quality and performance.
Level 3	Changes that are likely to have a significant impact on formulation quality and performance.

- Assessment of the effect of a change on bioequivalence (may include multipoint and/or multimedia dissolution profiles and/or an *in vivo* bioequivalence study)
- Evaluation of extractables from new packaging components or moisture permeability of a new container closure system

Equivalence

The manufacturer usually assesses the extent to which the manufacturing change has affected the identity, strength, quality, purity, or potency of the drug product by comparing test results from *pre-* and *postchange* material and then determining if the test results are equivalent. The drug product after any changes should be equivalent to the product made before the change. An exception to this general approach is that when bioequivalence should be redocumented for certain Abbreviated New Drug Application (ANDA) postapproval changes, the comparator should be the reference listed drug. Equivalence does not necessarily mean identical. Equivalence may also relate to maintenance of a quality characteristic (eg, stability) rather than a single performance of a test.

Critical Manufacturing Variables

Critical manufacturing variables (CMVs, sometimes referred to as *critical manufacturing attributes*, CMAs) include items in the formulation, process, equipment, materials, and methods for the drug product that can significantly affect *in vitro* dissolution. If possible, the manufacturer should determine whether there is a relationship between CMV, *in vitro* dissolution, and *in vivo* bioavailability.[4] The goal is to develop product specifications that will ensure bioequivalence of future batches prepared within limits of acceptable dissolution specifications. One approach to obtaining this relationship is to compare the bioavailability of test products with slowest and fastest dissolution characteristics to the bioavailability of the marketed drug product. Dissolution specifications for the drug product are then established so that future production batches do not fall outside the bioequivalence of the marketed drug product.

Adverse Effect

Sometimes manufacturing changes have an adverse effect on the identity, strength, quality, purity, or potency of the drug product. For example, a type of process change could cause a new degradant to be formed that requires qualification and/or quantification. The manufacturer must show that the new degradant will not affect the safety or efficacy of the product. Changes in the qualitative or quantitative formulation, including inactive ingredients, are considered major changes and are likely to have a significant impact on formulation quality and performance. However, the deletion or reduction of an ingredient intended to affect only the color of a product is considered to be a minor change that is unlikely to affect the safety of the drug product.

Postapproval Changes of Drug Substance

Manufacturing changes of the *active pharmaceutical ingredient* (API)—also known as the drug substance or bulk active—may change its quality attributes. These quality attributes include chemical purity, solid-state properties, and residual solvents. Chemical purity is dependent on the synthetic pathway and purification process. Solid-state properties include particle size, polymorphism, hydrate/solvate, and solubility. Small amounts of residual solvents such as dichloromethane may remain in the API after extraction and/or purification. Changes in the solid-state properties of the API may affect the manufacture of the dosage form or product performance. For example, a change in particle size may affect API bulk density and tablet hardness, whereas different polymorphs may affect API solubility and stability. Changes in particle size and/or polymorph may affect the drug's bioavailability *in vivo*. Moreover, the excipient(s) and vehicle functionality and possible pharmacologic properties may affect product quality and performance.

> **Frequently Asked Question**
> ▶ *Does a change in the manufacturing process require FDA approval?*

---

[4]*In vitro* dissolution/drug release studies that relate to the *in vivo* drug bioavailability may be considered a drug product performance test.

PRACTICAL FOCUS

Quantitative Change in Excipients

A manufacturer would like to increase the amount of starch by 2% (w/w) in an immediate-release drug product.

- Would you consider this change in an excipient to be a Level 1, 2, or 3 change? Why?

The FDA has determined that small changes in certain excipients for immediate-release drug products may be considered Level 1 changes. Table 18-9 lists the changes in excipients, expressed as percentage (w/w) of the total formulation, less than or equal to the following percent ranges that are considered Level 1 changes. According to this table, a 2% increase in starch would be considered a Level 1 change.

The total additive effect of all excipient changes should not be more than 5%. For example, in a drug product containing the active ingredient lactose, mirocrystalline cellulose, and magnesium stearate, the lactose and microcrystalline cellulose should not vary by more than an absolute total of 5% (eg, lactose increases 2.5% and microcrystalline cellulose decreases by 2.5%) relative to the target dosage form weight if it is to stay within the Level 1 range. The examples are for illustrations only and the latest official guidance should be consulted for current views.

It should be noted that a small change in the amount of excipients is less likely to affect the bioavailability of a highly soluble, highly permeable drug in an immediate-release drug product compared to a drug that has low solubility and low permeability.

Changes in Batch Size (Scale-Up/Scale-Down)

For commercial reasons, a manufacturer may increase the batch size of a drug product from 100,000 units to 5 million units. Even though similar equipment is used and the same Standard Operating Procedures (SOPs) are used, there may be problems in manufacturing a very large batch. This problem is similar to a chef's problem of cooking the main entrée for two persons versus cooking the same entrée for a banquet of 200 persons using the same recipe. The FDA has generally considered that a change in batch size greater than tenfold is a Level 2 change and requires the manufacturer to notify the FDA and provide documentation for all testing before marketing this product.

TABLE 18-9   Level 1—Allowable Changes in Excipients

Excipient	Percent Excipient (W/W) of Total Target Dosage Form Weight
Filler	±5
Disintegrant	±3
Starch	±1
Other	
Binder	±0.5
Lubricant	±0.25
Calcium stearate	±0.25
Magnesium stearate	±1
Other	
Glidant	±1
Talc	±0.1
Other	
Film coat	±1

These percentages are based on the assumption that the drug substance in the product is formulated to 100% of label/potency.

Source: FDA Guidance, 1995.

PRODUCT QUALITY PROBLEMS

The FDA and industry are working together to establish a set of quality attributes and acceptance criteria for certain approved drug substances and drug products that would indicate less manufacturing risk. Table 18-10 summarizes some of the quality attributes for these products. However, all approved drug products must be manufactured under current Good Manufacturing Practices.

Drug substances and drug products that have more quality risk are generally those products that are more complex to synthesize or manufacture (Fig. 18-4). For example, biotechnology-derived drugs (eg, proteins) made by fermentation may have more quality risk than chemically synthesized small molecules. Extended-release and delayed-release drug products may also present a greater quality risk than an immediate-release drug product. Drug products

TABLE 18-10   Quality Attributes and Criteria for Certain Approved Drug Substances and Drug Products

| Drug Substances | | Drug Products | |
Attribute	Criteria	Attribute	Criteria
Chemical structure	Well characterized	Dosage form	Oral (immediate release), simple solutions, others
Synthetic process	Simple process		
Quality	No toxic impurities; adequate specifications	Manufacturing process Quality	Easy to manufacture (TBD) Adequate specifications
Physical properties	Polymorphic forms, particle size are well controlled	Biopharmaceutic Classification Systems (BCS)	Highly permeable and highly soluble drugs
Stability	Stable drug substance	Stability	Stable drug product (TBD)
Manufacturing history	TBD		
Others	TBD	Manufacturing history	TBD
		Others	TBD

TBD, to be defined.

Adapted from Chui, 2000.

that have a very small ratio of active drug substance to excipients are more difficult to blend uniformly and thus may have a greater quality risk. Good Manufacturing Practices and control of the critical manufacturing operations help maintain the quality of the finished product. Complex operations can have consistent outcome quality as long as the manufacturer maintains control of the process and builds in quality during manufacturing operations.

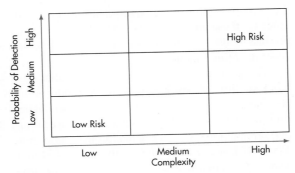

FIGURE 18-4   General principles to define low-risk drugs. (Adapted from Chui, 2002.)

POSTMARKETING SURVEILLANCE

Pharmaceutical manufacturers are required to file periodic postmarket reports for an approved ANDA to the FDA through its *Postmarketing Surveillance Program*. The main component of the requirement is the reporting of adverse drug experiences. This is accomplished by reassessing drug risks based on data learned after the drug is marketed. In addition, labeling changes may occur after market approval. For example, a new adverse reaction discussed by postmarketing surveillance is required for both branded and generic drug products.

GLOSSARY

BioRAM: The biopharmaceutics risk assessment roadmap (BioRAM) optimizes drug product development and performance by using therapy-driven target drug delivery profiles as a framework to achieve the desired therapeutic outcome.

Continuous process verification: An alternative approach to process validation in which manufacturing process performance is continuously monitored and evaluated.

Critical quality attribute (CQA): A physical, chemical, biological, or microbiological property or characteristic that should be within an appropriate limit, range, or distribution to ensure the desired product quality.

Design space: The multidimensional combination and interaction of input variables (eg, material attributes) and process parameters that have been demonstrated to provide quality assurance. Working within the design space is not considered a change. Movement out of the design space is considered to be a change and would normally initiate a regulatory postapproval change process. Design space is proposed by the applicant and is subject to regulatory assessment and approval.

Formal experimental design: A structured, organized method for determining the relationship between factors affecting a process and the output of that process. Also known as "design of experiments."

Life cycle: All phases in the life of a product from the initial development through marketing until the product's discontinuation.

Process analytical technology (PAT): A system for designing, analyzing, and controlling manufacturing through timely measurements (ie, during processing) of critical quality and performance attributes of raw and in-process materials and processes with the goal of ensuring final product quality.

Process robustness: Ability of a process to tolerate variability of materials and changes in the process and equipment without negative impact on quality.

Quality: The suitability of either a drug substance or a drug product for its intended use. This term includes such attributes as the identity, strength, and purity (from ICH Q6A specifications: test procedures and acceptance criteria for new drug substances and new drug products: chemical substances).

Quality by design (QbD): A systematic approach to development that begins with predefined objectives and emphasizes product and process understanding and process control, based on sound science and quality risk management.

Quality target product profile (QTPP): A prospective summary of the quality characteristics of a drug product that ideally will be achieved to ensure the desired quality, taking into account safety and efficacy of the drug product.

Specified impurity: An identified or unidentified impurity that is selected for inclusion in the new drug substance or new drug product specification and is individually listed and limited in order to ensure the quality of the new drug substance or new drug product.

Unidentified impurity: An impurity that is defined solely by qualitative analytical properties (eg, chromatographic retention time).

CHAPTER SUMMARY

The pharmaceutical development process must design a quality drug product (QbD, quality by design) using a manufacturing process that provides consistent drug product performance and achieves the desired therapeutic objective. Drug product quality and drug product performance are important for patient safety and therapeutic efficacy. Drug product quality and drug product performance relate to the biopharmaceutic and physicochemical properties of the drug substance and the drug product and to the manufacturing process. The development of a drug product requires a systematic, scientific, risk-based, holistic, and proactive approach that begins with predefined objectives and emphasizes product and processes understanding and process control (QbD). Quality cannot be tested into drug products. Quality should be built in the design and confirmed by testing. Quality control (QC) and quality assurance (QA) help ensure that drug products are manufactured with quality and have consistent performance throughout their life cycle. Manufacturers must demonstrate that any changes in the formulation after FDA approval (SUPAC) does not alter drug product quality and performance compared to the initial formulation. Excipients that have no inherent pharmacodynamic activity may affect drug product performance. Drug products may be recalled due to deficiencies in drug product quality. Product quality defects are controlled through Good Manufacturing Practices, monitoring, and surveillance. The QTPP approach is an approach commonly recommended for drug development. The need for "learn and confirm" is an important approach evaluating different quality systems balancing risk and need for progress.

LEARNING QUESTIONS

1. Three batches of ibuprofen tablets, 200 mg, are manufactured by the same manufacturer using the same equipment. Each batch meets the same specifications. Does meeting specifications mean that each batch of drug product contains the identical amount of ibuprofen?

2. What should a manufacturer of a modified-release tablet consider when making a qualitative or quantitative change in an excipient?

3. Explain how a change in drug product quality may affect drug product performance. Provide at least three examples.

4. For solid oral drug products, a change in the concentration of which of the following excipients is more likely to influence the bioavailability of a drug? Why?
   Starch
   Magnesium stearate
   Microcrystalline cellulose
   Talc
   Lactose

5. How does the polymorphic form of the active drug substance influence the bioavailability of a drug? Can two different polymorphs of the same active drug substance have the same bioavailability?

ANSWERS

Learning Questions

Three batches of ibuprofen tablets, 200 mg, are manufactured by the same manufacturer using the same equipment. Each batch meets the same specifications. Does meeting specifications mean that each batch of drug product contains the identical amount of ibuprofen?

- Specifications provide a quantitative limit (acceptance criteria) to a test product (eg, the total drug content must be within ±5% or the amount of impurities in the drug substance must not be more than [NMT] 1%). Thus, one batch of nominally 200-mg ibuprofen tablets may contain an average content of 198 mg, whereas the average content for another batch of 200-mg ibuprofen tablets may have an average content of 202 mg. Both batches meet a specification of ±5% and would be considered to meet the label claim of 200 mg of ibuprofen per tablet.

What should a manufacturer of a modified-release tablet consider when making a qualitative or quantitative change in an excipient?

- The manufacturer must consider whether the excipient is critical or not critical to drug release. If the excipient (eg, starch) is not critical to drug release (ie, a non-release-controlling excipient), then small changes in the starch concentration, generally less than 3% of the total target dosage form weight, is unlikely to affect the formulation quality and performance. A qualitative change in the excipient may affect drug release and thus will have significant effect on the formulation performance.

REFERENCES

Amidon GE, Peck GE, Block LH, Moreton RC, Katdare A, Lafaver R, Sheehan C: Proposed new USP general information chapter, Excipient performance <1059>. *Pharm Forum* **33**(6):1311–1323, 2007.

Chui Y: Risk-Based CMC Review, An Update, Advisory Committee for Pharmaceutical Sciences Meeting, FDA, October 21, 2002.

CMC initiative: Risk-Based CMC Reviews, PhRMA-Dialog, Oct 27, 2000. The critical path initiative—Transforming the way FDA-regulated products are developed, evaluated, manufactured, and used. FDA, April 2009 (www.fda.gov/downloads/ScienceResearch/SpecialTopics/CriticalPathInitiative/UCM186110.pdf).

FDA, CDER Report to the Nation: 2005.

FDA, CDER 2007 Update.

FDA Guidance: Immediate Release Solid Oral Dosage Forms: Scale-Up and Postapproval Changes, 1995.

FDA Guidance for Industry: Changes to an Approved NDA or ANDA, April 2004 http://www.fda.gov/drugs/guidancecomplianceregulatoryinformation/guidances/ucm121568.htm.

FDA Guidance for Industry: PAT—A Framework for Innovative Pharmaceutical Development, Manufacturing, and Quality Assurance, September 2004.

FDA Guidance for Industry: Q8(R1) Pharmaceutical Development, June 2009.

FDA Quality Guidances for Industry, http://www.fda.gov/Drugs/GuidanceComplianceRegulatoryInformation/Guidances/ucm065005.htm.

International Conference on Harmonisation (ICH) Guidances: http://www.ich.org.

Lionberger RL: FDA critical path initiatives: Opportunities for generic drug development. *AAPS J* **10**(1):103–109, 2008.

Risk-Based CMC Review; Advisory Committee for Pharmaceutical Sciences, FDA, Oct 21, 2002.

Selen A: Office of New Drug Quality Assessment/CDER/FDA, 32nd Annual Midwest Biopharmaceutical Statistics Workshop, Ball State University, Muncie, Indiana, May 18–20, 2009.

Selen A, et al: The biopharmaceutics risk assessment roadmap for optimizing clinical drug product performance. *J Pharm Sci* **103**(11):3377–3397, 2014. Also published online in Wiley Online Library (wileyonlinelibrary.com). DOI 10.1002/jps.24162, August 22, 2014.

Shargel L: Drug product performance and interchangeability of multisource drug substances and drug products. *Pharm Forum* **35**:744–749, 2010.

US Code of Federal Regulations (CFR), 21 CFR Part 211. http://www.fda.gov/drugs/guidancecomplianceregulatoryinformation/guidances/ucm121568.htm. Accessed August 10, 2011.

Yu LX: Pharmaceutical quality by design: Product and process development, understanding, and control. *Pharm Res* **25**:781–791, 2008.

BIBLIOGRAPHY

http://www.fda.gov/Drugs/GuidanceComplianceRegulatoryInformation/Guidances/ucm065005.htm (source of regulatory documents for quality systems and QbD discussions).

Sood, R: Question-Based Review—A Vision, 9-Jun-2014, http://www.fda.gov/downloads/aboutfda/centersoffices/officeofmedicalproductsandtobacco/cder/ucm410433.pdf. Accessed June 10, 2015.

Yu LX, Amidon G, Khan MA, Hoag SW, Polli J, Raju GK, Woodcock J: Understanding pharmaceutical quality by design. *AAPS J* **6**(4):771–783, 2014.

Yu, LX: Regulatory Assessment of Pharmaceutical Quality for Generic Drugs, http://www.fda.gov/downloads/aboutfda/centersoffices/officeofmedicalproductsandtobacco/cder/ucm119204.pdf. Accessed June 10, 2015.

19

Modified-Release Drug Products and Drug Devices

Hong Ding

Chapter Objectives

► Define modified-release drug products.

► Differentiate between conventional, immediate-release, extended-release, delayed-release, and targeted drug products.

► Explain the advantages and disadvantages of extended-release drug products.

► Describe the kinetics of extended-release drug products compared to immediate-release drug products.

► Explain when an extended-release drug product should contain an immediate-release drug dose.

► Explain why extended-release beads in capsule formulation may have a different bioavailability profile compared to an extended-release tablet formulation of the same drug.

► Describe several approaches for the formulation of an oral extended-release drug product.

► Explain why a transdermal drug product (patch) may be considered an extended-release drug product.

MODIFIED-RELEASE (MR) DRUG PRODUCTS AND CONVENTIONAL (IMMEDIATE-RELEASE, IR) DRUG PRODUCTS

Most conventional (also named as immediate-release, IR) oral drug products, such as tablets and capsules, are formulated to release the active pharmaceutical ingredient (API) immediately after oral administration. In the formulation of conventional drug products, no deliberate effort is made to modify the drug release rate. Usually, immediate-release products generally result in relatively rapid drug absorption and onset of accompanying pharmacodynamic (PD) effects, but not always. In the case of conventional oral products containing prodrugs, the pharmacodynamic activity may be altered due to the time consumption with conversion from prodrugs to the active drug by hepatic or intestinal metabolism or by chemical hydrolysis. Alternatively, in the case of conventional oral products containing poorly soluble (lipophilic drugs), drug absorption may be gradual due to slow dissolution in or selective absorption across the GI tract, also resulting in a delayed onset time.

In order to achieve a desired therapeutic objective or better patient compliance, the pattern of drug release from modified-release (MR) dosage forms is deliberately changed from that of a conventional (immediate-release, IR) dosage formulation. MR drug products have always been more effective therapeutic alternative to conventional or IR dosage forms. The objective of MR drug products for oral administration is to control the release of the therapeutic agent and thus control drug absorption from gastrointestinal tract. Types of MR drug products include, but not limited to, delayed-release (eg, enteric-coated), extended-release (ER), and orally disintegrating tablets (ODT).

The term *modified-release (MR) drug product* is used to describe products that alter the timing and/or rate of release of the drug substance in the formulation. A modified-release dosage form is a formulation in which the drug-release characteristics of time course and/or location are chosen to accomplish therapeutic or

▶ Describe the components of a transdermal drug delivery system.

▶ Explain why an extended-release formulation of a drug may have a different efficacy profile compared to the same dose of drug given in as a conventional, immediate-release, oral dosage form in multiple doses.

▶ List the studies that might be required for the development of an extended-release drug product.

▶ List the several achievements on the drug devices based on the modified-release drug design.

convenience objectives, which is not offered by conventional dosage forms such as solutions, ointments, or promptly dissolving dosage forms. Several types of modified-release oral drug products are recognized:

1. *Extended-release drug products.* A dosage form that allows at least a twofold reduction in dosage frequency as compared to that drug presented as an immediate-release (conventional) dosage form. Examples of extended-release dosage forms include controlled-release, sustained-release, and long-acting drug products.
2. *Delayed-release drug products.* A dosage form that releases a discrete portion/portions of drug at a time other than the promptly release after administration. An initial portion may be released promptly after administration. Enteric-coated dosage forms are common delayed-release products (eg, enteric-coated aspirin and other NSAID products).
3. *Targeted-release drug products.* A dosage form that releases drug at or near the intended physiologic site of action (see Chapter 20). Targeted-release dosage forms may have either immediate- or extended-release characteristics.
4. *Orally disintegrating tablets* (ODTs). ODTs have been developed to disintegrate rapidly in the saliva after oral administration. ODTs may be used without the addition of water. The drug is dispersed in saliva and swallowed with little or no water.

The term *controlled-release drug product* was previously used to describe various types of oral extended-release-rate dosage forms on the action firm applied, including sustained-release, sustained-action, prolonged-action, long-action, slow-release, and programmed drug delivery. Other terms, such as ER (extended-release), SR (sustained-release), XL (another abbreviation for extended-release), XR (extended-release), and CR (controlled-release), are also used to indicate the mechanism of the extended-release drug product employed. Retarded release is an older term for a slow-release drug product. Many of these terms for modified-release drug products were introduced by drug companies to reflect a special design either for an extended-release drug product or for use in marketing.

Modified-release drug products are designed for different routes of administration based on the physicochemical, pharmacodynamic (PD), and pharmacokinetic (PK) properties of the drug and on the properties of the materials used in the dosage form (Table 19-1). Several different terms are now defined to describe the available types of modified-release drug products based on the drug release characteristics of the products.

TABLE 19-1   Modified Drug Delivery Products

Route of Administration	Drug Product	Examples	Comments
Oral drug products	Extended release	Diltiazem HCl extended release	Once-a-day dosing.
	Delayed release	Diclofenac sodium delayed-release	Enteric-coated tablet for drug delivery into small intestine.
	Delayed (targeted) drug release	Mesalamine delayedrelease	Coated for drug release in terminal ileum.
	Oral mucosal drug delivery	Oral transmucosal fentanyl citrate	Fentanyl citrate is in the form of a flavored sugar lozenge that dissolves slowly in the mouth.
	Oral soluble film	Ondansetron	The film is placed top of the tongue. Film will dissolve in 4 to 20 seconds.
	Orally disintegrating tablets (ODT)	Aripiprazole	ODT is placed on the tongue. Tablet disintegration occurs rapidly in saliva.
Transdermal drug delivery systems	Transdermal therapeutic system (TTS)	Clonidine transdermal therapeutic system	Clonidine TTS is applied every 7 days to intact skin on the upper arm or chest.
	Iontophoretic drug delivery		Small electric current moves charged molecules across the skin.
Ophthalmic drug delivery	Insert	Controlled-release pilocarpine	Elliptically shaped insert designed for continuous release of pilocarpine following placement in the cul-de-sac of the eye.
Intravaginal drug delivery	Insert	Dinoprostone vaginal insert	Hydrogel pouch containing prostaglandin within a polyester retrieval system.
Parenteral drug delivery	Intramuscular drug products	Depot injections	Lyophylized microspheres containing leuprolide acetate for depot suspension.
		Water-immiscible injections (eg, oil)	Medroxyprogesterone acetate (Depo-Provera).
	Subcutaneous drug products	Controlled-release insulin	Basulin is a controlled-release, recombinant human insulin delivered by nanoparticulate technology.
Targeted delivery systems	IV injection	Daunorubicin citrate liposome injection	Liposomal preparation to maximize the selectivity of daunorubicin for solid tumors *in situ*.
Implants	Brain tumor	Polifeprosan 20 with carmustine implant (Gliadel wafer)	Implant designed to deliver carmustine directly into the surgical cavity when a brain tumor is resected.
	Intravitreal implant	Fluocinolone acetonide intravitreal implant	Sterile implant designed to release fluocinolone acetonide locally to the posterior segment of the eye.

Examples of Modified-Release Oral Dosage Forms

The pharmaceutical industry uses various terms to describe modified-release drug products. New and novel drug delivery systems are being developed by the pharmaceutical industry to alter the drug release profile, which in turn results in a unique plasma drug concentration-versus-time profile and pharmacodynamic effect. In many cases, the industry will patent their novel drug delivery systems. Due to the proliferation of these modified-release dosage forms, the following terms are general descriptions and should not be considered definitive.

An *enteric-coated* tablet is one kind of delayed-release type within the modified-release dosage family designed to release drug in the small intestine. Different from the film coating on tablets or capsules to prevent bitter taste from medicine or protect tablets from microbial growth as well as color alteration, usually the enteric-coating materials are polymer-based barrier applied on oral medicine. This coating may delay release of the medicine until after it leaves the stomach, either for the purpose of drug protection under harsh pH circumstance or for alleviation of irritation on cell membrane from the drug itself. For example, aspirin irritates the gastric mucosal cells of the stomach. Then the enteric coating on the aspirin tablet may prevent the tablet from disintegration promptly and releasing its contents at the low pH in the stomach. The coating and the tablet later dissolve and release the drug in the relative mild pH of the duodenum, where the drug is rapidly absorbed with less irritation to the mucosal cells. Mesalamine (5-aminosalicylic acid) tablets (Asacol, Proctor & Gamble) are also a delayed-release tablet coated with acrylic-based resin that delays the release of mesalamine until it reaches the terminal ileum and colon. Mesalamine tablets could also be considered as a *targeted-release* dosage form.

The advantage for certain drugs is that the dosage form contains a sufficient amount of medication to last all day or all night. A *repeat-action tablet* is a type of modified-release drug product that is designed to release one dose of drug initially, followed by a second or more doses of drug at a later time. It provides the required dosage initially and then maintains or repeats it at desired intervals.

For the *repeat-action tablets*, such as prolonged, sustained, delayed, and timed-release dosage forms, may generally be considered as having the property of prolonged-action. This dosage form purports to describe just when and how much of a drug is released, and simplified curves of blood levels or clinical response claim to depict how the preparation will act *in vivo*. Since these products usually contain the equivalent of 2–3 times the normal dose of the drug, it is of considerable importance to the physician to know that the drug will actually be released in the designed manner.

A *prolonged-action drug product* is a formulation whose drug activity can continue for a longer time than conventional drugs. It is also one kind of modified-release drug product. The prolonged-release drug product prevents very rapid absorption of the drug, which could result in extremely high peak plasma drug concentration. Most prolonged-release products extend the duration of action but do not release drug at a constant rate. A prolonged-action tablet is similar to a first-order-release product except that the peak is delayed differently. A prolonged-action tablet typically results in peak and trough drug levels in the body. The product releases drug without matching the rate of drug elimination, resulting in uneven plasma drug levels in the body.

A *sustained-release drug product* is designed to release a drug at a predetermined rate for the constant drug concentration maintaining during a specific period of time. Usually, the drug may be delivered in an initial therapeutic dose, followed by a slower and constant release. The purpose of a loading dose is to provide immediate or fast drug release to quickly provide therapeutic drug concentrations in the plasma. The rate of release of the maintenance dose is designed so that the amount of drug loss from the body by elimination is constantly replaced. With the sustained-release product, a constant plasma drug concentration is maintained with minimal fluctuations.

Sustained-release and extended-release drug products look similar since both of them have the same release drugs in which those drugs dissolve and release in the body over a period of time. The difference is that for the sustained-release drug product, the drug may release its medication properties over a controlled mode within a certain period where the drug is released bit by bit in the body. The extended-release drug product is more toward an instant effect medication where once administrated, the effects took place immediately and its extended effect would be often happened at an hourly basis. When the drug concentration goes down, the extended-release drug product may have the capability to maintain the effectiveness by the formulation itself. Besides the tablets or capsules, other formulations including liposomes and drug-loaded polymeric nano-formulations (eg, micelles, drug–polymer conjugates and hydrogels, etc) can also be counted as the sustained-release drug product. Figure 19-1 shows the dissolution rate of three sustained-release products without loading dose. The plasma concentrations resulting from the sustained-release products are shown in Fig. 19-2.

Various terms for extended-release drug products often imply that drug release is at a constant or zero-order drug release rate. However, many of these drug products release the drug at a first-order rate. Some modified-release drug products are formulated with materials that are more soluble at a specific pH, and the product may release the drug depending on the pH of a particular region of the gastrointestinal (GI) tract. Ideally, an extended-release drug product should release the drug at a constant rate, independent of the pH, the ionic content, and other contents within the entire segment of the gastrointestinal tract.

An extended-release dosage form with zero- or first-order drug absorption is compared to drug absorption from a conventional dosage form given in

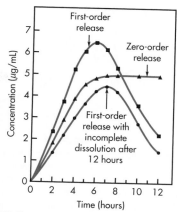

FIGURE 19-2   Simulated plasma drug concentrations resulting from three different sustained-release products in Fig. 19-1.

multiple doses in Figs. 19-3 and 19-4, respectively. Drug absorption from conventional (immediate-release) dosage forms generally follows first-order drug absorption.

Frequently Asked Questions

▶ *What is the difference between extended release, delayed release, sustained release, modified release, and controlled release?*

▶ *Why does the drug bioavailability from some conventional, immediate-release, drug products resemble an extended-release drug product?*

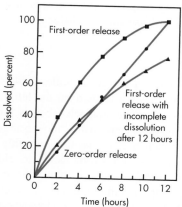

FIGURE 19-1   Drug dissolution rates of three different extended-release products *in vitro*.

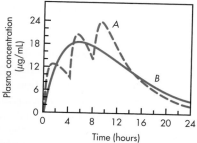

FIGURE 19-3   Plasma level of a drug from a conventional tablet containing 50 mg of drug given at 0, 4, and 8 hours (*A*) compared to a single 150-mg drug dose given in an extended-release dosage form (*B*). The drug absorption rate constant from each drug product is first order. The drug is 100% bioavailable and the elimination half-life is constant.

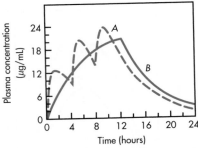

FIGURE 19-4 Bioavailability of a drug from an immediate-release tablet containing 50 mg of drug given at 0, 4, and 8 hours compared to a single 150-mg drug dose given in an extended-release dosage form. The drug absorption rate constant from the immediate-release drug product is first order, whereas the drug absorption rate constant from the extended-release drug product is zero order. The drug is 100% bioavailable and the elimination half-life is constant.

BIOPHARMACEUTIC FACTORS

Some drugs are well-established medicine in the treatment of specific diseases because of its effectiveness and well tolerance; however, the relatively short plasma half-life requires frequent dosing associated with a poor compliance. The poor pharmacokinetic (PK) of this drug in IR formulation refrains its broader application. Modified-release drug products should produce a pharmacokinetic profile that provides the desired therapeutic efficacy and minimizes adverse events. In the case of delayed-release drug products, the enteric coating minimizes gastric irritation of the drug in the stomach. The major objective of extended-release drug products is to achieve a prolonged therapeutic effect while minimizing unwanted side effects due to fluctuating plasma drug concentrations.

An ideal extended-release (ER) drug product should demonstrate complete bioavailability, minimal fluctuations in drug concentration at steady state, reproducibility of release characteristics independent of food, and minimal diurnal variation. Hence, ER drug product should release the drug at a constant or zero-order rate. As the drug is released from the drug product, the drug is rapidly absorbed, and the drug absorption rate should follow zero-order kinetics similar to an intravenous drug infusion. The drug product is designed so that the rate of systemic drug absorption is limited by the rate of drug release from the drug delivery system. Unfortunately, most ER drug products that release a drug by zero-order kinetics *in vitro* do not demonstrate zero-order drug absorption, *in vivo*. The lack of zero-order drug absorption from these ER drug products after oral administration may be due to a number of unpredictable events happening in the gastrointestinal tract during drug absorption.

The ER oral drug products remain in the gastrointestinal (GI) tract longer than conventional, immediate-release, drug products. Thus, drug release from an ER drug product is more subject to be affected by the anatomy and physiology of the GI tract, GI transit, pH, and its contents such as food compared to an immediate-release oral drug product. The physiologic characteristics of the GI tract, including variations in pH, blood flow, GI motility, presence of food, enzymes and bacteria, etc, affect the local action of the extended-release drug product within the GI tract and may affect the drug release rate from the product. In some cases, there may be a specific absorption site or location within the GI tract in which the extended-release drug product should release the drug. This specific drug absorption site or location within the GI tract is referred to as an *absorption window*. The absorption window is the optimum site for drug absorption. If drug is not released and available for absorption within the absorption window, the extended-release tablet moves further distally in the GI tract and incomplete drug absorption may occur and may give rise to unsatisfactory drug absorption *in vivo* despite excellent *in vitro* release characteristics.

Stomach

The stomach is a muscular, hollow, dilated part of the digestive system located on the left side of the upper abdomen. The stomach receives food or liquids from the esophagus. In this "mixing and secreting" organ, stomach secretes protein-digesting enzymes called proteases and strong acids to aid in food digestion, through smooth muscular contortions before sending partially digested food (chyme) periodically to the small intestines. However, the movement of food or drug product in the stomach and small intestine is very different depending on the physiologic state. In the presence of food, the stomach is in the *digestive phase*; in the absence of food, the stomach is in the *interdigestive phase* (Chapter 14). During the digestive phase, food particles or solids larger than 2 mm are retained in the stomach, whereas smaller particles are emptied through the pyloric sphincter at a first-order rate depending on the content and size of the meals. During the interdigestive phase, the stomach rests for a period of up to 30–40 minutes, coordinated with an equal resting period in the small intestine. Peristaltic contractions then occur, which end with strong *housekeeper contractions* that move everything in the stomach through to the small intestine. Similarly, large particles in the small intestine are moved along only in the housekeeper contraction period.

A drug may remain for several hours in the stomach if it is administered during the digestive phase. Fatty material, nutrients, and osmolality may further extend the time of the drug staying in the stomach. When the drug is administered during the interdigestive phase, the drug may be swept along rapidly into the small intestine. The drug release rates from some extended-release drug products are affected by mechanism of drug release (Sujjaareevath et al, 1998), viscosity (Rahman et al, 2011), pH and ironic strength (Asare-Addo et al, 2011), and food (Abrahamsson et al, 2004). Dissolution of drugs in the stomach may also be affected by the presence or absence of food. When food and nutrients are present, the stomach pH may change from 1 to 2 by stomach acid (usually HCl) secretion about 3–5 because of the food and nutrients neutralization.

In one example, drug release from various theophylline ER formulations could be influenced (either increased or decreased) by concomitant intake of food compared to fasting conditions (Jonkman, 1989). Food intake can influence the rate of drug release from the dosage form, the rate of drug absorption, the amount of drug absorbed, or all of these parameters simultaneously. The rate of drug release of various ER formulations can be affected by the composition of the coadministered meal. This effect may result in both "positive" and "negative." Positive food effects usually come with drug release

speeding up from ER formulation, which may cause high risk for patients at extreme cases by tablets coating erosion (Jonkman, 1987). The solubilization effect by bile micelles in the presence of food may have a positive effect on drug absorption (Kawai et al, 2011). Negative food effects may take effect at an opposite direction by increasing the viscosity in the upper GI tract, delay the absorption rate, and prolong the passage time of ER drug product in GI tract (Marasanapalle et al, 2009). A longer time of retention in the stomach may expose the drug to stronger agitation in the acid environment. The stomach has been described as having "jet mixing" action, which sends mixture at up to -50 mm Hg pressure toward the pyloric sphincter, causing it to open and periodically release chyme to the small intestine.

Small Intestine and Transit Time

The small intestine is about 10–14 ft in length. The duodenum is sterile, while the terminal part of the small intestine that connects the cecum contains some bacteria. The proximal part of the small intestine has a pH of about 6, because of neutralization of acid by bicarbonates secreted into the lumen by the duodenal mucosa and the pancreas. The small intestine provides an enormous surface area for drug absorption because of the presence of microvilli. The small-intestine transit time of a solid preparation has been concluded to be about 3 hours or less in 95% of the population (Hofmann et al, 1983). As Table 19-2 summarizes, the small intestinal transit time is more reproducible around 3–4 hours. The transit time from mouth to cecum ranges from 3 to 7 hours. Colonic transit time has the highest variation, which is typically from 10 to 20 hours (Shareef et al, 2003; Ritschel, 1991; Yu et al, 1996). Various investigators have used the lactulose hydrogen test, which measures the appearance of hydrogen in a patient's breath, to estimate transit time. Lactulose is metabolized rapidly by bacteria in the large intestine, yielding hydrogen that is exhaled. Hydrogen is normally absent in a person's breath. These results and the use of gamma-scintigraphy studies confirm a relatively short GI transit time from mouth to cecum of 4–6 hours (Shareef et al, 2003). This technique has

TABLE 19-2   pH Values against Transit Time at Different Segments of GI Tract

Anatomical location	Fasting condition		Food condition	
	pH	Transition time (h)	pH	Transition time (h)
Stomach	1-3	0.5-0.7	4.3-5.4	1
Duodenum	~6	<0.5	5.4	<0.5
Jejunum	6-7	1.7	5.4-5.6	1.7
Heum	6.6-7.4	1.3	6.6-7.4	1.3
Cecum	6.4	4.5	6.4	4.5
Colon	6.8	13.5	6.8	13.5

been applied in the exploring of extended oro-cecal transit time in the intestine (Eisenmann et al, 2008).

This transit time interval was concluded to be too short for extended-release dosage forms that last up to 12 hours, unless the drug is to be absorbed in the colon. The colon has little fluid and the abundance of bacteria may make drug absorption erratic and incomplete.

In a Phase I study, 12 healthy males were given a controlled-release, new gastro-resistant, extended-release tablets with multimatrix structure (ie, MMX®-tablets containing 9 mg budesonide). The noninvasive technique of gamma-scintigraphy was employed to monitor the gastrointestinal transit of orally ingested dosage forms for the purpose of identification of the exact time and region of disintegration and to follow the release of the active ingredient from the extended-release formulation. The effect of food was tested by comparing plasma pharmacokinetics after intake of a high-fat and high-calorie breakfast with fasting controls. The results showed that [153]Sm-labeled MMX-budesonide extended-release tablets reached the colonic region after a mean of 9.8 hours. Initial tablet disintegration was observed in the ileum in 42% of subjects, whereas in 33% the main site of disintegration was either the ascending or the transverse colon. The budesonide plasma concentrations were first detected after 6.8 ± 3.2 h (Brunner et al, 2006).

Large Intestine

The large intestine is about 4–5 ft long. It consists of the cecum, the ascending and descending colons, and eventually ends at the rectum. Little fluid is in the colon, and drug transit is slow. Not much is known about drug absorption in this area, although unabsorbed drug that reaches this region may be metabolized by bacteria. Incompletely absorbed antibiotics may affect the normal flora of the bacteria. The rectum has a pH of about 6.8–7.0 and contains more fluid compared to the colon. Drugs are absorbed rapidly when administered as rectal preparations. However, the transit rate through the rectum is affected by the rate of defecation. Presumably, drugs formulated for 24-hour duration must remain in this region to be absorbed.

Several extended-release and delayed-release drug products, such as mesalamine delayed-release tablets (Asacol), are formulated to take advantage of the physiologic conditions of the GI tract (Shareef et al, 2003). Enteric-coated beads have been found to release drug over 8 hours when taken with food, because of the gradual emptying of the beads into the small intestine. Specially formulated "floating tablets" that remain in the top of the stomach have been used to extend the residence time of the product in the stomach. None of these methods, however, is consistent enough to perform reliably for potent medications. More experimental research is needed in this area. In 2012, Dr. Zhu et al (2012) designed a large intestine–targeted oral delivery with pH-dependent nanoparticles containing vaccine nanoparticles to control genitorectal viral infection. This new type of extended-release drug system can induce colorectal immunity in mice comparably to colorectal vaccination and protected against rectal and vaginal viral challenge. Their conclusion showed that using this oral vaccine delivery system to target the large intestine, but not the small intestine, may represent a feasible new strategy for immune protection of rectal and vaginal mucosa (Qiu et al, 2014).

DOSAGE FORM SELECTION

The properties of the drug and the size of the required dosage are important in formulating an extended-release product. These properties will also influence the selection of appropriate dissolution media, apparatus, and test parameters to obtain *in vitro* drug release data that will reflect *in vivo* drug absorption. For example, a drug with low aqueous solubility generally should not be formulated into a nondisintegrating tablet, because the risk of incomplete drug dissolution is high. Instead, a drug with low solubility at neutral pH should be formulated as an erodible tablet, so that most of the drug is released before it reaches the colon. The lack of fluid in the colon may make complete drug dissolution difficult. Erodible tablets are more reliable for these drugs because the entire tablet eventually dissolves.

A drug that is highly water soluble in the acid pH in the stomach but very insoluble at intestinal pH may be very difficult to formulate into an ER drug product. An ER drug product with too much coating protection may result in low drug bioavailability, while too little coating protection may result in rapid drug release or dose-dumping in the stomach. A moderate extension of duration with enteric-coated beads may be possible. However, the risk of erratic performance is higher than with a conventional dosage form. The osmotic type of controlled drug release system may be more suitable for this type of drug.

With most single-unit dosage forms, there is a risk of erratic performance due to variable stomach emptying and GI transit time. The size and shape of the single-unit dosage form will also influence GI transit time. Selection of a pellet or bead dosage form may minimize the risk of erratic stomach emptying, because pellets are usually scattered soon after ingestion. Disintegrating tablets have the same advantages because they break up into small particles soon after ingestion. The ultimate goal of the dissolution test is used to predict the *in vivo* performance of products from *in vitro* test by a proper *in vitro–in vivo*

correlation (IVIVC) (see also Chapter 15). These tests may not be pharmacopeial standard; however, they should be sensitive, reliable, and discriminatory with regard to the *in vitro* drug release characteristics. This technique is applied not only to immediate-release drug products but also to extended-release drug products with promising future (Cheng et al, 2014; Honório et al, 2013; Meulenaar et al, 2014).

ADVANTAGES AND DISADVANTAGES OF EXTENDED-RELEASE PRODUCTS

To maintain a long therapeutic effect, frequent administration of conventional formulations of many drugs with short half-life is necessary. Otherwise, concentration under therapeutic window occurs frequently in the course treatment, which may induce drug resistance. Extended-release dosage forms may solve these issues by having a number of advantages in safety and efficacy over immediate-release drug products in that the frequency of dosing can be reduced, drug efficacy can be prolonged, and the incidence and/or intensity of adverse effects can be decreased.

Advantages

1. Sustained therapeutic blood levels of the drug

   Extended-release drug products offer several important advantages over conventional dosage forms of the same drug by optimizing biopharmaceutic, pharmacokinetic, and pharmacodynamic properties of drugs. Extended release allows for sustained therapeutic blood levels of the drug; sustained blood levels provide for a prolonged and consistent clinical response in the patient. Moreover, if the drug input rate is constant, the blood levels should not fluctuate between a maximum and a minimum compared to a multiple-dose regimen with an immediate-release drug product (Chapter 8). Highly fluctuating blood concentrations of drug may produce unwanted side effects in the patient if the drug level is too high, or may fail to exert the proper therapeutic effect if the drug level is too low. In such a way, extended-release drug products may maintain a constant plasma drug concentration within therapeutic window for a prolonged period; extended-release dosage forms maximize the therapeutic effect of drugs while minimizing possible resistance.

2. Improved patient compliance

Another undoubted advantage of extended-release formulation is improved patient compliance. It may provide the convenience of supplying additional doses without the need of re-administration. It may reduce dosing frequency to an extent that once-daily dose is sufficient for therapeutic management through uniform plasma concentration providing maximum utility of drug with reduction in local and systemic side effects and cure or control condition in shortest possible time by smallest quantity of drug to assure greater patient compliance. For example, if the patient needs to take the medication only once daily, he or she will not have to remember to take additional doses at specified times during the day. Furthermore, because the dosage interval is longer, the patient's sleep may not be interrupted to take another drug dose. With longer therapeutic drug concentrations, the patient awakes without having subtherapeutic drug levels.

3. Reduction in adverse side effects and improvement in tolerability

Drug plasma levels are maintained within a narrow window with no sharp peaks and with the AUC of plasma concentration-versus-time curve equivalent to the AUC from multiple dosing with immediate-release dosage form. Because of the well-controlled drug concentration in therapeutic and safe window, the possible side effects can be significantly decreased due to the absence of drug plasma levels higher than toxic level. Meanwhile, the tolerability of drug can be improved due to no drug level lower than the minimum effective level.

4. Reduction in healthcare cost

The patient may also derive an economic benefit in using an extended-release drug product. A single dose of an extended-release product may cost less than an equivalent drug dose given several times a day in rapid-release tablets. For patients under nursing care, the cost of nursing time required to administer medication is decreased if only one drug dose is given to the patient each day.

For some drugs with long elimination half-lives, such as chlorpheniramine, the inherent duration of pharmacologic activity is long. Minimal fluctuations in blood concentrations of these drugs are observed after multiple doses are administered. Therefore, there is no rationale for extended-release formulations of these drugs. However, such drug products are marketed with the justification that extended-release products minimize toxicity, decrease adverse reactions, and provide patients with more convenience and, thus, better compliance. In contrast, drugs with very short half-lives need to be given at frequent dosing intervals to maintain therapeutic efficacy. For drugs with very short elimination half-lives, an extended-release drug product maintains the efficacy over a longer duration.

Disadvantages

Beyond the advantages, there are also some disadvantages of using extended-release medication, such as the following:

1. Dose-dumping

Dose-dumping is defined either as the release of more than the intended fraction of drug or as the release of drug at a greater rate than the customary amount of drug per dosage interval, such that potentially adverse plasma levels may be reached. Dose-dumping is a phenomenon whereby relatively large quantity of drug in a controlled-release formulation is rapidly released, introducing potentially toxic quantity of the drug into systemic circulation (Dighe and Adams, 1988). Dose-dumping can lead to a severe condition for patients, especially for a drug with narrow therapeutic index. Usually, the dose-dumping comes from the fault of formulation design.

2. Less flexibility in accurate dose adjustment

If the patient suffers from an adverse drug reaction or accidentally becomes intoxicated, the removal of drug from the system is more difficult with an extended-release drug product. In conventional dosage forms, dose adjustments are much simpler, for example, tablets can be divided into two fractions.

3. Less possibility for high dosage

Orally administered extended-release drug products may yield erratic or variable drug absorption as a result of various drug interactions with the contents of the GI tract and changes in GI motility. The formulation of extended-release drug products may not be practical for drugs that are usually given in large single doses (eg, 500 mg) in conventional dosage forms. Because the extended-release drug product may contain two or more times the dose given at more frequent intervals, the size of the extended-release drug product may have to be quite large, too large for the patient to swallow easily.

Besides the above-mentioned disadvantages, other issues including increased potential for first-pass clearance and poor IVIVC correlation are also the challenges. For example, with delayed release or enteric drug products, two possible problems may occur if the enteric coating is poorly formulated. First, the enteric coating may become degraded in the stomach, allowing for early release of the drug, possibly causing irritation to the gastric mucosal lining. Second, the enteric coating may fail to dissolve at the proper site, and therefore, the tablet may be lost from the body prior to drug release, resulting in incomplete absorption (Nagaraju et al, 2010; Wilson et al, 2013).

KINETICS OF EXTENDED-RELEASE DOSAGE FORMS

The amount of drug required in an extended-release dosage form to provide a sustained drug level in the body is determined by the pharmacokinetics of the drug, the desired therapeutic level of the drug, and the intended duration of action. In general, the total dose required (D_{tot}) is the sum of the maintenance dose (D_m) and the initial dose (D_I) released immediately to provide a therapeutic blood level.

$$D_{tot} = D_I + D_m \qquad (19.1)$$

In practice, D_m (mg) is released over a period of time and is equal to the product of t_d (the duration of drug release) and the zero-order rate k_r^0 (mg/h). Therefore, Equation 19.1 can be expressed as

$$D_{tot} = D_I + k_r^0 t_d \qquad (19.2)$$

Ideally, the maintenance dose (D_m) is released after D_I has produced a blood level equal to the therapeutic drug level (C_p). However, due to the limits of formulations, D_m actually starts to release at $t = 0$. Therefore, D_I may be reduced from the calculated amount to avoid "topping."

$$D_{tot} = D_I - k_r^0 t_p + k_r^0 t_d \qquad (19.3)$$

Equation 19.3 describes the total dose of drug needed, with t_p representing the time needed to reach peak drug concentration after the initial dose.

For a drug that follows a one-compartment open model, the rate of elimination (R) needed to maintain the drug at a therapeutic level (C_p) is

$$R = kV_D C_p \qquad (19.4)$$

where k_r^0 must be equal to R in order to provide a stable blood level of the drug. Equation 19.4 provides an estimation of the release rate (k_r^0) required in the formulation. Equation 19.4 may also be written as

$$R = C_p Cl_T \qquad (19.5)$$

where Cl_T is the clearance of the drug. In designing an extended-release product, D_I would be the loading dose that would raise the drug concentration in the body to C_p, and the total dose needed to maintain therapeutic concentration in the body would be simply

$$D_{tot} = D_I + C_p Cl_T \tau \qquad (19.6)$$

For many sustained-release drug products, there is no built-in loading dose (ie, $D_I = 0$). The dose needed to maintain a therapeutic concentration for τ hours is

$$D_0 = C_p \tau Cl_T \qquad (19.7)$$

where τ is the dosing interval.

TABLE 19-3   Release Rates for Extended-Release Drug Products as a Function of Elimination Half-Life[a]

$t_{1/2}$ (h)	k (h⁻¹)	R (mg/h)	Total (mg) to Achieve Duration			
			6 h	8 h	12 h	24 h
1	0.693	69.3	415.8	554.4	831.6	1663
2	0.347	34.7	208.2	277.6	416.4	832.8
4	0.173	17.3	103.8	138.4	207.6	415.2
6	0.116	11.6	69.6	92.8	139.2	278.4
8	0.0866	8.66	52.0	69.3	103.9	207.8
10	0.0693	6.93	41.6	55.4	83.2	166.3
12	0.0577	5.77	34.6	46.2	69.2	138.5

[a]Assume $C_{desired}$ is 5 μg/mL and the V_D is 20,000 mL; $R = kV_DC_p$: no immediate-release dose.

EXAMPLE ▶▶▶

What dose is needed to maintain a therapeutic concentration of 10 μg/mL for 12 hours in a sustained-release product? (a) Assume that $t_{1/2}$ for the drug is 3.46 hours and V_D is 10 L. (b) Assume that $t_{1/2}$ of the drug is 1.73 hours and V_D is 5 L.

a.
$$k = \frac{0.693}{3.46} = 0.2/h$$

$$Cl_T = kV_D = 0.2 \times 10 = 2\,L/h$$

From Equation 19.7,
$$D_0 = (10\ \mu g/mL)(1000\ mL/L)(12\ h)(2\ L/h)$$
$$= 240{,}000\ \mu g\ or\ 240\ mg$$

b.
$$k = \frac{0.693}{1.73} = 0.4h$$

$$Cl_T = 0.4 \times 5 = 2\ L/h$$

From Equation 19.7,
$$D_0 = 10 \times 2 \times 1000 \times 12 = 240{,}000\ \mu g\ or\ 240\ mg$$

In this example, the amount of drug needed in a sustained-release product to maintain therapeutic drug concentration is dependent on both V_D and the elimination half-life. In part **b** of the example, although the elimination half-life is shorter, the volume of distribution is also smaller. If the volume of distribution is constant, then the amount of drug needed to maintain C_p is dependent simply on the elimination half-life.

Table 19-3 shows the influence of $t_{1/2}$ on the amount of drug needed for an extended-release drug product. Table 19-3 was constructed by assuming that the drug has a desired serum concentration of 5 μg/mL and an apparent volume of distribution of 20,000 mL. The release rate needed to achieve the desired concentration, R, decreases as the elimination half-life increases. Because elimination is slower for a drug with a long half-life, the input rate should be slower. The total amount of drug needed in the extended-release drug product is dependent on both the release rate R and the desired duration of activity for the drug. For a drug with an elimination half-life of 4 hours and a release rate of 17.3 mg/h, the extended-release product must contain 207.6 mg to provide a duration of activity of 12 hours. The bulk weight of the extended-release product will be greater than this amount, due to the presence of excipients needed in the formulation. The values in Table 19-3 show that, in order to achieve a long duration of activity ($\geq$12 hours) for a drug with a very short half-life (1–2 hours), the extended-release drug product becomes quite large and impractical for most patients to swallow.

PHARMACOKINETIC SIMULATION OF EXTENDED-RELEASE PRODUCTS

The plasma drug concentration profiles of many extended-release products fit an oral one-compartment model assuming first-order absorption and elimination.

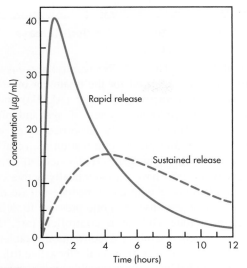

FIGURE 19-5 Plasma drug concentration of a sustained-release and a regular-release product. Note the difference of peak time and peak concentration of the two products.

Compared to an immediate-release product, the extended-release product typically shows a smaller absorption rate constant, because of the slower absorption of the extended-release product. The time for peak concentration (t_{max}) is usually longer (Fig. 19-5), and the peak drug concentration (C_{max}) is reduced. If the drug is properly formulated, the area under the plasma drug concentration curve should be the same. Parameters such as C_{max}, t_{max}, and area under the curve (AUC) conveniently show how successfully the extended-release product performs *in vivo*. For example, a product with a t_{max} of 3 hours would not be very satisfactory if the product is intended to last 12 hours. Similarly, an excessively high C_{max} is a sign of dose-dumping due to inadequate formulation. The pharmacokinetic analysis of single- and multiple-dose plasma data has been used by regulatory agencies to evaluate many sustained-release products. The analysis is practical because many products can be fitted to this model even though the drug is not released in a first-order manner. The limitation of this type of analysis is that the absorption rate constant may not relate to the rate of drug dissolution *in vivo*. If the drug strictly follows zero-order release and absorption, the model may not fit the data.

Various other models have been used to simulate plasma drug levels of extended-release products (Welling, 1983). The plasma drug levels from a zero-order, extended-release drug product may be simulated with Equation 19.8.

$$C_p = \frac{R}{kV_D}(1 - e^{-kt}) \qquad (19.8)$$

where R = rate of drug release (mg/min), C_p = plasma drug concentration, k = overall elimination constant, and V_D = volume of distribution. In the absence of a loading dose, the drug level in the body rises slowly to a plateau with minimum fluctuations (Fig. 19-6). This simulation assumes that (1) rapid drug release occurs without delay, (2) perfect zero-order release and absorption of the drug takes place, and (3) the drug is given exactly every 12 hours. In practice, the above assumptions are not precise, and fluctuations in drug level do occur.

When a sustained-release drug product with a loading dose (rapid release) and a zero-order maintenance dose is given, the resulting plasma drug concentrations are described by

$$C_p = \frac{D_i k_a}{V_D(k_a - k)}(e^{-kt} - e^{-k_a t}) + \frac{D_s}{kV_D}(1 - e^{-kt}) \quad (19.9)$$

where D_i = immediate-release (loading dose) dose and D_s = maintenance dose (zero-order). This expression is the sum of the oral absorption equation

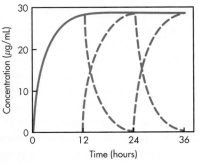

FIGURE 19-6 Simulated plasma drug level of an extended-release product administered every 12 hours. The plasma level shows a smooth rise to steady-state level with no fluctuations.

(first part) and the intravenous infusion equation (second part).

Extended-Release Drug Product with Immediate-Release Component

Extended-release drug products may be formulated with or without an immediate-release loading dose. Extended-release drug products that are given to patients in daily multiple doses to maintain steady-state therapeutic drug concentrations do not need a built-in loading dose when given subsequent doses. Pharmacokinetic models have been proposed for extended-release drug products that have a rapid first-order drug release component and a slow zero-order release maintenance dose component. This model assumes a long elimination $t_{1/2}$ in which drug accumulation occurs until steady state is attained. The model predicts spiking peaks due to the loading dose component when the extended-release drug product is given continuously in multiple doses. In this model, a rapid-release loading dose along with the extended-release drug dose given in a daily multiple-dose regimen introduces more drug into the body than is necessary. This is observed by a *"topping"* effect. As shown in the example, amoxicillin extended-release tablets (Moxatag®) is designed to consist of three components, one immediate-release and two delayed-release parts, each containing amoxicillin. The three components are combined in a specific ratio to prolong the release of amoxicillin from Moxatag compared to immediate-release amoxicillin.

When a loading dose is necessary, a rapid- or immediate-release drug product may be given separately as a loading dose to initially bring the patient's plasma drug level to the desired therapeutic level. In certain clinical situations, an extended-release drug product with an immediate-release component along with a controlled-release core can provide a specific pharmacokinetic profile that provides rapid onset and prolonged plasma drug concentrations that relates to the time course for the desired pharmacodynamic activity. For these extended-release drug products with initial immediate-release components, the active drug must have a relatively short elimination $t_{1/2}$ so that the drug does not accumulate between dosing.

CLINICAL EXAMPLES

Methylphenidate HCl Extended-Release Tablets (Concerta®)

Methylphenidate HCl is a CNS (central nervous system) stimulant indicated for the treatment of attention deficit hyperactivity disorder (ADHD) and is often used in children 6 years of age and older. Methylphenidate is readily absorbed after oral administration and has an elimination $t_{1/2}$ of about 3.5 hours. Methylphenidate HCl extended-release tablets (Concerta) have an osmotically active controlled-release core with an immediate-release drug overcoat. Concerta uses osmotic pressure to deliver methylphenidate HCl at a controlled rate. The system, which resembles a conventional tablet in appearance, comprises an osmotically active trilayer core surrounded by a semipermeable membrane with an immediate-release drug overcoat. The trilayer core is composed of two drug layers containing the drug and excipients, and a push layer containing osmotically active components. Each extended-release tablet for once-a-day oral administration contains 18, 27, 36, or 54 mg of methylphenidate HCl USP and is designed to have 12-hour duration of effect. After oral administration of Concerta, the plasma methylphenidate concentration increases rapidly reaching an initial maximum at about 1 hour, followed by gradual ascending concentrations over the next 5–9 hours after which a gradual decrease begins. Mean t_{max} occurs between 6 and 10 hours. When the patient takes this product in the morning, the patient receives an initial loading dose followed by a maintenance dose that is eliminated by the evening when the patient wants to go to sleep. Due to the short elimination $t_{1/2}$, the drug does not accumulate.

Oxymorphone Extended-Release Tablets (Opana® ER)

Oxymorphone extended-release tablets (Opana ER) are approved for the management of chronic pain. The pharmacokinetic profile of oxymorphone ER is predictable, linear, and dose-proportional. Opana ER may maintain steady plasma levels over 12-hour period with $t_{1/2}$ of about 9–11 hours. It has a low fluctuation index of less than 1 after achieving steady state, as do its two metabolites. Oxymorphone is metabolized primarily via hepatic glucuronidation to one active metabolite (6-OH-oxymorphone) and to one inactive metabolite (oxymorphone-3-glucuronide). It is neither metabolized by cytochrome P-450 (CYP) enzymes nor inhibited or induced by CYP substrates. And since oxymorphone ER has minimal potential for pharmacokinetic interactions, its use with sedatives, tranquilizers, hypnotics, phenothiazines, and other central nervous system (CNS) depressants can produce additive effects. Hence, as with other opioids, vigilance is required in preventing pharmacodynamic interactions during therapy with oxymorphone ER (Craig, 2010).

Zolpidem Tartrate Extended-Release Tablets (Ambien® CR)

Zolpidem tartrate extended-release tablets are indicated for the treatment of insomnia characterized by difficulties with sleep onset and/or sleep maintenance. Zolpidem has a mean elimination $t_{1/2}$ of 2.5 hours. Zolpidem tartrate extended-release tablets exhibit biphasic absorption characteristics, which results in rapid initial absorption from the gastrointestinal tract similar to zolpidem tartrate immediate release and then provides extended plasma concentrations beyond 3 hours after administration.[1] Patients who use this product have a more rapid onset of sleep due to the initial dose and are able to maintain sleep due to the maintenance dose. Due to the short elimination $t_{1/2}$, the drug does not accumulate. In adult and elderly patients treated with zolpidem tartrate extended-release tablets, there was no evidence of accumulation after repeated once-daily dosing for up to 2 weeks. A food-effect study compared the pharmacokinetics of zolpidem tartrate extended-release tablets 12.5 mg when administered while fasting or within 30 minutes after a meal. Results demonstrated that with food, mean AUC and C_{max} were decreased by 23% and 30%, respectively, while median T_{max} was increased from 2 to 4 hours. The half-life was not changed. These results suggest that, for faster sleep onset, zolpidem tartrate extended-release tablets should not be administered with or immediately after a meal.

---

[1]Approved label for Ambien CR, April 2010.

Divalproex Sodium Extended-Release Tablets (Depakote® ER)

Divalproex sodium is used to treat seizure disorders and mental/mood conditions (such as manic phase of bipolar disorder), and to prevent migraine headaches. It works by restoring the balance of certain natural substances (neurotransmitters) in the brain. The mechanisms by which valproate exerts its therapeutic effects have not been established. It has been suggested that its activity in epilepsy is related to increased brain concentrations of gamma-aminobutyric acid (GABA). The absolute bioavailability of divalproex sodium extended-release tablets administered as a single dose after a meal was approximately 90% relative to intravenous infusion. The median time to maximum plasma valproate concentrations (C_{max}) after divalproex sodium extended-release tablet administration ranged from 4 to 17 hours. Mean terminal $t_{1/2}$ for valproate monotherapy ranged from 9 to 16 hours depending on the dosage applied.

TYPES OF EXTENDED-RELEASE PRODUCTS

The pharmaceutical industry has been developing newer modified-release drug products at a very rapid pace. Many of these modified-release drug products have patented drug delivery systems. This chapter provides an overview of some of the more widely used methods for the manufacture of modified drug products.

The extended-release drug product is designed to contain a drug dose that will release drug at a desired rate over a specified period of time. As discussed previously, the extended-release drug product may also contain an immediate-release component. The general approaches to manufacturing an extended-release drug product include the use of a matrix structure in which the drug is suspended or dissolved, the use of a rate-controlling membrane through which the drug diffuses, or a combination of both. None of the extended-release drug products works by a single drug-release mechanism. Most extended-release products release drug by a combination of processes involving drug dissolution, permeation, erosion, and diffusion. The single most important factor is water permeation into the drug product, without which none of the product release mechanisms would operate. Controlling the rate of water influx into the product generally dictates the rate at which the drug dissolves in the gastrointestinal tract. Once the drug is dissolved, the rate of drug diffusion may be further controlled to a desirable rate. Table 19-4 describes some common extended-release product examples and the mechanisms for controlling drug release. Table 19-5 lists the composition for some drugs.

TABLE 19-4   Examples of Oral Modified-Release Drug Products

	Type	Trade Name	Rationale
Extended-Release Drug Products	Erosion tablet	Constant-T Tenuate Dospan	Theophylline Diethylpropion HCl dispersed in hydrophilic matrix
		Tedral SA	Combination product with a slow-erosion component (theophylline, ephedrine HCl) and an initial-release component theophylline, ephedrine HCl, phenobarbital
	Waxy matrix tablet	Kaon *Cl*	Slow release of potassium chloride to reduce GI irritation
	Coated pellets in capsule	Ornade spansule	Combination phenylpropanolamine HCl and chlorpheniramine with initial- and extended-release component
	Pellets in tablet Leaching	Theo-Dur Ferro-Gradumet (Abbott)	Theophylline Ferrous sulfate in a porous plastic matrix that is excreted in the stool; slow release of iron decreases GI irritation
		Desoxyn gradumet tablet (Abbott)	Methamphetamine methylacrylate methylmethacrylate copolymer, povidone, magnesium stearate; the plastic matrix is porous
	Coated ion exchange	Tussionex	Cation ion-exchange resin complex of hydrocodone and phenyltoloxamine
	Flotation–diffusion	Valrelease	Diazapam
	Osmotic delivery	Acutrim	Phenylpropanolamine HCl (Oros delivery system)
		Procardia-XL	GITS—Gastrointestinal therapeutic system with NaCl-driven (osmotic pressure) delivery system for nifedipine
	Microencapsulation	Bayer timed-release Nitrospan Micro-K Extencaps	Aspirin Microencapsulated nitroglycerin Potassium chloride microencapsulated particles
Delayed-release drug products		diclofenac sodium enteric-coated tablets mesalamine) delayed-release tablets	Enteric coating dissolves at pH >5 for release of drug in duodenum
			Delayed-release tablets are coated with acrylic-based resin, Eudragit S (methacrylic acid copolymer B, NF), which dissolves at pH 7 or greater, releasing mesalamine in the terminal ileum and beyond for topical anti-inflammatory action in the colon
Orally disintegrating tables			

TABLE 19-5 Composition and Examples of Some Modified-Release Products

K-Tab (Abbott)	750 mg or 10 mEq of potassium chloride in a film-coated matrix tablet. The matrix may be excreted intact, but the active ingredient is released slowly without upsetting the GI tract. Inert ingredients: Cellulosic polymers, castor oil, colloidal silicon dioxide, polyvinyl acetate, paraffin. The product is listed as a waxy/polymer matrix tablet for release over 8–10 h.
Toprol-XL tablets (Astra)	Contains metoprolol succinate for sustained release in pellets, providing stable beta-blockade over 24 h with one daily dose. Exercise tachycardia was less pronounced compared to immediate-release preparation. Each pellet separately releases the intended amount of medication. Inert ingredients: Paraffin, PEG, povidone, acetyltributyl citrate, starch, silicon dioxide, and magnesium stearate.
Quinglute Dura tablets (Berlex)	Contains 320 mg quinidine gluconate in a prolonged-action matrix tablet lasting 8–12 h and provides PVC protection. Inert ingredients: Starch, confectioner's sugar and magnesium stearate.
Brontil Slow-Release capsules (Carnrick) Slow Fe tablets (Ciba)	Phendimetrazine tartrate 105 mg sustained pellet in capsule. Slow-release iron preparation (OTC medication) with 160 mg ferrous sulfate for iron deficiency. Inert ingredients: HPMC, PEG shellac, and cetostearyl alcohol.
Tegretol-XR tablets (Ciba Geneva)	Carbamazepine extended-release tablet. Inert ingredients: Zein, cetostearyl alcohol, PEG, starch, talc, gum tragacanth, and mineral oil.
Sinemed CR tablets (Dupont pharma)	Contains a combination of carbidopa and levodopa for sustained-release delivery. This is a special erosion polymeric tablet for Parkinson's disease treatment.
Pentasa capsules (Hoechst Marion/Roussel)	Contains mesalamine for ulcerative colitis in a sustained-release mesalamine coated with ethylcellulose. For local effect mostly, about 20% absorbed versus 80% otherwise.
Isoptin SR (Knoll)	Verapamil HCI sustained-release tablet. Inert ingredients: PEG, starch, PVP, alginate, talc, HPMC, methylcellulose, and microcrystalline cellulose.
Pancrease capsules (McNeil)	Enteric-coated microspheres of pancrelipase. Protects the amylase, lipase, and protease from the action of acid in the stomach. Inert ingredients: CAP, diethyl phthalate, sodium starch glycolate, starch, sugar, gelatin, and talc.
Cotazym-S (Organon)	Enteric-coated microspheres of pancrelipase.
Eryc (erythromycin delayed-release capsules) (Warner-Chilcott)	Erythromycin enteric-coated tablet that protects the drug from instability and irritation.
Dilantin Kapseals (Parke-Davis)	Extended-release phenytoin capsule which contains beads of sodium phenytoin, gelatin, sodium lauryl sulfate, glyceryl monooleate, PEG 200, silicon dioxide, and talc.
Micro-K Extencaps (Robbins)	Ethylcellulose forms semipermeable film surrounding granules by microencapsulation for release over 8–10 h without local irritation. Inert ingredients: Gelatin and sodium lauryl sulfate.
Quinidex Extentabs (Robbins)	300-mg dose, 100-mg release immediately in the stomach and is absorbed in the small intestine. The rest is absorbed later over 10–12 h in a slow-dissolving core as it moves down the GI tract. Inert ingredients: White wax, carnauba wax, acacia, acetylated monoglyceride, guar gum, edible ink, calcium sulfate, corn derivative, and shellac.
Compazine Spansules (GSK)	Initial dose of prochlorperazine release first, then release slowly over several hours. Inert ingredients: Glycerylmonostearate, wax, gelatin, sodium lauryl sulfate.
Slo-bid Gyrocaps (Rhone-Poulenc Rorer)	A controlled-release 12–24-h theophylline product.
Theo-24 capsules (UCB Pharma)	A 24-h sustained-release theophylline product. Inert ingredients: Ethylcellulose, edible ink, talc, starch, sucrose, gelatin, silicon dioxide, and dyes.
Sorbitrate SA (Zeneca)	The tablet contains isosorbide dinitrate 10 mg in the outer coat and 30 mg in the inner coat. Inert ingredients: Carbomer 934P, ethylcellulose, lactose magnesium stearate, and Yellow No. 10.

Drug Release from Matrix

A *matrix* is an inert solid vehicle in which a drug is uniformly suspended. A variety of excipients based on wax, lipid, as well as natural and synthetic polymers have been used as carrier material in the preparation of such matrix type of drug delivery systems. The drug release from such matrix systems is mainly controlled by the diffusion process, concomitant swelling, and/or erosion processes. A matrix may be formed by compressing or fusing the drug and the matrix material together. When an erodible or swellable polymer matrix is involved, the drug release kinetics is further complicated by the presence of a second moving boundary, namely, the swelling or eroding front, which moves either opposite to or in the same direction as the diffusion front. Generally, the drug is present in a small percentage, so that the matrix protects the drug from rapid dissolution and the drug slowly diffuses out over time. Most matrix materials are water insoluble, although some matrix materials may swell slowly in water. Drug release using a matrix dosage form may be achieved using tablets or small beads, depending on the formulation composition and therapeutic objective (Lee, 2011). Figure 19-7 shows three common approaches by which matrix mechanisms are employed. In Fig. 19-7A, the drug is coated with a soluble coating, so drug release relies solely on the regulation of drug release by the matrix material. If the matrix is porous, water penetration will be rapid and the drug will diffuse out rapidly. A less porous matrix may give a longer duration of release. Unfortunately, drug release from a simple matrix tablet is not zero order. Five decades ago, Professor Takeru Higuchi was the first one in the pharmaceutical field to tackle this moving boundary mathematical problem for drug release from matrix systems. The Higuchi equation was originally derived to describe the drug release from an ointment layer containing suspended drug at an initial concentration (or amount of drug loading per unit volume), which is substantially greater than the solubility of the drug per unit volume in the vehicle matrix. The *Higuchi equation* describes the release rate of a matrix tablet:

$$Q = DS\left(\frac{P}{\lambda}\right)(A - 0.5SP)1/2\sqrt{t} \qquad (19.10)$$

where Q = amount of drug release per cm² of surface at time t, S = solubility of drug in g/cm³ in the dissolution medium, A = content of drug in insoluble matrix, P = porosity of matrix, D = diffusion coefficient of drug, and λ = tortuosity factor.

Figure 19-7B represents a matrix enclosed by an insoluble membrane, so the drug release rate is regulated by the permeability of the membrane as well as the matrix. Figure 19-7C represents a matrix tablet enclosed with a combined film. The film becomes porous after dissolution of the soluble part of the film. An example of this is the combined film formed by ethylcellulose and methylcellulose. Close to zero-order release has been obtained with this type of release mechanism.

Classification of Matrix Tablets

Based on the retarded materials used, matrix tablets can be divided into five types: (1) hydrophobic matrix (plastic matrix); (2) lipid matrix; (3) hydrophilic matrix; (4) biodegradable matrix; and (5) mineral matrix. Matrix system can also be classified according to their porosity situation, including macroporous, microporous, and nonporous system. By the usage frequency, matrix tablets can also be categorized as follows.

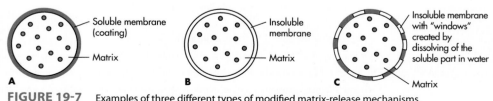

FIGURE 19-7   Examples of three different types of modified matrix-release mechanisms.

Gum-Type Matrix Tablets

Some excipients have a remarkable ability to swell in the presence of water and form a substance with a gel-like consistency. When this happens, the gel provides a natural barrier to drug diffusion from the tablet. Natural gum polysaccharides consisting of multiple sugar units linked together to create large molecules. Natural gums are biodegradable and nontoxic, which hydrate and swell on contact with aqueous media, and these have been used for the preparation of dosage form. They are used in pharmaceuticals for their diverse properties and applications. They can receive modification for the purpose of hydration rate control, pH-dependent solubility adjustment, thickness alteration and viscosity change, etc (Pachuau and Mazumder, 2012; Rana et al, 2011).

Because the gel-like material is quite viscous and may not disperse for hours, this approach provides a means for maintaining the drug for hours until all the drug has been completely dissolved and diffused into the intestinal fluid. Gelatin is a common gelling material. However, gelatin dissolves rapidly after the gel is formed. Drug excipients such as methylcellulose, gum tragacanth, Veegum, and alginic acid form a viscous mass and provide a useful matrix for controlling drug release and dissolution. Drug formulations with these excipients provide extended drug release for hours.

Polymeric Matrix Tablets

Various polymeric materials have been used to prolong the rate of drug release. The most important characteristic of this type of preparation is that the prolonged release may last for days or weeks rather than for a shorter duration (as with other techniques). An early example of an oral polymeric matrix tablet was *Gradumet* (Abbott Laboratories), which was marketed as an iron preparation. The nonbiodegradable plastic matrix provides a rigid geometric surface for drug diffusion, so that a relatively constant rate of drug release is obtained. In the case of the iron preparation, the matrix reduces the exposure of the irritating drug to the GI mucosal tissues. The matrix is usually expelled unchanged in the feces after all the drug has leached out.

Polymeric matrix tablets for oral use can be regarded as release-controlling excipients, which can be divided into water soluble (or hydrophilic) and insoluble carriers (or hydrophobic) (Grund et al, 2014). Considering the application in formulation, they should be quite safe. However, for certain patients with reduced GI motility caused by disease, polymeric matrix tablets should be avoided, because accumulation or obstruction of the GI tract by matrix tablets has been reported (Franek et al, 2014). As an oral sustained-release product, the matrix tablet has not been popular. In contrast, the use of the matrix tablet in implantation has been more popular.

The use of biodegradable polymeric material for extended release has been the focus of more recent research. Chitosan–carrageenan matrix tablets were characterized and used for the controlled release of highly soluble drug of trimetazidine hydrochloride (Li et al, 2013). One such example is poly(lactic acid-co-glycolic acid) copolymer, which degrades to lactic/glatic acid and eliminates the problem of retrieval after implantation (Clark et al, 2014). And the associated mathematical modeling is used for the advanced analysis on the release/delivery process of polymeric-based matrix tablets, including porous, microporous, and nonporous matrix. With generating more and more complex models or a parametric fitting process, these modeling efforts can help practitioners to achieve a better formulation design and understanding (Peppas and Narasimhan, 2014).

Other polymers for drug formulations include polyacrylate, methacrylate, polyester, ethylene–vinyl acetate copolymer (EVA), polyglycolide, polylactide, and silicone. Of these, the hydrophilic polymers, such as polylactic acid and polyglycolic acid, erode in water and release the drug gradually over time (Clark et al, 2014). Polymer properties may affect the integrity and drug release from insoluble matrices. Typical examples of insoluble carriers are Kollidon® SR (co-processed polyvinyl acetate and polyvinylpyrrolidone, ratio 8:2), Eudragit® RS (ammonium methacrylate copolymer), and ethylcellulose. A hydrophobic and also a non-degradable polymer such as EVA release the drug over a longer duration time of weeks or months. The rate of release may be controlled by blending two polymers and increasing the proportion of the more hydrophilic polymer, thus increasing the rate of drug release. The addition of a low-molecular-weight polylactide to a polylactide polymer formulation increased the release rate of the drug and enabled the preparation of an extended-release system (Kleiner et al, 2014; Krivoguz et al, 2013). The type of plasticizer and the degree of cross-linking provide additional means for modifying the release rate of the drug. Many drugs are incorporated into the polymer as the polymer is formed chemically from its monomer. Light, heat, and other agents may affect the polymer chain length, degree of cross-linking, and other properties. This may provide a way to modify the release rate of the polymer matrices prepared. Drugs incorporated into polymers may have release rates that last over days, weeks, or even months. These vehicles have been often recommended for protein and peptide drug administration. For example, EVA is biocompatible and was shown to prolong insulin release in rats.

Hydrophobic polymers with water-labile linkages are prepared so that partial breakdown of the polymers allows for desired drug release without deforming the matrix during erosion. And hydrophilic polymer such as hypromellose (hydroxypropyl methylcellulose, HPMC) may be integrated with hydrophobic block, for example, polyacrylate polymers, Eudragit RL100, and Eudragit RS100 with or without incorporating ethylcellulose on a matrix-controlled metformin hydrochloride drug delivery system (Jain et al, 2014; Viridén et al, 2009). For oral drug delivery, the problem of incomplete drug release from the matrix is a major hurdle that must be overcome with the polymeric matrix dosage form. Another problem is that drug release rates may be affected by the amount of drug loaded. For implantation and other uses, the environment is more stable compared to oral routes, so a stable drug release from the polymer matrix may be attained for days or weeks.

Slow-Release Pellets, Beads, or Granules

Pellets or beads are small spherical particles that can be formulated to provide a variety of modified drug release properties. The size of these beads can be very small (microencapsulation) for injections or larger for oral drug delivery. Several approaches have been used to manufacture beaded formulations including pan coating, spray drying, fluid-bed drying, and extrusion-spheronization.

An early approach to the manufacture of ER drug products was the use of encapsulated drugs in a beaded or pellet formulation. In general, the beads are prepared by coating the powdered drug onto preformed cores known as *nonpareil seeds*. The nonpareil seeds are made from slurry of starch, sucrose, and lactose. The drug-coated beads are then coated by a variety of materials that act as a barrier to drug release. The beads may have a blend of different thicknesses to provide the desired drug release. The beads may be placed in a capsule (eg, amphetamine ER capsules, Adderall XR) or with the addition of other excipients compressed into tablets (eg, metoprolol succinate extended-release tablets, Toprol XL).

Pan coating is a modified method adopted from candy manufacturing. Cores or nonpareil seeds of a given mesh size are slowly added to known amount of fine drug powder and coating solution and rounded for hours to become coated drug beads. The drug-coated beads are then coated with a polymeric layer, which regulates drug release rate by changing either the thickness of the film or the composition of the polymeric material. Coatings may be aqueous or nonaqueous. Aqueous coatings are generally preferred. Nonaqueous coatings may leave residual solvents in the product, and the removal of solvents during manufacture presents danger to workers and the environment. Cores are coated by either sprayed pan coating or air-suspension coating. Once the drug beads are prepared, they may be further coated with a protective coating to allow a sustained or prolonged release of the drug. *Spray dry coating* or *fluid-bed coating* is a more recent approach and has several advantages over pan coating. Drug may be dissolved in a solution that is sprayed or dispersed in small droplets in a chamber. A stream of hot air evaporates the solvent and the drug becomes a dry powder. The powdered material, which is aerated, may be coated with a variety of excipients to achieve the desired drug release. Several experimental process variables for fluid-bed coating include inlet air temperature, spray rate (g/min), atomizing air pressure, solid content, and curing time. Pelletization may also be obtained by *extrusion-spheronization* in which the powdered drug and excipients are mixed in a mixer/granulator. The moist mixture is then fed through an extruder at a specified rate and becomes spheronized on exit through small-diameter dies. A wide range of extrusion screen sizes and configurations are available for optimization of pellet diameter.

The use of various amounts of coating solution can provide beads with various coating protection. A careful blending of beads is used to achieve a desired drug release profile. The finished drug product (eg, beads in capsule or beads in tablet) may contain a blend of beads coated with materials of different solubility rates to provide a means of controlling drug release and dissolution.

The orally administered extended-release drug products may display in single or multiple-unit dosage forms. In single-unit formulations, they contain the active ingredient within the single tablet or capsule, whereas multiple-unit dosage forms comprise of a number of discrete particles that are combined into one dosage unit. Both of them may exist as pellets, granules, sugar seeds (nonpareil), minitablets, ion-exchange resin particles, powders, and crystals, with drugs being entrapped in or layered around cores. In this way, multiple-unit dosage forms offer several advantages over single-unit systems such as nondisintegrating tablets or capsules, although the drug release profiles are similar. Once multiple-unit systems are taken orally, the subunits of multiple-unit preparations distribute readily over a large surface area in the gastrointestinal tract. And because of the small particles in sizes (<2 mm), multiple-unit preparations can enable them to be well distributed along the gastrointestinal tract, which could improve the bioavailability (Kambayashi et al, 2014; Rosiaux et al, 2014). Some products take advantage of bead blending to provide two doses of drug in one formulation. For example, a blend of rapid-release beads with some pH-sensitive enteric-coated material may provide a second dose of drug release when the drug reaches the intestine.

The pellet dosage form can be prepared as a capsule or tablet. When pellets are prepared as tablets, the beads must be compressed lightly so that they do not break. This process is called as compaction of pellets, which is also a challenging area. Only a few multiple-unit-containing tablet products are available, such as Beloc® ZOK, Antra® MUPS, and Prevacid® SoluTab™. Compaction of multiparticulates into tablets could result in either a disintegrating tablet providing a multiparticulate system during gastrointestinal transit or intact tablets due to the fusion of the multiparticulates in a larger compact. Usually, a disintegrant is included in the tablet, causing the beads to be released rapidly after administration. Formulation of a drug into pellet form may reduce gastric irritation, because the drug is released slowly over a period of time, therefore avoiding high drug concentration in the stomach (Abdul et al, 2010). Figure 19-8 shows the two types of multiple-unit pellets in tablets, coated by polymer (reservoir-type) (a) compaction of matrix and/or uncoated drug pellets (b). The drug release from both of the pellets shows significant extended characterization, regardless the polymer coating or matrix dispersion. For the reservoir-type coated-pellet dosage forms, the polymeric coating must be able to withstand the compaction force. It may deform but should not rupture since any crack on the coating layer may cause unexpected drug release. The type and amount of coating agent, the size of subunits, selection of external additives,

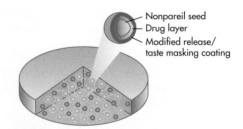

(a) MUPS containing polymer-coated pellets

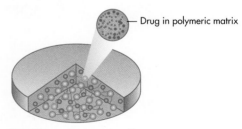

(b) MUPS containing matrix pellets

FIGURE 19-8   Schematic representation of types of multiple unit pellets system (MUPS) in tablets—(a) comprising of coated pellets, and (b) uncoated/matrix pellets.

and the rate and magnitude of pressure applied must be considered carefully to maintain the desired drug release properties.

Dextroamphetamine sulfate formulated as timed-release pellets in capsules (Dexedrine Spansule) is an early example of a beaded dosage form. Another older product is a pellet-type extended-release product of theophylline (Gyrocap). Table 19-6 shows the frequency of adverse reactions after theophylline is administered as a solution or as pellets. If theophylline is administered as a solution, a high drug concentration is reached in the body due to rapid drug absorption. Some side effects may be attributed to the high concentration of theophylline. Pellet dosage forms allow drug to be absorbed gradually, therefore reducing the incidence of side effects by preventing a high C_{max}.

Potassium chloride is irritating to the GI tract. Studies reported reduced gastrointestinal side effects of the drug potassium chloride in pellet or microparticulate form. Formulation of potassium chloride in pellet form reduces the chance of exposing high concentrations of potassium chloride to the mucosal cells in the GI tract.

Many extended-release cold products also employ the bead formulation approach. A major advantage of pellet dosage forms is that the pellets are less affected by stomach emptying. Because numerous pellets are within a capsule, some pellets will gradually reach the small intestine each time the stomach empties, whereas a single extended-release tablet may be delayed in the stomach for a long time as a result of erratic stomach emptying. Stomach emptying time is particularly important in the formulation and *in vivo* behavior of enteric-coated products. Enteric-coated tablets may be delayed for hours by the presence of food in the stomach, whereas enteric-coated pellets are relatively unaffected by the presence of food.

Prolonged-Action Tablets

An alternate approach to prolong the action of a drug is to reduce the aqueous solubility of the drug, so that the drug dissolves slowly over a period of several hours. The solubility of a drug is dependent on the salt form used. An examination of the solubility of the various salt forms of the drug is performed in early drug development. In general, the nonionized base or acid form of the drug is usually much less soluble than the corresponding salt. For example, sodium phenobarbital is more water soluble than phenobarbital, the acid form of the drug. Diphenhydramine hydrochloride is more soluble than the base form, diphenhydramine.

In cases where it is inconvenient to prepare a less soluble form of the drug, the drug may be granulated with an excipient to slow dissolution of the drug. Often, fatty or waxy lipophilic materials are employed in formulations. Stearic acid, castor wax, high-molecular-weight polyethylene glycol (Carbowax), glycerylmonosterate, white wax, and spermaceti oil are useful ingredients in providing an oily barrier to slow water penetration and the dissolution of the tablet. Many of the lubricants used in tableting may also be used as lipophilic agents to slow dissolution. For example, magnesium stearate and hydrogenated vegetable oil (Sterotex) are actually used in high percentages to cause sustained drug release in a preparation. The major disadvantage of this type of preparation is the difficulty in maintaining a reproducible drug release from patient to patient, because oily materials may be subjected to digestion, temperature, and mechanical stress, which may affect the release rate of the drug.

TABLE 19-6   Incidence of Adverse Effects of Sustained-Release Theophylline Pellet Versus Theophylline Solution[a]

Side Effects	Volunteers Showing Side Effects	
	Using Solution	Using Sustained-Release Pellets
Nausea	10	0
Headache	4	0
Diarrhea	3	0
Gastritis	2	0
Vertigo	5	0
Nervousness	3	1

[a]After 5-day dosing at 600 mg theophylline/24 h, adverse reaction points on fifth day: solution, 135; pellets, 18.

From Breimer and Dauhof (1980), with permission.

Another application of prolong-action tablets is also called as pulsatile drug delivery system. This chrono-pharmaceutical formulation is usually used in the treatment of circadian rhythm dysfunction diseases. This effort may improve the therapeutic efficacy of oral drug administration for some specific chrono-treatment. In one of the studies, drug was compressed into regular tablets with ingredients of starch, lactose, magnesium stearate, etc. Then the tablet was put at a lower position into capsule with another erodible plug composed by hydroxypropyl methylcellulose (HPMC): lactose, whose erodible process was controlled by osmotic extent from outer water. After determined time point, the drug-contained tablet was ejected from this pulsincap capsule by the mechanism of osmotic control (Ranjan et al, 2013; Wu et al, 2006). The time-controlled devices can also be prepared by tablet surface coating with different compositions in order to defer the onset of its release (Zhang et al, 2003). According to the coating agent(s) employed, various release mechanisms can be involved, such as in the case of erodible, reputable, or diffusive reservoir systems (Maroni et al, 2010).

Ion-Exchange Products

Ion-exchange technique has been popularly applied in water purification and chemical extraction. Ion-exchange preparations usually involve an insoluble resin capable of reacting with either an anionic or a cationic drug. An anionic resin is negatively charged so that a positively charged cationic drug may attach the resin to form an insoluble nonabsorbable resin–drug complex. Upon exposure in the GI tract, cations in the gut, such as potassium and sodium, may displace the drug from the resin, releasing the drug, which is absorbed freely. Researchers already applied the combination technique of iontophoresis and cation-exchange fibers as drug matrices for the controlled transdermal delivery of antiparkinsonian drug apomorphine (Malinovskaja et al, 2013). The main disadvantage of ion-exchange preparations is that the amount of cation–anion in the GI tract is not easily controllable and varies among individuals, making it difficult to provide a consistent mechanism or rate of drug release. A further disadvantage

is that resins may provide a potential means of interaction with nutrients and other drugs.

Ion exchange may be used in extended-release liquid preparations. An added advantage is that the technique provides some protection for very bitter or irritating drugs. Ion exchange has been combined with a coating to obtain a more effective sustained-release product. Examples include dextromethorphan polistirex (Delsyn®), an oral suspension formulated as an ion-exchange complex to mask the bitter taste and to prolong the duration of drug action, and TussionexPennkinetic®, an oral suspension containing chlorpheniramine polistirex and hydrocodone polistirex.

A general mechanism for the formulation of cationic drugs is

$$H^+ + resin - SO_3^- drug \rightleftharpoons resin - SO_3^- H^+ + drug^+$$

Insoluble drug complex   Soluble drug

For anionic drugs, the corresponding mechanism is

$$Cl^- + resin - N^+(CH_3)_3\, drug^- \rightleftharpoons resin - N^+(CH_3)_3\, Cl^- + drug^-$$

Insoluble drug complex   Soluble drug

The insoluble drug complex containing the resin and drug dissociates in the GI tract in the presence of the appropriate counterions. The released drug dissolves in the fluids of the GI tract and is rapidly absorbed.

Core Tablets

A core tablet is a tablet within a tablet. The inner core is usually used for the slow-drug-release component, and the outside shell contains a rapid-release dose of drug. Formulation of a core tablet requires two granulations. The core granulation is usually compressed lightly to form a loose core and then transferred to a second die cavity, where a second granulation containing additional ingredients is compressed further to form the final tablet.

The core material may be surrounded by hydrophobic excipients so that the drug leaches out over a prolonged period of time. This type of preparation is sometimes called a *slow-erosion core tablet*, because the core generally contains either no disintegrant or insufficient disintegrant to fragment the tablet. The composition of the core may range from wax to gum or polymeric material. Numerous slow-erosion tablets have been patented and are sold commercially under various trade names.

The success of core tablets depends very much on the nature of the drug and the excipients used. As a general rule, this preparation is very much hardness dependent in its release rate. Critical control of hardness and processing variables are important in producing a tablet with a consistent release rate. OSDrC®OptiDose™ is a new commercial core tablet whose manufacture was conducted in a solvent-free, dry compression single process operation. Its single- or multi-cored tablets with a range of dose forms including fixed-dose combination tablets offer differentiated controlled-release functionality. This product is produced by Catalent partnering with Sanwa Kagaku Kenkyusho Co., Ltd.

Core tablets are occasionally used to avoid incompatibility in preparations containing two physically incompatible ingredients. For example, buffered aspirin has been formulated into a core and shell to avoid a yellowing discoloration of the two ingredients upon aging (Desai et al, 2013).

Microencapsulation

Microencapsulation is a process of encapsulating microscopic drug particles with a special coating material, therefore making the drug particles more desirable in terms of physical and chemical characteristics. A common drug that has been encapsulated is aspirin. Aspirin has been microencapsulated with ethylcellulose, making the drug superior in its flow characteristics; when compressed into a tablet, the drug releases more gradually compared to a simple compressed tablet (Dash et al, 2010). Usually, biodegradable polymers such as dextran, collagen, chitosan, poly(lactide), ethylcellulose, and casein are natural materials applied in microencapsulation. After forming the encapsulation materials as flowing powder, it is suitable for formulation as compressed tablets, hard gelatin capsules, suspensions, and other dosage forms (Baracat et al, 2012; Singh et al, 2010).

Many techniques are used in microencapsulating a drug. One process used in microencapsulating acetaminophen involves suspending the drug in an aqueous solution while stirring. The coating material, ethylcellulose, is dissolved in cyclohexane, and the two liquids are added together with stirring and heating. As the cyclohexane is evaporated by heat, the ethylcellulose coats the microparticles of the acetaminophen. The microencapsulated particles have a slower dissolution rate because the ethylcellulose is not water soluble and provides a barrier for diffusion of drug. The amount of coating material deposited on the acetaminophen determines the rate of drug dissolution. The coating also serves as a means of reducing the bitter taste of the drug. In practice, microencapsulation is not consistent enough to produce a reproducible batch of product, and it may be necessary to blend the microencapsulated material in order to obtain a desired release rate.

Osmotic Drug Delivery Systems

Osmotic drug delivery systems have been developed for both oral extended-release products known as gastrointestinal therapeutic systems (GITS) and for parenteral drug delivery as an implantable drug delivery (eg, osmotic minipump). Drug delivery is controlled by the use of an osmotically controlled device in which a constant amount of water flows into the system causing the dissolving and releasing of a constant amount of drug per unit time. Drug is released via a single laser-drilled hole in the tablet.

Figure 19-9A describes an osmotic drug delivery system in the form of a tablet that contains an outside semipermeable membrane and an inner core filled with a mixture of drug and osmotic agent (salt solution).

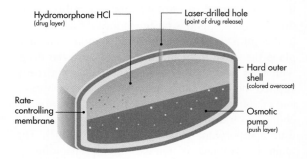

FIGURE 19-9A   Cross section of the extended-release hydromorphone tablet. (Adapted with permission from Gupta S, Sathyan G: Providing constant analgesia with OROS® hydromorphone. *J Pain Symptom Manage* **33**(2 suppl):S19–S24, 2007.)

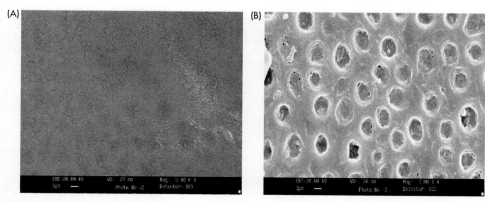

FIGURE 19-9B   SEM micrograph of the membrane of controlled porosity osmotic pump (CPOP) tablet containing diltiazem hydrochloride (A) before and (B) after dissolution studies.

When the tablet is placed in water, osmotic pressure is generated by the osmotic agent within the core. Water moves into the device, forcing the dissolved drug to exit the tablet through an orifice. The rate of drug delivery is relatively constant and unaffected by the pH of the environment. Figure 19-9B provides the surface electronic micrograph (SEM) images of the membrane of controlled porosity osmotic pump (CPOP) tablet containing diltiazem hydrochloride (A) before and (B) after dissolution studies, which can clearly find the drug-release mechanism under microscopic domain (Adibkia et al, 2014).

Newer osmotic drug delivery systems are considered "push-pull" systems. Nifedine (Procardia XL) extended-release tablets have the appearance of a conventional tablet. Procardia XL ER tablets have a semipermeable membrane surrounding an osmotically active drug core. The core itself is divided into two layers: an "active" layer containing the drug and a "push" layer containing pharmacologically inert (but osmotically active) components. As water from the gastrointestinal tract enters the tablet, pressure increases in the osmotic layer and "pushes" against the drug layer, releasing drug through a laser-drilled tablet orifice in the active layer. Drug delivery is essentially constant (zero order) as long as the osmotic gradient remains constant, and then gradually falls to zero. Upon swallowing, the biologically inert components of the tablet remain intact during gastrointestinal transit and are eliminated in the feces as an insoluble shell.

Methylphenidate HCl (Concerta) extended-release tablet uses osmotic pressure to deliver methylphenidate HCl at a controlled rate. The system, which resembles a conventional tablet in appearance, comprises an osmotically active trilayer core surrounded by a semipermeable membrane with an immediate-release drug overcoat. The trilayer core is composed of two drug layers containing the drug and excipients, and a push layer containing osmotically active components. A laser-drilled orifice on the drug-layer end of the tablet allows for exit of the drug. This product is similar to the gastrointestinal therapeutic systems discussed earlier. The biologically inert components of the tablet remain intact during gastrointestinal transit and are eliminated in the stool as an insoluble tablet shell.

The frequency of side effects experienced by patients using gastrointestinal therapeutic systems was considerably less than that with conventional tablets. When the therapeutic system was compared to the regular 250-mg tablet given twice daily, ocular pressure was effectively controlled by the osmotic system. The blood level of acetazolanine using gastrointestinal therapeutic systems, however, was considerably below that from the tablet. In fact, the therapeutic index of the drug was measurably increased by using the therapeutic system. The use of extended-release drug products, which release drug consistently, may provide promise for administering many drugs that previously had frequent adverse side effects because of the drug's narrow

TABLE 19-7   OROS Osmotic Therapeutic Systems[a]

Trade Name	Manufacturer	Generic Name	Description
Acutrim	Ciba	Phenylpropanolamine	Once-daily, over-the-counter appetite suppressant
Covera-HS	Searle	Verapamil	Controlled-Onset Extended-Release (COER-24) system for hypertension and angina pectoris
DynaCirc CR	Sandoz Pharmaceuticals	Isradipine	Treatment of hypertension
Efidac 24	Ciba Self-Medication		Over-the-counter, 24-hour extended-release tablets providing relief of allergy and cold symptoms, containing either chlorphenira-mine maleate, pseudoephedrine hydrochlo-ride, or a combination of pseudoephedrine hydrochloride/brompheniramine maleate
Glucotrol XL	Pfizer	Glipizide	Extended-release tablets indicated as an adjunct to diet for the control of hyperglyce-mia in patients with non-insulin-dependent diabetes
Minipress XL	Pfizer	Prazosin	Extended-release tablets for treatment of hypertension
Procardia XL	Pfizer	Nifedipine	Extended-release tablets for treatment of angina and hypertension
Adalat CR	Bayer AG	Nifedipine	An Alza-based OROS system of nifedipine introduced internationally
Volmax	Glaxo-Wellcome	Albuterol	Extended-release tablets for the relief of bronchospasm in patients with reversible obstructive airway disease

[a]Alza's OROS Osmotic Therapeutic Systems use osmosis to deliver drug continuously at controlled rates for up to 24 h.

therapeutic index. The osmotic drug delivery system has become a popular drug vehicle for many products that require an extended period of drug delivery for 12–24 hours (Table 19-7).

A newer osmotic delivery system is the L-OrosSoftcap (Alza), which claims to enhance bioavailability of poorly soluble drug by formulating the drug in a soft gelatin core and then providing extended drug delivery through an orifice drilled into an osmotic-driven shell (Fig. 19-10). The soft gelatin capsule is surrounded by the barrier layer, the expanding osmotic layer, and the release-rate-controlling membrane. A delivery orifice is formed through the three outer layers but not through the gelatin shell. When the system is administered, water permeates through the rate-controlling membrane and activates the osmotic engine. As the engine expands, hydrostatic pressure inside the system builds up, thereby forcing the liquid formulation to break through the hydrated gelatin capsule shell at the delivery orifice and be pumped out of the system. At the end of the operation, liquid drug fill is squeezed out, and the gelatin capsule shell becomes flattened. The osmotic layer, located between the inner layer and the rate-controlling membrane, is the driving force for pumping the liquid formulation out of the system. This layer can gel when it hydrates. In addition, the high osmotic pressure can be sustained to achieve a constant release. This layer should comprise, therefore, a high-molecular-weight hydrophilic polymer and an osmotic agent. It is a challenge to develop a coating solution for a high-molecular-weight hydrophilic polymer. A mixed solvent of water and ethanol was used for this coating composition.

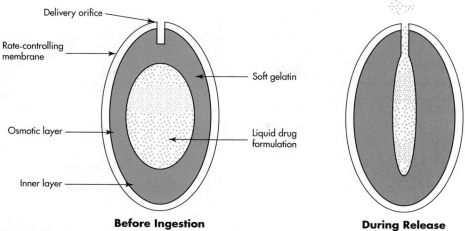

FIGURE 19-10   Configuration of L-OrosSoftcap. (From Dong et al, 2002, with permission.)

Gastroretentive System

The extended-release drug product should release the drug completely within the region in the GI tract in which the drug is optimally absorbed. Due to GI transit, the extended-release drug product continuously moves distally down the GI tract. In some cases, the extended-release drug product containing residual drug may exit from the body. Pharmaceutical formulation developers have used various approaches to retain the dosage form in the desired area of the gastrointestinal tract. One such approach is a *gastroretentive system* that can remain in the gastric region for several hours and prolong the gastric residence time of drugs (Arora et al, 2005). Usually, the gastroretentive systems can be classified into several types based on the mechanism applied such as (i) high-density systems; (ii) floating systems; (iii) expandable systems; (iv) superporous hydrogels; (v) mucoadhesive or bioadhesive systems; (vi) magnetic systems; and (vii) dual working systems (Adibkia et al, 2011).

One of the most commonly used gastroretentive systems is *floating* drug delivery systems (FDDS). For example, diazepam (Valium) was formulated using methylcellulose to provide sustained release (Valrelease). The manufacturer of Valrelease claimed that the hydrocolloid (gel) floated in the stomach to give sustained-release diazepam. In other studies, however, materials of various densities were emptied from the stomach without any difference as to whether the drug product was floating on top or sitting at the bottom of the stomach (Adibkia et al, 2011; Eberle et al, 2014). Another gastroretentive system is mucoadhesive or bioadhesive drug delivery systems. These systems permit a given drug delivery system to be incorporated with the bio/mucoadhesive agents, enabling the device to adhere to the stomach (or other gastrointestinal) walls, thus resisting gastric emptying (Bhattarai et al, 2010). Sometimes, bio/mucoadhesive substance is a natural or synthetic polymer capable of adhering to biological membrane (bioadhesive polymer) or the mucus lining of the GIT (mucoadhesive polymer).

The most important consideration in this type of formulation appears to be the gelling strength of the gum material and the concentration of gummy material. Modification of the release rates of the product may further be achieved with various amounts of talc or other lipophilic lubricant. However, the gastroretentive system is not feasible for drugs having solubility or stability problems in gastric fluid or having irritation on gastric mucosa. Drugs such as nifedipine, which is well absorbed along the entire GIT and which undergoes significant first-pass metabolism, may not be desirable candidates for FDDS since the slow gastric emptying may lead to reduced systemic bioavailability.

Transdermal Drug Delivery Systems

Skin represents the largest and most easily accessible organ of the body. A transdermal drug delivery system (patch) is a dosage form intended for delivering drug across the skin for systemic drug absorption (see Chapters 7 and 13). Transdermal drug absorption also avoids presystemic metabolism or "first-pass" effects. The transdermal drug delivery systems deliver the drug through the skin in a controlled rate over an extended period of time (Chapter 15, Table 15-12). Examples of transdermal drug delivery systems are listed in Tables 19-8 and 19-9. Transdermal delivery drug products vary in patch design (Fig. 19-11). Generally, the transdermal patch consists of (i) a backing or support layer that protects the patch, (ii) a drug layer that might be in the form of a solid gel reservoir or in a matrix, (iii) a pressure-sensitive adhesive layer, and (iv) a release liner or protective strip that is removed before placing the patch on the skin. In some cases, the adhesive layer may also contain the active drug (Gonzalez and Cleary, 2010).

The skin is a natural barrier to prevent the influx of foreign chemicals (including water) into the body

TABLE 19-8   Examples of Transdermal Delivery Systems

Type	Trade Name	Rationale
Membrane-controlled system	Transderm-Nitro (Novartis)	Drug in reservoir, drug release through a rate-controlling polymeric membrane
Adhesive diffusion-controlled system	Deponit system (Pharma-Schwartz)	Drug dispersed in an adhesive polymer and in a reservoir
Matrix-dispersion system	Nitro-Dur (Key)	Drug dispersed into a rate-controlling hydrophilic or hydrophobic matrix molded into a transdermal system
Microreservoir system	Nitro-Disc (Searle)	Combination reservoir and matrix-dispersion system

TABLE 19-9   Transdermal Delivery Systems

Trade Name	Manufacturer	Generic Name	Description
Catapres-TTS	Boehringer Ingelheim	Clonidine	Once-weekly product for the treatment of hypertension
Duragesic	Janssen Pharmaceutical	Fentanyl	Management of chronic pain in patients who require continuous opioid analgesia for pain that cannot be managed by lesser means
Estraderm	Ciba-Geigy	Estradiol	Twice-weekly product for treating certain postmenopausal symptoms and preventing osteoporosis
Nicoderm CQ	Hoechst Marion	Nicotine	An aid to smoking cessation for the relief of nicotine-withdrawal symptoms
Testoderm	Alza	Testosterone	Replacement therapy in males for conditions associated with a deficiency or absence of endogenous testosterone
Transderm-Nitro	Novartis	Nitroglycerin	Once-daily product for the prevention of angina pectoris due to coronary artery disease; contains nitroglycerin in a proprietary, transdermal therapeutic system
Transderm Scop		Scopolamine	Prevention of nausea and vomiting associated with motion sickness

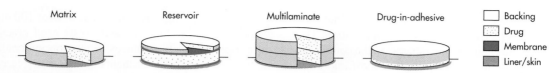

Matrix   Reservoir   Multilaminate   Drug-in-adhesive   ☐ Backing
                                                                                    ☐ Drug
                                                                                    ■ Membrane
                                                                                    ▨ Liner/skin

FIGURE 19-11   The four basic configurations for transdermal drug delivery systems.

and the loss of water from the body (Guy, 1996). To be a suitable candidate for transdermal drug delivery, the drug must possess the right combination of physicochemical and pharmacodynamic properties. The drug must be highly potent so that only a small systemic drug dose is needed and the size of the patch (dose is also related to surface area) need not be exceptionally large, not greater than 50 cm^2 (Guy, 1996). Physicochemical properties of the drug include a small molecular weight (<500 Da), and high lipid solubility. The elimination half-life should not be too short, to avoid having to apply the patch more frequently than once a day.

To enhance transdermal permeation, there are two main category techniques already recognized as effective: (i) physical methods, including iontophoresis, electroporation, sonophoresis, and microneedles; (ii) chemical methods, including prodrug, salt formation, ion pairs, and chemical enhancers. Among these approaches, microneedles and chemical enhancers look like more promising. For microneedles technique, it can disrupt skin barrier and inject drug directly. For chemical enhancer, it may decrease the barrier function of stratum corneum (SC) for molecules (Subedi et al, 2010).

Microneedles were first reported to deliver calcein by permeation improvement in 1998 (Henry et al, 1998). It can painlessly disrupt skin barrier and create pores inside the skin to increase drug penetration. In the recent years, microneedles have been extensively investigated for the delivery of compounds like diclofenac, desmopressin, and even vectors for gene therapy (Badran et al, 2009). Despite the possible problems such as low dosage, accurate dose administration and patient compliance can be solved by introducing development of dissolvable/degradable and hollow microneedles to deliver drugs at a higher dose and to engineer drug release. Besides the steel, microneedles may be fabricated from micro-electromechanical systems employing silicon,

metals, polymers, or polysaccharides. Solid-coated microneedles can be used to pierce the superficial skin layer followed by delivery of the drug. Microneedles can be used to deliver macromolecules such as insulin, growth hormones, immunobiologicals, proteins, and peptides (Bariya et al, 2012).

Transdermal drug delivery system has been extensively studied for 40 years. By now, only about forty drug products were commercialized from twenty drug substances source, due to the drug diffusion problem since all drug delivery approaches need to overcome the barrier function of skin. Drug diffusion may be controlled by a semipermeable membrane next to the reservoir layer. In other cases, drug diffusion is controlled by passage through the epidermis layer of the skin. The transdermal delivery system generally contains large drug concentrations to produce the ideal drug delivery with a zero-order rate. The patch may contain residual drug when the patch is removed from the application site.

Nitroglycerin is commonly administered by transdermal delivery (eg, Nitro-Dur, Transderm-Nitro®). Transdermal delivery systems of nitroglycerin may provide hours of protection against angina, whereas the duration of nitroglycerin given in a sublingual tablet (Nitrostat®) or sublingual spray (Nitrolingual) may be only a few minutes. The nitroglycerin patch is placed over the chest area and provides up to 12 hours of angina protection. In a study comparing these three dosage forms in patients, no substantial difference was observed among the three preparations. In all cases, the skin was found to be the rate-limiting step in nitroglycerin absorption. There were fewer variations among products than of the same product among different patients.

After the application of a transdermal patch, there is generally a lag time before the onset of the drug action, because of the drug's slow diffusion into the dermal layers of the skin. When the patch is removed, diffusion of the drug from the dermal layer to the systemic circulation may continue for some time until the drug is depleted from the site of application. The solubility of drug in the skin rather than the concentration of drug in the patch layer is the most important factor controlling the rate of drug absorption through the skin. Humidity, temperature, and other factors have been shown to affect the rate of drug absorption through the skin. With most drugs, transdermal delivery provides a more stable blood level of the drug than oral dosing. However, with nitroglycerin, the sustained blood level of the drug provided by transdermal delivery is not desirable, due to induced tolerance to the drug not seen with sublingual tablets.

Transdermal therapeutic systems (TTS) consist of a thin, flexible composite of membranes, resembling a small adhesive bandage, which is applied to the skin and delivers drug through intact skin into the bloodstream. Some examples of products delivered using this system are shown in Table 19-8. Transderm-Nitro consists of several layers: (1) an aluminized plastic backing that protects nitroglycerin from loss through vaporization; (2) a drug reservoir containing nitroglycerin adsorbed onto lactose, colloidal silicon dioxide, and silicone medical fluid; (3) a diffusion-controlling membrane consisting of ethylene–vinyl acetate copolymer; (4) a layer of silicone adhesive; and (5) a protective strip.

Other transdermal delivery manufacturers have made transdermal systems in which the adhesive functions both as a pressure-sensitive adhesive and as a controlling matrix. Dermaflex (Elan) is a uniquely passive transdermal patch system that employs a hydrogel matrix into which the drug is incorporated. Dermaflex regulates both the availability and absorption of the drug in a manner that allows for controlled and efficient systemic delivery of many drugs.

An important limitation of transdermal preparation is the amount of drug that is needed in the transdermal patch to be absorbed systemically to provide the optimum therapeutic response. The amount of drug absorbed transdermally is related to the amount of drug in the patch, the size of the patch, and the method of manufacture. A dose–response relationship is obtained by applying a proportionally larger transdermal patch that differs only in surface area. For example, a 5-cm^2 transdermal patch will generally provide twice as much drug absorbed systemically as a 2.5-cm^2 transdermal patch.

In general, drugs given at a dose of over 100 mg would require too large a patch to be used practically. However, new advances in pharmaceutic solvents may provide a mechanism for an increased amount of drug to be absorbed transdermally. Ideally, the increase in permeation enhancement should not cause skin irritation or any other kind of damage to the skin. To achieve this goal, the localization of the enhancer's effect only to the stratum corneum is necessary, though it is very difficult. Azone, one of the chemical permeation enhancers, is a solvent that increases the absorption of many drugs through the skin. Azone is usually composed by organic solvents such as dimethyl formamide, dimethylacetamide, etc (Chen et al, 2014). These solvents can only be regarded as relatively nontoxic.

Among physical transdermal permeation enhancers, for ionic drugs, absorption may be enhanced transdermally by *iontophoresis*, a method in which an electric field is maintained across the epidermal layer with special miniature electrodes. Some drugs, such as lidocaine, verapamil, insulin, and peptides, have been absorbed through the skin by iontophoresis. A process in which transdermal drug delivery is aided by high-frequency sound is called *sonophoresis*. Sonophoresis has been used with hydrocortisone cream applied to the skin to enhance penetration for treating "tennis elbow" and other mild inflammatory muscular problems. Characteristic drug delivery enhancements in drug transport induced by therapeutic ultrasound have been approximately tenfold compared to passive drug delivery. Many such novel systems are being developed by drug delivery companies (Azagury et al, 2014).

Panoderm XL patch technology (Elan) is a new system that delivers a drug through a concealed miniature probe, which penetrates the stratum corneum. Panoderm XL is fully disposable and may be programmed to deliver drugs as a preset bolus, in continuous or pulsed regimen. The complexity of the device is hidden from the patient and is simple to use. Panoderm (Elan) is an electrotransdermal drug delivery system that overcomes the skin diffusion barriers through the use of low-level electric current to transport the drug through the skin. Several transdermal products, such as fentanyl, hydromorphone, calcitonin, and LHRH (luteinizing hormone–releasing hormone), are in clinical trials. More improvements in transdermal delivery of larger molecules and the use of absorption enhancers will be available in future transdermal delivery systems.

Several additional studies that are unique to the development of a transdermal drug delivery system include (1) wear and adhesiveness of the patch, (2) skin irritation, (3) skin sensitization, and (4) residual drug in the patch after removal. The FDA is asking drug companies to consider minimizing the amount of residual drug left in transdermal patches. Marketed products that use transdermal and transmucosal drug delivery systems can contain between 10% and 95% of the initial active drug even after use, according to the FDA's draft guidance published in the Federal Register, August 3, 2010. Adverse events have been reported after patients have failed to remove a patch, resulting in increased or prolonged effects of the drug (eg, fentanyl patch).

Combination Products

Combination products are defined in 21 CFR 3.2(e).[2] The term *combination product* includes the following:

1. A product comprised of two or more regulated components, that is, drug/device, biologic/device, drug/biologic, or drug/device/biologic, that are physically, chemically, or otherwise combined or mixed and produced as a single entity
2. Two or more separate products packaged together in a single package or as a unit and comprised of drug and device products, device and biological products, or biological and drug products
3. A drug, device, or biological product packaged separately that, according to its investigational plan or proposed labeling, is intended for use only with an approved individually specified drug, device, or biological product where it is required to achieve the intended use, indication, or effect and where, upon approval of the proposed product, the labeling of the approved product would need to be changed, for example,

to reflect a change in intended use, dosage form, strength, route of administration, or significant change in dose
4. Any investigational drug, device, or biological product packaged separately that, according to its proposed labeling, is for use only with another individually specified investigational drug, device, or biological product where it is required to achieve the intended use, indication, or effect

Examples of combination products where the components are physically, chemically, or otherwise combined:

- Monoclonal antibody combined with a therapeutic drug
- Device coated or impregnated with a drug or biologic
- Drug-eluting stent; pacing lead with steroid-coated tip; catheter with antimicrobial coating; condom with spermicide
- Skin substitutes with cellular components; orthopedic implant with growth factors
- Prefilled syringes, insulin injector pens, metered dose inhalers, transdermal patches
- Drug or biological product packaged with a delivery device
- Surgical tray with surgical instruments, drapes, and lidocaine or alcohol swabs
- Photosensitizing drug and activating laser/light source
- Iontophoretic drug delivery patch and controller

In summary, combination products consist of the drug in combination with a device that is physically, chemically, or otherwise combined or mixed and produced as a single entity. The device and/or biologic is intended for use with the approved drug and influences the route of administration and pharmacokinetics of the drug.

Modified-Release Parenteral Dosage Forms

Modified-release parenteral dosage forms are parenteral dosage forms that maintain plasma drug concentrations through rate-controlled drug release from the formulation over a prolonged period of time (Martinez et al, 2008; Patil and Burgess, 2010).

[2]http://www.fda.gov/CombinationProducts/AboutCombination Products/ucm118332.htm.

Some examples of modified-release parenteral dosage forms include microspheres, liposomes, drug implants, inserts, drug-eluting stents, and nanoparticles. These formulations are designed by entrapment or microencapsulation of the drug into inert polymeric or lipophilic matrices that slowly release the drug, *in vivo*, for the duration of several days or up to several years. Modified-release parenteral dosage forms may be biodegradable or nonbiodegradable. Nonbiodegradable implants need to be surgically removed at the end of therapy.

Implants and Inserts

Despite the fact that oral route ought to be considered as highly desirable by the patients, it still represents a huge challenge, such as low bioavailability for peptides or proteins after oral administration. Alternative routes of administration (pulmonary, nasal, buccal, transdermal, ocular, and rectal) have also shown drawbacks such as enzymatic degradation or low/variable absorption. As a result, there is a renewed interest in parenteral administration because of the more and more innovation on new inactive ingredient development, especially as many improvements have been done in pain reduction. Among these approaches, biodegradable polymer-based implant and insert display excellent drug delivery characters and very good compatibility (Ding et al, 2006; Zhang et al, 2013).

In situ forming implants based on phase separation by solvent exchange are conventional preformed implants and microparticles for parenteral applications. After administration, the polymeric solutions may precipitate at the site of injection and thus forming a drug-eluting depot. Then drug release may initiate in three phases: (i) burst during precipitation of the depot, (ii) diffusion of drug through the polymeric matrix, and (iii) finally drug release by implants degradation at an extended style. They are easier to manufacture and their administration does not require surgery, therefore improving patient compliance. The drawbacks of this drug delivery system are lack of reproducibility in depot shape, burst during solidification, and potential toxicity (Parent et al, 2013).

Polymeric drug implants can deliver and sustain drug levels in the body for an extended period of time. Both biodegradable and nonbiodegradable polymers can be impregnated with drugs in a controlled drug delivery system. For example, levonorgestrel implants (Norplant system, Wyeth-Ayerst) are a set of six flexible closed capsules made of silastic (dimethylsiloxane–methylvinylsiloxane copolymer), each containing 36 μg of the progestin levonorgestrel. The capsules are sealed with silastic adhesive and sterilized. The Norplant system is available in an insertion kit to facilitate subdermal insertion of all six capsules in the mid-portion of the upper arm. The dose of levonorgestrel is about 85 μg/day, followed by a decline to about 50 μg/day by 9 months and to about 35 μg/day by 18 months, declining further to about 30 μg/day. The levonorgestrel implants are effective for up to 5 years for contraception and then must be replaced. An intrauterine progesterone contraceptive system (Progestasert, Alza) is a T-shaped unit that contains a reservoir of 38 μg of progesterone. Contraceptive effectiveness for Progestasert is enhanced by continuous release of progesterone into the uterine cavity at an average rate of 65 μg/day for 1 year.

A dental insert available for the treatment of peridontitis is the doxycycline hyclate delivery system (Atrigel®). This is a subgingival controlled-release product consisting of two-syringe mixing systems that, when combined, form a bioabsorbable, flowable polymeric formulation. After administration under the gum, the liquid solidifies and then allows for controlled release of doxycycline for a period of 7 days.

Nanotechnology-Derived Drugs

Nanotechnology is the manufacture of materials in the nanometer size range, usually less than 100–200 nm. Nanotechnology has been applied to drug development, food, electronics, biomaterials, and other applications. Nanoscale materials have chemical, physical, or biological properties that are totally different with comparison to those of their larger counterparts. Such differences may include altered surface area, magnetic properties, altered electrical or optical activity, increased structural integrity, or altered chemical or biological activity (Nanotechnology, FDA 2007). Because of these properties, nanoscale materials have great potential for use in a variety of therapeutic agents. Because of some of their special properties, nanoscale materials may pose different safety and efficacy issues compared to their larger or smaller (ie, molecular) counterparts.

According to the materials composition, the nanoparticles can be categorized into two main aspects: organic and inorganic. Organic-based nanoparticles may be composed from biodegradable materials, such as polylactide (PLA), polyglycolide (PGA), poly(lactide-co-glycolide) (PLGA), polyethylene glycol (PEG), etc, and some biocompatible materials, for example, poly(propylene oxide) (PPO), polyvinylpyrrolidone (PVP), etc. Inorganic-based nanoparticles may come from gold, iron oxide, etc. All of them displayed bright future in the area of controlled drug delivery (Ding et al, 2007, 2011, 2013).

In addition to the large surface area of nanoparticles, surface modification of the nanoparticles such as binding different chemical groups to the surface with surfactants or biocompatible polymers (eg, polyethylene glycol, PEG) changes the pharmacokinetics, toxicity, and surface reactivity of the nanoparticles, *in vivo*. Therefore, nanoparticles can have a wide variety of properties that are markedly different from the same materials in larger particle forms (Couvreur and Vauthier, 2006) (see also Chapter 18).

Liposomes

A liposome is a microvesicle composed of a bilayer of lipid amphipathic molecules enclosing an aqueous compartment (FDA Guidance for Industry, 2002). Liposomes may be nanoparticle size or larger. Its outer size can be controlled by the process of filter pore, from 50 to 200 nm. Liposome drug products are formed when a liposome is used to encapsulate a drug substance within the lipid bilayer or in the interior aqueous space of the liposome depending on the physicochemical characteristics of the drug. Liposomes can be composed of naturally derived phospholipids with mixed lipid chains (like egg phosphatidylethanolamine) or other surfactants. Liposome drug products exhibit a different pharmacokinetic and/or tissue distribution profile from the same drug substance (or active moiety) in a nonliposomal formulation given by the same route of administration.

Daunorubicin has been used for the treatment of ovarian cancer, AIDS-related Kaposi's sarcoma, and multiple myeloma. Two different liposomal formulations of daunorubicin are currently marketed. DaunoXome® contains an aqueous solution of the citrate salt of daunorubicin encapsulated within lipid vesicles (liposomes) composed of a lipid bilayer of distearoylphosphatidylcholine and cholesterol, whereas Doxil® is doxorubicin HCl encapsulated in liposomes that are formulated with surface-bound methoxypolyethylene glycol (MPEG). The use of MPEG is a process often referred to as pegylation, to protect liposomes from detection by the mononuclear phagocyte system (MPS) and to increase blood circulation time. Each of these products has different pharmacokinetics, and they are not interchangeable.

Another application of liposome is to change the pharmacokinetic profile and optimize the immunogenicity of loaded protein drugs. In one study, PEGylated phosphatidylinositol (PI) containing liposome was designed to load recombinant FVIII by reducing immunogenicity and prolonging the circulating half-life. Reduced activity *in vitro* and improved retention of activity in the presence of antibodies suggested strong shielding of FVIII by the particle; thus, *in vivo* studies were conducted in hemophilia A mice showing that the apparent terminal half-life was improved *versus* both free FVIII and FVIII–PI, but exposure determined by area under the curve was reduced. The formation of inhibitory antibodies after subcutaneous immunization with FVIII–PI/PEG was lower than free FVIII but resulted in a significant increase in inhibitors following intravenous administration (Peng et al, 2012).

Liposomes were first described in 1965 and soon proposed as drug delivery systems, with numerous important chemical structure improvements such as remote drug loading, size homogeneity, long-circulating (PEGylated) modification, triggered release, combination drugs loading, etc. Liposomes have been led tonumerous clinical trials in such diverse areas as the delivery of anticancer, antifungal, and antibiotic drugs, the delivery of gene medicines, and the delivery of anesthetics and anti-inflammatory drugs. Some of liposome products are on the market, and many more are in the pipeline. These lipidic

TABLE 19-10   Marketed and in Clinic Trial Liposomal and Lipid-Based Drug Products

Trade Name	Manufacturer	Generic Name	Description
Marketed			
Doxil/Caelyx	Johnson & Johnson	Doxorubicin	Kaposi's sarcoma, Ovarian cancer, Breast cancer, Multiple myeloma + Velcade
Myocet	Cephalon	Doxorubicin	Breast cancer + cyclophosphamide
DaunoXome	Galen	Daunorubicin	Kaposi's sarcoma
Amphotec	Intermune	Amphotericin B	Invasive aspergillosis
DepoDur	Pacira	Morphine sulfate	Pain following surgery
DepoCyt	Pacira	Cytosine + Arabinoside	Lymphomatous, meningitis, Neoplastic
Diprivan	AstraZeneca	Propofol	Anesthesia
Estrasorb	King	Estrogen	Menopausal therapy
Marqibo	Talon	Vincristine	Acute lymphoblastic leukemia
Clinic trials			
SPI-077	Alza	Cisplatin	Solid tumors (Phase II)
CPX-351	Celator	Cytarabine: daunorubicin	Acute myeloid leukemia (Phase II)
MM-398	Merrimack	CPT-11	Gastric and pancreatic cancer (Phase II)
Lipoplatin	Regulon	Cisplatin	Non-small cell lung cancer (Phase III)
ThermoDox	Celsion	Thermosensitive doxorubicin	Primary hepatocellular, carcinoma, Refractory chest wall breast cancer, Colorectal liver metastases (Phase III)
Stimuvax	Oncothyreon/Merck	Anti-MUC1 cancer vaccine	Non-small cell lung cancer (Phase III)
Exparel	Pacira	Bupivacaine	Nerve block (Phase II)

nanoparticles are the first nanomedicine delivery system to make the transition from concept to clinical application, and they are now an established technology platform with considerable clinical acceptance (Allen and Cullis, 2013). Table 19-10 lists the liposomal or lipid-based drug products in the market or still in the clinical trials. From this table, not only the chemical drugs but also the antibodies, vaccine, nucleic acids, and gene medicine can be loaded into liposome, for treatment of infections and for cancer treatment, for lung disease, and for skin conditions. With surface bioconjugating of targeting molecules on the long-circulating liposome, the common "passive" liposomal drug delivery system may evolve to "active" system in the coming future.

Polymer-Based Nano Drug Delivery System

The term "polymer therapeutics" was coined to describe the therapeutics associated with polymer, including polymeric drugs, polymer conjugates of proteins, drugs, and aptamers, together with those block copolymer micelles and multicomponent nonviral vectors. These nonviral vectors may display as micelles, implants, inserts, and nanoparticles.

Poly(lactic-co-glycolic) acid (PLGA), poly(lactic acid) (PLA), and polyglycolic acid (PGA) are perhaps the most commonly studied polymers due to their versatility in tuning biodegradation time and high biocompatibility arising from their natural by-products, lactic acid, and glycolic acid. Now polylactide has been commonly used in the surgery, while polyglycolide or its drug conjugates are being increasingly used as a drug carrier. Their molecular weight can be tailored to the expected extent upon the clinic requirement. Because of the unique property of biodegradability and integration of quality-by-design approach (QbD) concept during the development, this polymer therapeutics can be applied to preclinical structure optimization of and to manufacturing process control.

Lupron Depot® is the first US Food and Drug Administration (FDA)-approved microparticle-based depot drug delivery system. Lupron Depot consists of leuprolide encapsulated in PLGA microspheres. In order to improve the compliance of leuprolide injection, Takeda-Abbott Products developed this new class of controlled-release polymeric drug delivery system for the treatment of advanced prostate cancer. Lupron Depot has been approved for management of endometriosis and also for the treatment of central precocious puberty. Lupron Depot has been commercially successful, reaching annual sales of nearly $1 billion (Anselmo and Mitragotri, 2014). Lupron Depot can be intramuscularly injected, having dosage schedule as 7.5 mg 1×/month, 22.5 mg 1× for every 3 months or 30 mg 1× for every 4 months. The peptide drug is released from these depot formulations at a functionally constant daily rate for 1, 3, or 4 months, depending on the polymer type (polylactic/glycolic acid [PLGA] for a 1-month depot and polylactic acid [PLA] for depot of >2 months), with doses ranging between 3.75 and 30 mg. Mean peak plasma leuprorelin concentrations (C_{max}) of 13.1, 20.8 to 21.8, 47.4, 54.5, and 53 μg/L occur within 1–3 hours of depot subcutaneous administration of 3.75, 7.5, 11.25, 15, and 30 mg, respectively, compared with 32–35 μg/L at 36–60 minutes after a subcutaneous injection of 1 mg of a non-depot formulation. Sustained drug release from the PLGA microspheres maintains plasma concentrations between 0.4 and 1.4 μg/L over 28 days after single 3.75, 7.5, or 15 mg depot injections. Mean areas under the concentration–time curve (AUCs) are similar for subcutaneous or intravenous injection of short-acting leuprorelin. A 3-month depot PLA formulation of leuprorelin acetate 11.25 mg ensures a C_{max} of around 20 μg/L at 3 hours after subcutaneous injection and continuous drug concentrations of 0.43–0.19 μg/L from day

7 until before the next injection (Dreicer et al, 2011; Periti et al, 2002).

In the area of polymer therapeutics, polymeric drugs, polymeric sequestrants, and PEG conjugates (both protein conjugates and the PEG-aptamer conjugate) have progressed to market or under clinic trials. Table 19-11 shows the marketed and clinical trial polymeric therapeutics. Particular success stories include Copaxone as a treatment for multiple sclerosis (a complex random copolymer of three amino acids), the PEGylated interferons (Pegasys; Peg-Intron), and the PEGylated rhG-CSF (Neulasta) as a more convenient once-a-cycle adjunct to cancer chemotherapy (Duncan and Vicent, 2013).

> **Frequently Asked Questions**
>
> ▶ *How do patient-specific variables influence performance of modified-release dosage forms?*
>
> ▶ *What is the difference between the different types of modified-release dosage forms?*

CONSIDERATIONS IN THE EVALUATION OF MODIFIED-RELEASE PRODUCTS

The development of a modified-release formulation has to be based on a well-defined clinical need and on an integration of physiological, pharmacodynamic (PD), and pharmacokinetic (PK) considerations. The two important requirements in the development of extended-release products are (1) demonstration of safety and efficacy and (2) demonstration of controlled drug release.

Safety and efficacy data are available for many drugs given in a conventional or immediate-release dosage form. Bioavailability data of the drug from the extended-release drug product should demonstrate sustained plasma drug concentrations and bioavailability equivalent to giving the conventional dosage in the same total daily dose in two or more multiple doses. The bioavailability data requirements are specified in the Code of Federal

TABLE 19-11   Marketed and Clinical Trials Polymeric Therapeutics

Trade Name	Sub Class	Composition	Market/Clinic Trial
Copaxone		Glu, Ala, Tyr copolymer	Market
Vivagel	Polymeric drugs	Lysine-based dendrimer	Phase III
Hyaluronic acid		Hyalgal, Synvisc	Market
Zinostatin Stimaler	Polymer–protein conjugates	Styrene maleic anhydride-neocarzinostatin, (SMANCS)	Market (Japan)
Cimzia		PEG-anti-TNF Fab	Market
Peg-intron	PEGylated proteins	PEG-Interferon alpha 2b	Market
Neulasta		PEG-hrGCSF	Market
Macugen	PEGylated-aptamer	PEG-aptamer (apatanib)	Market
CT-2103; Xyotax	Polymer–drug conjugate	Poly-glutamic acid (PGA)-paclitaxel	Phase II/III
NKTR-118		PEG-naloxone	Phase III
IT-101	Self-assembled polymer conjugate nanoparticles	Polymer conjugated-cyclodextrin nanoparticle-camptothecin	Phase II
NK-6004	Block copolymer micelles	Cisplatin block copolymer micelle	Phase II

Regulations, 21 CFR 320.25(f). The important points are as follows.

1. The product should demonstrate sustained release, as claimed, without dose-dumping (abrupt release of a large amount of the drug in an uncontrolled manner).
2. The drug should show steady-state levels comparable to those reached using a conventional dosage form given in multiple doses, and which was demonstrated to be effective.
3. The drug product should show consistent pharmacokinetic performance between individual dosage units.
4. The product should allow for the maximum amount of drug to be absorbed while maintaining minimum patient-to-patient variation.
5. The demonstration of steady-state drug levels after the recommended doses are given should be within the effective plasma drug levels for the drug.
6. An *in vitro* method and data that demonstrate the reproducible extended-release nature of the product should be developed. The *in vitro* method usually consists of a suitable dissolution

procedure that provides a meaningful *in vitro–in vivo* correlation.
7. *In vivo* pharmacokinetic data consist of single and multiple dosing comparing the extended-release product to a reference standard (usually an approved non-sustained-release or a solution product).

The pharmacokinetic data usually consist of plasma drug data and/or drug excreted into the urine. Pharmacokinetic analyses are performed to determine such parameters as $t_{1/2}$, V_D, t_{max}, AUC, and k.

Pharmacodynamic and Safety Considerations

Pharmacokinetic and safety issues must be considered in the development and evaluation of a modified-release dosage form. The most critical issue is to consider whether the modified-release dosage form truly offers an advantage over the same drug in an immediate-release (conventional) form. This advantage may be related to better efficacy, reduced toxicity, or better patient compliance. However, because the cost of manufacture of a modified-release dosage form is generally higher than the cost for a conventional dosage form, economy or cost savings for patients also may be an important consideration.

Ideally, the extended-release dosage form should provide a more prolonged pharmacodynamic effect compared to the same drug given in the immediate-release form. However, an extended-release dosage form of a drug may have a different pharmacodynamic activity profile compared to the same drug given in an acute, intermittent, rapid-release dosage form. For example, transdermal patches of nitroglycerin, which produce prolonged delivery of the drug, may produce functional tolerance to vasodilation that is not observed when nitroglycerin is given sublingually for acute angina attacks. Certain bactericidal antibiotics such as penicillin may be more effective when given in intermittent (pulsed) doses compared to continuous dosing. The continuous blood level of a hormone such as a corticosteroid might suppress adrenocorticotropic hormone (ACTH) release from the pituitary gland, resulting in atrophy of the adrenal gland. Furthermore, drugs that act indirectly or cause irreversible toxicity may be less efficacious when given in an extended-release rather than in conventional dosage form.

Because the modified-release dosage form may be in contact with the body for a prolonged period, the recurrence of sensitivity reactions or local tissue reactions due to the drug or constituents of the dosage form are possible. For oral modified-release dosage forms, prolonged residence time in the GI tract may lead to a variety of interactions with GI tract contents, and the efficiency of absorption may be compromised as the drug moves distally from the duodenum to the large intestine.

Moreover, dosage form failure due to either dose-dumping or the lack of drug release may have important clinical implications. Another possible unforeseen problem with modified-release dosage forms is an alteration in the metabolic fate of the drug, such as nonlinear biotransformation or site-specific disposition.

Design and selection of extended-release products are often aided by dissolution tests carried out at different pH units for various time periods to simulate the condition of the GI tract. This *in vitro–in vivo* correlation is also called as IVIVC for oral

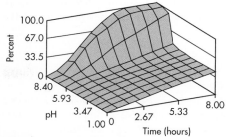

FIGURE 19-12 Topographical dissolution characterization of theophylline controlled release. Topographical dissolution characterization (as a function of time and pH) of Theo-24, a theophylline controlled-release preparation, which has been shown to have a greater rate and extent of bioavailability when dosed after a high-fat meal than when dosed under fasted conditions. (From Skelly and Barr, 1987, with permission.)

extended-release drug product (will discuss further at the next section in this chapter). The supporting documents have been involved in the FDA submission of New Drug Application (NDA), Abbreviated New Drug Application (ANDA), or Antibiotic Drug Application (AADA). Topographical plots of the dissolution data may be used to graph the percent of drug dissolved versus two variables (time, pH) that may affect dissolution simultaneously. For example, Skelly and Barr have shown that extended-release preparations of theophylline, such as Theo-24, have a more rapid dissolution rate at a higher pH of 8.4 (Fig. 19-12), whereas Theo-Dur is less affected by pH (Fig. 19-13) (Skelly and Barr 1987).

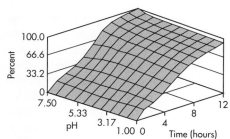

FIGURE 19-13 Topographical dissolution characterization of theophylline extended release. Topographical dissolution characterization (as a function of time and pH) of Theo-Dur, a theophylline controlled-release preparation, the bioavailability of which was essentially the same whether administered with food or under fasted conditions. (From Skelly and Barr, 1987, with permission.)

These dissolution tests *in vitro* may help predict the *in vivo* bioavailability performance of the dosage form.

> **Frequently Asked Question**
> ▶ *Does the extended-release drug product have the same safety and efficacy compared to a conventional dosage form of the same drug?*

EVALUATION OF MODIFIED-RELEASE PRODUCTS

Dissolution Studies

Dissolution requirements for each of the three types of modified-release dosage form are published in the USP-NF. Some of the key elements for the *in vitro* dissolution/drug release studies are listed in Table 19-12. Dissolution studies may be used together with bioavailability studies to predict *in vitro–in vivo* correlation of the drug release rate of the dosage forms.

In Vitro–In Vivo *Correlations (IVIVC)*

A general discussion of correlating *in vitro* drug product performance (eg, dissolution rate) to an *in vivo* biologic response (eg, blood-level-versus-time profile) is discussed in Chapter 15. Ideally, the *in vitro* drug release of the extended-release drug product should relate to the bioavailability of the drug *in vivo*, so that changes in drug dissolution rates will correlate directly to changes in drug bioavailability.

From the consideration of European Medicines Agency (EMA) and the Food and Drug Administration (FDA) on the quality control of oral modified-release drug products, *in vitro* profile for drug products has relationship with pharmacokinetics (PK), pharmacodynamics (PD), and clinical efficacy/safety. *In vitro* dissolution testing is important as a necessary quality assurance not only for batch-to-batch consistency but also to indicate consistency within a batch (ie, that individual dosage units will have the desired *in vivo* performance). By establishing a meaningful correlation between *in vitro* release characteristics and *in vivo*

TABLE 19-12 Suggested Dissolution/Drug Release Studies for Modified-Release Dosage Forms

Dissolution studies

1. Reproducibility of the method.
2. Proper choice of medium.
3. Maintenance of sink conditions.
4. Control of solution hydrodynamics.
5. Dissolution rate as a function of pH, ranging from pH 1 to pH 8 and including several intermediate values.
6. Selection of the most discriminating variables (medium, pH, rotation speed, etc) as the basis for the dissolution test and specification.

Dissolution procedures

1. Lack of dose dumping, as indicated by a narrow limit on the 1-h dissolution specification.
2. Controlled-release characteristics obtained by employing additional sampling windows over time. Narrow limits with an appropriate Q value system will control the degree of first-order release.
3. Complete drug release of the drug from the dosage form. A minimum of 75%–80% of the drug should be released from the dosage form at the last sampling interval.
4. The pH dependence/independence of the dosage form as indicated by percent dissolution in water, appropriate buffer, simulated gastric juice, or simulated intestinal fluid.

Data from Skelly and Barr, 1987.

bioavailability parameters, the *in vitro* dissolution test can serve as a surrogate marker for *in vivo* behavior and thereby confirm consistent therapeutic performance of batches from routine production. The variability of the data should be reported and discussed when establishing a correlation. In general, the higher the variability in the data used to generate the IVIVC, the less confidence can be placed on the predictive power of the correlation (Guidance for Industry, 1997; Guideline on Quality of Oral Modified Release Products, 2012).

For modified-release dosage forms, IVIVC is highly desirable in that it provides a critical linkage between product quality and clinical performance. With an established IVIVC, an *in vitro* test, such as dissolution test, can serve as a critical tool for product and process understanding; aid product/process development, manufacturing, and control; provide significantly increased assurance for consistent product performance; and predict *in vivo* performance throughout the life cycle of a modified-release product (Qiu et al, 2014).

A well-established IVIVC (Level A) is a point-to-point correlation and may apply deconvolution technique, in which *in vivo* absorption or *in vivo* dissolution can be predicted from *in vitro* data and not C_{max} and AUC. IVIVC may reduce the number of *in vivo* studies during product development, be helpful in setting specifications, and be used to facilitate certain regulatory decisions (eg, scale-up and postapproval variations). Other correlation such as Level B, the mean *in vitro* dissolution time is compared either to the mean residence time or to the mean *in vivo* dissolution time. It is not a point-to-point correlation. Level C IVIVC establishes a single-point relationship between a dissolution parameter, for example, $t_{50\%}$. Its correlation does not reflect the complete shape of the plasma concentration time curve. Multiple Level C correlation relates one or several pharmacokinetic parameters of interest to the amount of drug dissolved at several time points of the dissolution profile. In general, AUC and C_{max} of a complex modified-release product are dependent not only on the input rate and extent but also on drug properties and product design characteristics. Therefore, an attempt to develop such an IVIVC should be considered by the applicant.

Pharmacokinetic Studies

In many cases, the active drug is first formulated in an immediate-release drug product. After market experience with the immediate-release drug product, a manufacturer may design a modified or an extended-release drug product based on the pharmacokinetic profile of the immediate-release drug product as discussed earlier in this chapter. Various types of pharmacokinetic studies may be required by the Food and Drug Administration (FDA) for marketing approval of the modified-release drug product, depending on knowledge of the drug, its clinical pharmacokinetics and pharmacodynamics, and its biopharmaceutic properties (Skelley et al, 1990). Usually, a complete pharmacokinetic data package is required for a new chemical entity

developed as modified-release formulation. Additional documentation specific to the modified-release dosage form includes studies evaluating factors affecting the biopharmaceutic performance of the modified-release formulation. Moreover, the extended-release dosage form should be available in several dosage strengths to allow flexibility for the clinician to adjust the dose for the individual patient.

Single-dose ranging studies and multiple-dose steady-state crossover studies using the highest strength of the dosage form may be performed. In addition, a food intervention bioavailability study is also performed since food interactions may be related to the drug substance itself and/or the formulation, the latter being most important in the case of modified-release products. The reference dosage form may be a solution of the drug or the full NDA-approved conventional, immediate-release, dosage form given in an equal daily dose as the extended-release dosage form. If the dosage strengths differ from each other only in the amount of the drug–excipient blend, but the concentration of the drug–excipient blend is the same in each dosage form, then the FDA may approve the NDA or ANDA on the basis of single- and multiple-dose studies of the highest dosage strength, whereas the other lower-strength dosage forms may be approved on the basis of comparative *in vitro* dissolution studies (Chapter 15). The latest FDA Guidance for Industry should be consulted for regulatory requirements (www.fda.gov/cder/guidance/index.htm). Skelly et al (1990, 1993) have described several types of such pharmacokinetic studies.

Clinical Considerations of Modified-Release Drug Products

Clinical efficacy and safety may be altered when drug therapy is changed from a conventional, immediate-release (IR) drug product given several times a day to a modified, extended-release drug product given once or twice a day. Usually, the original marketed drug is a conventional, IR drug product. After experience with the IR drug product, a pharmaceutical manufacturer (sponsor) may develop an extended-release product containing the same drug. In this case, the sponsor needs to demonstrate that the pharmacokinetic profile of the extended-release drug product has sustained plasma drug concentrations compared to the conventional drug product. In addition, the sponsor may perform a clinical safety and efficacy study comparing both drug products.

Bupropion hydrochloride (Wellbutrin), an antidepressant drug, is available as an immediate-release (IR) drug product given three times a day, a sustained-release[3] (SR) drug product given twice a day, and an extended-release (XL) drug product given once a day. Jefferson et al reviewed the pharmacokinetics of these three products. These investigators reported that although the pharmacokinetic profiles are different for each drug product, the clinical efficacy for each drug product is similar if bupropion hydrochloride is given in equal daily doses. According to the approved label information for Wellbutrin XL, patients who are currently being treated with Wellbutrin tablets at 300 mg/day (eg, 100 mg 3 times a day) may be switched to Wellbutrin XL 300 mg once daily. Patients who are currently being treated with Wellbutrin SR sustained-release tablets at 300 mg/day (eg, 150 mg twice daily) may be switched to Wellbutrin XL 300 mg once daily. Thus, for buprion HCl, the fluctuations in plasma drug concentration-versus-time profiles do not affect clinical efficacy as long as the patient is given the same daily dose of drug (Jefferson et al, 2005).

Generic Substitution of Modified-Release Drug Products

Generic extended-release drug products may have different drug-release mechanisms compared to the brand-drug product. The different drug-release mechanisms may lead to slightly different pharmacokinetic profiles. Generic extended-release drug products are approved by the FDA and are bioequivalent based on AUC and C_{max} criteria and therapeutic equivalence to the brand name equivalent (Chapter 16). For some drugs, several different modified-release products containing exactly the same active ingredient are commercially available. These modified-release drug products have different pharmacokinetic profiles and may have different clinical efficacy compared to the conventional form

of the drug given in the same daily dose and compared to other extended-release products containing the same active drug. Since the pharmacokinetic profiles may differ, the practitioner needs to consult the FDA publication, *Approved Drug Products with Therapeutic Equivalence Evaluations* (Orange Book),[4] to determine which of these drug products may be substituted.

EXAMPLE ▶▶▶

Methylphenidate Drug Products

Methylphenidate hydrochloride is a central nervous system (CNS) stimulant indicated for the treatment of attention deficit hyperactivity disorder (ADHD). Numerous conventional and modified-release drug products containing methylphenidate hydrochloride are available (Table 19-13). Although each of these methylphenidate hydrochloride drug products has the same indication, the prescriber needs to understand which product would be most appropriate for the patient.

EVALUATION OF *IN VIVO* BIOAVAILABILITY DATA

The data from a properly designed *in vivo* bioavailability study are evaluated using both pharmacokinetic and statistical analysis methods. The evaluation may include a pharmacokinetic profile, steady-state plasma drug concentrations, rate of drug absorption, occupancy time, and statistical evaluation of the computed pharmacokinetic parameters.

Pharmacokinetic Profile

The plasma drug concentration–time curve should adequately define the bioavailability of the drug from the dosage form. The bioavailability data should include a profile of the fraction of drug absorbed (Wagner–Nelson) and should rule out

---

[3]A sustained-release drug product may also be called an extended-release drug product.

[4]www.fda.gov/Drugs/InformationOnDrugs/ucm129662.htm.

TABLE 19-13   Various Methylphenidate Hydrochloride Drug Products

Drug Product	Formulation	Comments
Ritalin	Immediate release	Conventional drug product
Ritalin SR	Extended release	ER drug product with no initial dose
Ritalin LA	Extended release with an initial IR dose	Produces a bi-modal plasma concentration-time profile when given orally; not interchangeable with Concerta
Concerta	Extended release with an initial IR dose	Not interchangeable for Ritalin LA
Daytrana	Film, extended release; transdermal	Provides extended release via transdermal drug absorption
Methylin	Solution; oral	Immediate release drug product
Methylin	Tablet, chewable; oral	Immediate release drug product

dose-dumping or lack of a significant food effect. The bioavailability data should also demonstrate the extended-release characteristics of the dosage form compared to the reference or immediate-release drug product.

Steady-State Plasma Drug Concentration

The fluctuation between the C_{max}^{∞} (peak) and C_{min}^{∞} (trough) concentrations should be calculated:

$$\text{Fluctation} = \frac{C_{max}^{\infty} - C_{min}^{\infty}}{C_{av}^{\infty}} \qquad (19.11)$$

where C_{av}^{∞} is equal to $[AUC]/\tau$.

An ideal extended-release dosage form should have minimum fluctuation between C_{max} and C_{min}. A true zero-order release will have no fluctuation. In practice, the fluctuation in plasma drug levels after the extended-release dosage form should be less than the fluctuation after the same drug given in an immediate-release dosage form.

Rate of Drug Absorption

For the extended-release drug product to claim zero-order absorption, an appropriately calculated input function such as used in the Wagner–Nelson approach should substantiate this claim. The difference between first-order and zero-order absorption of a drug is shown in Fig. 19-14. The rate of drug absorption from the conventional or immediate-release dosage form is generally first order, as shown by Fig. 19-14A. Drug absorption after an extended-release dosage form may be zero order (Fig. 19-14B), first order (see Fig. 19-14A), or an indeterminate order (Fig. 19-14C). For many extended-release dosage forms, the rate of drug absorption is first order, with an absorption rate constant k_a smaller than the elimination rate constant k. The pharmacokinetic model when $k_a > k$ is termed *flip-flop pharmacokinetics* and is discussed in Chapter 7.

Occupancy Time

Drugs for which the therapeutic window is known, the plasma drug concentrations should be maintained above the minimum effective drug concentration (MEC) and below the minimum toxic drug concentration (MTC). The time required to obtain plasma

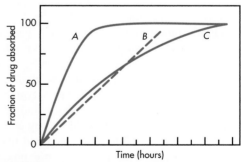

FIGURE 19-14   The fraction of drug absorbed using the Wagner–Nelson method may be used to distinguish between the first-order drug absorption rate of a conventional (immediate-release) dosage form (A) and an extended-release dosage form (C). Curve B represents an extended-release dosage form with zero-order absorption rate.

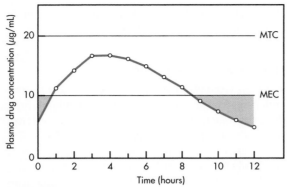

FIGURE 19-15   Occupancy time.

drug levels within the therapeutic window is known as *occupancy time* (Fig. 19-15).

Bioequivalence Studies

Bioequivalence studies for extended-release drug products are discussed in detail in Chapter 15. Bioequivalence studies may include (1) a fasting study, (2) a food-intervention study, and (3) a multiple-dose study. The FDA's Center for Drug Evaluation and Research (CDER) maintains a website (www .fda.gov/cder) that lists regulatory guidances to provide the public with the FDA's latest submission requirements for NDAs and ANDAs.

Statistical Evaluation

Variables subject to statistical analysis generally include plasma drug concentrations at each collection time, AUC (from zero to last sampling time), AUC (from zero to time infinity), C_{max}, t_{max}, and elimination half-life $t_{1/2}$. Statistical testing may include an analysis of variance (ANOVA), computation of 90% and 95% confidence intervals on the difference in formulation means, and the power of ANOVA to detect a 20% difference from the reference mean.

Frequently Asked Questions

▶ *Are extended-release drug products always more efficacious than immediate-release drug products containing the same drug?*

▶ *Why do some extended-release formulations of a drug have a different efficacy profile compared to a conventional dosage form, given in multiple doses?*

▶ *What are the advantages and disadvantages of a zero-order rate design for drug absorption?*

CHAPTER SUMMARY

The goal of modified-release (MR) formulations is to reduce the peak-to-trough fluctuations of drug concentrations and, consequently, enable the less frequent administration of the drug. This is generally accomplished by lowering the rate of drug release with better patient compliance and thereby that of drug absorption. In this drug product, the timing and the rate of drug release can be adjusted according to clinic requirement along with efficacy and safety consideration, which cannot be achieved by conventional dosage forms. Within the modified-release formulations, extended-release (ER) drug products are one of the most important compositions not only minimizing the possible side effects derived from fluctuating plasma drug concentrations but also offering a prolonged therapeutic effect. Oral modified-release drug products are easily affected by the anatomy and physiology of the gastrointestinal tract, gastrointestinal transit, pH, and its contents compared to conventional oral drug products. Modified-release drug products may also have a different pharmacodynamic and safety profile compared to immediate-release drug products containing the same drug. With help from the more and more biodegradable materials developed, various approaches have been used to manufacture modified- and extended-release drug products including matrix tablets, coated beads, osmotic release, ion-exchange, liposome, polymeric therapeutics, etc. The administration method may not only limit in the area of oral route but also includes transdermal, injection, nasal, etc. Although the route of administration and pharmacokinetic parameters may be different, the bioequivalence should be equal or improved between immediate-release formulations with modified-release drug products. More and more pharmacometrics have been applied to the *in vivo* and clinic prediction, including single-dose studies, steady-state studies, partial AUC calculation, *in vitro–in vivo* correlation (IVIVC) assay, etc. Overall, modified-release products may have different clinical efficacy compared to other extended-release products containing the same active drug. The practitioner needs to consult the FDA publication *Approved Drug Products with Therapeutic Equivalence Evaluations* (Orange Book) to determine which of these drug products may be substituted.

LEARNING QUESTIONS

1. The design for most extended-release or sustained-release oral drug products allows for the slow release of the drug from the dosage form and subsequent slow absorption of the drug from the gastrointestinal tract.
   a. Why does the slow release of a drug from an extended-release drug product produce a longer-acting pharmacodynamic response compared to the same drug prepared in a conventional, oral, immediate-release drug product?
   b. Why do manufacturers of sustained-release drug products attempt to design this dosage form to have a zero-order rate of systemic drug absorption?
2. The dissolution profiles of three drug products are illustrated in Fig. 19-16.
   a. Which of the drug products in Fig. 19-16 releases drug at a zero-order rate of about 8.3% every hour?
   b. Which of the drug products does not release drug at a zero-order rate?
   c. Which of the drug products has an almost zero rate of drug release during certain hours of the dissolution process?
   d. Suggest a common cause of slowing drug dissolution rate of many rapid-release drug products toward the end of dissolution.
   e. Suggest a common cause of slowing drug dissolution of a sustained-release product toward the end of a dissolution test.

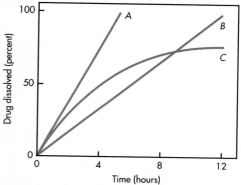

FIGURE 19-16   Dissolution profile of three different drug products. Drug dissolved (percent).

3. A drug is normally given at 10 mg 4 times a day. Suggest an approach for designing a 12-hour, zero-order release product.
   a. Calculate the desired zero-order release rate.
   b. Calculate the concentration of the drug in an osmotic pump type of oral dosage form that delivers 0.5 mL/h of fluid.
4. An industrial pharmacist would like to design a sustained-release drug product to be given every 12 hours. The active drug ingredient has an apparent volume of distribution of 10 L, an elimination half-life of 3.5 hours, and a desired therapeutic plasma drug concentration of 20 μg/mL. Calculate the zero-order release rate of the sustained-release drug product and the total amount of drug needed, assuming no loading dose is required.

REFERENCES

Abdul S, Chandewar AV, Jaiswal SB: A flexible technology for modified-release drugs: Multiple-unit pellet system (MUPS). *J Control Rel* **147**(1):2–16, 2010. doi: http://dx.doi.org/10.1016/j.jconrel.2010.05.014.

Abrahamsson B, Albery T, Eriksson A, Gustafsson I, Sjöberg M: Food effects on tablet disintegration. *Eur J Pharm Sci* **22**(2–3):165–172, 2004. doi: http://dx.doi.org/10.1016/j.ejps.2004.03.004.

Adibkia K, Ghanbarzadeh S, Shokri MH, Arami Z, Arash Z, Shokri J: Micro-porous surfaces in controlled drug delivery systems: Design and evaluation of diltiazem hydrochloride controlled porosity osmotic pump using non-ionic surfactants as pore-former. *Pharm Dev Technol* **19**(4):507–512, 2014. doi: doi:10.3109/10837450.2013.805774.

Adibkia K, Hamedeyazdan S, Javadzadeh Y: Drug release kinetics and physicochemical characteristics of floating drug delivery systems. *Expert Opin Drug Deliv* **8**(7):891–903, 2011. doi: doi :10.1517/17425247.2011.574124.

Allen TM, Cullis PR: Liposomal drug delivery systems: From concept to clinical applications. *Adv Drug Deliv Rev* **65**(1):36–48, 2013. doi: http://dx.doi.org/10.1016/j.addr .2012.09.037.

Anselmo AC, Mitragotri S: An overview of clinical and commercial impact of drug delivery systems. *J Control Rel* **190**(0):15–28, 2014. doi: http://dx.doi.org/10.1016/j.jconrel.2014.03.053.

Arora S, Ali J, Ahuja A, Khar RK, Baboota S: Floating drug delivery systems: A review. *AAPS PharmSciTech* **6**(3):E372–E390, 2005.

Arora S, Ali J, Ahuja A, Khar RK, Baboota S: Floating drug delivery systems: A review. [Review]. *AAPS PharmSciTech* **6**(3):E372–E390, 2005. doi: 10.1208/pt060347.

Asare-Addo K, Levina M, Rajabi-Siahboomi AR, Nokhodchi A: Effect of ionic strength and pH of dissolution media on theophylline release from hypromellose matrix tablets—Apparatus USP III, simulated fasted and fed conditions. *Carbohydr Polym* **86**(1):85–93, 2011. doi: http://dx.doi.org/10.1016/j.carbpol.2011.04.014.

Azagury A, Khoury L, Enden G, Kost J: Ultrasound mediated transdermal drug delivery. *Adv Drug Deliv Rev* **72**(0):127–143, 2014. doi: http://dx.doi.org/10.1016/j.addr.2014.01.007.

Badran MM, Kuntsche J, Fahr A: Skin penetration enhancement by a microneedle device (Dermaroller®) in vitro: Dependency on needle size and applied formulation. *Eur J Pharm Sci* **36**(4–5):511–523, 2009. doi: http://dx.doi.org/10.1016/j.ejps.2008.12.008.

Baracat M, Nakagawa A, Casagrande R, Georgetti S, Verri W, Jr, de Freitas O: Preparation and characterization of microcapsules based on biodegradable polymers: Pectin/Casein complex for controlled drug release systems. *AAPS PharmSciTech* **13**(2):364–372, 2012. doi: 10.1208/s12249-012-9752-0.

Bariya SH, Gohel MC, Mehta TA, Sharma OP: Microneedles: An emerging transdermal drug delivery system. *J Pharm Pharmacol* **64**(1):11–29, 2012. doi: 10.1111/j.2042-7158.2011.01369.x.

Bhattarai N, Gunn J, Zhang M: Chitosan-based hydrogels for controlled, localized drug delivery. *Adv Drug Deliv Rev* **62**(1): 83–99, 2010. doi: http://dx.doi.org/10.1016/j.addr.2009.07.019.

Breimer DD, Dauhof M: *Towards Better Safety of Drugs and Pharmaceutical Products*. Amsterdam, Elsevier/North-Holland, 1980, pp 117–142.

Brunner M, Ziegler S, Di Stefano AFD, et al: Gastrointestinal transit, release and plasma pharmacokinetics of a new oral budesonide formulation. *British Journal of Clinical Pharmacology* **61**(1):31–38, 2006. doi: 10.1111/j.1365-2125 .2005.02517.x.

Chen Y, Cun D, Quan P, Liu X, Guo W, Peng L, Fang L: Saturated long-chain esters of isopulegol as novel permeation enhancers for transdermal drug delivery. *Pharm Res* **31**(8):1907–1918, 2014. doi: 10.1007/s11095-013-1292-0.

Cheng C, Wu P-C, Lee H-Y, Hsu K-Y: Development and validation of an in vitro–in vivo correlation (IVIVC) model for propranolol hydrochloride extended-release matrix formulations. *Journal of Food and Drug Analysis* **22**(2):257–263, 2014. doi: http://dx.doi.org/10.1016/j.jfda.2013.09.016.

Clark A, Milbrandt TA, Hilt JZ, Puleo DA: Mechanical properties and dual drug delivery application of poly(lactic-co-glycolic acid) scaffolds fabricated with a poly(β-amino ester) porogen. *Acta Biomaterialia* **10**(5):2125–2132, 2014. doi: http://dx.doi.org/10.1016/j.actbio.2013.12.061.

Couvreur P, Vauthier C: Nanotechnology: Intelligent design to treat complex disease. *Pharm Res* **23**:1417–1450, 2006.

Craig D: Oxymorphone extended-release tablets (Opana ER) for the management of chronic pain. *Pharm Therap* **35**(6): 324–329, 2010.

Dash V, Mishra SK, Singh M, Goyal AK, Rath G: Release kinetic studies of aspirin microcapsules from ethyl cellulose, cellulose acetate phthalate and their mixtures by emulsion solvent evaporation method. *Sci Pharm* **78**(1):93–101, 2010. doi: 10.3797/scipharm.0908-09.

Desai D, Wang J, Wen H, Li X, Timmins P: Formulation design, challenges, and development considerations for fixed dose combination (FDC) of oral solid dosage forms. *Pharmaceutical Development and Technology* **18**(6):1265–1276, 2013. doi: doi:10.3109/10837450.2012.660699.

Dighe SV, Adams WP: Bioavailability and bioequivalence of oral extended-release products: A regulatory perspective. In Welling PG, Tse FLS (eds). *Pharmacokinetics: Regulatory, Industrial, Academic Perspectives*. New York, Marcel Dekker, 1988.

Ding H, Wu F, Huang Y, Zhang Z, Nie Y: Synthesis and characterization of temperature-responsive copolymer of PELGA modified poly(N-isopropylacrylamide). *Polymer* **47**(5):1575–1583, 2006. doi: http://dx.doi.org/10.1016/j.polymer.2005.12.018.

Ding H, Wu F, Nair MP: Image-guided drug delivery to the brain using nanotechnology. *Drug Discov Today* **18**(21–22): 1074–1080, 2013. doi: http://dx.doi.org/10.1016/j.drudis .2013.06.010.

Ding H, Yong K, Roy I, Pudavar H, Law W, Bergey E, Prasad P: Gold nanorods coated with multilayer polyelectrolyte as contrast agents for multimodal imaging. *The Journal of Physical Chemistry C* **111**(34):12552–12557, 2007. doi: 10.1021 /jp0733419.

Ding H, Yong KT, Roy I, et al: Bioconjugated PLGA-4-arm-PEG branched polymeric nanoparticles as novel tumor targeting carriers. [Research Support, N.I.H., Extramural]. *Nanotechnology* **22**(16):165101, 2011. doi: 10.1088/0957-4484/22/16/165101.

Dong L, Shafi K, Wong P, Wan J: L-OROS® SOFTCAP™ for controlled release of non-aqueous liquid formulation. *Drug Deliv Technol* **2**(1):52–55, 2002.

Dreicer R, Bajorin DF, McLeod DG, Petrylak DP, Moul JW: New data, new paradigms for treating prostate cancer patients—VI: Novel hormonal therapy approaches. *Urology* **78**(5):S494–S498, 2011.

Duncan R, Vicent MJ: Polymer therapeutics-prospects for 21st century: The end of the beginning. *Advanced Drug Delivery Reviews* **65**(1):60–70, 2013. doi: http://dx.doi.org/10.1016/j.addr.2012.08.012.

Eberle VA, Schoelkopf J, Gane PAC, Alles R, Huwyler J, Puchkov M: Floating gastroretentive drug delivery systems: Comparison of experimental and simulated dissolution profiles and floatation behavior. *Eur J Pharm Sci* **58**(0):34–43, 2014. doi: http://dx.doi.org/10.1016/j.ejps.2014.03.001.

Eisenmann A, Amann A, Said M, Datta B, Ledochowski M: Implementation and interpretation of hydrogen breath tests. *J Breath Res* **2**:046002–046009, 2008.

FDA Guidance for Industry: Liposome Drug Products-Chemistry, Manufacturing, and Controls; Human Pharmacokinetics and Bioavailability; and Labeling Documentation, Draft, August, 2002.

Franek F, Holm P, Larsen F, Steffansen B: Interaction between fed gastric media (Ensure Plus®) and different hypromellose based caffeine controlled release tablets: Comparison and mechanistic study of caffeine release in fed and fasted media versus water using the USP dissolution apparatus 3. *Int J Pharm* **461**(1–2):419–426, 2014. doi: http://dx.doi.org/10.1016/j.ijpharm.2013.12.003.

Gonzalez MA, Cleary GW: Transdermal dosage forms. In Shargel L, Kanfer I (eds). *Generic Drug Product Development–Specialty Dosage Forms*. New York, Informa Healthcare, 2010, Chap 8.

Grund J, Koerber M, Walther M, Bodmeier R: The effect of polymer properties on direct compression and drug release from water-insoluble controlled release matrix tablets. *International Journal of Pharmaceutics* **469**(1):94–101, 2014. doi: http://dx.doi.org/10.1016/j.ijpharm.2014.04.033.

Guidance for Industry. Extended Release Oral Dosage Forms: Development, Evaluation, and Application of In Vitro/In Vivo Correlations. Food and Drug Administration (FDA), 1997.

Guideline on Quality of Oral Modified Release Products. European Medicines Agency, 2012.

Guy RH: Current status and future prospects of transdermal drug delivery. *Pharm Res* **13**:1765–1769, 1996.

Henry S, McAllister DV, Allen MG, Prausnitz MR: Microfabricated microneedles: A novel approach to transdermal drug delivery. [In Vitro Research Support, Non-U.S. Gov't Research Support, U.S. Gov't, Non-P.H.S.]. *J Pharm Sci* **87**(8):922–925, 1998. doi: 10.1021/js980042+.

Hofmann AF, Pressman JH, Code CF, Witztum KF: Controlled entry of orally administereddrugs: Physiological considerations. *Drug Dev Ind Pharm* **9**(7):1077–1109, 1983. doi: 10.3109/03639048309046314.

Honório TS, Pinto E, Rocha H, et al: In vitro–in vivo correlation of efavirenz tablets using GastroPlus®. *AAPS PharmSciTech* **14**(3):1244–1254, 2013. doi: 10.1208/s12249-013-0016-4.

Jain AK, Söderlind E, Viridén A, et al: (2014). The influence of hydroxypropyl methylcellulose (HPMC) molecular weight, concentration and effect of food on in vivo erosion behavior of HPMC matrix tablets. *J Control Rel* **187**(0):50–58, 2014. doi: http://dx.doi.org/10.1016/j.jconrel.2014.04.058.

Jefferson JW, Pradko JF, Muir KT: Bupropion for major depressive disorder: Pharmacokinetic and formulation considerations. *Clin Ther* **27**(11):1685–1695, 2005.

Jonkman JHG: Food interactions with once-a-day theophylline preparations: A review. *Chronobiology International* **4**(3):449–458, 1987. doi: 10.3109/07420528709083533.

Jonkman JHG: Food interactions with sustained-release theophylline preparations. *Clin Pharmacokinet* **16**(3):162–179, 1989. doi: 10.2165/00003088-198916030-00003.

Kambayashi A, Blume H, Dressman JB: Predicting the oral pharmacokinetic profiles of multiple-unit (pellet) dosage forms using a modeling and simulation approach coupled with biorelevant dissolution testing: Case example diclofenac sodium. *Eur J Pharm Biopharm* **87**(2):236–243, 2014. doi: http://dx.doi.org/10.1016/j.ejpb.2014.01.007.

Kawai Y, Fujii Y, Tabata F, et al: Profiling and trend analysis of food effects on oral drug absorption considering micelle interaction and solubilization by bile micelles. *Drug Metab Pharmacokinet* **26**(2):180–191, 2011. doi: 10.2133/dmpk.DMPK-10-RG-098.

Kleiner LW, Wright JC, Wang Y: Evolution of implantable and insertable drug delivery systems. *J Control Rel* **181**(0):1–10, 2014. doi: http://dx.doi.org/10.1016/j.jconrel.2014.02.006.

Krivoguz YM, Guliyev AM, Pesetskii SS: Free-radical grafting of trans-ethylene-1,2-dicarboxylic acid onto molten ethylene-vinyl acetate copolymer. *J Appl Polym Sci* **127**(4):3104–3113, 2013. doi: 10.1002/app.37703.

Lee PI: Modeling of drug release from matrix systems involving moving boundaries: Approximate analytical solutions. *Int J Pharm* **418**(1):18–27, 2011. doi: http://dx.doi.org/10.1016/j.ijpharm.2011.01.019.

Li L, Wang L, Shao Y, et al: Elucidation of release characteristics of highly soluble drug trimetazidine hydrochloride from chitosan–carrageenan matrix tablets. *J Pharm Sci* **102**(8): 2644–2654, 2013. doi: 10.1002/jps.23632.

Malinovskaja K, Laaksonen T, Kontturi K, Hirvonen J: Ion-exchange and iontophoresis-controlled delivery of apomorphine. *Eur J Pharm Biopharm* **83**(3):477–484, 2013. doi: http://dx.doi.org/10.1016/j.ejpb.2012.11.014.

Marasanapalle VP, Crison JR, Ma J, Li X, Jasti BR: Investigation of some factors contributing to negative food effects. *Biopharm Drug Dispos* **30**(2):71–80, 2009. doi: 10.1002/bdd.647.

Maroni A, Zema L, Curto MDD, Loreti G, Gazzaniga A: Oral pulsatile delivery: Rationale and chronopharmaceutical formulations. *Int J Pharm* **398**(1–2):1–8, 2010. doi: http://dx.doi.org/10.1016/j.ijpharm.2010.07.026.

Martinez M, Rathbone M, Burgess D, Huynh M: In vitro and in vivo considerations associated with parenteral sustained release products: A review based upon information presented and points expressed at the 2007 Controlled Release Society Annual Meeting. *J Control Rel* **129**:79–87, 2008.

Meulenaar J, Keizer RJ, Beijnen JH, Schellens JHM, Huitema ADR, Nuijen B: Development of an extended-release formulation of capecitabine making use of in vitro–in vivo correlation modelling. *J Pharm Sci* **103**(2):478–484, 2014. doi: 10.1002/jps.23779.

Nagaraju R, Swapna Y, Baby RH, Kaza R: Design and evaluation of delayed and extended release tablets of mesalamine. *J Pharm Technol* **2**(1):103–110, 2010.

Nanotechnology, A Report of the U.S. Food and Drug Administration Nanotechnology Task Force, July 25, 2007 (http://www.fda.gov/downloads/ScienceResearch/SpecialTopics/Nanotechnology/ucm110856.pdf).

Pachuau L, Mazumder B: Albizia procera gum as an excipient for oral controlled release matrix tablet. *Carbohydr Polym* **90**(1):289–295, 2012. doi: http://dx.doi.org/10.1016/j.carbpol.2012.05.038.

Parent M, Nouvel C, Koerber M, Sapin A, Maincent P, Boudier A: PLGA in situ implants formed by phase inversion: Critical physicochemical parameters to modulate drug release. *J Control Rel* **172**(1):292–304, 2013. doi: http://dx.doi.org/10.1016/j.jconrel.2013.08.024.

Patil SD, Burgess DJ: Pharmaceutical development of modified release parenteral dosage forms using bioequivalence (BE), quality by design (QBD) and in vitro in vivo correlation (IVIVC) principles. In Shargel I, Kanfer I (eds). *Generic Drug Product Development–Specialty Dosage Forms*. New York, Informa Healthcare, 2010, Chap 9.

Peng A, Kosloski M, Nakamura G, Ding H, Balu-Iyer S: PEGylation of a factor VIII–phosphatidylinositol complex: Pharmacokinetics and immunogenicity in hemophilia a mice. *AAPS J* **14**(1):35–42, 2012. doi: 10.1208/s12248-011-9309-2.

Peppas NA, Narasimhan B: Mathematical models in drug delivery: How modeling has shaped the way we design new drug delivery systems. *J Control Rel* **190**(0):75–81, 2014. doi: http://dx.doi.org/10.1016/j.jconrel.2014.06.041.

Periti P, Mazzei T, Mini E (2002). Clinical pharmacokinetics of depot leuprorelin. *Clin Pharmacokinet* **41**(7):485–504, 2002. doi: 10.2165/00003088-200241070-00003.

Qiu Y, Li X, Duan JZ: Influence of drug property and product design on in vitro–in vivo correlation of complex modified-release dosage forms. *J Pharm Sci* **103**(2):507–516, 2014. doi: 10.1002/jps.23804.

Rahman M, Roy S, Das SC, et al: Evaluation of various grades of hydroxypropyl methylcellulose matrix systems as oral sustained release drug delivery systems. *J Pharm Sci Res* **3**(1): 930–938, 2011.

Rana V, Rai P, Tiwary AK, Singh RS, Kennedy JF, Knill CJ: Modified gums: Approaches and applications in drug delivery. *Carbohydrate Polymers* **83**(3):1031–1047, 2011. doi: http://dx.doi.org/10.1016/j.carbpol.2010.09.010.

Ranjan OP, Nayak UY, Reddy MS, Dengale SJ, Musmade PB, Udupa N: Osmotically controlled pulsatile release capsule of montelukast sodium for chronotherapy: Statistical optimization, in vitro and in vivo evaluation. *Drug Deliv* **0**(0): 1–10, 2013. doi: doi:10.3109/10717544.2013.853209.

Ritschel WA: Targeting in the gastrointestinal tract: new approaches, method and find. *Exp Clin Pharmacol* **13**(5):313–336, 1991.

Rosiaux Y, Velghe C, Muschert S, Chokshi R, Leclercq B, Siepmann F, Siepmann, J: Mechanisms Controlling Theophylline Release from Ethanol-Resistant Coated Pellets. *Pharmaceutical Research* **31**(3):731–741, 2014. doi: 10.1007/s11095-013-1194-1.

Shareef MA, Ahuja A, Ahmad FJ, Raghava S: Colonic drug delivery: An updated review. *AAPS PharmSci* **5**:161–186, 2003.

Shareef MA, Khar RK, Ahuja A, Ahmad FJ, & S., R. (2003). Colonic drug delivery: an updated review. *AAPS PharmSci* **5**(2), E17.

Singh MN, Hemant KS, Ram M, Shivakumar HG: (2010). Microencapsulation: A promising technique for controlled drug delivery. *Res Pharm Sci* **5**(2):65–77, 2010.

Skelley JP, Amidon GL, Barr WH, et al: Report of the workshop on in vitro and in vivo testing and correlation for oral controlled/modified-release dosage forms. *J Pharm Sci* **79**(9):849–854, 1990. doi: 10.1002/jps.2600790923.

Skelly JP, Barr WH: Regulatory assessment. In Robinson JR, Lee VHL (eds). *Controlled Drug Delivery: Fundamentals and Applications*, 2nd ed. New York, Marcel Dekker, 1987.

Skelly JP, Van Buskirk GA, Arbit HM, et al: Scaleup of oral extended-release dosage forms. *Pharm Res* **10**(12): 1800–1805, 1993. doi: 10.1023/a:1018946819849.

Subedi R, Oh S, Chun M-K, Choi H-K: (2010). Recent advances in transdermal drug delivery. *Arch Pharmacol Res* **33**(3):339–351, 2010. doi: 10.1007/s12272-010-0301-7.

Sujja-areevath J, Munday DL, Cox PJ, Khan KA (1998). Relationship between swelling, erosion and drug release in hydrophillic natural gum mini-matrix formulations. *Eur J Pharm Sci* **6**(3):207–217, 1998. doi: http://dx.doi.org/10.1016/S0928-0987(97)00072-9.

Viridén A, Wittgren B, Larsson A: Investigation of critical polymer properties for polymer release and swelling of HPMC matrix tablets. *Eur J Pharm Sci* **36**(2–3):297–309, 2009. doi: http://dx.doi.org/10.1016/j.ejps.2008.10.021.

Welling PG: Oral controlled drug administration pharmacokinetic considerations. *Drug Dev Ind Pharm* **9**:1185–1225, 1983.

Wilson B, Babubhai PP, Sajeev MS, Jenita JL, SRB P: Sustained release enteric coated tablets of pantoprazole: Formulation, in vitro and in vivo evaluation. *Acta Pharmaceutica* **63**(1): 131–140, 2013.

Wu F, Ding H, ZR Z: Investigation of the in vivo desintegration and transit behavior of tetramethylpyrazine phosphate pulsincap capsule in the GI tract of dogs by gamma scintigraphy. *Journal of Biomedical Engineering* **23**(4):790–794, 2006.

Yu, LX, Crison JR, Amidon GL: (1996). Compartmental transit and dispersion model analysis of small intestinal transit flow in humans. *Int J Pharm* **140**(1):111–118, 1996. doi: http://dx.doi.org/10.1016/0378-5173(96)04592-9.

Zhang X, Zhang C, Zhang W, et al: Feasibility of poly (ε-caprolactone-co-DL-lactide) as a biodegradable material for in situ forming implants: Evaluation of drug release and in vivo degradation. *Drug Dev Ind Pharm* **0**(0):1–11, 2013. doi: doi:10.3109/03639045.2013.866140.

Zhang Y, Zhang Z, Wu F: A novel pulsed-release system based on swelling and osmotic pumping mechanism. *J Control Rel* **89**(1):47–55, 2003. doi: http://dx.doi.org/10.1016/S0168-3659 (03)00092-0.

Zhu Q, Talton J, Zhang G, et al: Large intestine-targeted, nanoparticle-releasing oral vaccine to control genitorectal viral infection. *Nat Med* **18**(8):1291–1296, 2012. doi: 10.1038/nm.2866..

BIBLIOGRAPHY

Akala EO, Collett JH: Influence of drug loading and gel structure on in-vitro release kinetics from photopolymerized gels. *Ind Pharm* **13**:1779–1798, 1987.

Arnon R: In Gregoriadis G, Senior J, Trouet A (eds). *Targeting of Drugs*. New York, Plenum, 1982, pp 31–54.

Arnon R, Hurwitz E: In Goldberg EP (ed). *Targeted Drugs*. New York, Wiley, 1983, pp 23–55.

Bayley H, Gasparro F, Edelson R: Photoactive drugs. *TIPS* **8**: 138–144, 1987.

Boxenbaum HG: Physiological and pharmacokinetic factors affecting performance of sustained release dosage forms. *Drug Dev Ind Pharm* **8**:1–25, 1982.

Brodsky FM: Monoclonal antibodies as magic bullets. *Pharm Res* **5**:1–9, 1988.

Bruck S (ed): *Controlled Drug Delivery*. Boca Raton, FL, CRC Press, 1983.

Cabana BE: Bioavailability regulations and biopharmaceutic standard for controlled release drug delivery. *Proceedings of 1982 Research and Scientific Development Conference.* Washington, DC, The Proprietary Association, 1983, pp 56–69.

Chien YW: *Novel Drug Delivery Systems*. New York, Marcel Dekker, 1982.

Chien YW: Oral controlled drug administration. *Drug Dev Ind Pharm* **9**: 1983.

Chien YW, Siddiqui O, Shi WM, et al: Direct current iontophoretic transdermal delivery of peptide and protein drugs. *J Pharm Sci* **78**:376–383, 1989.

Chu BCF, Whiteley JM: High molecular weight derivatives of methotrexate as chemotherapeutic agents. *Mol Pharmacol* **13**:80, 1980.

Fiume L, Busi C, Mattioli A: Targeting of antiviral drugs by coupling with protein carriers. *FEBS Lett* **153**:6, 1983.

Fiume L, Busi C, Mattioli A, et al: In Gregoriadis G, Senior J, Trouet A (eds). *Targeting of Drugs*. New York, Plenum, 1982.

Friend DR, Pangburn S: Site-specific drug delivery. *Med Res Rev* **7**:53–106, 1987.

Gros L, Ringsdorf H, Schupp H: *Angew Chem Int Ed Engl* **20**:312, 1981.

Heller J: Controlled drug release from monolithic bioerodible polymer devices. *Pharm Int* **7**:316–318, 1986.

Hunter E, Fell JT, Sharma H: The gastric emptying of pellets contained in hard gelatin capsules. *Drug Dev Ind Pharm* **8**: 151–157, 1982.

Joshi HN: Recent advances in drug delivery systems: Polymeric prodrugs. *Pharm Technol* **12**:118–125, 1988.

Langer R: New methods of drug delivery. *Science* **249**: 1527–1533, 1990.

Levy G: Targeted drug delivery: Some pharmacokinetic considerations. *Pharm Res* **4**:3–4, 1987.

Malinowski HJ: Biopharmaceutic aspects of the regulatory review of oral controlled release drug products. *Drug Dev Ind Pharm* **9**:1255–1279, 1983.

Miyazaki S, Ishii K, Nadai T: Controlled release of prednisolone from ethylene-vinyl acetate copolymer matrix. *Chem Pharm Bull* **29**:2714–2717, 1981.

Mueller-Lissner SA, Blum AL: The effect of specific gravity and eating on gastric emptying of slow-release capsules. *N Engl J Med* **304**:1365–1366, 1981.

Okabe K, Yamoguchi H, Kawai Y: New ionotophoretic transdermal administration of the beta-blocker metoprolol. *J Control Rel* **4**:79–85, 1987.

Park H, Robinson JR: Mechanisms of mucoadhesion of poly(acrylic acid) hydrogels. *Pharm Res* **4**:457–464, 1987.

Pozansky MJ, Juliano RL: Biological approaches to the controlled delivery of drugs: A critical review. *Pharmacol Rev* **36**: 277–336, 1984.

Robinson JR: *Sustained and Controlled Release Drug Delivery Systems*. New York, Marcel Dekker, 1978.

Robinson JR: Oral drug delivery systems. *Proceedings of 1982 Research and Scientific Development Conference*. Washington, DC, The Proprietary Association, 1983, pp 54–69.

Robinson JR, Eriksen SP: Theoretical formulation of sustained release dosage forms. *J Pharm Sci* **53**:1254–1263, 1966.

Robinson JR, Lee VHL (eds): *Controlled Drug Delivery: Fundamentals and Applications*, 2nd ed. New York, Marcel Dekker, 1987.

Rosement TJ, Mansdorf SZ: *Controlled Release Delivery Systems*. New York, Marcel Dekker, 1983.

Schechter B, Wilchek M, Arnon R: Increased therapeutic efficacy of cis-platinum complexes of poly L-glutamic acid against a murine carcinoma. *Int J Cancer* **39**:409–413, 1987.

Urquhart J: *Controlled-Release Pharmaceuticals*. Washington, DC, American Pharmaceutical Association, 1981.

Guidance for Industry: Extended Release Oral Dosage Forms: Development, Evaluation, and Application of In Vitro/In Vivo Correlations. Food and Drug Administration (FDA), Center for Drug Evaluation and Research (CDER) September, 1997, BP 2.

20 Targeted Drug Delivery Systems and Biotechnological Products

Susanna Wu-Pong

Chapter Objectives

▶ Compare and contrast biologic and small-molecule drugs in terms of their mechanism of action, design, and development hurdles.

▶ Discuss why biologic drugs may require delivery and/or targeting systems.

▶ Describe the main methods used to deliver and target biologic drugs and give examples.

▶ Explain the difference between active and passive targeting.

▶ State whether generic biologics exist, and if not, describe why.

▶ Explain in general terms the pharmacokinetic differences between small-molecule and biologic drugs and why these differences exist.

Many diseases occur as a result of variability in the genes involved in producing essential enzymes or proteins in the body. The genes are coded in *deoxyribonucleic acid* (DNA), helical double-stranded molecules folded into chromosomes in the nucleus of cells. The Human Genome Project was created more than a decade ago to sequence the human genome. This national effort is continuing to yield information on the role of genetics in congenital defects, cancer, disorders involving the immune system, and other diseases that have a genetic link.

The ever-evolving genetic basis of disease will continue to provide novel opportunities for the development of new drugs to treat these disorders, particularly in the field of biotechnology. The discovery of recombinant DNA (rDNA) technology and its application to new drug development has revolutionized the biopharmaceutical industry. Previously, the pharmaceutical industry relied on the use of relatively simple small drug molecules to treat disease. Modern molecular techniques have changed the face of new drug development to include larger, more sophisticated and complex drug molecules. These large biopharmaceuticals have enormous potential to treat disease in ways previously unavailable to small drug molecules. As a result, *biotechnology,* or the use of biological materials to create a specific product, in this case pharmaceuticals, has become an important sector of the pharmaceutical industry and accounts for the fastest growing class of new drugs in the market. Nucleic acid, protein and peptide drugs, and diagnostics are the main drug products emerging from the biopharmaceutical industry.

BIOTECHNOLOGY

Protein Drugs

The human genome produces thousands of gene products that prevent disease and maintain health. Many may have therapeutic applications if supplemented to normal or supraphysiologic levels in the body. Most of the biologic molecules listed in Table 20-1 are normally present in the body in small concentrations but are used

TABLE 20-1   A Sample of Approved Recombinant Drugs

Drug	Indication	Pharmacokinetics	Year Introduced, Company (Trade Name)
Aldesleukin; interleukin-2	Renal cell carcinoma	Half-life = 85 min; Cl = 268 mL/min	1992 Chiron (Proleukin)
Alteplase	Acute myocardial infarction Acute pulmonary embolism	Half-life < 5 min; Cl = 380–570 mL/min; V_d ≈ plasma volume	1987 Genentech (Activase) 1990 Genentech (Activase)
Antihemophilic factor	Hemophilia B		1992 Armour (Mononine)
Antihemophilic factor	Hemophilia A	Half-life = 13 h	1992 Genetics Institute, Baxter Healthcare, Bayer (ReFacto, Recombinate, Kogenate, Helixate FS)
Agalsidase-beta; α-galactosidase A	Fabry's disease	Half-life = 45–102 min; nonlinear kinetics	2003 Genzyme (Fabrazyme)
Anakinara; IL-1 receptor antagonist	Rheumatoid arthritis	Half-life = 4–6 h	2001 Amgen (Kineret)
β-Glucocerebrosidase	Type I Gaucher's disease		1991 Genzyme (Ceredase)
β-Glucocerebrocidase	Type I Gaucher's disease		1994 Genzyme (Cerezyme)
CMV immune globulin	CMV prevention in kidney transplant		1990 Medimmune (CytoGam)
DNase	Cystic fibrosis		1993 Genentech (Pulmozyme)
Drotrecogin-α; activated protein C	Severe sepsis	Cl = 40 L/h	2001 Lilly (Xigris)
Erythropoietin	Anemia associated with chronic renal failure Anemia associated with AIDS/AZT Anemia associated with cancer and chemotherapy	Half-life = 4–13 h	1989 Amgen; Johnson & Johnson; Kirin (Epogen); 1990 Ortho Biotech (Procrit) 1990 Amgen; Ortho Biotech (Procrit) 1993 Amgen; Ortho Biotech (Procrit)
Factor VIII	Hemophilia A		1993 Genentech; Miles (Kogenate)
Filgrastim; G-CSF	Chemotherapy-induced neutropenia Bone marrow transplant	Half-life = 3.5 h; V_d = 150 mL/kg; Cl = 0.5–0.7 mL/kg/min	1991 Amgen (Neupogen) 1994 Amgen (Neupogen)
Human insulin	Diabetes		1982 Eli Lilly, Genentech (Humulin)
Interferon-α-2a	Hairy cell leukemia;	Half-life = 5.1 h; V_d = 0.4 L/kg; Cl = 2.9 mL/min/kg	1986 Hoffmann-La Roche (Roferon-A)
	AIDS-related Kaposi's sarcoma		1988 Hoffmann-La Roche (Roferon-A)

TABLE 20-1   A Sample of Approved Recombinant Drugs (Continued)

Drug	Indication	Pharmacokinetics	Year Introduced, Company (Trade Name)
Interferon-α-2b	Hairy cell leukemia;	Half-life = 2–3 h	1986 Schering-Plough; Biogen (Intron A)
	AIDS-related Kaposi's sarcoma		1991 Schering-Plough; Biogen (Intron A)
Interferon-α-n3	Genital warts		1989 Interferon Sciences (Alferon N injection)
Interferon-β-1b	Relapsing/remitting multiple sclerosis	Half-life = 8 min–4.3 h; Cl = 9.4–28.9 mL/kg/min; V_d = 0.25–2.9 L/kg	1993 Chiron; Berlex (Betaseron)
Interferon-β-1a	Multiple sclerosis	Half-life = 8.6–10 h	1996 Biogen (Avonex); 2002 Serano (Rebif)
Interferon-γ-1b	Management of chronic granulomatous disease		1990 Genentech (Actimmune)
Human growth hormone	Short stature caused by human growth hormone deficiency		1994 Genentech (Nutropin)
Hepatitis B vaccine, MSD	Hepatitis B prevention		1986 Merck; Chiron (Recombivax HB) Smith Kline 1989 Beecham; Biogen (Engerix-B)
Laronidase; α-L-iduronidase	Mucopolysaccharidosis I	Half-life = 1.5–3.6 h; Cl = 1.7–2.7 mL/min/kg; V_d = 0.24–0.6 L/kg	2003 Biomarin (Aldurazyme)
Pegadamase (PEG-adenosin)	ADA-deficient SCID		1990 Enzon; Eastman Kodak (Adagen)
PEG-L-asparaginase	Refractory childhood acute lymphoblastic leukemia		1994 Enzon (Oncaspar)
Reteplase; plasminogen activator	Acute myocardial infarction	Half-life = 0.2–0.3 h; Cl = 7.5–9.7 mL/min/kg	1996 Boehringer Mannheim (Retavase)
Sargramostim (GM-CSF)	Autologous bone marrow transplantation		1991 Hoechst-Roussel; Immunex (Prokine)
	Neutrophil recovery following bone marrow transplantation		1991 Immunex; Hoechst-Roussel (Leukine)
Somatropin, somatrem	hGH deficiency in children		1987 Eli Lilly (Humatrope) 1985 Genentech (Protropin)
Tenecteplase	Acute myocardial infarction	Half-life = 90–130 min; Cl = 99–119 mL/min; $V_d \approx$ plasma vol.	2002 Genentech (TNKase)

From Yu and Fong, 1997, and www.fda.gov.cber/appr2003.

for certain therapeutic indications. For example, some diseases such as insulin-dependent diabetes result from insufficient production of a natural product, in this case insulin. For these patients, the treatment is to supplement the patient's own insulin production with recombinant human insulin (eg, Humulin). Similarly, human recombinant growth hormone (Protropin, Nutropin) and glucocerebrocidase (Ceredase, Cerezyme) are used to treat growth hormone deficiency and Gaucher's disease, respectively.

In contrast, *interferons* are proteins produced by the immune system in response to viral infection and other biologic inducers. When infection or cancer surpasses the capacity of the body's immune system, recombinant interferons (Roferon-A, Intron A, Alferon N, Actimmune, Infergen, Rebif) or other immune-enhancing molecules can be used to boost immunity. Recombinant interferons and interleukins (Proleukin, Neumega) are therefore used to strengthen the immune system during infection, immunosuppression, cancer, and multiple sclerosis. Erythropoietin and derivatives (Epogen, Procrit, Aronesp) and growth factors (Prokine, Leukine, Neupogen, Becaplermin) are also used to stimulate red and white cell production for anemia or immune suppression following chemotherapy. These molecules were originally available only by purification from human or animal sources. Biotechnology, bioengineering, and the use of cell banks have enabled the large-scale and reproducible production of these naturally occurring biologically derived drugs (Table 20-1).

The size and complexity of protein and nucleic acid drugs require extensive design and engineering of the manufacturing and control processes to produce the drug in large quantities with consistent quality. The size of a protein or peptide drug can range from a few hundred to several hundred thousand daltons. The three-dimensional structure of a protein or peptide drug is important for its pharmacodynamic activity, so the corresponding specific primary amino acid, secondary (alpha helix or beta sheet), tertiary (special relationship of secondary structures), or even quaternary orientation of subunits must be considered. A biotechnology-derived drug (also referred to as a *biologic drug* or *biopharmaceutical*) must be designed such that the structure is stable, reproducible, and accurate during manufacture, storage, and administration. The manufacturing process and product are intricately linked. Small changes in the manufacturing process may affect the sequence of the resulting protein, but more likely will affect the structure, yield, or activity of the protein. Therefore, pharmaceutical controls and testing must be carefully designed, controlled, and monitored, and must also be able to distinguish minor chemical or structural changes that could affect the safety or efficacy in the product during each of these stages.

Drug delivery of biologics can be a problem for therapeutic use because the protein drug must reach the site of action physically and structurally intact. Biologic drugs are notoriously unstable in plasma and the gastrointestinal tract, so modifications to improve drug delivery or stability are often required. Currently, most biologic drugs are generally too unstable for oral delivery and must usually be administered by parenteral routes, though a number of protein and peptide drug candidates including calcitonin, lactoferrin, and glucocerebrocidase are in clinical trials for oral delivery. However, other, nonparenteral routes of administration, such as intranasal and inhalation, are being investigated for biologic drug and vaccine delivery. The first recombinant for inhalation, insulin (Exubera) was approved in 2006, only to be withdrawn from the market 2 years later because of poor patient and physician acceptance. More recently in 2014, another inhaled short-acting insulin product named Afrezza has been approved by the FDA. Lung function must be measured before the drug can be prescribed for the patient. Fortunately, because many of these recombinant protein drugs are designed to act extracellularly, transmembrane delivery may not be required once the drug reaches the plasma.

Monoclonal Antibodies

Another class of protein drugs is *monoclonal antibodies* (mAbs). Antibodies are produced by the body's immune system for specific recognition and removal of foreign bodies. The power of mAbs lies in their highly specific binding of only one antigenic determinant. As a result, mAb drugs, targeting agents, and diagnostics are creating new ways to treat and diagnose previously untreatable diseases and to detect extraordinarily low concentrations of protein or other molecules (Table 20-2).

TABLE 20-2   Applications of Monoclonal Antibodies

Cancer treatment

mAbs against leukemia and lymphomas have been used in treatment with variable results. Regression of tumor is produced in about 25%, although mostly transient.

Imaging diagnosis

mAbs may be used together with radioactive markers to locate and visualize the location and extent of the tumors.

Target-specific delivery

mAbs may be conjugated to drugs or other delivery systems such as liposomes to allow specific delivery to target sites. For example, urokinase was conjugated to an antifibrin mAb to dissolve fibrin clots. The carrier system would seek fibrin sites and activate the conversion of plasmogen to plasmin to cause fibrin to degrade.

Transplant rejection suppression

In kidney transplants, an mAb against CD3, a membrane protein of cytotoxic T cells that causes a rejection reaction, was very useful in suppressing rejection and allowing the transplant to function. The drug was called OKT3. mAbs are also used for kidney and bone marrow transplants.

Theoretically, an almost infinite amount and number of antibodies can be produced by the body to respond immunologically to foreign substances containing antigenic sites. These antigenic sites are usually on protein molecules, but nonprotein material or *haptens* may be conjugated to a protein to form an epitope, or the part of the molecule that binds an antibody. Periodic injections of an antigen into an animal result in production of antibodies that bind epitope. The serum of the animal will also contain antibodies to antigens to which the animal has been previously exposed. Though these mixtures of antibodies in the serum (*polyclonal antibodies*) are now considered too impure for therapeutic use, they can be used for diagnostic immunoassays.

In contrast to polyclonal antibodies, mAbs are preparations that contain many copies of a single antibody that will therefore bind to and only detect one antigenic site. The purity of these preparations makes them very useful as diagnostics, targeting agents, and new therapeutic agents. However, the techniques for the preparation of mAbs are quite complicated. In mAb production, normal antibody-producing cells, such as a mouse spleen cell, are fused with a myeloma

cell and allow the hybrid cells (*hybridoma*) to grow in a test tube. The nonfused cells will die, and the myeloma cells will be selectively destroyed with an antitumor drug such as aminopterin (Fig. 20-1), whereas the hybridoma cells will continue to grow. Each hybridoma cell is then separated into a separate growth chamber or well in which they are allowed to multiply. Each cell and its clones in the respective growth chamber will make antibodies to only one antigen (mAb). The cells producing the desired antibody are selected by testing each well for mAb binding to the desired antigen. The desired cells (clones) are then expanded for mAb production. Since the resulting mAb is of murine origin, often genetic engineering is used to "humanize" the mAb, thus minimizing an immune response to the therapeutic mAb.

Monoclonal antibodies may be used therapeutically to neutralize unwanted cells or molecules. Several mAbs with proven indications are listed in Tables 20-1, 20-2, and 20-3. Monoclonal antibodies are used as antivenoms (CroFab), for overdose of digoxin (DigiFab), or to neutralize endotoxin (investigative) or viral antigen (Nabi-HB). Monoclonal antibodies (mAbs) are named by a source identifier preceding "-mab," for example, -**u**mab (human), -**o**mab (mouse), -**zu**mab (humanized), and -**xi**mab (chimeric). Other common indications for mAb drugs include imaging (ProstaScint, Myocint, Verluma), cancer (Campath, Ontak, Zevalin, Rituxan, Herceptin), rheumatoid arthritis (Humira, Remicade), and transplant immunosuppression (Simulect, Thymoglobulin). Monoclonal antibodies are also used for more novel indications. For example, Abciximab (c7E3 Fab, ReoPro) is a chimeric mAb Fab (humanized) fragment specific for platelet glycoprotein IIb-IIIa receptors. This drug is extremely effective in reducing fatalities (0.50%) in subjects with unstable angina after angioplasty treatment.

Monoclonal antibodies can also target and deliver toxins specifically to cancer cells and destroy them while sparing normal cells (see below), and they are important detectors used in laboratory diagnostics.

Gene Therapy

Gene therapy refers to a pharmaceutical product that delivers a recombinant gene to somatic cells *in vivo* (Ledley, 1996). In turn, the gene within the patients'

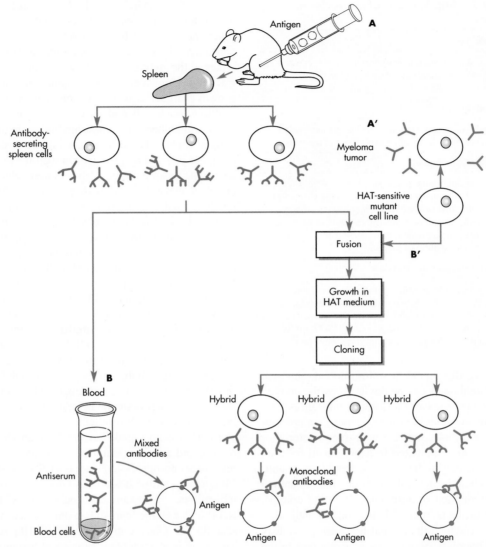

FIGURE 20-1   Monoclonal antibody production. (**A**) A mouse is immunized with an antigen bearing three antigenic determinants (distinct sites that can be recognized by an antibody). Antibodies to each determinant are produced in the spleen. One spleen cell produces a single type of antibody. A spleen cell has a finite lifetime and cannot be cultured indefinitely *in vitro*. (**B**) In the mouse, the antibody-producing cells from the spleen secrete into the blood. The liquid portion of the blood (serum) therefore contains a mixture of antibodies reacting with all three sites on the antigen (antiserum). (**A'**) A mutant cell derived from a mouse myeloma tumor of an antibody-producing cell that has stopped secreting antibody and is selected for sensitivity to the drug aminopterin (present in HAT medium). This mutant tumor cell can grow indefinitely *in vitro* but is killed by HAT medium. (**B'**) The mutant myeloma cell is fused by chemical means with spleen cells from an immunized mouse. The resulting hybrid cells can grow indefinitely *in vitro* due to properties of the myeloma cell parent and can grow in HAT medium because of an enzyme provided by the spleen cell parent. The unfused myeloma cells die because of their sensitivity to HAT, and unfused spleen cells cannot grow indefinitely *in vitro*. The hybrid cells are cloned so that individual cultures are grown from a single hybrid cell. These individual cells produce a single type of antibody because they derive from a single spleen cell. The monoclonal antibody isolated from these cultures is specific for only one antigenic determinant on the original antigen. (From Brodsky FM: Monoclonal antibodies as magic bullets. *Pharm Res* **5**(1):1–9, January 1988, with permission.)

TABLE 20-3 Approved Monoclonal Antibody Drugs and *In Vivo* Diagnostics

mAb Product (Trade Name)	Target		Indication
Abciximab (ReoPro)	Platelet surface glycoprotein	Half-life < 10 min	Unstable angina, coronary angioplasty or atherectomy (PCTA), antiplatelet prevention of blood clots
Adalimumab (Humira)	Tumor necrosis factor	V_d = 4–6 L; Cl = 12 mL/h; half-life = 2 wk	Rheumatoid arthritis
Alefacept (Amevive)	CD2 (LFA) on lymphocytes	Half-life = 270 h; Cl = 0.25 mL/kg/h; V_d = 94 mL/kg	Psoriasis
Alemtuzumab (Campath)	CD52 on blood cells	Half-life = 12 d	B-cell chronic lymphocytic leukemia
Antithymocyte globulin (rabbit) thymoglobulin	T-lymphocyte antigens	Half-life = 2–3 d	Acute rejection in renal transplant patients
Basiliximab (Simulect)	Interleukin-2	Half-life = 7.2 d; V_d = 8.6 L; Cl = 41 mL/h	Renal transplantation immunosuppression
Capromab pendetide (ProstaScint)	Prostate glycoprotein	Half-life = 67 h; Cl = 42 mL/h; V_d = 4 L	Diagnosing imaging agent in prostate cancer
Daclizumab (Zenapax)	Interleukin-2 receptor	Half-life = 20 d; Cl = 15 mL/h; V_d = 6 L	Renal transplants immunosuppression
Denileukin diftitox (Ontak)	Interleukin-2 mAb conjugate to diptheria toxin	Half-life = 70–80 min; Cl = 1.5–2 mL/min/kg; V_d = 0.06–0.08 L/kg	Cutaneous T-cell lymphoma
Digoxin immune Fab—Ovine (DigiFab)	Digoxin	Half-life = 15–20 h; V_d = 0.3–0.4 L/kg	Digoxin toxicity or overdose
Etanercept (Enbrel)	Tumor necrosis factor receptor	Half-life = 115 h; Cl = 89 mL/h	Rheumatoid arthritis
Hepatitis B immune globulin—human (Nabi-HB)	Hepatitis B	Half-life = 25 d; Cl = 0.4 L/d; V_d = 15 L	Acute exposure to hepatitis B
Ibritumomab tiuxetan (Zevalin)	CD28 on B cells	Half-life = 30 h	Follicular or transformed B-cell non-Hodgkin's lymphoma
Imciromab pentetate (Myoscint)	Myosin	Half-life = 20 h	Imaging agent for detecting myocardial injury
Infliximab (Remicade)	Tumor necrosis factor	Half-life = 9.5 d; V_d = 3 L	Crohn's disease Rheumatoid arthritis
Nofetumomab (Verluma)	Carcinoma-associated antigen, ^{99m}Tc labeled	Half-life = 10.5 h	Detection of small cell lung cancer

(Continued)

TABLE 20-3   Approved Monoclonal Antibody Drugs and *In Vivo* Diagnostics (Continued)

mAb Product (Trade Name)	Target		Indication
Muromonab-CD3 (Orthoclone OKT3)	CD3 on T cells		Reversal of acute kidney transplant rejection
Palivizumab (Synagis)	RSV antigens	Half-life = 197 h; Cl = 0.33 mL/h/kg; V_d = 90 mL/kg	RSV disease
Rituximab (Rituxan)	CD20 on B cells	Half-life = 60 h	Follicular, B-cell non-Hodgkin's lymphoma
Trastuzumab (Herceptin)	Human epidermal growth factor receptor	Half-life = 1.7–12 d; V_d = 44 mL/kg	Metastatic breast cancer whose tumors overexpress the HER-2 protein

cell produces a protein that has therapeutic benefit to the patient. The therapeutic approach in gene therapy is often the restoration of defective biologic function within cells or enhancing existing functions such as immunity, as is frequently seen in inherited disorders and cancer.

Gene therapy has been applied to the rare genetic disorder lipoprotein lipase (LPL) deficiency. Patients who suffer from LPL deficiency have abnormally high levels of triglycerides and very low-density lipoproteins (VLDL) causing pancreatitis and cardiovascular disease. The LPL gene has been incorporated into a recombinant adeno-associated virus by uniQure, a Dutch biotechnology company, which has been approved in the European Union (EU) as the LPL gene therapy product Glybera. The drug is expected to be launched in the United States in the near future.

Despite the recent approval in the EU, gene therapy continues to face several challenges. These challenges include gene delivery, sufficient extent and duration of stable gene expression, and safety. Because the gene coding the therapeutic protein (*transgene*) must also contain gene control regions such as the promoter, the actual rDNA (*recombinant DNA*) to be delivered to target cells' nucleus can easily be 10–20 kilobases (kb) in size.

Two main approaches have been used for *in vivo* delivery of rDNA. The first is a virus-based approach that involves replacing viral replicative genes with the transgene, and then packaging the rDNA into the viral particle. The recombinant virus can then infect target cells, and the transgene is expressed, though the virus is not capable of replicating. Both retroviruses, RNA viruses that have the ability to permanently insert their genes into the chromosomes of the host cells, and DNA viruses (which remain outside host chromosomes) have been used successfully in viral gene delivery. Most of the gene therapy trials worldwide involve the use of such viral delivery systems.

In addition to viral delivery systems (*vectors*), nonviral approaches have been used with some success for *in vivo* gene delivery. The transgene is engineered into a plasmid vector, which contains gene-expression control regions. These naked DNA molecules may enter cells and express product in some cell types, such as muscle cells to produce small amounts of antigen that stimulate immunity to the antigen. This naked DNA delivery technique has been approved for veterinary use for West Nile virus. However, usually either polymeric nanoparticles or lipid delivery systems (see below) are required in most other cell types to produce measurable levels of transgene expression. Such vesicles or particles result in intracellular delivery of DNA to cells.

An alternative to direct *in vivo* delivery is a cell-based approach that involves the administration of transgenes to cells that have been removed from a patient. For example, cells (usually bone marrow cells) are removed from the patient; genes encoding a therapeutic product are then introduced into these cells *ex vivo* using a viral or nonviral delivery system, and then the cells are returned into the patient. The advantage of *ex vivo* approaches is that systemic toxicity of viral or nonviral delivery systems is avoided.

Effective gene therapy depends on several conditions. The vector must be able to enter the target cells efficiently and deliver the corrective gene to the nucleus without damaging the target cell. The corrective gene should be stably expressed in the cells, to allow continuous production of the functional protein. Neither the vector nor the functional protein produced from it should cause an immune reaction in the patient. It is also difficult to control the amount of functional protein produced after gene therapy, and excess production of the protein could cause side effects, although insufficient production is more typically observed. Additional problems in gene therapy include the physical and chemical properties of DNA and RNA molecules, such as size, shape, charge, surface characteristics, and the chemical stability of these molecules and delivery systems. *In vivo* problems may include bioavailability, distribution, and cellular and nuclear uptake of these macromolecules into cells. Moreover, naked DNA and RNA molecules are rapidly degraded in the body (Ledley, 1996).

Antisense Drugs

Antisense drugs are drugs that seek to block DNA transcription or RNA translation in order to moderate many disease processes. Antisense drugs consist of nucleotides linked together in short DNA or RNA sequences known as *oligonucleotides*. Oligonucleotides are designed knowing the sequence of target DNA/RNA (eg, messenger RNA) to block transcription or translation of that targeted protein. An oligonucleotide that binds complementary ("sense") mRNA sequences and blocks translation is referred to as *antisense*. To further stabilize the drug, many chemical modifications have been made to the oligonucleotide structure. The most common modification used involves substitution of nonbridging oxygen in the phosphate backbone with sulfur, resulting in a phosphorothioate-derived antisense oligonucleotide. Some of these drugs have been designed to target viral disease and cancer cells in

the body. Vitravene (ISIS Pharmaceuticals), an oligonucleotide targeted to cytomegalovirus, was the first antisense oligonucleotide drug approved by the US Food and Drug Administration (FDA). The cost of a second oligonucleotide drug, Macugen, has made the treatment prohibitive given the availability of cheaper, equally effective drugs. Both drugs act locally (in the eye) but several other antisense drugs administered intravenously have also been approved such as Alicaforsen and Mipomirsen.

For this approach to be useful, the etiology and genetics of the disease must be known. For example, in the case of viral infection, known sequences belonging to vital genes can be targeted and inhibited by antisense drugs. Many antisense sequences are usually tested to find the best candidate, since intra- and intermolecular interactions can affect oligonucleotide activity and delivery. Though oligonucleotides are relatively well internalized compared to rDNA molecules, cellular uptake is often low enough to require delivery systems, such as liposomes. Antisense and gene therapy approaches have also been combined using viral vectors to deliver an antisense sequence. In this case, the transgene is transcribed into an mRNA molecule that is antisense and, therefore, binds to the target mRNA. The resulting RNA–RNA interaction is high affinity and results in inhibition of translation of that mRNA molecule.

RNAi

Like antisense oligonucleotides, RNAis, or RNA interferences, are effective and potent sequence-specific inhibitors of gene expression. RNAi molecules can be either single stranded (miRNAs, or micro-RNAs) or double-stranded (siRNAs or small, interfering RNAs) (for review, see Li and Rana, 2014). The single-stranded RNA molecules are based on the naturally occurring, cellular regulatory micro-RNA molecules involved in gene regulation. Like antisense technology, RNAi sequence-specific gene inhibition is mediated by complementary binding to the target mRNA, but translation inhibition occurs through target strand degradation via a molecular complex called RISC (RNA-induced silencing complex). siRNAs require high homology in target base-pairing but miRNA can occur even with mismatches.

RNAis are important therapeutically from two perspectives. First, miRNAs may be involved in the pathogenesis of certain diseases and, therefore, may make useful therapeutic targets. Antisense molecules targeted to miRNAs are in preclinical and early clinical testing to determine whether miRNAs are viable therapeutic targets. Second, RNAis themselves may be a useful alternative to antisense oligonucleotides as sequence-specific inhibitory therapeutic molecules. siRNAs provide an advantage compared to antisense molecules because of the involvement of RISC, which allows degradation of multiple target molecules upon activation of a single siRNA molecule.

Chemical modification and delivery technologies that have been used for antisense oligonucleotides are also applied to miRNA and siRNA drugs because of their comparable stability and transport issues. miRNA and siRNA drugs are currently in clinical testing for diseases involving cancer, viral infection, and cardiovascular disease.

> ### Frequently Asked Questions
>
> ▶ *What is the most frequent route of administration of biologic compounds?*
>
> ▶ *What is the effect of glycosylation on the activity of a biologic compound? Give an example.*
>
> ▶ *What kinds of biologic drugs are available and how are they used? Are they similar or different from small-molecule drugs?*

DRUG CARRIERS AND TARGETING

Formulation and Delivery of Protein Drugs

Advances in biotechnology have resulted in the commercial production of naturally produced active drug substances for drug therapy (Table 20-1). These substances hold great potential for more specific drug action with fewer side effects. However, many naturally produced substances are complex molecules, such as large-molecular-weight proteins and peptides. Conventional delivery of protein and peptide drugs is generally limited to injectables and implantable dosage forms. Insulin pumps for implantation have been developed for precise control of sugar levels for diabetes, as well as other novel delivery methods

such as inhalers such as Afrezza, which delivers rapid acting insulin to the lung.

Formulating protein drugs for systemic use by oral, or even any extravascular, route of administration is extremely difficult due to drug degradation and absorption from the site of administration. There are several requirements for effective oral drug delivery of protein and peptide drugs: (1) protection of the drug from degradation while in the harsh environment of the digestive tract, (2) consistent absorption of the drug in a manner that meets bioavailability requirements, (3) consistent release of the drug so that it enters the bloodstream in a reproducible manner, (4) nontoxicity, and (5) delivery of the drug through the GI tract or other organ and maintenance of pharmacologic effect similar to IV injection.

Designing, evaluating, and improving protein and peptide drug stability is considerably more complex than for small conventional drug molecules. A change in quaternary structure, such as aggregation or deaggregation of the protein, may result in loss of activity. Changes in primary structure of proteins frequently occur and include deamidation of the amino acid chains, oxidation of chains with sulfhydryl groups, and cleavage by proteolytic enzymes present throughout the body and that may be present due to incomplete purification. Because of protein drugs' complex structures, impurities are much harder to detect and quantify. In addition, proteins may be recognized as foreign substances in the body and become actively phagocytized by the reticuloendothelial system (RES), resulting in the inability of these proteins to reach the intended target. Proteins may also have a high allergenic or immunogenic potential, particularly when nonhuman genes or production cells are used.

Because of the many stability and delivery problems associated with protein and nucleic acid drugs, new delivery systems are being tested to improve their *in vivo* properties. Carriers can be used to protect the drug from degradation, improve transport or delivery to cells, decrease clearance, or a combination of the above. In this chapter, carriers used for both small traditional drug and biopharmaceutical drug delivery are reviewed. Carriers may be covalently bound to the drug, where drug release is usually required for pharmacologic activity. Noncovalent drug carriers such as

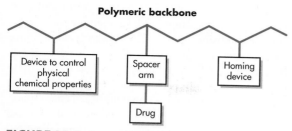

FIGURE 20-2   Site-specific polymeric carrier.

liposomes typically require uncoating of the drug for biologic activity to occur.

Polymeric Delivery Systems

Polymers can be designed to include a wide range of physical and chemical properties and are popularly used in drug formulations because of their versatility. Polymers initially were used to prolong drug release in controlled-release dosage forms. The development of site-specific polymer or macromolecular carrier systems is a more recent extension of earlier research. The basic components of site-specific polymer carriers are (1) the polymeric backbone (Fig. 20-2), (2) functional chains to enhance the physical characteristics of the carrier system, (3) the drug covalently or electrostatically attached to the polymer chain, and possibly (4) a site-specific component (homing device) for recognizing the target. Improved physical characteristics may include improved aqueous solubility. In the case of polymeric prodrugs, a spacer group may be present, bridging the drug and the carrier. The spacer chain may influence the rate at which the drug will hydrolyze from the prodrug system. At present, most site-specific polymeric drug carriers are limited to parenteral administration and primarily utilize soluble polymers.

Positively charged polymers such as polyethylenediamine (PEI), polylysine, cyclodextrin, dendrimers, and chitosan (Fig. 20-3) are used in noncovalent complexes for macromolecular drugs, such as gene or oligonucleotide therapy. For example, polymer–DNA complexes improve DNA delivery to cells in part by providing some protection from nuclease degradation *in vivo*. An added advantage of complexed cationic polymers is that targeting agents such as receptor ligands can be covalently attached to the polymer rather than the drug to provide cell-specific targeting. Cationic polymer use *in vivo* is limited because of polymer toxicity, stability, efficacy, and dissociation of the complex.

Polymers may also be covalently conjugated to drugs to improve their solubility or pharmacokinetic properties. Polymers with molecular weights greater than 30–50 kDa bypass glomerular filtration, thereby extending the duration of drug circulation in the body. Polyethylene glycol (PEG) is used to improve the clearance of some drugs, such as adenosine deaminase (PEG-ADA), filgrastim (Neulasta), pegaptanib (Macugen), interferon (PEG-Intron and PEGASYS), asparaginase (Oncospar), and several others. Dextrans are large polysaccharide molecules (MW 2000 to 1 million Da) with good water solubility, stability, and low toxicity. Drugs with a free amino or hydroxyl group may be linked chemically to hydroxyl groups in dextrans by activation of the dextran with periodate, azide, or other agents.

The molecular weight of the polymer carrier is an important consideration in designing these dosage forms. Generally, large-molecular-weight polymers have longer residence time and diffuse more slowly. However, large polymers are also more prone to capture by the reticuloendothelial system. To gain specificity, a monoclonal antibody, a recognized

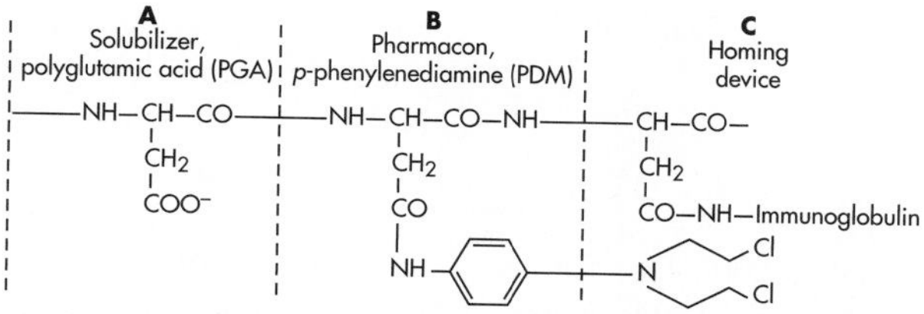

FIGURE 20-3   An example of a drug-polymer conjugate. A = solubilizer, IG = immunoglobulin; polyglutamic acid (PGA); B = Pharmacon, *p*-phenylenediamine (PDM); C = homing device. (Reproduced with permission from Shaikh R, Raj Singh TR, Garland MJ, Woolfson AD, Donnelly RF. Mucoadhesive drug delivery systems. *J Pharm Bioall Sci* **3**(1):89–100, February 5, 2011.)

sugar moiety, or a small cell-specific ligand may be incorporated as a targeting agent into the delivery system. For example, exposed galactose residues are recognized by hepatocytes, whereas mannose or L-fructose is recognized by surface receptors in macrophages.

In addition to use as regular carriers, polymers may also be formulated into *microparticles* and *nanoparticles*. In such delivery systems, the therapeutic agent is encapsulated within a biodegradable polymeric and/or lipid colloidal particle that is in the micrometer or nanometer size range, respectively. Micro- and nanosphere formulations are useful for solubilizing poorly soluble drugs, improving oral bioavailability, protecting against degradation, or providing sustained drug delivery. The small size of nanospheres generally allows good tissue penetration while providing protection or sustained release.

The size of the microsphere and nanosphere has a profound impact on an encapsulated drug's *in vivo* properties and disposition. At over 12 μm, particles are lodged in the capillary bed at the site of the injection. From 2 to 12 μm, particles are retained at the lung, spleen, or liver. Particles less than 0.5 μm (500 nm) deposit into the spleen and bone marrow. In gene therapy, particles smaller than 100 nm demonstrate higher gene expression *in vitro* compared to larger particles (Panyam and Labhasetwar, 2003). More recently, nanoparticles are believed to accumulate in cancer tissue because of hyperpermeability of the permeating vascular endothelia due to fenestrations in the micrometer range, also known as the enhanced permeation and retention (EPR) effect. Delivery systems may be used to differentially target certain cancer cell types or stage of disease based on such permeabilities (see Ferrari, 2010). Though some peptides and nucleic acids have been successfully formulated into nanospheres, protein denaturation and degradation can be significant during encapsulation.

Albumin

Albumin is a large protein (MW 69,000 Da) that is distributed in the plasma and extracellular water. Albumin has been experimentally conjugated or complexed with many drugs to improve site-specific drug delivery for controlled release or oral delivery. Many anticancer drugs such as methotrexate, cytosine arabinoside, and 6-fluorodeoxyuridine have each been conjugated with albumin. Paclitaxel has been formulated into an albumin-bound nanoparticle (Abraxane) to allow increased drug accumulation into breast cancer tissue without the use of Cremophor, a toxic solvent frequently associated with adverse reactions such as hypersensitivity and demyelination, and possibly decreased drug penetration. In a novel approach, Levemir insulin and Victoza glucagon are chemically modified specifically to create high-affinity binding to endogenous albumin, resulting in the prolongation of the respective half-lives from minutes to hours. ^{99m}Tc aggregated to albumin is also commonly used as an imaging agent.

Liposomes

Liposomes have an aqueous, drug- or imaging agent-containing interior surrounded by an exterior lipid bilayer, and typically range in size from 0.5 to 100 μm. Liposomes have been used successfully to reduce side effects of antitumor drugs and antibiotics. For example, doxorubicin liposomes (Doxil) have reduced cardiotoxicity and emetic side effects. Amphotericin B may have reduced nephrotoxicity side effects when formulated with liposomes. An innovative liposome-related product (Abelcet) consists of amphotericin B complexed with two phospholipids, L-a-dimyristoylphosphatidylcholine and L-a-dimyristoylphosphatidylglycerol (Liposome Company, www.lipo.com). The lipid drug complex releases the drug at the site of infection and reduces renal toxicity of amphotericin B without altering its antifungal activity. A more representative liposome product is AmBisome (NeXstar), which consists of very fine liposomes of amphotericin B. The product significantly reduces the side effects of amphotericin B. Daunorubicin citrate liposome (DaunoXome, NeXstar) is an aqueous solution of the citrate salt of the antineoplastic daunorubicin encapsulated within lipid vesicles. The distearoylphosphotidylcholine and cholesterol (2:1 molar ratio) liposome formulation in DaunoXome attempts to maximize the selectivity of daunorubicin into solid brain tumors. Once in the tumor, daunorubicin is released and exerts its

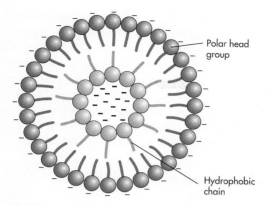

FIGURE 20-4 Diagrammatic representation of a liposome showing polar head group and hydrophobic chain.

antineoplastic activity. Liposome formulations have also been prepared with cytarabine (Depocyte) and other drugs.

There are three general ways of preparing conventional liposomes: (1) phase separation, (2) spray or shear method through orifice, and (3) coacervation. The choice of method depends on the drug, the yield requirements, and the nature of the lipids. Formation of the liposome bilayer depends on the hydrophobic and hydrophilic orientation of the lipids (Fig. 20-4).

Liposomes have different electrical surface charges depending on the type of material used. Common anionic lipid materials are phosphatidylcholine and cholesterol. The phosphatidyl group is amphiphilic, with the choline being the polar group. This structure allows each molecule to attach to others through hydrophobic and hydrophilic interactions. Thermodynamically, liposomes are in equilibrium between different membrane conformations or structures (lipid polymorphism). Thus, some seemingly stable liposome systems exhibit leakage and generally do not have long shelf lives.

Liposomes can be engineered to be site specific. Generally, site specificity is conferred by the type of lipid or by inclusion of a targeting agent, such as a monoclonal antibody or a tumor-specific antigen, into the liposome bilayer (see Targeted Drug Delivery, below) or just above a protective polymer layer, such as PEG. Magneto-, light- and thermosensitive liposomes have also been developed to enable site-specific drug release.

Liposomes may be used to improve intracellular delivery, in which case the liposome must also be designed to fuse with the plasma or endosome membrane. Lipids or fusogenic peptides that facilitate membrane fusion, such as phosphatidylethanolamine or arginine-containing or amphipathic cell-penetrating peptides, respectively, have been used to improve liposome intracellular delivery. Peptides such as tat or octa-arginine have also been used for intracellular targeting and increased uptake of genes. Cationic lipids, such as N-[1-(2,3-dioleyloxy)propyl]-N,N,N-trimethylammonium chloride (DOTMA), or oleoyl-phoshphatidylethanolamine (DOPE), are also commonly used for *in vitro* delivery of DNA. When cationic lipids are mixed with DNA, a particle forms from DNA–lipid charge interactions. The cationic lipid is believed to destabilize biological membranes resulting in improved intracellular DNA delivery. The *in vivo* use of cationic lipids is limited by systemic toxicity due to the positive charge of the lipid. Combinations of modifications to liposomes may also be employed to increase residence time in the body including PEG to make the liposome invisible (ie, "stealth" liposomes) to macrophages combined with a targeting antibody and/or cationic lipids. However, PEG coatings may prevent recognition of targeting agents when placed simultaneously on nanoparticle delivery systems (see Ferrari, 2010).

Frequently Asked Questions

▶ What is meant by targeted drug delivery? How does gene therapy differ from targeted drug delivery?

▶ Why are macromolecular carrier systems used for targeted drug delivery?

TARGETED DRUG DELIVERY

Most conventional dosage forms deliver drug into the body that eventually reaches the site of action by distribution and passive diffusion. In addition, the drug also distributes to nontarget site tissues. Because of nonselective distribution, a much larger dose is given to the patient to achieve therapeutic concentrations in the desired tissue. However, drug action at nontarget sites may result in toxicity or other adverse reactions. Delivery systems that target the drug only to the desired site of drug action allow for more selective, safe, and effective therapeutic activity. For biopharmaceuticals, selective and targeted drug therapy could result in a significant reduction in toxicity, dose, and cost.

Targeted drug delivery or *site-specific drug delivery* refers to drug carrier systems that place the drug at or near the receptor site. Friend and Pangburn (1987) have classified site-specific drug delivery into three broad categories or drug targeting: (1) first-order targeting, which refers to drug delivery systems that deliver the drug to the capillary bed of the active site; (2) second-order targeting, which refers to the specific delivery of drug to a special cell type such as the tumor cells and not to the normal cells; and (3) third-order targeting, which refers to drug delivery specifically to the internal (intracellular) site of cells. An example of third-order drug targeting is the receptor-mediated entry of a drug complex into the cell by endocytosis followed by lysosomal release of the lysosomally active drug. Numerous techniques have been developed for site-specific delivery. Ideally, site-specific carriers guide the drug to the intended target site (tissues or organ) in which the receptor is located without exposing the drug to other tissues, thereby avoiding adverse toxicity. Much of the research in targeted drug delivery has been in cancer chemotherapy.

Site-specific drug delivery has also been characterized as passive or active targeting (Takakura and Hashida, 1996). *Passive targeting* refers to the exploitation of the natural (passive) disposition profiles of a drug carrier, which are passively determined by its physicochemical properties relative to the anatomic and physiologic characteristics of the body. *Active targeting* refers to alterations of the natural disposition of a drug carrier, directing it to specific cells, tissues, or organs. Active targeting employing receptor-mediated endocytosis is a saturable, nonlinear process that depends on the drug–carrier concentration, whereas passive targeting is most often a linear process over a large range of doses.

One approach to active targeting is the use of ligands or monoclonal antibodies, which can target specific cells. Monoclonal antibodies were discussed more fully earlier in this chapter. To date three antibody-drug conjugates have been FDA approved including brentuximab vedotin (Adcetris) to treat Hodgkin's lymphoma and anaplastic large cell lymphoma and trastuzumab emtansine (Kadcyla) to treat breast cancer. Gemtuzumab ozogamicin (Mylotarg) to treat acute myelogenous leukemia was also previously approved, though later withdrawn from the market in 2010 due to marginal clinical benefit.

General Considerations in Targeted Drug Delivery

Considerations in the development of site-specific or targeted drug delivery systems include (1) the anatomic and physiologic characteristics of the target site, including capillary permeability to macromolecules and cellular uptake of the drug (Molema et al, 1997); (2) the physicochemical characteristics of the therapeutically active drug; (3) the physical and chemical characteristics of the carrier; (4) the selectivity of the drug–carrier complex; (5) any impurities introduced during the conjugation reaction linking the drug and the carrier that may be immunogenic, be toxic, or produce other adverse reactions.

Target Site

The accessibility of the drug–carrier complex to the target site may present bioavailability and pharmacokinetic problems, which also include anatomic and/or physiologic considerations. For example, targeting a drug into a brain tumor requires a different route of drug administration (intrathecal injection) than targeting a drug into the liver or spleen. Moreover, the permeability of the blood vessels or biologic membranes to macromolecules or drug–carrier complex may be a barrier preventing delivery and intracellular uptake of these drugs (Molema et al, 1997).

Site-Specific Carrier

To target a drug to an active site, one must consider whether there is a unique property of the active site that makes the target site differ from other organs or tissue systems in the body. The next consideration is to take advantage of this unique difference so that the drug goes specifically to the site of action and not to other tissues in which adverse toxicity may occur. In many cases the drug is complexed with a carrier that targets the drug to the site of action. For example, one of the first approved drugs developed using pharmacogenomic principles is Herceptin (trastuzumab), a monoclonal antibody designed to bind to the human epidermal growth factor receptor. This receptor is overexpressed on HER-2 positive breast cancer cells. Therefore, the drug will preferentially bind HER-2 positive breast cancer cells, though other noncancerous cells may also express the receptor. Trastuzumab has also been approved as a drug conjugate as discussed above, where the antibody is linked to anticancer/antimicrotubule agents that may, for example, be released in the lysosome after internalization. Similarly, trastuzumab has also been used as targeting agents for anticancer drug-encapsulated nanoparticles in clinical studies. The successful application of these delivery systems requires the drug–carrier complex to have both affinity for the target site and favorable pharmacokinetics for delivery to the organ, cells, and subcellular target sites. An additional problem, particularly in the use of protein carriers, is the occurrence of adverse immunological reactions—an occurrence that is partially overcome by designing less immunoreactive proteins. Humanized mAbs are an example of a therapeutic protein engineered to be less immunoreactive.

Drugs

Most of the drugs used for targeted drug delivery are highly reactive drugs that have potent pharmacodynamic activities with a narrow therapeutic range. These drugs are often used in cancer chemotherapy. Many of these drugs may be derived from biologic sources, made by a semisynthetic process using a biologic source as a precursor, or produced by recombinant DNA techniques. The drugs may also be large macromolecules, such as proteins, and are prone to instability and inactivation problems during processing, chemical manipulation, and storage.

Targeting Agents

Properly applied, drug targeting can improve the therapeutic index of many toxic drugs. However, monoclonal antibodies (see discussion above) are

not the "magic bullet" for drug targeting that many people had hoped. One difficulty encountered is that the large molecule reduces the total amount of active drug that can be easily dosed (ie, the ratio of drug to carrier). In contrast, conventional carriers or targeting agents that are not specific are often many orders of magnitude smaller in size, and a larger effective drug dose may be given more efficiently. Antibody fragments comprised of either the double- or single-chain variable regions are also being tested as smaller drug targeting agents (see Srivastava et al, 2014, and van der Meel et al, 2013, for review).

In addition to employing monoclonal antibodies in liposomes and other delivery systems as described above, mAbs may be conjugated directly to drugs as mentioned above. The resulting conjugate can theoretically deliver the drug directly to a cell that expresses a unique surface marker. For example, a tumor cell may overexpress the interleukin-2 receptor. In this case, a cytotoxic molecule such as recombinant diptheria toxin is coupled to an mAb specific for the interleukin-2 receptor (Ontak). The conjugate delivers the toxin preferentially to these tumor cells. An overall tumor response rate for Ontak is 38%, with side effects including acute hypersensitivity reaction (69%) and vascular leak syndrome (27%) (Foss, 2001). Zolimomab aritox (Orthozyme-CD5, Xoma/Ortho Biotech) is an investigational immunoconjugate of monoclonal anti-CD5 murine IgG and the ricin A-chain toxin. This conjugate is used in the treatment of steroid-resistant graft-versus-host disease after allogeneic bone marrow transplants for hematopoietic neoplasms, such as acute myelogenous leukemia. Myoscint is an ^{111}In-labeled mAb targeted to myosin that is used to image myocardial injury in patients with suspected myocardial infarction. An immune response to mAb drugs may develop, since mAbs are produced in mouse cells. "Humanized" mAbs are genetically engineered to produce molecules that are less immunogenic.

Oral Immunization

Antigens or fragmented antigenic protein may be delivered orally and stimulate gut-associated lymphoid tissue (GALT) in the gastrointestinal tract. This represents a promising approach for protecting many secretory surfaces against a variety of infectious pathogens, but products have not yet reached clinical trials. Immunization against salmonella and *Escherichia coli* in chickens was investigated for agricultural purposes. Particulate antigen delivery systems, including several types of microspheres, have been shown to be effective orally inducing various types of immune response. Encapsulation of antigens with mucosal adjuvants can protect both the antigen and the adjuvant against gastric degradation and increase the likelihood that they will reach the site of absorption.

PHARMACOKINETICS OF BIOPHARMACEUTICALS

The unusual nature of biopharmaceuticals compared to traditional drugs presents development challenges for scientists in the biotechnology industry. Because of the size and complexity of biopharmaceuticals, stability and delivery are major developmental issues with these new drugs. The prerequisite of the maintenance of higher-order structure adds a new dimension to formulation, drug delivery, and stability testing of biologic drugs. Pharmacokinetic studies are often complicated by bioanalytic challenges, since preservation of primary structure or an isotope label alone does not necessarily coincide with biologic activity, and effective concentrations are often much lower compared to conventional drugs.

Once in the body, protein and nucleic acid drugs are subject to rapid degradation by endogenous proteases and nucleases that are present in the serum, tissues, and cells. Unmodified phosphodiester DNA and RNA are extremely labile in the body, with half-lives of the order of a few minutes. Houk et al (2001) report that naked DNA clearance in rats is rapid and depends on the conformation of the plasmid: supercoiled, open circular, versus linear. Many of the early recombinant protein drugs also have half-lives of the order of a few minutes, such as alteplase (Activase) and interleukin-2 (Proleukin) (Table 20-1). However, if immediate stability or immunigenicity concerns can be remedied by chemical modification or bioengineering, the biopharmaceutical may be large enough to escape glomerular filtration and enjoy a prolonged circulation in the body (Table 20-1). In addition, since biologics are typically eliminated from the body by non-cytochrome-mediated mechanisms, drug–drug interactions with small-molecule drugs is less likely to occur.

The size and generally hydrophilic nature of the nucleic acid and protein molecules also often preclude the use of diffusional and paracellular transport pathways available to small drug molecules. The capillary wall in most organs and tissues limits passage of macromolecules such as albumin. A typical vector is 20–150 nm, and monoclonal antibodies are composed of four polypeptide chains (over 1200 amino acids in total). Such compounds would be expected to have limited diffusional access to most tissues, except the liver, spleen, bone marrow, and tumor tissues, which have higher vascular permeability. As a result, the volume of drug distribution is often smaller for the larger protein and nucleic acid drugs because of vascular confinement or binding to specific tissues. Indeed, the volume of distribution for some of these drugs approximates plasma volume: the apparent volume of distribution at steady state of the mAb Nebacumab is 0.11 ± 0.03 L/kg (Romano et al, 1993), and of Simulect is approximately 7.5 L.

Because of the stability and distribution limitations of large biologic drugs, delivery systems such as conjugates, nanoparticles, liposomes, and viral vectors as described above have been used to improve activity and delivery. The pharmacokinetics of recombinant viral gene delivery systems have been difficult to measure because of the relatively low doses given and often inefficient transgene expression. As a result, gene expression and transgene persistence in tissues are used to determine pharmacokinetic profiles (NIH Report, 2002). Nonviral and naked DNA delivery systems are relatively well characterized in comparison to viral delivery systems. Hengge et al (2001), using polymerase chain reaction (PCR), demonstrate that intramuscular or cutaneous injection of a DNA vaccine resulted in gene expression primarily in surrounding tissues unless extremely high doses were administered. Zhou et al (2009) used real-time PCR (RT-PCR) to demonstrate two-compartment pharmacokinetic profiles of naked DNA and simple and reversibly stabilized DNA (rSDN) polymer nanoparticles, with mean retention time increasing from 4.5 minutes with naked DNA to almost 23 minutes with the reversibly rSDN.

Liposome delivery systems are fairly well characterized in terms of their pharmacokinetic properties. Liposome encapsulation may reduce the V_D (Minchin et al, 2001), and may (Houk et al, 2001) or may not (Minchin et al, 2001) improve upon DNA half-life by several hours. However, lipid delivery systems are also rapidly cleared by the mononuclear phagocyte system (spleen and liver) unless injected intratumorally (Nomura et al, 1997). In addition, liposomes may enhance an immune response to the drug and complement activation, also resulting in rapid clearance.

Alternatively, liposomes can be designed to evade phagocyte detection and improve circulation time by coating with polyethylene glycol (PEG), which minimizes opsonin-dependent clearance. *In vivo,* the PEG provides a "bulky" head group that serves as a barrier to prevent interaction with the plasma opsonins. The hydrated groups sterically inhibit hydrophobic and electrostatic interaction of a variety of blood components at the liposome surface, thereby evading recognition by the reticuloendothelial system. An example of this concept is the stealth liposome, which led to reduction in the volume of distribution, half-life extension (Gabizon et al, 2003), and eventual marketing (Doxil) in the United States. Optimal formulation of a PEGylated liposome can improve liposome stability from 1% to 31% of dose remaining in the body at 24 hours postinjection (Allen et al, 2002).

The pharmacokinetics of a liposomal formulation can be different from those of a nonliposomal product given by the same route of administration. For new liposome products, the FDA (draft guidance, see http://www.fda.gov/downloads/Drugs /GuidanceComplianceRegulatoryInformation /Guidances/ucm070570.pdf) recommends a comparative mass balance study be performed to assess the differences in systemic exposure and pharmacokinetics between liposome and nonliposome drug products when (1) the two products have the same active moiety, (2) the two products are given by the same route of administration, and (3) one of the products is already approved for marketing. If satisfactory mass balance information is already available for the approved drug product, a limited mass balance study can be undertaken for the new drug product. Comparison of the absorption, distribution, metabolism, and excretion (ADME) of the liposome and nonliposome drug product forms should be made, using a crossover or a parallel noncrossover study design that employs an appropriate number of subjects.

BIOEQUIVALENCE OF BIOTECHNOLOGY-DERIVED DRUG PRODUCTS

The dosage form or formulation of a drug product may change during the course of drug development. In addition, since the product quality (number and type of contaminants for example) and even product microheterogeneities (degree of glycosylation, post-translational modifications, genetic variants, etc) are a function of the manufacturing process, the protein or nucleic acid drug itself will continue to evolve prior to approval of the biologics licence agreement (BLA). Likewise, the initial drug formulation used in early clinical studies (eg, Phase I/II) may not be the same formulation as the drug formulation used in later clinical trials (Phase III) or the marketed formulation. Therefore, even genetically "identical" recombinant drugs will differ because of differences in variables such as cell, cell clone, manufacturing, purification and storage, formulation, expression system, or raw chemicals. Such variations may result in profound differences in bioavailability, immunogenicity, adverse reactions, and efficacy. Because of such differences, biological "generics" are instead referred to as "biosimilars." A pathway for FDA approval of biosimilars has been defined as part of the 2009 Biologics Price Competition and Innovation Act (BPCI Act). Under this Act, companies may submit a 351(k) application for their biosimilar candidate. The FDA then considers the "totality of the evidence" in terms of the interchangability between the candidate and reference drug. The candidate should be "highly similar" and have "no clinically meaningful difference" between the two. Product immunogenicity should be evaluated via at least one clinical study, and variability between lots of the innovator product should be determined as a guide to the candidate's product variability. The FDA now also provides recommendations regarding development of biosimilars and quality considerations of analytical factors that should be considered when submitting a 351(k) application. Also see Chapter 15 for more details on bioequivalence.

Frequently Asked Questions

▶ *What are the major differences in drug distribution and elimination between conventional molecules and biotechnological compounds?*

▶ *What are the many ways antibodies are used therapeutically?*

LEARNING QUESTIONS

1. Explain why most drugs produced by biotechnology cannot be given orally. What routes of drug administration would you recommend for these drugs? Why?
2. What is meant by site-specific drug delivery? Describe several approaches that have been used to target a drug to a specific organ.
3. Doxorubicin (Adriamycin) is available as a conventional solution and as a liposomal preparation. What effect would the liposomal preparation have on the distribution of doxorubicin compared to an injection of the conventional doxorubicin injection?

ANSWERS

Frequently Asked Questions

What is the most frequent route of administration of biologic compounds?

• The most frequent route of administration for biologic compounds is parenteral (eg, IM or IV). For example, β-interferon for multiple sclerosis is given IM to allow gradual drug release into the systemic circulation.

What is the effect of glycosylation on the activity of a biologic compound? Give an example.

• Glycosylation is the addition of a carbohydrate group to the molecule. For example, Betaseron (interferon-β-1a) is not glycosylated, whereas Avonex (interferon-β-1b) is glycosylated. Glycosylation will increase the water solubility and the molecular weight of the drug. Although both drugs are β-interferons, glycosylation affects the pharmacokinetics, the stability, and the efficacy of these drugs.

What kind of biologic drugs are available and how are they used? Are they similar or different from small-molecule drugs?

• The distribution of a biotechnology compound depends on its physicochemical characteristics. Many peptides, proteins, and nucleotides have polar chains so that a major portion of the drug is distributed in the extracellular fluid with a volume of 7–15 L. Drugs that easily penetrate into the cell have higher volumes of distribution, about 15–45 L, due to the larger volume of intracellular fluid.

REFERENCES

Allen C, Dos Santos N, Gallagher R: Controlling the physical behavior and biological performance of liposome formulations through use of surface grafted poly(ethylene glycol). *Biosci Rep* **22**:225–250, 2002.

Ferrari, M. Frontiers in cancer nanomedicine: Directing mass transport through biological barriers. *Trends Biotech* **28**(4): 181–188, 2010.

Foss FM, Bacha P, Osann KE, Demicre MF, Bell T, Kuzel T: Biological correlates of acute hypersensitivity events with DAB(389) IL-2(deni leukin diftitox, ONAK) in cutaneous T-cell lymphoma: decreased frequency & severity with steroid premedication. *Clin Lymphoma* **1**:298–302, 2001.

Friend DR, Pangburn S: Site-specific drug delivery. *Med Res Rev* **7**:53–106, 1987.

Gabizon A, Shmeeda H, Barenholz Y, et al: Pharmacokinetics of pegylated liposomal doxorubicin—Review of animal and human studies. *Clin Pharmacokinet* **42**(45):419–436, 2003.

Gros L, Ringsdorf H, Schupp H: Polymeric antitumor agents on a molecular & cellular level. *Angew Chem Int Ed Engl* **20**:312, 1981.

Hengge UR, Dexling B, Mirmohammadsadegh A: Safety and pharmacokinetics of naked plasmid DNA in the skin: Studies on dissemination and ectopic expression. *J Invest Dermatol* **116**:979, 2001.

Houk BE, Martin R, Hochhaus G, Hughes JA: Pharmacokinetics of plasmid DNA in the rat. *Pharm Res* **18**:67–74, 2001.

Ledley, FD: Pharmaceutical approaches to somatic cell therapy. *Pharm Res* **13**:1595–1614, 1996.

Li Z, Rana TM: Therapeutic targeting of microRNAs: Current status and future challenges. *Nature* **13**:622–638, 2014.

Minchin RF, Carpenter D, Orr RJ: Polyinosinic acid and poly-cationic liposomes attenuate the hepatic clearance of circulating plasmid DNA. *J Pharmacol Exp Ther* **296**:1006–1012, 2001.

Molema G, de Leij LFMH, Meijer DKE: Tumor vascular endothelium: Barrier or target in tumor directed drug delivery and immunotherapy. *Pharm Res* **14**:2–10, 1997.

NIH Report: Assessment of adenoviral vector safety and toxicity: Report of the National Institutes of Health Recombinant DNA Advisory Committee. *Hum Gene Ther* **13**:3–13, 2002.

Nomura T, Nakajima S, Kawabata K, et al: Intratumoral pharma-cokinetics and *in vivo* gene expression of naked plasmid DNA and its cationic liposome complexes after direct gene transfer. *Cancer Res* **57**:2681–2686, 1997.

Panyam J, Labhasetwar V: Biodegradable nanoparticles for drug and gene delivery to cells and tissue. *Adv Drug Del Rev* **55**: 329–347, 2003.

Romano MJ, Kearns GL, Kaplan SL, et al: Single-dose pharmaco-kinetics and safety of HA-1A, a human IgM anti-lipid-A mono-clonal antibody, in pediatric patients with sepsis syndrome. *J Pediatr* **122**(6):974–984, 1993.

Srivastava A, O'Connor IB, Pandit A, Wall JG: Polymer-antibody fragment conjugates for biomedical applications. *Prog Polym Sci* **39**:308–329, 2014.

Takakura Y, Hashida M: Macromolecular carrier systems for tar-geted drug delivery: Pharmacokinetic considerations on bio-distribution. *Pharm Res* **13**:820–831, 1996.

van der Meel R, Vehmeijer LJC, Kok RJ, Storm G, van Gaal. Ligand-targeted particulate nanomedicines undergoing clinical evaluation: Current status. *Adv Drug Deliv Rev* **65**:1284–1298, 2013.

Yu ABC, Fong GW: Biotechnologic products. In Shargel L, Mutnick AH, Souney PF and Swanson LN (eds). *Comprehen-sive Pharmacy Review*, 3rd ed. Baltimore, Williams & Wilkins, 1997, chap 10.

Zhou QH, Wu C, Manickam DS, Oupicky D. Evaluation of phar-macokinetics of bioreducible gene delivery vectors by real-time PCR. *Pharm Res* **26**:1581–1589, 2009.

BIBLIOGRAPHY

Akala EO, Collett JH: Influence of drug loading and gel structure on in-vitro release kinetics from photopolymerized gels. *Ind Pharm* **13**:1779–1798, 1987.

Bayley H, Gasparro F, Edelson R: Photoactive drugs. *TIPS* **8**: 138–144, 1987.

Body A, Aarons L: Pharmacokinetic and pharmacodynamic aspects of site specific drug delivery. *Adv Drug Deliv Rev* **3**:155–163, 1989.

Borchardt RT, Repta AJ, Stella VJ (eds): *Directed Drug Delivery*. Clifton, NJ, Humana, 1985.

Boxenbaum HG: Physiological and pharmacokinetic factors affecting performance of sustained release dosage forms. *Drug Dev Ind Pharm* **8**:1–25, 1982.

Breimer DD, Dauhof M: *Towards Better Safety of Drugs and Pharmaceutical Products*. Amsterdam, Elsevier/North-Holland, 1980, pp 117–142.

Brester ME, Hora MS, Simpkins JW, Bodor N: Use of 2-hydroxypropyl-b-cyclodextrin as a solubilizing and stabi-lizing excipient for protein drugs. *Pharm Res* **8**:792–795, 1991.

Brodsky FM: Monoclonal antibodies as magic bullets. *Pharm Res* **5:**1–9, 1988.

Bruck S (ed): *CRC Controlled Drug Delivery.* Boca Raton, FL, CRC Press, 1983.

Chien YW: *Novel Drug Delivery Systems.* New York, Marcel Dekker, 1982.

Dighe SV, Adams WP: Bioavailability and bioequivalence of oral controlled-release products: A regulatory perspective. In Welling PG, Tse FLS (eds). *Pharmacokinetics: Regulatory, Industrial, Academic Perspectives.* New York, Marcel Dekker, 1988.

Eckhardt BM, Oeswein JQ, Bewley TA: Effect of freezing on aggregation of human growth hormone. *Pharm Res* **8:** 1360–1364, 1991.

Emisphere literature: Mucosal immunization with derivatized μ- and non-μ-amino acid delivery agents. Presented at the American Association of Pharmaceutical Scientists (AAPS) Annual Meeting, Seattle, WA, October 1996.

Emisphere literature: Oral delivery of interferon in rats and primates. Presented at the American Association of Pharmaceutical Scientists (AAPS) Annual Meeting, San Diego, CA, 1994. *Pharm Res* **11**(10):S-298, 1994.

Galeone M, Nizzola L, Cacioli D, Moise G: *In vivo* demonstration of delivery mechanisms from sustained-release pellets. *Curr Ther Res* **29:**217–234, 1981.

Heller J: Controlled drug release from monolithic bioerodible polymer devices. *Pharm Int* **7:**316–318, 1986.

Jensen JD, Jensen LW, Madsen JK, Poulsen L: The metabolism of erythropoietin in liver cirrhosis patients compared with healthy volunteers. *Eur J Haematol* **54**(2):111–116, 1995.

Langer R: New methods of drug delivery. *Science* **249:**1527–1533, 1990.

Le-Cotonnec JY, Porchet HC, Betrami V, et al: Comprehensive pharmacokinetics of urinary human follicle stimulating hormone in healthy female volunteers. *Pharm Res* **12**(6):844–850, 1995.

Lee VH, Hashida M, Mizushima Y: *Trends and Future Perspectives in Peptide and Protein Drug Development.* Langhorne, PA, Harwood Academic, 1995.

Levy G: Targeted drug delivery: Some pharmacokinetic considerations. *Pharm Res* **4:**3–4, 1987.

Oeswein JA: Formulation considerations in polypeptide delivery. Presented at Biotech 87. Pinner, UK, Online Publications, 1987.

Ostro MJ: *Liposome: From Biophysics to Therapeutics.* New York, Marcel Dekker, 1987.

Park H, Robinson JR: Mechanisms of mucoadhesion of poly(acrylic acid) hydrogels. *Pharm Res* **4:**457–464, 1987.

Pozansky MJ, Juliano RL: Biological approaches to the controlled delivery of drugs: A critical review. *Pharmacol Rev* **36:**277–336, 1984.

Robinson JR: Oral drug delivery systems. *Proceedings of 1982 Research and Scientific Development Conference.* Washington, DC, The Proprietary Association, 1983, pp 54–69.

Rodwell JD (ed): *Antibody Mediated Delivery Systems.* New York, Marcel Dekker, 1988.

Salmonson T, Danielson BG, Wikstrom B: The pharmacokinetics of recombinant erythropoietin after intravenous and subcutaneous administration to healthy subjects. *Br J Clin Pharm* **29:**709, 1990.

Silverman HS, Becker LC, Siddoway LA, et al: Pharmacokinetics of human recombinant superoxide dismutase. *J Am Coll Cardiol* **11:**164A, 1988.

Sobel BE, Fields LE, Robinson AK, et al: Coronary thrombolysis with facilitated absorption of intramuscular injected tissue-type plasminogen activator. *Proc Natl Acad Sci USA* **82:**4258, 1985.

Spenlehauer G, Vert M, Benoit JP, et al: Biodegradable cisplatin microspheres prepared by the solvent evaporation method: Morphology and release characteristics. *J Control Rel* **7:** 217–229, 1988.

21

Relationship Between Pharmacokinetics and Pharmacodynamics

Mathangi Gopalakrishnan, Vipul Kumar, and Manish Issar

Chapter Objectives

▶ Quantitatively describe the relationship between drug, receptor, and the pharmacologic response.

▶ Explain why the intensity of the pharmacologic response increases with drug concentrations and/or dose up to a maximum response.

▶ Explain the difference between an agonist, a partial agonist, and an antagonist.

▶ Describe the difference between a reversible and a nonreversible pharmacologic response.

▶ Define the term biomarker and explain how biomarkers may be used in the clinical development of drugs.

▶ Show how the E_{max} and sigmoidal E_{max} model describe the relationship of the pharmacodynamic response to drug concentration.

▶ Define the term pharmacokinetic–pharmacodynamic model and provide equations that quantitatively simulates the time course of drug action.

PHARMACOKINETICS AND PHARMACODYNAMICS

The role of pharmacokinetics (PK) to derived dosing regimens to achieve therapeutic drug concentrations for optimal safety and efficacy will be discussed in the next two chapters. A more objective approach for designing a drug's dosing regimen would need to link the exposure of the drug within the body to the desirable (efficacy) and undesirable (safety/toxicity) effects of the drug. At the site of action, the drug interacts with a receptor that may be located within a cell or on special cell membranes. This drug–receptor interaction initiates a cascade of events resulting in a pharmacodynamic response or effect. Thus, *pharmacodynamics (PD)* refers to the relationship between drug concentration at the site of action (receptor) and the observed pharmacologic response. This chapter describes how the exposure of a drug over time (dose, concentrations, dosing regimens) can be related to the desirable and undesirable effects of the drug. Just as the PK of a drug has been described via mathematical models such as a one- or two-compartmental model, the relationship between drug concentration and effect can also be described using mathematical models. These PK-PD models can further be applied for simulations and prediction of drug action. This chapter is organized as follows: First, formal definitions of terms and those used interchangeably in the PK-PD literature are provided. Second, an introduction to how the PK-PD principles are integrated into drug development is provided. In addition, the chapter briefly describes the drug receptor theory and the use of biomarkers. This is followed by the theoretical basis of PK-PD relationship. Lastly, the chapter describes the different types of possible PK-PD relationships showing how the time course of drug action relates to drug concentration in the body. Examples and case studies are provided in the chapter to integrate therapeutic concepts and drug development perspectives.

▶ Explain the effect compartment in the pharmacodynamic model and name the underlying assumptions.

▶ Describe the effect of changing drug dose and/or drug elimination half-life on the duration of drug response.

▶ Describe how observed drug tolerance or unusual hysteresis-type drug response may be explained using PD models based on simple drug receptor theory.

▶ Define the term drug exposure and explain how it is used to improve drug therapy and safety.

Definitions for Exposure, Response, and Effect

Various terminologies have been used to describe PK and PD. To avoid confusion, current correct terminology and definitions of these terms are provided and such definitions will be followed throughout this chapter.

The relationship between PK and PD is also referred to as exposure-response relationship or concentration-response relationship or concentration–effect relationship. Exposure-response information is used to determine the safety and efficacy of drugs in the process of drug approval, more importantly to understand the benefit–risk of drugs during the drug approval process and to derive dosing information.

Exposure

The term *exposure* can be defined as any dose or drug input to the body or various measures of acute or integrated drug concentrations in plasma or other biological fluid (eg, C_{max}, C_{min}, C_{ss}, AUC). Exposure is related to a measure of drug amount at a particular site in the body from which it elicits a response. Commonly used exposure measures are dose of a drug and plasma concentrations (C_p). Any input to characterize the pharmacokinetic aspect of the drug is a measure of exposure.

Response

A *response (R)* refers to a direct measure of the pharmacologic observation. For example, measure of diastolic blood pressure (DBP) at some time point is considered as a response.

$$R(t) = \text{Response at time, } t : \text{Diastolic blood pressure}$$

Effect

Effect, E refers to a change in the biological response from one time to another. In other words, an effect is a derived or calculated value from an observed response. For example, change from baseline in diastolic blood pressure is the effect.

$$E = \text{Effect} : \text{Change from baseline in DBP at 8 weeks}$$

To further illustrate, let us consider the DBP measured at the beginning of a clinical trial in a subject as 92 mm Hg, denoted as $R(t = 0)$, and DBP measured at the end of 8 weeks of the trial, $R(t = 8)$ is 82 mm Hg. Here, $R(t = 0)$ and $R(t = 8)$ are the responses. The effect, E, which is of interest, is change from baseline in DBP at 8 weeks calculated as –10 mm Hg and is denoted below:

$$E = R(t = 8) - R(t = 0) = 82 \text{ mm Hg} - 92 \text{ mm Hg} = -10 \text{ mm Hg}$$

Effects include a broad range of endpoints or biomarkers ranging from clinically remote biomarkers (eg, receptor occupancy) to a presumed mechanistic effect (eg, % angiotensin converting enzyme [ACE] inhibition) to a potential surrogate (eg, change from baseline in blood pressure or change in lipids etc). Often, the scientific community uses response and effect interchangeably.

PK-PD Information Flow in Drug Development

The role of PK and PD in the drug development process is considered to be impactful and scientists have reiterated its importance in drug development and decision making (Derendorf et al, 2000; Sheiner and Steimer, 2000; Gobburu and Marroum, 2001;

Kimko and Pinheiro, 2014). In general, the current drug development process is a series of developmental and evaluative steps carried out from the stage of an Investigational New Drug Application (IND) leading to the submission of New Drug Application (NDA). The regulatory bodies like the Food and Drug administration (FDA) and the European Medicines Agency (EMA) review the NDA and provide approval/disapproval for the new drugs to be used in the market. The applicable process as it pertains to the US FDA is illustrated as an example in Fig. 21-1.

There are predominantly four phases in the drug development process as shown in Fig. 21-1. The details of the four phases in drug development and how the PK-PD information at each of the phases can be useful are described briefly here and

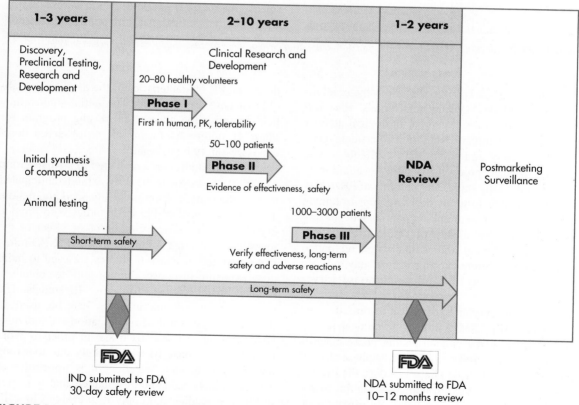

FIGURE 21-1 New drug development process. (Adapted from Peck et al, 1994.)

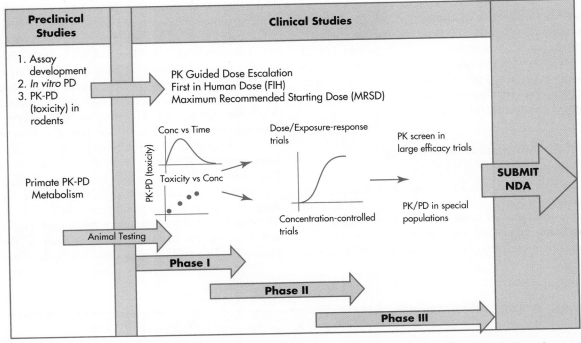

FIGURE 21-2   PK, PD, and toxicity information during the drug development process. (Adapted from Peck et al, 1994.)

shown in Fig. 21-2. The initial phase is the preclinical testing phase. During this phase, the new molecular entities are tested for biological activity in experimental animals from mice to primate models. The toxicity and safety data available at this stage are used to proceed for safety evaluation in humans at the IND stage. The preclinical PK-safety information is helpful in deriving first-in-human (FIH) doses or maximum recommended starting dose (MRSD) by means of allometric scaling. Moreover, preclinical studies on pharmacodynamic activity from different exposures/dose may indicate the likely steepness of the dose–response curves in humans.

After discovery and preclinical testing, the new molecular entity (NME) enters the clinical testing phase. Typically, the clinical testing phase consists of early phase (Phase I and II) and late phase clinical trials (Phase III). During Phase I studies, the PK and tolerability of the NME are studied in healthy volunteers by means of dose escalation. Information on initial parameters of toxicity, maximum tolerated dose, and PK characteristics of the drug and metabolite (if any) are obtained. The initial studies may help establish the appropriate dosing program for Phase II studies by means of the observed dose/ exposure-safety relationship.

Phase II studies are conducted in a small group of patients to assess if the drug exhibits anticipated therapeutic benefit or not in the intended population. The principal goal of Phase II studies is to provide evidence for the efficacy or proof of effect of the investigational drug. Additionally, the PK-PD information gained in Phase-II studies are used to build dose-exposure-response relationship to obtain a rational dosing strategy for Phase III studies. The exposure-response relationships can be used to design strategies for dose optimization and individualized dosing in Phase III trials. In order to avoid failure in the Phase III trials mainly due to wrong dose/dosing regimen selection, it is imperative to accrue/leverage valuable information that is gained in Phase II studies and apply it to design Phase III trials to increase likelihood of success.

Phase III studies used for drug approval are considered pivotal trials and typically two adequate and well-controlled clinical trials are submitted for drug approval. Phase III studies are conducted in a larger patient population and are designed to document the clinical efficacy and safety of the investigational drug and further refine the dose-exposure-response relationship. The information gained in preclinical and clinical studies become part of the drug label that ultimately reaches the prescriber and hence the patient.

The preceding section discussed the implications of PK-PD relationship in the drug development process. To understand how a drug elicits a response, it is necessary to understand the process at a cellular and a molecular level. The following section describes the interaction of a drug molecule with a receptor, resulting in a pharmacodynamic response.

Drug–Receptor Interaction

Receptors are cellular proteins that interact with endogenous ligands (such as neurotransmitters and hormones) to elicit a physiological response thereby regulating cellular functions (Blumenthal and Garrison, 2011). Understanding the role of receptor–endogenous ligands interaction in physiology and pathophysiology enables targeting of specific receptors for therapeutic benefit. There are different types of receptors that are located either outside or inside of cell membranes. Various types of receptors, their localization, and some representative examples are listed in Table 21-1.

The drug–receptor interactions involve weak chemical forces or bonds (eg, hydrogen bonding, ionic electrostatic bonds, Van der Waals forces).

Typically, the drug–receptor interaction results in a cascade of downstream events eliciting a PD response. The interaction of drug with a receptor follows the law of mass action (Clark, 1927), which can be described as per the receptor occupancy theory, which is described in greater detail under the section E_{max} Drug-Concentration Effect Model.

Typically, a single drug molecule interacts with a receptor with a single binding site to produce a pharmacologic response, as illustrated below.

[Drug] + [Receptor] $\Leftrightarrow$
[Drug – receptor complex] $\rightarrow$ Response

where the brackets [ ] denote molar concentrations.

This scheme illustrates the *occupation theory* for the interaction of a drug molecule with a receptor molecule. More recent schemes consider a drug that binds to macromolecules as a *ligand*. Thus, the reversible interaction of a ligand (drug) with a receptor may be written as follows (Neubig et al, 2003):

$$L + R \underset{}{\overset{K_1}{\rightleftharpoons}} LR \underset{}{\overset{K_2}{\rightleftharpoons}} LR^*$$

where L is generally referred to as ligand concentration (since many drugs are small molecules) and LR is analogous to the (drug–receptor complex). LR^* is the activated form that results in the effect.

The last step is written to accommodate different modes of how LR leads to a drug effect. For example, the interaction of a subsequent ligand with the receptor may involve a conformation change of the receptor or simply lead to an additional effect. In this chapter, effect and response are used interchangeably.

TABLE 21-1   Selected Examples of Drug Receptors

Type	Description	Examples
Ion channels	Located on cell surface or transmembrane; governs ion flux	Acetylcholine (nicotinic)
G-protein coupled receptor	Located on cell surface or transmembrane; GTP involved in receptor action	Acetylcholine (muscarinic) α- and β-adrenergic receptor proteins Eicosanoids
Transcription factors	Within cell in cytoplasm, activate or suppress DNA transcription	Steroid hormones Thyroid hormone

Partially adapted from Moroney (2011) and Katzung et al (2011).

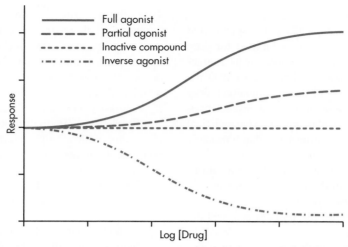

FIGURE 21-3   Representation of different drug–receptor interactions. (Adapted from Goodman Gilman, Chapter 3, 12th edition.)

This model makes the following assumptions:

1. The drug molecule combines with the receptor molecule as a bimolecular association, and the resulting drug–receptor complex disassociates as a unimolecular entity.
2. The binding of drug with the receptor is fully reversible.
3. The basic model assumes a single type of receptor binding site, with one binding site per receptor molecule. It is also assumed that a receptor with multiple sites may be modeled after this (Cox, 1990).
4. The occupancy of the drug molecule at one receptor site does not change the affinity of more drug molecules to complex at additional receptor sites.
5. Each receptor has equal affinity for the drug molecule.

The model is not suitable for drugs with allosteric binding to receptors, in which the binding of one drug molecule to the receptor affects the binding of subsequent drug molecules, as in the case of oxygen molecules binding to iron in hemoglobin. As more receptors are occupied by drug molecules, a greater pharmacodynamic response is obtained until a maximum response is reached.

Based on the interaction of the drug with the receptor, a drug can be classified as an agonist, partial agonist, inverse agonist, or antagonist. Agonist is an agent that interacts with a receptor producing effects similar to that of an endogenous ligand (eg, stimulation of the μ opioid receptor by morphine [Yaksh and Wallace, 2011]). Antagonist on the other hand is an agent that blocks the effect of an agonist by binding to the receptor, thereby inhibiting the effect of an endogenous ligand or agonist (eg, atenolol, a blood pressure-lowering agent is a β_1-receptor antagonist) (Westfall and Westfall, 2011). A partial agonist is an agent that produces a response similar to an agonist but cannot reach a maximal response as that of an agonist (eg, buspirone, an anxiolytic agent is a partial agonist of 5-HT$_{1a}$ receptor) (O'Donnell and Shelton, 2011). An inverse agonist selectively binds to the inactive form of the receptor and shifts the conformational equilibrium toward the inactive state (eg, famotidine, a gastric acid production inhibitor is an inverse agonist of H$_2$ receptor) (Skidgel et al, 2011). The manner in which different drugs/ligands interact with the receptors can be represented graphically as shown in Fig. 21-3.

RELATIONSHIP OF DOSE TO PHARMACOLOGIC EFFECT

The onset, intensity, and duration of the pharmacologic effect depend on the dose and the pharmacokinetics of the drug. As the dose increases, the drug

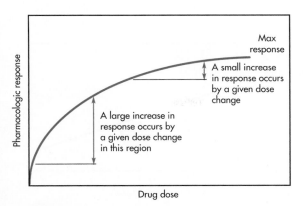

FIGURE 21-4   A plot of pharmacologic response versus dose on a linear scale.

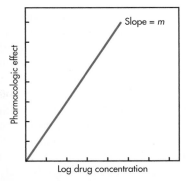

FIGURE 21-6   Graph of log drug concentration versus pharmacologic effect. Only the linear portion of the curve is shown.

concentration at the receptor site increases, and the pharmacologic response (effect) increases up to a maximum effect. A plot of the pharmacologic effect to dose on a linear scale generally results in a hyperbolic curve with maximum effect at the plateau (Fig. 21-4). The same data may be compressed and plotted on a log-linear scale and result in a sigmoid curve (Fig. 21-5).

For many drugs, the graph of the log dose–response curve shows a linear relationship at a dose range between 20% and 80% of the maximum response, which typically includes the therapeutic dose range for many drugs. For a drug that follows one-compartment pharmacokinetics, the volume of distribution is constant; therefore, the pharmacologic

response is also proportional to the log plasma drug concentration within a therapeutic range, as shown in Fig. 21-6.

Mathematically, the relationship in Fig. 21-6 may be expressed by the following equation, where m is the slope, e is an extrapolated intercept, and E is the drug effect at drug concentration C:

$$E = m \log C + e \qquad (21.1)$$

Solving for log C yields

$$\log C = \frac{E - e}{m} \qquad (21.2)$$

However, after an intravenous dose, the concentration of a drug in the body in a one-compartment open model is described as follows:

$$\log C = \log C_0 - \frac{kt}{2.3} \qquad (21.3)$$

By substituting Equation 21.2 into Equation 21.3, we get Equation 21.4, where E_0 = effect at concentration C_0:

$$\frac{E - e}{m} = \frac{E_0 - e}{m} - \frac{kt}{2.3}$$

$$\qquad (21.4)$$

$$E = E_0 - \frac{kmt}{2.3}$$

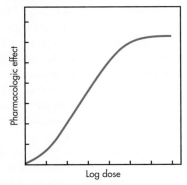

FIGURE 21-5   A typical log dose-versus-pharmacologic response curve.

The theoretical pharmacologic response at any time after an intravenous dose of a drug may be calculated using Equation 21.4. Equation 21.4 predicts that the pharmacologic effect will decline linearly with time for a drug that follows a one-compartment model, with a linear log dose–pharmacologic response. From this equation, the pharmacologic effect declines with a slope of $km/2.3$. The decrease in pharmacologic effect is affected by both the elimination constant k and the slope m. For a drug with a large m, the pharmacologic response declines rapidly and multiple doses must be given at short intervals to maintain the pharmacologic effect.

The relationship between pharmacokinetics and pharmacologic response can be demonstrated by observing the percent depression of muscular activity after an IV dose of ± tubocurarine. The decline of pharmacologic effect is linear as a function of time (Fig. 21-7). For each dose and resulting pharmacologic response, the slope of each curve is the same. Because the values for each slope, which include km (Equation 21.4), are the same, the sensitivity of the receptors for ± tubocurarine is assumed to be the same at each site of action. Note that a plot

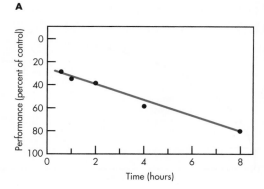

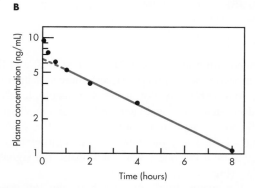

FIGURE 21-8   Mean plasma concentrations of LSD and performance test scores as a function of time after IV administration of 2 μg LSD per kilogram to five normal human subjects. (Data from Aghajanian and Bing, 1964.)

of the log concentration of drug versus time yields a straight line.

A second example of the pharmacologic effect declining linearly with time was observed with lysergic acid diethylamide (LSD) (Fig. 21-8). After an IV dose of the drug, log concentrations of drug decreased linearly with time except for a brief distribution period. Furthermore, the pharmacologic effect, as measured by the performance score of each subject, also declined linearly with time. Because the slope is governed in part by the elimination rate constant, the pharmacologic effect declines much more rapidly when the elimination rate constant is increased as a result of increased metabolism or renal excretion. Conversely, a longer pharmacologic response is experienced in patients when the drug has a longer half-life.

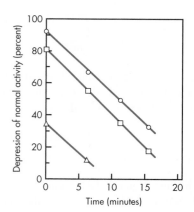

FIGURE 21-7   Depression of normal muscle activity as a function of time after IV administration of 0.1–0.2 mg ± tubocurarine per kilogram to unanesthetized volunteers, presenting mean values of six experiments on five subjects. Circles represent head lift; squares, hand grip; and triangles, inspiratory flow. (Adapted from Johansen et al, 1964, with permission.)

RELATIONSHIP BETWEEN DOSE AND DURATION OF ACTIVITY (t_{eff}), SINGLE IV BOLUS INJECTION

The relationship between the duration of the pharmacologic effect and the dose can be inferred from Equation 21.3. After an intravenous dose, assuming a one-compartment model, the time needed for any drug to decline to a concentration C is given by the following equation, assuming the drug takes effect immediately:

$$t = \frac{2.3(\log C_0 - \log C)}{k} \qquad (21.5)$$

Using C_{eff} to represent the minimum effective drug concentration, the duration of drug action can be obtained as follows:

$$t_{eff} = \frac{2.3[\log(D_0/V_D) - \log C_{eff}]}{k} \qquad (21.6)$$

Some practical applications are suggested by this equation. For example, a doubling of the dose will not result in a doubling of the effective duration of pharmacologic action. On the other hand, a doubling of $t_{1/2}$ or a corresponding decrease in k will result in a proportional increase in duration of action. A clinical situation is often encountered in the treatment of infections in which C_{eff} is the bactericidal concentration of the drug, and, in order to double the duration of the antibiotic, a considerably greater increase than simply doubling the dose is necessary.

PRACTICE PROBLEM

The minimum effective concentration (MEC or C_{eff}) in plasma for a certain antibiotic is 0.1 μg/mL. The drug follows a one-compartment open model and has an apparent volume of distribution, V_d, of 10 L and a first-order elimination rate constant of 1.0 h^{-1}.

a. What is the t_{eff} for a single 100-mg IV dose of this antibiotic?

b. What is the new t_{eff} or t'_{eff} for this drug if the dose were increased tenfold, to 1000 mg?

Solution

a. The t_{eff} for a 100-mg dose is calculated as follows. Because $V_d = 10,000$ mL,

$$C_0 = \frac{100 \text{ mg}}{10,000 \text{ mL}} = 10 \ \mu\text{g/mL}$$

For a one-compartment-model IV dose, $C = C_0 e^{-kt}$. Then,

$$0.1 = 10 e^{-(1.0)t_{eff}}$$

$$t_{eff} = 4.61 \text{ h}$$

b. The t'_{eff} for a 1000-mg dose is calculated as follows (prime refers to a new dose). Because $V_d = 10,000$ mL,

$$C'_0 = \frac{1000 \text{ mg}}{10,000 \text{ mL}} = 100 \ \mu\text{g/mL}$$

and

$$C'_{eff} = C'_0 e^{-kt'_{eff}}$$

$$0.1 = 100 e^{-(1.0)t'_{eff}}$$

$$t'_{eff} = 6.91 \text{ h}$$

The percent increase in t_{eff} is, therefore, found as

$$t_{eff} = \frac{t'_{eff} - t_{eff}}{t_{eff}} \times 100$$

Percent increase in t_{eff}

$$= \frac{6.91 - 4.61}{4.61} \times 100$$

$$= 50\%$$

This example shows that a tenfold increase in the dose increases the duration of action of a drug (t_{eff}) by only 50%.

EFFECT OF BOTH DOSE AND ELIMINATION HALF-LIFE ON THE DURATION OF ACTIVITY

A single equation can be derived to describe the relationship of dose (D_0) and the elimination half-life ($t_{1/2}$) on the effective time for therapeutic activity

(t_{eff}). This expression is derived below:

$$\ln C_{eff} = \ln C_0 - kt_{eff}$$

Because $C_0 = D_0/V_D$,

$$\ln C_{eff} = \ln\left[\frac{D_0}{V_d}\right] - kt_{eff}$$

$$kt_{eff} = \ln\left[\frac{D_0}{V_d}\right] - \ln C_{eff} \tag{21.7}$$

$$t_{eff} = \frac{1}{k}\ln\left[\frac{D_0/V_d}{C_{eff}}\right]$$

Substituting $0.693/t_{1/2}$ for k,

$$t_{eff} = 1.44 t_{1/2}\ln\left(\frac{D_0}{V_d C_{eff}}\right) \tag{21.8}$$

From Equation 21.8, an increase in $t_{1/2}$ will increase the t_{eff} in direct proportion. However, an increase in the dose, D_0, does not increase the t_{eff} in direct proportion. The effect of an increase in V_D or C_{eff} can be seen by using generated data. Only the positive solutions for Equation 21.8 are valid, although mathematically a negative t_{eff} can be obtained by increasing C_{eff} or V_D. The effect of changing dose on t_{eff} is shown in Fig. 21.9 using data generated with Equation 21.8. A nonlinear increase in t_{eff} is observed as dose increases.

EFFECT OF ELIMINATION HALF-LIFE ON DURATION OF ACTIVITY

Because elimination of drugs is due to the processes of excretion and metabolism, an alteration of any of these elimination processes will affect the $t_{1/2}$ of

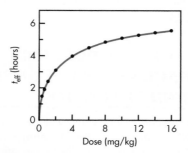

FIGURE 21-9   Plot of t_{eff} versus dose.

the drug. In certain disease states, pathophysiologic changes in hepatic or renal function will decrease the elimination of a drug, as observed by a prolonged $t_{1/2}$. This prolonged $t_{1/2}$ will lead to retention of the drug in the body, thereby increasing the duration of activity of the drug (t_{eff}) as well as increasing the possibility of drug toxicity.

To improve antibiotic therapy with the penicillin and cephalosporin antibiotics, clinicians have intentionally prolonged the elimination of these drugs by giving a second drug, probenecid, which competitively inhibits renal excretion of the antibiotic. This approach to prolonging the duration of activity of antibiotics that are rapidly excreted through the kidney has been used successfully for a number of years. Similarly, Augmentin is a combination of amoxicillin and clavulanic acid; the latter is an inhibitor of β-lactamase. This β-lactamase is a bacterial enzyme that degrades penicillin-like drugs. The data in Table 21-2 illustrate how a change in the elimination $t_{1/2}$ will affect the t_{eff} for a drug. For all doses, a 100% increase in the $t_{1/2}$ will result in a 100% increase in the t_{eff}. For example, for a drug whose $t_{1/2}$ is 0.75 hour and that is given at a dose of 2 mg/kg, the t_{eff} is 3.24 hours. If the $t_{1/2}$ is increased to 1.5 hours, the t_{eff} is increased to 6.48 hours, an increase of 100%. However, the effect of doubling the dose from 2 to 4 mg/kg (no change in elimination processes) will only increase the t_{eff} to 3.98 hours, an increase of 22.8%. The effect of prolonging the elimination half-life has an extremely important effect on the treatment of infections, particularly in patients with high metabolism, or clearance, of the antibiotic. Therefore, antibiotics must be dosed with full consideration of the effect of alteration of the $t_{1/2}$ on the t_{eff}. Consequently, a simple proportional increase in dose will leave the patient's blood concentration below the effective antibiotic level most of the time during drug therapy. The effect of a prolonged t_{eff} is shown in lines *a* and *c* in Fig. 21-10, and the disproportionate increase in t_{eff} as the dose is increased tenfold is shown in lines *a* and *b*.

SUBSTANCE ABUSE POTENTIAL

The rate of drug absorption has been associated with the potential for substance abuse. Drugs taken by the oral route have the lowest abuse potential. For example,

TABLE 21-2 **Relationship between Elimination Half-Life and Duration of Activity**

Dose (mg/kg)	$t_{1/2} = 0.75$ h t_{eff} (h)	$t_{1/2} = 1.5$ h t_{eff} (h)
2.0	3.24	6.48
3.0	3.67	7.35
4.0	3.98	7.97
5.0	4.22	8.45
6.0	4.42	8.84
7.0	4.59	9.18
8.0	4.73	9.47
9.0	4.86	9.72
10	4.97	9.95
11	5.08	10.2
12	5.17	10.3
13	5.26	10.5
14	5.34	10.7
15	5.41	10.8
16	5.48	11.0
17	5.55	11.1
18	5.61	11.2
19	5.67	11.3
20	5.72	11.4

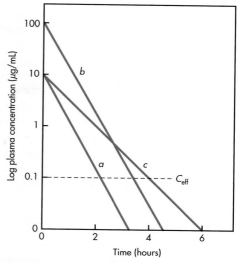

FIGURE 21-10 Plasma level–time curves describing the relationship of both dose and elimination half-life on duration of drug action. C_{eff} = effective concentration. Curve a = single 100-mg IV injection of drug; $k = 1.0$ h^{-1}. Curve b = single 1000-mg IV injection; $k = 1.0$ h^{-1}. Curve c = single 100-mg IV injection; $k = 0.5$ h^{-1}. V_D is 10 L.

DRUG TOLERANCE AND PHYSICAL DEPENDENCY

The study of drug tolerance and physical dependency is of particular interest in understanding the actions of abused drug substances, such as opiates and cocaine. Drug tolerance is a quantitative change in the sensitivity of the drug at the receptor site and is demonstrated by a decrease in pharmacodynamic effect after repeated exposure to the same drug. The degree of tolerance may vary greatly (Cox, 1990). Drug tolerance has been well described for organic nitrates, opioids, and other drugs. For example, the nitrates relax vascular smooth muscle and have been used for both acute angina (eg, nitroglycerin sublingual spray or transmucosal tablet) or angina prophylaxis (eg, nitroglycerin transdermal, oral controlled-release isosorbide dinitrate). Well-controlled clinical studies have shown that tolerance to the vascular and antianginal effects of nitrates may develop. For nitrate therapy, the use of a low nitrate or nitrate-free periods has been advocated as part of the therapeutic approach. The magnitude of drug tolerance is a function of both the

coca leaves containing cocaine alkaloid have been chewed by South American Indians for centuries (Johanson and Fischman, 1989). Cocaine abuse has become a problem as a result of the availability of cocaine alkaloid ("crack" cocaine) and because of the use of other routes of drug administration (intravenous, intranasal, or smoking) that allow a very rapid rate of drug absorption and onset of action (Cone, 1995). Studies on diazepam (de Wit et al, 1993) and nicotine (Henningfield and Keenan, 1993) have shown that the rate of drug delivery correlates with the abuse liability of such drugs. Thus, the rate of drug absorption influences the abuse potential of these drugs, and the route of drug administration that provides faster absorption and more rapid onset leads to greater abuse.

dosage and the frequency of drug administration. Cross-tolerance can occur for similar drugs that act on the same receptors. Tolerance does not develop uniformly to all the pharmacologic or toxic actions of the drug. For example, patients who show tolerance to the depressant activity of high doses of opiates will still exhibit "pinpoint" pupils and constipation.

The mechanism of drug tolerance may be due to (1) disposition or pharmacokinetic tolerance or (2) pharmacodynamic tolerance. Pharmacokinetic tolerance is often due to enzyme induction (discussed in earlier chapters), in which the hepatic drug clearance increases with repeated drug exposure. Pharmacodynamic tolerance is due to a cellular or receptor alteration in which the drug response is less than what is predicted in the patient given subsequent drug doses. Measurement of serum drug concentrations may differentiate between pharmacokinetic tolerance and pharmacodynamic tolerance.

Acute tolerance, or tachyphylaxis, which is the rapid development of tolerance, may occur due to a change in the sensitivity of the receptor or depletion of a cofactor after only a single or a few doses of the drug. Drugs that work indirectly by releasing norepinephrine may show tachyphylaxis. Drug tolerance should be differentiated from genetic factors that account for normal variability in the drug response.

Physical dependency is demonstrated by the appearance of withdrawal symptoms after cessation of the drug. Workers exposed to volatile organic nitrates in the workplace may initially develop headaches and dizziness followed by tolerance with continuous exposure. However, after leaving the workplace for a few days, the workers may demonstrate nitrate withdrawal symptoms. Factors that may affect drug dependency may include the dose or amount of drug used (intensity of drug effect), the duration of drug use (months, years, and peak use), and the total dose (amount of drug × duration). The appearance of withdrawal symptoms may be abruptly precipitated in opiate-dependent subjects by the administration of naloxone (Suboxone®), an opioid antagonist that has no agonist properties.

Frequency Asked Question

▶ *How does the rate of systemic drug absorption affect the abuse potential of drugs such as cocaine or heroin?*

HYPERSENSITIVITY AND ADVERSE RESPONSE

Many drug responses, such as hypersensitivity and allergic responses, are not fully explained by pharmacodynamics and pharmacokinetics. Allergic responses generally are not dose related, although some penicillin-sensitive patients may respond to threshold skin concentrations, but otherwise no dose–response relationship has been established. Skin eruption is a common symptom of drug allergy. Allergic reactions can occur at extremely low drug concentrations. Some urticaria episodes in patients have been traced to penicillin contamination in food or to penicillin contamination during dispensing or manufacturing of other drugs. A patient's allergic reactions are important data that must be recorded in the patient's profile along with other adverse reactions. Penicillin allergic reaction in the population is often detected by skin test with benzylpenicilloyl polylysine (PPL). The incidence of penicillin allergic reaction occurs in about 1%–10% of patients. The majority of these reactions are minor cutaneous reactions such as urticaria, angioedema, and pruritus. Serious allergic reactions such as anaphylaxis are rare, with an incidence of 0.021%–0.106% for penicillins (Lin, 1992). For cephalosporins, the incidence of anaphylactic reaction is less than 0.02%. Anaphylactic reaction for cefaclor was reported to be 0.001% in a postmarketing survey. There are emerging trends showing that there may be a difference between the original and the new generations of cephalosporins (Anne and Reisman, 1995). Cross-sensitivity to similar chemical classes of drugs can occur.

Allergic reactions may be immediate or delayed and have been related to IgE mechanisms. In β-lactam (penicillin) drug allergy, immediate reactions occur in about 30–60 minutes, but either a delayed reaction or an accelerated reaction may occur from 1 to 72 hours after administration. Anaphylactic reaction may occur in both groups. Although some early evidence of cross-hypersensitivity between penicillin and cephalosporin was observed, the incidence in patients sensitive to penicillin shows only a twofold increase in sensitivity to cephalosporin compared with that of the general population. The report rationalized that it is safe to administer cephalosporin to penicillin-sensitive patients and that the penicillin skin test is not useful in identifying patients who are allergic to cephalosporin, because of the low incidence of cross-reactivity (Anne and Reisman, 1995). In practice, the clinicians should evaluate the risk of drug allergy against the choice of alternative medication. Some earlier reports showed that cross-sensitivity between penicillin and cephalosporin was due to the presence of trace penicillin present in cephalosporin products.

Biological Markers (Biomarkers)

As described previously, the interaction of the drug with the receptor results in a cascade of events ultimately leading to a PD response. The PD response measured could be a biomarker level that could be linked to a clinical endpoint. This section provides an overview of biomarkers and surrogate endpoints and its application in drug development.

Biomarkers are a set of parameters that can be measured quantitatively to represent a healthy or a pathological process within the body. It could be as simple as a physical measurement like blood pressure or a biochemical such as blood glucose to greater complex situations that involves genomic markers such as Taq1B polymorphism in the cholesteryl ester transfer protein (*CETP*) gene that code for cholesterol ester transfer protein (Kuivenhoven et al, 1998) or the *HER2* (a tyrosine kinase that is a member of the epidermal growth factor receptor [EGFR] family) expression in metastatic breast cancer (Shak, 1999). Lesko and Atkinson (2001) have proposed a working definition of a biological marker, referring to it as a physical sign or laboratory measurement that occurs in association with a pathological process and that has putative diagnostic and/or prognostic utility.

Biomarkers when utilized in a logical and rational way could help accelerate clinical drug development by fostering informed decision making and can bridge preclinical mechanistic studies and empirical clinical trials. Some examples where use of biomarkers leads to accelerated drug development are described below. The number of fractures is considered as a primary response variable for approving drugs to treat osteoporosis, and such trials are typically lengthy and hence very costly. To approve a different dosing regimen for drugs already approved based on the number of fractures as the primary endpoint, changes in the bone mineral density can be utilized as a biomarker for drug approval. Bone mineral density is relatively simpler and easier to measure, and hence shorter trials are required. Aminobisphosphonate, risedronate 5 mg once daily (Actavis, 1998) was approved based on fracture as the endpoint. Subsequently 35 mg once weekly and two 75-mg tablets monthly were approved based on changes in bone mineral density.

Along similar lines, if we assume that the progression of disease and treatment intervention is similar among adults and children populations, then drug approvals in pediatric population can be based on PK studies (exposure) and/or biomarker data. For example, sotalol (a beta-blocker) that was approved for ventricular tachycardia in adults using atrial fibrillation and flutter as endpoints was approved in the pediatric population based on a PK study and its effect on QTc and heart rate (Gobburu, 2009).

Besides bridging preclinical and clinical phases of development, biomarkers can also be used as (i) a diagnostic tool to detect and diagnose disease conditions in patients (eg, elevated blood glucose levels are indicative of onset of diabetes mellitus), (ii) a tool for the staging of disease (eg, levels of prostate-specific antigen concentration in blood that is correlated to tumor growth and metastasis), (iii) an indicator of disease prognosis (anatomically measuring size of tumors), and (iv) a predictive and monitoring tool to assess the extent of clinical response to a therapeutic intervention (eg, measuring blood cholesterol as a means to assess cardiac disease or viral load used to assess the efficacy of an antiviral therapy) (Biomarkers Definitions Working, 2001).

A *surrogate endpoint* is a biomarker that is intended to substitute a clinically meaningful endpoint. Thus, a surrogate endpoint is expected to predict the presence or absence of clinical benefit or harm based on epidemiologic, therapeutic, pathophysiologic, or other forms of scientific evidence (Lesko and Atkinson, 2001). In a way, a surrogate endpoint is a subset of biomarkers; however, it should be realized that not all biomarkers could achieve the status of a surrogate endpoint. Whereas, a clinical endpoint relates a clinically meaningful measure of how a patient feels, functions, or survives (Strimbu and Tavel, 2010). Blood pressure is probably one of the well-studied surrogates that correlates well to the cardiovascular health of the individual.

Elevated blood pressure (also called hypertension) is known to be a direct cause of stroke, heart failure, renal failure, and accelerated coronary artery disease, and lowering blood pressure can lead to reduction in the rates of morbidity and mortality outcomes (Temple, 1999). Another example where a surrogate endpoint that has created immense interest is the CD4+ count in the treatment of AIDS and HIV infections (Weiss and Mazade, 1990). The surrogate endpoints not only reduce the overall cost of the trial but also allow shorter follow-up periods than would be possible during clinical endpoint studies.

Among the successes of surrogate endpoints in predicting clinical outcomes, certain failures of perceived surrogate endpoints not predicting meaningful clinical outcomes have created controversies doubting whether surrogate markers should be a principal driver for making decisions for drug approvals (Colburn, 2000). To this context, one of many examples where surrogate endpoints that have been proven to mislead clinical outcomes posing greater threat to health and safety of thousands of patients happened to be in the Cardiac Arrhythmia Suppression Trial (CAST). In this trial, three antiarrhythmic drugs flecainide, ecainide, and moricizine were compared to a placebo treatment in patients with myocardial infarction who frequently experienced premature ventricular contractions where sudden death was considered as a primary outcome. These drugs were successful in suppressing arrhythmias but, on the contrary, were responsible to increase the risk of death from other causes (Echt et al, 1991). In this case the surrogate endpoint "arrhythmia" was unable to capture the effect of the treatment on the true outcome "death" of the treatment.

In the drug development process, the rationale to introduce a biomarker or surrogate endpoint should begin as early as possible, typically as a receptor or enzyme-based high-throughput screening rationale during the preclinical phases. As newer technologies develop through genomics and proteomics, these existing biomarkers would evolve further as correct clinical targets get identified. The ability of a surrogate endpoint to predict clinical outcome is equally good as the intermediate bridge that is developed to link the surrogate to the clinical endpoint. As long as the mechanism of drug action to efficacy and toxicity is thoroughly studied, the surrogate endpoints would be predictive of clinical outcomes. Examples of biomarkers described in Table 21-3 that substitute for specific clinical endpoints may differ from one another in their predictive

TABLE 21-3   Examples of Biomarkers/Surrogate Endpoints and Their Respective Clinical Endpoints

Therapeutic Class	Biomarker/Surrogate	Clinical Endpoint
Physiological markers		
Antihypertensive drugs	Reduced blood pressure	Reduced stroke
Drugs for glaucoma	Reduced intraocular pressure	Preservation of vision
Drugs for osteoporosis	Increased bone density	Reduced fracture rate
Antiarrhythmic drugs	Reduced arrhythmias	Increased survival
Laboratory markers		
Antibiotics	Negative culture	Clinical cure
Antiretroviral drugs	Increased CD4 counts and reduced viral RNA	Increased survival
Antidiabetic drugs	Reduced blood glucose	Reduced morbidity
Lipid-lowering drugs	Reduced cholesterol	Reduced coronary artery disease
Drugs for prostate cancer	Reduced prostate specific antigen	Tumor response

Adapted from Atkinson (2001).

ability; nonetheless, their clinical utility cannot be underestimated.

Frequently Asked Questions

▶ *What is a drug receptor?*

▶ *Explain why a drug that binds to a receptor may be an agonist, a partial agonist, or an antagonist.*

▶ *If we need to develop a drug where only 25% of maximal activation is needed to achieve therapeutic benefit, what type of agent among the four classes will you pick and why?*

▶ *What are the other utilities of biomarkers besides being used as a bridging tool to link preclinical and clinical drug development?*

Types of Pharmacodynamic Response

PD responses can be continuous, discrete (categorical), and time-to-event outcomes. Continuous PD responses can take any value in a range such as blood glucose levels, blood pressure readings, or enzyme levels. Categorical or discrete responses are either binary, for example, death or no death, or ordinal, for example, graded pain scores or counts over a time period, such as the number of seizures in a month. Time-to-event outcomes constitute continuous measures of time but with censoring, for example, time to relapse or time until transplant. In this chapter, we will deal with continuous PD responses only.

Components of PK-PD Models

The use of mathematical modeling to link the PK of the drug to the time course of drug effects (PD) has evolved greatly since the pioneering work of Gerhard Levy in the mid-1960s (Levy, 1964, 1966). Today, PK-PD modeling is a scientific discipline in its own, which characterizes the PK of a drug, relates PK to the PD, and is then applied for predictions of the response under new conditions (eg, new dose or dosing regimen). For any PK-PD model, the conceptual framework of the relationship is depicted in Fig. 21-11 (Jusko et al, 1995; Mager et al, 2003). The scheme describes that there may be at least four intermediary components between drug in plasma (C_p) and the measured response (R).

The first component of the PK-PD framework is the administration of the drug and the time course of drug in the relevant biological fluid (plasma, C_p). The drug gets eliminated from the body depending on its disposition kinetics. The concentration–time profile of the drug in plasma is typically represented by a PK model or function given as

$$C_p = f(\theta_{PK}, X, t) \qquad (21.9)$$

The PK model or function can be thought as a one-compartment model after an intravenous bolus administration described as

$$C_p = \frac{\text{Dose}}{V} \cdot e^{-\frac{CL}{V} \cdot t} \qquad (21.10)$$

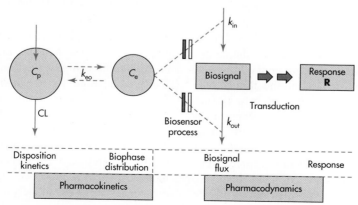

FIGURE 21-11 Basic components of PD models of drug action. (Adapted from Jusko et al, 1995).

Here, θ_{PK} denotes the fundamental PK parameters namely, clearance (Cl), and volume of distribution (V_D). X refers to the subject variables such as dose, dosing regimen, and t is the time. The drug concentration in plasma then distributes to the site of action or the effect site referred to as biophase concentrations, C_e. The plasma concentrations, C_p, are assumed to be proportional to the biophase concentrations, C_e, and the distribution of the drug to the effect site is governed by a distributional rate constant namely, k_{e0}. The effect site or the biophase concentrations then serve as the driving function responsible for pharmacodynamic response, R, by influencing the production or degradation of the biosignal. The formation rate constant for the biosignal is denoted as k_{in} and the degradation rate constant is denoted as k_{out}. Analogous to PK Equation 21.9 above, the time course of response is described by a mathematical function as

$$R = f(\theta_{PD}, C_p \ or \ C_e, Z) \qquad (21.11)$$

The mathematical function can be thought of as an equation linking the pharmacodynamic response to the drug concentrations. Here, θ_{PD} represents the fundamental pharmacodynamic parameters, namely maximum effect, E_{max} and potency of the drug, EC_{50}, which are described in detail in later sections; C_p and C_e are the concentrations of the drug in plasma or at the biophase, and Z represents a vector of drug-independent system parameters. As seen from Fig. 21-11, the effect site concentrations affect formation or degradation of the biosignal via a biosensor process, and further undergo a transduction process to elicit the response. Thus, biosignal can be considered as a biomarker and is related to clinical endpoint or the response. Depending on the nature of the experiment, either only data on the biosignal is measured or both biosignals and the clinical outcome information may be available. In a typical situation, it might not be possible to capture all components of PK-PD framework; rather the manifestation of the response will depend on which of the processes dominate the overall response. For example, there are three rate constants involved, namely k_{e0}, which controls the distribution of the

drug concentration between plasma and the biophase, and k_{in} and k_{out}, which are formation and degradation rate constants of the biosignal, and the role of these three rate constants may influence the type of the PK-PD relationship. When the biophase distribution represents a rate-limiting step (ie, k_{e0} is slow compared to k_{in} or k_{out}) for drugs in producing their response, a distributional delay or a link compartment model is used to explain the PK-PD relationship. The drug elicits a direct response, but there is a delay in the response due to distributional delay in the drug to reach the biophase. On the other hand, if the distribution of the drug to effect site is very fast, then the process involving the formation or degradation of the biosignal may take over. Such instances occur when the drug acts via an indirect mechanism and the biosensor process (depicted in Fig. 21-11) may stimulate or inhibit the production or degradation of the biosignal. In such a case, an indirect response model is used to describe the PK-PD relationship. The biosensor process involves interaction between the drug and the pharmacological target and can be explained by the receptor theory.

In summary, the conceptual PK-PD framework can be considered broadly applicable to various drugs with different mechanism of action and the final PK-PD model chosen to describe should encompass principles of pharmacology of the drug and the system. The various PD models described here in this section are dealt with in detail with examples in the following sections.

Pharmacodynamic Models

PD models involve complex mechanisms that may not be easily simplified. Researchers have employed empirical, semi-mechanistic, or mechanistic models to explain the complex mechanisms of drug action. The predictive ability of empiric models might be limited under new scenarios such as new dose or dosing regimen. The understanding of drug response is greatly enhanced when PK modeling techniques are combined with clinical pharmacology, resulting in the development of mechanism-based PK-PD models. In this section, we will explore in details different types of PD models with examples.

Noncompartmental PK-PD Models

Under this approach, PK parameters like peak plasma drug concentrations (C_{max}), area under the curve (AUC), and half-life ($t_{1/2}$) are often correlated to PD parameters like half maximal inhibitory concentration (IC_{50}). Such PK-PD relationship has been applied successfully among antimicrobials where the minimum inhibitory concentration (MIC) is often the PD parameter. The PK parameters C_{max}, AUC, and $t_{1/2}$ are considered because they are often influenced by the choice of drug or by the manner the antibiotics are administered (route and dosing regimen). Large doses of antibiotics when administered via intravenous route can produce high C_{max}, whereas a large AUC can be achieved by administering a large dose that has a relatively longer plasma half-life or by multiple dosing. A longer half-life drug will persist in the plasma for an extended time compared to a drug with shorter half-life. Thus, the manner by which these PK parameters relate to the MIC of the infecting pathogen becomes a key factor to the observed effect. Hence, the MIC is then designated to play an important role as a PD parameter. Usually, the PK parameters C_{max} and AUC are divided by the MIC yielding PK-PD indices, namely C_{max}/MIC, AUC/MIC (or AUIC), whereas the time over which drug concentrations remain above its MIC is another PK-PD index referred to as $T >$ MIC. It may be worth realizing that better predictions of clinical efficacy using PK-PD indices can be sought if protein binding is adequately factored into these considerations as the therapeutic effect of a drug is often produced by the free fraction of the drug rather than the total drug concentrations in plasma. Thus the most relevant concentrations are the free drug concentrations at the site of action, and it has been shown that antibiotics that distribute to the interstitial fluid may in fact have much lower tissue concentrations compared to plasma (Lorentzen et al, 1996). Figure 21-12 shows the three MIC-based PK-PD indices for a hypothetical antimicrobial drug.

Now let's understand what these indices really are and how they relate to the two distinct patterns associated with killing of antimicrobials (Craig, 2002), viz: (a) concentration-dependent and (b) time-dependent killing patterns.

Concentration-dependent killing pattern is associated with a *higher rate and extent* of killing with increasing concentrations of the drug above the MIC of the pathogen. Hence, drugs that follow this pattern can maximize killing by maximizing their systemic drug exposure that is often represented by peak plasma drug concentration (C_{max}) and the extent of exposure (AUC). The C_{max}/MIC ratio relates to the

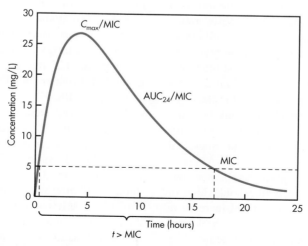

FIGURE 21-12   MIC-based PK-PD indices for the evaluation of a hypothetical anti-infective agent. MIC: minimum inhibitory concentrations; PD: pharmacodynamics; PK: pharmacokinetics. (Adapted from Schuck and Derendorf, 2005.)

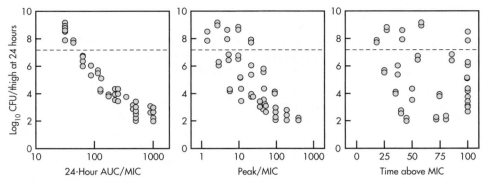

FIGURE 21-13   Relationship between three PD parameters (24-hour AUC/MIC ratio, C_{max}/MIC ratio, and percentage of time that serum levels exceed above MIC) and the number of *S. pneumoniae* ATCC 10813 in the thighs of neutropenic mice after 24 hours of therapy with temafloxacin. Each point represents one data for one mouse. The dotted line reflects the number of bacteria at the time of therapy initiation.

efficacy of drugs that exhibit a concentration-dependent killing pattern. Figure 21-13 shows a plot of colony-forming units (CFUs) against three PK-PD indices: AUC/MIC ratio, C_{max}/MIC ratio, and time above MIC in a mouse infection model where an infection in the thigh due to *Streptococcus pneumoniae* was treated with temafloxacin (Craig, 2002). It was interesting to note that there was no correlation between CFU/thigh and the percentage of time the drug levels exceeded the MIC in the serum. However, an excellent relationship was evident between CFU/thigh and the AUC/MIC ratio followed by C_{max}/MIC. The AUC/MIC and C_{max}/MIC ratios have been the PK-PD indices that often well correlate with the therapeutic efficacy of aminoglycoside and fluoroquinolone antimicrobials. Most often and so in the above example, the AUC/MIC ratio shows a better correlation to efficacy compared to the C_{max}/MIC ratio. However, the latter index may be more relevant and thus important where there is a significant risk of emergence of a resistant microbial subpopulation.

Time-dependent killing produces higher systemic concentrations beyond a threshold value or MIC and does not cause a proportional increase in the killing rate of the microbes. In fact the killing proceeds at a *zero-order rate* when systemic drug concentrations are above the MIC for its pathogen, and under such conditions, a minimal correlation is expected between C_{max}/MIC and the pathogen

survival rates. However, the PK-PD index that would most likely correlate to the killing would be the %T > MIC; which is the percentage of time within the dosing interval during which the systemic drug concentrations remain above the MIC of the drug for the pathogen. In contrast to aminoglycosides and fluoroquinolones, all β-lactam antibiotics and macrolides (Vogelman et al, 1988; Craig, 1995) follow a time-dependent bactericidal activity. To illustrate this killing pattern, Craig (1995) studied the activity of cefotaxime against the standard strain of *Klebseilla pneumoniae* in the lungs of a neutropenic mice model. In this study, pairs of mice were treated with multiple dose regimens that varied by the dose and the dosing interval (ie, a 500-mg single oral dose, 250 mg bid, 125 mg qid, and so on). Lungs were assessed for remaining CFUs after 24 hours of therapy and the PK-PD indices C_{max}/MIC, AUC/MIC, and %T > MIC were determined for each dosing regimen. Figure 21-14A and 21-14B showed poor relationship between the CFU per lung and the C_{max}/MIC, AUC/MIC ratios. A highly significant correlation between the CFU remaining per lung and the duration of time that serum levels were above the MIC (%T > MIC) was evident. Thus depending upon the type of antimicrobial, there would be one PK-PD index that would be highly correlated to its antimicrobial efficacy. It may be worth considering that percent time above MIC could be enhanced by dose fractionation such that the total daily dose

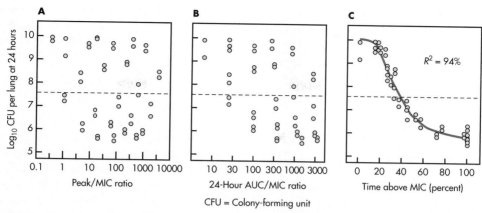

FIGURE 21-14   (A–C). Relationship between three PD parameters (C_{max}/MIC ratio, 24-hour AUC/MIC ratio, and percentage of time that serum levels exceed above MIC) and the number of *K. pneumoniae* ATCC 43816 in the lungs of neutropenic mice after 24 hours of therapy with cefotaxime. Each point represents one mouse. Animals were infected by a 45-minute aerosol given 14 hours prior to therapy. The dotted line reflects the number of bacteria at the time of therapy initiation (7.5 $\log_{10}$ colony forming units [CFU]/lung). The R^2 value in (**C**) represents the percentage of variation in bacterial numbers that could be attributed to differences in time above MIC. (Adapted from Craig, 1995.)

remains constant. Table 21-4 illustrates some of the specific PK-PD indices that correlate with efficacy in the animal infection models for different class of antimicrobials.

E_{max} Drug-Concentration Effect Model

Receptor occupancy theory forms the basis of pharmacodynamic response evaluation and is routinely employed to describe concentration–effect/exposure-response relationship in drug discovery and development. The origins of the fundamental PD models can

TABLE 21-4   PK-PD Indices Determining the Efficacy for Different Antimicrobials

PK-PD Index	Antimicrobial
% Time above MIC	Penicillins, cephalosporins, aztreonam, carbapenems, tribactams, macrolides, clindamycin, oxazolidinones, flucytosine
Peak/MIC ratio	Aminoglycosides, fluoroquinolones, daptomycin, vancomycin, amphotericin B
AUC/MIC ratio	Aminoglycosides, fluoroquinolones, daptomycin, vancomycin, ketolides, quinupristin/dalfopristin, tetracyclines, fluconazole

be derived using the receptor occupancy theory. The theory and derivation are described in detail as follows.

In general, as the drug is administered, one or more drug molecules may interact with a receptor to form a complex that in turn elicits a pharmacodynamic response.

$$R + C \leftrightarrow RC \qquad (21.12)$$

The rate of change of the drug–receptor (RC) complex is given by the following equation:

$$\frac{d[RC]}{dt} = k_{on} \cdot (R_T - RC) \cdot C - k_{off} \cdot RC \qquad (21.13)$$

where R_T is the maximum receptor density, C is the concentration of the drug at the site of action, k_{on} is the second-order association rate constant, and k_{off} is the first-order dissociation rate constant. The term $(R_T - RC)$ represents the free receptors, R, available as the total number of receptors, or the maximum receptor density can be written as $R_T = R + RC$. Under equilibrium conditions, that is, when $\frac{d[RC]}{dt} = 0$, the above equation becomes:

$$k_{on} \cdot (R_T - RC) \cdot C = k_{off} \cdot RC \qquad (21.14)$$

Upon further rearrangement we get

$$k_{on} \cdot R_T \cdot C = RC \cdot (k_{on} \cdot C + k_{off}) \tag{21.15}$$

$$RC = \frac{k_{on} \cdot R_T \cdot C}{k_{off} + k_{on} \cdot C} \tag{21.16}$$

$$RC = \frac{R_T \cdot C}{\dfrac{k_{off}}{k_{on}} + C} \tag{21.17}$$

$$RC = \frac{R_T \cdot C}{K_D + C} \tag{21.18}$$

where K_D is the equilibrium dissociation constant ($\frac{k_{off}}{k_{on}}$). Under the assumption that the magnitude of effect, E, is proportional to the $[RC]$ complex, the fraction of maximum possible effect, E_{max}, is equal to the fractional occupancy, $f_b = \dfrac{E}{E_{max}}$, of the receptor, which can be described as

$$f_b = \frac{E}{E_{max}} = \frac{[RC]}{R_T} \tag{21.19}$$

Hence,

$$E = E_{max} \cdot \frac{\dfrac{R_T \cdot C}{K_D + C}}{R_T} \tag{21.20}$$

$$E = \frac{E_{max} \cdot C}{k_D + C} \tag{21.21}$$

Here, K_D has the units of concentration and represents the concentration at which 50% of E_{max} is achieved. On substituting $K_D = EC_{50}$ yields the classical E_{max} concentration–effect relationship as below:

$$E = \frac{E_{max} \cdot C}{EC_{50} + C} \tag{21.22}$$

E_{max} refers to the maximum possible effect that can be produced by a drug and EC_{50} is the sensitivity parameter or the potency parameter representing the drug concentration producing 50% of E_{max}. As the fundamental PK parameters of a drug are clearance (Cl) and volume of distribution (V_D), E_{max} and EC_{50} are the fundamental PD parameters for a drug, and hence they define the pharmacodynamic properties of the drug. From Equation 21.22, it can be inferred that the typical effect–concentration relationship is curvilinear as shown in Fig. 21-15 with parameters as $E_{max} = 100$ and $EC_{50} = 50 \ \mu g/mL$.

The Hill equation or the sigmoidal E_{max} model contains an additional parameter, typically represented as γ and called as the Hill coefficient. The sigmoidal E_{max} model is shown in Equation 21.23 below:

$$E = \frac{E_{max} \cdot C^{\gamma}}{EC_{50}^{\gamma} + C^{\gamma}} \tag{21.23}$$

The Hill coefficient, γ (or the slope term), describes the steepness of the effect–concentration relationship.

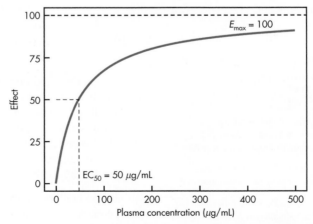

FIGURE 21-15   The E_{max} concentration–effect relationship. Fifty percent of the maximum effect is achieved at the EC_{50} concentration.

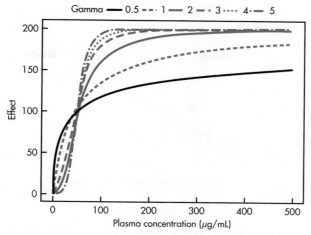

FIGURE 21-16   Effect of varying Hill coefficients on the E_{max} concentration–effect relationship.

Some researchers also describe γ as the number of drug molecules binding to a receptor. When more drug molecules bind (typically $\gamma > 5$), the effect–concentration relationship is very steep. Figure 21-16 shows the sigmoidal E_{max} model for different Hill coefficient values. As seen from Fig. 21-16, values of γ less than or equal to unity have broader slopes, and as γ increases, the steepness of the relationship increases with values of $\gamma > 4$ signifying an all-or-none response. The utility of the Hill coefficient in model building is usually considered as an empirical device to provide improved model fit for the data. However, the value of Hill coefficient potentially is from its real application in terms of treatment adherence. For example, if a drug has a steep concentration–effect relationship, then missing a dose can have greater impact on the response for a subject as compared to a drug for which the Hill coefficient is around unity. Examples of drugs where an E_{max} model was used to describe the PK-PD relationships will be discussed in detail in a later section on direct effect models.

Linear Concentration-Effect Model

Linear concentration-effect model is based on the assumption that the effect (E) is proportional to the drug concentration, typically the plasma drug concentration (C). This model can be derived from the E_{max} model under the conditions that drug concentration (C) << EC_{50}, reducing Equation 21.22 to the following:

$$E = S \cdot C \qquad (21.24)$$

where mathematically S is defined as the slope of linear concentration–effect relationship line (Holford and Sheiner, 1981). Pharmacodynamically, S is the effect produced by 1 unit of drug concentration. This relationship can be observed visually in Fig. 21-15, when the concentration is <<EC_{50}, the concentration–effect (C-E) follows approximately linear relationship. This model assumes that effect will continue to increase as the drug concentration is increased, although as we know there is always a maximal pharmacological effect (E_{max}) beyond which increasing drug concentrations does not yield further increase in the effect. Also, the concentration–effect relationship is seldom linear over a broad range of drug concentrations. Thus, this simple model has limited application in PD modeling. Nonetheless, a specific PD effect where linear C-E model is utilized extensively is in evaluation of drug effects on cardiac repolarization (as measured by QT interval from an electrocardiogram [ECG]) in humans (Garnett et al, 2008; Russell et al, 2008; Florian et al, 2011). Linear C-E model has been applied to describe the concentration–QTc relationship for moxifloxacin (Florian et al, 2011)

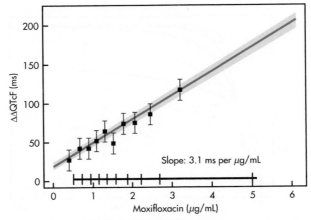

FIGURE 21-17   ΔΔQTcF versus concentration predictions with 90% confidence interval (CI). Data points depict quantile means ±90% CI. Decile ranges are displayed along the *x* axis.

as shown in Fig. 21-17 and also applied for modeling concentration–QTc relationship for new drugs under development. Furthermore, the concentration–QTc relationship and analysis has played a key role in the US FDA regulatory review of new drugs for pro-arrhythmic risk evaluation (Garnett et al, 2008).

Log-Linear Concentration-Effect Model

The log-linear model is based on the assumption that effect is proportional to the log of drug concentration and can be described as:

$$E = S \cdot \log C + E_0 \qquad (21.25)$$

where S is the same as that described for the linear concentration-effect model previously and E_0 is the baseline effect. This model is also a special case of E_{max} model as the log C versus effect follows a nearly linear relationship between 20% and 80% of E_{max} (Meibohm and Derendorf, 1997). The limitation of this model is that it can predict neither the effect when drug concentrations are zero nor the maximal effect (E_{max}). This model has been used to describe concentration–effect relationship for (i) synthesis rate of prothrombin complex activity in relation to warfarin plasma concentrations (Nagashima et al, 1969) and (ii) propranolol concentration and reduction of exercise-induced tachycardia (Coltart and Hamer, 1970) (Fig. 21-18).

Additive and Proportional Drug Effect Models

The fundamental E_{max} model (Equation 21.22) or the linear effect model (Equation 21.24) signifies that when the drug concentration is not present, then there is no effect. But often, there exists a baseline response, which implies that even when the drug is not present, there exists a baseline response. The effect of baseline can be additive or proportional to the drug effect leading to additive or proportional drug response model.

Additive Drug Effect Model

When a drug exhibits additive drug effect, it implies that the drug response is independent of the baseline as represented by the equation below:

$$R(t) = R(0) + E \qquad (21.26)$$

where $R(t)$ is the drug response at time t, $R(0)$ is the response at baseline or time = 0, and E represents the drug effect, which could be linear as in Equation 21.27, or E_{max} type of relationship as shown in Equation 21.28:

Additive linear drug effect model:

$$R(t) = R(0) + S \cdot C \qquad (21.27)$$

Additive E_{max} drug effect model:

$$R(t) = R(0) + \frac{E_{max} \cdot C}{EC_{50} + C} \qquad (21.28)$$

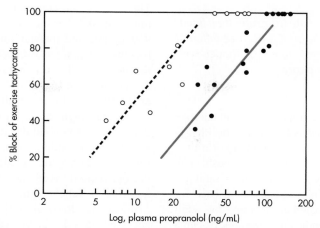

FIGURE 21-18   Log plasma concentration/response relationship for orally administered (°) and intravenously administered (•) propranolol.

Here, C is the plasma concentration at any time t. The interpretation of E_{max} is the maximal drug effect that can be obtained and has the same units as the response. Based on the equations above, it can be inferred that there is a constant baseline response added to the drug effect, or in other words, the drug effect is independent of the baseline response. The baseline response in mathematical terms can be considered similar to an intercept term. The additive drug effect for the linear and the E_{max} drug effect model, where the slope is positive, is shown in Fig. 21-19. The slopes for the different baseline responses remain the same. Depending on whether it is a stimulatory (positive slope: $S > 0$ or $E_{max} > 0$) or an inhibitory effect (negative slope: $S < 0$ or $E_{max} < 0$), the graphs have an increasing or a decreasing trend with increasing concentrations.

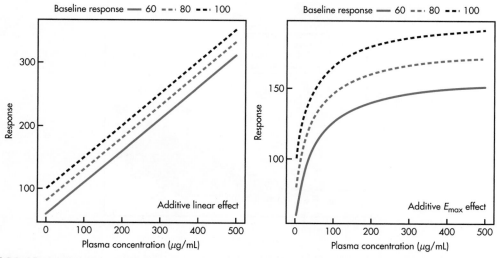

FIGURE 21-19   Additive drug effect (linear and E_{max}) upon varying baseline values. For the linear effect model, $S = 0.5$ units was used. For the E_{max} model, the drug effect parameters are $E_{max} = 100$ units and $EC_{50} = 50$ μg/mL.

> **Exercise:** *Using Excel, create the graph for a linear effect model with a slope of –0.3 at three different baseline values. Similarly for E_{max} model with negative E_{max} value, inhibitory.*

Application: One of the examples where an additive E_{max} effect model was used is to explain the PK-PD relationship of activated plasma thromboplastin time (aPTT) to argatroban concentrations (Madabushi et al, 2011). Argatroban is a synthetic thrombin inhibitor and is approved in the United States to be used for prophylaxis or as anticoagulant therapy for adult subjects with heparin-induced thrombocytopenia (HIT). Initially, there was no dosing recommendations for argatroban in pediatric subjects with HIT and often extrapolated from adult dose. Madabushi et al used PK (argatroban concentrations) and PD (aPTT) data from healthy adults and pediatric patients to derive dosing recommendations of argatroban in pediatric subjects with HIT. They used a direct additive E_{max} model to describe the argatroban concentration–aPTT relationship as shown below:

$$\text{aPTT } (t, \text{seconds}) = \text{aPTT } (t = 0, \text{seconds})$$

$$+ \frac{E_{max}(\text{seconds}) \cdot C}{EC_{50} + C} \qquad (21.29)$$

The argatroban concentration producing 50% of maximal aPTT response (EC_{50}) was estimated as 959 ng/mL and the maximal aPTT response from baseline (E_{max}) was estimated as 84.4 seconds, and the baseline aPTT response is estimated at 32 seconds as evident from Fig. 21-20. The article also considered different subject-specific factors, such as hepatic status, that might explain the variability seen in the data, which is beyond the scope of this chapter. The PK-PD relationship developed was used for simulations based on which pediatric dosing recommendations were derived and are currently available in argatroban label (http://www.accessdata.fda.gov /drugsatfda_docs/label/2014/020883s016lbl.pdf, accessed, June 17, 2014, section 8.4).

Proportional Drug Effect Model

As the name suggests, the response at any time depends proportionally on the baseline response. If the baseline response is higher, depending on whether we have stimulatory or inhibitory drug effect, a greater stimulation or inhibition can be expected. The general form of a proportional drug effect model is given as

$$R(t) = R(0) \cdot (1 + E) \qquad (21.30)$$

where $R(t)$ is the drug response at time t, $R(0)$ is the response at baseline or time $= 0$, and E represents the drug effect, which could be linear or E_{max} type of relationship as shown below:

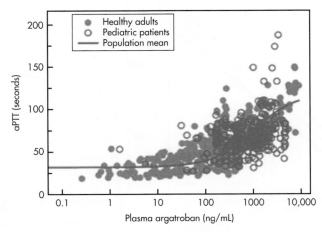

FIGURE 21-20   Predicted argatroban plasma concentration–aPTT relationship. Filled circles: healthy adults; open circles: pediatric patients (Madabushi et al, 2011).

Proportional linear drug effect model (stimulatory)

$$R(t) = R(0) \cdot (1 + S \cdot C) \qquad (21.31)$$

Proportional E_{max} drug effect model (stimulatory)

$$R(t) = R(0) \cdot \left(1 + \frac{S_{max} \cdot C}{SC_{50} + C}\right) \qquad (21.32)$$

Proportional E_{max} drug effect model (Inhibitory)

$$R(t) = R(0) \cdot \left(1 - \frac{I_{max} \cdot C}{IC_{50} + C}\right) \qquad (21.33)$$

where C is the plasma concentration of the drug at time t. However, the interpretation of S_{max} or I_{max} is different from that of an additive effect model. They represent fractional stimulation or inhibition from the baseline response or, in other words, represents proportional change (increase or decrease) of the response from baseline and hence a unitless quantity. The drug concentrations at which 50% of S_{max} or I_{max} is obtained refer to SC_{50} and IC_{50}, respectively, and these have the units of concentration. The proportional drug effect for three different baseline values of a response is depicted in Fig. 21-21.

As seen from Fig. 21-21, the response is dependent on the baseline value with a steeper decrease for the largest baseline as compared to small baseline. For both linear (proportional increase) and the inhibitory I_{max} effect, for a baseline of 150 units, the decrease in response is much higher as compared to the baseline value of 60 units, but the fractional decrease from the baseline value is the same. For example, let us consider the right graph in Fig. 21-21, with the baseline value as 150 and 60. When baseline is 150 units, the response decreased to 95 units upon increase in drug concentrations, whereas when baseline is 60 units, the maximum inhibitory response in the presence of drug reaches 38 units. Thus, the absolute difference in the response is 55 units for higher baseline and 22 units for lower baseline, whereas the fractional decrease in response (I_{max}) is $\dfrac{150 - 95}{150} = 0.37$ for the higher baseline and $\dfrac{60 - 38}{60} = 0.37$ for the lower baseline. Hence, the general expression for $I_{max} = \dfrac{R_0 - R_{min}}{R_0}$, where R_0 is the response at time $t = 0$ or at baseline and R_{min} is the maximum inhibitory response.

The same argument can be applied when there is a stimulatory effect on the baseline. Typically such

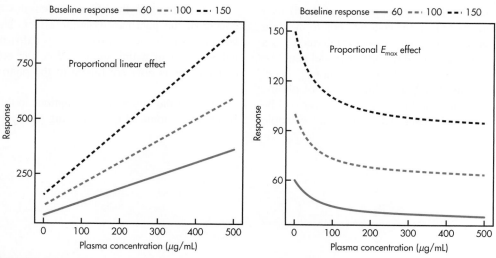

FIGURE 21-21   Proportional drug effect (linear and E_{max}) model upon varying baseline values. For the linear effect, a proportional increase of 0.01 ($s = 0.01$) was used and for the I_{max} effect model, the value of $I_{max} = 0.40$ (40% decrease from baseline).

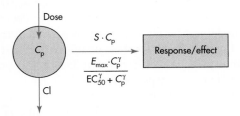

FIGURE 21-22   Schematic diagram for a direct effect model.

a proportional drug effect model is employed for drugs wherever baseline response plays an important role (eg, blood pressure–lowering drugs).

The model description so far dealt with the different types of the drug concentration–effect relationships (eg, linear, E_{max}, additive drug effect, proportional drug effect). As described in the section (Components of PK-PD models), the site at which the concentration–effect relationship drives the PD process leads to further PD models that are used for describing the different mechanisms by which the drug acts. For this section, the notation "C_p" is used to refer to plasma concentrations of the drug.

Direct Effect Model

When the distribution of the drug to the site of action is very rapid and when the drug elicits the response by a direct mechanism (no biosensor process involved), then a model directly linking the concentration to the drug response can be used. Such a model is referred to as a direct effect model. The direct effect model could be linearly related to concentrations or via an E_{max} model as shown in Fig. 21-22. The time course of plasma concentrations and the time course of effect will be in parallel to each other. The argatroban example

discussed previously is an example of a direct effect where the argatroban plasma concentrations were directly related to aPTT response via an E_{max} model.

Effect Compartment or Link Model

Some drugs may produce a delayed pharmacologic response that may not directly parallel the time course of the plasma drug concentration. The maximum pharmacologic response produced by the drug may be observed after the plasma drug concentration has peaked. In such cases, the drug distribution to the site of action or biophase may represent a rate-limiting step for drugs to elicit the biological response. The delay could be caused due to convection transport and diffusion processes that deliver the drug to the site of action. To describe the delay in effect, Sheiner et al (1979) proposed a hypothetical effect compartment as a mathematical link between the time course of plasma concentrations and the pharmacodynamic effect. The effect compartment models account for this delay by representing it as an additional compartment between the plasma concentration and the effect defined by a first-order equilibrium rate constant, k_{e0} as shown in Fig. 21-23. The hypothetical effect site concentration is represented as C_e. The equilibrium rate constant, k_{e0}, accounts for the delay in the drug concentrations reaching the effect site or the biophase, and therefore, the time course of concentration at the effect site mimics the time course of the pharmacodynamic effect. The effect compartment model is also called as a distributional delay model or a link model, since the effect site concentrations now are linked to the pharmacodynamic effect.

One of the important assumptions in this model is that the amount of drug entering the hypothetical

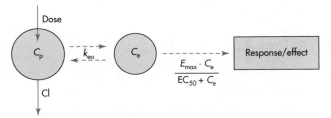

FIGURE 21-23   Schematic diagram for effect compartment model.

effect compartment is considered negligible and hence need not be reflected in the PK of the drug. The rate of change of drug concentration at the effect site is then given as

$$\frac{dC_e}{dt} = k_{e0} \cdot (C_p - C_e) \qquad (21.34)$$

The effect site concentration, C_e, profile is governed by the plasma concentration, C_p, and the equilibration rate constant, k_{e0}. A large value of k_{e0} would imply that the effect site concentrations closely follow the plasma concentration profile and the effect compartment is rapidly equilibrating, whereas a smaller k_{e0} value would signify that the effect compartment equilibrates slowly with C_e profile and hence the effect is delayed as compared to C_p. The effect is then linked to the effect site concentrations typically via an E_{max} model as

$$E = \frac{E_{max} \cdot C_e}{EC_{50} + C_e} \qquad (21.35)$$

Figure 21-24 depicts the C_p, C_e, and response profile for a hypothetical drug with two different k_{e0} values. As seen from the figure, the C_e profile mimics the time course of PD and the delay between the PK and

PD is accounted by the equilibration rate constant k_{e0}. When there is a temporal difference between the PK and the PD, and when time-matched response and plasma concentrations are plotted, the plot depicts a *hysteresis* loop, which is anticlockwise in nature as seen in Fig. 21-25. Another feature of the effect compartment models is, though the peak effects will be delayed relative to plasma concentrations, the times at which peak C_e occurs and hence the peak effect occurs are dose independent. Another type of time-dependent pharmacologic response may occur due to development of tolerance, induced metabolite deactivation, reduced response, or translocation of receptors at the site of action. This type of time-dependent pharmacological response is characterized by a clockwise profile when the pharmacological response is plotted versus the plasma drug concentration over time (Fig. 21-26). Drugs like fentanyl (lipid soluble, opioid anesthetic) and alfentanyl (a closely related drug) display a clockwise hysteresis loop apparently due to lipid partitioning effect of these drugs. Similarly, euphoria produced by cocaine also displayed a clockwise profile when responses were plotted versus plasma cocaine concentration (Fig. 21-27).

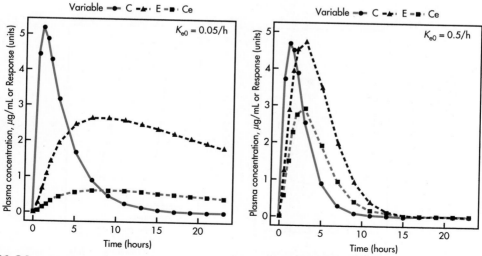

FIGURE 21-24   Simulated concentration–response time profiles obtained using effect compartment model to describe the influence of k_{e0}: distributional delay rate constant. C: plasma concentration; C_e: concentrations at the hypothetical effect site; E: drug effect. Drug concentrations from a one-compartment model is used to derive the effect using the effect compartment model, with $E_{max} = 20$ units, $EC_{50} = 4$ μg/mL.

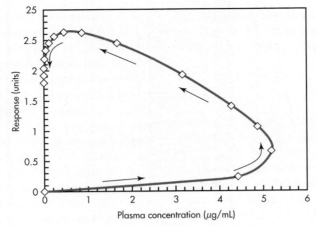

FIGURE 21-25 Anticlockwise hysteresis loop to describe the temporal difference between PK and PD.

Application: One of the early examples where an effect compartment model was used to describe the PK-PD relationship is to compare the PD effects of midazolam and diazepam using a surrogate measure for psychomotor performance (Mould et al, 1995). In the study, the PK and PD of midazolam and diazepam were compared after two intravenous infusions of 0.03 and 0.07 mg/kg of midazolam and 0.1 and 0.2 mg/kg of diazepam on four occasions in healthy adults. The Digit Symbol Substitution Test (DSST) was used as the pharmacodynamic response as it was thought to be a sensitive measure for drug-induced changes in psychomotor performances than electroencephalogram (EEG). Plasma concentrations of diazepam, midazolam, and DSST were measured at different times up to 180 minutes. The authors described the PK-DSST relationship using an effect compartment model with additive baseline effect,

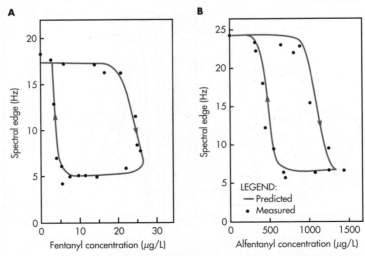

FIGURE 21-26 Response of the EEG spectral edge to changing fentanyl (A) and alfentanyl (B) serum concentrations. Plots are data from single patients after rapid drug infusion. Time is indicated by arrows. The clockwise hysteresis indicates a significant time lag between blood and effect site.

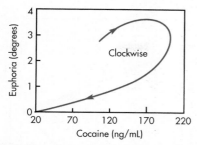

FIGURE 21-27   Clockwise hysteresis loop typical of tolerance is seen after intranasal administration of cocaine when related to degree of euphoria experienced in volunteers.

as there was a slight delay in the pharmacodynamic effect as compared to the plasma concentrations of the drugs. The estimated distributional delay half-life $(t_{1/2} - k_{e0})$ of midazolam was 3.2 minutes and of diazepam was 1.2 minutes. The use of effect compartment model was able to collapse the temporal difference between the PK and DSST as seen from the hysteresis plots in a representative subject (Figs. 21-28 and 21-29). Based on this analysis, the authors were able to confirm the fact that midazolam has a delayed onset of peak effect and the potency of midazolam was 6 times higher than that of diazepam. Moreover, the use of DSST as a surrogate measure instead of EEG was supported by this analysis.

Indirect Response Models

When the pharmacological response is seen immediately in parallel to the plasma drug concentrations, pharmacodynamic models such as linear model, E_{max} model, or sigmoid E_{max} models are used to model PK-PD relationship. When there is a delay in the pharmacological response as compared to the drug concentrations, an effect compartment or the link model is used. The use of an effect compartment model is justified when the delay in the pharmacodynamic response can be attributed to the distribution of the drug to the effect site characterized by a hypothetical effect compartment. The equilibrium between the plasma and the effect site is characterized by the equilibration rate constant as described under the section Effect Compartment or Link Model.

Many drugs, however, exhibit pharmacological response via an indirect mechanism. The drugs might induce their effects not by direct interaction with the receptors, but rather the interaction with receptors might affect the production or degradation of an endogenous compound and the subsequent response is mediated by those substances. The earliest reference to a PK-PD model using an indirect mechanism of action for a drug was described for the anticoagulant effect of warfarin by Nagashima et al (1969). A systematic modeling approach for characterizing diverse types of indirect response models into four basic models was described by Sharma et al (Sharma and Jusko, 1996). The context where the use of an indirect response model may arise was briefly explained in the section on conceptual PK-PD framework. The characteristics of four basic indirect response models that are most commonly used are described in detail.

The four basic indirect response models arise when the factors controlling the input or production (k_{in}) of the response variable is either stimulated or inhibited, or the loss or degradation (k_{out}) of an endogenous compound or the response variable is either stimulated or inhibited. The rate of change of a response variable in the *absence of the drug* is given as

$$\frac{dR}{dt} = k_{in} - k_{out} \cdot R \qquad (21.36)$$

where k_{in} represents the zero-order production rate constant of the response and k_{out} represents the first-order degradation rate constant of the response variable. It is assumed that k_{in} and k_{out} fully account for the production and degradation of the response. In the presence of the drug, inhibition of k_{in} or k_{out} by the drug concentration gives rise to the model I and model II and stimulation of k_{in} or k_{out} in the presence of drug leads to model III and model IV. Model I is the inhibition of k_{in} and model II is the inhibition of k_{out} as shown in Fig. 21-30.

Inhibition of Production of Response, k_{in} (Model I) and Inhibition of Degradation of Response, k_{out} (Model II)

The rate of change of response in model I is described as

$$\frac{dR}{dt} = k_{in} \cdot (1 - E) - k_{out} \cdot R \qquad (21.37)$$

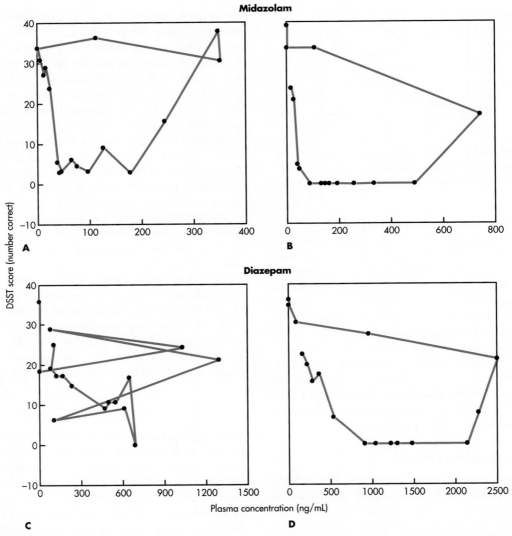

FIGURE 21-28   Plasma concentration versus effect (DSST score) in subject 6 after 0.03 mg/kg midazolam (a), 0.07 mg/kg midazolam (b), 0.1 mg/kg diazepam (c), and 0.2 mg/kg diazepam (d).

and the rate of change of response in model II is explained by

$$\frac{dR}{dt} = k_{in} - k_{out} \cdot (1 - E) \cdot R \qquad (21.38)$$

where the inhibitory action of the drug is given by $E = \dfrac{I_{max} \cdot C_p}{IC_{50} + C_p}$. Here, C_p represents the plasma concentration of the drug as a function of time, I_{max} refers

to the maximal fractional inhibition of production or degradation of the response by the drug and always takes a value between 0 and 1 ($0 < I_{max} \leq 1$), and IC_{50} is the plasma concentration producing 50% of the maximal inhibition achieved at the effect site. Since stationarity is assumed for all models, in the absence of drug at steady state, $\dfrac{dR}{dt} = 0$; hence

$$k_{in} = k_{out} \cdot R_0 \qquad (21.39)$$

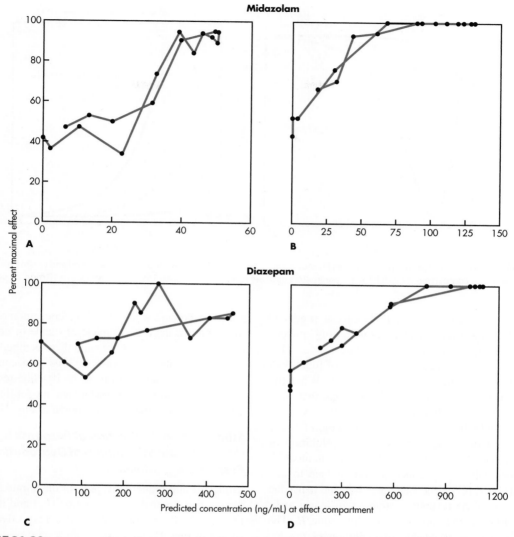

FIGURE 21-29   Percent maximal effect versus predicted concentration at the effect site after determination of k_{e0} and collapse of hysteresis loop in subject 6 after 0.03 mg/kg midazolam (a), 0.07 mg/kg midazolam (b), 0.1 mg/kg diazepam (c), and 0.2 mg/kg diazepam (d).

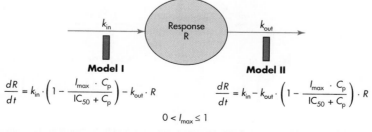

FIGURE 21-30   Schematic diagram for basic indirect response models I and II. In model I, the drug inhibits the production of response. In model II, the drug inhibits the degradation of the response.

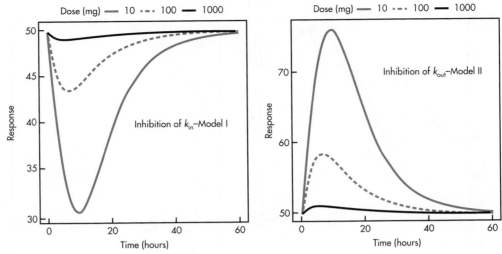

FIGURE 21-31   Simulated response profiles for model I and model II. Three intravenous doses were used and plasma concentrations follow a one-compartment model. The PD parameters used are $k_{in} = 5$ mg/h; $k_{out} = 0.1/h$; $I_{max} = 5$; and $IC_{50} = 10$ mg/L or μg/mL.

Thus the response variable, R, begins at predetermined baseline value R_0, changes with drug concentrations, and returns to the baseline value. This assumption further reduces the number of functional parameters in the models described above. When the plasma drug concentrations are very high, that is, at steady state ($C_p \gg IC_{50}$), the value of IC_{50} is insignificant, and when $I_{max} = 1$, then the value of $E = 1$ (C_p cancels out), and hence complete inhibition of production of the response variable occurs in model I.

Later, when drug concentrations reduce to low values ($C_p \ll IC_{50}$), the value of $E = 0$, and hence the production of the response variable will return to k_{in} and the PD system returns to its baseline value, R_0. The same concept is applicable to inhibition of the k_{out}

model, wherein, when the drug concentrations are much higher, there is complete blockade of degradation of the response variable and there is a buildup of response to its maximum, and as concentrations decrease, the system returns to its baseline response. The response profiles for model I and model II at three different doses of the drug are shown in Fig. 21-31.

Stimulation of Production of Response k_{in} (Model III) and Stimulation of Degradation of Response k_{out} (Model IV)

Model III and model IV represent the stimulation of factors that control the production (k_{in}) and dissipation (k_{out}) of the drug response, respectively, as shown in Fig. 21-32.

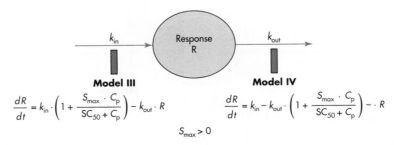

$$\frac{dR}{dt} = k_{in} \cdot \left(1 + \frac{S_{max} \cdot C_p}{SC_{50} + C_p}\right) - k_{out} \cdot R$$

Model III

$$\frac{dR}{dt} = k_{in} - k_{out} \cdot \left(1 + \frac{S_{max} \cdot C_p}{SC_{50} + C_p}\right) - \cdot R$$

Model IV

$$S_{max} > 0$$

FIGURE 21-32   Schematic diagram for basic indirect response models III and IV. In model III, the drug stimulates the production of response. In model IV, the drug stimulates the degradation of the response.

The rate of change of drug response in model III is given as

$$\frac{dR}{dt} = k_{in} \cdot (1+E) - k_{out} \cdot R \qquad (21.40)$$

whereas in the case of model IV, the differential equation corresponds to

$$\frac{dR}{dt} = k_{in} - k_{out} \cdot (1+E) \cdot R \qquad (21.41)$$

Here, the drug effect E is described as $E = \dfrac{S_{max} \cdot C_p}{SC_{50} + C_p}$, providing a stimulatory effect for the factors controlling the response. S_{max} refers to the maximal fractional stimulation of production or degradation of the response by the drug and always takes a value greater than 0 ($S_{max} > 0$), and SC_{50} is the plasma concentration producing 50% of the maximal stimulation achieved at the effect site. As described in the inhibitory models, in the absence of drug, the drug response is at its baseline value as expressed in Equation 21.40. As drug concentrations become much higher ($C_p \gg SC_{50}$), there is maximal buildup of response (model III) based on the value of S_{max}, and as drug concentrations decrease, the response returns to its baseline value. In the case of model IV, the steady-state concentrations of the drug produce maximal stimulation of the loss of factors controlling the drug response. The response profiles for model III and model IV at three different doses of the drug are shown in Fig. 21-33.

In general, the characteristics of the four basic indirect response models can be summarized as follows:

1. There is a delay in the maximal PD response (R_{max}) as compared to the peak plasma concentrations of the drug (C_{max}), which is attributed to the indirect mechanism by which the drug acts.

2. The response time profiles show a slow decline or rise in the response variable to a maximum value (R_{max}) dictated by the steady-state concentrations of the drug followed by a gradual return to baseline conditions ($\dfrac{k_{in}}{k_{out}}$ or R_0) as drug concentrations decline below IC_{50} or SC_{50} values.

3. Typically, the initial rate of decline or rise in the response profiles is governed by k_{out}, independent of dose. The gradual return to baseline after R_{max} is reached is governed by both k_{in} and the elimination rate constant of the drug ($k_{el} = \dfrac{CL}{V}$).

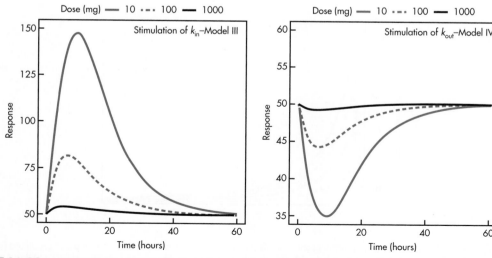

FIGURE 21-33 Simulated response profiles for model III and model IV. Three intravenous doses were used and plasma concentrations follow a one-compartment model. The PD parameters used are $k_{in} = 5$ mg/h; $k_{out} = 0.1$/h; $S_{max} = 5$; $SC_{50} = 10$ mg/L or μg/mL.

4. The time to peak pharmacodynamic response ($t_{R_{\max}}$) occurs at later times for larger doses owing to the increased duration of the plasma drug concentrations above IC_{50} or SC_{50} values.

Complete reviews of the basic properties of these models and the application of these models for different drugs are described in literature (Jusko and Ko, 1994; Sharma and Jusko, 1998). Two applications of the indirect response models in the context of drug development are described here.

Application: Indirect response models have been used in the context of making decisions on dosing recommendations or selection of drug candidates early in the drug development process. A physiologic indirect response model was developed to characterize the time course of the flare area (cm²) after oral administration of single ascending doses of mizolastine, a new H_1-receptor antagonist in healthy volunteers (Nieforth et al, 1996). The *in vivo* test in which histamine-induced skin wheal and flare reactions are inhibited by H_1-receptor antagonist is considered a predictive test for demonstrating the clinical antiallergic activity of investigative H_1-receptor antagonists. In this study, mizolastine was orally administered to healthy volunteers at 4 different doses (5, 10, 15, and 20 mg) including placebo. The pharmacodynamic response was measured in terms of histamine-induced flare area (cm²) and wheal area (cm²) at different time points till 24 hours after administration of the mizolastine. A PK-PD model was developed to predict the mizolastine pharmacodynamics and further use the model for prediction purposes. The authors used an indirect response model to describe the flare area response over time considering inhibition of the production of histamine (model I) in the presence of mizolastine concentrations as given below.

$$\frac{d\text{Flare}_{\text{area}}}{dt} = k_{\text{in}} \cdot \left(1 - \frac{I_{\max} \cdot C}{IC_{50} + C}\right) - k_{\text{out}} \cdot \text{Flare}_{\text{area}}$$

$$(21.42)$$

where C refers to the plasma mizolastine concentrations, $\text{Flare}_{\text{area}}$ refers to the area of the histamine-induced flare on the skin, $I_{\max}$ is the maximum fractional inhibition (k_{in}) of production of histamine response indicated by area of flare, IC_{50} is the plasma concentration of mizolastine producing 50% of the $I_{\max}$, and k_{out} is the first-order rate constant for the flare disappearance. The PK-PD model provided adequate fit of the data as seen in Fig. 21-34. As seen from Fig. 21-34, there is a dose-dependent inhibition in the flare area with inhibition sustained at higher doses, which are indicative of indirect mechanism of action of the drug.

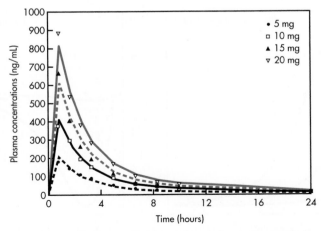

FIGURE 21-34 Plasma time–concentration profiles of mizolastine at 4 different doses and observed and predicted flare area–time course profiles after oral administration of 5, 10, 15, and 20 mg of mizolastine. An indirect response model with inhibition of production of response (model I) was used to predict the flare area responses.

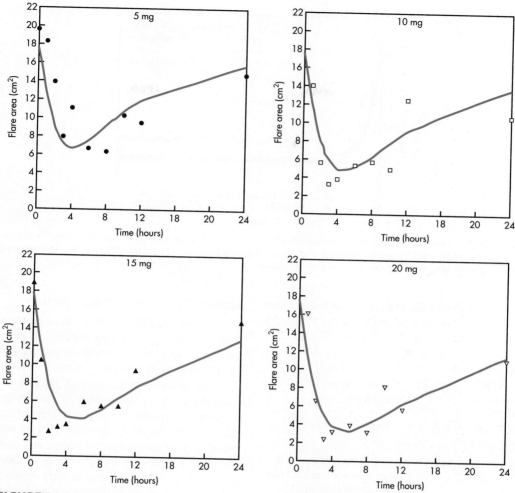

FIGURE 21-34   (*Continued*)

The authors reported 92% maximal inhibition (I_{max}) of flare area by the drug with 50% of the maximal inhibition (IC_{50}) obtained at 21 ng/mL of mizolastine.

Another application of an indirect response model is in deciding the dosing regimen for abatacept, a recombinant soluble fusion protein, used in the treatment of rheumatoid arthritis (RA) (Roy et al, 2007). The pharmacodynamic response to abatacept was measured in terms of a biomarker, interleukin-6 (IL-6), as abatacept causes reduction of IL-6 levels, and increased IL-6 levels are indicated in RA disease pathology. The authors utilized data from Phase II and Phase III studies of abatacept (at doses, 2 and 10 mg/kg) to characterize

the abatacept–IL-6 suppression relationship and to predict IL-6 suppressions at different doses not studied in clinical studies by clinical trial simulations. An indirect response model where there is stimulation of IL-6 degradation (model IV) was used to describe the abatacept-IL-6 relationship as shown below:

$$\frac{dC_{IL-6}}{dt} = k_{in} - k_{out} \cdot \left(1 + \frac{S_{max} \cdot C_p}{SC_{50} + C_p}\right) \cdot C_{IL-6} \quad (21.43)$$

where C_{IL-6} represents serum IL-6 concentrations. The developed PK-PD model adequately described the IL-6 data, and further simulations using the

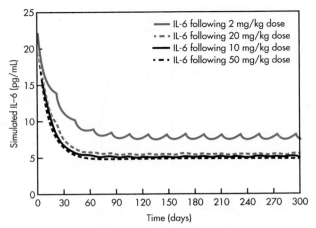

FIGURE 21-35   Simulated average serum interleukin-6 (IL-6) concentrations versus time by abatacept dose. Simulated median IL-6 concentrations over time for 2 mg/kg abatacept (solid line), 10 mg/kg abatacept (long dashed line), 20 mg/kg abatacept (intermediate dashed line), and 50 mg/kg abatacept (short dashed line).

model at doses unstudied in the clinical studies revealed that the studied 10 mg/kg doses produced increased suppression than 2 mg/kg dose (Fig. 21-35). But higher than 10 mg/kg did not offer any additional therapeutic benefit, and hence the PK-PD analysis and simulations supported the recommended abatacept doses studied in the clinical trials.

Frequently Asked Questions

▶ *Explain why the log-linear model cannot be used to determine effect when concentration is zero. Describe which simple model could be used in such situation.*

▶ *Explain why doubling the dose of a drug does not double the pharmacodynamic effect of the drug.*

▶ *What is meant by a hysteresis loop? Why do some drugs follow a clockwise hysteresis loop and other drugs follow a counterclockwise hysteresis loop?*

▶ *What is meant by an effect compartment? How does the effect compartment differ from pharmacokinetic compartments, such as the central compartment and the tissue compartment?*

▶ *Why are in vitro or ex vivo biomarkers not useful for monitoring the clinical progress of drug treatment? What are the main considerations for using biomarkers to monitor drug treatment or disease progression?*

Systems Pharmacodynamic Models

The field of PK-PD modeling has made tremendous progress over the last two decades in progressing from empirical PK-PD models to mechanism-based PK-PD models. Although mechanistic PK-PD modeling incorporates drug–receptor interaction and/or physiology into consideration, these models still focus on the specific subsystem of physiology that is impacted by the drug. Systems pharmacodynamic models aim to incorporate all known and understood biological processes that control body events into the model (Jusko, 2013). These models capture multitude of processes via mathematical equations incorporating homeostasis as well as feedback mechanisms that are hallmark of complex biological systems. Thus, systems pharmacology models represent probably the most complex models in the area of PK-PD modeling. The greatest advantage of systems models is that they can be used to assess impact of perturbing one process on the overall biological system under consideration. The challenge that still remains with systems models includes multitude of mathematical equations, functions, and parameter values for each step of biological process. In the interim, models that are more mature than mechanism-based PK-PD model but somewhat less than the complete systems pharmacology models are being employed as depicted by Fig. 21-36.

Levels of modeling complexity

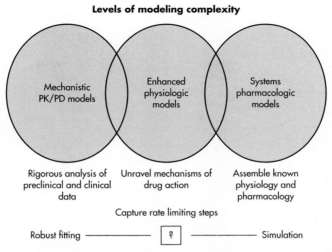

FIGURE 21-36   Range and types of modeling complexity at three modeling levels of quantitative and systems pharmacology (QSP) (Jusko, 2013).

This hybrid approach was utilized by Earp et al's PK-PD model for dexamethasone effects in rat model of collagen-induced arthritis as shown in Fig. 21-37.

PK-PD Models and Their Role in Drug Approval and Labeling

The impact of PK-PD modeling in regulatory decision making has been increasing over the last many years. The US FDA has been utilizing PK-PD modeling and simulation for drug approval as well as labeling-related decisions (Bhattaram et al, 2005, 2007). To illustrate the role of PK-PD in regulatory decision making and approval, two examples from approved drugs are described below.

Case 1: Nesiritide

Case 1 demonstrates how PK-PD modeling and simulation can be applied to learn from an existing set of clinical trials result and design the future clinical trials with greater probability of success, which in this example resulted in the approval of drug by the FDA (Bhattaram et al, 2005). Nesiritide (Natrecor®), a recombinant human brain natriuretic peptide, was being developed for the treatment of acute decompensated congestive heart failure (CHF). The New Drug Application (NDA) for nesiritide

was rejected after review by the FDA in April 1999 on the basis that at a given dose, (a) the desired maximal effect (change in pulmonary capillary wedge pressure [PCWP]) was not achieved instantaneously and (b) the PCWP could not be achieved without the undesired effect of hypotension. The FDA recommended the sponsor to optimize nesiritide dosing regimen that would result in instantaneous effect on PCWP (benefit) and minimize the hypotension (risk). As part of the regulatory review, nesiritide exposure–response data were modeled to develop a PK-PD model. The PK-PD model was then applied to evaluate different dosing regimens via simulations. The analysis suggested that a loading dose followed by a maintenance infusion should result in faster onset of desired action. Additionally, the simulations suggested that the lower infusion rates might result in smaller effect on undesired side effect of hypotension. The analysis indicated that a loading bolus dose of 2 μg/kg with a maintenance dose of 0.01 μg/min/kg infusion could provide optimal risk–benefit profile. The sponsor investigated this PK-PD simulations-based modeling dosing regimen in an actual clinical trial for management of acute CHF and submitted the results for supporting a modified dosing regimen (Publication Committee for the, 2002). The modeled and actual results are

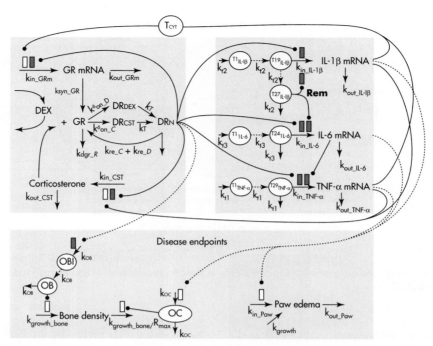

FIGURE 21-37   Model schematic for corticosteroid and cytokine inter-regulation during arthritis progression. Lines with arrows indicate conversion to or turnover of the indicated responses. Lines ending in closed circles indicate an effect is being exerted by the connected factors.

shown in Fig. 21-38. The drug was subsequently approved by the FDA for treatment of acute CHF in May 2001.

Case 2: Micafungin

This example focuses on how the US FDA as a regulatory authority recommended approval for a particular dosage for micafungin, a semisynthetic lipopeptide formulated as an intravenous infusion for the treatment of esophageal candidiasis (Bhattaram et al, 2007). The review involved dose optimization by quantifying the exposure-response relationship by performing a benefit-to-risk assessment over a dynamic range of doses. Micafungin is an antifungal agent that belongs to the echinocandin class of compounds. The proposed dosage for treatment of esophageal candidiasis was 150 mg given every 24 hours for a period of 2–3 weeks (FUJISAWA, 2005). During the review a thorough assessment of the dose to the clinical effectiveness was performed from two available Phase II trials and a registration study where the endoscopic

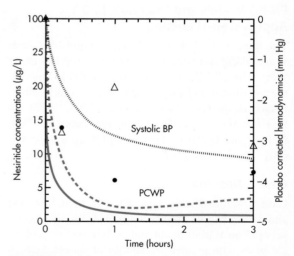

FIGURE 21-38   Typical time course of nesiritide plasma concentrations (—), and the effects on the PCWP (• indicates observed; - - - - indicates model predicted), and systolic blood pressure (systolic BP; Δ indicates observed; ..... indicates model predicted) after a 2 mg/kg bolus followed by a fixed-dose infusion of 0.01 mg/kg/min. Data for the initial 3 hours are being shown here.

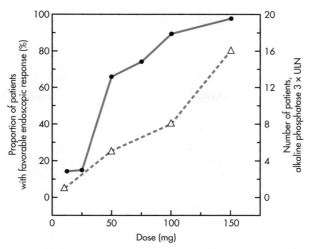

FIGURE 21-39   Benefit–risk plot for micafungin. The solid line represents the proportion of patients with endoscopic response increased with dose. The dotted like represents incidence of elevations in alkaline phosphatase levels (>3 × ULN) with dose.

response rate (proportion of patients that were cleared of the infection at the end of the therapy) was the primary endpoint. A clinical response endpoint was considered as a secondary parameter for effectiveness. Biochemical markers like alkaline phosphatase, serum glutamic oxaloacetic transaminase (SGOT), serum glutamic pyruvic transaminases (SGPT), and total bilirubin were assessed for a relationship between enzymatic elevations to the dose of antifungal agent. It was observed that both 100- and 150-mg doses of micafungin were able to achieve a maximal response as the primary endpoint (Fig. 21-39). Interestingly patients who were treated with higher dose (150 mg) had a 15% lower relapse compared to the lower dose that was associated with a much lower clinical cure rate. Of all biochemical markers the alkaline phosphatase was correlated to the entire dynamic range of dose studied (12.5–150 mg). These elevations in the liver enzymes were transient, which returned to normal levels upon discontinuation of the treatment.

CHAPTER SUMMARY

Both agonist and antagonist drug effects can be quantitatively simulated by PK-PD models. The most common models are E_{max} models mechanistically based on drug receptor theory. Although most drug responses are complex, pharmacologic response versus log dose type of plots have been shown to follow sigmoid type of curve (*S*-curve) with maximum response peaking when all receptors become saturated. *In vitro* screening preparations are useful to study EC_{50}, potency, and mechanism of a drug. However, pharmacologic response in a patient is generally far more complicated. Physiologically based PD models must consider how the drug is delivered to the active site and the effect of various drug disposition processes, as well as plasma and tissue drug binding. In addition, pharmacogenomics of the drug and disease processes must be considered in the model. Appropriately developed PK-PD models may be applied to predict onset, intensity, and duration of action of a drug. Toxicokinetics may also be applied to explain the side effects or drug–drug interactions.

The progress of a disease or its response to a therapeutic agent is often accompanied by biologic changes (markers or biomarkers) that are observable and/or measurable. Biomarkers (BMs) may be selected and validated to monitor the course of drug response in the body. BMs should be mechanistically based and fulfill a number of clinically relevant criteria in order to be useful as potential clinical endpoints. BM together with PK-PD could be a very useful tool in expediting drug development, and many reviews and discussions are available about this application.

LEARNING QUESTIONS

1. On the basis of the graph in Fig. 21-40, answer "true" or "false" to statements (a) through (e) and state the reason for each answer.
   a. The plasma drug concentration is more related to the pharmacodynamic effect of the drug compared to the dose of the drug.
   b. The pharmacologic response is directly proportional to the log plasma drug concentration.
   c. The volume of distribution is not changed by uremia.
   d. The drug is exclusively eliminated by hepatic biotransformation.
   e. The receptor sensitivity is unchanged in the uremic patient.

2. How would you define a response and an effect? Identify whether the following is a pharmacodynamic response or a pharmacodynamic effect:
   a. Change from baseline in HbA1c at the end of 26 weeks
   b. Blood histamine levels
   c. Number of sleep awakenings at week 4
   d. Percent reduction in seizures at the end of 8 weeks
   e. Measure of body weight at the end of 52 weeks

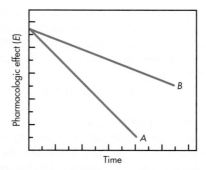

FIGURE 21-40   Graph of pharmacologic response E as a function of time for the same drug in patients with normal **(A)** and uremic **(B)** kidney function, respectively.

3. What is the difference between a partial and an inverse agonist? Name a drug its therapeutic class that behaves like a (i) partial agonist and (ii) inverse agonist?

4. What is the difference between biomarkers and surrogate endpoints? Elaborate your answer by giving an example.

5. Explain why subsequent equal doses of a drug do not produce the same pharmacodynamic effect as the first dose of a drug.
   a. Provide an explanation based on pharmacokinetic considerations.
   b. Provide an explanation based on pharmacodynamic considerations.

6. How are the parameters AUC and t_{eff} used in pharmacodynamic models?

7. What class of drug tends to have a lag time between the plasma and the effect compartment?

8. Name an example of a pharmacodynamic response that does not follow a drug dose–response profile?

9. What is AUIC with regard to an antibiotic?

10. What is the difference between IC_{50} and EC_{50}? Are the values reproducible from one lab to another? In functional studies, the antagonist IC_{50} is most useful if the concentration of the agonist is below maximal. Higher concentrations of the agonist will increase the IC_{50} of the competitive antagonist well above its equilibrium dissociation constant. Even with low agonist concentrations, the IC_{50} from functional studies, like an agonist EC_{50} or maximal response, is dependent on the conditions of the experiment (tissue, receptor expression, type of measurement, etc). True or false?

11. K_i refers to the equilibrium dissociation constant of a ligand determined in inhibition studies. The K_i for a given ligand is typically determined in a competitive radioligand binding study by measuring the inhibition of

the binding of a reference radioligand by the inhibiting ligand under equilibrium conditions. Why?

12. What is the dissociation constant K in the following interaction between a drug ligand L and a drug receptor R:

$$L + R \underset{k_{-1}}{\overset{k_{+1}}{\rightleftharpoons}} LR$$

$$P_{LR} = \frac{|L|}{|L| + K}$$

where K is expressed as k_{-1}/k_{+1} and P_{LR} is the proportion of receptor occupied by L.
How many binding sites are assumed in the above model?

13. Which one of the following would you select as a biomarker for a type 2 diabetic patient? State the reasons that support your selection.
    a. Blood sugar level
    b. Blood insulin level
    c. HbA1C

14. What are the three types of pharmacodynamic responses? Give an example for each type of PD responses that will help to differentiate between them.

15. Explain the principal difference between concentration-dependent and time-dependent killing patterns associated with the use of antibiotics. What PK-PD index would be most appropriate to predict the therapeutic efficacy of antibiotics associated with respect to these two killing patterns?

16. For an investigative antibiotic under early discovery, a series of efficacy studies in mice thigh infection model were conducted. Following are the results for three PK-PD indices of AUC/MIC ratio, C_{max}/MIC ratio, and (%) time above MIC. Analyze these results and determine what PK-PD index is best correlated to the log CFU reduction. Explain why you picked the particular PK-PD index.

17. The below graph shows a concentration–effect relationship for three hypothetical drugs.

AUC/MIC Ratio	Log (CFU) Reduction	C_{max}/MIC Ratio	Log (CFU) Reduction	(%) Time above MIC	Log (CFU) Reduction
31	8.9	1.4	7.8	18	7.7
32	8.4	2.6	8.8	25	5.7
40	7.5	2.7	9.1	27	8.8
61	6.7	4.7	8.6	35	3.9
64	5.9	4.9	7.9	35	4.2
88	5.8	5.7	6.8	36	5.3
93	5.3	9.4	6.7	37	6.0
108	5.6	9.7	6.4	39	2.7
122	5.0	10.8	5.0	41	8.6
125	4.2	11.1	3.5	45	2.2
168	3.7	12.6	4.3	50	4.3
172	3.9	20.3	6.0	55	6.8
210	4.2	21.4	7.6	58	8.9

226	3.4	34.3	3.0	71	2.2
250	4.2	37.2	3.3	75	4.1
328	3.6	44.3	5.7	75	3.8
488	3.5	47.8	5.4	81	2.0
488	2.3	50.7	3.0	85	6.5
500	3.1	91.8	4.0	99	8.8
841	2.5	97.6	1.9	99	2.5
862	3.2	99.1	3.9	99	3.8
952	2.6	183.5	2.7	100	3.0
975	2.0	190.5	2.5	100	3.1
975	2.8	383.6	2.2	100	3.2
1025	2.2	398	1.9	100	3.5

(Hint: Plot each PK-PD index against log CFU reduction.)

Assuming all drugs produce a maximum effect of 5 units, determine EC_{50} for each drug X, Y, and Z. What does EC_{50} signify?

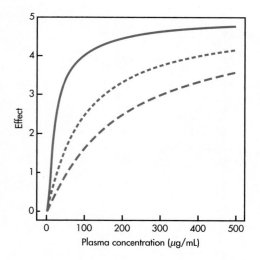

18. Assume a drug exhibits a proportional drug effect which is stimulatory in nature. Derive the expression for S_{max} the fractional stimulation

from baseline. (Hint: Use the same approach as for I_{max}, but in opposite direction.)

19. Based on the graphs below, identify what kind of a PK-PD relationship can be assumed for this hypothetical drug.

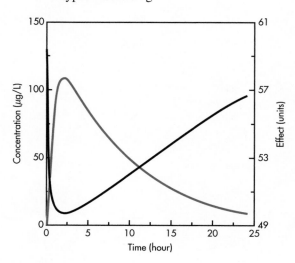

20. Hysteresis: what is the rationale for observing hysteresis in drug therapeutics?

ANSWERS

Learning Questions

1. **a.** *True.* Drug concentration is more precise because an identical dose may result in different plasma drug concentration in different subjects due to individual differences in pharmacokinetics.

   b. *True.* The kinetic relationship between drug response and drug concentration is such that the response is proportional to log concentration of the drug.

   c. *True.* The data show that after IV bolus dose, the response begins at the same point, indicating that the initial plasma drug concentration is the same. In uremic patients, the volume of distribution may be affected by changes in protein binding and electrolyte levels, which may range from little or no effect to strongly affecting the V_D.

   d. *False.* The drug is likely to be excreted through the kidney, since the slope (elimination) is reduced in uremic patients.

   e. *True.* Assuming that the volume of distribution is unchanged, the starting pharmacologic response should be the same if the receptor sensitivity is unchanged. In a few cases, receptor sensitivity to the drug can be altered in uremic patients. For example, the effect of digoxin will be more intense if the serum potassium level is depleted.

2. **a.** Effect
   b. Response
   c. Response
   d. Effect
   e. Response

3. A partial agonist is an agent that produces a response similar to an agonist but cannot reach a maximal response as that of an agonist. However, an inverse agonist selectively binds to the inactive form of the receptor and shifts the conformational equilibrium toward the inactive state. An example of a partial agonist is buspirone and famotidine being an inverse agonist.

5. **a.** Pharmacokinetic considerations: Subsequent doses induce the hepatic drug-metabolizing enzymes (autoinduction), thereby decreasing the elimination half-life, resulting in lower steady-state drug concentrations.

   b. Pharmacodynamic considerations: The patient develops tolerance to the drug, resulting in the need for a higher dose to produce the same effect.

7. CNS drugs.

8. An allergic response to a drug may be unpredictable and does not generally follow a dose–response relationship.

9. AUC/MIC or AUIC is a pharmacokinetic parameter incorporating MIC together in order to provide better prediction of antibiotic response (cure percent). An example is ciprofloxacin. AUIC is a good predictor of percent cure in infection treated at various dose regimens.

14. Continuous, categorical, and time-to-event responses are the three types of responses. Blood pressure measurement is an example of continuous response. Mild, moderate, and severe status of an adverse event like diarrhea is an example for a discrete response. Time until relapse is an example of a time-to-event outcome. Here time to relapse is a continuous response, but not all patients would have relapse. Therefore, patients who do not have relapse are censored, hence the distinction from continuous response.

17. EC_{50} signifies the concentration of the drug at which 50% of E_{max} (maximum effect is achieved or also referred to as the potency of the drug). Smaller the EC_{50} value, more potent is the drug. For X (solid line), E_{max} is approximately 5 units, and EC_{50} approximately 25 μg/mL. This can be obtained by eyeballing the concentration corresponding to an effect of 2.5 units. For Y (short dotted line), EC_{50} is approximately 100 μg/mL. For Z (long dotted line), EC_{50} is approximately 250 μg/mL.

19. The maximal drug concentrations are achieved at about 2.5 hours and the corresponding PD response occurs at the same time indicat-

ing that the drug–effect relationship can be explained by a direct effect model.

20. Hysteresis occurs when there is time lag between the concentration and the corresponding effect. It could be manifested when there is a distributional delay of the drug reaching the effect site, or it could be based on the mechanism of action of the drug. Typically hysteresis plots are observed when the maximum effect occurs later than the maximum concentrations.

REFERENCES

Actavis: Risedronate prescribing label, 1998.

Aghajanian GK, Bing OH: Persistence of Lysergic Acid Diethylamide in the Plasma of Human Subjects. *Clin Pharmacol Ther* **5**:611–614, 1964.

Anne S, Reisman RE: Risk of administering cephalosporin antibiotics to patients with histories of penicillin allergy. *Ann Allergy Asthma Immunol* **74**(2):167–170, 1995.

Atkinson AJJ: *Physiological and Laboratory Markers of Drug Effect*. New York, Academic Press, 2001.

Bhattaram VA, Bonapace C, Chilukuri DM, et al: Impact of pharmacometric reviews on new drug approval and labeling decisions—A survey of 31 new drug applications submitted between 2005 and 2006. *Clin Pharmacol Ther* **81**(2):213–221, 2007.

Bhattaram VA, Booth BP, Ramchandani RP, et al: Impact of pharmacometrics on drug approval and labeling decisions: A survey of 42 new drug applications. *AAPS J* **7**(3):E503–E512, 2005.

Biomarkers Definitions Working G: Biomarkers and surrogate endpoints: Preferred definitions and conceptual framework. *Clin Pharmacol Ther* **69**(3):89–95, 2001.

Blumenthal DK, Garrison JC: Pharmacodynamics: Molecular mechanisms of drug action. In Brunton LL (ed). *The Pharmacological Basis of Therapeutics*. McGraw-Hill, 2011, pp 41–72.

Clark AJ: The reaction between acetyl choline and muscle cells: Part II. *J Physiol* **64**(2):123–143, 1927.

Colburn WA: Optimizing the use of biomarkers, surrogate endpoints, and clinical endpoints for more efficient drug development. *Journal of Clinical Pharmacology* **40**(12 Pt 2):1419–1427, 2000.

Coltart DJ, Hamer J: A comparison of the effects of propranolol and practolol on the exercise tolerance in angina pectoris. *Br J Pharmacol* **40**(1):147P–148P, 1970.

Cone EJ: Pharmacokinetics and pharmacodynamics of cocaine. *J Anal Toxicol* **19**(6):459–478, 1995.

Cox BM: Drug tolerance and physical dependence. In Pratt WB, Taylor P (eds). *The Basis of Pharmacology*. New York, Churchill Livingstone, 1990.

Craig WA: Interrelationship between pharmacokinetics and pharmacodynamics in determining dosage regimens for broadspectrum cephalosporins. *Diagn Microbiol Infect Dis* **22**(1–2):89–96, 1995.

Craig WA: Pharmacodynamics of antimicrobials: General concepts and applications. In Nightingale CH, Murakawa T, Ambrose PG (eds). *Antimicrobial Pharmacodynamics in Theory and Clinical Practice*. New York, Mercel Dekker, 2002. **28:**1–22.

de Wit H, Dudish S, Ambre J: Subjective and behavioral effects of diazepam depend on its rate of onset. *Psychopharmacology (Berl)* **112**(2–3):324–330, 1993.

Derendorf H, Lesko LJ, Chaikin P, et al: Pharmacokinetic/pharmacodynamic modeling in drug research and development. *J Clin Pharmacol* **40**(12 Pt 2):1399–1418, 2000.

Echt DS, Liebson PR, Mitchell LB, et al: Mortality and morbidity in patients receiving encainide, flecainide, or placebo. The cardiac arrhythmia suppression trial. *New Eng J Med* **324**(12):781–788, 1991.

Florian JA, Tornoe CW, Brundage R, Parekh A, Garnett CE: Population pharmacokinetic and concentration—QTc models for moxifloxacin: Pooled analysis of 20 thorough QT studies. *J Clin Pharmacol* **51**(8):1152–1162, 2011.

FUJISAWA: Mycamine Prescribing Label, FDA, 2005.

Garnett CE, Beasley N, Bhattaram VA, et al: Concentration-QT relationships play a key role in the evaluation of proarrhythmic risk during regulatory review. *J Clin Pharmacol* **48**(1):13–18, 2008.

Gobburu JV: Biomarkers in clinical drug development. *Clin Pharmacol Ther* **86**(1):26–27, 2009.

Gobburu JV, Marroum PJ: Utilisation of pharmacokinetic-pharmacodynamic modelling and simulation in regulatory decision-making. *Clin Pharmacokinet* **40**(12):883–892, 2001.

Henningfield JE, Keenan RM: Nicotine delivery kinetics and abuse liability. *J Consult Clin Psychol* **61**(5):743–750, 1993.

Holford NH, Sheiner LB: Understanding the dose-effect relationship: clinical application of pharmacokinetic-pharmacodynamic models. *Clin Pharmacokinet* **6**(6):429–453, 1981.

Johanson CE, Fischman MW: The pharmacology of cocaine related to its abuse. *Pharmacol Rev* **41**(1):3–52, 1989.

Johansen SH, Jorgensen M, Molbech S: Effect of Tubocurarine on Respiratory and Nonrespiratory Muscle Power in Man. *J Appl Physiol* **19**:990–994, 1964.

Jusko WJ: Moving from basic toward systems pharmacodynamic models. *J Pharm Sci* **102**(9):2930–2940, 2013.

Jusko WJ, Ko HC: Physiologic indirect response models characterize diverse types of pharmacodynamic effects. *Clin Pharmacol Ther* **56**(4):406–419, 1994.

Jusko WJ, Ko HC, Ebling WF: Convergence of direct and indirect pharmacodynamic response models. *J Pharmacokinet Biopharm* **23**(1):5–8, 1995; discussion 9–10.

Katzung BG, Masters SB, Trevor AJ: Drug receptors & pharmacodynamics. *Basic & Clinical Pharmacology*. McGraw-Hill, 2011.

Kimko H, Pinheiro J: Model-based clinical drug development in the past, present & future: A commentary. *Br J Clin Pharmacol* **79**(1):108–116, 2015.

Kuivenhoven JA, Jukema JW, Zwinderman AH, et al: The role of a common variant of the cholesteryl ester transfer protein gene in the progression of coronary atherosclerosis. The Regression Growth Evaluation Statin Study Group. *N Engl J Med* **338**(2):86–93, 1998.

Lesko LJ, Atkinson AJ, Jr: Use of biomarkers and surrogate endpoints in drug development and regulatory decision making: Criteria, validation, strategies. *Annu Rev Pharmacol Toxicol* **41**:347–366, 2001.

Levy G: Relationship between elimination rate of drugs and rate of decline of their pharmacologic effects. *J Pharm Sci* **53**: 342–343, 1964.

Levy G: Kinetics of pharmacologic effects. *Clin Pharmacol Ther* **7**(3):362–372, 1966.

Lin RY: A perspective on penicillin allergy. *Arch Intern Med* **152**(5):930–937, 1992.

Lorentzen H, Kallehave F, Kolmos HJ, Knigge U, Bulow J, Gottrup F: Gentamicin concentrations in human subcutaneous tissue. *Antimicrob Agents Chemother* **40**(8):1785–1789, 1996.

Madabushi R, Cox DS, Hossain M, et al: Pharmacokinetic and pharmacodynamic basis for effective argatroban dosing in pediatrics. *J Clin Pharmacol* **51**(1):19–28, 2011.

Mager DE, Wyska E, Jusko WJ: Diversity of mechanism-based pharmacodynamic models. *Drug Metab Dispos* **31**(5):510–518, 2003.

Meibohm B, Derendorf H: Basic concepts of pharmacokinetic/pharmacodynamic (PK/PD) modelling. *Int J Clin Pharmacol Ther* **35**(10):401–413, 1997.

Moroney AC, PharmD (2011). Drug–Receptor Interactions. The MERCK Manual of Diagnosis and Therapy. MERCK SHARP & DOHME CORP., A SUBSIDIARY OF MERCK & CO., INC. Whitehouse Station, NJ.

Mould DR, DeFeo TM, Reele S, et al: Simultaneous modeling of the pharmacokinetics and pharmacodynamics of midazolam and diazepam. *Clin Pharmacol Ther* **58**(1):35–43, 1995.

Nagashima R, O'Reilly RA, Levy G: Kinetics of pharmacologic effects in man: the anticoagulant action of warfarin. *Clin Pharmacol Ther* **10**(1):22–35, 1969.

Neubig RR, Spedding M, Kenakin T, Christopoulos A: International Union of Pharmacology Committee on Receptor Nomenclature and Drug Classification. XXXVIII. Update on terms and symbols in quantitative pharmacology. *Pharmacol Rev* **55**(4):597–606, 2003.

Nieforth KA, Nadeau R, Patel IH, Mould D: Use of an indirect pharmacodynamic stimulation model of MX protein induction to compare in vivo activity of interferon alfa-2a and a polyethylene glycol-modified derivative in healthy subjects. *Clin Pharmacol Ther* **59**(6):636–646, 1996.

O'Donnell JM, Shelton RC: Drug therapy of depression and anxiety disorders. In Brunton LL (ed). *The Pharmacological Basis of Therapeutics*. McGraw-Hill, 2011.

Peck CC, Barr WH, Benet LZ, et al: Opportunities for integration of pharmacokinetics, pharmacodynamics, and toxicokinetics in rational drug development. *J Clin Pharmacol* **34**(2):111–119, 1994.

Publication Committee for the, V. I: Intravenous nesiritide vs nitroglycerin for treatment of decompensated congestive heart failure: a randomized controlled trial. *JAMA* **287**(12): 1531–1540, 2002.

Roy A, Mould DR, Wang XF, Tay L, Raymond R, Pfister M: Modeling and simulation of abatacept exposure and interleukin-6 response in support of recommended doses for rheumatoid arthritis. *J Clin Pharmacol* **47**(11):1408–1420, 2007.

Russell T, Riley SP, Cook JA, Lalonde RL: A perspective on the use of concentration-QT modeling in drug development. *J Clin Pharmacol* **48**(1):9–12, 2008.

Schuck EL, Derendorf H: Pharmacokinetic/pharmacodynamic evaluation of anti-infective agents. *Expert Rev Anti Infect Ther* **3**(3):361–373, 2005.

Shak S: Overview of the trastuzumab (Herceptin) anti-HER2 monoclonal antibody clinical program in HER2-overexpressing metastatic breast cancer. Herceptin Multinational Investigator Study Group. *Semin Oncol* **26**(4 Suppl 12):71–77, 1999.

Sharma A, Jusko WJ: Characterization of four basic models of indirect pharmacodynamic responses. *J Pharmacokinet Biopharm* **24**(6):611–635, 1996.

Sharma A, Jusko WJ: Characteristics of indirect pharmacodynamic models and applications to clinical drug responses. *Br J Clin Pharmacol* **45**(3):229–239, 1998.

Sheiner LB, Stanski DR, Vozeh S, Miller RD, Ham J: Simultaneous modeling of pharmacokinetics and pharmacodynamics: application to d-tubocurarine. *Clin Pharmacol Ther* **25**(3): 358–371, 1979.

Sheiner LB, Steimer JL: Pharmacokinetic/pharmacodynamic modeling in drug development. *Annu Rev Pharmacol Toxicol* **40**:67–95, 2000.

Skidgel RA, Kaplan AP, Erdös EG: Histamine, bradykinin, and their antagonists. In Brunton LL (ed). *The Pharmacological Basis of Therapeutics*. McGraw-Hill, 2011.

Strimbu K, Tavel JA: What are biomarkers? *Curr Opin HIV AIDS* **5**(6):463–466, 2010.

Temple R: Are surrogate markers adequate to assess cardiovascular disease drugs? *JAMA* **282**(8):790–795, 1999.

Vogelman B, Gudmundsson S, Leggett J, Turnidge J, Ebert S, Craig WA: Correlation of antimicrobial pharmacokinetic parameters with therapeutic efficacy in an animal model. *J Infect Dis* **158**(4):831–847, 1988.

Weiss R, Mazade L: *Surrogate Endpoints in Evaluating the Effectiveness of Drugs against HIV Infection and AIDS*. Institute of Medicine, Washington DC, National Academy Press, 1990.

Westfall TC, Westfall DP: Adrenergic agonists and antagonists. In Brunton LL (ed). *The Pharmacological Basis of Therapeutics*. McGraw-Hill, 2011.

Yaksh TL, Wallace MS: Opioids, analgesia, and pain management. In Brunton LL (ed). *The Pharmacological Basis of Therapeutics*. McGraw-Hill, 2011.

22 Application of Pharmacokinetics to Clinical Situations

Vincent H. Tam

Chapter Objectives

▶ Define Medication Therapy Management (MTM) and explain how MTM can improve the success of drug therapy.

▶ Explain what "critical-dose drugs" are and name an example.

▶ Define therapeutic drug monitoring and explain which drugs should be monitored through a therapeutic drug monitoring service.

▶ Calculate a drug dosage regimen in an individual patient for optimal drug therapy for a drug that has complete pharmacokinetic information and for a drug that has incomplete pharmacokinetic information.

▶ Explain the relationship of changing the dose and/or the dosing interval on the C_{max}^{∞}, C_{min}^{∞}, and C_{av}^{∞}.

▶ Define drug–drug interactions and the mechanisms of drug–drug interactions, and provide examples.

▶ Provide instructions to a patient who has missed a dose and discuss the therapeutic implications.

The success of drug therapy is highly dependent on the choice of the drug, the drug product, and the design of the dosage regimen. The choice of the drug is generally made by the physician after careful patient diagnosis and physical assessment. The choice of the drug product (eg, immediate release vs modified release) and dosage regimen is based on the patient's individual characteristics and known pharmacokinetics of the drug as discussed in earlier chapters. Ideally, the dosage regimen is designed to achieve a desired drug concentration at a receptor site to produce an optimal therapeutic response with minimum adverse effects. Individual variation in pharmacokinetics and pharmacodynamics makes the design of dosage regimens difficult. Therefore, the application of pharmacokinetics to dosage regimen design must be coordinated with proper clinical evaluation of the patient. For certain critical-dose drugs, monitoring both the patient and drug regimen is important for proper efficacy.

MEDICATION THERAPY MANAGEMENT

Medication Therapy Management (MTM) was officially recognized by the US Congress in the Medicare Prescription Drug, Improvement, and Modernization Act of 2003.[1] The objective of this act is to improve the quality, effectiveness, and efficiency of healthcare delivery including prescription drugs. An MTM program is developed in cooperation with pharmacists and physicians to optimize therapeutic outcomes through improved medication use. MTM provides consultative, educational, and monitoring services to patients to obtain better therapeutic outcomes from medications by the enhanced understanding of medication therapy, improved compliance, control of costs, and prevention of adverse events and drug interactions. MTM programs have been developed for specific practice areas such as elderly care, diabetes, and asthma (Barnett et al, 2009).

[1] www.cms.gov/PrescriptionDrugCovContra/082_MTM.asp.

- ► Explain how the pharmacokinetics of a drug may be altered in special populations, such as the elderly, infants, obese patients, and patients with renal or hepatic disease.

- ► Explain how Bayesian theory can help determine the probability of a diagnostic test to give accurate results.

- ► Define population pharmacokinetics and explain how population pharmacokinetics enables the estimate of pharmacokinetic parameters from relatively sparse data obtained from study subjects.

INDIVIDUALIZATION OF DRUG DOSAGE REGIMENS

Not all drugs require rigid individualization of the dosage regimen. Many drugs have a large margin of safety (ie, exhibit a wide therapeutic window), and strict individualization of the dose is unnecessary. For a number of drugs generally recognized as safe and effective (GRAS), the US Food and Drug Administration (FDA) has approved an *over-the-counter* (OTC) classification for drugs that the public may buy without prescription. In addition, many prescription drugs, such as ibuprofen, loratidine, omeprazole, naproxen, nicotine patches, and others, that were originally prescription drugs have been approved by the FDA for OTC status. These OTC drugs and certain prescription drugs, when taken as directed, are generally safe and effective for the labeled indications without medical supervision. For drugs that are relatively safe and have a broad safety-dose range, such as the penicillins, cephalosporins, and tetracyclines, the antibiotic dosage is not dose titrated precisely but is based rather on the clinical judgment of the physician to maintain an effective plasma antibiotic concentration above a minimum inhibitory concentration. Individualization of the dosage regimen is very important for drugs with a narrow therapeutic window (also known as *critical-dose drugs* and *narrow therapeutic index* [NTI] drugs), such as digoxin, aminoglycosides, antiarrhythmics, anticoagulants, anticonvulsants, and some antiasthmatics, such as theophylline. Critical-dose drugs are defined as those drugs where comparatively small differences in dose or concentration lead to dose- and concentration-dependent, serious therapeutic failures and/or serious adverse drug reactions. These adverse reactions may be persistent, irreversible, slowly reversible, or life threatening, or could result in inpatient hospitalization or prolongation of existing hospitalization, persistent or significant disability or incapacity, or death. Adverse reactions that require significant medical intervention to prevent one of these outcomes are also considered to be serious (Guidance for Industry, 2006).

The objective of the dosage regimen design is to produce a safe plasma drug concentration that does not exceed the minimum toxic concentration or fall below a critical minimum drug concentration below which the drug is not effective. For this reason, the dose of these drugs is carefully individualized to avoid plasma drug concentration fluctuations due to intersubject variation in drug absorption, distribution, or elimination processes. For drugs such as phenytoin, a critical-dose drug that follows nonlinear pharmacokinetics at therapeutic plasma drug concentrations, a small change in the dose may cause a huge increase in the therapeutic response and possible adverse effects.

THERAPEUTIC DRUG MONITORING

Many drugs, such as nonsteroidal anti-inflammatory drugs (NSAIDs) such as ibuprofen, and calcium channel-blocking agents, such as nifedipine, have a wide therapeutic range and do not need therapeutic drug monitoring. In addition, OTC drugs such as various cough and cold remedies, analgesics, and other products are also generally safe when used as directed. Therapeutic monitoring of plasma drug concentrations is valuable only if a relationship exists between the plasma drug concentration and the desired clinical effect or between the plasma drug concentration and an adverse effect. For those drugs in which plasma drug concentration and clinical effect are not directly related, other pharmacodynamic or "surrogate" parameters may be monitored. For example, clotting time may be measured directly in patients on warfarin anticoagulant therapy. Glucose concentrations are often monitored in diabetic patients using insulin products. Asthmatic patients may use the bronchodilator, albuterol taken by inhalation via a metered-dose inhaler. For these patients, FEV_1 (forced expiratory volume) may be used as a measure of drug efficacy. In cancer chemotherapy, dose adjustment for individual patients may depend more on the severity of side effects and the patient's ability to tolerate the drug. For some drugs that have large inter- and intrasubject variability, clinical judgment and experience with the drug are needed to dose the patient properly.

The therapeutic range for a drug is an approximation of the average plasma drug concentrations that are safe and efficacious in most patients. When using published therapeutic drug concentration ranges, such as those in Table 22-1, the clinician must realize that the therapeutic range is essentially a probability concept and should never be considered as absolute values (Evans et al, 1992; Schumacher, 1995). For example, the accepted therapeutic range for theophylline is 10–20 μg/mL. Some patients may exhibit signs of theophylline intoxication such as central nervous system excitation and insomnia at serum drug concentrations below 20 μg/mL (Fig. 22-1),

TABLE 22-1 **Therapeutic Range for Commonly Monitored Drugs**

Amikacin	20–30 μg/mL
Carbamazepine	4–12 μg/mL
Digoxin	1–2 ng/mL
Gentamicin	5–10 μg/mL
Lidocaine	1–5 μg/mL
Lithium	0.6–1.2 mEq/L
Phenytoin	10–20 μg/mL
Procainamide	4–10 μg/mL
Quinidine	1–4 μg/mL
Theophylline	10–20 μg/mL
Tobramycin	5–10 μg/mL
Valproic acid	50–100 μg/mL
Vancomycin	20–40 μg/mL

From Schumacher (1995), with permission.

whereas other patients may show drug efficacy at serum drug concentrations below 10 μg/mL.

In administering potent drugs to patients, the physician must maintain the plasma drug level within

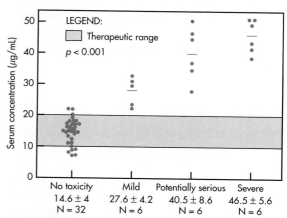

FIGURE 22-1   Correlation between the frequency and severity of adverse effects and plasma concentration of theophylline (mean ± SD) in 50 adult patients. Mild symptoms of toxicity included nausea, vomiting, headache, and insomnia. A potentially serious effect was sinus tachycardia, and severe toxicity was defined as the occurrence of life-threatening cardiac arrhythmias and seizures. (Adapted from Hendeles and Weinberger, 1980, with permission.)

a narrow range of therapeutic concentrations (see Table 22-1). Various pharmacokinetic methods (or nomograms) may be used to calculate the initial dose or dosage regimen. Usually, the initial dosage regimen is calculated based on body weight or body surface after a careful consideration of the known pharmacokinetics of the drug, the pathophysiologic condition of the patient, and the patient's drug history including nonprescription drugs and nutraceuticals.

Because of interpatient variability in drug absorption, distribution, and elimination as well as changing pathophysiologic conditions in the patient, *therapeutic drug monitoring* (TDM) or clinical pharmacokinetic (laboratory) services (CPKS) have been established in many hospitals to evaluate the response of the patient to the recommended dosage regimen. The improvement in the clinical effectiveness of the drug by TDM may decrease the cost of medical care by preventing untoward adverse drug effects. The functions of a TDM service are listed below.

- Select drug.
- Design dosage regimen.
- Evaluate patient response.
- Determine need for measuring serum drug concentrations.
- Assay for drug concentration in biological fluids.
- Perform pharmacokinetic evaluation of drug concentrations.
- Readjust dosage regimen, if necessary.
- Monitor serum drug concentrations.
- Recommend special requirements.

Drug Selection

The choice of drug and drug therapy is usually made by the physician. However, many practitioners consult with the clinical pharmacist in drug product selection and dosage regimen design. Increasingly, clinical pharmacists in hospitals and nursing care facilities are closely involved in prescribing, monitoring, and substitution of medications as part of a total MTM program. The choice of drug and the drug product is made not only on the basis of therapeutic consideration but also based on cost and therapeutic equivalency.

Hospitals and various prescription reimbursement plans have a drug formulary.[2] Pharmacokinetics

TABLE 22-2 Factors Producing Variability in Drug Response

Patent Factors	Drug Factors
Age	Bioavailability and biopharmaceutics
Weight	Pharmacokinetics (including absorption, distribution, and elimination)
Pathophysiology	Drug interactions
Nutritional status	Receptor sensitivity
Genetic variability Gender	Rapid or slow metabolism

and pharmacodynamics are part of the overall considerations in the selection of a drug for inclusion in the drug formulary. An Institutional Pharmacy and Therapeutic Committee (IPTC) periodically reviews clinical efficacy data on new drug products for inclusion in the formulary and on older products for removal from the formulary. Drugs with similar therapeutic indications may differ in dose and pharmacokinetics. The pharmacist may choose one drug over another based on therapeutic, adverse effect, pharmacokinetic (dosing convenience), and cost considerations. Other factors include patient-specific information such as medical history, pathophysiologic states, concurrent drug therapy, known allergies, drug sensitivities, and drug interactions; all are important considerations in drug selection (Table 22-2). As discussed in Chapter 13, the use of pharmacogenetic data may become another tool in assisting in drug selection for the patient.

Dosage Regimen Design

The main objective of designing an appropriate dosage regimen for the patient is to provide a drug dose and dosing interval that achieve a *target* drug concentration at the receptor site. Once the proper drug is selected for the patient, a number of factors must be considered

---

[2]A drug formulary contains a list of prescription drug products that will be reimbursed fully or partially by the prescription plan provider. Drug products not listed in the formulary may be reimbursed if specially requested by the physician.

when designing a therapeutic dosage regimen. Usually, the manufacturer's dosing recommendations in the package insert will provide guidance on the initial starting dose and dosing interval in the typical patient population. These recommendations are based upon clinical trials performed during and after drug development. The package insert containing the FDA-approved label suggests an average dose and dosage regimen for the "average" patient who was enrolled in these studies. Genetic variation, drug interactions, or physiologic conditions such as disease or pregnancy may change the pharmacokinetics and/or pharmacodynamics of a drug, therefore requiring dosing regimen individualization. First, the known pharmacokinetics of the drug, including its absorption, distribution, and elimination profile, are considered in the patient who is to be treated. Some patients may have unusual first-pass metabolism (eg, fast or slow metabolizers) that will affect bioavailability after oral administration and the elimination half-life after systemic dug absorption. Second, the physiology of the patient, age, weight, gender, and nutritional status will affect the disposition of the drug and should be considered. Third, any pathophysiologic conditions, such as renal dysfunction, hepatic disease, or congestive heart failure, may change the normal pharmacokinetic profile of the drug, and the dose must be carefully adjusted. Fourth, the effect of long-term exposure to the medication in the patient must be considered including the possibility of drug abuse by the patient. In addition, personal lifestyle factors, such as cigarette smoking, alcohol abuse, and obesity, are other issues that are known to alter the pharmacokinetics of drugs. Lastly, lack of patient compliance (ie, patient noncompliance) in taking the medication can also be a problem in achieving effective therapeutic outcomes.

An optimal dosing design can greatly improve the safety and efficacy of the drug, including reduced side effects and a decrease in frequency of TDM and its associated costs. For some drugs, TDM will be necessary because of the unpredictable nature of their pharmacodynamics and pharmacokinetics. Changes in drug or drug dose may be required after careful patient assessment by the pharmacist, including changes in the drug's pharmacokinetics, drug tolerance, cross-sensitivity, or history of unusual reactions to related drugs. The pharmacist must develop competency and experience in clinical pharmacology and therapeutics in addition to the necessary pharmacokinetic skills. Several mathematical approaches to dosage regimen design are given in later sections of this chapter and in Chapter 24.

Dosage regimen guidelines obtained from the literature and from approved product labeling are often based upon average patient response. However, substantial individual variation to drug response can occur. The design of the dosage regimen must be based upon clinical assessment of the patient. Labeling for recently approved drugs provides information for dosing in patients with renal and/or hepatic disease. Frequently, drug dose adjustment of another coadministered drug may be necessary due to drug–drug interactions. For example, an elderly patient who is on haloperidol (Haldol®) may require a reduction of his usual morphine dose. With many new drugs, pharmacogenetic information is also available and should be considered for dosing individual patients. For example, the extents of drug resistance are important considerations during dosage regimen design in cancer and anti-infective chemotherapy.

Pharmacokinetics of the Drug

Various popular drug references list pharmacokinetic parameters such as clearance, bioavailability, and elimination half-life. The values for these pharmacokinetic parameters are often obtained from small clinical studies. Therefore, it is difficult to determine whether these reported pharmacokinetic parameters are reflected in the general population or in a specific patient group. Differences in study design, patient population, and data analysis may lead to conflicting values for the same pharmacokinetic parameters. For example, values for the apparent volume of distribution and clearance can be estimated by different methods, as discussed in previous chapters.

Ideally, the effective target drug concentration and the therapeutic window for the drug should be obtained. When using the target drug concentration in the development of a dosage regimen, the clinical pharmacist should know whether the reported target drug concentration represents an average steady-state drug concentration, a peak drug concentration, or a trough concentration.

Drug Dosage Form (Drug Product)

The dosage form of the drug will affect drug bio-availability and the rate of absorption and thus the subsequent pharmacodynamics of the drug in the patient (see also Chapter 15). The choice of drug dosage form may be based on the desired route of drug administration, the desired onset and duration of the clinical response, cost, and patient compliance. For example, an extended-release drug product instead of an immediate-release drug product may provide a longer duration of action and better patient compliance. An orally disintegrating tablet (ODT) may be easier for the patient who has difficulty in swallowing a conventional tablet. Patients with profuse vomiting may prefer the use of a transdermal delivery system rather than an oral drug product. Available dosage forms and strengths are usually listed under the *How Supplied section* in the package insert.

Patient Compliance

Factors that may affect patient compliance include the cost of the medication, complicated instructions, multiple daily doses, difficulty in swallowing, type of dosage form, and adverse drug reactions. The patient who is in an institution may have different issues compared to an ambulatory patient. Patient compliance in institutions is maintained by the healthcare personnel who provides/administers the medication on schedule. Ambulatory patients must remember to take the medication as prescribed to obtain the optimum clinical effect of the drug. It is very important that the prescriber or clinical pharmacist consider the patient's lifestyle and personal needs when developing a drug dosage regimen. The FDA-approved labeling in the package insert contains *Patient Counseling Information* to improve patient compliance. There are also sections on *Information for Patients* and *Medication Guide*.

Evaluation of Patient's Response

After the drug and drug products are chosen and the patient receives the initial dosage regimen, the practitioner should evaluate the patient's clinical response. If the patient is not responding to drug therapy as expected, then the drug and dosage regimen should be reviewed. The dosage regimen should be reviewed for adequacy, accuracy, and patient compliance with the drug therapy. In many situations, sound clinical judgment may preclude the need for measuring serum drug concentrations.

Measurement of Drug Concentrations

Before biological samples are taken from the patient, the need to determine serum drug concentrations should be assessed by the practitioner. In some cases, adverse events may not be related to the serum drug concentration but preclude the patient from using the prescribed drug. For example, allergy or mild nausea may not be dose related. Plasma, serum saliva, urine, and occasionally tissue drug concentrations may be measured for (1) clinical drug monitoring to improve drug therapy, (2) drug abuse screening, and (3) toxicology evaluation such as poisoning and drug overdose. Examples of common drugs that may be measured are listed in Table 22-3. In addition, many prescription medications (eg, opiates, benzodiazepines, NSAIDs, anabolic steroids) and nonprescription drugs (eg, dextromethorphan, NSAIDs) can also be abused. Analyses have been used for measurement of the presence of abused drugs in blood, urine, saliva, hair, and breath (alcohol).

A major assumption made is that serum drug concentrations relate to the therapeutic and/or toxic effects of the drug. For many drugs, clinical studies have demonstrated a therapeutically effective range of serum concentrations. Knowledge of the serum drug concentration may clarify why a patient is not responding to the drug therapy or why the drug is having an adverse effect. In some cases, the practitioner may want to verify the accuracy of the dosage regimen.

The timing of the blood sample and the number of blood samples to be taken from the patient must be considered. In many cases, a single blood sample gives insufficient information. Occasionally, more than one blood samples are needed to clarify the adequacy of the dosage regimen. When ordering serum drug concentrations to be measured, a single serum drug concentration may not yield useful information unless other factors are considered. For example, the dosage regimen of the drug should be known, including the dose and the dosage interval, the route of drug administration, the time

TABLE 22-3   Drugs Commonly Measured in Serum, Plasma, or Other Tissues

Therapeutic Drug Monitoring	Drug Abuse Screen	Drug Overdose or Poisoning
Anticonvulsants	*Alcohol*	*Alcohol*
Carbamazepine, phenytoin, valproic acid, primidone	*Cotinine*	Ethyl alcohol, methanol
Antibiotics	*Anabolic steroids*	*Opiates*
Aminglycosides (gentamicin), vancomycin	*Opiates*	Heroin, morphine, codeine derivatives, methadone, buprenorphine
	Heroin, morphine, codeine derivatives, methadone, buprenorphine	*Stimulants*
Cardiovascular agents Digoxin, lidocaine, procainamide, quinidine	*Stimulants* Cocaine, amphetamine, methamphetamine	Cocaine, amphetamine, methamphetamine, pseudoephedrine
Immunosupressants Cyclosporine, tacrolimus, sirolimus	*Cannabinoids* Marijuana, hashish	*Hallucinogens and related drugs* These drugs are subject to overdose and/or poisoning
Antipsychotics Clozapine		*Other drugs* Barbiturates, benzodiazepines, tricyclics
Other drugs Lithium, theophylline	*Hallucinogens and related drugs* Phencyclidine, PCP, ketamine, MDMA (ecstasy, 3,4-methylenedioxy-N-methylamphetamine)	*Inhalants* Nitrous oxide, paint thinners, solvents
Hormonal drugs TSH, thyroxin, estrogens	*Other drugs* Barbiturates, benzodiazepines, various hypnotics and sedatives	*Heavy metals* Lead, mercury, arsenic, chromium
		Various nonprescription medications such as acetaminophen

Nicotine from tobacco is often included in some drug abuse literature, but is not usually part of a drug abuse screen.

of sampling (peak, trough, or steady state), and the type of drug product (eg, immediate-release or extended-release drug product).

In practice, trough serum concentrations are easier to obtain than peak or C_{av}^{∞} samples under a multiple-dose regimen. In addition, there are limitations in terms of the number of blood samples that may be taken, total volume of blood needed for the assay, and time to perform the drug analysis. Schumacher (1985) has suggested that blood sampling times for TDM should be taken during the postdistributive phase for loading and maintenance doses, but at steady state for maintenance doses. After distribution equilibrium has been achieved, the plasma drug concentration during the postdistributive phase is better correlated with the tissue concentration and, presumably, the drug concentration at the site of action. In some cases, the clinical pharmacist may want an early-time sample that approximates the peak drug level, whereas a blood sample taken at three or four elimination half-lives during multiple dosing will approximate the steady-state drug concentration. The practitioner who orders the measurement of serum concentrations should also consider the cost of the assays, the risks and discomfort for the patient, and the utility of the information gained.

Assay for Drug

Drug analyses are usually performed either by a clinical chemistry laboratory or by a clinical pharmacokinetics laboratory. A variety of analytic techniques are available for drug measurement, such as high-pressure liquid chromatography coupled with mass spectrometry (LCMS), immunoassay, and other methods. The methods used by the analytic laboratory may depend on such factors as the physicochemical characteristics of the drug, target drug concentration, amount (volume) and nature of the biologic specimen (serum, urine, saliva), available instrumentation, cost for each assay, and analytical skills of the laboratory personnel. The laboratory should have a standard operating procedure (SOP) for each drug analysis method and follow good laboratory practices (GLP). Moreover, analytic methods used for the assay of drugs in serum or plasma should be validated with respect to specificity, linearity, sensitivity, precision, accuracy, stability, and ruggedness. The times to perform the assays and receive the results are important factors that should be considered if the clinician needs this information to make a quick therapeutic decision.

Specificity

Chromatographic evidence is generally required to demonstrate that the analytic method is specific for detection of the drug and other analytes, such as an active metabolite. The method should demonstrate that there is no interference between the drug and its metabolites and endogenous or exogenous substances such as other drugs that the patient may have taken. In addition, the internal standard should be resolved completely and also demonstrate no interference with other compounds. Immunoassays depend on an antibody and antigen (usually the drug to be measured) reaction. The antibody should be specific for the drug analyte, but may instead also cross-react with drugs that have similar structures, including related compounds (endogenous or exogenous chemicals) and metabolites of the drug. Colorimetric and spectrophotometric assays are usually less specific. Interference from other materials may inflate the results.

Sensitivity

Sensitivity is the minimum detectable level or concentration of drug in serum that may be approximated as the lowest drug concentration that is two to three times the background noise. A *minimum quantifiable level* (MQL) or *minimum detectable limit* (MDL) is a statistical method for the determination of the precision of the lower level.

Linearity and Dynamic Range

Dynamic range refers to the relationship between the drug concentration and the instrument response (or signal) used to measure the drug. Many assays show a linear drug concentration–instrument response relationship. Immunoassays generally have a nonlinear dynamic range. High serum drug concentrations, above the dynamic range of the instrument response, must be diluted before assay. The dynamic range is determined by using serum samples that have known (standard) drug concentrations (including a blank serum sample or zero drug concentration). Extrapolation of the assay results above or below the measured standard drug concentrations may be inaccurate if the relationship between instrument response and extrapolated drug concentration is unknown.

Precision

Precision is a measurement of the variability or reproducibility of the data. Precision measurements are obtained by replication of various drug concentrations and by replication of standard concentration curves prepared separately on different days. A suitable statistical measurement of the dispersion of the data, such as standard deviation or coefficient of variation, is then performed.

Accuracy

Accuracy refers to the difference between the average assay values and the true or known drug concentrations. Control (known) drug serum concentrations should be prepared by an independent technician using such techniques to minimize any error in their preparation. These samples, including a "zero" drug concentration, are assayed by the technician assigned to the study along with a suitable standard drug concentration curve.

Stability

Standard drug concentrations should be maintained under the same storage conditions as the unknown serum samples and assayed periodically. The stability study should continue for at least the same length of time as the patient samples are to be stored. Freeze–thaw stability studies are performed to determine the effect of thawing and refreezing on the stability of the drug in the sample. On occasion, a previously frozen biologic sample must be thawed and reassayed if the first assay result is uncertain.

Plasma samples obtained from subjects on a drug study are usually assayed along with a minimum of three standard processed serum samples containing known standard drug concentrations and a minimum of three control plasma samples whose concentrations are unknown to the analyst. These control plasma samples are randomly distributed in each day's run. Control samples are replicated in duplicate to evaluate both within-day and between-day precision. The concentration of drug in each plasma sample is based on each day's processed standard curve.

Ruggedness

Ruggedness is the degree of reproducibility of the test results obtained by the analysis of the same samples by different analytical laboratories or by different instruments. The determination of ruggedness measures the reproducibility of the results under normal operational conditions from laboratory to laboratory, instrument to instrument, and analyst to analyst.

Because each method for drug assay may have differences in sensitivity, precision, and specificity, the clinical pharmacokineticist should be aware of which drug assay method the laboratory used.

Pharmacokinetic Evaluation

After the serum or plasma drug concentrations are measured, the clinical pharmacokineticist must evaluate the data. Many laboratories report total drug (free plus bound drug) concentrations in the serum. The pharmacokineticist should be aware of the usual therapeutic range of serum drug concentrations from the literature. However, the literature may not indicate whether the reported values were trough, peak serum, or average drug levels. Moreover, the methodology for the drug assay used in the analytical laboratory may be different in terms of accuracy, specificity, and precision.

The assay results from the analytical laboratory may show that the patient's serum drug levels are higher, lower, or similar to the expected serum levels. The pharmacokineticist should evaluate these results while considering the patient and the patient's pathophysiologic condition. Table 22-4 lists a number of factors the pharmacokineticist should consider when interpreting serum drug concentration. Often, additional data, such as a high serum creatinine and high blood urea nitrogen (BUN), may help verify that an observed high serum drug concentration in a patient is due to lower renal drug clearance because of compromised kidney function. In another case, a complaint by the patient of overstimulation and insomnia might corroborate the laboratory's finding of higher-than-anticipated serum concentrations of theophylline. Therefore, the clinician or pharmacokineticist should evaluate the data using sound clinical judgment and observation. The therapeutic decision should not be based solely on serum drug concentrations.

Dosage Adjustment

From the serum drug concentration data and patient observations, the clinician or pharmacokineticist may recommend an adjustment in the dosage regimen. Ideally, the new dosage regimen should be calculated using the pharmacokinetic parameters derived from the *patient's* serum drug concentrations. Although there may not be enough data for a complete pharmacokinetic profile, the pharmacokineticist should still be able to derive a new dosage regimen based on the available data and the pharmacokinetic parameters in the literature that are based on average population data.

Monitoring Serum Drug Concentrations

In many cases, the patient's pathophysiology may be unstable, either improving or deteriorating further. For example, proper therapy for congestive heart failure will improve cardiac output and renal perfusion,

TABLE 22-4   Pharmacokinetic Evaluation of Serum Drug Concentrations

Serum Concentrations Lower Than Anticipated
Patient compliance
Error in dosage regimen
Wrong drug product (controlled release instead of immediate release)
Poor bioavailability
Rapid elimination (efficient metabolizer)
Reduced plasma–protein binding
Enlarged apparent volume of distribution
Steady state not reached
Timing of blood sample
Improving renal/hepatic function
Drug interaction due to stimulation of elimination enzyme autoinduction
Changing hepatic blood flow
Serum Concentrations Higher Than Anticipated
Patient compliance
Error in dosage regimen
Wrong drug product (immediate release instead of controlled release)
Rapid bioavailability
Smaller-than-anticipated apparent volume of distribution
Slow elimination (poor metabolizer)
Increased plasma–protein binding
Deteriorating renal/hepatic function
Drug interaction due to inhibition of elimination
Serum Concentration Correct but Patient Does Not Respond to Therapy
Altered receptor sensitivity (eg, tolerance)
Drug interaction at receptor site
Changing hepatic blood flow

thereby increasing renal drug clearance. Therefore, continuous monitoring of serum drug concentrations is necessary to ensure proper drug therapy for the patient. For some drugs, an acute pharmacologic response can be monitored in lieu of actual serum drug concentration. For example, prothrombin time might be useful for monitoring anticoagulant therapy and blood pressure monitoring for antihypertensive agents.

Special Recommendations

At times, the patient may not be responding to drug therapy because of other factors. For example, the patient may not be following instructions for taking the medication (patient noncompliance). The patient may be taking the drug after a meal instead of before or may not be adhering to a special diet (eg, low-salt diet). Therefore, the patient may need special instructions that are simple and easy to follow. It may be necessary to discontinue the drug and prescribe another drug from the same therapeutic class.

> **Frequently Asked Questions**
> ▶ *Can therapeutic drug monitoring be performed without taking blood samples?*
>
> ▶ *What are the major considerations in therapeutic drug monitoring?*

CLINICAL EXAMPLE

Dosage and Administration of Lanoxin® (Digoxin) Tablets, USP

In the new package insert, dosing information is available under *Dosage and Administration*. In addition, the section under *Clinical Pharmacology* provides valuable information for therapeutic considerations such as:

- Mechanism of action
- Pharmacodynamics
- Pharmacokinetics

Lanoxin (digoxin) is one of the cardiac (or digitalis) glycosides indicated for the treatment of congestive heart failure and atrial fibrillation. According to the approved label[3] for Lanoxin, the recommended

---

[3]Lanoxin (digoxin) tablets, USP, NDA 20405/S-004, GlaxoSmith-Kline, August 2009.

dosages of digoxin may require considerable modification because of individual sensitivity of the patient to the drug, the presence of associated conditions, or the use of concurrent medications. In selecting a dose of digoxin, the following factors must be considered:

1. The body weight of the patient. Doses should be calculated based upon lean (ie, ideal) body weight.
2. The patient's renal function, preferably evaluated on the basis of estimated creatinine clearance.
3. The patient's age: Infants and children require different doses of digoxin than adults. Also, advanced age may be indicative of diminished renal function even in patients with normal serum creatinine concentration (ie, below 1.5 mg/dL).
4. Concomitant disease states, concurrent medications, or other factors likely to alter the pharmacokinetic or pharmacodynamic profile of digoxin.

Serum Digoxin Concentrations

In general, the dose of digoxin used should be determined based on clinical grounds. However, measurement of serum digoxin concentrations can be helpful to the clinician in determining the adequacy of digoxin therapy and in assigning certain probabilities to the likelihood of digoxin intoxication. About two-thirds of adults considered adequately digitalized (without evidence of toxicity) have serum digoxin concentrations ranging from 0.8 to 2.0 ng/mL; lower serum trough concentrations of 0.5–1 ng/mL may be appropriate in some adult patients. About two-thirds of adult patients with clinical toxicity have serum digoxin concentrations greater than 2.0 ng/mL. Since one-third of patients with clinical toxicity have concentrations less than 2.0 ng/mL, values below 2.0 ng/mL do not rule out the possibility that a certain sign or symptom is related to digoxin therapy. Rarely, there are patients who are unable to tolerate digoxin at serum concentrations below 0.8 ng/mL. Consequently, the serum concentration of digoxin should always be interpreted in the overall clinical context, and an isolated

measurement should not be used alone as the basis for increasing or decreasing the dose of the drug.

To allow adequate time for equilibration of digoxin between serum and tissue, sampling of serum concentrations should be done just before the next scheduled dose of the drug (trough level). If this is not possible, sampling should be done at least 6–8 hours after the last dose, regardless of the route of administration or the formulation used. On a once-daily dosing schedule, the concentration of digoxin will be 10%–25% lower when sampled at 24 versus 8 hours, depending upon the patient's renal function. On a twice-daily dosing schedule, there will be only minor differences in serum digoxin concentrations whether sampling is done at 8 or 12 hours after a dose.

If a discrepancy exists between the reported serum concentration and the observed clinical response, the clinician should consider the following possibilities:

1. Analytical problems in the assay procedure.
2. Inappropriate serum sampling time.
3. Administration of a digitalis glycoside other than digoxin.
4. Conditions causing an alteration in the sensitivity of the patient to digoxin.
5. Serum digoxin concentration may decrease acutely during periods of exercise without any associated change in clinical efficacy due to increased binding of digoxin to skeletal muscle.

An important statement in the approved label for Lanoxin is the following, which is in bold for emphasis: **"It cannot be overemphasized that both the adult and pediatric dosage guidelines provided are based upon average patient response and substantial individual variation can be expected. Accordingly, ultimate dosage selection must be based upon clinical assessment of the patient."**

Adverse Events and Therapeutic Monitoring

An *adverse drug reaction*, also called a *side effect* or *adverse event* (AE), is any undesirable experience associated with the use of a medicine in a patient. AEs can range from mild to severe. Serious AEs are those that can cause disability, are life threatening, result in hospitalization or death, or cause birth defects.[4] Some AEs are expected and are documented in the literature and in the approved labeling for the drug. Other AEs may be unexpected. The severity of these AEs and whether the AE is related to the patient's drug therapy should be considered. The FDA maintains safety information and an AE reporting program (MedWatch) that provides important and timely medical product information to healthcare professionals, including information on prescription and over-the-counter drugs, biologics, medical devices, and special nutritional products.

It is sometimes difficult to determine whether the AE in the patient is related to the drug, due to progression of the disease or other pathology, or due to some unknown source. There are several approaches to determining whether the observed AE is due to the drug:

1. Check that the correct drug product and dose was ordered and given to the patient.
2. Verify that the onset of the AE was after the drug was taken and not before.
3. Determine the time interval between the beginning of drug treatment and the onset of the event.
4. Discontinue the drug and monitor the patient's status, looking for improvement.
5. Rechallenge or restart the drug, if appropriate, and monitor for recurrence of the AE.

For some drugs, there may be an AE due to the initial exposure to the drug. However, the patient may become desensitized to the AE after longer drug treatment or drug dose titration. The clinician should be familiar with the drug and relevant literature concerning AEs. Generally, the manufacturer of the drug can also be a resource to consult.

Frequently Asked Questions

▶ *Why are drugs that demonstrate high intrasubject variability generally safer than critical-dose drugs?*

▶ *What type of drugs should be monitored?*

▶ *How does one determine whether an adverse event is drug related?*

---

[4]FDA Consumer Health Information, April 11, 2008 (http://www.fda.gov/downloads/ForConsumers/ConsumerUpdates/ucm107976.pdf).

CLINICAL EXAMPLE

Serum Vancomycin Concentrations

Vancomycin is a glycopeptide antibiotic commonly used in the treatment of serious Gram-positive infections. Nephrotoxicity is often cited as an adverse effect, especially when high dose therapy is used for a prolonged duration. The feasibility of using vancomycin as a continuous infusion has been examined recently in a variety of settings (eg, in intensive care units and as outpatient parenteral therapy).

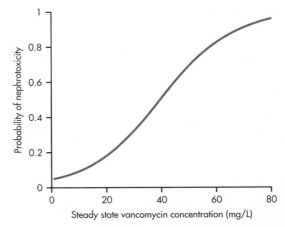

(From Ingram PR: *JAC* 2008; Spapen: *Ann Intensive Care*, 2011; Norton K: *JAC*, 2014.)

Regardless of the clinical setting, the likelihood of nephrotoxicity was found to be significantly higher if the steady-state vancomycin concentrations were >25–32 μg/mL. Unless there is a compelling clinical reason to do otherwise, it would be prudent to adjust dosing and maintain serum vancomycin concentrations to below 25 μg/mL.

DESIGN OF DOSAGE REGIMENS

Several methods may be used to design a dosage regimen. Generally, the initial dosage of the drug is estimated using average population pharmacokinetic parameters obtained from the literature and modified according to the patient's known diagnosis, pathophysiology, demographics, allergy, and any other known factor that might affect the patient's response to the dosage regimen.

After initiation of drug therapy, the patient is then monitored for the therapeutic response by clinical and physical assessment. After evaluation of the patient, adjustment of the dosage regimen may be needed. If necessary, measurement of plasma drug concentrations may be used to obtain the patient's individual pharmacokinetic parameters from which the data are used to modify the dosage regimen. Further TDM in the patient may be needed.

Various clinical pharmacokinetic software programs are available for dosage regimen calculations. The dosing strategies are based generally on pharmacokinetic calculations that were previously performed manually. Computer automation and pharmacokinetic software packages improve the accuracy of the calculation, make the calculations "easier," and have an added advantage of maintaining proper documentation (see Appendix A). However, the use of these software programs should not replace good clinical judgment.

- The package insert (PI) is a useful source for dose regimen. The section *Use in Specific Populations* provides information that may apply to individual patients.
- Pregnancy
- Labor and delivery
- Nursing mothers
- Pediatric use
- Geriatric use
- Hepatic impairment
- Renal impairment
- Gender effect

Individualized Dosage Regimens

The most accurate approach to dosage regimen design is to calculate the dose based on the pharmacokinetics of the drug in the individual patient. This approach is not feasible for calculation of the initial dose. However, once the patient has been medicated, the readjustment of the dose may be calculated using pharmacokinetic parameters derived from measurement of the serum drug levels from the patient after the initial dose. Most dosing programs record the patient's age and weight and calculate the individual dose based on creatinine clearance and lean body weight.

Dosage Regimens Based on Population Averages

The method most often used to calculate a dosage regimen is based on average pharmacokinetic parameters obtained from clinical studies published in the drug literature. This method may be based on a fixed or an adaptive model (Greenblatt, 1979; Mawer, 1976).

The *fixed model* assumes that population average pharmacokinetic parameters may be used directly to calculate a dosage regimen for the patient, without any alteration. Usually, pharmacokinetic parameters such as absorption rate constant k_a, bioavailability factor F, apparent volume of distribution V_D, and elimination rate constant k are assumed to remain constant. Most often the drug is assumed to follow the pharmacokinetics of a one-compartment model. When a multiple-dose regimen is designed, multiple-dosage equations based on the principle of superposition (see Chapter 9) are used to evaluate the dose. The practitioner may use the usual dosage suggested by the literature and then make a small adjustment of the dosage based on the patient's weight and/or age.

The *adaptive model* for dosage regimen calculation uses patient variables such as weight, age, sex, body surface area, and known patient pathophysiology, such as renal disease, as well as the known population average pharmacokinetic parameters of the drug. In this case, calculation of the dosage regimen takes into consideration any changing pathophysiology of the patient and attempts to adapt or modify the dosage regimen according to the needs of the patient. In some cases, pharmacogenetic data may be helpful in determining dosing. For example, clopidogrel (Plavix) has a black box warning cautioning use in patients who have slow CYP2D6 metabolism and who will, therefore, have slower activation of the prodrug to the active metabolite. However, an appropriate dose regimen has not been established for these patients. The adaptive model generally assumes that pharmacokinetic parameters such as drug clearance do not change from one dose to the next. However, some adaptive models allow for continuously adaptive change with time in order to simulate more closely the changing process of drug disposition in the patient, especially during a disease state (Whiting et al, 1991).

Dosage Regimens Based on Partial Pharmacokinetic Parameters

For many drugs, the entire pharmacokinetic profile of the drug is unknown or unavailable. Therefore, the pharmacokineticist needs to make some assumptions in order to calculate the dosage regimen in the absence of pharmacokinetic data in animals or humans. For example, a common assumption is to let the bioavailability factor F equal 1 or 100%. Thus, if the drug is less than fully absorbed systemically, the patient will be undermedicated rather than overmedicated. Some of these assumptions will depend on the safety, efficacy, and therapeutic range of the drug. The use of population pharmacokinetics (discussed later in this chapter) employs average patient population characteristics and only a few serum drug concentrations from the patient. Population pharmacokinetic approaches to TDM have increased with the increased availability of computerized databases and the development of statistical tools for the analysis of observational data (Schumacher, 1985).

Nomograms and Tabulations in Dosage Regimen Designs

For ease of calculation of dosage regimens, many clinicians rely on nomograms to calculate the proper dosage regimen for their patients. The use of a nomogram may give a quick dosage regimen adjustment for patients with characteristics requiring adjustments, such as age, body weight, and physiologic state. In general, the nomogram of a drug is based on population pharmacokinetic data collected and analyzed using a specific pharmacokinetic model. In order to keep the dosage regimen calculation simple, complicated equations are often solved and the results displayed diagrammatically on special scaled axes or as a table to produce a simple dose recommendation based on patient information. Some nomograms make use of certain physiologic parameters, such as serum creatinine concentration, to help modify the dosage regimen according to renal function (see Chapter 24).

Pharmaceutical manufacturers provide dosage recommendations in the approved label for many marketed drugs in the form of a table or as a nomogram. These are general guidelines to aid the clinician in establishing an initial dosage regimen for patients. The tables may include loading and maintenance doses that are modified for the demographics of the patient (eg, age, weight) and for certain disease states (eg, renal insufficiency).

For drugs with a narrow therapeutic range, such as theophylline, a guide for monitoring serum drug concentrations is given. Another example is the aminoglycoside antibiotic, tobramycin sulfate USP (Nebcin, Eli Lilly), which is eliminated primarily by renal clearance. Thus, the dosage of tobramycin sulfate should be reduced in direct proportion to a reduction in creatinine clearance (see Chapter 24). The manufacturer provides a nomogram for estimating the percent of the normal dose of tobramycin sulfate assuming the serum creatinine level (mg/100 mL) has been obtained.

Empirical Dosage Regimens

In many cases, the physician selects a dosage regimen for the patient without using any pharmacokinetic variables. In such a situation, the physician makes the decision based on empirical clinical data, personal experience, and clinical observations. The physician characterizes the patient as representative of a similar well-studied clinical population that has used the drug successfully.

CONVERSION FROM INTRAVENOUS INFUSION TO ORAL DOSING

After the patient's dosing is controlled by intravenous infusion, it is often desirable to continue to medicate the patient with the same drug using the oral route of administration. When intravenous infusion is stopped, the serum drug concentration decreases according to first-order elimination kinetics (see Chapter 6). For most oral drug products, the time to reach steady state depends on the first-order elimination rate constant for the drug. Therefore, if the patient starts the dosage regimen with the oral drug product at the same time as the intravenous infusion is stopped, then the exponential decline of serum levels from the intravenous infusion should be matched by the exponential increase in serum drug levels from the oral drug product.

The conversion from intravenous infusion to a controlled-release oral medication given once or twice daily has become more common with the availability of more extended-release drug products, such as theophylline (Stein et al, 1982) and quinidine. Computer simulation for the conversion of intravenous theophylline (aminophylline) therapy to oral controlled-release theophylline demonstrated that oral therapy should be started at the same time as intravenous infusion is stopped (Iafrate et al, 1982). With this method, minimal fluctuations are observed between the peak and trough serum theophylline levels. Moreover, giving the first oral dose when IV infusion is stopped may make it easier for the nursing staff or patient to comply with the dosage regimen.

Either of these methods may be used to calculate an appropriate oral dosage regimen for a patient whose condition has been stabilized by an intravenous drug infusion. Both methods assume that the patient's plasma drug concentration is at steady state.

Method 1

Method 1 assumes that the steady-state plasma drug concentration, C_{ss}, after IV infusion is identical to the desired C_{av}^{∞} after multiple oral doses of the drug. Therefore, the following equation may be used:

$$C_{av}^{\infty} = \frac{SFD_0}{kV_D\tau} \tag{22.1}$$

$$\frac{D_0}{\tau} = \frac{C_{av}^{\infty}kV_D}{SF} \tag{22.2}$$

where S is the salt form of the drug and D_0/τ is the dosing rate.

EXAMPLE ▶▶▶

An adult male asthmatic patient (age 55 years, 78 kg) has been maintained on an intravenous infusion of aminophylline at a rate of 34 mg/h. The steady-state theophylline drug concentration was 12 μg/mL and total body clearance was calculated as 3.0 L/h. Calculate an appropriate oral dosage regimen of theophylline for this patient.

Solution

Aminophylline is a soluble salt of theophylline and contains 85% theophylline ($S = 0.85$). Theophylline is 100% bioavailable ($F = 1$) after an oral dose. Because total body clearance, $Cl_T = kV_D$, Equation 22.2 may be expressed as

$$\frac{D_0}{\tau} = \frac{C_{av}^{\infty}Cl_T}{SF} \tag{22.3}$$

The dose rate, D_0/τ (34 mg/h), was calculated on the basis of aminophylline dosing. The patient, however, will be given theophylline orally. To convert to oral theophylline, S and F should be considered.

$$\text{Theophylline dose rate} = \frac{SFD_0}{\tau}$$

$$= \frac{(0.85)(1)(34)}{1} = 28.9 \, \text{mg/h}$$

The theophylline dose rate of 28.9 mg/h must be converted to a reasonable schedule for the patient with a consideration of the various commercially available theophylline drug products. Therefore, the total daily dose is 28.9 mg/h × 24 h or 693.6 mg/d. Possible theophylline dosage schedules might be 700 mg/d, 350 mg every 12 hours, or 175 mg every 6 hours. Each of these dosage regimens would achieve the same C_{av}^{∞} but different C_{max}^{∞} and C_{min}^{∞}, which should be calculated. The dose of 350 mg every 12 hours could be given in sustained-release form to avoid any excessive high drug concentration in the body.

Method 2

Method 2 assumes that the rate of intravenous infusion (mg/h) is the same desired rate of oral dosage.

EXAMPLE ▶▶▶

Using the example in method 1, the following calculations may be used.

Solution

The aminophylline is given by IV infusion at a rate of 34 mg/h. The total daily dose of aminophylline is 34 mg/h × 24 h = 816 mg. The equivalent daily dose in terms of theophylline is 816 × 0.85 = 693.6 mg. Thus, the patient should receive approximately 700 mg of theophylline per day or 350 mg controlled-release theophylline every 12 hours.

DETERMINATION OF DOSE

The calculation of the starting dose of a drug and dosing interval is based on the objective of delivering a desirable (target) therapeutic level of the drug in the body. For many drugs, the desirable therapeutic drug levels and pharmacokinetic parameters are available in the literature. However, the literature in some cases may not yield complete drug information, or some of the information available may be equivocal. Therefore, the pharmacokineticist must make certain necessary assumptions in accordance with the best pharmacokinetic information available.

For a drug that is given in multiple doses for an extended period of time, the dosage regimen is usually calculated to maintain the average steady-state blood level within the therapeutic range. The dose can be calculated with Equation 22.4, which expresses the C_{av}^{∞} in terms of dose (D_0), dosing interval (τ), volume of distribution (V_D), and the elimination half-life of the drug. F is the fraction of drug absorbed and is equal to 1 for drugs administered intravenously.

$$C_{av}^{\infty} = \frac{1.44 D_0 t_{1/2} F}{V_D \tau} \qquad (22.4)$$

PRACTICE PROBLEMS

1. Pharmacokinetic data for clindamycin were reported by DeHaan et al (1972) as follows:

$$k = 0.247 \, \text{h}^{-1}$$
$$t_{1/2} = 2.81 \, \text{h}$$
$$V_D = 43.9 \, \text{L}/1.73 \, \text{m}^2$$

What is the steady-state concentration of the drug after 150 mg of the drug is given orally every 6 hours for a week? (Assume the drug is 100% absorbed.)

Solution

$$\begin{aligned}
C_{av}^{\infty} &= \frac{1.44 D_0 t_{1/2} F}{V_D \tau} \\
&= \frac{1.44 \times 150,000 \times 2.81 \times 1}{43,900 \times 6} \, \mu\text{g/mL} \\
&= 2.3 \, \mu\text{g/mL}
\end{aligned}$$

2. According to Regamey et al (1973), the elimination half-life of tobramycin was reported to be 2.15 hours and the volume of distribution was reported to be 33.5% of body weight.

   a. What is the dose for an 80-kg individual if a steady-state level of 2.5 μg/mL is desired? Assume that the drug is given by intravenous bolus injection every 8 hours.

Solution

Assuming the drug is 100% bioavailable as a result of IV injection,

$$\begin{aligned}
C_{av}^{\infty} &= \frac{1.44 D_0 t_{1/2} F}{V_D \tau} \\
2.5 &= \frac{1.44 \times 2.15 \times 1 \times D_0}{80 \times 0.335 \times 1000 \times 8} \\
D_0 &= \frac{2.5 \times 80 \times 0.335 \times 1000 \times 8}{1.44 \times 2.15} \, \mu\text{g} \\
D_0 &= 173 \, \text{mg}
\end{aligned}$$

The dose should be 173 mg every 8 hours.

b. The manufacturer has suggested that in normal cases, tobramycin should be given at a rate of 1 mg/kg every 8 hours. With this dosage regimen, what would be the average steady-state level?

Solution

$$C_{av}^{\infty} = \frac{1.44 \times 1 \times 1000 \times 2.15}{0.335 \times 1000 \times 8}$$

$$C_{av}^{\infty} = 1.16 \mu g/mL$$

Because the bactericidal concentration of an antibiotic varies with the organism involved in the infection, the prescribed dose may change. The average plasma drug concentration is used to indicate whether optimum drug levels have been reached. With certain antibiotics, the steady-state peak and trough levels are sometimes used as therapeutic indicators. (See Chapter 21 for discussion of time above minimum effective concentration [MIC].) For example, the effective concentration of tobramycin was reported to be around 4–5 $\mu g/mL$ for peak levels and around 2 $\mu g/mL$ for trough levels when given intramuscularly every 12 hours (see Table 22-1). Although peak and trough levels are frequently reported in clinical journals, these drug levels are only transitory in the body. Peak and trough drug levels are less useful pharmacokinetically, because peak and trough levels fluctuate more and are usually reported less accurately than average plasma drug concentrations. When the average plasma drug concentration is used as a therapeutic indicator, an optimum dosing interval must be chosen. The dosing interval is usually set at approximately one to two elimination half-lives of the drug, unless the drug has a very narrow therapeutic index. In this case the drug must be given in small doses more frequently or by IV infusion. Of note, once the average plasma drug concentration is known, the overall daily drug exposure can be easily transformed and represented by the area under concentration–time curve (AUC).

EFFECT OF CHANGING DOSE AND DOSING INTERVAL ON C_{max}^{∞}, C_{min}^{∞}, AND C_{av}^{∞}

During intravenous infusion, C_{ss} may be used to monitor the steady-state serum concentrations. In contrast, when considering TDM of serum concentrations after the initiation of a multiple-dosage regimen, the trough serum drug concentrations or C_{min}^{∞} may be used to validate the dosage regimen. The blood sample withdrawn just prior to the administration of the next dose represents C_{min}^{∞}. To obtain C_{max}^{∞}, the blood sample must be withdrawn exactly at the time for peak absorption, or closely spaced blood samples must be taken and the plasma drug concentrations graphed. In practice, an approximate time for maximum drug absorption is estimated and a blood sample is withdrawn. Because of differences in rates of drug absorption, C_{max}^{∞} measured in this manner is only an approximation of the true C_{max}^{∞}.

The C_{av}^{∞} is used most often in dosage calculation. The advantage of using C_{av}^{∞} as an indicator for deciding therapeutic blood level is that C_{av}^{∞} is determined on a set of points and generally fluctuates less than either C_{max}^{∞} or C_{min}^{∞}. Moreover, when the dosing interval is changed, the dose may be increased proportionally, to keep C_{av}^{∞} constant. This approach works well for some drugs. For example, if the drug diazepam is given either 10 mg TID (three times a day) or 15 mg BID (twice daily), the same C_{av}^{∞} is obtained, as shown by Equation 22.1. In fact, if the daily dose is the same, the C_{av}^{∞} should be the same (as long as clearance is linear). However, when monitoring serum drug concentrations, C_{av}^{∞} cannot be measured directly but may be obtained from AUC/τ during multiple-dosage regimens. As discussed in Chapter 9 the C_{av}^{∞} is not the arithmetic average of C_{min}^{∞} and C_{max}^{∞} because serum concentrations decline exponentially.

The dosing interval must be selected while considering the elimination half-life of the drug; otherwise, the patient may suffer the toxic effect of a high C_{max}^{∞} or subtherapeutic effects of a low C_{min}^{∞} even if the C_{av}^{∞} is kept constant. For example, using the same example of diazepam, the same C_{av}^{∞} is achieved at 10 mg TID or 60 mg every other day. Obviously, the C_{max}^{∞} of the latter dose regimen would produce a C_{max}^{∞} several times larger than that achieved with 10-mg-TID dose regimen. In general, if a drug has a relatively wide therapeutic index and a relatively long elimination half-life, then flexibility exists in changing the dose or dosing interval, τ, using C_{av}^{∞} as an indicator. When the drug has a narrow therapeutic index, C_{max}^{∞} and C_{max}^{∞} must be monitored to ensure safety and efficacy.

As the dose or dosage intervals change proportionately, the C_{av}^{∞} may be the same but the steady-state peak, C_{max}^{∞}, and trough, C_{min}^{∞}, drug levels will change. C_{max}^{∞} is influenced by the dose and the dosage interval. An increase in the dose given at a longer dosage interval will cause an increase in C_{max}^{∞} and a decrease in C_{min}^{∞}. In this case C_{max}^{∞} may be very close or above the minimum toxic drug concentration (MTC). However, the C_{min}^{∞} may be lower than the minimum effective drug concentration (MEC). In this latter case the low C_{min}^{∞} may be subtherapeutic and dangerous for the patient, depending on the nature of the drug.

DETERMINATION OF FREQUENCY OF DRUG ADMINISTRATION

The drug dose is often related to the frequency of drug administration. The more frequently a drug is administered, the smaller the dose is needed to obtain the same C_{av}^{∞}. Thus, a dose of 250 mg every 3 hours can be changed to 500 mg every 6 hours without affecting the average steady-state plasma concentration of the drug. However, as the dosing intervals get longer, the dose required to maintain the average plasma drug concentration gets correspondingly larger. When an excessively long dosing interval is chosen, the larger dose may result in peak plasma levels that are above toxic drug concentration and trough plasma concentrations that are below the minimum effective concentration, even though C_{av}^{∞} will remain the same (see Chapter 9).

In general, the dosing interval for most drugs is determined by the elimination half-life. Drugs such as the penicillins, which have relatively low toxicity, may be given at intervals much longer than their elimination half-lives without any toxicity problems. Drugs having a narrow therapeutic range, such as digoxin and phenytoin, must be given relatively frequently to minimize excessive "peak-and-trough" fluctuations in blood levels. For example, the common maintenance schedule for digoxin is 0.25 mg/d and the elimination half-life of digoxin is 1.7 days. In contrast, penicillin G is given at 250 mg every 6 hours, while the elimination half-life of penicillin G is 0.75 hour. Penicillin is given at a dosage interval equal to 8 times its elimination half-life, whereas digoxin is given at a dosing interval only 0.59 times its elimination half-life. The toxic plasma concentration of penicillin G is over 100 times greater than its effective concentration, whereas digoxin has an effective concentration of 1–2 ng/mL and a toxicity level of 3 ng/mL. The toxic concentration of digoxin is only 1.5 times effective concentration. Therefore, a drug with a large therapeutic index (ie, a large margin of safety) can be given in large doses and at relatively long dosing intervals.

DETERMINATION OF BOTH DOSE AND DOSAGE INTERVAL

Both the dose and the dosing interval should be considered in the dosage regimen calculations. For intravenous multiple-dosage regimens, the ratio of $C_{max}^{\infty}/C_{min}^{\infty}$ may be expressed by

$$\frac{C_{max}^{\infty}}{C_{min}^{\infty}} = \frac{C_p^0/(1-e^{-k\tau})}{C_p^0 e^{-k\tau}(1-e^{-k\tau})} \qquad (22.5)$$

which can be simplified to

$$\frac{C_{max}^{\infty}}{C_{min}^{\infty}} = \frac{1}{e^{-k\tau}} \qquad (22.6)$$

From Equation 22.6, a maximum dosage interval, τ, may be calculated that will maintain the serum concentration between desired C_{min}^{∞} and C_{max}^{∞}. After the dosage interval is calculated, then a dose may be calculated.

PRACTICE PROBLEM

The elimination half-life of an antibiotic is 3 hours with an apparent volume of distribution equivalent to 20% of body weight. The usual therapeutic range for this antibiotic is between 5 and 15 μg/mL. Adverse toxicity for this drug is often observed at serum concentrations greater than 20 μg/mL. Calculate a dosage regimen (multiple IV doses) that will just maintain the serum drug concentration between 5 and 15 μg/mL.

Solution

From Equation 22.6, determine the maximum possible dosage interval τ.

$$\frac{15}{5} = \frac{1}{e^{-(0.693/3)\tau}}$$

$$e^{-0.231\tau} = 0.333$$

Take the natural logarithm (ln) on both sides of the equation.

$$-0.231\tau = -1.10$$

$$\tau = 4.76 \text{ h}$$

Then determine the dose required to produce from $C_{\max}^{\infty}$ Equation 22.7 after substitution of $C_p^0 = D_0/V_D$:

$$C_{\max}^{\infty} = \frac{D_0/V_D}{1-e^{-k\tau}} \qquad (22.7)$$

Solve for dose D_0, letting $V_D = 200$ mL/kg (20% body weight).

$$15 = \frac{D_0/200}{1-e^{-(0.231)(4.76)}}$$

$$D_0 = 2 \text{ mg/kg}$$

To check this dose for therapeutic effectiveness, calculate $C_{\min}^{\infty}$ and C_{av}^{∞}.

$$C_{\min}^{\infty} = \frac{(D_0/V_D)e^{-k\tau}}{1-e^{-k\tau}} = \frac{(2000/200)e^{(-0.231)(4.76)}}{1-e^{-(0.231)(4.76)}}$$

$$C_{\min}^{\infty} = 4.99\mu g/mL$$

As a further check on the dosage regimen, calculate C_{av}^{∞}.

$$C_{av}^{\infty} = \frac{D_0}{V_D k\tau} = \frac{2000}{(200)(0.231)(4.76)}$$

$$C_{av}^{\infty} = 9.09\mu g/mL$$

By calculation, the dose of this antibiotic should be 2 mg/kg every 4.76 hours to maintain the serum drug concentration between 5 and 15 μg/mL.

In practice, rather than a dosage interval of 4.76 hours, the dosage regimen and the dosage interval should be made as convenient as possible for the patient, and the size of the dose should take into account the commercially available drug formulation. Therefore, the dosage regimen should be recalculated to have a convenient value (below the maximum possible dosage interval) and the dose adjusted accordingly.

DETERMINATION OF ROUTE OF ADMINISTRATION

Selection of the proper route of administration is an important consideration in drug therapy. The rate of drug absorption and the duration of action are influenced by the route of drug administration. However, the use of certain routes of administration is precluded by physiologic and safety considerations. For example, intra-arterial and intrathecal drug injections are less safe than other routes of drug administration and are used only when absolutely necessary. Drugs that are unstable in the gastrointestinal tract such as proteins or drugs that undergo extensive first-pass effect are not suitable for oral administration. For example, insulin is a protein that is degraded in the gastrointestinal tract by proteolytic enzymes. Drugs such as xylocaine and nitroglycerin are not suitable for oral administration because of high first-pass effect. These drugs, therefore, must be given by an alternative route of administration.

Intravenous administration is the fastest and most reliable way of delivering a drug into the circulatory system. Drugs administered by intravenous bolus are delivered to the plasma immediately and the entire dose is immediately subject to elimination. Consequently, more frequent drug administration is required. Drugs administered extravascularly must be absorbed into the bloodstream, and the total absorbed dose is eliminated more slowly. The frequency of administration can be lessened by using routes of administration that give a sustained rate of drug absorption. Intramuscular injection generally provides more rapid systemic absorption than oral administration of drugs that are not very soluble.

Certain drugs are not suitable for administration intramuscularly because of erratic drug release, pain, or local irritation. Even though the drug is injected into the muscle mass, the drug must reach the circulatory system or other body fluid to become bioavailable. The anatomic site of drug deposition following intramuscular injection will affect the rate of drug absorption. A drug injected into the deltoid muscle is more rapidly absorbed than a drug injected similarly into the gluteus maximus, because there is better blood flow in the former. In general, the method of drug administration that provides the most consistent and greatest bioavailability should be used to ensure maximum therapeutic effect. The various routes of drug administration can be classified as either *extravascular* or *intravascular* and are listed in Table 22-5.

Precipitation of an insoluble drug at the injection site may result in slower absorption and a delayed response. For example, a dose of 50 mg of chlordiazepoxide (Librium) is more quickly absorbed

TABLE 22-5   Common Routes of Drug Administration

Parenteral	Extravascular
Intravascular	Enteral
Intravenous injection (IV bolus)	Buccal
Intravenous infusion (IV drip)	Sublingual
Intra-arterial injection	Oral
Intramuscular injection	Rectal
Intradermal injection	Inhalation
Subcutaneous injection	Transdermal
Intrathecal injection	

after oral administration than after intramuscular injection. Some drugs, such as haloperidol decanoate, are very oil-soluble products that release very slowly after intramuscular injection.

DOSING INFANTS AND CHILDREN

Infants and children have different dosing requirements than adults (Bartelink et al, 2006; FDA Guidance for Industry, 2000; Leeder et al, 2010). Information for pediatric dosings was generally lacking in the past. In December 1994, the FDA required drug manufacturers to determine whether existing data were sufficient to support information on pediatric use for drug labeling purposes and implemented a plan to encourage the voluntary collection of pediatric data. The FDA Modernization (FDAMA) authorized an additional 6 months of patent protection for manufacturers that conducted pediatric clinical trials. As a consequence of various legislative initiatives later, the results of pediatric studies conducted on 322 drugs and biological products are available to help dosing in children.[5] The studies reveal important new information regarding dosing and pharmacokinetic differences between children and adults (Leeder et al, 2010). Dosing of drugs in this population requires a thorough consideration of the differences in the pharmacokinetics and pharmacology of a specific drug in the preterm newborn infant, newborn infant (birth to 28 days), infant (28 days–23 months), young child (2–5 years), older child (6–11 years), adolescent (12–18 years), and adult. Unfortunately, the pharmacokinetics and pharmacodynamics of most drugs are still not well known in children under 12 years of age.[6] The variation in body composition and the maturity of liver, kidney, and other organ functions are potential sources of differences in pharmacokinetics with respect to age. For convenience, "infants" are here

---

[5]http://www.fda.gov/downloads/ScienceResearch/SpecialTopics/PediatricTherapeuticsResearch/UCM163159.pdf; accessed July 2, 2009.

[6]The FDA issued a Guidance for Industry, Qualifying for Pediatric Exclusivity under Section 505(A) of the Federal Food, Drug, and Cosmetic Act (June 1998), to encourage drug manufacturers to develop dosage guidelines for children.

arbitrarily defined as children of 0–2 years of age. However, within this group, special consideration is necessary for infants less than 4 weeks (1 month) old, because their ability to handle drugs often differs from that of more mature infants.

In addition to different dosing requirements for the pediatric population, there is a need to select pediatric dosage forms that permit more accurate dosing and patient compliance. For example, liquid pediatric drug products may have a calibrated dropper or a premeasured teaspoon (5 mL) for more accurate dosing and also have a cherry flavor for pediatric patient compliance. Pediatric drug formulations may also contain different drug concentrations compared to the adult drug formulation and must be considered in order to prevent dosage errors. Because of the small muscle mass in an infant, alternative drug delivery such as an intramuscular antibiotic drug injection into the gluteus medius may be considered for a pediatric patient, as opposed to the deltoid muscle for an adult patient. However, body composition is different in infants compared to adults.

In general, complete hepatic function is not attained until the third week of life. Oxidative processes are fairly well developed in infants, but there is a deficiency of conjugative enzymes, in particular, glucuronidation. For example, kernicterus is a form of jaundice in the newborn characterized by very high levels of unconjugated bilirubin in the blood. Since the tissues protecting the brain (the blood–brain barrier) are not well formed in newborns, unconjugated bilirubin may enter the brain and cause brain damage. In addition to reduced liver function in infants, altered drug distribution may occur due to reduction in drug binding to plasma albumin and to different body composition, especially water and fat content.

Newborns show only 30%–50% of the renal function of adults on the basis of activity per unit of body weight (Table 22-6). Drugs that are heavily dependent on renal excretion will have a sharply decreased elimination half-life. For example, the penicillins are excreted for the most part through the kidneys. The elimination half-lives of such drugs are much increased in infants, as shown in Table 22-7.

When dosage guidelines are not available for a drug, empirical dose adjustment methods are often used. These empirical dose adjustment methods are based on body surface area or body weight. Dosage based on the child's age and body weight, and normalized to drug dosages in adults, was used in the past. However, pharmacokinetic parameters may vary as a function of age. Dosage based on body

TABLE 22-6   Comparison of Newborn and Adult Renal Clearances[a]

	Average Infant	Average Adult
Body weight (kg)	3.5	70
Body water		
(%)	77	58
(L)	2.7	41
Inulin clearance		
(mL/min)	Approx 3	130
k (min^{-1})	$3/2700 = 0.0011$	$130/41,000 = 0.0032$
$t_{1/2}$ (min)	630	220
PAH clearance		
(mL/min)	Approx 12	650
k (min^{-1})	$12/2800 = 0.0043$	$650/41,000 = 0.016$
$t_{1/2}$ (min)	160	43

[a]Computations are for a drug distributed in the whole body water, but any other V_D would give the same relative values.

TABLE 22-7   Elimination Half-Lives of Drugs in Infants and Adults

Drug	Half-Life in Neonates[a] (h)	Half-Life in Adults (h)
Penicillin G	3.2	0.5
Ampicillin	4	1–1.5
Methicillin	3.3/1.3	0.5
Carbenicillin	5–6	1–1.5
Kanamycin	5–5.7	3–5
Gentamicin	5	2–3

[a]0–7 days old.

surface area has the advantage of avoiding some bias due to obesity or unusual body weight, because the height and the weight of the patient are both considered. The body surface area method gives only a rough estimation of the proper dose, because the pharmacokinetic differences between patients of the same body surface area are not considered. Dosage regimens for the newborn, infant, and child must consider the changing physiologic development of the patient and the pharmacokinetics of the specific drug for that age group. In the package insert of new drugs, under the section on *Use in Specific Populations*, pediatric use information should be consulted for drug-specific information.

PRACTICE PROBLEM

The elimination half-life of penicillin G is 0.5 hour in adults and 3.2 hours in neonates (0–7 days old). Assuming that the normal adult dose of penicillin G is 4 mg/kg every 4 hours, calculate the dose of penicillin G for an 11-lb infant.

Solution

$$\frac{\tau_1}{\tau_2} = \frac{(t_{1/2})_1}{(t_{1/2})_2}$$

$$t_{1/2} = 0.5\ \text{h}$$

$$\tau_2 = \frac{4 \times 3.2}{0.5} = 25.6\ \text{h}$$

Therefore, this infant may be given the following dose:

$$\text{Dose} = 4\ \text{mg/kg} = \frac{11\ \text{lb}}{2.2\ \text{lb/kg}} = 20\ \text{mg every 24 h}$$

Alternatively, 10 mg every 12 hours would achieve the same C_{av}^{∞}.

DOSING THE ELDERLY

Elderly subjects are considered as specific populations and a formal discussion is given in Chapter 23. However, some relevant basic information is introduced below for discussion in clinical situations. Defining "elderly" is difficult. The geriatric population is often arbitrarily defined as patients who are older than 65 years, and many of these people live active and healthy lives. In addition, there is an increasing number of people who are living beyond 85 years old, who are often considered the "older elderly" population. The aging process is more often associated with physiologic changes during aging rather than purely chronological age. Chronologically, the elderly have been classified as the *young old* (ages 65–75 years), the *old* (ages 75–85 years), and the *old old* (ages >85 years) (Abernethy, 2001).

Performance capacity and the loss of homeostatic reserve decrease with advanced age but occur to a different degree in each organ and in each patient. Physiologic and cognitive functions tend to change with the aging process and can affect compliance, therapeutic safety, and efficacy of a prescribed drug. The elderly also tend to be on multiple drug therapy due to concomitant illness(es). Decreased cognitive function in some geriatric patients, complicated drug dosage schedules, and/or the high cost of drug therapy may result in poor drug compliance, resulting in lack of drug efficacy, possible drug interactions, and/or drug intoxication.

Several objectively measured vital physiologic functions related to age show that renal plasma flow, glomerular filtration, cardiac output, and breathing capacity can drop from 10% to 30% in elderly subjects compared to those at age 30 years. The physiologic changes due to aging may necessitate special considerations in administering drugs in the elderly. For some drugs, an age-dependent increase in adverse drug reactions or toxicity may be observed. This apparent increased drug sensitivity in the elderly may be due to pharmacodynamic and/or pharmacokinetic changes (Mayersohn, 1994; Schmucker, 1985).

The pharmacodynamic hypothesis assumes that age causes alterations in the quantity and quality of target drug receptors, leading to altered drug response. Quantitatively, the number of drug receptors may decline with age, whereas qualitatively, a change in the affinity for the drug may occur. Alternatively, the pharmacokinetic hypothesis assumes that age-dependent increases in adverse drug reactions are due to physiologic changes in drug absorption, distribution, and elimination, including renal excretion and hepatic clearance.

In the elderly, age-dependent alterations in drug absorption may include a decline in the splanchnic blood flow, altered gastrointestinal motility, increase in gastric pH, and alteration in the gastrointestinal absorptive surface. The incidence of achlorhydria in the elderly may have an effect on the dissolution of certain drugs such as weak bases and certain dosage forms that require an acid environment for disintegration and release (Mayersohn, 1994). From a distribution consideration, drug–protein binding in the plasma may decrease as a result of decrease in the albumin concentration, and the apparent volume of distribution may change due to a decrease in muscle mass and an increase in body fat. Renal drug excretion generally declines with age as a result of decrease in the glomerular filtration rate (GFR) and/or active tubular secretion. Moreover, the activity of the enzymes responsible for drug biotransformation may decrease with age, leading to a decline in hepatic drug clearance.

Elderly patients may have several different pathophysiologic conditions that require multiple drug therapy that increases the likelihood for a drug interaction. Moreover, increased adverse drug reactions and toxicity may result from poor patient compliance. Both penicillin and kanamycin show prolonged $t_{1/2}$ in the aged patient, as a consequence of an age-related gradual reduction in the kidney size and function. The Gault–Cockroft rule for calculating creatinine clearance clearly quantitates a reduction in clearance with increased age (see Chapter 24). Age-related changes in plasma albumin and α_1-acid glycoprotein may also be a factor in the binding of drugs in the body.

PRACTICE PROBLEMS

1. An aminoglycoside has a normal elimination half-life of 107 minutes in young adults. In patients 70–90 years old, the elimination half-life of the aminoglycoside is 282 minutes. The normal dose of the aminoglycoside is 15 mg/kg per day divided into two doses. What is the dose for a 75-year-old patient, assuming that the volume of distribution per body weight is not changed by the patient's age?

Solution

The longer elimination half-life of the aminoglycoside in elderly patients is due to a decrease in renal function. A good inverse correlation has been obtained of elimination half-life to the aminoglycoside and creatinine clearance. To maintain the same average concentration of the aminoglycoside in the elderly as in young adults, the dose may be reduced.

$$C_{av}^\infty = \frac{1.44 D_N (t_{1/2})_N}{\tau_N V_N} = \frac{1.44 D_0 (t_{1/2})_0}{\tau_0 V_0}$$

$$\frac{D_N (t_{1/2})_N}{\tau_N} = \frac{D_0 (t_{1/2})_0}{\tau_0}$$

Keeping the dose constant,

$$D_N = D_0$$

where D_N is the new dose and D_0 is the old dose.

$$\frac{\tau_0}{\tau_N} = \frac{(t_{1/2})_0}{(t_{1/2})_N}$$

$$\tau_0 = 12 \times \frac{282}{107} = 31.6\,\text{h}$$

Therefore, the same dose of the aminoglycoside may be administered every 32 hours without affecting the average steady-state level of the aminoglycoside.

2. The clearance of lithium was determined to be 41.5 mL/min in a group of patients with an average age of 25 years. In a group of elderly patients with an average age of 63 years, the clearance of lithium was 7.7 mL/min. What percentage of the normal dose of lithium should be given to a 65-year-old patient?

Solution

The dose should be proportional to clearance; therefore,

$$\text{Dose reductions (\%)} = \frac{7.7 \times 100}{41.5} = 18.5\%$$

The dose of lithium may be reduced to about 20% of the regular dose in the 65-year-old patient without affecting the steady-state blood level.

CLINICAL EXAMPLE

Hypertension is common in elderly patients. The pharmacokinetics of felodipine (Plendil), a calcium channel antagonist for hypertension, was studied in young and elderly subjects. After a dose of 5 mg oral felodipine, the AUC and C_{max} in the elderly patients (67–79 years of age, mean weight 71 kg) were three times that of the young subjects (20–34 years of age, mean weight 75 kg), as shown in Fig. 22-2. Side effects of felodipine in the elderly patients, such as flushing, were reported in 9 of 11 subjects, and palpitation was reported in 3 of 11 subjects, whereas only 1 of 12 of the young subjects reported side effects. Systemic clearance in the elderly was 248 ± 108 L/h compared to 619 ± 214 L/h in the young subjects. The bioavailability of felodipine was reported to be about 15.5% in the elderly and 15.3% in the young subjects. (Concomitant medications included a diuretic and a beta-blocker.)

a. What is the main cause for the difference in the observed AUC between the elderly and young subjects?

b. What would be the steady-state level of felodipine in the elderly if dose and dosing interval are unchanged?

c. Can felodipine be given safely to elderly patients?

Solution

a. The higher AUC in the elderly compared to young adults is due to the decreased drug clearance in the older subjects.

b. The elderly have more side effects with felodipine compared to young adults. Factors that may have increased side effects in the elderly could be (1) reduced hepatic blood flow, (2) potassium depletion in the body, (3) increased bioavailability, or (4) reduced clearance.

c.
$$C_{av}^{\infty} = \frac{FD_0}{Cl_{\tau}} \tag{22.8}$$

If D_0, F, and τ are the same, the steady-state drug concentration, C_{av}^{∞}, will be inversely proportional to clearance:

$$\frac{C_{av\ elderly}^{\infty}}{C_{av\ young}^{\infty}} = \frac{Cl_{young}}{Cl_{elderly}}$$

$$\frac{C_{av\ elderly}^{\infty}}{C_{av\ young}^{\infty}} = \frac{619}{248} = 2.5$$

(*Note:* Cl is in the denominator in Equation 22.8 and is inversely related to concentration.) The steady concentration of felodipine will be 250% or 2.5 times that in the young subjects.

Changes in Renal Function with Age

Many studies have shown a general decline in GFR with age. Lindeman (1992) reported that the GFR as measured by creatinine clearance (see Chapter 24) decreases at a mean rate of 1% per year after 40 years of age. However, there is considerable variation in this rate of decline in normal healthy aging adults. In a previous study by Lindeman et al (1985), approximately two-thirds of the subjects (162 of 254) had declining creatinine clearances, whereas about one-third of the subjects (92 of 254) had no decrease in creatinine clearance. Since muscle mass and urinary

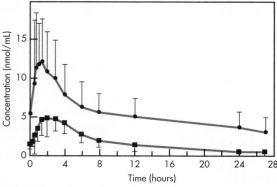

FIGURE 22-2   Plasma concentrations (mean ± SD) of felodipine after an oral dose during steady-state treatment with 5 mg twice daily in healthy subjects ($n = 12$) [■] and elderly hypertensive patients ($n = 1$] [●]. (From Landahl et al, 1988, with permission.)

creatinine excretion decrease at nearly the same rate in the elderly, mean serum concentrations may stay relatively constant. Creatinine clearance measured by serum creatinine concentrations only (see Chapter 24) may yield inaccurate GFR function if urinary creatinine excretion is not measured.

EXAMPLES ▶ ▶ ▶

1. An elderly 85-year-old adult patient with congestive heart failure has a serum creatinine of 1.0 mg/dL. The 24-hour urinary creatinine excretion was 0.7 g. Based on the serum creatinine only, this patient has normal renal function, whereas based on both serum creatinine concentration and total 24-hour urinary creatinine excretion, the patient has a GFR of less than 50 mL/min. In practice, serum creatinine clearance is often estimated from serum creatinine concentration alone for dose adjustment. In elderly subjects, the clinician should carefully assess the patient, since substantial deviation from the true clearance may occur in some elderly subjects.

2. Diflunisal pharmacokinetics was studied in healthy young and old subjects. After a single dose of diflunisal, the terminal plasma half-life, mean residence time, and apparent volume of distribution were higher in elderly subjects than in young adults (Erikson et al, 1989). This study shows that renal function in elderly subjects is generally reduced somewhat compared to younger patients because of a diminished rate of glomerular filtration.

DOSING THE OBESE PATIENTS

Obesity is a major problem in the United States and is discussed formally under specific population in Chapter 23. Only simple points regarding dosing in clinical situations are introduced below. Obesity has been associated with increased mortality resulting from increases in the incidence of hypertension, atherosclerosis, coronary artery disease, diabetes, and other conditions compared to nonobese patients (Blouin and Warren, 1999; National Institutes of Health, National Heart, Lung and Blood Institute 2003).

A patient is considered obese if actual body weight exceeds ideal or desirable body weight by 20%, according to Metropolitan Life Insurance Company data (latest published tables). Ideal or desirable body weights are based on average body weights and heights for males and for females considering age. Athletes who have a greater body weight due to greater muscle mass are not considered obese. Obesity often is defined by *body mass index* (BMI), a value that normalizes body weight based on height. BMI is expressed as body weight (kg) divided by the square of the person's height (meters) or kg/m². BMI is calculated according to the following two equations:

$$\text{BMI} = \left[\frac{\text{weight (lb)}}{\text{height (in)}^2}\right] \times 703$$

$$\text{BMI} = \left[\frac{\text{weight (kg)}}{\text{height (cm)}^2}\right] \times 10,000$$

An extensive study on obesity has been published by the National Institutes of Health, National Heart, Lung and Blood Institute (2003), giving five weight classifications based on BMI:

Classification	BMI (kg/m²)
Underweight	<18.5
Normal body weight	18.5–24.9
Overweight	25–29.9
Obese	30–39.9
Extreme obesity	>40

BMI correlates strongly with total body fat in nonelderly adults; it is commonly used as a surrogate for total body fat. Excess body fat increases the risk of death and major comorbidities such as type 2 diabetes, hypertension, dyslipidemia, cardiovascular disease, osteoarthritis of the knee, sleep apnea, and some cancers. An obese patient (BMI > 30) has a greater accumulation of fat tissue than is necessary for normal body functions. Adipose (fat) tissue has a smaller proportion of water compared to muscle tissue. Thus, the obese patient has a smaller proportion of total body water to total body weight compared to the patient of ideal body weight, which could affect the apparent volume of distribution of the drug. For example, Abernethy and Greenblatt (1982) showed a significant difference in the apparent volume of distribution of antipyrine in obese patients (0.46 L/kg) compared to ideal-body-weight patients (0.62 L/kg) based on actual total body weight. *Ideal body weight* (IBW) refers to the appropriate or normal weight for a male or female based on age, height, weight, and frame size; ideal body weights are generally obtained from the latest table of desirable weights for men and women compiled by the Metropolitan Life Insurance Company.

BMI is not a very accurate measure of adiposity in certain individual patients, particularly in people with elevated lean body mass, such as athletes, and in children. Other approaches have been used to predict the relationship of obesity to cardiovascular risk, such as waist circumference, waist-to-hip ratio, and the waist-to-hip-to-height index (Green and Duffull, 2004).

In addition to differences in total body water per kilogram body weight in the obese patient, the greater proportion of body fat in these patients could lead to distributional changes in the drug's pharmacokinetics due to partitioning of the drug between lipid and aqueous environments (Blouin and Warren, 1999). Drugs such as digoxin and gentamicin are very polar and tend to distribute into water rather than into fat tissue. Although lipophilic drugs are associated with larger volumes of distribution in obese patients compared to hydrophilic drugs, there are exceptions and the effect of obesity on specific drugs must be considered for accurate dosing strategy.

Other pharmacokinetic parameters may be altered in the obese patient as a result of physiologic alterations, such as fatty infiltration of the liver affecting biotransformation and cardiovascular changes that may affect renal blood flow and renal excretion (Abernethy and Greenblatt, 1982).

Dosing by actual body weight may result in overdosing of drugs such as aminoglycosides (eg, gentamicin), which are very polar and are distributed in extracellular fluids. Dosing of these drugs is based on ideal body weight. *Lean body weight* (LBW) has been estimated by several empirical equations based on the patient's height and actual (total) body weight.

The following equations have been used for estimating LBW, particularly for adjustment of dosage in renally impaired patients:

$$LBW(males) = 50 \text{ kg} + 2.3 \text{ kg}$$
$$\text{for each inch over 5 ft} \qquad (22.9)$$

$$LBW(females) = 45.5 \text{ kg} + 2.3 \text{ kg}$$
$$\text{or each inch over 5 ft} \qquad (22.10)$$

where LBW is lean body weight.

EXAMPLE ▶ ▶ ▶

Calculate the lean body weight for an adult male patient who is 5 ft 9 in (175.3 cm) tall and weighs 264 lb (120 kg).

Solution
Using Equation 22.9,
   LBW = 50 + (2.3 × 9) = 70.7 kg

PHARMACOKINETICS OF DRUG INTERACTIONS

A *drug interaction* generally refers to a modification of the expected drug response in the patient as a result of exposure of the patient to another drug or substance. Some unintentional drug interactions produce adverse reactions in the patient, whereas some drug interactions may be intentional, to provide an improved therapeutic response or to decrease adverse drug effects. Drug interactions may include drug–drug interactions, food–drug interactions, or chemical–drug interactions, such as the interaction of a drug with alcohol or tobacco. A listing of food interactions is given in Chapter 14. A drug–laboratory test interaction pertains to an alteration in a diagnostic clinical laboratory test result because of the drug.

Drug interactions may cause an alteration in the pharmacokinetics of the drug due to an interaction in drug absorption, distribution, or elimination (Tables 22-8 and 22-9). Drug interactions can also be pharmacodynamic interactions at the receptor site in which the competing drug potentiates or antagonizes the action of the first drug. Pharmaceutical drug

TABLE 22-8   **Sources of Drug Interactions**

Type of Drug Interaction	Source	Example
Pharmacokinetic	Absorption	Drug interactions can affect the rate and the extent of systemic drug absorption (bioavailability) from the absorption site, resulting in increased or decreased drug bioavailability.
	Distribution	Drug distribution may be altered by displacement of the drug from plasma protein or other binding sites due to competition for the same binding site.
	Hepatic elimination	Drugs that share the same drug-metabolizing enzymes have a potential for a drug interaction.
	Renal clearance	Drugs that compete for active renal secretion may decrease renal clearance of the first drug. Probenecid blocks the active renal secretion of penicillin drugs.
Pharmacodynamic	Drug receptor site	Pharmacodynamic drug interactions at the receptor site in which the competing drug potentiates or antagonizes the action of the first drug.
Pharmaceutical compounding	Pharmaceutical interactions are caused by a chemical or physical incompatibility when two or more drugs are mixed together	An IV solution of aminophylline has an alkaline pH and should not be mixed with such drugs as epinephrine which decompose in an alkaline pH.

interaction occurs when physical and/or chemical incompatibilities arise during extemporaneous pharmaceutical compounding. Pharmaceutical drug interactions, such as drug–excipient interactions, are considered during the development and manufacture of new and generic drug products.

The risk of a drug interaction increases with multiple drug therapy, multiple prescribers, poor patient compliance, and patient risk factors, such as predisposing illness (diabetes, hypertension, etc) or advancing age. Multiple drug therapy has become routine in most acute and chronic care settings. Elderly patients and patients with various predisposing illnesses tend to be a population using multiple drug therapy. A recent student survey found an average of 8–12 drugs per patient used in a group of hospital patients.

An important source of drug interactions is the combination of herbal remedies (sometimes referred to as *neutraceuticals* or dietary supplements) with drug therapy. Although many herbal products are safe when taken alone, many drug–herbal interactions have been reported (Izzo and Ernst, 2009). For example, St. John's wort is an inducer of cytochrome P-450, which is involved in the metabolism of many drugs.

St. John's wort reduces the plasma drug concentrations of indinavir, a protease inhibitor used to treat HIV infection and AIDS.

Screening for drug interactions is generally performed whenever multiple drug products are dispensed to the patient. However, the pharmacist should ask the patient when dispensing any medication whether the patient is taking over-the-counter (OTC) drugs, herbal supplements, or contraceptive drugs. Some patients do not realize that these products may interact with their drug therapy. There are many computer programs that will "flag" a potential drug interaction. However, the pharmacist needs to determine the clinical significance of the interaction and whether there is an alternate drug or alternate dosage regimen design that will prevent the drug interaction. The clinical significance of a potential drug interaction should be documented in the literature. The likelihood of a drug interaction may be classified as an established drug interaction, probable drug interaction, possible drug interaction, or unlikely drug interaction. The dose and the duration of therapy, the onset (rapid, delayed), the severity (major, minor) of the potential interaction, and extrapolation to related drugs should also be considered.

TABLE 22-9   Pharmacokinetic Drug Interactions

Drug Interaction	Examples (Precipitant Drugs)	Effect (Object Drugs)
Bioavailability		
Complexation/chelation	Calcium, magnesium, or aluminum and iron salts	Tetracycline complexes with divalent cations, causing a decreased bioavailability
Adsorption binding/ionic interaction	Cholestyramine resin (anionexchange resin binding)	Decreased bioavailability of thyroxine, and digoxin; binds anionic drugs and reduces absorption. Some antacid may cause HCl salt to precipitate out in stomach.
Adsorption	Antacids (adsorption) Charcoal, antidiarrheals	Decreased bioavailability of antibiotics Decreased bioavailability of many drugs
Increased GI motility	Laxatives, cathartics	Increases GI motility, decreases bioavailability for drugs which are absorbed slowly; may also affect the bioavailability of drugs from controlled-release products
Decreased GI motility	Anticholinergic agents	Propantheline decreases the gastric emptying of acetaminophen (APAP), delaying APAP absorption from the small intestine
Alteration of gastric pH	H-2 blockers, antacids	Both H-2 blockers and antacids increase gastric pH; the dissolution of ketoconazole is reduced, causing decreased drug absorption
Alteration of intestinal flora	Antibiotics (eg, tetracyclines, penicillin)	Digoxin has better bioavailability after erythromycin; erythromycin administration reduces bacterial inactivation of digoxin
Inhibition of drug metabolism in intestinal cells	Monoamine oxidase inhibitors (MAO-I) (eg, tranylcypromine, phenelzine)	Hypertensive crisis may occur in patients treated with MAO-I and foods containing tyramine
Distribution		
Protein binding	Warfarin–phenylbutazone Phenytoin–valproic acid	Displacement of warfarin from binding Displacement of phenytoin from binding
Hepatic Elimination		
Enzyme induction	Smoking (polycyclic aromatic hydrocarbons) Barbiturates	Smoking increases theophylline clearance Phenobarbital increases the metabolism of warfarin
Enzyme inhibition	Cimetidine	Decreased theophylline, diazepam metabolism
Mixed-function oxidase		
	Fluvoxamine	Diazepam $t_{1/2}$ longer
	Quinidine	Decreased nifedipine metabolism
	Fluconazole	Increased levels of phenytoin, warfarin
Other enzymes	Monoamine oxidase inhibitors, MAO-I (eg, pargyline, tranylcypromine)	Serious hypertensive crisis may occur following ingestion of foods with a high content of tyramine or other pressor substances (eg, cheddar cheese, red wines)
Inhibition of biliary secretion	Verapamil	Decreased biliary secretion of digoxin causing increased digoxin levels

(Continued)

TABLE 22-9   **Pharmacokinetic Drug Interactions (Continued)**

Drug Interaction	Examples (Precipitant Drugs)	Effect (Object Drugs)
Renal Clearance		
Glomerular filtration rate (GFR) and renal blood flow	Methylxanthines (eg, caffeine, theobromine)	Increased renal blood flow and GFR will decrease time for reabsorption of various drugs, leading to more rapid urinary drug excretion
Active tubular secretion	Probenecid	Probenecid blocks the active tubular secretion of penicillin and some cephalosporin antibiotics
Tubular reabsorption and urine pH	Antacids, sodium bicarbonate	Alkalinization of the urine increases the reabsorption of amphetamine and decreases its clearance
		Alkalinization of urine pH increases the ionization of salicylates, decreases reabsorption, and increases its clearance
Diet		
Charcoal hamburgers	Theophylline Terfenadine, cyclosporin	Increased elimination half-life of theophylline decreases due to increased metabolism Blood levels of terfenadine and cyclosporine increase due to decreased metabolism
Grapefruit juice	Lovastatin, simvastatin, nifedipine	Grapefruit juice is a moderate CYP3A inhibitor and increases plasma drug concentrations
Alcohol (ethanol)	Acetaminophen	Possible hepatotoxicity
Alcohol (ethanol)		May increase or decrease absorption of many drugs
Environmental		
Smoking	Theophylline	Cigarette smoke contains aromatic hydrocarbons that induce cytochrome isozymes involved in metabolism of theophylline, thereby shortening the elimination $t_{1/2}$
Pharmacodynamic		
Alcohol (ethanol)	Antihistamines, opioids	Increased drowsiness
Virus Drug Interactions		
Reye's syndrome	Aspirin	Aspirin in children exposed to certain viral infections such as influenza B virus leads to Reye's syndrome

Preferably, drugs that interact should be avoided or doses of each drug should be given sufficiently far apart so that the interaction is minimized. In situations involving two drugs of choice that may interact, dose adjustment based on pharmacokinetic and therapeutic considerations of one or both of the drugs may be necessary. Dose adjustment may be based on clearance or elimination half-life of the drug. Assessment of the patient's renal function, such as serum creatinine concentration, and liver function indicators, such as alkaline phosphatase, alanine aminotransferase (ALT), aspartate aminotransferase (AST), or other markers of hepatic metabolism (see Chapter 24), should be undertaken. In general, if the therapeutic response is predictable from serum drug concentration, dosing at regular intervals may be based on a steady-state concentration equation such as Equation 22.1. When the elimination half-life is lengthened by drug interaction, the dosing interval may be extended or the dose reduced according to Equation 22.4. Some examples of pharmacokinetic drug interactions are listed in Table 22-9. A more complete discussion of pharmacologic and therapeutic drug interactions of drugs is available in standard textbooks on clinical pharmacology.

Many drugs affect the cytochrome P-450 (CYP) family of hemoprotein enzymes that catalyze drug biotransformation (see also Chapters 12 and 13). Dr. David A. Flockhart, Indiana University School of Medicine, has compiled an excellent website that lists various drugs that may be substrates or inhibitors of cytochrome P-450 isozymes (http://medicine. iupui.edu/flockhart). Some examples of substrates of CYPs are:

CYP1A2	Amitriptyline, fluvoxamine
CYP2B6	Cyclophosphamide
CYP2C9	Ibuprofen, fluoxetine, tolbutamide, amitriptyline
CYP2C19	Omeprazole, S-methenytoin, amitriptyline
CYP2D6	Propanolol, amitriptyline, fluoxetine, paroxetine
CYP2E1	Halothane
CYP3A4	Erythromycin, clarithromycin, midazolam, diazepam
CYP3A5	Clarithromycin, simvastatin, indinavir
CYP3A6	Erythromycin, clarithromycin, diltiazem

Many calcium channel blockers, macrolides, and protease inhibitors are substrates of CYP3A4, CYP3A5, or CYP3A6. An enzyme substrate may competitively interfere with other substrates' metabolism if coadministered. Drug inducers of CYPs may also result in drug interactions by accelerating the rate of drug metabolism. When an unusually high plasma level is observed as a result of coadministration of a second drug, pharmacists should check whether the two drugs share a common CYP metabolic pathway. New substrates are still being discovered. For example, many proton pump inhibitors are substrates of CYP2C19, and many calcium channel blockers are CYP3A4 substrates. It is important to assess the clinical significance with the prescriber before alarming the patient. It is also important to suggest an alternative drug therapy to the prescriber if a clinically significant drug interaction is likely to be occurring.

Some examples of pharmacokinetic drug interactions are discussed in more detail below and in Chapters 12 and 13. Many side effects occur as a result of impaired or induced (enhanced) drug metabolism. Changes in pharmacokinetics due to impaired drug metabolism should be evaluated quantitatively. For example, acetaminophen is an OTC drug that has been used safely for decades, but incidences of severe hepatic toxicity leading to coma have occurred in some subjects with impaired liver function because of chronic alcohol use. Drugs that have reactive intermediates, active metabolites, and/or metabolites with a longer half-life than the parent drug need to be considered carefully if there is a potential for a drug interaction. A polar metabolite may also distribute to a smaller fluid volume, leading to high concentration in some tissues. Drug interactions involving metabolism may be temporal, observed as a delayed effect. Temporal drug interactions are more difficult to detect in a clinical situation.

INHIBITION OF DRUG METABOLISM

Numerous clinical instances of severe adverse reactions as a result of drug interaction involving a change in the rate of drug metabolism have been reported. Knowledge of pharmacokinetics allows the clinical pharmacist to evaluate the clinical significance of the drug interaction. Pharmacokinetic models help determine the need for dose reduction or discontinuing a drug. In assessing the situation, the pathophysiology of the patient and the effect of chronic therapy on drug disposition in the patient must be considered. A severe drug reaction in a patient with liver impairment has resulted in near-fatal reaction in subjects taking otherwise safe doses of acetaminophen. In some patients with traumatic injury or severe cardiovascular disease, blood flow may be impaired, resulting in delayed drug absorption and distribution. Many incidents of serious toxicity or accidents are caused by premature administration of a "booster dose" when the expected response is not immediately observed. Potent drugs such as morphine, midazolam, lidocaine, sodium thiopental, and fentanyl can result in serious adverse reactions if the kinetics of multiple dosing are not carefully assessed.

EXAMPLES ▶ ▶ ▶

1. *Fluvoxamine doubles the half-life of diazepam*: The effect of fluvoxamine on the pharmacokinetics of diazepam was investigated in healthy volunteers (Perucca et al, 1994). Concurrent fluvoxamine intake increased mean peak plasma diazepam concentrations from 108 to 143 ng/mL, and oral diazepam clearance was reduced from 0.40 to 0.14 mL/min/kg. The half-life of diazepam increased from 51 to 118 hours. The area under the plasma concentration–time curve for the diazepam metabolite *N*-desmethyldiazepam was also significantly increased during fluvoxamine treatment. These data suggest that fluvoxamine inhibits the biotransformation of diazepam and its active *N*-demethylated metabolite.

   In this example, the dosing interval, τ, may be increased twofold to account for the doubling of elimination half-life to keep average steady-state concentration unchanged based on Equation 22.4. The rationale for this recommendation may be demonstrated by sketching a diagram showing how the steady-state plasma drug level of diazepam differs after taking 10 mg orally twice a day with or without taking fluvoxamine for a week.

$$C_{av}^{\infty} = \frac{1.44 D_0 t_{1/2} F}{V_D \tau}$$

2. *Quinidine inhibits the metabolism of nifedipine and other calcium channel-blocking agents*: Quinidine coadministration significantly inhibited the aromatization of nifedipine to its major first-pass pyridine metabolite and prolonged the elimination half-life by about 40% (Schellens et al, 1991). The interaction between quinidine and nifedipine supports the involvement of a common cytochrome P-450 (P450 3A4) in the metabolism of the two drugs. Other calcium channel antagonists may also be affected by a similar interaction. What could be a potential problem if two drugs metabolized by the same isozyme are coadministered?

3. *Theophylline clearance is decreased by cimetidine*: Controlled studies have shown that cimetidine can decrease theophylline plasma clearance by 20%–40% (apparently by inhibiting demethylation) (Loi et al, 1997). Prolongation of half-life by as much as 70% was found in some patients. Elevated theophylline plasma concentrations with toxicity may lead to nausea, vomiting, cardiovascular instability, and even seizure. What could happen to an asthmatic patient whose meals are high in protein and low in carbohydrate, and who takes Tagamet 400 mg BID? (*Hint:* Check the effect of food on theophylline, below.)

4. *Interferon-β reduces metabolism of theophylline*: Theophylline pharmacokinetics was also examined before and after interferon treatment (Okuno et al, 1993). Interferon-β treatment reduced the activities of both O-dealkylases by 47%. The total body clearance of theophylline was also decreased (from 0.76 to 0.56 mL/kg/min) and its elimination half-life was increased (from 8.4 to 11.7 hours; $p < 0.05$). This study provided the first direct evidence that interferon-β can depress the activity of drug-metabolizing enzymes in the human liver. What percent of steady-state theophylline plasma concentration would be changed by the interaction? (Use Equation 22.8.)

5. *Torsades de pointes interaction*: A life-threatening ventricular arrhythmia associated with prolongation of the QT interval, known as torsades de pointes, caused the removal of the antihistamine terfenadine (Seldane) from the market because of drug interactions with cisapride, astemizole, and ketoconazole. Clinical symptoms of torsades de pointes include dizziness, syncope, irregular heartbeat, and sudden death. The active metabolite of terfenadine is not cardiac toxic and is now marked as fexofenadine (Allegra), a nonsedative antihistamine.

6. *Cimetidine and diazepam interaction*: The administration of 800 mg of cimetidine daily for 1 week increased the steady-state plasma diazepam and

nordiazepam concentrations due to a cimetidine-induced impairment in microsomal oxidation of diazepam and nordiazepam. The concurrent administration of cimetidine caused a decrease in total metabolic clearance of diazepam and its metabolite, nordiazepam (Lima et al, 1991). How would the following pharmacokinetic parameters of diazepam be affected by the coadministration of cimetidine?

a. Area under the curve in the dose interval ($AUC_{0-24\,h}$)
b. Maximum plasma concentration (C_{max})
c. Time to peak concentration (t_p)
d. Elimination rate constant (k)
e. Total body clearance (Cl_T)
f. Inhibition of monoamine oxidase (MAO)

INHIBITION OF MONOAMINE OXIDASE (MAO)

Nonhepatic enzymes can be involved in drug interactions. For example, drug interactions have been reported for patients taking the antibacterial drug linezolid (Zyvox) who are concurrently taking certain psychiatric medications that work through the serotonin system of the brain (serotonergic psychiatric medications). Linezolid is a reversible monoamine oxidase inhibitor (MAOI). Serotonergic psychiatric medications may include antidepressant drugs such as citalopram, paroxetine, fluoxetine, sertraline, and other drugs that affect the serotonergic pathway in the brain. MAOIs, such as phenelzine and isocarboxazid, are also contraindicated. Although the exact mechanism of this drug interaction is unknown, linezolid inhibits the action of monoamine oxidase A—an enzyme responsible for breaking down serotonin in the brain. It is believed that when linezolid is given to patients taking serotonergic psychiatric medications, high levels of serotonin can build up in the brain, causing toxicity. This is referred to as *serotonin syndrome*. Its signs and symptoms include mental changes (confusion, hyperactivity, memory problems), muscle twitching, excessive sweating, shivering or shaking, diarrhea, trouble

with coordination, and/or fever. A complete list is posted on the FDA website, http://www.fda.gov/Drugs/DrugSafety/ucm265305.htm (accessed August 26, 2011).

INDUCTION OF DRUG METABOLISM

Cytochrome P-450 isozymes are often involved in the metabolic oxidation of many drugs (see Chapter 12). Many drugs can stimulate the production of hepatic enzymes. Therapeutic doses of phenobarbital and other barbiturates accelerate the metabolism of coumarin anticoagulants such as warfarin and substantially reduce the hypoprothrombinemic effect. Fatal hemorrhagic episodes can result when phenobarbital is withdrawn and warfarin dosage maintained at its previous level. Other drugs known to induce drug metabolism include carbamazepine, rifampin, valproic acid, and phenytoin. Enzymatic stimulation can shorten the elimination half-life of the affected drug. For example, phenobarbital can result in lower levels of dexamethasone in asthmatic patients taking both drugs. St. John's wort, a herbal supplement, also induces cytochrome P-450 isozymes and is known to reduce plasma drug concentrations of digoxin, indinavir, and other drugs.

INHIBITION OF DRUG ABSORPTION

Various drugs and dietary supplements can decrease the absorption of drugs from the gastrointestinal tract. Antacids containing magnesium and aluminum hydroxide often interfere with absorption of many drugs. Coadministration of magnesium and aluminum hydroxide caused a decrease of plasma levels of perfloxacin. The drug interaction is caused by the formation of chelate complexes and is possibly also due to adsorption of the quinolone to aluminum hydroxide gel. Perfloxacin should be given at least 2 hours before the antacid to ensure sufficient therapeutic efficacy of the quinolone.

Sucralfate is an aluminum glycopyranoside complex that is not absorbed but retards the oral absorption of ciprofloxacin. Sucralfate is used in the local treatment of ulcers. Cholestyramine is an anion-exchange resin that binds bile acid and many drugs in the gastrointestinal tract. Cholestyramine can bind digitoxin in the GI tract and shorten the elimination half-life of digitoxin by approximately 30%–40%. Absorption of thyroxine may be reduced by 50% when it is administered closely with cholestyramine.

INHIBITION OF BILIARY EXCRETION

The interaction between digoxin and verapamil (Hedman et al, 1991) was studied in six patients (mean age 61 ± 5 years) with chronic atrial fibrillation. The effects of adding verapamil (240 mg/d) on steady-state plasma concentrations of digoxin were studied. Verapamil induced a 44% increase in steady-state plasma concentrations of digoxin. The biliary clearance of digoxin was determined by a duodenal perfusion technique. The biliary clearance of digoxin decreased by 43%, from 187 ± 89 to 101 ± 55 mL/min, whereas the renal clearance was not significantly different (153 ± 31 vs 173 ± 51 mL/min).

ALTERED RENAL REABSORPTION DUE TO CHANGING URINARY pH

The normal adult urinary pH ranges from 4.8 to 7.5 but can increase due to chronic antacid use. This change in urinary pH affects the ionization and reabsorption of weak electrolyte drugs (see Chapter 12). An increased ionization of salicylate due to an increase in urine pH reduces salicylate reabsorption in the renal tubule, resulting in increased renal excretion. Magnesium aluminum hydroxide gel (Maalox), 120 mL/d for 6 days, decreased serum salicylate levels from 19.8 to 15.8 mg/dL in 6 subjects who had achieved a control serum salicylate level of 0.10 mg/dL with the equivalent of 3.76 g/d aspirin (Hansten et al, 1980). Single doses of magnesium aluminum hydroxide gel did not alter urine pH significantly. Five milliliters of Titralac (calcium carbonate with glycine) 4 times a day or magnesium hydroxide for 7 days also increased urinary pH. In general, drugs with pK_a values within the urinary pH range are affected the most. Basic drugs tend to have longer half-lives when urinary pH is increased, especially near its pK_a.

PRACTICAL FOCUS

Some drugs can change urinary pH and, thereby, affect the rate of excretion of weak electrolyte drugs in the urine. Which of the following treatments would be most likely to decrease the elimination $t_{1/2}$ of aspirin? Explain the rationale for your answer.

1. Calcium carbonate PO
2. Sodium carbonate PO
3. IV sodium bicarbonate

EFFECT OF FOOD ON DRUG DISPOSITION

Diet–Theophylline Interaction

Theophylline disposition is influenced by diet. A protein-rich diet will increase theophylline clearance. Average theophylline half-lives in subjects on a low-carbohydrate, high-protein diet increased from 5.2 to 7.6 hours when subjects were changed to a high-carbohydrate, low-protein diet. A diet of charcoal-broiled beef, which contains polycyclic aromatic hydrocarbons from the charcoal, resulted in a decrease in theophylline half-life of up to 42% when compared to a control non-charcoal-broiled-beef diet. Irregular intake of vitamin K may modify the anticoagulant effect of warfarin. Many foods, especially green, leafy vegetables such as broccoli and spinach, contain high concentrations of vitamin K. In one study, warfarin therapy was interfered with inpatients receiving vitamin K, broccoli, or spinach daily for 1 week (Pedersen et al, 1991).

Grapefruit–Drug Interactions

The ingredients in a common food product, grapefruit juice, taken in usual dietary quantities, can significantly inhibit the metabolism by gut-wall cytochrome P-450 3A4 (CYP3A4) (Spence, 1997). For example, grapefruit juice increases average felodipine levels about threefold, increases cyclosporine levels, and increases the levels of terfenadine, a common antihistamine. In the case of terfenadine, Spence (1997) reported the death of a 29-year-old man who had been taking terfenadine and drinking grapefruit juice 2–3 times per week. Death was attributed to terfenadine toxicity. Grapefruit juice can also affect P-gp-mediated efflux of some drugs.

ADVERSE VIRAL DRUG INTERACTIONS

Recent findings have suggested that some interactions of viruses and drugs may predispose individuals to specific disease outcomes (Haverkos et al, 1991). For example, Reye's syndrome has been observed in children who had been taking aspirin and were concurrently exposed to certain viruses, including influenza B virus and varicella zoster virus. The mechanism by which salicylates and certain viruses interact is not clear. However, the publication of this interaction has led to the prevention of morbidity and mortality due to this complex interaction (Haverkos et al, 1991).

POPULATION PHARMACOKINETICS

Population pharmacokinetics (PopPK) is the study of variability in plasma drug concentrations between and within patient populations receiving therapeutic doses of a drug. Traditional pharmacokinetic studies are usually performed on healthy volunteers or highly selected patients, and the average behavior of a group (ie, the mean plasma concentration–time profile) is the main focus of interest. PopPK examines the relationship of the demographic, genetic, pathophysiological, environmental, and other drug-related factors that contribute to the variability observed in safety and efficacy of the drug. The PopPK approach encompasses some of the following features (FDA Guidance for Industry, 1999):

- The collection of relevant pharmacokinetic information in patients who are representative of the target population to be treated with the drug
- The identification and measurement of variability during drug development and evaluation
- The explanation of variability by identifying factors of demographic, pathophysiological, environmental, or concomitant drug-related origin that may influence the pharmacokinetic behavior of a drug
- The quantitative estimation of the magnitude of the unexplained variability in the patient population

The resolution of the issues causing variability in patients allows for the development of an optimum dosing strategy for a population, subgroup, or individual patient. The importance of developing optimum dosing strategies has led to an increase in the use of PopPK approaches in new drug development.

Introduction to Bayesian Theory

Bayesian theory was originally developed to improve forecast accuracy by combining subjective prediction with improvement from newly collected data. In the diagnosis of disease, the physician may make a preliminary diagnosis based on symptoms and physical examination. Later, the results of laboratory tests are received. The clinician then makes a new diagnostic forecast based on both sets of information. Bayesian theory provides a method to weigh the prior information (eg, physical diagnosis) and new information (eg, results from laboratory tests) to estimate a new probability for predicting the disease.

In developing a drug dosage regimen, we assess the patient's medical history and then use average or population pharmacokinetic parameters appropriate for the patient's condition to calculate the initial dose. After the initial dose, plasma or serum drug concentrations are obtained from the patient that provide new information to assess the adequacy of the dosage. The dosing approach of combining old information with new involves a "feedback" process and is, to some degree, inherent in many dosing methods involving some parameter readjustment when new serum drug concentrations become known. The advantage of the Bayesian approach is the improvement in estimating the patient's pharmacokinetic parameters based on Bayesian probability versus an ordinary least-squares-based program. An example comparing the Bayesian method with an alternative method for parameter estimation from some simulated theophylline data will be shown in the next section. The method is particularly useful when only a few blood samples are available.

Because of inter- and intrasubject variability, the pharmacokinetic parameters of an individual patient must be estimated from limited data in the presence of unknown random error (assays, etc), known covariates and variables such as clearance, weight, and disease factor, etc, and possible structural (kinetic model) error. From the knowledge of mean population pharmacokinetic parameters and their variability, Bayesian methods often employ a special *weighted least-squares* (WLS) approach and allow improved estimation of patient pharmacokinetic parameters when there is a lot of variation in data. The methodology is discussed in more detail under the Bayes estimator in the next section and also under pharmacokinetic analysis.

EXAMPLE ▶▶▶

After diagnosing a patient, the physician gave the patient a probability of 0.4 of having a disease. The physician then ordered a clinical laboratory test. A positive laboratory test value had a probability of 0.8 of positively identifying the disease in patients with the disease (true positive) and a probability of 0.1 of positive identification of the disease in subjects without the disease (false positive). From the prior information (physician's diagnosis) and current patient-specific data (laboratory test), what is the posterior probability of the patient having the disease using the Bayesian method?

Solution

Prior probability of having the disease (positive) = 0.4

Prior probability of not having the disease (negative) = 1 − 0.4 = 0.6

Ratio of disease positive to disease negative = 0.4/0.6 = 2/3, or the physician's evaluation shows a 2/3 chance for the presence of the disease

The probability of the patient actually having the disease can be better evaluated by including the laboratory findings. For this same patient, the probability of a positive laboratory test of 0.8 for the detection of disease in positive patients (with disease) and the probability of 0.1 in negative patients (without disease) are equal to a ratio of 0.8/0.1 or 8/1. This ratio is known as the *likelihood ratio*. Combining with the prior probability of 2/3, the posterior probability ratio is

Posterior probability ratio = (2/3) (8/1) = 16/3

Posterior probability = 16/(16 + 3) = 84.2%

Thus, the laboratory test that estimates the likelihood ratio and the preliminary diagnostic evaluation are both used in determining the posterior probability. The results of this calculation show that with a positive diagnosis by the physician and a positive value for the laboratory test, the probability that the patient actually has the disease is 84.2%.

Bayesian probability theory when applied to dosing of a drug involves a given pharmacokinetic parameter (P) and plasma or serum drug concentration (C), as shown in Equation 22.11. The probability of a patient with a given pharmacokinetic parameter P, taking into account the measured concentration, is Prob(P/C):

$$\text{Prob}(P/C) = \frac{\text{Prob}(P) \cdot \text{Prob}(C/P)}{\text{Prob}(C)} \quad (22.11)$$

where Prob(P) = the probability of the patient's parameter within the assumed population distribution, Prob(C/P) = the probability of measured concentration within the population, and Prob (C) = the unconditional probability of the observed concentration.

EXAMPLE ▶▶▶

Theophylline has a therapeutic window of 10–20 μg/mL. Serum theophylline concentrations above 20 μg/mL produce mild side effects, such as nausea and insomnia; more serious side effects, such as sinus tachycardia, may occur at drug concentrations above 40 μg/mL; at serum concentrations above 45 μg/mL, cardiac arrhythmia and seizure may occur (see Fig. 22-1). However, the probability of some side effect occurring is by no means certain. Side effects are not determined solely by plasma concentration, as other known or unknown variables (called covariates) may affect the side effect outcome. Some patients have initial side effects of nausea and restlessness (even at very low drug concentrations) that later disappear when therapy is continued. The clinician should therefore assess the probability of side effects in the patient, order a blood sample for serum theophylline determination, and then estimate a combined (or posterior) probability for side effects in the patient.

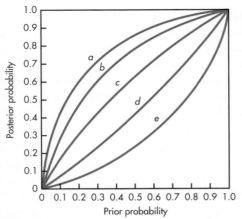

FIGURE 22-3 Conditional probability curves relating prior probability of toxicity to posterior probability of toxicity of STC, theophylline serum concentrations: (*a*) 27–28.9; (*b*) 23–24.9; (*c*) 19–20.9; (*d*) 15–16.9; and (*e*) 11–12.9 (all STC in μg/mL). (From Schumacher GE et al: Applying decision analysis in therapeutic drug monitoring: using decision trees to interpret serum theophylline. *Clin Pharm* **5**(4):325–333, 1986, with permission.)

The decision process is illustrated graphically in Fig. 22-3. The probability of initial (prior) estimation of side effects is plotted on the *x* axis, and the final (posterior) probability of side effects is plotted on the *y* axis for various serum theophylline concentrations. For example, a patient was placed on theophylline and the physician estimated the chance of side effects to be 40%, but therapeutic drug monitoring showed a theophylline level of 27 μg/mL. A vertical line of prior probability at 0.4 intersects curve *a* at about 0.78 or 78%. Hence, the Bayesian probability of having side effects is 78% taking both the laboratory and physician assessments into consideration. The curves (*a–e* in Fig. 22-3) for various theophylline concentrations are called *conditional probability curves*. Bayesian theory does not replace clinical judgment, but it provides a quantitative tool for incorporating subjective judgment (human) with objective (laboratory assay) in making risk decisions. When complex decisions involving several variables are involved, this objective tool can be very useful.

Bayesian probability is used to improve forecasting in medicine. One example is its use in the diagnosis of healed myocardial infarction (HMI) from a 12-lead electrocardiogram (ECG) by artificial neural networks using the Bayesian concept. Bayesian results were comparable to those of an experienced electrocardiographer (Heden et al, 1996). In pharmacokinetics, Bayesian theory is applied to "feed-forward neural networks" for gentamicin concentration predictions (Smith and Brier, 1996). A brief literature search of Bayesian applications revealed over 400 therapeutic applications between 1992 and 1996. Bayesian parameter estimations were most frequently used for drugs with narrow therapeutic ranges, such as the aminoglycosides, cyclosporin, digoxin, anticonvulsants (especially phenytoin), lithium, and theophylline. The technique has now been extended to cytotoxic drugs, factor VIII, and warfarin. Bayesian methods have also been used to limit the number of samples required in more conventional pharmacokinetic studies with new drugs (Thomson and Whiting, 1992). The main disadvantage of Bayesian methods is the subjective selection of prior probability. Therefore, it is not considered to be unbiased by many statisticians for drug approval purposes.

Adaptive Method or Dosing with Feedback

In dosing drugs with narrow therapeutic ratios, an initial dose is calculated based on mean population pharmacokinetic parameters. After dosing, plasma drug concentrations are obtained from the patient. As more blood samples are drawn from the patient, the calculated individualized patient pharmacokinetic parameters become increasingly more reliable. This type of approach has been referred to as *adaptive* or *Bayesian adaptive method* with feedback when a special extended least-squares algorithm is used. Many ordinary least-squares (OLS) computer software packages are available to clinical practice for parameter and dosage calculation (see Appendix A). Some software packages record medical history and provide adjustments for weight, age, and in some cases, disease factors. A common approach is to estimate the clearance and volume of distribution from intermittent infusion (see Chapter 6). Abbottbase Pharmacokinetic Systems (1986 and 1992) is an example of patient-oriented software that records patient information and dosing history based on 24-hour clock time. An adaptive-type algorithm is used to estimate pharmacokinetic parameters. The average population clearance and volume of distribution of drugs are used for initial estimates, and the program computes patient-specific Cl and V_D as serum drug concentrations are entered. The program accounts for renal dysfunction based on creatinine clearance, which is estimated from serum creatinine concentration using the Cockroft–Gault equation (see Chapter 24). The software package allows specific parameter estimation for digoxin, theophylline, and aminoglycosides, although other drugs can also be analyzed manually.

Many *least-squares* (LS) and *weighted least-squares* (WLS) algorithms are available for estimating patient pharmacokinetic parameters. Their common objective involves estimating the parameters with minimum bias and good prediction, often as evaluated by mean predictive error. The advantage of the Bayesian method is the ability to input known information into the program, so that the search for the real pharmacokinetic parameter is more efficient and, perhaps, more precise. For example, a drug is administered by intravenous infusion at a rate, R, to a patient. The drug is infused over t hours (t may be 0.5–2 hours for a typical infusion). The patient's clearance, Cl_T, may be estimated from plasma drug concentration taken at a known time according to a one-compartment model equation. Sheiner and Beal (1982) simulated a set of theophylline data and estimated parameters from the data using one- and two-serum concentrations, assuming different variabilities. These investigators tested the method with a Bayesian approach and with an OLS method, OBJ_{OLS}.

$$C_i = f(P, t_i)\varepsilon_i \qquad (22.12)$$

$$OBJ_{OLS} = \sum_{i=1}^{n} \frac{\left(C_i - \widehat{C_i}\right)^2}{\sigma_i^2} \qquad (22.13)$$

The Bayes Estimator

When the pharmacokinetic parameter, P, is estimated from a set of plasma drug concentration data (C_i) having several potential sources of error with different variance, the OLS method for parameter estimation is no longer adequate (it yields trivial estimates). The intersubject variation, intrasubject variance, and random error must be minimized properly to allow efficient parameter estimation.

The weighted least-squares function in Equation 22.14 was suggested by Sheiner and Beal (1982). The equation represents the least-squares estimation of the concentration by minimizing deviation squares (first summation term of Equation 22.14), and deviation of population parameter squares (second summation term). Equation 22.14 is called the *Bayes estimator*. This approach is frequently referred to as *extended least-squares* (ELS).

$$\text{Intrasubject } C_i = f(P, X_i) + \varepsilon_i$$
$$\text{Intersubject } P_k = \widehat{P}_k + \eta_k \qquad (22.14)$$

$$OBJ_{BAYES} = \sum_{i=1}^{n} \frac{\left(C_i - \widehat{C_i}\right)^2}{\sigma_i^2} + \sum_{k=1}^{S} \frac{\left(P_k - \widehat{P}_k\right)^2}{\omega_k^2}$$

For n number of drug plasma concentration data, i is an index to refer to each data item, C_i is the ith concentration, $\widehat{C}_i$ is the ith model-estimated concentration, and σ^2 is the variance of random error, ε_i (assay errors, random intrasubject variation, etc). There is a series of population parameters in the model for the kth population parameter, $P_k \cdot \widehat{P}_k$ is the estimated population parameter and η_k is the kth parameter random error with variance of ω_k^2.

To compare the performance of the Bayesian method to other methods in drug dosing, Sheiner and Beal (1982) generated some theophylline plasma drug concentrations based on known clearance. They added various error levels to the data and divided the patients into groups with one and two plasma drug samples. The two pharmacokinetic parameters used were based on population pharmacokinetics for theophylline derived from the literature: (1) for P_1, a V_D of 0.5 L/kg and coefficient of variation of 32%; and (2) for P_2, clearance of 0.052 L/kg/h and coefficient of variation of 44%.

The data were then analyzed using the Bayesian method and a second (alternative) approach in determining the pharmacokinetic parameter (Cl_T). In the presence of various levels of error, the Bayesian approach was robust and resulted in better estimation of clearance in both the one- and two-sample groups (Fig. 22-4 and Table 22-10). The success of the Bayesian approach is due to the ability of the

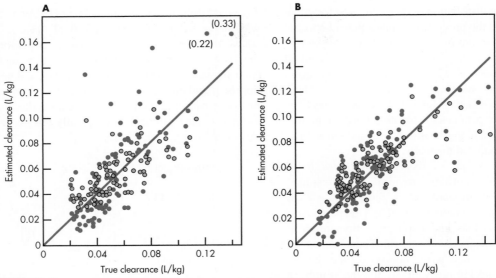

FIGURE 22-4   Plots of predicted clearance versus true (simulated) clearance for predictions by the Bayesian (<inline>) and alternative (<inline>) methods. The diagonal line on each graph is the line of identity. **A** shows results for one-sample group; **B** shows results for two-sample group. (From Sheiner and Beal, 1982, with permission.)

algorithm to minimize the total mean square terms of errors. A more precise clearance estimation will lead to more accurate dose estimation in the patient.

The implementation of the Bayesian (ELS) approach uses the NONMEM computer software,

facilitated by response criteria defined through a first-order (FO) Taylor series expansion. Among other computer software packages available, the NPEM2 (USC*PACK) is a nonparametric maximum expectation maximization method that makes no parametric

TABLE 22-10   Performance of Clearance Estimation Methods

| Method | $\frac{\omega_{Cl}{}^a}{\sigma}$ | $\frac{\omega_{V_D}{}^a}{\sigma}$ | Mean Clearance Error (±SEM) as Percent of Mean Clearance | | | |
| | | | Error | | Absolute Error | |
			Example 1	Example 2	Example 1	Example 2
Alternative	—	—	−5.77 (5.8)	−2.82 (3.3)	37.1 (4.5)	26.4 (2.1)
Bayesian	1	1	−1.02 (3.0)	−1.08 (3.1)	22.2 (2.0)[b]	21.7 (2.2)[b]
	3/2	1	−4.94 (3.4)	−3.77 (3.0)	25.6 (2.3)[b]	23.1 (2.1)[b]
	2/3	1	5.02 (3.2)	2.52 (3.4)	23.7 (2.2)[b]	23.5 (2.4)
	1	3/2	0.44 (3.0)	−0.26 (3.1)	22.5 (2.1)[b]	21.4 (2.2)[b]
	1	2/3	−0.76 (3.0)	−1.56 (3.1)	22.5 (1.9)[b]	21.7 (2.2)

[a]Ratio of standard deviation of clearance (or V_D) to σ used in the Bayesian method. All ratios are divided by the correct ratio so that a value of unity signifies that the correct ratio itself was used.

[b]Mean absolute error of Bayesian method less than that of alternative ($p < 0.05$).

From Sheiner and Beal (1982), with permission.

assumptions about the mean and standard deviation of the distribution. The program can also discover unrecognized subpopulations. NONMEM also features FOEM, a first-order expectation maximization method. Generally, finding a set of best parameter estimates to describe the data involves minimizing the error terms; alternatively, another paradigm that maximizes the probability of the parameter estimates in the distribution serves the same purpose equally well or better. Thus, the first-order expectation maximization (FOEM) paradigm is also available in NONMEM and in other programs, such as P-PHARM (Mentre and Gomeni, 1995).

Comparison of Bayes, Least-Squares, Steady-State, and Chiou Methods

For theophylline dosing, the Bayes method and others, including the conventional steady-state method, were compared by Hurley and McNeil (1988). The Bayes method compared favorably with other methods (Tables 22-11 and 22-12). The steady-state method was also useful, but none of the methods was sufficiently accurate, probably due to other variables, such as saturation kinetics or the use of an inappropriate compartment model.

Model fitting in pharmacokinetics often involves the search for a set of parameters that fits the data, a situation analogous to finding a point within a large geometric space. The OLS approach of iteratively minimizing the error terms may not be adequate when data are sparse, but are fine when sufficient data and good initial estimates are available. The Bayesian approach uses prior information, and, in essence, guides the search pointer to a proximity in the geometric space where the estimates are more likely to be found (reducing variability but increasing subjectivity). Many algorithms use some form of gradient- or derivative-based method; other algorithms use a variable sequential simplex method.

TABLE 22-11   Pharmacokinetic Parameter Estimates (Mean ± SD)

Method	Cl^a (L/h/kg IBW)	k^b(h^{-1})	V_D (L/kg IBW)
Least-squares			
Day 1	0.0383 ± 0.0129	0.105 ± 0.014	0.519 ± 0.291
Final	0.0391 ± 0.0117	0.095 ± 0.064	0.511 ± 0.239
Chiou			
1	0.0399 ± 0.0306		
2	0.0437 ± 0.0193		
3	0.0438 ± 0.0212		
Steady-state clearance			
	0.0408 ± 0.0174		
Bayesian			
1	0.0421 ± 0.0143	0.081 ± 0.030	0.534 ± 0.0745
2	0.0424 ± 0.0158	0.082 ± 0.035	0.532 ± 0.0802
3	0.0408 ± 0.0182	0.078 ± 0.037	0.531 ± 0.0820
4	0.0403 ± 0.0147	0.077 ± 0.027	0.530 ± 0.0787
Final	0.0372 ± 0.0113	0.070 ± 0.026	0.536 ± 0.0741

Cl = total body clearance, k = elimination rate constant, V_D = volume of distribution, IBW = ideal body weight.

[a]Calculated from least-squares estimates.

[b]Calculated by Bayesian estimates.

From Hurley and McNeil (1988), with permission.

TABLE 22-12   Predictive Accuracy at the End of Infusion 1[a]

Method	Mean Prediction Error (mg/L)	Mean Percent Absolute Prediction Error (%)
Least-squares		
Day 1	−0.06 (−1.1, 0.95)	17.6 (13.4, 21.7)
Chiou		
1	0.96 (−1.7, 3.60)	36.8 (27.3, 46.3)
2	−1.7 (−3.3, −0.08)	20.8 (14.1, 27.5)
3	−1.5 (−3.7, 0.80)	27.7 (17.8, 37.5)
Bayesian		
1	−0.61 (−1.7, 0.50)	18.8 (14.1, 23.6)
2	−0.65 (−2.0, 0.69)	22.7 (16.3, 29.2)
3	0.16 (−1.1, 1.40)	21.7 (16.1, 27.2)
4	−0.15 (−1.2, 0.96)	19.8 (15.6, 24.1)

[a]Figures in parentheses are 95% confidence intervals.

From Hurley and McNeil (1988), with permission.

A discussion of the pharmacokinetic estimation methods was given by D'Argenio and Schumitzky (1979). Some common pharmacokinetic algorithms for parameter estimation are (1) Newton–Raphson with first and second derivatives, (2) Gauss–Newton method, (3) Levenberg–Marquardt method, and (4) Nelder–Mead simplex method. The Gauss–Newton method was used in the early versions of NONLIN. As discussed in relation to the mixed-effect models in later sections, assuming a relationship such as Cl_R proportional to Cl_{cr} (technically called linearization) reduces the minimum number of data necessary for parameter estimation.

Analysis of Population Pharmacokinetic Data

Traditional pharmacokinetic studies involve taking multiple blood samples periodically over time in a few individual patients, and characterizing basic pharmacokinetic parameters such as k, V_D, and Cl; because the studies are generally well designed, there are fewer parameters than data points (ie, that provide sufficient degree of freedom to reflect lack of fit of the model), and the parameters are efficiently estimated from the model with most least-squares programs. Traditional pharmacokinetic parameter estimation is very accurate, provided that enough samples can be taken for the individual patient. The disadvantage is that only a few relatively homogeneous healthy subjects are included in pharmacokinetic studies, from which dosing in different patients must be projected.

In the clinical setting, patients are usually less homogeneous; patients vary in sex, age, and body weight; they may have concomitant disease and may be receiving multiple drug treatments. Even the diet, lifestyle, ethnicity, and geographic location can differ from a selected group of "normal" subjects. Further, it is often not possible to take multiple samples from the same subject, and, therefore, no data are available to reflect intrasubject difference, so that iterative procedures for finding the maximum likelihood estimate can be complex and unpredictable due to incomplete or missing data. However, the vital information needed about the pharmacokinetics of drugs in patients at different stages of their disease with various therapies can only be obtained from the same population, or from a collection of pooled blood samples. The advantages of population pharmacokinetic analysis using pooled data were reviewed by Sheiner and Ludden (1992) and included a summary of population pharmacokinetics for dozens of drugs. Pharmacokinetic analysis of pooled data of plasma drug concentration from a large group of subjects may reveal much information about the disposition of a drug in a population. Unlike data from an individual subject collected over time, inter- and intrasubject variations must be considered. Both pharmacokinetic and nonpharmacokinetic factors, such as age, weight, sex, and creatinine concentration, should be examined in the model to determine the relevance to the estimation of pharmacokinetic parameters.

The *nonlinear mixed-effect model* (or NONMEM) is so called because the model uses both fixed and random factors to describe the data. Fixed factors such as patient weight, age, gender, and creatinine clearance are assumed to have no error, whereas random factors include inter- and intraindividual differences.

NONMEM is a statistical program written in Fortran (see Appendix A) that allows Bayesian pharmacokinetic parameters to be estimated using an efficient algorithm called the *first-order* (FO) method. The parameters may now be estimated also with a *first-order conditional estimate* (FOCE) algorithm. In addition, to pharmacokinetic parameters, many examples of population plasma data have been analyzed to determine population factors. Multiplicative coefficients or parameters for patient factors may also be estimated.

NONMEM fits plasma drug concentration data for all subjects in the groups simultaneously and estimates the population parameter and its variance. The parameter may be clearance and/or V_D. The model may also test for other fixed effects on the drug due to factors such as age, weight, and creatinine clearance.

The model describes the observed plasma drug concentration (C_i) in terms of a model with:

1. P_k = fixed effect parameters, which include pharmacokinetic parameters or patient factor parameters. For example, P_1 is Cl, P_2 is the multiplicative coefficient including creatinine factor, and P_3 is the multiplicative coefficient for weight.
2. Random effect parameters, including (a) the variance of the structural (kinetic) parameter, P_k, or intersubject variability within the population, ω_k^2; and (b) the residual intrasubject variance or variance due to measurement errors, fluctuations in individual parameter values, and all other errors not accounted for by the other parameters.

There are generally two reliable and practical approaches to population pharmacokinetic data analysis. One approach is the *standard two-stage* (STS) *method*, which estimates parameters from the plasma drug concentration data for an individual subject during the first stage. The estimates from all subjects are then combined to obtain an estimate of the parameters for the population. The method is useful because unknown factors that affect the response in one patient will not carry over and bias parameter estimates of the others. The method works well when sufficient drug concentration–time data are available.

A second approach, the *first-order* (FO) *method*, is also used but is perhaps less well understood. The estimation procedure is based on minimization of an extended least-squares criterion, which was defined through an FO Taylor series expansion of the response vector about the fixed effects and which utilized a Newton–Raphson-like algorithm (Beal and Sheiner, 1980). This method attempts to fit the data and partition the unpredictable differences between theoretical and observed values into random error terms. When this model includes concomitant effects, it is called a *mixed-effect statistical model* (Beal and Sheiner, 1985).

The advantage of the FO model is that it is applicable even when the amount of time–concentration data obtained from each individual is small, provided that the total number of individuals is sufficiently large. For example, in the example cited by Beal and Sheiner (1985), 116 plasma concentrations were collected from 39 patients with various weight, age, gender, serum creatinine, and congestive heart failure conditions. The two-stage method was not suitable, but the FO method was useful for analyzing this set of data. With a large number of factors and only limited data, and with hidden factors possibly affecting the pharmacokinetics of the drug, the analysis may sometimes be misleading. Beal and Sheiner (1985) suggested that the main concomitant factor should be measured whenever possible. Several examples of population pharmacokinetic data analysis using clinical data are listed below. Typically, a computer method is used in the data analysis based on a statistical model using either the weighted least-squares (WLS) or the extended least-squares (ELS) method in estimating the parameters. In the last few years, NONMEM has been regularly updated and improved. Many drugs have been analyzed with population pharmacokinetics to yield the information not obtainable using the traditional two-stage method (Sheiner and Ludden, 1992). An added feature is the development of a population model involving both pharmacokinetics and pharmacodynamics, the so-called population PK/PD models.

One example involving analysis of population plasma concentration data involved the drug procainamide. The drug clearance of an individual in a group may be assumed to be affected by several factors (Whiting et al, 1986). These factors include body weight, creatinine clearance, and a clearance factor P_1 described in the following equation:

$$Cl_{\text{drug}\, j} = P_1 + P_2(C_{\text{creatinine}\, j})$$
$$+ P_3(\text{weight}_j) + \eta_{Clj} \qquad (22.15)$$

where η_{Clj} is the intersubject error of clearance and its variance is ω^2_{Clj}.

In another mixed-effect model involving the analysis of lidocaine and mexiletine, Vozeh et al (1984) tested age, sex, time on drug therapy, and congestive heart failure (CHF) for effects on drug clearance. The effects of CHF and weight on V_D were also examined. The test statistic, DELS (*difference extended least-squares*), was significant for CHF and moderately significant for weight on lidocaine clearance.

Population pharmacokinetics may be analyzed from various clinical sites. The information content is better when sampling is strategically designed. Proper sampling can yield valuable information about the distribution of pharmacokinetic parameters in a population. Pooled clinical drug concentrations taken from hospital patients are generally not well controlled and are much harder to analyze. A mixed-effect model can yield valuable information about various demographic and pathophysiologic factors that may influence drug disposition in the patient population.

Model Selection Criteria

Data analysis in pharmacokinetics frequently selects either a monoexponential or a polyexponential that will better describe the concentration–time relationship. The selection criteria for the better model are determined by the goodness-of-fit, taking into account the number of parameters involved. Three common model selection criteria are (1) the Akaike Information Criterion (AIC), (2) the Schwarz Criterion (SC), and (3) the F test ($\alpha = 0.05$). The performance characteristics of these criteria were examined by Ludden et al

(1994) using Monte Carlo (random or stochastic) simulations. The precision and bias of the estimated parameters were considered. The Akaike Information Criterion and the Schwarz Criterion lead to selection of the most appropriate model more often than does the F test, which tends to choose the simpler model even when the more complex model is informative. The F test is also more sensitive to deficient sampling designs. Clearance was quite robust among the different methods and generally well estimated. Other pharmacokinetic parameters are more sensitive to model choice, particularly the apparent elimination rate constant. Prediction of concentrations is generally more precise when a suitable model is chosen.

Decision Analysis Involving Diagnostic Tests

Diagnostic tests may be performed to determine the presence or absence of a disease. A scheme for the predictability of a disease by a diagnostic test is shown in Table 22-13. A true positive, represented by *a,* indicates that the laboratory test correctly predicted the disease, whereas a false positive, represented by *b,* shows that the laboratory test incorrectly predicted that the patient had the disease when, in fact, the patient did not have the disease. In contrast, a true negative, represented by *d,* correctly gave a negative test in patients without the disease, whereas a false negative, represented by *c,* incorrectly gave a negative test when, in fact, the patient did have the disease.

CLINICAL EXAMPLE

A new diagnostic test for HIV$^+$/AIDS was developed and tested in 5772 intravenous drug users. The results of this study are tabulated in Table 22-14. From the results in Table 22-14, a total of 2863 subjects had a positive diagnostic test for HIV$^+$/AIDS and 2909 subjects had a negative diagnostic test for HIV$^+$/AIDS. Further tests on these subjects showed that 2967 subjects actually had HIV$^+$/AIDS, although 211 of these subjects had negative diagnostic test results. Moreover, 107 subjects who had a positive

TABLE 22-13   Errors in Decision Predictability

Decision	Diagnostic Test Result		Totals
	Disease Present	**Disease Absent**	
Accept disease	Test positive	Test positive	
Present	(True positive) a	(False positive) b	$a + b$
Reject disease	Test negative	Test negative	
Present	(False negative) c	(True negative) d	$c + d$
Totals	$a + c$	$b + d$	$a + b + c + d$

TABLE 22-14   Results of HIV⁺/AIDS Test

Decision	Diagnostic Test Result		Totals
	Disease Present	**Disease Absent**	
Accept HIV⁺/AIDS present	2756	107	2863
Reject HIV⁺/AIDS present	211	2698	2909
Totals	2967	2805	5772

diagnostic test result did not, in fact, have HIV⁺/AIDS after further tests were made.

1. The *positive predictability* of the test is the likelihood that the test will correctly predict the disease if the test is positive and is estimated as

$$\text{Positive predictability} = \frac{a}{a+b} = \frac{2756}{2863}$$

$$= 0.963 \ (96.3\%)$$

2. The *negative predictability* of the test is the likelihood that the patient will not have the disease if the test is negative and is estimated as

$$\text{Negative predictability} = \frac{d}{c+d} = \frac{2698}{2909}$$

$$= 0.927 \ (92.7\%)$$

3. The *total predictability* of the test is the likelihood that the patient will be predicted correctly and is estimated as

$$\text{Total predictability} = \frac{a+d}{a+b+c+d}$$

$$= \frac{2756 + 2698}{5772}$$

$$= 0.945 \ (94.5\%)$$

4. The *sensitivity* of the test is the likelihood that a test result will be positive in a patient with the disease and is estimated as

$$\text{Sensitivity} = \frac{a}{a+c} = \frac{2756}{2967} = 0.929 \ (92.9\%)$$

5. The *specificity* of the test is the likelihood that a test result will be negative in a patient without the disease and is estimated as

$$\text{Specificity} = \frac{d}{b+d} = \frac{2698}{2805} = 0.962 \ (96.2\%)$$

Analysis of the results in Table 22-14 shows that a positive result from the new test for HIV⁺/AIDS will only predict the disease correctly 94.5% of the time. Therefore, the clinician must use other measures to predict whether the patient has the disease. These other measures may include physical diagnosis of the patient, other laboratory tests, normal incidence of the disease in the patient population (in this case, intravenous drug users), and the experience of the clinician. Each test has different predictive values.

REGIONAL PHARMACOKINETICS

Pharmacokinetics is the study of the time course of drug concentrations in the body. Pharmacokinetics is based generally on the time course of drug concentrations in systemic blood sampled from either a vein or an artery. This general approach is useful as long as the drug concentrations in the tissues of the body are well reflected by drug concentrations in the blood. Clinically, the blood drug concentration may not be proportional to the drug concentration in tissues. For example, after IV bolus administration, the distributive phase is attributed to temporally different changes in mixing and redistribution of drug in organs such as the lung, heart, and kidney (Upton, 1990). The time course for the pharmacodynamics of the drug may have no relationship to the time course for the drug concentrations in the blood. The pharmacodynamics of the drug may be related to local tissue drug levels and the status of homeostatic physiologic functions. After an IV bolus dose, Upton (1990) reported that lignocaine (lidocaine) rapidly accumulates in the spleen and kidney but is slowly sequestered into fat. More than 30 minutes were needed before the target-site (heart and brain) drug levels established equilibrium with drug concentrations in the blood. These *regional equilibrium factors* are often masked in conventional pharmacokinetic models that assume rapid drug equilibrium.

Regional pharmacokinetics is the study of pharmacokinetics within a given tissue region. The tissue region is defined as an anatomic area of the body between specified afferent and efferent blood vessels. For example, the myocardium includes the region perfused by the coronary arterial (afferent) and coronary sinus (efferent) blood vessels. The selection of a region bounded by its network of blood vessel is based on the movement of drug between the blood vessels and the interstitial and intracellular spaces of the region. The conventional pharmacokinetic approach for calculating systemic clearance and volume of distribution tends to average various drug distributions together, such that the local perturbations are neglected. Regional pharmacokinetics (see Mather, 2001, Chapter 10) supplement systemic pharmacokinetics when inadequate information is provided by conventional pharmacokinetics.

Various homeostatic physiologic functions may be responsible for the nonequilibrium of drug concentrations between local tissue regions and the blood. For example, most cells have an electrochemical difference across the cell membrane consisting of a membrane potential of negative 70 mV inside the membrane relative to the outside. Moreover, regional differences in pH normally exist within a cell. For example, the pH within the lysosome is between 4 and 5, which could allow a basic drug to accumulate within the lysosome with a concentration gradient of 400-fold to 160,000-fold over the blood. Other explanations for regional drug concentration differences have been reviewed by Upton (1990), who also considers that dynamic processes may be more important than equilibrium processes in affecting dynamic response. Thus, regional pharmacokinetics is another approach in applying pharmacokinetics to pharmacodynamics and clinical effect.

Frequently Asked Questions

▶ *What is meant by population pharmacokinetics? What advantages does population pharmacokinetics have over classical pharmacokinetics?*

▶ *Why is it possible to estimate individual pharmacokinetic parameters with just a few data points using the Bayesian method?*

▶ *Why is pharmacokinetics important in studying drug interactions?*

CHAPTER SUMMARY

Successful drug therapy involves the selection of the drug, the drug product, and the development of a dosage regiment that meets the needs of the patient. Often, drug dosage regimens are based on average population pharmacokinetics. Ideally, the dosage regimen can be developed for the individual patient by taking into consideration the patient's demographics, genetics, pathophysiology, environmental issues, possible drug–drug interactions, known variability in drug response, and other drug-related issues. The development of Medication Therapy Management (MTM) and therapeutic drug monitoring services can improve patient compliance and the success of drug therapy. Drug dosage regimens may be calculated in an individual patient based on complete or incomplete pharmacokinetic information. Changes in the dose and/or in the dosing interval can affect the $C_{max}^{\infty}, C_{min}^{\infty}$, and C_{av}^{∞}.

Pharmacokinetics of a drug may be altered in special populations, such as the elderly, infants, obese patients, and patients with renal or hepatic disease. Elderly patients may have several different pathophysiologic conditions that require multiple drug therapy that increases the likelihood for a drug interaction. Infants and children have different dosing requirements than adults. Dosing of drugs in this population requires a thorough consideration of the differences in the pharmacokinetics and pharmacology of a specific drug in the preterm newborn infant, newborn infant, infant, young child, older child, adolescent, and the adult. Unfortunately, the pharmacokinetics and pharmacodynamics of most drugs are not well known in children under 12 years of age. Obesity often is defined by *body mass index* (BMI). For some drugs, dosing is based on ideal body weight. A drug interaction generally refers to a modification of the expected drug response in the patient as a result of exposure of the patient to another drug or substance. Drug–drug interactions may cause an alteration in the pharmacokinetics of the drug due to an interaction in drug absorption, distribution, or elimination. Bayesian theory can help determine the probability of a diagnostic test to give accurate results. Population pharmacokinetics (PopPK) is the study of variability in plasma drug concentrations between and within patient populations receiving therapeutic doses of a drug and enables the estimate of pharmacokinetic parameters from relatively sparse data obtained from study subjects.

LEARNING QUESTIONS

1. Why is it harder to titrate patients with a drug whose elimination half-life is 36 hours compared to a drug whose elimination is 6 hours?

2. Penicillin G has a volume of distribution of 42 L/1.73 m² and an elimination rate constant of 1.034 h⁻¹. Calculate the maximum peak concentration that would be produced if the drug was given intravenously at a rate of 250 mg every 6 hours for a week.

3. Dicloxacillin has an elimination half-life of 42 minutes and a volume of distribution of 20 L. Dicloxacillin is 97% protein bound. What would be the steady-state free concentration of dicloxacillin if the drug was given intravenously at a rate of 250 mg every 6 hours?

4. The normal elimination half-life of cefamandole is 1.49 hours and the apparent volume of distribution (V_D) is 39.2% of body weight. The elimination half-life for a patient with a creatinine clearance of 15 mL/min was reported by Czerwinski and Pederson (1979) to be 6.03 hours, and cefamandole's V_D is 23.75% of body weight. What doses of cefamandole should be given to the normal and the uremic patient (respectively) if the drug is administered intravenously every 6 hours and the desired objective is to maintain an average steady concentration of 2 μg/mL?

5. The maintenance dose of digoxin was reported to be 0.5 mg/d for a 60-kg patient with normal renal function. The half-life of digoxin is 0.95 days and

the volume of distribution is 306 L. The bioavailability of the digoxin tablet is 0.56.

   a. Calculate the steady-state concentration of digoxin.

   b. Determine whether the patient is adequately dosed (effective serum digoxin concentration is 1–2 ng/mL).

   c. What is the steady-state concentration if the patient is dosed with the elixir instead of the tablet? (Assume the elixir to be 100% bioavailable.)

6. An antibiotic has an elimination half-life of 2 hours and an apparent volume of distribution of 200 mL/kg. The minimum effective serum concentration is 2 μg/mL and the minimum toxic serum concentration is 16 μg/mL. A physician ordered a dosage regimen of this antibiotic to be given at 250 mg every 8 hours by repetitive intravenous bolus injections.

   a. Comment on the appropriateness of this dosage regimen for an adult male patient (23 years, 80 kg) whose creatinine clearance is 122 mL/min.

   b. Would you suggest an alternative dosage regimen for this patient? Give your reasons and suggest an alternative dosage regimen.

7. Gentamycin (Garamycin, Schering) is a highly water-soluble drug. The dosage of this drug in obese patients should be based on an estimate of the lean body mass or ideal body weight. Why?

8. Why is the calculation for the loading dose (D_L) for a drug based on the apparent volume of distribution, whereas the calculation of the maintenance dose is based on the elimination rate constant?

9. A potent drug with a narrow therapeutic index is ordered for a patient. After making rounds, the attending physician observes that the patient is not responding to drug therapy and orders a single plasma-level measurement. Comment briefly on the value of measuring the drug concentration in a single blood sample and on the usefulness of the information that may be gained.

10. Calculate an oral dosage regimen for a cardiotonic drug for an adult male (63 years old, 68 kg) with normal renal function. The elimination half-life for this drug is 30 hours and its apparent volume of distribution is 4 L/kg. The drug is 80% bioavailable when given orally, and the suggested therapeutic serum concentrations for this drug range from 0.001 to 0.002 μg/mL.

   a. This cardiotonic drug is commercially supplied as 0.075-mg, 0.15-mg, and 0.30-mg white, scored, compressed tablets. Using these readily available tablets, what dose would you recommend for this patient?

   b. Are there any advantages for this patient to give smaller doses more frequently compared to a higher dosage less frequently? Any disadvantages?

   c. Would you suggest a loading dose for this drug? Why? What loading dose would you recommend?

   d. Is there a rationale for preparing a controlled-release product of this drug?

11. The dose of sulfisoxazole (Gantrisin, Roche) recommended for an adult female patient (age 26 years, 63 kg) with a urinary tract infection was 1.5 g every 4 hours. The drug is 85% bound to serum proteins. The elimination half-life of this drug is 6 hours and the apparent volume of distribution is 1.3 L/kg. Sulfisoxazole is 100% bioavailable.

   a. Calculate the steady-state plasma concentration of sulfisoxazole in this patient.

   b. Calculate an appropriate loading dose of sulfisoxazole for this patient.

   c. Gantrisin (sulfisoxazole) is supplied in tablets containing 0.5 g of drug. How many tablets would you recommend for the loading dose?

   d. If no loading dose was given, how long would it take to achieve 95%–99% of steady state?

12. The desired plasma level for an antiarrhythmic agent is 5 μg/mL. The drug has an apparent volume of distribution of 173 mL/kg and an elimination half-life of 2 hours. The kinetics of the drug follow the kinetics of a one-compartment open model.

   a. An adult male patient (75 kg, 56 years of age) is to be given an IV injection of this drug. What loading dose (D_L) and infusion rate (R) would you suggest?

b. The patient did not respond very well to drug therapy. Plasma levels of drug were measured and found to be 2 μg/mL. How would you readjust the infusion rate to increase the plasma drug level to the desired 5 μg/mL?

c. How long would it take to achieve 95% of steady-state plasma drug levels in this patient assuming no loading dose was given and the apparent V_D was unaltered?

13. An antibiotic is to be given to an adult male patient (75 kg, 58 years of age) by intravenous infusion. The elimination half-life for this drug is 8 hours and the apparent volume of distribution is 1.5 L/kg. The drug is supplied in 30-mL ampules at a concentration of 15 mg/mL. The desired steady-state serum concentration for this antibiotic is 20 mg/mL.

a. What infusion rate (R) would you suggest for this patient?

b. What loading dose would you suggest for this patient?

c. If the manufacturer suggests a starting infusion rate of 0.2 mL/h/kg of body weight, what is the expected steady-state serum concentration in this patient?

d. You would like to verify that this patient received the proper infusion rate. At what time after the start of the IV infusion would you take a blood sample to monitor the serum antibiotic concentration? Why?

e. Assume that the serum antibiotic concentration was measured and found to be higher than anticipated. What reasons, based on sound pharmacokinetic principles, would account for this situation?

14. Nomograms are frequently used in lieu of pharmacokinetic calculations to determine an appropriate drug dosage regimen for a patient. Discuss the advantages and disadvantages for using nomograms to calculate a drug dosage regimen.

15. Based on the following pharmacokinetic data for drugs A, B, and C: **(a)** Which drug takes the longest time to reach steady state? **(b)** Which drug would achieve the highest steady-state drug concentration? **(c)** Which drug has the largest apparent volume of distribution?

	Drug A	Drug B	Drug C
Rate of infusion (mg/h)	10	20	15
k (h^{-1})	0.5	0.1	0.05
Cl (L/h)	5	20	5

16. The effect of repetitive administration of phenytoin (PHT) on the single-dose pharmacokinetics of primidone (PRM) was investigated by Sato et al (1992) in three healthy male subjects. The peak concentration of unchanged PRM was achieved at 12 and 8 hours after the administration of PRM in the absence and the presence of PHT, respectively. The elimination half-life of PRM was decreased from 19.4 ± 2.2 (mean ± SE) to 10.2 ± 5.1 hours ($p < 0.05$), and the total body clearance was increased from 24.6 ± 3.1 to 45.1 ± 5.1 mL/h/kg ($p < 0.01$) in the presence of PHT. No significant change was observed for the apparent volume of distribution between the two treatments. Based on pharmacokinetics of the two drugs, what are the possible reasons for phenytoin to reduce primidone elimination half-life and increase its renal clearance?

17. Itraconazole (Sporanox, Janssen) is a lipophilic drug with extensive lipid distribution. The drug levels in fatty tissue and organs contain 2–20 times the drug levels in the plasma. Little or no drug was found in the saliva and in the cerebrospinal fluid, and the half-life is 64 ± 32 hours. The drug is 99.8% bound. How do (a) plasma drug–protein binding, (b) tissue drug distribution, and (c) lipid tissue partitioning contribute to the long elimination half-life for itraconazole?

18. JL (29-year-old man, 180 kg) received oral ofloxacin 400 mg twice a day for presumed bronchitis due to *Streptococcus pneumoniae*. His other medications were the following: 400 mg cimetidine, orally, 3 times a day; 400 mg metronidazole, as directed. JL was still having a fever of 100.1°C a day after taking the quinolone antibiotic. Comment on any appropriate action.

ANSWERS

Frequently Asked Questions

Can therapeutic drug monitoring be performed without taking blood samples?

- Therapeutic drug monitoring (TDM) may be performed by sampling other biologic fluids, such as saliva or, when available, tissue or ear fluids. However, the sample must be correlated to blood or special tissue level. Urinary drug concentrations generally are not reliable. Saliva is considered an ultrafiltrate of plasma and does not contain significant albumin. Saliva drug concentrations represent free plasma drug levels and have been used with limited success to monitor some drugs.
  Pharmacodynamic endpoints such as prothrombin clotting time for warfarin, blood glucose concentrations for antidiabetic drugs, blood pressure for antihypertensive drugs, and other clinical observations are useful indications that the drug is dosed correctly.

What are the major considerations in therapeutic drug monitoring?

- The major considerations in TDM include the pathophysiology of the patient, the blood sample collection, and the data analysis. Clinical assessment of patient history, drug interaction, and demographic factors are all part of a successful program for therapeutic drug monitoring.

What is meant by population pharmacokinetics? What advantages does population pharmacokinetics have over classical pharmacokinetics?

- Most pharmacokinetic models require well-controlled studies in which many blood samples are taken from each subject and the pharmacokinetic parameters estimated. In patient care situations, only a limited number of blood samples is collected, which does not allow for the complete determination of the drug's pharmacokinetic profile in the individual patient. However, the data from blood samples taken from a large demographic sector are more reflective of the disease states and pharmacogenetics of the patients treated. Population pharmacokinetics allow data from previous patients to be used in addition to the limited blood sample from the individual patient. The type of information obtained is less constrained and is sometimes dependent on the model and algorithm used for analysis. However, many successful examples have been reported in the literature.

Why is it possible to estimate individual pharmacokinetic parameters with just a few data points using the Bayesian method?

- With the Bayesian approach, the estimates of patient parameters are constrained more narrowly, to allow easier parameter estimation based on information provided from the population. The information is then combined with one or more serum concentrations from the patient to obtain a set of final patient parameters (generally Cl and V_D). When no serum sample is taken, the Bayesian approach is reduced to *a priori* model using only population parameters.

Why is pharmacokinetics important in studying drug interactions?

- Pharmacokinetics provides a means of studying whether an unusual drug action is related to pharmacokinetic factors, such as drug disposition, distribution, or binding, or is related to pharmacodynamic interaction, such as a difference in receptor sensitivity, drug tolerance, or some other reason. Many drug interactions involving enzyme inhibition, stimulation, and protein binding were discovered as a result of pharmacokinetic, pharmacogenetic, and pharmacodynamic investigations.

Learning Questions

1. Steady-state drug concentrations are achieved in approximately 5 half-lives. For a drug with a half-life of 36 hours, steady-state drug

concentrations are achieved in approximately 180 hours (or 7.5 days). Thus, dose adjustment in patients is difficult for drugs with very long half-lives. In contrast, steady-state drug concentrations are achieved in approximately 20–30 hours (or 1 day) for drugs whose half-lives are 4–6 hours.

2. $C_{max}^{\infty} = \dfrac{D_0}{V_D}\left(\dfrac{1}{1-e^{-k\tau}}\right)$

$C_{max}^{\infty} = \dfrac{250,000}{42,000}\left(\dfrac{1}{1-e^{-(6)(1.034)}}\right)$

$C_{max}^{\infty} = \dfrac{250,000}{42,000}\left(\dfrac{1}{0.998}\right) = 5.96\ \mu g/mL$

At steady state, the peak concentration of penicillin G will be 5.96 μg/mL.

3. $C_{av}^{\infty} = \dfrac{D}{kV_D\tau} = \dfrac{250,000}{(0.99)(20,000)(6)} = 2.10\ \mu g/mL$

Free drug concentration at steady state = 2.10 $(1-0.97) = 0.063\ \mu g/mL$.

4. $C_{av}^{\infty} = \dfrac{1.44 D_0 F t_{1/2}}{V_D\tau}$

For the Normal Patient:

$V_D = (0.392)(1)(1000) = 392\ mL/kg$

$C_{av}^{\infty} = \dfrac{(1.44)(D_0)(1)(1.49)}{(392)(6)} = 2\ \mu g/mL$

$D_0 = \dfrac{(392)(6)(2)}{(1.44)(1.49)} = 2192\ \mu g/kg = 2.2\ mg/kg$

For the Uremic Patient:

$V_D = (23.75)(1)(1000) = 237.5\ mL/kg$

$C_{av}^{\infty} = \dfrac{(1.44)(D_0)(1)(6.03)}{(237.5)(6)} = 2\ \mu g/mL$

$D_0 = \dfrac{(2)(237.5)(6)}{(1.44)(6.03)} = 328.2\ \mu g/mL$

$= 0.3\ mg/kg$

5. a.

Dose = 0.5×10^6 ng

$C_{av}^{\infty} = \dfrac{(1.44)(DFt_{1/2})}{V_D\tau}$

$= \dfrac{(1.44)(0.5\times 10^6)(0.56)(0.95)}{(306,000)(1)}$

$= 1.25\ ng/mL$

b. The patient is adequately dosed.

c. $F = 1$; using the above equation, the C_{av}^{∞} is 2.2 ng/mL; although still effective, the C_{av}^{∞} will be closer to the toxic serum concentration of 3 ng/mL.

6. The Cl_{Cr} for this patient shows normal kidney function.

$t_{1/2} = 2\ h \quad k = 0.693/2 = 0.3465\ h^{-1}$
$V_D = 0.2\ L/kg \times 80\ kg = 16\ L$

a. $C_{max}^{\infty} = \dfrac{D_0/V_D}{1-e^{-k\tau}} = \dfrac{250/16}{1-e^{-(0.3465)(8)}} = 16.68\ mg/L$

$C_{min}^{\infty} = C_{max}^{\infty}e^{-k\tau} = 16.68e^{-(0.3465)(8)} = 1.04\ mg/L$

The dosage regimen of 250 mg every 8 hours gives a C_{max}^{∞} above 16 mg/L and a C_{min}^{∞} below 2 mg/L. Therefore, this dosage regimen is not correct.

b. Several trials might be necessary to obtain a more optimal dosing regimen. One approach is to change the dosage interval, τ, to 6 hours and to calculate the dose, D_0:

$D_0 = C_{max}^{\infty}V_D(1-e^{-k\tau})$
$= (16)(16)(1-e^{-(0.3465)(6)}) = 224\ mg$

$C_{min}^{\infty} = C_{max}^{\infty}e^{-k\tau} = 16e^{-(0.3465)(6)} = 2\ mg/L$

A dose of 224 mg given every 6 hours should achieve the desired drug concentrations.

10. Assume desired $C_{av}^{\infty} = 0.0015\ \mu g/mL$ and $\tau = 24\ h$.

$C_{av}^{\infty} = \dfrac{FD_0 1.44 t_{1/2}}{V_D\tau}$

$D_0 = \dfrac{C_{av}^{\infty}V_D\tau}{F 1.44 t_{1/2}}$

$D_0 = \dfrac{(0.0015)(4)(68)(24)}{(0.80)(1.44)(30)} = 0.283\ mg$

Give 0.283 mg every 24 hours.

a. For a dosage regimen of one 0.30-mg tablet daily

$$C_{av}^{\infty} = \frac{(0.80)(0.3)(1.44)(30)}{(4)(68)(24)} = 0.0016 \,\mu g/mL$$

which is within the therapeutic window.

b. A dosage regimen of 0.15 mg every 12 hours would provide smaller fluctuations between C_{max}^{∞} and C_{min}^{∞} compared to a dosage regimen of 0.30 mg every 24 hours.

c. Since the elimination half-life is long (30 hours), a loading dose is advisable.

$$D_L = D_m \left(\frac{1}{1-e^{-k\tau}} \right)$$

$$D_L = 0.30 \left(\frac{1}{1-e^{-(0.693/30)(24)}} \right) = 0.70 \text{ mg}$$

For cardiotonic drugs related to the digitalis glycosides, it is recommended that the loading dose be administered in several portions with approximately half the total as the first dose. Additional fractions may be given at 6- to 8-hour intervals, with careful assessment of the clinical response before each additional dose.

d. There is no rationale for a controlled-release drug product because of the long elimination half-life of 30 hours inherent in the drug.

11. a. $C_{av}^{\infty} = \dfrac{FD_0 1.44 t_{1/2}}{V_D \tau}$

$$C_{av}^{\infty} = \frac{(1500)(1.44)(6)}{(1.3)(63)(4)} = 39.6 \,\mu g/mL$$

b. $D_L = D_M \left(\dfrac{1}{1-e^{-k\tau}} \right)$

c. A D_L of 4.05 g is needed, which is equivalent to 8 tablets containing 0.5 g each.

d. The time to achieve 95%–99% of steady state is, approximately, $5t_{1/2}$ without a loading dose. Therefore,

$$5 \times 6 = 30 \text{ h}$$

12. a. $C_{ss} = \dfrac{R}{kV_D}$ $R = C_{ss}kV_D$

$$R = (5)\left(\frac{0.693}{2} \right)(0.173)(75) = 22.479 \text{ mg/h}$$

$$D_L = C_{ss}V_D = (5)(0.173)(75) = 64.875 \text{ mg}$$

b.
$$\frac{R_{old}}{C_{ss,\,old}} = \frac{R_{new}}{C_{ss,\,new}}$$

$$\frac{22.479}{2} = \frac{R_{new}}{5} \qquad R_{new} = 56.2 \text{ mg/h}$$

c. $4.32 t_{1/2} = 4.32 \,(2) = 8.64 \text{ h}$

13. $t_{1/2} = 8 \text{ h} \quad k = 0.693/8 = 0.0866 \text{ h}^{-1}$

$$V_D = (1.5 \text{ L/kg})\,(75 \text{ kg}) = 112.5 \text{ L}$$

$$C_{ss} = 20 \,\mu g/mL$$

a. $R = C_{ss}V_D = (20)(0.0866)(112.5)$

$$= 194.85 \text{ mg/h}$$

b. $D_L = C_{ss}V_D = (20)\,(112.5) = 2250 \text{ mg}$
Alternatively, $D_L = R/k = 194.85/0.0866 = 2250$ mg

c. 0.2 mL of a 15-mg/mL solution contains 3 mg.

$$R = 3 \text{ mg/h/kg} \times 75 \text{ kg} = 225 \text{ mg/h}$$

$$C_{ss} = \frac{R}{kV_D} = \frac{225}{(0.0866)(112.5)} = 23.1 \text{ mg/L}$$

The proposed starting infusion rate given by the manufacturer should provide adequate drug concentrations.

REFERENCES

Abernethy DR: Drug therapy in the elderly. In Atkinson AJ, Daniels C, Dedrick R, et al (eds). *Principles of Clinical Pharmacology.* New York, Academic, 2001, Chap 24.

Abernethy DR, Greenblatt DJ: Pharmacokinetics of drugs in obesity. *Clin Pharmacokinet* **7:**108–124, 1982.

Barnett, M, Frank J, Wehring, H, et al: Analysis of pharmacist-provided medication therapy management (MTM) services in community pharmacies over 7 years. *J Manag Care Pharm* **15**(1):18–31, 2009.

Bartelink IH, Rademaker CMA, Schobben AFAM, van den Anker JN: Guidelines on paediatric dosing on the basis of developmental physiology and pharmacokinetic considerations. *Clin Pharmacokinet* **45**(11):1077–1097, 2006.

Beal SL, Sheiner LB: The NONMEM system, AM. *Statistics* **34:**118–119, 1980.

Beal SL, Sheiner LB: Methodology of population pharmacokinetics. In Garrett ER, Hirtz JL (eds). *Drug Fate and Metabolism: Methods and Techniques,* Vol 5. New York, Marcel Dekker, 1985.

Blouin RA, Warren GW: Pharmacokinetic considerations in obesity. *J Pharm Sci* **88:**1–7, 1999.

Czerwinski AW, Pederson JA: Pharmacokinetics of cefamandole in patients with renal impairment. *Antimicrob Agents Chemother* **15:**161–164, 1979.

D'Argenio DZ, Schumitzky A: A program package for simulation and parameter estimation in pharmacokinetic systems. *Comput Prog Biomed* **9:**115–134, 1979.

DeHaan RM, Metzler CM, Schellenberg D, et al: Pharmacokinetic study of clindamycin hydrochloride in humans. *Int J Clin Pharmacol Biopharm* **6:**105–119, 1972.

Erikson LO, Wahlin Boll-E, Odar Cederlof I, Lindholm L, Melander A: Influence of renal failure, rheumatoid arthritis and old age on the pharmacokinetics of diflunisal. *Eur J Clin Pharmacol* **36**(2):165–174, 1989.

Evans WE, Schentag JJ, Jusko WJ: *Applied Pharmacokinetics. Principles of Therapeutic Drug Monitoring.* San Francisco, Applied Therapeutics, 1992.

FDA Guidance for Industry: Population Pharmacokinetics, 1999.

FDA Guidance for Industry: E11 Clinical Investigation of Medicinal Products in the Pediatric Population. ICH, December, 2000.

Green B, Duffull SB. What is the best descriptor to use for pharmacokinetic studies in the obese? *Br J Clin Pharmacol* **8:** 119–133, 2004.

Greenblatt DJ: Predicting steady state serum concentration of drugs. *Annu Rev Pharmacol Toxicol* **19:**347–356, 1979.

Guidance for Industry: Bioequivalence Requirements: Critical Dose Drugs, Minister of Health, Therapeutic Products Directorate (TPD, 2006-05-31 (http://www.hc-sc.gc.ca/dhp-mps /alt_formats/pdf/prodpharma/applic-demande/guide-ld/bio /critical_dose_critique-eng.pdf).

Hansten PD, Hayton WI: Effect of antacid and ascorbic acid on serum salicylate concentration. *J Clin Pharmacol* **20:** 326–331, 1980.

Haverkos HW, Amsel Z, Drotman DP: Adverse virus–drug interactions. *Rev Infect Dis* **13:**697–704, 1991.

Heden B, Ohlsson M, Rittner R, et al: Agreement between artificial neural networks and experienced electrocardiographer on electrocardiographic diagnosis of healed myocardial infarction. *J Am Coll Cardiol* **28**(4): 1012–1016, 1996.

Hedman A, Angelin B, Arvidsson A, et al: Digoxin–verapamil interaction: Reduction of biliary but not renal digoxin clearance in humans. *Clin Pharmacol Ther* **49**(3):256–262, 1991.

Hendeles L, Weinberger M: Avoidance of adverse effects during chronic therapy with theophylline. *Drug Intell Clin Pharm* **14:**523, 1980.

Hurley SF, McNeil JF: A comparison of the accuracy of a least-squares regression, a Bayesian, Chiou's and the steady state clearance method of individualizing theophylline dosage. *Clin Pharmacokinet* **14:**311–320, 1988.

Iafrate RP, Glotz VP, Robinson JD, Lupkiewicz SM: Computer simulated conversion from intravenous to sustained-release oral theophylline drug. *Intell Clin Pharm* **16:**19–25, 1982.

Ingram PR, Lye DC, Tambyah PA, et al: Risk factors for nephrotoxicity associated with continuous vancomycin infusion in outpatient parenteral antibiotic therapy. *J Antimicrob Chemother* **62:**168–71, 2008.

Izzo AA, Ernst E: Interactions between herbal medicines and prescribed drugs: An updated systematic review. *Drugs* **69**(13):1777–1798, 2009.

Landahl S, Edgar B, Gabrielsson M, et al: Pharmacokinetics and blood pressure effects of felodipine in elderly hypertensive patients–A comparison with the young healthy subjects. *Clin Pharmacokinet* **14:**374–383, 1988.

Leeder JS, Kearns GL, Spielberg, SP, Anker JV: Understanding the relative roles of pharmacogenetics and ontogeny in pediatric drug development and regulatory science. *J Clin Pharmacol* **50**(12):1377–1387, 2010.

Lima DR, Santos RM, Werneck E, Andrade GN: Effect of orally administered misoprostol and cimetidine on the steady-state pharmacokinetics of diazepam and nordiazepam in human volunteers. *Eur J Drug Metab Pharmacokinet* **16**(3):61–70, 1991.

Lindeman RD: Changes in renal function with aging. Implications for treatment. *Drugs Aging* **2:**423–431, 1992.

Lindeman RD, Tobin J, Shock NW: Longitudinal studies on the rate of decline in renal function with age. *J Am Geriatr Soc* **33:**278–285, 1985.

Loi CM, Parker BM, Cusack BJ: Aging and drug interactions. III. Individual and combined effects of cimetidine and cimetidine and ciprofloxacin on theophylline metabolism in healthy male and female nonsmokers. *J Pharmacol Exp Ther* **280**(2): 627–637, 1997.

Ludden TM, Beal SL, Sheiner LB: Comparison of the Akaike Information Criterion, the Schwarz criterion and the *F* test as guides to model selection. *J Pharmacokinet Biopharm* **22**(5):431–445, 1994.

Mather LE: Anatomical-physiological approaches in pharmacokinetics and pharmacodynamics. *Clin Pharmacokinet* **40**: 707–22, 2001.

Mawer GE: Computer assisted prescribing of drugs. *Clin Pharmacokinet* **1**:67–78, 1976.

Mayersohn M: Pharmacokinetics in the elderly. *Environ Health Perspect Suppl* **102**(s11), 1994 (http://ehp.niehs.nih.gov/members /1994/Suppl-11/mayersohn-full.html).

Medicare Prescription Drug, Improvement, and Modernization Act of 2003 (/www.fda.gov/ohrms/dockets/dockets/04s0170 /04s-0170-bkg0001-108s1013.pdf).

Mentre F, Gomeni R: A two-step iterative algorithm for estimation in nonlinear mixed-effect models with an evaluation in population pharmacokinetics. *J Biopharm Stat* **5**(2):141–158, 1995.

National Institutes of Health, National Heart, Lung and Blood Institute: Clinical guidelines on the identification, evaluation and treatment of overweight and obesity in adults: The evidence report, 2003 (www.nhlb.nih.gov/obesity/ob-home.htm).

Norton K, Ingram PR, Heath CH, Manning L: Risk factors for nephrotoxicity in patients receiving outpatient continuous infusions of vancomycin in an Australian tertiary hospital. *J Antimicrob Chemother* **69**:805–8, 2014.

Okuno H, Takasu M, Kano H, Seki T, Shiozaki Y, Inoue K: Depression of drug metabolizing activity in the human liver by interferon-beta. *Hepatology* **17**(1):65–69, 1993.

Pedersen FM, Hamberg O, Hess K, Ovesen L: The effect of dietary vitamin K on warfarin-induced anticoagulation. *J Intern Med* **229**:517–20, 1991.

Perucca E, Gatti G, Cipolla G, et al: Inhibition of diazepam metabolism by fluvoxamine: A pharmacokinetic study in normal volunteers. *Clin Pharmacol Ther* **56**(5):471–476, 1994.

Regamey C, Gordon RC, Kirby WMM: Comparative pharmacokinetics of tobramycin and gentamicin. *Clin Pharmacol Ther* **14**:396–403, 1973.

Sato J, Sekizawa Y, Yoshida A, et al: Single-dose kinetics of primidone in human subjects: Effect of phenytoin on formation and elimination of active metabolites of primidone, phenobarbital and phenylethylmalonamide. *J Pharmacobiodyn* **15**(9): 467–472, 1992.

Schellens JH, Ghabrial H, van-der-Wart HH, Bakker EN, Wilkinson GR, Breimer DD: Differential effects of quinidine on the disposition of nifedipine, sparteine, and mephenytoin in humans. *Clin Pharmacol Ther* **50**(5 pt 1):520–528, 1991.

Schmucker DL: Aging and drug disposition: An update. *Pharmacol Rev* **37**:133–148, 1985.

Schumacher GE: Choosing optimal sampling times for therapeutic drug monitoring. *Clin Pharm* **4**:84–92, 1985.

Schumacher GE: *Therapeutic Drug Monitoring.* Norwalk, CT, Appleton & Lange, 1995.

Schumacher GE, Barr JT: Applying decision analysis in therapeutic drug monitoring: Using decision trees to interpret serum theophylline concentrations. *Clin Pharm* **5**:325–333, 1986.

Sheiner LB, Beal SL: Bayesian individualization of pharmacokinetics. Simple implementation and comparison with non-Bayesian methods. *J Pharm Sci* **71**:1344–1348, 1982.

Sheiner LB, Ludden TM: Population pharmacokinetics/dynamics. *Annu Rev Pharmacol Toxicol* **32**:185–209, 1992.

Smith BP, Brier ME: Statistical approach to neural network model building for gentamicin peak predictions. *J Pharm Sci* **85**(1):65–69, 1996.

Spapen HD, Janssen van Doorn K, Diltoer M, et al: Retrospective evaluation of possible renal toxicity associated with continuous infusion of vancomycin in critically ill patients. *Ann Intensive Care* **1**:26, 2011.

Spence JD: Drug interactions with grapefruit: Whose responsibility is it to warn the public? *Clin Pharmacol Ther* **61**: 395–400, 1997.

Stein GE, Haughey DB, Ross RJ, Vakoutis J: Conversion from intravenous to oral dosing using sustained release theophylline tablets. *Clin Pharm* **1**:772–773, 1982.

Thomson AH, Whiting B: Bayesian parameter estimation and population pharmacokinetics. *Clin Pharmacokinet* **22**(6): 447–467, 1992.

Upton RN: Regional pharmacokinetics, I. Physiological and physicochemical basis. *Biopharm Drug Disp* **11**:647–662, 1990.

Vozeh S, Wenk M, Follath F: Experience with NONMEM: Analysis of serum concentration data in patients treated with mexiletine and lidocaine. *Drug Metab Rev* **15**:305–315, 1984.

West JR, Smith HW, Chasis H: Glomerular filtration rate, effective blood flow and maximal tubular excretory capacity in infancy. *J Pediatr* **32**:10, 1948.

Whiting B, Kelman AW, Grevel J: Population pharmacokinetics: Theory and clinical application. *Clin Pharmacokinet* **11**: 387–401, 1986.

Whiting B, Niven AA, Kelman AW, Thomson AH: A Bayesian kinetic control strategy for cyclosporin in renal transplantation. In D'Argenio DZ (ed). *Advanced Methods of Pharmacokinetic and Pharmacodynamic Systems Analysis.* New York, Plenum, 1991.

BIBLIOGRAPHY

Abernethy DR, Azarnoff DL: Pharmacokinetic investigations in elderly patients. Clinical and ethical considerations. *Clin Pharmacokinet* **19**:89–93, 1990.

Abernethy DR, Greenblatt DJ, Divoll M, et al: Alterations in drug distribution and clearance due to obesity. *J Pharmacol Exp Ther* **217**:681–685, 1981.

Anderson KE: Influences of diet and nutrition on clinical pharmacokinetics. *Clin Pharmacokinet* **14**:325–346, 1988.

Aranda JV, Stern L: Clinical aspects of developmental pharmacology and toxicology. *Pharmacol Ther* **20**:1–51, 1983.

Atkinson AJ, Daniels CE, Dedrick RL, Grudzinskas CV, Markey SP: *Principles of Clinical Pharmacology.* New York, Academic, 2001.

Bartelink IH, Rademaker CMA, Schobben AFAM, van den Anker JN: Guidelines on paediatric dosing on the basis of developmental physiology and pharmacokinetic considerations. *Clin Pharmacokinet* **45**(11): 1077–1097, 2006.

Beal SL: *NONMEM Users Guide VII: Conditional Estimation Methods*. San Francisco, NONMEM Project Group, University of California, San Francisco, 1992.

Benet LZ (ed): *The Effect of Disease States on Drug Pharmacokinetics*. Washington, DC, American Pharmaceutical Association, 1976.

Benowitz NL, Meister W: Pharmacokinetics in patients with cardiac failure. *Clin Pharmacokinet* **1**:389–405, 1976.

Besunder JB, Reed MD, Blumer JL: Principles of drug biodisposition in the neonate: A critical evaluation of the pharmacokinetic–pharmacodynamic interface, Part I. *Clin Pharmacokinet* **14**:189–216, 1988.

Chiou WL, Gadalla MAF, Pang GW: Method for the rapid estimation of total body clearance and adjustment of dosage regimens in patients during a constant-rate infusion. *J Pharmacokinet Biopharm* **6**:135–151, 1978.

Chrystyn H, Ellis JW, Mulley BA, Peak MD: The accuracy and stability of Bayesian theophylline predictions. *Ther Drug Monit* **10**:299–303, 1988.

Clinical Symposium on Drugs and the Unborn Child. *Clin Pharmacol Ther* **14**:621–770, 1973.

Crooks J, O'Malley K, Stevenson IH: Pharmacokinetics in the elderly. *Clin Pharmacokinet* **1**:280–296, 1976.

Crouthamel WG: The effect of congestive heart failure on quinidine pharmacokinetics. *Am Heart J* **90**:335, 1975.

DeVane CL, Jusko WJ: Dosage regimen design. *Pharmacol Ther* **17**:143–163, 1982.

Dimascio A, Shader RI: Drug administration schedules. *Am J Psychiatry* **126**:6, 1969.

Friis-Hansen B: Body-water compartments in children: Changes during growth and related changes in body composition. *Pediatrics* **28**:169–181, 1961.

Giacoia GP, Gorodisher R: Pharmacologic principles in neonatal drug therapy. *Clin Perinatol* **2**:125–138, 1975.

Gillis AM, Kates R: Clinical pharmacokinetics of the newer antiarrhythmic agents. *Clin Pharmacokinet* **9**:375–403, 1984.

Godley PJ, Black JT, Frohna PA, Garrelts JC: Comparison of a Bayesian program with three microcomputer programs for predicting gentamicin concentrations. *Ther Drug Monit* **10**:287–291, 1988.

Gomeni R, Pineau G, Mentre F: Population kinetics and conditional assessment of the optimal dosage regimen using the P-pharm software package. *Cancer Res* **14**:2321–2326, 1994.

Grasela TH, Sheiner LB: Population pharmacokinetics of procainamide from routine clinical data. *Clin Pharmacokinet* **9**:545, 1984.

Gross G, Perrier CV: Intrahepatic portasystemic shunting in cirrhotic patients. *N Engl J Med* **293**:1046, 1975.

Harnes HT, Shiu G, Shah VP: Validation of bioanalytical methods. *Pharm Res* **8**:421–426, 1991.

Holloway DA: Drug problems in the geriatric patient. *Drug Intell Clin Pharm* **8**:632–642, 1974.

Jaehde U, Sorgel F, Stephan U, Schunack W: Effect of an antacid containing magnesium and aluminum on absorption, metabolism, and mechanism of renal elimination of pefloxacin in humans. *Antimicrob Agents Chemother* **38**(5):1129–1133, 1994.

Jensen EH: Current concepts for the validation of compendial assays. *Pharm Forum* March–April:1241–1245, 1986.

Jusko WJ: Pharmacokinetic principles in pediatric pharmacology. *Pediatr Clin N Am* **19**:81–100, 1972.

Kamimori GH, Somani SM, Kawlton, et al: The effects of obesity and exercise on the pharmacokinetics of caffeine in lean and obese volunteers. *Eur J Clin Pharmacol* **31**:595–600, 1987.

Klotz U, Avant GR, Hoyumpa A, et al: The effects of age and liver disease on the disposition and elimination of diazepam in adult man. *J Clin Invest* **55**:347, 1975.

Krasner J, Giacoia GP, Yaffe SJ: Drug–protein binding in the newborn infant. *Ann NY State Acad Sci* **226**:102–114, 1973.

Kristensen M, Hansen JM, Kampmann J, et al: Drug elimination and renal function. *Int J Clin Pharmacol Biopharm* **14**:307–308, 1974.

Latini R, Bonati M, Tognoni G: Clinical role of blood levels. *Ther Drug Monit* **2**:3–9, 1980.

Latini R, Maggioni AP, Cavalli A: Therapeutic drug monitoring of antiarrhythmic drugs. Rationale and current status. *Clin Pharmacokinet* **18**:91–103, 1990.

Lehmann K, Merten K: Die Elimination von Lithium in Abhängigkeit vom Lebensalten bei Gesunden und Niereninsuffizienten. *Int J Clin Pharmacol Biopharm* **10**:292–298, 1974.

Levy G (ed): *Clinical Pharmacokinetics: A Symposium*. Washington, DC, American Pharmaceutical Association, 1974.

Ludden TM: Population pharmacokinetics. *J Clin Pharmacol* **28**:1059–1063, 1988.

Matzke GR, St Peter WL: Clinical pharmacokinetics 1990. *Clin Pharmacokinet* **18**:1–19, 1990.

Maxwell GM: Paediatric drug dosing. Body weight versus surface area. *Drugs* **37**:113–115, 1989.

Meister W, Benowitz NL, Melmon KL, Benet LZ: Influence of cardiac failure on the pharmacokinetics of digoxin. *Clin Pharmacol Ther* **23**:122, 1978.

Mentre F, Pineau G, Gomeni R: Population kinetics and conditional assessment of the optimal dosage regimen using the P-Pharm software package. *Anticancer Res* **14**:2321–2326, 1994.

Morley PC, Strand LM: Critical reflections on therapeutic drug monitoring. *J Pharm Pract* **2**:327–334, 1989.

Morselli PL: Clinical pharmacokinetics in neonates. *Clin Pharmacokinet* **1**:81–98, 1976.

Mungall DR: *Applied Clinical Pharmacokinetics*. New York, Raven, 1983.

Neal EA, Meffin PJ, Gregory PB, Blaschke TF: Enhanced bioavailability and decreased clearance of analgesics in patients with cirrhosis. *Gastroenterology* **77**:96, 1979.

Niebergall PJ, Sugita ET, Schnaare RL: Potential dangers of common drug dosing regimens. *Am J Hosp Pharm* **31**:53–58, 1974.

Rane A, Sjoquist F: Drug metabolism in the human fetus and newborn infant. *Pediatr Clin N Am* **19**:37–49, 1972.

Rane A, Wilson JT: Clinical pharmacokinetics in infants and children. *Clin Pharmacokinet* **1:**2–24, 1976.

Richey DP, Bender DA: Pharmacokinetic consequences of aging. *Annu Rev Pharmacol Toxicol* **17:**49–65, 1977.

Roberts J, Tumer N: Age and diet effects on drug action. *Pharmacol Ther* **37:**111–149, 1988.

Rowland M, Tozer TN: *Clinical Pharmacokinetics Concepts and Applications.* Philadelphia, Lea & Febiger, 1980.

Schumacher GE, Barr JT: Pharmacokinetics in drug therapy. Bayesian approaches in pharmacokinetic decision making. *Clin Pharm* **3:**525–530, 1984.

Schumacher GE, Barr JT: Making serum drug levels more meaningful. *Ther Drug Monit* **11:**580–584, 1989.

Schumacher GE, Griener JC: Using pharmacokinetics in drug therapy II. Rapid estimates of dosage regimens and blood levels without knowledge of pharmacokinetic variables. *Am J Hosp Pharm* **35:**454–459, 1978.

Sheiner LB, Benet LZ: Premarketing observational studies of population pharmacokinetics of new drugs. *Clin Pharmacol Ther* **35:**481–487, 1985.

Sheiner LB, Rosenberg B, Marathe V: Estimation of population characteristics of pharmacokinetic parameters from routine clinical data. *J Pharmacokinet Biopharm* **9:**445–479, 1977.

Shirkey HC: Dosage (dosology). In Shirkey HC (ed). *Pediatric Therapy.* St. Louis, Mosby, 1975, pp 19–33.

Spector R, Park GD, Johnson GF, Vessell ES: Therapeutic drug monitoring. *Clin Pharmacol Ther* **43:**345–353, 1988.

Thompson PD, Melmon KL, Richardson JA, et al: Lidocaine pharmacokinetics in advanced heart failure, liver disease, and renal failure in humans. *Ann Intern Med* **78:**499–508, 1973.

Thomson AH: Bayesian feedback methods for optimizing therapy. *Clin Neuropharmacol* **15**(suppl 1, part A):245A–246A, 1992.

Uematsu T, Hirayama H, Nagashima S, et al: Prediction of individual dosage requirements for lignocaine. A validation study for Bayesian forecasting in Japanese patients. *Ther Drug Monit* **11:**25–31, 1989.

Vestel RE: Drug use in the elderly: A review of problems and special considerations. *Drugs* **16:**358–382, 1978.

Vonesh EF, Carter RL: Mixed-effects nonlinear regression for unbalanced repeated measures. *Biometrics* **48:**1–17, 1992.

Williams RW, Benet LZ: Drug pharmacokinetics in cardiac and hepatic disease. *Annu Rev Pharmacol Toxicol* **20:**289, 1980.

Winter ME: *Basic Clinical Pharmacokinetics.* San Francisco, Applied Therapeutics, 1980.

Yuen GJ, Beal SL, Peck CC: Predicting phenytoin dosages using Bayesian feedback. A comparison with other methods. *Ther Drug Monit* **5:**437–441, 1983.

23

Application of Pharmacokinetics to Specific Populations: Geriatric, Obese, and Pediatric Patients

S.W. Johnny Lau*, Lily K. Cheung, and
Diana Shu-Lian Chow

SPECIFIC AND SPECIAL POPULATIONS

The biggest issue in PK/PD and drug therapy is variability in response. Variability factors that affect pharmacokinetics and pharmacodynamics influence clinical trials and dose regimen designs. Early in drug development, the term "pharmacokinetics in disease states" was used to describe disease factors that affect PK. This term is concise but proved inadequate in the regulatory and clinical environment. The term "population" pharmacokinetics was then used to emphasize that the PD response can be quite different dependent on the demographic of the subjects. In the clinical trial and labeling environment, the term "specific populations" may be used to convey important specific medical conditions such as cancer or other pathophysiologic conditions that greatly influence the patient's outcome. The terms "specific" and "special" have been used in different occasions referring to different subject populations or patient conditions.

A population approach refers to the many factors that influence PK/PD as both intrinsic and extrinsic. Some of these factors were also discussed in Chapter 22. For example, PK differences in systemic exposure as a result of changes in age, gender, racial, weight, height, disease, genetic polymorphism, and organ impairment are well known clinically. These influences may be summarized as *intrinsic factors*.

Extrinsic factors summarize information associated with the patient environment. *Extrinsic factors* are quite numerous and diverse. Details are discussed in *International Conference on Harmonisation* (ICH–E5, http://ich.org/) for clinical trials and evaluations. Some examples that are referenced in this guidance include the medical environment, use of other drugs (interaction), tobacco, alcohol, and food habits.

*Disclaimer: The geriatric section of this chapter reflects the views and opinions of this author and does not represent the views and opinions of the Food and Drug Administration. This author declares no conflict of interest.

The term "specific populations" in this chapter is conveniently chosen to refer to populations that have important differences in pharmacokinetics due to age (pediatric, young adult, and elderly patients) or weight (obesity). Additional alterations in pharmacokinetics may occur due to renal impairment, hepatic impairment (Chapter 24), pregnancy, various pathophysiologic conditions, and drug–drug interactions discussed elsewhere.

This chapter focuses on three specific populations, which are divided into the following modules:

Module I   Application of Pharmacokinetics to the Geriatric Patients

Module II   Application of Pharmacokinetics to the Obese Patients

Modula III   Application of Pharmacokinetics to the Pediatric Patients

MODULE I: APPLICATION OF PHARMACOKINETICS TO THE GERIATRIC PATIENTS

Objectives

- List the demographic changes in the coming decades.
- Describe the effects of age on pharmacokinetics in older adults.
- Describe the effects of age on pharmacodynamics in older adults.
- Describe the confounders of pharmacokinetics and pharmacodynamics in older adults.
- Describe the emerging approaches to avoid adverse drug events in older adults.
- Describe the measures to help older adults adhere to taking their medications.
- Describe the emerging methods to study pharmacology in older adults.

Demographic Changes in the Coming Decades

The age group of 65 and over will be the fastest growing segment of the population in the United States for the next 4 decades due primarily to the migration of the Baby Boom generation into this age group. In 2050, the projected number of people in the United States aged 65 and over will be 88.5 million, more than double the population estimate of 40.2 million in 2010 (U.S. Census Bureau, 2010). Figure 23.1-1 shows the age distribution of the US population in the next 4 decades (U.S. Census Bureau, 2010).

This aging phenomenon is consistent with that of other countries like Canada, Denmark, France, Germany, Italy, Japan, and the United Kingdom (Christensen et al, 2009). Figure 23.1-2 shows the age distribution of the German population in the next 4 decades (Christensen et al, 2009).

Aging is a complex and multifactorial process that is an outcome of the accumulation of various functional deficits of multiorgan systems occurring over time at varying rates. No reliable biological marker for aging currently exists despite numerous research efforts. We rely on the chronological age to stratify the aging population. Due to the expected increase in the aging population, it may be advisable to divide the older population into 3 subgroups: young-old, age 65–75 years; old, age 75–85 years; and old-old, age ≥85 years, to better understand the processes and changes of aging as well as its impact on drug therapy (Klotz, 2008).

Drug therapy is an important medical intervention for the care of older patients. Persons aged 65 and older are the most medicated group of patients and receive the highest proportion of medications (Schwartz and Abernethy, 2009). Older patients usually have more disease burden and thus take multiple drug therapies that result in polypharmacy. Polypharmacy is commonly defined as the use of multiple medications or the use of a medication that is not indicated (Bushardt et al, 2008). Polypharmacy can cause multiple drug interactions and results in adverse drug events (Hilmer and Gnjidic, 2009).

Underrepresentation of the older population in clinical trials is very common across multiple therapeutic areas such as cancer, dementia, epilepsy, incontinence, transplantation, and cardiovascular disease. This underrepresentation phenomenon is also common to the pharmacokinetic and pharmacodynamic trials (Chien and Ho, 2011; Mangoni et al, 2013). Understanding the effect of aging on pharmacokinetics and pharmacodynamics is important since it can help maximize the therapeutic effects and minimize the adverse effects of medications for better care of older patients.

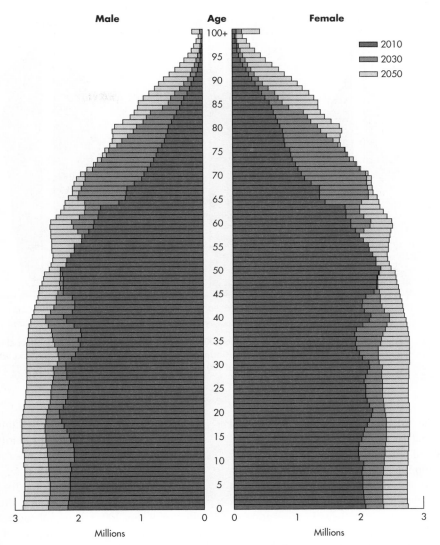

FIGURE 23.1-1   Age and sex structure of the population for the United States: 2010, 2030, and 2050. (U.S Census Bureau)

Effects of Age on Pharmacokinetics in Older Adults

Drug Absorption

Gastrointestinal. The most common route of drug administration is oral. Aging results in many physiological changes in the gastrointestinal tract such as increased gastric pH, delayed gastric emptying, decreased splanchnic blood flow, decreased absorption surface, and decreased gastrointestinal motility. Despite these changes, drug absorption upon oral administration does not appear to alter in advancing age especially for drugs that show passive diffusion-mediated absorption (Schwartz, 2007; Klotz, 2009).

Transdermal. The transdermal route of drug delivery has good potential for application in older patients since it is simple to use by the patients or their caregivers and may reduce adverse effects especially for the management of pain and neurological conditions that require sustained

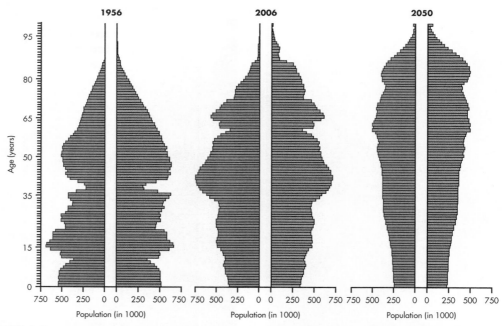

FIGURE 23.1-2   Population pyramids for Germany in 1956, 2006, and 2050. Horizontal bars are proportional to number of men (grey) and women (green). Data for 2050 are based on the German Federal Statistical Office's 1-W1 scenario, which assumes a roughly constant total fertility rate of 1.4, yearly net migration of 100,000 and life expectancy in 2050 reaching 83.5 years for men and 88.0 years for women. (Christensen et al, 2009)

effective plasma drug concentrations. Age-related changes in hydration and lipids result in increased barrier function of the stratum corneum for relatively hydrophilic compounds. Highly lipophilic chemicals may be able to dissolve readily into the stratum corneum even when the available lipid medium is reduced. No significant differences in absorption of drugs from transdermal delivery systems appear to exist between young and old individuals (Kaestli et al, 2008). Transdermal absorption of fentanyl was suggested to be reduced in the older patients resulting in dose adjustments, whereas transdermal absorption of buprenorphine is little affected because of age (Vadivelu and Hines, 2008). Nevertheless, more research is necessary to better understand how age-related changes in skin may affect transdermal drug absorption.

Subcutaneous. Subcutaneous drug absorption is through the vascular capillaries and lymphatic channels. Molecular size primarily determines the passage across the capillary endothelium. Polypeptides of less than about 5000 g/mole primarily pass through the capillary pathway, whereas those of greater than about 20,000 g/mole primarily enter blood via the lymphatic pathway (Rowland and Tozer, 2011). The skin blood supply and lymphatic drainage change with age (Ryan, 2004). Thus, subcutaneous absorption of drugs may be affected with aging and has clinical consequences. The subcutaneous route is of particular interest since it is the most common route of administration for therapeutic peptides and proteins, which become increasingly important in the therapeutic arena.

Pulmonary. Lung anatomy and physiology change with age. Older individuals show a decrease of the alveolar surface, a variation of lung elasticity, a decrease of the alveolar capillary volume combined with a decline of the ventilation/perfusion ratio, a decrease of the pulmonary diffusion capacity for carbon monoxide, and an increase of the pulmonary residual volume. Thus, age is an important parameter that affects the pharmacokinetics of inhaled drugs (Siekmeier and Scheuch, 2008).

In a study of young (18–45 years of age) and older (over 65 years) patients with type 2 diabetes, absorption was comparable among the 2 groups following a single inhalation of insulin but the older patients had less glucose reduction suggesting the need for higher doses in the older patients. There were no statistically significant differences for the mean insulin AUC and C_{max} values between the young and older patients (Henry et al, 2003). To the contrary, the concentrations of isoflurane and sevoflurane (inhalation anesthetic drugs) necessary to maintain adequate depth of anesthesia are less in older age (Matsuura et al, 2009).

There has been very little research for the pharmacokinetic and pharmacodynamic characteristics of new inhaled drugs in older patients and the effects of lung aging and copathologies are not known, particularly in the very old. Moreover, decrements in cognition, praxis, and executive function that are highly prevalent in frail older individuals have a profoundly detrimental effect on inhaler technique. Thus, it is likely that a large proportion of older patients may be unable to use drugs targeted for alveolar absorption because accurate and reliable inhalation performance may not be achievable. However, cognitively intact older individuals with good neurological, pulmonary, and musculoskeletal performance may be able to use inhaled treatments in the same manner as younger individuals (Allen, 2008).

Intramuscular. The intramuscular drug absorption is very similar to the subcutaneous drug absorption (Rowland and Tozer, 2011). Intramuscular absorption of the two benzodiazepines, diazepam and midazolam, does not appear to alter with older age (Divoll et al, 1988; Holazo et al, 1988). However, the effect of advancing age on the absorption of drugs upon intramuscular administration in older patients has not been adequately evaluated.

Ocular. Cornea shows decreases in permeability to a variety of compounds with different physicochemical properties between young and old rabbits (Ke et al, 1999). Human and rabbit eyes are very similar; their anatomical and physiological differences are well documented (Francoeur et al, 1983). Choroidal thickness becomes thinner with older age, whereas Bruch's membrane thickens with older age in humans. Thickness changes of choroid and Bruch's membrane may affect drug permeability from subconjunctiva or episcleral space into the retina and the vitreous (Kuno and Fujii, 2011). More research is necessary for better ocular drug delivery in older patients who suffer from age-related macular degeneration, cataract, glaucoma, and diabetic retinopathy (Harvey, 2003).

Drug Distribution

Factors such as plasma protein concentration, body composition, blood flow, tissue-protein concentration, and tissue fluid pH are important for drug distribution. Of these factors, the changes in plasma protein concentration and in body composition are the two major factors of aging on drug distribution (Mayersohn, 1994).

Albumin and α1-acid glycoprotein are the major drug binding proteins in plasma (see Chapter 11). In general, the blood albumin concentration is about 10% lower in older people but α1-acid glycoprotein is higher in older people (McLean and Le Couteur, 2004). These changes in plasma proteins are generally not due to aging itself but to the pathophysiological changes or disease states that may occur more frequently in older patients. Also these changes in plasma proteins may not affect the clinical exposure of a patient to a drug. Thus, no adjustments in dosing regimens may be necessary in general except in rare case of a drug with a high extraction ratio and narrow therapeutic index that is parenterally administered such as intravenous dosing of lidocaine or, rarer, a drug with a narrow therapeutic index that is administered orally and has a very rapid pharmacokinetic–pharmacodynamic equilibration time (Benet and Hoener, 2002).

In contrast to plasma protein binding, we know little about the binding processes of drugs with tissues and their responses to aging. This phenomenon may be due to the experimental difficulty to measure tissue binding *in vitro* without disrupting the integrity of the tissue and its protein content (Mayersohn, 1994).

With advancing age, the decrease in lean body mass includes a decrease in total body water. The total body water for an 80-year-old is 10%–20% lower than a 20-year-old (Vestal, 1997; Beaufrère and Morio, 2000). Thus, the distribution volume of hydrophilic drugs such as digoxin, theophylline, and aminoglycosides will decrease with aging (Shi and Klotz, 2011).

With advancing age, in contrast, body fat is 18%–36% higher in men and 33%–45% higher in women (Vestal, 1997; Beaufrère and Morio, 2000). This increase in body fat may provide partial explanation for the increase in volume of distribution for lipophilic drugs such as benzodiazepines (Greenblatt et al, 1991). Thus, plasma drug concentrations will decrease with equivalent doses in the absence of changes in drug elimination.

Assuming that the therapeutic goal is to achieve the same plasma drug concentration in the older patient, the changes in volume of distribution of a drug will only be relevant for drugs that are administered as single doses or for determining the loading doses of drugs in which the use of a loading dose is appropriate. For safety concerns, the loading doses of drugs or drugs for one-time use should generally be lower in older patients than younger patients. Thus, weight-based loading regimens should be routinely used (Schwartz, 2007).

Hepatic and Extrahepatic Drug Metabolism

Human liver, gastrointestinal tract, kidneys, lung, and skin contain quantitatively important amounts of enzymes for drug metabolism. However, almost all organs have some metabolic activity. *In vivo* drug metabolism usually consists of two processes, namely, the degradative and synthetic processes (also known as the Phase I and Phase II metabolism, respectively). Phase I metabolism is catalyzed by membrane-bound enzymes in the endoplasmic reticulum and Phase II metabolism occurs primarily in the cytosol, with the exception of the UDP-glucuronosyltransferases that are also bound to the endoplasmic reticulum membranes. Phase I metabolism is primarily catalyzed by enzymes of the cytochrome P450 monoxygenase system (CYP450), and the key members in this family of drug-metabolizing isozymes are CYP3A, CYP2D6, CYP2C9, CYP2C19, CYP1A2, CYP2B6, and CYP2E1.

In vitro data showed that the content and activities of various CYP isozymes from liver microsomal preparations did not decline with advancing age in the range of 10–85 years (Parkinson et al, 2004). Figure 23.1-3 shows the effects of age on CYP activities *in vitro* from nearly 150 samples of human liver microsomes (Parkinson et al, 2004). The samples represent 3 age groups, namely, <20 years, 20–60 years, and 60+ years. The liver microsomal CYP activity is highly variable but not significantly different in the CYP activities between the age group of 20–60 years and the age group of 60+ years (Parkinson et al, 2004).

Hepatic drug clearance via CYP metabolism that is studied for many drugs in older individuals is either unchanged or modestly decreased with reductions in clearance reported to be in the range of 10%–40%. These data usually originate from the young-old and old individuals, who were generally in good health. The clearance of two CYP3A substrates, amlodipine and erythromycin, was evaluated in the old and old-old frail as well as nursing home patients and was not changed compared to younger individuals in these patient groups (Kang et al, 2006; Schwartz, 2006). However, a study of old-old patients and nursing home residents showed that the oral clearance of atorvastatin, a CYP3A substrate, decreased in men (Schwartz and Verotta, 2009). A more recent study identified age as a significant factor in predicting the concentrations of atorvastatin for patients up to 86 years of age and recommended dose reduction (DeGorter et al, 2013). These observations are consistent with early pharmacokinetic studies that old age was associated with increased exposure of atorvastatin (Gibson et al, 1996).

Phase II drug metabolism does not seem to change with age based on the following studied reactions and prototype substrates (Benedetti et al, 2007):

- Glucuronidation—lorazepam, oxazepam, and acetaminophen
- Sulfation—acetaminophen
- Acetylation—isoniazid and procainamide

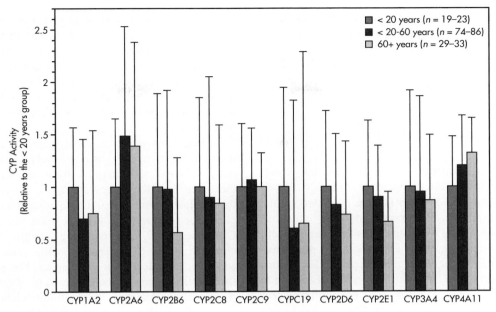

FIGURE 23.1-3   The effects of age on CYP activities *in vitro* with nearly 150 samples of human liver microsomes. The CYPC19 on the horizontal axis means CYP2C19.

No general approach has been developed to estimate age-related changes in hepatic and extrahepatic drug metabolism, perhaps partly because hepatic and extrahepatic drug metabolism processes are affected by complex and heterogeneous factors that involve genetic and environmental influences (Klotz, 2009).

The liver undergoes many changes with aging that includes reduction in blood flow and size of the liver. The reduction in blood flow suggests a reduction in clearance of high extraction ratio or nonrestrictively cleared drugs. It is more difficult to interpret the effect of changes in liver size on drug clearance (McLean and Le Couteur, 2004).

In general, the reduction of drug metabolism with advancing age appears modest.

Drug Excretion

Renal drug clearance is the most consistent and predictable age-related change in pharmacokinetics. Renal function including renal blood flow, glomerular filtration rate (GFR; measured as mean inulin clearance decreased from 122.8 to 65.3 mL/min/1.73 m² between 20 and 90 years of age in 70 men), and active renal tubular secretory processes, all decline with increasing age (Davies and Shock, 1950). Renal tubular reabsorption also decreases, at least measured as glucose reabsorption, and appears to parallel the decline in GFR (Miller et al, 1952).

Measured GFR is the best overall indicator of renal function but it is cumbersome to collect urine for extended period of time (24 hours) and is more prone to error of measurement. Diurnal variation in GFR and day-to-day variation in creatinine excretion may also contribute to the errors for GFR estimation with timed urine collection. Thus, the following two formulas are commonly used to estimate GFR based on serum creatinine:

The Cockcroft–Gault (CG) equation for creatinine clearance as GFR estimate (Cockcroft and Gault, 1976):

$$Cl_{cr} \text{ (mL/min)} = \frac{(140 - \text{age in years}) \times (\text{weight in kg})}{72 \times (\text{serum creatinine in mg/dL})}$$

$$(23.1.1)$$

For women, the Cl_{cr} estimate should be reduced by 15%.

The Modification of Diet in Renal Disease (MDRD) equation for GFR estimate (Levey et al, 2006):

GFR (mL/min/1.73 m²)
$$= 175 \times (\text{standardized serum creatinine})^{-1.154}$$
$$\times (\text{age})^{-0.203} \times (0.742 \text{ if female})$$
$$\times (1.212 \text{ if African American}) \qquad (23.1.1)$$

The CG equation-estimated creatinine clearance predicts a linear decrease with age that is steeper than the nonlinear decline predicted via the MDRD equation. Either one of these equations gives a reasonable estimate that is sufficiently accurate to determine drug dose for drugs that have predominant renal clearance. Extensive discussions for the merits of CG equation and MDRD equation to estimate renal function exist but with no clear resolution (Spruill et al, 2009; Stevens and Levey, 2009; Nyman et al, 2011). The major disadvantage of the MDRD equation is the limited information available on dosage adjustments as many of the age-adjusted recommendations are based on the CG equation. Both CG and MDRD equations were not derived from significant numbers of people over the age of 70 years, which may be the greatest limitation of these equations (Schwartz and Abernethy, 2009).

Serum creatinine concentration is a common endogenous glomerular filtration marker in clinical practice. Creatinine is predominantly produced from creatine and phosphocreatine in skeletal muscle with small contribution from ingestion of meat (Sandilands et al, 2013). Lean muscle mass declines at a rate of about 1% a year after 30 years of age with multiple causes (Morley et al, 2010). Creatinine is freely filtered at the glomerulus and is not reabsorbed, but up to 15% is actively secreted by the tubules (Traynor et al, 2006). For renally impaired patients, the age-associated decrease in creatinine production may significantly blunt an increase of serum creatinine concentration despite a marked decrease in the GFR and creatinine clearance. This is a particular issue with small women or in malnourished individuals whose creatinine production is well below normal (Perrone et al, 1992). Thus, serum creatinine concentration alone may lead to serious errors in assessing the severity of renal disease in the older population. A retrospective medical record review study showed that serum creatinine concentration is an inadequate screening test for renal failure in older patients as well as it leads to underinvestigation and underrecognition of renal failure in the older population (Swedko et al, 2003).

Drugs that are eliminated primarily via glomerular filtration, including aminoglycoside antibiotics, lithium, and digoxin, have an elimination clearance that decreases with age in parallel with the decline in measured or calculated creatinine clearance (Ljungberg and Nilsson-Ehle, 1987; Cusack et al, 1979; Sproule et al, 2000). The renal clearance of drugs undergoing active renal tubular secretion also decreases with aging. For example, the decrease in renal tubular secretion of cimetidine parallels the decrease in creatinine clearance in older patients (Drayer et al, 1982). Conversely, the ratios of renal drug clearance/creatinine clearance of both procainamide and N-acetylprocainamide decrease in the older patients, suggesting that with aging the renal tubular secretion of these drugs declines more rapidly than creatinine clearance (Reidenberg et al, 1980).

The Baltimore Longitudinal Study of Aging followed 254 healthy volunteers for up to 25 years and prospectively found that creatinine clearance via 24-hour urine collection decreased 0.75 mL/min/year (Lindeman et al, 1985). However, one-third of these participants had no decrease in creatinine clearance in about 20 years. Later studies showed that aging itself may have a minor effect on kidney function but the confounding factors such as hypertension and chronic heart diseases account for the decline of kidney function (Fliser et al, 1997a, 1997b). The recent Italian Longitudinal Study on Aging also showed that the age-related reduction of kidney function was associated with coexisting cardiovascular diseases and other risk factors (Baggio et al, 2005).

Age-Related Changes in Transporters

Transporters such as P-glycoprotein, organic anion transporting peptide, organic cation transporter, and organic anion transporter involve in drug absorption, distribution, metabolism, and excretion (see Chapters 11 and 12). However, very few published data exist for the effect of aging on the expression and function of drug transporters. P-glycoprotein is one of the better characterized drug transporters. The relatively few published articles so far provided conflicting results on the impact of advancing age on P-glycoprotein activity and expression (Mangoni, 2007). For example, an *ex vivo* uptake study of MDR1-encoded P-glycoprotein in leukocytes from healthy older and frail older participants as well as healthy young participants showed that aging and frailty had minor impact on this validated cellular P-glycoprotein model (Brenner and Klotz, 2004). However, a positron emission tomography study showed that older participants have significantly reduced P-glycoprotein function in the internal capsule and corona radiata white matter and in orbito-frontal regions, which may partly explain the vulnerability of aging brain to white matter degeneration (Bartels et al, 2009).

Effects of Age on Pharmacodynamics in Older Adults

Age-related pharmacokinetic changes are generally well characterized as discussed above. However, limited information exists for age-related changes in pharmacodynamics. This may be partly due to the relatively simpler bioanalytical methods that involve determining drug concentrations in serial samples of biomaterial versus the challenge to develop and validate appropriate measures of drug responses.

Majority of information for the age-related differences in human pharmacodynamics originate from cross-sectional studies. Cross-sectional studies assume that the mean differences observed between age groups reflect the change that occurs in study participants with the passage of time without directly observing the same participants in longitudinal studies. This assumption may be invalid because of the following (Bowie and Slattum, 2007; Trifirò and Spina, 2011):

- Difficulties to differentiate chronological age versus biological age or physiological effects versus pathological effects
- Selective mortality effects since the oldest study cohort includes only those participants who

survived to reach old age and these participants may be unique regarding the variable of interest

These limitations may prevent the generalizability of the results for the pharmacodynamic studies to the entire older population. Anyhow, longitudinal pharmacodynamic studies that measure individual rates of aging for the specified variable are rare.

The following are examples to illustrate the effect of aging on the pharmacodynamics of specific therapeutic areas. For more comprehensive listings, the readers can refer to other published articles (Bowie and Slattum, 2007; Trifirò and Spina, 2011; Corsonello et al, 2010).

Drugs That Act on the Central Nervous Systems

Benzodiazepines. Changes in pharmacodynamics rather than pharmacokinetics with increasing age can be more relevant to explain the altered response to benzodiazepines. Many studies documented a greater sensitivity to the clinical action of benzodiazepines in older people, which is not attributable to the differences in plasma concentrations, half-life, or apparent volume of distribution of drugs. The exact mechanisms responsible for the increased sensitivity to benzodiazepines with aging are unknown. No significant age-related differences in GABA receptor binding properties or GABA receptor number are observable, both in animal models (Bickford and Breiderick, 2000) and in humans (Sundman et al, 1997). Diazepam, flurazepam, flunitrazepam, nitraze, midazolam, and triazolam show age-related increase in sensitivity to cognitive and sedative effects of benzodiazepines in the absence of significant pharmacokinetic changes (Swift et al, 1985; Castleden et al, 1977; Greenblatt et al, 1981, 2004; Kanto et al, 1981; Albrecht et al, 1999).

Drugs That Act on the Cardiovascular System

Beta-adrenergic Receptors. Pharmacodynamic sensitivity to beta-adrenergic drugs declines with age. A reduced response to both agonist and antagonist of cardiac β_1 and bronchial β_2 receptors is observable (Vestal et al, 1979; Scott et al, 1995). These age-related changes in response to beta-adrenergic drugs are not attributable to reduced beta receptor density or affinity, but it may be the result of impaired signal transduction of beta receptor in older people (Doyle et al, 1982; Landmann et al, 1981). Beta-adrenoreceptors are coupled with Gs proteins, which in turn are linked to adenylate cyclase. Age-associated decreases in Gs activity are observed *in vitro* from human heart beta receptors (White et al, 1994). A downregulation of beta-adrenergic receptors may also explain the higher systemic drug concentration necessary with increasing age to reach the desired effect (Scarpace et al, 1991). The reduced beta receptor sensitivity does not imply the absence of safety issues for both beta agonists and beta antagonists in older patients. The risk–benefit ratio for the treatment of beta receptor antagonists needs careful evaluation because higher doses may be more effective but with safety concerns (Dobre et al, 2007).

Drugs That Act on Blood Clotting

Warfarin. Evidence exists of a greater inhibition of synthesis of vitamin K-dependent clotting factors at similar plasma warfarin concentrations in older patients than young patients. However, the exact mechanism of this age-related change in sensitivity is unknown. Age is one of the strongest predictors of the anticoagulant effects of warfarin (Miao et al, 2007; Schwartz, 2007).

Confounders of Pharmacokinetics and Pharmacodynamics in Older Adults

Factors such as pharmacogenetic polymorphisms, nutrition, concomitant medications, smoking, and drinking habits can influence the disposition and action of drugs in older patients. Another confounding factor for drug disposition and action in older patients can be frailty (Shi and Klotz, 2011; Sitar, 2012). Wynne reported that frailty may impair conjugation pathways (sulfation and glucuronidation) for metoclopramide (Wynne et al, 1993). However, the definition of frailty is still being developed. Nevertheless, frailty is associated with higher inflammatory markers such as C-reactive protein, interleukin-6, or tumor necrosis factor-alpha (Fried et al, 2009; Clegg et al, 2013).

The function of different neurotransmitters in dopaminergic, serotonergic, and cholinergic systems may be influenced not only by the aging process itself but also by the psychopathology of psychiatric disorders, including schizophrenia, depression, or dementia (Meltzer, 1999). Thus, the effects of psychotropic drugs in the older patients may differ between patients with and without these mental diseases.

The arrhythmogenic potential of antipsychotic and antidepressant drugs, which may lead to QTc interval prolongation as well as polymorphic ventricular tachycardia, torsade de pointes, and sudden cardiac death, is significantly higher in older patients with preexisting cardiovascular disease or who are treated with concomitant QTc prolonging drugs (Vieweg et al, 2009).

In general, the interindividual pharmacokinetic variability is prominent, which is usually due not only to the influence of age-related physiological changes but also to the impact of comorbidities and drug interactions (Shi and Klotz, 2011). Mallet et al recommend a multiprofessional team approach to manage drug interactions and optimize drug therapy in older patients (Mallet et al, 2007).

Effect of Age on Dosing the Older Adults

Based on the limited knowledge for the impact of aging on pharmacokinetic and pharmacodynamic properties, it is difficult to make definite dosage recommendations for older patients. The complex interactions among comorbidity, polypharmacy, changes in pharmacodynamic sensitivity, and relatively modest pharmacokinetic changes in the older patients warrant the dosing recommendation to follow the conventional wisdom of "start low and go slow" (Schwartz and Abernethy, 2009; Shi and Klotz, 2011).

Emerging Approaches to Avoid Adverse Drug Events in Older Adults

The Beers list (also known as Beers criteria) has been widely used as a reference for pharmacists and physicians in the United States to improve the use of medication in older patients. A gerontologist, Mark H. Beers, advocated the use of explicit criteria developed through consensus panels for identifying inappropriate use of medications in older patients.

The Beers list was originally developed for frail older individuals living in nursing homes. Subsequently, it was updated and expanded to include new medical conditions and generalized to the older population regardless of their frailty status or place of residence. The current Beers list is the fourth rendition after revision of the 1991, 1997, and 2003 editions (The American Geriatrics Society 2012 Beers Criteria Update Expert Panel, 2012). The Europeans also compiled a list that guides the prevention of inappropriate use of medications in older patients (Laroche et al, 2007). Some of Beers list's limitations were obsolete drugs, drug–drug interactions, and prescribing omission errors. There were also attempts to improve the limitations of Beers list such as the STOPP/START criteria (O'Mahony et al, 2010). STOPP and START stand for "Screening Tool of Older Persons' Prescriptions" and "Screening Tool to Alert doctors to Right Treatment."

An estimated one-third to more than one half of the most commonly prescribed medications for older patients have anticholinergic (conventional with published literature but antimuscarinic for pharmacological accuracy) effects (Tune et al, 1992; Chew et al, 2008). These anticholinergic effects have been linked with cognitive impairment in older patients (Cancelli et al, 2008). Drugs with sedative adverse effects are also of concern for older patients since these sedative effects can cause falls and bone fractures (Leipzig et al, 1999; Ensrud et al, 2002), which may further cause older patients to lose independence.

Scientists and clinicians have developed at least the following methods to quantitate the overall anticholinergic effects of medications for older patients:

- Serum anticholinergic activity
- Anticholinergic risk scale
- Drug burden index

Serum anticholinergic activity, as measured via a radioreceptor assay, quantifies a patient's overall anticholinergic burden caused by all drugs and their metabolites (Mulsant et al, 2003; Chew et al, 2008). Serum anticholinergic activity measurement is expensive and is not readily available to practitioners, and interpretation of the results in clinical practice is difficult (Bostock et al, 2010).

The anticholinergic risk scale method ranks medications for anticholinergic potential on a 3-point scale (0, no or low risk; 3, high anticholinergic potential). The anticholinergic risk scale score for a patient is the sum of points for the patient's number of medications (Rudolph et al, 2008). The list of rated medication was selected in 2005, so newer medications will not apply. No allowance is included for drug dosage or potentially important factors such as renal and hepatic function (Bostock et al, 2010).

The drug burden index method characterizes medications with respect to risk in two risk groups: (1) drugs with anticholinergic effects and (2) drugs with sedative effects. Medications with both anticholinergic and sedative effects were classified as anticholinergic (Hilmer et al, 2007, 2009). The following factors were used in the equation for total drug burden (TDB):

$$TDB = B_{AC} + B_s \qquad (23.1.3)$$

where B_{AC} and B_S each represent the linear additive sum of $D/(\delta + D)$ for every anticholinergic (AC) or sedative (S) drug to which the person is exposed, D is the daily dose taken by the person, and δ is the minimum efficacious daily dose (minimum daily dose approved by the Food and Drug Administration). Both prescription and over-the-counter drugs are included in the analysis. The major limitation of the drug burden index method is the lack of consideration for patient's factors such as renal and hepatic function, which may have major impact on the anticholinergic adverse effects and clinical outcomes (Bostock et al, 2010).

A recent article advocates the application of pharmacokinetic and pharmacodynamic mechanisms of anticholinergic drugs for safer use of these drugs in older patients (de Leon, 2011).

Measures to help Older Adults Adhere to Taking Their Medications

The errors of drug administration are high in many older patients, and these errors can cause both efficacy and safety concerns. Older patients may likely have the following unique set of needs for taking their medications:

- The ability to remember and organize the medications especially for multiple medications with different dosing regimens
- The reduced visual abilities to accurately measure the medications or to read the instruction on the label of medications
- Instability of their hands to hold medications
- Dexterity of their fingers to accurately measure the dose especially for liquid formulations or to open the medications' container

Scientists discussed measures such as organizer for medications, devices with improved visualization of graduation for measurement, eye-drop applicator, and deblistering machine for oral dosage forms in blister packs to help older patients adhere to taking their medications (Breitkreutz and Boos, 2007). Alternative formulations, delivery methods, and administration options for psychotropic medications may be necessary for older patients with behavioral and psychological symptoms of dementia (Muramatsu et al, 2010).

For the future, scientists, engineers, clinicians, and businesspersons need to work together to develop age-appropriate products that can better deliver the medications to meet older patients' needs.

Emerging Methods to Study Pharmacology in Older Adults

The current regulatory environment has the following two publications for the study of drugs in the older population:

- "Guideline for the Study of Drugs Likely to Be Used in the Elderly" published in November 1989 by the United States Food and Drug Administration (Food and Drug Administration, 1989)
- "Guideline for Industry: Studies in Support of Special Populations: Geriatrics" and "ICH Topic E7, Studies in Support of Special Populations: Geriatrics. Questions and Answers" published on August 1994 and July 2011, respectively, by the European Medicines Agency (European Medicines Agency, 1994, 2011)

Currently, the inclusion of older individuals in clinical trials of drugs under evaluation for registration in the United States is guided by the "Guideline for the Study of Drugs Likely to Be Used in the Elderly" published in November 1989. Approaches to clinical trial design have been further informed in Europe and the United States by the European Medicines Agency documents "Studies in Support of Special Populations: Geriatrics" and "ICH Topic E7, Studies in Support of Special Populations: Geriatrics. Questions and Answers." An underlying theme of these documents, as stated in the November 1989 Food and Drug Administration guideline, is that "drugs should be studied in all age groups, including the older population, for which they will have significant utility."

In 1997, the Food and Drug Administration established the Geriatric Use subsection, as a part of the PRECAUTIONS section, in the labeling for human prescription drugs to include more comprehensive information about the use of a drug or biological product in persons aged 65 years and older (Food and Drug Administration, 1997).

Population pharmacokinetic and pharmacodynamic approach with sparse sampling through covariate analysis in clinical efficacy and safety trials is an option to evaluate the effects of age on pharmacokinetics and pharmacodynamics. Some scientists refer this approach as the "top-down approach" (Tsamandouras et al, 2015). The population pharmacokinetic and pharmacodynamic approach is particularly suitable for the older patients since extensive blood sampling for the older patients may be too invasive and the studied patients more resemble the intended patient population than a dedicated pharmacokinetic or pharmacodynamic study that requires extensive blood sampling in rather healthy older participants. A recent example is the application of population pharmacokinetics to study participants living in the community and in nursing homes and found that advancing age (relevant only to men) and concomitant medications with cytochrome 3A4 inhibitors lowered the apparent clearance of orally administered atorvastatin (Schwartz and Verotta, 2009). The Food and Drug Administration has a guidance on the design, execution, and analysis of population pharmacokinetics (Food and Drug Administration, 1999).

Physiologically based pharmacokinetic modeling is another tool that has potential to study drug disposition and action in the older population (Rowland et al, 2011). Some scientists refer this approach as the "bottom-up" approach, which is more mechanistic in nature (Food and Drug Administration, 1997). Recent examples of the application of the physiologically based pharmacokinetic modeling approach include understanding the effect of renal impairment on the pharmacokinetics of diltiazem, paroxetine, and repaglinide as well as pharmacometrics in pregnancy (Rowland Yeo et al, 2011; Ke et al, 2014).

Scientists have compiled physiological parameters for healthy and health-impaired people 65 years of age and older for the physiologically based pharmacokinetic models (Thompson et al, 2009). Others used the physiologically based pharmacokinetic modeling approach to predict metabolic drug clearance with advancing age (Polasek et al, 2013). Scientists are applying the physiologically based pharmacokinetic modeling approach to estimate drug dosing in children (Barrett et al, 2012). Thus, applying the physiologically based pharmacokinetic modeling approach to understand drug disposition and action for the older patients seems appropriate (Della Casa Alberighi, 2013; Johnston et al, 2013).

Scientists have been working on the systems biology of aging, which is intrinsically complex, being driven by multiple causal mechanisms (Kirkwood, 2011). In general, the systems biology approach combines the following:

- Data-driven modeling, often using the large volumes of data generated by functional genomics technologies
- Hypothesis-driven experimental studies to investigate causal pathways and identify their parameter values in an unusually quantitative manner, which enables us to better understand the contributions of individual mechanisms and their interactions as well as allows for the design of experiments to explicitly test the complex predictions arising from such models

The learning from these systems biology studies will help us understand healthier aging. Healthier aging is aimed at the compression of morbidity in older age (Myint and Welch, 2012). The compression of morbidity hypothesis states that the age of onset of chronic illness may be postponed more than the age at death, squeezing most of the morbidity in life into a shorter period with less lifetime disability (Fries, 1980; Fries et al, 2011).

Clinical Examples of Concomitant Medication in Older Patients

The following two examples are modified from a reference (Mallet et al, 2007). Example 1 illustrates an older patient's multiple drug interaction potentials. Example 2 illustrates another older patient's prescribing cascade and drug interactions.

EXAMPLE 1 ▶▶▶

An 82-year-old man was hospitalized for general deterioration. His medical history included renal transplant 18 years ago, type 2 diabetes mellitus, atrial fibrillation, congestive heart failure, and early Alzheimer's dementia. He was taking cyclosporine, prednisone, warfarin, digoxin, furosemide, levothyroxine, losartan, glyburide, donepezil, lactulose, calcium carbonate, vitamin D, and ginkgo biloba. A week before admission, clarithromycin was started to treat bronchitis.

Discussion of this 82-year-old patient's medications:

- Potential drug–drug interactions:
  - Clarithromycin + warfarin: Clarithromycin is a CYP3A4 inhibitor. Warfarin is a CYP3A4 substrate. This combination has risk of increased warfarin exposure and anticoagulant effect.
  - Clarithromycin + cyclosporine: Clarithromycin is a CYP3A4 inhibitor. Cyclosporine is a CYP3A4 substrate. This combination has risk of increased cyclosporine exposure and nephrotoxicity.
  - Calcium carbonate + levothyroxine: decreased absorption of levothyroxine.
  - Ginkgo biloba + warfarin: increased risk of hemorrhage.
  - Donepezil, cyclosporine, and losartan: All are CYP3A4 substrates with potential risk of interaction.
  - Losartan and glyburide: All are CYP2C9 substrates with potential risk of interaction.
- Potential drug–disease interactions:
  - Prednisone in patient with congestive heart failure to cause fluid and electrolyte disturbances.

– Prednisone in diabetic patient to increase requirements for insulin or oral hypoglycemic agents.

Indiana University, School of Medicine, Department of Medicine, Division of Clinical Pharmacology, P450 Drug Interaction Table. http://medicine.iupui.edu/clinpharm/ddis/main-table/Indianapolis, IN 46202

Therapeutic plan for this 82-year-old patient: Management of drug interactions in older patients needs a team effort and communication is pivotal to achieve this goal. Several clinicians may take care of this patient, such as nephrologist, endocrinologist, cardiologist, neurologist, geriatrician, and family practice physician to prescribe medications. The pharmacist is likely to have access to this patient's most complete medication records and may help the following:

- Communicate with clarithromycin's prescriber for the potential interaction between clarithromycin and cyclosporine as well as warfarin. May need to recommend azithromycin or other antibiotic as alternative to minimize the potential CYP3A4 inhibition for cyclosporine and warfarin.
- Communicate with the patient or caregiver to take calcium carbonate and levothyroxine at least 4 hours apart to prevent the potential of calcium carbonate interfering with the absorption of levothyroxine.
- Communicate with the nurse or caregiver to watch for signs of worsening congestive heart failure such as shortness of breath and fluid retention as well as signs of fall from hypotension or hypoglycemia for further evaluation.

EXAMPLE 2 ▶ ▶ ▶

A 75-year-old man was taking paroxetine and haloperidol for the treatment of psychotic depression. His primary-care physician sent him for a neurological consult of his new-onset tremors. The neurologist started him with carbidopa and levodopa for probable Parkinson's disease. He was eventually hospitalized after several recurrent falls. The initial assessment attributed his falls to worsening instability secondary to suboptimally treated Parkinson's disease. Thus, his carbidopa and levodopa dose was increased. Risperidone was prescribed for nighttime agitated behavior (haloperidol was discontinued). He was still taking paroxetine.

Discussion of this 75-year-old patient's medications: Paroxetine and haloperidol can both cause extrapyramidal adverse effects leading to this patient's tremors. Moreover, these two drugs are CYP2D6 substrates with potential risk of mutual interaction to increase exposure of paroxetine and haloperidol, which leads to the extrapyramidal adverse effects. A prescribing cascade started with the prescription of carbidopa and levodopa. Carbidopa and levodopa's possible central nervous system adverse effects may cause the prescription of risperidone, which itself can cause extrapyramidal adverse effects. Also, risperidone and paroxetine are CYP2D6 substrates with potential risk of interaction.

Indiana University, School of Medicine, Department of Medicine, Division of Clinical Pharmacology, P450 Drug Interaction Table. http://medicine.iupui.edu/clinpharm/ddis/main-table/Indianapolis, IN 46202

Therapeutic plan for this 75-year-old patient: The pharmacist is likely to have access to this patient's most complete medication records and may help the following:

- Communicate with the neurologist that the patient is taking paroxetine and haloperidol for the treatment of psychotic depression, which may cause the extrapyramidal adverse effects and tremors. This may alert the neurologist to recognize the prescribing cascade and stop it.
- Communicate with the primary-care physician that dose reduction for paroxetine and haloperidol may be necessary for this patient.
- Communicate with the nurse or caregiver for mouth, dental, and bowel hygiene to watch for potential anticholinergic adverse effects. Paroxetine has strong anticholinergic effect per the 2012's Beers list.

SUMMARY

The number of people 65 years of age and older in the United States will more than double to 88.5 million in the year 2050 from that in year 2010. A similar trend occurs in other developed countries in the world as well. Careful consideration of drug therapy is essential to take care of older patients, who usually have comorbidities and concurrently take multiple medications. Knowledge of age's effect on pharmacokinetics and pharmacodynamics will help maximize the therapeutic effects and minimize the adverse effects of drugs.

Oral absorption of drugs does not appear to alter with advancing age despite physiological changes in the gastrointestinal tract. Plasma albumin concentration decreases about 10% with advancing age, whereas plasma α_1-acid glycoprotein concentration increases due to comorbidities. These changes usually do not result in dose adjustments except for rare cases. Phase I or degradative process of drug metabolism decreases to some extent and may require dose adjustments, whereas Phase II or synthetic process of drug metabolism do not change with advancing age. In general, the overall decrease in drug metabolism due to advancing age seems modest. Renal drug clearance is the most consistent and predictable age-related change in pharmacokinetics. The decrease in renal function may not be due to aging itself but due to comorbidity such as hypertension and chronic heart diseases.

Age-related changes in pharmacodynamics are more difficult to study than age-related changes in pharmacokinetics due to difficulties in establishing validated drug responses for pharmacodynamics. In general, older patients have increased sensitivity to drugs that act in the central nervous system and blood clotting system. However, older patients have decreased sensitivity to drugs that act on the adrenergic receptors in autonomic nervous system.

In general, dosing recommendation in older patients should follow the conventional wisdom of "start low and go slow."

Tools such as the Beers list may help appropriate prescribing in the older population. Several approaches emerged such as the serum anticholinergic activity, anticholinergic risk scale, and drug burden index to quantitate the anticholinergic burden of certain drugs may assist prescribing medications for older patients to reduce adverse drug events. Older individuals also have unique needs for adherence to take their medications. Emerging methods also exist to study pharmacology in older patients such as the population pharmacokinetics/pharmacodynamics, physiologically based pharmacokinetics/pharmacodynamics, and systems biology.

LEARNING QUESTIONS

1. Which of the following is the most appropriate choice related to aging?
   a. Increased extracellular fluid volume
   b. Increased hepatic blood flow
   c. Increased amount of sleep required
   d. Increased subcutaneous fat as a percentage of total body mass
   e. Increased size of alveolar ducts in the lung
2. Which of the following is the most appropriate choice to describe age-associated changes that can affect pharmacokinetics in older patients?
   a. Changes in gastrointestinal function that lead to reduced drug absorption
   b. Increase in total body water
   c. Decrease in body fat
   d. Decrease in serum albumin concentrations with advancing age
   e. Decrease in creatinine clearance with advancing age

3. Which of the following statement regarding renal function and pharmacokinetics in older patients is most accurate?
   a. Decreased muscle mass is the reason for normal or low serum creatinine concentration in older patients even in the presence of decreased renal function.
   b. Renal tubular secretion is not changed with aging.
   c. Serum creatinine concentration of 1.5 mg/dL reflects normal renal function in older men.
   d. Glomerular function always declines with aging.
   e. Gentamicin can be used safely in older patients with serum creatinine concentrations of 1.7 mg/dL.
4. Which of the following regarding medication use by older patients in the United States is wrong?
   a. Older patients count about 13% of the United States population but consume 25%–30% of all medications.
   b. Institutionalized older residents usually take 3–8 medications a day.

c. Older patients regularly take about 4–5 medications.
d. Adverse drug reactions in older patients appear unrelated to the number of medications taken.
e. Taking over-the-counter medications and nutritional supplements other than those prescribed can contribute to polypharmacy.
5. Which of the following statements concerning the safety of medications used by older patients is wrong?
   a. Chlorpropamide can cause hypoglycemia.
   b. Benzodiazepines have large volume of distribution and are thus relatively safe for use in older people.
   c. Amantadine's excretion depends on renal function and may cause confusion and falls if the dose is not adjusted for renal impairment.
   d. Diphenhydramine may exacerbate urinary retention of older men.
   e. Meperidine is not an effective oral analgesic in dosages commonly used and may cause neurotoxicity.

ANSWERS

Learning Questions

1. The correct answer is **e**. The size of alveolar ducts increases with aging, which causes a decrease in the lung surface area. **a** and **b** are wrong statements. Older persons need less sleep but need short naps during the day. Increase of subcutaneous fat, as a percentage of total body mass, is not a change associated with aging. Fat as a percentage of total body mass increases in older persons. However, fat redistributes from subcutaneous to truncal areas. Thus, this leads to a net loss of subcutaneous fat and increases the risk of pressure ulcers.
2. The correct answer is **e**. **d** and **e** are correct but **d** is most likely not significantly enough that requires dose adjustment. **a**, **b**, and **c** are wrong statements.
3. The correct answer is **a**. **b** and **c** are wrong statements. Per longitudinal studies, renal function as reflected via glomerular function may not change with aging except with comorbidity

such as diabetes and chronic heart diseases. Gentamicin's elimination is via renal excretion and serum creatinine concentration of 1.7 mg/dL reflects renal impairment.
4. The correct answer is **d**. **d** is a wrong statement. **a**, **b**, **c**, and **e** are correct statements.
5. The correct answer is **b**. Benzodiazepines tend to distribute to fat tissues and thus have a large volume of distribution. With increasing age, we tend to gain body fat and thus need longer time to eliminate benzodiazepines than younger adults. Benzodiazepines show age-related increase in sensitivity to cognitive and sedative functions. Amantadine is primarily excreted unchanged in the urine via glomerular filtration and tubular secretion. All sulfonylurea drugs including chlorpropamide are capable of causing severe hypoglycemia. Diphenhydramine has high anticholinergic adverse effects, which can exacerbate the urinary retention issue of older men with prostate hypertrophy. **e** is a correct statement per the 2012's Beers list.

REFERENCES

Albrecht S, Ihmsen H, Hering W, et al: The effect of age on the pharmacokinetics and pharmacodynamics of midazolam. *Clin Pharmacol Ther* **65**:630, 1999.

Allen S: Are inhaled systemic therapies a viable option for the treatment of the elderly patient? *Drugs Aging* **25**:89, 2008.

Baggio B, Budakovic A, Perissinotto E, et al: Atherosclerotic risk factors and renal function in the elderly: The role of hyper-fibrinogenaemia and smoking. Results from the Italian Lon-gitudinal Study on Ageing (ILSA). *Nephrol Dial Transplant* **20**:114, 2005.

Barrett JS, Della Casa Alberighi O, Läer S, et al: Physiologically based pharmacokinetic (PBPK) modeling in children. *Clin Pharmacol Ther* **92**:40, 2012.

Bartels AL, Kortekaas R, Bart J, et al: Blood-brain barrier P-glycoprotein function decreases in specific brain regions with aging: A possible role in progressive neurodegeneration. *Neurobiol Aging* **30**:1818, 2009.

Brenner SS, Klotz U: P-glycoprotein function in the elderly. *Eur J Clin Pharmacol* **60**:97, 2004.

Beaufrère B, Morio B: Fat and protein redistribution with aging: Metabolic considerations. *Eur J Clin Nutr* **54**(suppl 3):S48, 2000.

Benet LZ, Hoener B-A: Changes in plasma protein binding have little clinical significance. *Clin Pharmacol Ther* **71**:115, 2002.

Benedetti MS, Whomsley R, Canning M: Drug metabolism in the paediatric population and in the elderly. *Drug Discov Today* **12**:599, 2007.

Bickford PC, Breiderick L: Benzodiazepine modulation of GAB-Aergic responses is intact in the cerebellum of aged F344 rats. *Neurosci Lett* **291**:187, 2000.

Bostock CV, Soiza RL, Mangoni AA: Association between pre-scribing of antimuscarinic drugs and antimuscarinic adverse effects in older people. *Expert Rev Clin Pharmacol* **3**:441, 2010.

Bowie MW, Slattum PW: Pharmacodynamics in older adults: A review. *Am J Geriatr Pharmacother* **5**:263, 2007.

Breitkreutz J, Boos J: Paediatric and geriatric drug delivery. *Expert Opin Drug Deliv* **4**:37, 2007.

Bushardt, RL, Massey, EB, Simpson, TW, Ariail, JC, Simpson, KN: Polypharmacy: Misleading, but manageable. *Clin Interv Aging* **3**:383, 2008.

Cancelli I, Gigli GL, Piani A, et al: Drugs with anticholinergic properties as a risk factor for cognitive impairment in elderly people: A population-based study. *J Clin Psychopharmacol* **28**:654, 2008.

Castleden CM, George CF, Marcer D, et al: Increased sensitivity to nitrazepam in old age. *Br Med J* **1**(6052):10, 1977.

Chew ML, Mulsant BH, Pollock BG, et al: Anticholinergic activ-ity of 107 medications commonly used by older adults. *J Am Geriatr Soc* **56**:1333, 2008.

Chien JY, Ho RJY: Drug delivery trends in clinical trials and trans-lational medicine: evaluation of pharmacokinetic properties in special populations. *J Pharm Sci* **100**:53, 2011.

Christensen K, Doblhammer G, Rau R, et al: Ageing populations: The challenges ahead. *Lancet* **374**:1196, 2009.

Clegg A, Young J, Iliffe S, et al: Frailty in elderly people. *Lancet* **381**:752, 2013.

Cockcroft DW, Gault MH: Prediction of creatinine clearance from serum creatinine. *Nephron* **16**:31, 1976.

Corsonello A, Pedone C, Incalzi RA: Age-related pharmaco-kinetic and pharmacodynamic changes and related risk of adverse drug reactions. *Curr Med Chem* **17**:571, 2010.

Cusack B, Kelly J, O'Malley K, et al: Digoxin in the elderly: Phar-macokinetic consequences of old age. *Clin Pharmacol Ther* **25**:772, 1979.

Davies DF, Shock NW: Age changes in glomerular filtration rate, effective renal plasma flow, and tubular excretory capacity in adult males. *J Clin Invest* **29**:496, 1950.

de Leon: Paying attention to pharmacokinetic and pharmacody-namic mechanisms to progress in the area of anticholinergic use in geriatric patients. *Curr Drug Metab* **12**:635, 2011.

DeGorter MK, Tirona RG, Schwarz UI, et al: Clinical and phar-macogenetic predictors of circulating atorvastatin and rosuv-astatin concentrations in routine clinical care. *Circ Cardiovasc Genet* **6**:400, 2013.

Della Casa Alberighi O, Barrett JS, Läer S, et al: Response to "Physiologically based pharmacokinetic modeling at the extremes of age." *Clin Pharmacol Ther* **93**:149, 2013.

Divoll M, Greenblatt DJ, Ochs HR, et al: Absolute bioavailability of oral and intramuscular diazepam: Effects of age and sex. *Anesth Analg* **62**:1, 1983.

Dobre D, Haaijer-Ruskamp FM, et al: beta-Adrenoceptor antago-nists in elderly patients with heart failure: A critical review of their efficacy and tolerability. *Drugs Aging* **24**:1031, 2007.

Doyle V, O'Malley K, Kelly JG: Human lymphocyte beta-adreno-ceptor density in relation to age and hypertension. *J Cardio-vasc Pharmacol* **4**:738, 1982.

Drayer DE, Romankiewicz J, Lorenzo B, et al: Age and renal clearance of cimetidine. *Clin Pharmacol Ther* **31**:45, 1982.

Ensrud KE, Blackwell TL, Mangione CM, et al: Central nervous system-active medications and risk for falls in older women. *J Am Geriatr Soc* **50**:1629, 2002.

European Medicines Agency: ICH Topic E7, Studies in Support of Special Population: Geriatrics. http://www.ema.europa.eu /docs/en_GB/document_library/Scientific_guideline/2009/09 /WC500002875.pdf. London, UK, 1994.

European Medicines Agency: ICH Topic E7, Studies in Support of Special Population: Geriatrics. Questions and Answers. http://www.ema.europa.eu/docs/en_GB/document_library /Scientific_guideline/2009/10/WC500005218.pdf. London, UK, 2011.

Fliser D, Franek E, Joest M, et al: Renal function in the elderly: Impact of hypertension and cardiac function. *Kidney Int* **51**:1196, 1997a.

Fliser D, Franek E, Ritz E: Renal function in the elderly—Is the dogma of an inexorable decline of renal function correct? *Nephrol Dial Transpl* **12**:1553, 1997b.

Food and Drug Administration: Guidance for Industry: Content and Format for Geriatric Labeling. http://www.fda.gov/downloads/Drugs/GuidanceComplianceRegulatoryInformation/Guidances/ucm075062.pdf. Rockville, MD 20857, 1997.

Food and Drug Administration: Guidance for Industry: Guideline for the Study of Drugs Likely to Be Used in the Elderly. http://www.fda.gov/downloads/Drugs/GuidanceComplianceRegulatoryInformation/Guidances/ucm072048.pdf. Rockville, MD 20857, 1989.

Food and Drug Administration: Guidance for Industry: Population Pharmacokinetics. http://www.fda.gov/downloads/Drugs/GuidanceComplianceRegulatoryInformation/Guidances/UCM072137.pdf. Rockville, MD 20857, 1999.

Francoeur M, Ahmed I, Sitek S, et al: Age-related differences in ophthalmic drug disposition III. Corneal permeability of pilocarpine in rabbits. *Int J Pharm* **16:**203, 1983.

Fried L, Walston J, Ferrucci L: Frailty. In Halter JB, Ouslander JG, Tinetti ME, et al (eds). *Hazzard's Geriatric Medicine and Gerontology.* New York, NY, McGraw-Hill Companies, Inc., 2009, p 631.

Fries JF: Aging, natural death, and the compression of morbidity. *N Engl J Med* **303:**130, 1980.

Fries JF, Bruce B, Chakravarty E: Compression of morbidity 1980-2011: A focused review of paradigms and progress. *J Aging Res* **2011:**1, 2011.

Gibson DM, Bron NJ, Richens A, et al: Effect of age and gender on pharmacokinetics of atorvastatin in humans. *J Clin Pharmacol* **36:**242, 1996.

Greenblatt DJ, Divoll M, Harmatz JS, et al: Kinetics and clinical effects of flurazepam in young and elderly noninsomniacs. *Clin Pharmacol Ther* **30:**475, 1981.

Greenblatt DJ, Harmatz JS, Shader RI: Clinical pharmacokinetics of anxiolytics and hypnotics in the elderly. Therapeutic considerations (Part I). *Clin Pharmacokinet* **21:**165, 1991.

Greenblatt DJ, Harmatz JS, von Moltke LL, et al: Age and gender effects on the pharmacokinetics and pharmacodynamics of triazolam, a cytochrome P450 3A substrate. *Clin Pharmacol Ther* **76:**467, 2004.

Harvey PT: Common eye diseases of elderly people: Identifying and treating causes of vision loss. *Gerontology* **49:**1, 2003.

Henry RR, Mudaliar S, Chu N, et al: Young and elderly type 2 diabetic patients inhaling insulin with the AERx® insulin diabetes management system: A pharmacokinetic and pharmacodynamic comparison. *J Clin Pharmacol* **43:**1228, 2003

Hilmer SN, Gnjidic D: The effects of polypharmacy in older adults. *Clin Pharmacol Ther* **85:**86, 2009.

Hilmer SN, Mager DE, Simonsick EM, et al: A drug burden index to define the functional burden of medications in older people. *Arch Intern Med* **167:**78, 2007.

Hilmer SN, Mager DE, Simonsick EM, et al: Drug burden index score and functional decline in older people. *Am J Med* **122:**1142, 2009.

Holazo YR, Winkler MB, Patel IH: Effects of age, gender and oral contraceptives on intramuscular midazolam pharmacokinetics. *J Clin Pharmacol* **28:**1040, 1988.

Johnston C, Kirkpatrick CM, McLachlan AJ, et al: Physiologically based pharmacokinetic modeling at the extremes of age. *Clin Pharmacol Ther* **93:**148, 2013.

Kaestli LZ, Wasilewski-Rasca AF, Bonnabry P, et al: Use of transdermal drug formulations in the elderly. *Drugs Aging* **25:**269, 2008.

Kang D, Verotta D, Schwartz JB: Population analyses of amlodipine in patients living in the community and patients living in nursing homes. *Clin Pharmacol Ther* **79:**114, 2006.

Kanto J, Kangas L, Altonen L, et al: Effect of age on the pharmacokinetics ad sedative effect of flunitrazepam. *J Clin Pharmacol* **19:**400, 1981.

Ke TL, Clark AF, Gracy RW: Age-related permeability changes in rabbit corneas. *J Ocul Pharmacol Ther* **15:**513, 1999.

Ke AB, Rostami-Hodjegan A, Zhao P, et al: Pharmacometrics in pregnancy: An unmet need. *Annu Rev Pharmacol Toxicol* **54:**53, 2014.

Kirkwood TB: Systems biology of ageing and longevity. *Phil Trans R Soc B* **366:**64, 2011.

Klotz U: The elderly—A challenge for appropriate drug treatment. *Eur J Clin Pharmacol* **64:**225, 2008.

Klotz U: Pharmacokinetics and drug metabolism in the elderly. *Drug Metab Rev* **41:**67, 2009.

Kuno N, Fujii S: Recent advances in ocular drug delivery systems. *Polymers* **3:**193, 2011.

Landmann R, Bittiger H, Buhler FR: High affinity beta-2-adrenergic receptors in mononuclear leucocytes: Similar density in young and old normal subjects. *Life Sci* **29:**1761, 1981.

Laroche ML, Charmes JP, Merle L: Potentially inappropriate medications in the elderly: A French consensus panel list. *Eur J Clin Pharmacol* **63:**725, 2007.

Lindeman RD, Tobin J, Shock NW: Longitudinal studies on the rate of decline in renal function with age. *J Am Geriatr Soc* **33:**278, 1985.

Leipzig RM, Cumming RG, Tinetti ME: Drugs and falls in older people: A systematic review and meta-analysis: II. Cardiac and analgesic drugs. *J Am Geriatr Soc* **47:**40, 1999.

Levey AS, Coresh J, Greene T, et al: Using standardized serum creatinine values in the modification of diet in renal disease study equation for estimating glomerular filtration rate. *Ann Intern Med* **145:**247, 2006.

Ljungberg B, Nilsson-Ehle I: Pharmacokinetics of antimicrobial agents in the elderly. *Rev Infect Dis* **9:**250, 1987.

Mallet L, Spinewine A, Huang A: The challenge of managing drug interactions in elderly people. *Lancet* **370:**185, 2007.

Mangoni AA: The impact of advancing age on P-glycoprotein expression and activity: Current knowledge and future directions. *Expert Opin Drug Metab Toxicol* **3:**315–320, 2007.

Mangoni AA, Jansen PAF, Jackson SHD: Under-representation of older adults in pharmacokinetic and pharmacodynamic studies: A solvable problem? *Expert Rev Clin Pharmacol* **6:**35, 2013.

Matsuura T, Oda Y, Tanaka K, et al: Advance of age decreases the minimum alveolar concentrations of isoflurane and sevoflurane for maintaining bispectral index below 50. *Br J Anaesth* **102:**331, 2009.

Mayersohn M: Pharmacokinetics in the elderly. *Environ Health Perspect* **102**(suppl):119, 1994.

McLean AJ, Le Couteur DG: Aging biology and geriatric pharmacology. *Pharmacol Rev* **56**:163, 2004.

Meltzer CC: Neuropharmacology and receptor studies in the elderly. *J Geriatr Psychiatry Neurol* **12**:137, 1999.

Miao L, Yang J, Huang C, et al: Contribution of age, body weight, and CYP2C9 and VKORC1 genotype to the anticoagulant response to warfarin: Proposal for a new dosing regimen in Chinese patients. *Eur J Clin Pharmacol* **63**:1135, 2007.

Miller JH, McDonald RK, Shock NW: Age changes in the maximal rate of renal tubular reabsorption of glucose. *J Gerontol* **7**:196, 1952.

Morley JE, Argiles JM, Evans WJ, et al: Nutritional recommendations for the management of sarcopenia. *J Am Med Dir Assoc* **11**:391, 2010.

Mulsant BH, Pollock BG, Kirshner M, et al: Serum anticholinergic activity in a community-based sample of older adults: Relationship with cognitive performance. *Arch Gen Psychiatry* **60**:198, 2003.

Muramatsu RS, Litzinger MH, Fisher E, et al: Alternative formulations, delivery methods, and administration options for psychotropic medications in elderly patients with behavioral and psychological symptoms of dementia. *Am J Geriatr Pharmacother* **8**:98, 2010.

Myint PK, Welch AA: Healthier ageing. *BMJ* **344**:42, 2012.

Nyman HA, Dowling TC, Hudson JQ, et al: Comparative evaluation of the Cockcroft-Gault equation and the Modification of Diet in Renal Disease (MDRD) study equation for drug dosing: An opinion of the Nephrology Practice and Research Network of the American College of Clinical Pharmacy. *Pharmacotherapy* **31**:1130, 2011.

O'Mahony D, Gallagher P, Ryan C, et al: STOPP & START criteria: A new approach to detecting potentially inappropriate prescribing in old age. *Eur Geriatr Med* **1**:45, 2010.

Parkinson A, Mudra DR, Johnson C, et al: The effects of gender, age, ethnicity, and liver cirrhosis on cytochrome P450 enzyme activity in human liver microsomes and inducibility in cultured human hepatocytes. *Toxicol Appl Pharmacol* **199**:193, 2004.

Perrone RD, Madias NE, Levey AS: Serum creatinine as an index of renal function: New insights into old concepts. *Clin Chem* **38**:1933, 1992.

Polasek TM, Patel F, Jensen BP, et al: Predicted metabolic drug clearance with increasing adult age. *Br J Clin Pharmacol* **75**:1019, 2013.

Reidenberg MM, Camacho M, Kluger J, et al: Aging and renal clearance of procainamide and acetylprocainamide. *Clin Pharmacol Ther* **28**:732, 1980.

Rowland M, Peck C, Tucker G: Physiologically-based pharmacokinetics in drug development and regulatory science. *Annu Rev Pharmacol Toxicol* **51**:45, 2011.

Rowland M, Tozer TN: Protein drugs. In Rowland M, Tozer TN (eds). *Clinical Pharmacokinetics and Pharmacodynamics: Concepts and Applications*. Philadelphia, PA, Lippincott Williams & Wilkins Publisher, 2011, p 633.

Rowland Yeo K, Aarabi M, Jamei M, Rostami-Hodjegan A: Modeling and predicting drug pharmacokinetics in patients with renal impairment. *Expert Rev Clin Pharmacol* **4**:261, 2011.

Rudolph JL, Salow MJ, Angelini MC, et al: The anticholinergic risk scale and anticholinergic adverse effects in older persons. *Arch Intern Med* **168**:508, 2008.

Ryan T: The ageing of the blood supply and the lymphatic drainage of the skin. *Micron* **35**:161, 2004.

Sandilands EA, Dhaun N, Dear JW, et al: Measurement of renal function in patients with chronic kidney disease. *Br J Clin Pharmacol* **76**:504, 2013.

Scarpace PJ, Tumer N, Mader SL: Beta-adrenergic function in aging. Basic mechanisms and clinical implications. *Drugs Aging* **1**:116, 1991.

Scott PJ, Meredith PA, Kelman AW, et al: The effects of age on the pharmacokinetics and pharmacodynamics of cardiovascular drugs: Application of concentration-effect modeling. 2. Acebutolol. *Am J Ther* **2**:537, 1995.

Schwartz JB: Erythromycin breath test results in elderly, very elderly, and frail elderly persons. *Clin Pharmacol Ther* **79**:440, 2006.

Schwartz JB: The current state of knowledge on age, sex, and their interactions on clinical pharmacology. *Clin Pharmacol Ther* **82**:87, 2007.

Schwartz JB, Abernethy DR: Aging and medications: Past, present, future. *Clin Pharmacol Ther* **85**:3, 2009.

Schwartz JB, Verotta D: Population analyses of atorvastatin clearance in patients living in the community and in nursing homes. *Clin Pharmacol Ther* **86**:497, 2009.

Shi S, Klotz U: Age-related changes in pharmacokinetics. *Curr Drug Metab* **12**:601, 2011.

Siekmeier R, Scheuch G: Inhaled insulin—Does it become reality? *J Physiol Pharmacol* **59**(suppl 6):81, 2008.

Sitar DS: Clinical pharmacology confounders in older adults. *Expert Rev Clin Pharmacol* **5**:397, 2012.

Spruill WJ, Wade WE, Cobb HH, 3rd: Continuing the use of the Cockcroft-Gault equation for drug dosing in patients with impaired renal function. *Clin Pharmacol Ther* **86**:468, 2009.

Sproule BA, Hardy BG, Shulman KI: Differential pharmacokinetics of lithium in elderly patients. *Drugs Aging* **16**:165, 2000.

Stevens LA, Levey AS: Use of the MDRD study equation to estimate kidney function for drug dosing. *Clin Pharmacol Ther* **86**:465, 2009.

Sundman I, Allard P, Eriksson A, et al: GABA uptake sites in frontal cortex from suicide victims and in aging. *Neuropsychobiology* **35**:11, 1997.

Swedko PJ, Clark HD, Paramsothy K, et al: Serum creatinine is an inadequate screening test for renal failure in elderly patients. *Arch Intern Med* **163**:356, 2003.

Swift CG, Ewen JM, Clarke P, et al: Responsiveness to oral diazepam in the elderly: Relationship to total and free concentrations. *Br J Clin Pharmacol* **20**:111, 1985.

The American Geriatrics Society 2012 Beers Criteria Update Expert Panel: American Geriatrics Society Updated Beers Criteria for Potentially Inappropriate Medication Use in Older Adults. *J Am Geriatr Soc* **60**:616, 2012.

Thompson CM, Johns DO, Sonawane B, et al: Database for physiologically based pharmacokinetic (PBPK) modeling: Physiological data for healthy and health-impaired elderly. *J Toxicol Environ Health B Crit Rev* **12:**1, 2009.

Traynor J, Mactier R, Geddes CC, et al: How to measure renal function in clinical practice. *BMJ* **333:**733, 2006.

Trifirò G, Spina E: Age-related changes in pharmacodynamics: Focus on drugs acting on central nervous and cardiovascular systems. *Curr Drug Metab* **12:**611, 2011.

Tsamandouras N, Rostami-Hodjegan A, Aarons L: Combining the "bottom-up" and "top-down" approaches in pharmacokinetic modelling: Fitting PBPK models to observed clinical data. *Br J Clin Pharmacol* **79:**48, 2015.

Tune L, Carr S, Hoag E, et al: Anticholinergic effects of drugs commonly prescribed for the elderly: potential means for assessing risk of delirium. *Am J Psychiatry* **149:**1393, 1992.

U.S. Census Bureau: The next four decades: The older population in the United States: 2010 to 2050. Current Population Reports, P25-1138, http://www.census.gov/prod/2010pubs/p25-1138.pdf. Washington, DC, 20233, 2010.

Vadivelu N, Hines RL: Management of chronic pain in the elderly: Focus on transdermal buprenorphine. *Clin Interv Aging* **3:**421, 2008.

Vestal RE: Aging and pharmacology. *Cancer* **80:**1302, 1997.

Vestal RE, Wood AJ, Shand DG: Reduced beta-adrenoceptor sensitivity in the elderly. *Clin Pharmacol Ther* **26:**181, 1979.

Vieweg WV, Wood MA, Fernandez A, et al: Proarrhythmic risk with antipsychotic and antidepressant drugs: Implications in the elderly. *Drugs Aging* **26:**997, 2009.

White M, Roden R, Minobe W, et al: Age-related changes in beta-adrenergic neuroeffector systems in the human heart. *Circulation* **90:**1225, 1994.

Wynne HA, Yelland C, Cope LH, et al: The association of age and frailty with the pharmacokinetics and pharmacodynamics of metoclopramide. *Age Ageing* **22:**354, 1993.

FURTHER READING

Cusack BJ: Pharmacokinetics in older persons. *Am J Geriatr Pharmacother* **2:**274, 2004.

Gronich N, Abernethy DR: Pharmacology across the aging continuum. In Waldman SA, Terzic A (eds). *Pharmacology and Therapeutics: Principles to Practice*. Philadelphia, PA, Saunders, 2009, p 257.

Hilmer SN, McLachlan AJ, Le Couteur DG: Clinical pharmacology in the geriatric patient. *Fundam Clin Pharmacol* **21:**217, 2007.

Katzung BG: Special aspects of geriatric pharmacology. In Katzung BG, Masters SB, Trevor AJ (eds). *Basic and Clinical Pharmacology*. New York, NY, McGraw-Hill Companies, Inc., 2012, p 1051.

Kim J, Mak M: Geriatric drug use. In Alldredge BK, Corelli RL, Ernst ME, et al (eds). *Koda-Kimble and Young's Applied Therapeutics: The Clinical Use of Drugs*. Philadelphia PA, Lippincott Williams & Wilkins, 2013, p 2359.

Lau SWJ, Abernethy DR: Drug therapy in the elderly. In Atkinson AJ, Huang S-M, Lertora JJ, et al (eds). *Principles of Clinical Pharmacology*. Waltham, MA, Academic Press, 2012, p 437.

Salles N: Basic mechanisms of the aging gastrointestinal tract. *Dig Dis* **25:**112, 2007.

Vestal RE, Gurwitz JH: Geriatric pharmacology. In Carruthers SG, Hoffman BB, Melmon KL, et al (eds). *Clinical Pharmacology: Basic Principles in Therapeutics*. New York, NY, McGraw-Hill Companies, Inc., 2000, p 1151.

MODULE II: APPLICATION OF PHARMACOKINETICS TO THE OBESE PATIENTS

Objectives

- Describe the prevalence and the impact of obesity on individuals and to the society.
- Classify obesity based on body mass index.
- Explain the differences of volume distribution in obese versus non-obese patients.
- Identify the differences in metabolism between obese and non-obese patients.
- Describe the differences in renal elimination between obese and non-obese patients.
- Apply pharmacokinetic principles in drug dosing for obesity.
- Estimate creatinine clearance for obese patients.

Introduction

Obesity, defined as body mass index (BMI) of 30 or higher, has been recognized as a "disease" in 2013 by the American Medical Association, requiring a range of medical interventions to advance treatment and prevention (AMA, 2013). The prevalence of obesity has increased substantially worldwide in recent years (Kopelman, 2000; Berghofer et al, 2008). The medical care costs related to obesity are staggering, and much of the cost is associated with obesity-related chronic conditions, including diabetes, hypertension, high cholesterol, stroke, heart disease, certain cancers, and arthritis (Malnick et al, 2006). In addition, obesity was associated with significantly increased mortality from cardiovascular diseases and obesity-related cancers (Flegal et al, 2007). Individuals with obesity also have significantly lower health-related quality-of-life scores than those individuals with normal weights (Jia et al, 2005), with or without the corresponding chronic diseases.

Individuals with severe obesity, defined as BMI ≥ 40, are a rapidly growing sector among the obese population in the United States. While the population of obesity in the US adults increased by 4.97% from 2003–2004 to 2007–2008 (Ogden et al, 2006), the population of severe obesity has increased by 18.75% during the same period of time.

Classification of obesity is most commonly using BMI, a value that normalizes body weight based on height (Table 23.2-1) (World Health Organization, 1998). It is calculated as body weight in kilograms divided by the height in meters squared.

Clinically, a patient may be considered obese when the total body weight (TBW) is equal to or greater than 20% of ideal body weight (IBW)

TABLE 23.2-1 Classification of Obesity Based on BMI

Classification	BMI (kg/m²)
Underweight	<18.5
Normal body weight	18.5–24.9
Overweight	25–29.9
Obese	30–39.9
Morbidly obese	≥40

(Winter, 2010). Some clinicians use 30% as their criteria for clinically obese. IBW is a weight with the lowest mortality (Metropolitan Life Insurance Company, 1959) derived from the data at Metropolitan Life Insurance Company. Morbidly obese may also refer to a patient's TBW at least 95% over the IBW. Table 23.2-2 details the weight descriptors and related formulas to estimate the weight descriptors.

In general, obese individuals have more fat tissue and less lean tissue per kilogram of TBW, as compared to their non-obese counterparts (Cheymol, 2000). Since the actual fat content in body tissues is difficult to measure in a clinical setting, the excess weight, or so-called fat weight, in an obese individual is commonly calculated as the difference between TBW and IBW.

TABLE 23.2-2 Weight Descriptors and Related Equations

Weight Descriptor	Equation	No.	Ref.
BMI	[Weight (kg)/height (cm)²] × 10,000 (cm²/m²)	23.2.1	World Health Organization (1998)
Ideal body weight (IBW), kg	Male: 50 + 2.3 × [Height (inches) – 60] Female: 45.5 + 2.3 × [Height (inches) – 60]	23.2.2	Devine (1974)
Total body weight (TBW), kg	Measured body weight	23.2.3	
Adjusted body weight (Adj. BW), kg	IBW + 0.4 × (TBW – IBW)	23.2.4	Bauer et al (1983)
Lean body weight (LBW2005), kg	Male: (9270 × TBW)/(6680 + 216 × BMI) Female: (9270 × TBW)/(8780 + 244 × BMI)	23.2.5 23.2.6	Janmahasatian et al (2005)

The excess fat tissue and its accompanying physiological changes in the obese individuals may have a significant impact on drug disposition.

Pharmacokinetic Changes in Obesity

Absorption

Information currently available on the absorption and bioavailability of medications in the obese population is scarce and inconclusive. Limited studies included a study comparing the absorption and bioavailability of metformin between patients underwent gastric bypass surgery and their BMI-matched (nonsurgery) cohorts showed a 50% increase of bioavailability in the surgery group after the surgery (Padwal et al, 2011). Another study comparing oral atorvastatin exposure before and after gastric bypass surgery in the same patient showed variable results (Skottheim et al, 2009).

Distribution

Drug distribution, measured as volume of distribution (V_D), is influenced by the size of the tissue, tissue perfusion, plasma protein binding, tissue membrane permeability, etc (Rowland and Tozer, 2011). The obese individuals have an increased total tissue mass and adipose tissue mass (Cheymol, 1993, 2000). Thus, the volume of distribution for many drugs may be increased in the obese population. However, studies have shown that physicochemical characteristics of the drug, namely, lipophilicity, plays a major role in the drug distribution (Cheymol, 1988; Medico and Walsh, 2010) in the obese population. Generally, in the obese patients, lipophilic medications showed a larger increased volume of distribution, and hydrophilic medications showed a less increased volume of distribution, as compared to the non-obese patients. Still, there are exceptions to this rule (Flechner et al, 1989; Wojcicki et al, 2003). For example, cyclosporine is highly lipophilic, its volume of distribution in non-obese patients was 295 L, but in obese patients, its volume of distribution was only 229 L. In addition, the concentrations of plasma binding proteins—albumin, α_1-acid glycoprotein, and lipoproteins—may be unchanged (albumin),

increased or decreased (α_1-acid glycoprotein) with obesity, resulted in an altered concentration of the unbound drug. At present, the impact of obesity on plasma protein binding of medications is still largely inconclusive.

Metabolism

Drug metabolism primarily occurs in the liver through Phase I reactions and Phase II conjugation. A majority of the obese patients have fatty infiltration in the liver (Moretto et al, 2003), resulted in nonalcoholic fatty liver disease (NAFLD), with or without inflammation of the liver. Therefore, the Phase I and II enzyme activities in obesity may be affected by the fatty infiltration of the liver and its associated changes.

1. Phase I Metabolism
   a. Cytochrome P450 (CYP) 3A4
      It has been reported that CYP 3A4 metabolic activity was reduced in the obese patients, either significantly, as for carbamazepine and triazolam (Abernethy et al, 1984; Caraco et al, 1995), or not significantly, as for midazolam and cyclosporine (Greenblatt et al, 1984; Yee, 1988), when compared to the non-obese patients. The weight-normalized clearances were invariably lower in the obese patients.
   b. CYP2E1
      Various studies showed consistent and significant increases in the clearance of CYP 2E1 substrates in the obese patients, including chlorzoxazone, enflurane, sevoflurane, and halothane (Miller et al, 1980; Bentley et al, 1982; Higuchi et al, 1993; Lucas et al, 1999; Emery et al, 2003). These data lead us to believe there is an increase of activity of CYP2E1 in obesity. When normalized for body weight, clearance values of these drugs are approximately equal among obese and non-obese individuals, which suggests that CYP2E1activity increases with body weight.
      CYP2E1 mediates the metabolism of fatty acids, ketones, and ethanol. Chronic exposure to the sesubstrates in large amounts

induces CYP2E1, leading to free-radical formation, lipid peroxidation, and liver injury (Lieber, 2004; Buechler and Weiss, 2011).

Fatty infiltration of the liver is likely to rise with increasing body weight, which may be the underlying cause of the increase in CYP2E1 enzyme activity (Brill et al, 2012).

c. CYP2D6

Studies on dexfenfluramine and nebivolol showed a trend toward increased CYP2D6 activity in the obese patients (Cheymol et al, 1995, 1997). However, its activity may vary based on its genetic polymorphisms (May, 1994; Van den Anker, 2010).

d. CYP1A2

Studies on caffeine and theophylline showed a trend of higher clearance in the obese group, indicating a slight increase in CYP1A2 activity in the obese patients (Jusko et al, 1979; Abernethy et al, 1985; Kamimori et al, 1987; Zahorska-Markiewicz et al, 1996).

e. CYP2C9

Studies on glimepiride and ibuprofen showed a small but significantly increased CYP2C9 activity in the obese patients (Abernethy and Greenblatt, 1985a; Shukla et al, 2004), and studies on glipizide and phenytoin showed an insignificant increase in the obese group (Abernethy and Greenblatt, 1985b; Jaber et al, 1996). While normalized for body weight, a lower enzyme activity of CYP2C9 was associated with the obese group.

f. CYP2C19

The only one study for CYP2C19 activities showed that the clearance of diazepam was significantly higher in the obese group, and no difference was shown for desmethyldiazepam (Abernethy et al, 1981a, 1982a). While adjusted for body weight, a lower enzyme activity was shown in the obese group for both drugs.

g. Xanthine oxidase

Studies in comparing xanthine oxidase activities using caffeine (Chiney et al, 2011)

and mercaptopurine (Balis, 1986) in the obese versus non-obese children showed significantly increased enzyme activity in the obese group.

B. Phase II Metabolism

a. Uridine diphosphate glucuronosyltransferase (UGT)

UGT enzymes catalyze the conjugation of endogenous substances and exogenous compounds, and are involved in approximately 50% of the Phase II metabolism for drugs. Since the liver is the main organ for UGT enzyme activities, liver disease or an increased size of the liver, as occurred in the obese patients, may correlate with UGT activities. Studies showed a significantly increased clearance in the obese group for medications metabolized via this pathway, including acetaminophen in adults (Brill et al, 2012), oxazepam, and lorazepam (Abernethy et al, 1982b, 1983). With the exception of oxazepam, the weight-normalized clearance values were either the same or slightly lower in the obese group.

b. Other Phase II metabolic enzymes

Besides UGT, other Phase II metabolic processes include N-acetyl-, methyl, glutathione, and sulfate conjugation of substrates. The study on procainamide, which is metabolized via N-acetylation, showed an increased, but not statistically significant, plasma clearance in the obese group (Christoff et al, 1983). The weight-normalized clearance for procainamide was lower in the obese group. As for studies with busulfan, which is metabolized via glutathione S-transferase, showed a significantly increased Cl/F in the obese group, while the weight-normalized clearance was significantly lower in the obese group (Gibbs et al, 1999).

c. Blood flow in the liver

Obesity is associated with absolute increases in cardiac output and blood volume, as compared to non-obese subjects (Alexander et al, 1962; Alexander, 1964). Yet the effect of obesity on liver blood flow is not fully determined, partly because nonalcoholic fatty liver disease increases fat deposition in the liver, resulting in sinusoidal narrowing and altered morphology of the liver (Farrell et al, 2008).

Drugs with high-extraction ratio, such as propofol, sufentanil, and paclitaxel, could potentially serve as markers of liver blood flow, because they are rapidly metabolized and sensitive to changes in the blood flow of the liver, and less sensitive to changes in enzyme activities. Studies of these drugs showed higher clearances in the obese subjects (Schwartz et al, 1991; Sparreboom et al, 2007; Cortinez et al, 2010; Van Kralingen et al, 2011). However, studies on propranolol, a drug with high-extraction ratio but less clearance rate, showed variable results (Cheymol et al, 1997; Wojcicki et al, 2003).

Renal Elimination

Many drugs are eliminated through kidney via glomerular filtration, tubular secretion, and tubular reabsorption. The size of the kidney, renal plasma flow, and urine flow rate may influence the function of the kidney.

A. Glomerular filtration

Studies comparing clearance of drugs that are primarily eliminated by glomerular filtration showed a significantly higher clearance in the obese group for vancomycin (Bauer et al, 1998), daptomycin (Dvorchik and Damphousse, 2005), and enoxaparin (Barras et al, 2009). Studies for carboplatin (Sparreboom et al, 2007) and dalteparin (Yee and Duffull, 2000) showed higher clearances in the obese group, but not statistically significant as compared to the non-obese group.

B. Tubular secretion

A significantly higher tubular secretion in the obese group was reported for procainamide, ciprofloxacin, and cisplatin (Christoff et al, 1983; Allard et al, 1993; Sparreboom et al, 2007). Studies for topotecan and digoxin (Abernethy et al, 1981b; Sparreboom et al, 2007) showed a trend toward higher tubular secretion in the obese group, but the difference was not statistically significant.

C. Tubular reabsorption

It appears that tubular reabsorption of lithium was significantly lower in the obese group as compared with the non-obese group in the one study available (Reiss et al, 1994). In this study, the renal clearance of lithium was significantly increased in the obese patients, while their glomerular filtration rates were not different between obese and non-obese groups.

Dosing Considerations in the Obese Patients

Studies for various drugs have been conducted to evaluate appropriate dosing regimens for obese patients. It is not possible to list all the studies and dosing recommendations in this text. However, based on the findings from the pharmacokinetic studies, principles of drug dosing for the obese patients may be adopted to calculate loading dose and maintenance dose.

A. Loading dose

The loading dose is primarily based on V_D. In general, the weight used to calculate the loading dose depends on how the drug is distributed in the lean and fat tissues in the body. If the drug is primarily distributed into the lean mass, IBW will be used to calculate the loading dose. In contrast, if the drug is largely distributed into the fat tissues, TBW will be used. If the distribution is somewhere in between, an adjusted weight may be used (Allen, 2008).

B. Maintenance dose

The maintenance dose primarily depends on drug clearance (Cl). The most commonly used equations to estimate glomerular filtration rate (GFR) are Cockcroft–Gault (CG) equation (Cockcroft and Gault, 1976) and Modification of Diet in Renal Disease (MDRD) equation (Levey et al, 1999). The MDRD equation was developed with six variables—age, gender, S_{cr}, blood urea nitrogen, albumin, and race—to estimate GFR in patients with chronic kidney disease.

The CG equation estimates creatinine clearance (Cl_{cr}) as a surrogate of GFR.

$$[(140 - age) \times (\text{Weight in kg})]/[72 \times \text{serum creatinine}] \times 0.85 \text{ if female} \quad (23.1.1)$$

Clearance of the endogenous creatinine in serum (S_{cr}) is dependent on GFR and renal tubular secretion. The production of the endogenous creatinine is affected by diet and muscle mass. To estimate Cl_{cr} by the CG equation, it is recommended to use TBW in underweight patients, IBW in patients with normal weight, and adjusted body weight for overweight, obese, and morbidly obese patients (Winter et al, 2012). A recent study (Pai, 2010) reported that using lean body weight (LBW) in the CG equation provides a practical estimation of GFR for drug dosing in obesity.

Applying the pharmacokinetic principles and using modified weight strategies may help with better drug dosing for the obese. However, due to limitations on published pharmacokinetic studies in obesity, and interindividual variations within the obese population, individualized therapeutic drug monitoring, especially for drugs with narrow therapeutic index, is warranted.

Clinical Examples on Estimating Creatinine Clearance in Obesity

EXAMPLE 1 ▶▶▶

A 50-year-old female, BT, was admitted to the hospital with sepsis. Her height is 5 feet and 5 inches, and weight was 350 lb. Her serum creatinine is 1.2 mg/dL. The team has decided to start BT on an antibiotic regimen.
Discussion:

- First, calculate BMI for BT using Equation 23.2.1:
  Her TBW in kilogram = 350 (lb)/2.2 (lb/kg), which is 159.1 kg

Her height in centimeter (cm) = 65 (inches) × 2.54 (cm/inch), which is 165.1 cm
Her BMI = 58.4 kg/m²
She is morbidly obese, according to the classification of obesity based on BMI (Table 23.2-1). It is recommended to use adjusted body weight to estimate Cl_{cr} from the CG equation for patients who are overweight, obese, or morbidly obese.

- In order to calculate Adj. BW, IBW needs to be calculated first, using Equation 23.2.3:
  IBW = 45.5 + 2.3 × [Height (inches) – 60] kg
  Her IBW = 57 kg

- Calculate Adj. BW using Equation 23.2.4:
  Adj. BW = IBW + 0.4 × (TBW – IBW) kg
  Her Adj. BW = 97.8 kg

- Calculate Cl_{cr} (mL/min) by CG equation (Equation 23.1.1) using Adj. BW:
  Cl_{cr} (mL/min) = [(140-age) × (Weight in kg)]/ [72 × serum creatinine] × 0.85
  Her estimated Cl_{cr} = 87 mL/min

EXAMPLE 2 ▶▶▶

A 45-year-old male was admitted to the hospital with chief complaints of shortness of breath, wheezing, chills, and fever. Past medical history included hypertension, arthritis, and asthma. The patient's weight and height were 300 lb and 5'-4", respectively, and his serum creatinine is 1.2 mg/dL.
Discussion:

- Calculate BMI as in Example 1; the answer is 51.6 kg/m².

- Calculate IBW using Equation 23.2.2:
  IBW = 50 + 2.3 × [Height (inches) – 60] kg
  His IBW = 59.2 kg

- Calculate Adj. BW as in Example 1:
  His Adj. BW = 90 kg

- Calculate Cl_{cr} (mL/min) using Adj. BW for weight:
  Cl_{cr} (mL/min) = [(140 – age) × (Weight in kg)]/ (72 × serum creatinine)
  His estimated Cl_{cr} = 99 mL/min

SUMMARY

Our understanding of obesity and its implications continues to improve, as more research has been devoted to this arena. However, the complexity of physiological changes in obesity combined with obesity-related comorbidities frequently incurred in the obese population may render pharmacokinetic studies challenging. More studies are needed on drug absorption in the obese population, as well as specific studies on drug distribution, metabolism, and elimination in obesity.

For Phase I metabolism, CYP3A4 activity was consistently lower in the obese group, while the enzyme activities of CYP2E1 and xanthine oxidase were consistently higher in the obese group. Other Phase I metabolism enzymes showed trends toward higher activities in the obese group, but the results were not conclusive. For Phase II metabolism, UGT-mediated drug clearances were significantly higher in the obese group. Liver blood flow may be increased in obesity, but the number of the drugs studied is small, and the weight difference between obese and non-obese groups was limited in these studies. As a note, the weight-normalized clearance values may provide quantitative difference information for clearance (Brill et al, 2012).

Renal clearance is increased in the obese patients due to increased glomerular filtration and tubular secretion. The impact of obesity on tubular reabsorption is currently inconclusive due to limited data. Weight-normalized clearances for all drugs studied for renal elimination showed similar or lower values in the obese group, as compared to the non-obese group.

In terms of drug dosing, even with the same BMI, individual obese patient may present with unique body composition and fat distribution. Thus, drug dosing for the obese patients remains to be elusive. Presently, in an effort to ensure optimal therapeutic outcome for drug therapies in obesity, we need to keep abreast with published pharmacokinetic data, apply the information to patients prudently, and provide individualized therapeutic monitoring as indicated.

LEARNING QUESTIONS

A 45-year-old female was admitted to the hospital with chief complaints of shortness of breath, wheezing, chills, and fever. Past medical history included hypertension, arthritis, and asthma. The patient's weight and height were 300 lb and 5′-4″, respectively.

1. Which of the following answers is correct for this patient's body mass index (BMI)?
   a. 35.0
   b. 39.3
   c. 60.9
   d. 54.2
   e. 51.6

2. If this patient has a serum creatinine of 1.0 mg/dL, calculate her estimated creatinine clearance in mL/min using adjusted body weight (Adj. BW) in the Cockcroft–Gault equation.
   a. 115.3
   b. 98.0
   c. 61.3
   d. 152.9
   e. 120.0

3. Which of the following CYP450 isoenzymes showed a reduced activity in the obese patients?
   a. CYP3A4
   b. CYP2E1
   c. CYP2C9
   d. CYP2D6
   e. Xanthine oxidase

4. Which of the following statements most accurately reflects the physiological changes commonly occurred with obesity?
   a. Glomerular filtration is usually increased in the obese patients.
   b. Tubular reabsorption is usually increased in the obese patients.
   c. Tubular secretion is usually decreased in the obese patients.
   d. The activity of uridine diphosphate glucuronosyltransferase is usually decreased in the obese patients.
   e. The size of the kidney is usually smaller in the obese patients.

5. Which of the following statements most accurately reflects an appropriate drug dosing strategy for the obese patients?
   a. The TBW should always be used to calculate the loading dose for the obese patients.
   b. The IBW should always be used to calculate the loading dose for the obese patients.
   c. The TBW should always be used to calculate the maintenance dose for the obese patients.
   d. The IBW should always be used to calculate the maintenance dose for the obese patients.
   e. Applying the pharmacokinetic principles and using modified weight strategies, combining with therapeutic drug monitoring.

ANSWERS

Learning Questions

1. a.
2. b.
3. a.
4. a.
5. e.

REFERENCES

Abernethy DR, Greenblatt DJ: Ibuprofen disposition in obese individuals. *Arthritis Rheum* **28:**1117, 1985a.

Abernethy DR, Greenblatt DJ: Phenytoin disposition in obesity: Determination of loading dose. *Arch Neurol* **42:**468, 1985b.

Abernethy DR, Greenblatt DJ, Divoll M, et al: Alterations in drug distribution and clearance due to obesity. *J Pharmacol Exp Ther* **217:**681, 1981a.

Abernethy DR, Greenblatt DJ, Smith TW: Digoxin disposition in obesity: Clinical pharmacokinetic investigation. *Am Heart J* **102:**740, 1981b.

Abernethy DR, Divoll M, Greenblatt DJ, et al: Obesity, sex, and acetaminophen disposition. *Clin Pharmacol Ther* **31:**783, 1982b.

Abernethy DR, Greenblatt DJ, Divoll M, et al: Prolongation of drug half-life due to obesity: Studies of desmethyldiazepam (clorazepate). *J Pharm Sci* **71:**942, 1982a.

Abernethy DR, Greenblatt DJ, Divoll M, et al: Enhanced glucuronde conjugation of drugs in obesity: Studies of lorazepam, oxazepam, and acetaminophen. *J Lab Clin Med* **101:**873, 1983.

Abernethy DR, Greenblatt DJ, Divoll M, et al: The influence of obesity on the pharmacokinetics of oral alprazolam and triazolam. *Clin Pharmacokinet* **9:**177, 1984.

Abernethy DR, Todd El, Schwartz JB: Caffeine disposition in obesity. *Br J Clin Pharmacol* **20:**61, 1985.

Alexander JK, Dennis EW, Smith WG, et al: Blood volume, cardiac output, and disposition of systemic blood flow in ectreme obesity. *Cardiovasc Res Cent Bull* **1:**39, 1962.

Alexander JK: Obesity and cardiac performance. *Am J Cardiol* **14:**860, 1964.

Allard S, Kinzig M, Boivin G, et al: Intravenous ciprofloxacin disposition in obesity. *Clin Pharmacol Ther* **54:**368, 1993.

AMA. Obesity as a disease. AMA Press Releases and Statements. June 18, 2013.

Balis FM: Pharmacokinetic drug interactions of commonly used anticancer drugs. *Clin Pharmacokinet* **11:**223, 1986.

Barras MA, Duffull SF, Atherton JJ, et al: Modelling the occurrence and severity of enoxaparin-induced bleeding and bruising events. *Br J Clin Pharmacol* **68:**700, 2009.

Bauer LA, Edwards WA, Dellinger EP, et al: Influence of weight on aminoglycoside pharmacokinetics in normal weight and morbidly obese patients. *Eur J Clin Pharmacol* **24:**643, 1983.

Bauer LA, Black DJ, Lill JS: Vancomycin dosing in morbidly obese patients. *Eur J Clin Pharmacol* **54:**621, 1998.

Bentley JB, Vaughan RW, Gandolfi AJ, et al: Halothane biotransformation in obese and nonobese patients. *Anesthesiology* **57:**94, 1982.

Berghofer A, Pischon T, Reinhold T, et al: Obesity prevalence from a European perspective: A systematic review. *BMC Public Health* **8:**200, 2008.

Brill MJ, Diepstraten J, van Rongen A, et al: Impact of obesity on drug metabolism and elimination in adults and children. *Clin Pharmacokinet* **51:**277, 2012.

Buechler C, Weiss TS: Does hepatic steatosis affect drug metabolizingenzymes in the liver? *Curr Drug Metab* **12:**24, 2011.

Caraco Y, Zylber-Katz E, Berry EM, et al: Carbamazepine pharmacokinetics in obese and lean subjects. *Ann Pharmacother* **29:**843, 1995.

Cheymol G: Drug pharmacokinetics in the obese. *Fundam Clin Pharmacol* **2:**239, 1988.

Cheymol G: Clinical pharmacokinetics of drugs in obesity. An update. *Clinical Pharmacokinet* **25:**103, 1993.

Cheymol G: Effects of obesity on pharmacokinetics implications for drug therapy. *Clin Pharmacokinet* **39:**215, 2000.

Cheymol G, Weissenburger J, Poirier JM, et al: The pharmacokinetics of dexfenfluramine in obese and non-obese subjects. *Br J Clin Pharmacol* **39:**684, 1995.

Cheymol G, Poirier JM, Carrupt PA, et al: Pharmacokinetics of beta-adrenoceptor blockers in obese and normal volunteers. *Br J Clin Pharmacol* **43:**563, 1997a.

Cheymol G, Woestenborghs R, Snoeck E, et al: Pharmacokinetic study and cardiovascular monitoring of nebivolol in normal and obese subjects. *Eur J Clin Pharmacol* **51:**493, 1997b.

Chiney MS, Schwarzenberg SJ, Johnson LA: Altered xanthine oxidase and N-acetyl transferase activity in obese children. *Br J Clin Pharmacol* **72:**109, 2011.

Cockcroft DW, Gault MH: Prediction of creatinine clearance from serum creatinine. *Nephron* **16:**31, 1976.

Cortinez LI, Anderson BJ, Penna A, et al: Influence of obesity on propofol pharmacokinetics: Derivation of a pharmacokinetic model. *Br J Anaesth* **105:**448, 2010.

Christoff PB, Conti DR, Naylor C, et al: Procainamide disposition in obesity. *Drug Intell Clin Pharm* **17:**516, 1983.

Devine BJ: Gentamicin therapy. *Drug Intell Clin Pharm* **7:**650, 1974.

Dvorchik BH, Damphousse D: The pharmacokinetics of daptomycin in moderately obese, morbidly obese, and matched non-obese subjects. *J Clin Pharmacol* **45:**48, 2005.

Emery MG, Fisher JM, Chien JY, et al: CYP2E1 activity before and after weight loss in morbidly obese subjects with nonalcoholic fatty liver disease. *Hepatology* **38:**428, 2003.

Farrell GC, Teoh NC, McCuskey RS: Hepatic microcirculation in fatty liver disease. *Anat Rec (Hoboken)* **291:**684, 2008.

Flegal KM et al: Cause-specific excess deaths associated with underweight, overweight, and obesity. *JAMA* **298:**2028, 2007.

Flechner SM, Kilbeinsson ME, Tam J, et al: The impact of body weight on cyclosporine pharmacokinetics in renal transplant recipients. *Transplantation* **47:**806, 1989.

Gibbs JP, Gooley T, Corneau B, et al: The impact of obesity and disease on busulfan oral clearance in adults. *Blood* **93:**4436, 1999.

Greenblatt DJ, Abernethy DR, Locniskar A, et al: Effect of age, gender, and obesity on midazolam kinetics. *Anesthesiology* **61:**27, 1984.

Higuchi H, Satoh T, Arimura S, et al: Serum inorganic fluoride levels in mildly obese patients during and after sevoflurane anesthesia. *Anesth Analg* **77:**1018, 1993.

Jaber LA, Ducharme MP, Halapy H: The effects of obesity on the pharmacokinetics and pharmacodynamics of glipizide in patients with non-insulin-dependent diabetes mellitus. *Ther Drug Monit* **18:**6, 1996.

Janmahasatian S, Duffull SB, Ash S, et al: Quantification of lean bodyweight. *Clin Pharmacokinet* **44:**1051, 2005.

Jia H et al: The impact of obesity on health-related quality-of-life in the general adult US population. *J Public Health* **27:**156, 2005.

Jusko WJ, Gardner MJ, Mangione A, et al: factors affecting theophylline clearances: Age, tobacco, marijuana, cirrhosis, congestive heart failure, obesity, oral contraceptives, benzodiazepines, barbiturates, and ethanol. *J Pharm Sci* **68:**1358, 1979.

Kamimori GH, Somani SM, Knowlton RG, et al: The effects of obesity and exercise on the pharmacokinetics of caffeine in lean and obese volunteers. *Eur J Clin Pharmacol* **31:**595, 1987.

Kopelman PG: Obesity as a medical problem. *Nature* **404:**635, 2000.

Levey AS, Bosch JP, Lewis JB, et al: A more accurate method to estimate glomerular filtration rate from serum creatinine: A new predicting equation. Modification of Diet in Lieber, C.S. CYP2E1: From ASH to NASH. *Hepatol Res* **28:**1, 2004.

Lucas D, Ferrara R, Gonzalez E, et al: Chlorzoxazone, a selective probe for phenotyping CYP2E1 in humans. *Pharmacogenetics* **9:**377, 1999.

Malnick SDH et al: The medical complications of obesity. *Q J Med* **99:**565, 2006.

May DG: Genetic differences in drug disposition. *J Clin Pharmacol* **34:**881, 1994.

Medico CJ, Walsh P: Pharmacotherapy in the critically ill obese patient. *Crit Care Clin* **26:**679, 2010.

Metropolitan Life Insurance Company. New weight standards for men and women. *Stat Bull Metrop Ins Co* **40:**1, 1959.

Miller MS, Gandolfi AJ, Vaughan RW, et al: Disposition of enflurane in obese patients. *J Pharmacol Exp Ther* **215:**292, 1980.

Moretto M, Kupski C, Mottin CC, et al: Hepatic steatosis in patients undergoing bariatric surgery and its relationship to body mass index and co-morbidities. *Obes Surg* **13:**622, 2003.

Ogden CL et al: Prevalence of overweight and obesity in the United States, 1999-2004. *JAMA* **295:**1549, 2006.

Padwal RS, Gabr RQ, Sharma AM, et al: Effect of gastric bypass surgery on the absorption and bioavailability of metformin. *Diabetes Care* **34:**1295, 2011.

Pai MP: Estimating the glomerular filtration rate in obese adult patients for drug dosing. *Adv Chronic Kidney Dis* **17:**e53, 2010.

Reiss RA, Haas CE, Karki SD, et al: Lithium pharmacokinetics in the obese. *Clin Pharmacol Ther* **55:**392, 1994.

Renal Disease Study Group. *Ann Intern Med* **130:**461, 1999.

Rowland M, Tozer TN: Membranes and distribution. In Rowland M and Tozer TN (eds). *Clinical Pharmacokinetics and Pharmacodynamics: Concepts and Applications.* Philadelphia, PA, Lippincott Williams & Wilkins Publisher, 2011, p 73.

Schwartz AE, matteo RS, Ornstein E, et al: Pharmacokinetics of sufentanil in obese patients. *Anesth Analg* **73:**790, 1991.

Shukla UA, Chi Em, Lehr KH: Glimepiride pharmacokinetics in obese versus non-obese diabetic patients. *Ann Pharmacother* **38:**30, 2004.

Skottheim IB, Stormark K, Christensen H, et al: Significantly altered systemic exposure to atorvastatin acid following gastric bypass surgery in morbidly obese patients. *Clin Pharmacol Ther* **86:**311, 2009.

Sparreboom A, Wolff AC, Mathijssen RH, et al: Evaluation of alternate size descriptors for dose calculation of anticancer drugs in the obese. *J Clin Oncol* **25:**4707, 2007.

Van den Anker JN: Developmental pharmacology. *Dev Disabil Res Rev* **16:**233, 2010.

Van Kralingen S, Diepstraten J, Peeters MYM, et al: Population pharmacokinetics and pharmacodynamics of propofol in morbidly obese patients. *Clin Pharmacokinet* **50:**739, 2011.

Winter MA, Guhr KN, Berg GM: Impact of various body weights and serum creatinine concentrations on the bias and accuracy of the Cockcroft-Gault equation. *Pharmacotherapy* **32:**604, 2012.

Winter ME: *Basic Clinical Pharmacokinetics*, 5th Ed. Philadelphia, PA, Lippincott Williams & Wilkins Publisher, 2010, p 100.

Wojcicki J, Jaroszynska M, Drozdzik M, et al: Comparative pharmacokinetics and pharmacodynamics of propranolol and atenolol in normolipaemic and hyperlipidaemic obese subjects. *Biopharm Drug Dispos* **24**:211, 2003.

World Health Organization: Report of a WHO Consultation on obesity: Preventing and managing the global epidemic. Geneva, WHO, June 3-5, 1998.

Yee GC, Lennon TP, Gmur DJ, et al: Effect of obesity on cyclosporine disposition. *Transplantation* **45**:649, 1988.

Yee JY, Duffull SB: The effect of body weight on dalteparin pharmacokinetics: A preliminary study. *Eur J Clin Pharmacol* **56**:293, 2000.

Zahorska-Markiewicz B, Waluga M, Zielinski M, et al: Pharmacokinetics of theophylline in obesity. *Int J Clin Pharmacol Ther* **34**:393, 1996.

MODULE III: APPLICATION OF PHARMACOKINETICS TO THE PEDIATRIC PATIENTS

Objectives

- List the demographic definition of pediatric population.
- Understand inadequacy of current guidance in dosing recommendation for pediatric patients.
- Describe the age-dependent differences in physiological functions and pharmacokinetic (ADME) consequences of drugs.
- Describe the effects of age on pharmacodynamics of drugs.
- Discuss the studies to help rational dosing in pediatric patients.
- Describe the emerging approaches to study pharmacology in pediatric population.

Pediatric Population

Pediatric subjects are not miniature adults, nor belong to a homogeneous population as their anatomical development and physiological functions vary depending on their age brackets. Therefore, the pharmacokinetic characteristics of medications differ among pediatric subpopulations. The pediatric subpopulations consist of preterm or term neonates, infants, children, and adolescents, with the age ranges defined in Food and Drug Administration (FDA) Guidance for Industry (Table 23.3-1) (FDA, 2014). The upper age limits used to define the pediatric subpopulations vary among experts (FDA, 1997; Rowland and Tozer, 2011; Murphy, 2012) as given in parentheses of Table 23.3-1, including for adolescents up to the age of 16, 18, 19, or 21 years

(Rowland and Tozer, 2011; Murphy, 2012). The age of 21 years is consistently used in several well-known sources (Avery, 1994; Kliegman et al, 2011; Rudolph et al, 2011).

Inadequate Guidance in Dosing Recommendation for Pediatric Patients

Pediatric patients have different dosing requirements from those for adults (ICH E11 Guideline, 2000; Bartelink et al, 2006; Leeder et al, 2010; Benavides et al, 2011). Information for pediatric dosing was generally lacking in the past. For most (75%) of drugs, pediatric patients are still dosed as "off-label" usage without specific pediatric dosing recommendations (Benavides et al, 2011).

When dosage guidelines are not available for a drug, empirical dose adjustment methods are often used. Dosage normalized based on the child's age or body weight from adult drug dosages was used through the Young's rule [Adult Dose × (Age ÷ (Age + 12)) = Child's Dose] and Clark's rule [Adult Dose × (Weight ÷ 150) = Child's Dose], respectively. Dosage based on body surface area has an advantage of avoiding bias

TABLE 23.3-1   Age Ranges of Pediatric Subpopulations

Premature (preterm) neonates	Born at gestational age <38 weeks
Neonates (term newborn)	0–4 weeks postnatal age
Infants	1 month to 2 years of age (1 month to <12 months old)
Children	2–12 years of age (1–12 years old)
Adolescents	12–21 years of age (13–16, 18, or 19 years old)

due to obesity or unusual body weight, because both the height and the weight of the patient are considered. However, these dosages are rough estimates and often inadequate to reflect the developmental and physiological differences that lead to pharmacokinetic consequences among the pediatric subpopulations, as well as between pediatric and adult populations. Therefore, pediatric subjects should not be considered as small adults in the aspect of pharmacokinetics. Pediatric drug use information should be consulted in the product label's *Use in Specific Populations* subsection.

In December 1994, the FDA required drug manufacturers to determine whether existing data were sufficient to support information on pediatric use for drug labeling purposes and implemented a plan to encourage the voluntary collection of pediatric data. The FDA Modernization Act (FDAMA) 505(A) authorized a pediatric exclusivity with an additional 6 months of patent protection for manufacturers who conducted pediatric clinical trials (FDA, 1997). As a consequence, the pediatric studies resulted in 202 product label changes in 2007–2012 with the inclusion of new indications and enhanced pediatric safety information for pediatric population (Leeder et al, 2010). These studies reveal significant new information regarding dosing and pharmacokinetic differences between children and adults (Maples et al, 2006).

The rational, effective, and safe dosing of drugs in the pediatric population requires a thorough understanding of the differences in developmental pharmacology, pharmacokinetics, and pharmacodynamics of a specific drug, among individual subpopulations, as well as between pediatric and adult subjects.

Age-Dependent Differences in Physiological Functions and Impacts on Pharmacokinetics of Drugs

Absorption

The physiological variables for oral absorption, such as gastric pH, gastric emptying time, intestinal transit time, and biliary function, are distinct among neonates, infants, and children. In neonates, the gastric pH is >4, and gastric emptying and intestinal transit are faster and irregular with immature biliary function (Murphy, 2012). In infants, the pH is 2–4

with increasing emptying and transit time, but biliary function is near the adult pattern. In children, the emptying and transit time is still increasing up to 4 years of age to mature, but pH and biliary function are similar to those of adults (Kearns et al, 2003). As a consequence, the higher pH in neonates and infants result in higher bioavailability (F) of acid-labile drugs, such as penicillin G, ampicillin, and nafcillin, but lower F of phenobarbital (weak acid) that may require a higher dose as compared to those for children and adults (O'Connor et al, 1965; Sliverio and Poole, 1973; Morselli, 1977). The fast GI transit reduces the rate and extent of absorption in neonates, infants, and young children. The neonates are difficult to absorb fat-soluble vitamins compared to infants and children due to the immature biliary function (Heubi et al, 1982).

Drug Distribution

Factors such as plasma protein concentration, body composition, blood flow, tissue-protein concentration, and tissue fluid pH are important for drug distribution. Of these factors, the changes in (a) plasma protein concentration, (b) total body fat, as well as (c) total body water and extracellular water are the three major factors exerting significant effects on drug distribution in pediatric population (Murphy, 2012).

The total body water is high, constituting 75%–90% of total body weight in neonates and infants up to the first 6 months of life, compared to about 60% in children and adults (O'Connor et al, 1965). As a result, the apparent volume of distribution (V) of hydrophilic drugs is age dependent, as illustrated in Table 23.3-2 with the well-documented case of gentamicin (Shevchuk and Taylor, 1990; Semchok et al, 1995). The extracellular fluid (ECF) is high in neonates, 45%, as compared to 25%–26% in adults, but approaching adult value in one year of life. The total body fat is less, 12% in neonates and infants, but peaks at 30% in one year, then decreasing gradually to adult value of 18%. Therefore, when we dose on a weight (kg) basis, lower plasma concentrations for hydrophilic drugs are expected in neonates and young infants, due to their higher percentage of total body water and ECF for drug distribution out of blood circulation. The age-dependent V of lipophilic drugs is less apparent (Table 23.3-2).

TABLE 23.3-2   Age-Dependent Apparent Volumes of Distribution of Gentamicin and Diazepam

Age	Gentamicin	V (L/kg) Diazepam
<34 weeks postnatal	0.67	
34–48 weeks postnatal	0.52	1.3–2.6
1–4.9 years	0.38	
5–9.9 years	0.33	
10–16 years	0.31	
Adults	0.30	1.6–3.2

The protein concentrations are low in the neonates and infants up to one year old. The changes in circulating plasma proteins, albumin and α-acid glycoprotein, affect the distribution of highly bound drugs. In neonates and young infants, phenytoin has a higher unbound fraction of the drug in circulation to exert activity (MacKichan, 1992). The competitive binding of bilirubin on albumin is also a relevant issue in neonates, in that a higher unbound fraction of a drug will be resulted from the displacement by bilirubin in binding of the drug to albumin (Allegaert et al, 2008).

Hepatic and Extrahepatic Drug Metabolism

The developmental differences in drug-metabolizing enzymes and transporters are still inadequately characterized (Allegaert et al, 2008; Murphy, 2012).

Phase I Enzymes-Related Metabolism. In neonates, Phase I enzymes of CYPs 3A4, 2D6, 2C9, and 2C19 are all reduced, with 30%–40%, 20%, 30%, and 30% of adult activities, respectively (Litterst et al, 1975; Neims et al, 1976). In infants, CYP2D6 remains reduced, but reaches adult pattern by the age of 1 year (Mortimer et al, 1990). Other CYP enzymes, CYP3A4, -2C9, and -2C19, reach adult levels by 6 months of life, peak in young children at ages of 3–10 years, and decline to adult levels at puberty (Morselli et al, 1973; Chiba et al,

1980; Payne et al, 1989; Burtin et al, 1994; Hines and McCarver, 2002).

Significant impacts of the age-dependent development of Phase I enzymes on the pharmacokinetics have been documented. The hepatic metabolism of carbamazepine (substrate of CYP3A4) is increased in infants and children as compared to neonates and adults (Korinthenberg et al, 1994). Phenytoin (substrate of CYP2C9) exhibits varying half-lives of 75 hours in preterm infants, 20 hours in first week of term infants, and 8 hours after the second week of life (Besunder et al, 1988). With diazepam (substrate of CYP2C19), the age-dependent changes in oxidative metabolism result in the shortest half-life in children, 7–37 hours, as compared to those of 25–100 hours in neonates and infants, and 20–50 hours in adults (Morselli et al, 1973).

Clinical observations are consistent that hepatic metabolism is age dependent in pediatric patients. Hepatic metabolism in children of 3–10 years of age is greater than that of adults. The greater hepatic clearance in this subpopulation remains significant even after the correction for the age-dependent liver weight (Murry et al, 1995). Therefore, the doses required for this subpopulation of children are often higher on the body weight basis, as compared to adolescents and adults.

Phase II Enzymes-Related Metabolism. The ontogeny of conjugation reactions is less well established than that involving Phase I drug-metabolizing enzymes. Among the Phase II drug-metabolizing enzymes, glucuronosyltransferase (UGT) has reduced activity in neonates and young children but approaches adult level by adolescents. For example, kernicterus is a form of jaundice in the newborn characterized by very high levels of unconjugated bilirubin in the blood. Since the tissues protecting the brain (the blood–brain barrier) are not well formed in newborns, unconjugated bilirubin may enter the brain and cause brain damage. Another example is that the glucuronide/sulfate ratios of acetaminophen increases as UGT system matures, with 0.34 in newborn and 0.8 in children of 3–10 years old, as compared to 1.61 and 1.8–2.3 in adolescents and adults (Miller et al, 1976). Sulfotransferase (SULT) has reduced activity in neonates, but higher activity in infants and children (Murphy, 2012). Methyltransferase in children has increased activities, 50% higher than that in adults (Maples et al, 2006).

Excretion

The rates of glomerular filtration, tubular secretion, and tubular reabsorption are slower at birth, but rapidly rise to adult levels in 8–12 months of age (van den Anker, 1995). Therefore, drugs of high f_e (fraction excreted in urine unchanged) require longer dosing intervals to accommodate the slower drug renal clearance. The prolonged dosing interval allows a longer period of time to excrete drug molecules into urine and minimize drug accumulation in circulation. As a result, similar systemic drug concentrations can be maintained as to those with more mature renal function. For example, the dosing interval of aminoglycoside is suitable as 24 hours for term newborns, but is required to be 36–48 hours for preterm newborn (Schwartz et al, 1987; Brion et al, 1991).

In summary, the understanding of differences in developmental changes and their impacts on pharmacokinetics (ADME) of medications is essential to interpret pharmacokinetic observations correctly and to recommend rational modification in dosing regimen for an effective and safe therapy in the pediatric population.

In recent years, antiretroviral therapy has been used in HIV-infected pediatric patients. An estimated 260,000 children were newly infected with HIV in 2012 (UNAIDS, 2013). The disposition of antiretroviral therapy is significantly affected by the differential pharmacokinetic characteristics among the pediatric subpopulations. The impacts can be drug specific.

The oral absorption of antiretrovirals is affected by the presence of food in GI tract of infants. For example, the F of nelfinavir (a weak acid drug) in newborns and infants <2 years of age is lower than those in older children, due to the food effect, higher gastric pH or both (Hirt et al, 2006). Decreased albumin contents in newborns and neonates cause increases in the unbound fraction of highly protein-bound anti-HIV drugs, such as enfuvirtide (>90% bound), that result in increased efficacy and toxicity (Bellibas et al, 2004). The current cocktail regimen with fixed-dose combinations of antiretrovirals for adults cannot be extrapolated to the pediatric population, because the varied metabolic changes among the pediatric subpopulations may result in subtherapeutic concentrations of one agent in young children, such as nevirapine (metabolized by CYP3A4 and CYP2B6), but overdosing of another agent, such as lamivudine of high $f_e = 0.7$ (eliminated by GFR and active tubular secretion), in neonates (Ellis et al, 2007). The recommended lamivudine dose for infants and children is 4 mg/kg twice daily, whereas the dose for neonates <28 days of age is halved due to the premature development of kidney functions (Panel on Antiretroviral Therapy and Medical Management of HIV-Infected Children, 2010).

Age-Dependent Differences on Pharmacodynamics of Drugs

In contrast to the current understanding of age-dependent pharmacokinetics, much less information is available for the developmental impacts on drug actions at the receptor level (pharmacodynamics) (Holford, 2010). Several age-dependent differences in treatment responses are recognized (Murphy, 2012), not related to the PK differences but in interaction between the drug and its corresponding receptor (warfarin and cyclosporine), or in the relation between the plasma drug concentration and the pharmacological effect (sedation effect of midazolam). The pediatric study decision tree (Fig. 23.3-1) from the FDA asks significant questions on potential age-dependent pharmacodynamics in each step, concerning disease progress, medical intervention, concentration response, and PK/PD to achieve target concentration between pediatric and adult populations (FDA Guidance to Industry, 2003).

Emerging Approaches to Study Pharmacology in Pediatric Population (Knibbe et al, 2011; Himebauch and Zuppa, 2014)

The awareness has grown in the past 20 years on the age-dependent pharmacokinetics of medications, resulting from physiological and pharmacological differences across the entire pediatric age range, and between pediatric and adult populations. With the legislative incentive from the FDA (Best

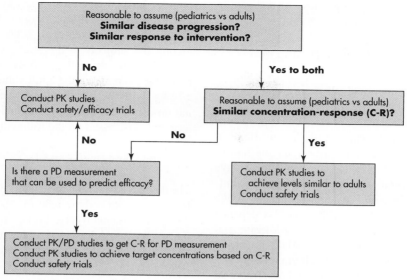

FIGURE 23.3-1   Pediatric study decision tree from FDA.

Pharmaceuticals for Children Act [BPCA] of 2002 (FDA, 2002) and Pediatric Research Equity Act [PREA] of 2003 (FDA, 2003), and EU [Pediatric Regulation 2007]), an increasing number of studies on pediatric PK and PD were conducted from both academic and industrial settings.

In general, the clinical pediatric PK data are scarce and often do not cover the entire pediatric age range. In addition, the study enrollment is small and the number of observations per pediatric subject is limited due to constraints in the volume and frequency of blood sampling. Advances have been made in descriptive pediatric population PK models for specific drugs and particular age range to overcome these constraints (Knibbe et al, 2011).

Two approaches are emerging to more efficiently study pharmacokinetics of drugs in pediatric population for trial design, execution, and data analysis. The approaches are allometric scaling (Knibbe et al, 2011; Wang et al, 2013) and physiological-based pharmacokinetic (PBPK) modeling (Leong et al, 2012; Himebauch and Zuppa, 2014).

In performing allometric scaling, the pharmacokinetic parameters of clearance (*Cl*) and volume distribution (*V*) of pediatric subjects are often predicted by scaling down from adult values with fixed

exponent values of 0.75 for *Cl* and of 1 for *V*. However, the allometric exponent for scaling *Cl* has been recognized to vary with ages in subpopulations of pediatric population (Wang et al, 2013). For example, the exponents for propofol to scale down from adults to neonates, infants, children, and adolescents are 1.11, 0.60, 0.70, and 0.74, respectively (Wang et al, 2013). Therefore, the current allometric scaling approach may be of value for scaling from adults to adolescents and perhaps children, while it is inadequate for scaling from adults to neonates, or between pediatric subpopulations (Wang et al, 2013).

On the other hand, the pediatric PBPK modeling and simulation have been increasingly employed in pediatric drug development, as well as in FDA regulatory review and decision making (Leong et al, 2012). The PBPK model is capable of integrating the factors that address developmental and maturational changes affecting ADME processes of PK in pediatric subpopulations (Barrett et al, 2012). The PBPK model is most commonly implemented in pediatric drug development, for first-time-in-pediatrics (FTIP) dose selection, which is a critical milestone and decision point in pediatric drug development (Edginton, 2011), simulation-based clinical trial design (Mouksassi et al, 2009), systemic exposure–response correlation, and safety assessments of target organ toxicity and in non-systemic biodistribution targets.

Clinical Example of Rational Dosing in Pediatric Patients

Busulfan is a bifunctional alkylating agent (MW 246.31 Da) and used for the preparative regimen before blood, bone marrow, or stem cell transplantation. Before the FDA approval of IV Busulfex® in 1999 for parenteral administration, patients had to receive 35 tablets q6h around the clock for 4 days (total 16 doses). Moreover, the drug triggered vomiting and resulted in erratic systemic exposure, AUC, in patients. However, the grafting success depends on reaching target AUC of 900–1500 μMol•min, and adverse effect is observed when AUC is >1500 μMol•min. Therefore, dosing busulfan precisely and effectively is challenged in adults, and even more so in pediatric patients due to the constraints in therapeutic drug monitoring in the pediatric population.

With the IV Busulfex, the age-dependent clearance is characterized based on 5 body weight strata from <9 kg to >34 kg (Fig. 23.3-2A; Vassal et al, 2008) for 55 pediatric patients 0.3–17.2 years old with 20 subjects younger than 4 years old. The

population total clearance (Cl_{tot}) in children is 3.96 L/h (Vassal et al, 2008), whereas that of adults is about 2.5 L/h (Nguyen et al, 2006). The Cl_{tot} varies among the subjects in the strata, with the greatest value for subjects of 9- to 16-kg body weight, and reducing to approach the adult value at body weight >34 kg. With the specifically derived Cl_{tot}, the rational doses are derived for individual subsets of pediatric patients, based on the following relationship:

$$\text{Total dose (mg/kg)} = Cl_{tot} \times (\text{Target AUC})$$

The dose levels adjusted are 1, 1.2, 1.1, and 0.95 mg/kg, for patients with body weights of <9, 9–16, 16–23, and 23–34 kg, respecitvely, higher than the dose of 0.8 mg/kg for adults. The resulting busulfan AUCs are all well within the theraputic range of 900–1500 μMol•min (Fig. 23.3-2B).

Other Considerations

In addition to different dosing requirements for the pediatric population, there is a need to select age-appropriate dosage forms that permit more accurate dosing and better patient compliance. For example, liquid pediatric drug products may have a calibrated

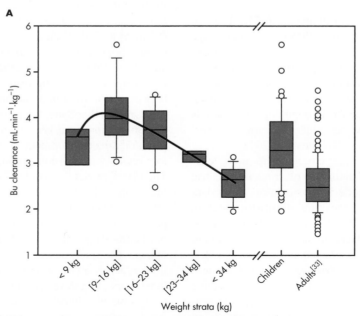

FIGURE 23.3-2   Busulfan clearance (**A**) and AUC with adjusted doses (**B**) among body weight strata.

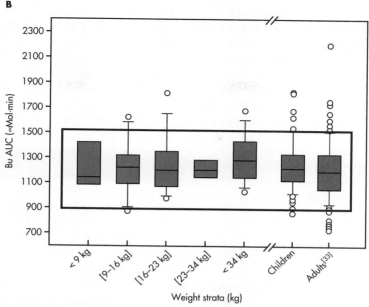

FIGURE 23.3-2   *(Continued)*

dropper or a premeasured teaspoon (5 mL) for more accurate dosing and also have a cherry flavor for pediatric patient compliance. Pediatric drug formulations may also contain different drug concentrations compared to the adult drug formulation and must be considered in order to prevent dosage errors. Moreover, the oral absorption of medications in neonates and infants may be well affected by the presence of milk or infant formula in GI tract.

SUMMARY

Pediatric subjects consist of four subpopulation groups, namely, neonates, infants, children, and adolescents. The pharmacokinetics of medications in pediatric patients is distinct from those of adult subjects, as well as among the pediatric subpopulations. Therefore, a thorough understanding of their developmental and physiological differences and the resulting impacts on pharmacokinetics (ADME) of medications is essential to interpret pharmacokinetic observations correctly and to recommend rational modification in dosing regimen for an effective and safe therapy in the pediatric population.

The absorptions in neonates and infants differ from those of children and adolescents, due to the high gastric pH, short gastric emptying time and intestinal transit time, and immature biliary function. The drug distribution (*V*) is affected by the composition of total body water and total body fat and plasma protein concentrations for highly bound drugs. The drug clearance (*Cl*) is affected by Phase I- and II-mediated metabolisms and renal excretion. The Phase I metabolisms in neonates and infants are lower than those in adults. However, these metabolisms in children of ages of 3–10 years are often higher than those in adults that require higher dose on body weight basis, than those for adolescents and adults. The Phase II metabolizing enzyme capacities approach adult levels in childhood. The renal function is immature in neonates but matures within the first year of life. The age-dependent variations in these clearance processes are unique among pediatric subpopulations. As a result, pediatric dose adjustment is challenging as it is drug specific and age dependent.

The current understanding in age-related pharmacodynamic variations between pediatric and adult populations, as well as those among pediatric subpopulations, is still limited, and requires more studies to fill the knowledge gap.

With the legislative incentive from the FDA and EU, an increasing number of studies on pediatric PK and PD have been performed from both academic and industrial settings. Emerging approaches of population PK, PBPK, and allometric scaling have been gaining acceptance in FTIP dose selection, rational clinical trial design, trial execution, and data analysis. It is anticipated that more useful PK/PD information will be generated in the next few decades to facilitate future rational and safe drug therapy in pediatrics.

LEARNING QUESTIONS

1. Which of the following groups belongs to the pediatric population?
   a. Children
   b. Infants
   c. Adolescents
   d. Neonates
   e. All of the above

2. Pediatric population has unique ADME characteristics from those of adults. In addition, the ADME are distinct among the subpopulations of pediatric subjects. Fill in the blanks in the following table, using ↓ (lower than adult capacity), ↑ (higher than adult capacity), and ↔ (similar or near [~ ↔] adult capacity).

Physiological or PK Characteristic	Neonate	Infant	Child	Adolescent
Absorption				
Gastric pH	_____	↑	↑	↔
GI transit time	_____	↓	_____	↔
Biliary function	↓	_____	↔	↔
Distribution				
Total water/ECF	_____	_____	↓~ ↔	↔
Total body fat	↓	↓	_____	_____
Plasma protein	↓	_____	↔	↔
Metabolism				
CYP enzymes	↓↓	_____	_____	↔
Phase II enzymes	↓	↓	_____	↔
Excretion				
Glomerular filtration	↓	_____	↔	↔
Tubular secretion	_____	~ ↔	↔	↔
Tubular reabsorption				

3. Temozolomide (Temodar®) is an antineoplastic alkylating agent, indicated for refractory (first relapse) anaplastic astrocytoma. The recommended treatment protocol is oral doses of 200 mg/m²/day for 5 days and repeated every 28 days. The F of temozolomide is 0.98 with an empty stomach and 0.6 when the drug is taken with fatty food. The Cl and $t_{1/2}$ of the drug are 100 mL/min/m² and 1.8 hours, respectively. The available capsule strengths are 5, 20, 100, and 250 mg.

   CB is a 15-month-old patient of 7-kg body weight (0.3 m²). (a) What is the Cl of temozolomide in CB? (b) Recommend a regimen for CB, which F is to be used? (c) Predict the $C_{ss,ave}$.

4. WS, an 8-year-old, 25-kg male, is receiving a 250-mg capsule of valproic acid (VA) q12h for the treatment of seizures. The Cls of VA are 13 mL/kg/h for children and 8 mL/kg/h for adults. The V and F of VA are 0.14 L/kg and 1, respectively. The therapeutic plasma VA concentrations are 50–100 mg/L. The toxicity is observed as >200 mg/L.

   WS has normal hepatic and renal functions. (a) Predict the steady state trough concentration ($C_{ss,min}$) for WS, and (b) comment on the adequacy of his current regimen, using a 1-compartment intravenous bolus model.

5. The elimination half-life of penicillin G is 0.5 hour in adults and 3.2 hours in neonates (0–7 days old). Assuming that the normal adult dose of penicillin G is 4 mg/kg every 4 hours, calculate the dose of penicillin G for an 11-lb infant.

ANSWERS

Learning Questions

1. E
2.

Physiological or PK Characteristic	Neonate	Infant	Child	Adolescent
Absorption				
Gastric pH	↑↑	↑	↑	↔
GI transit time	↓↓	↓	↔	↔
Biliary function	↓	~ ↔	↔	↔
Distribution				
Total water/ECF	↑	↑	↓~ ↔	↔
Total body fat	↓	↓	↑ by 1–10 yo	↔
Plasma protein	↓	↓~ ↔	↔	↔
Metabolism				
CYP enzymes	↓↓	↓ ~ ↔ by 1 yo	↑	↔
Phase II enzymes	↓	↓	↔	↔
Excretion				
Glomerular filtration	↓	↔	↔	↔
Tubular secretion	↓	~ ↔	↔	↔
Tubular reabsorption				

3. (a) $Cl = (100 \text{ mL/min/m}^2)(0.3 \text{ m}^2)$
$= 30 \text{ mL/min}$
$= [30 (60)/1000] \text{ L/h} = 1.8 \text{ L/h}$

The Cl in the infant is significantly lower than that of 10.3 L/h in adults with 1.73 m² of body surface area.

(b) $D/\tau = (200 \text{ mg/m}^2/\text{day})(0.3 \text{ m}^2)$
$= 60 \text{ mg/day} = 60 \text{ mg/24 hours}$
$= 20 \text{ mg/8 hours}$
The dose will be given with 3 × 20-mg capsules or in divided doses per day.

(c) $C_{ss,ave} = [F D]/[Cl \cdot \tau]$

Which F is to be used?

$F = 0.6$ (not 0.98) is used to predict the $C_{ss,ave}$, because infants are fed regularly; therefore, the medication is NOT given to the infant with empty stomach, and infant formula in general is rich in the fat content.

$C_{ss,ave} = [F D]/[Cl \cdot \tau]$
$= [(0.6)(60 \text{ mg})]/[(1.8 \text{ L/h})(24 \text{ h})]$
$= 0.83 \text{ mg/L}$

The $C_{ss,ave}$ will be overestimated by 1.6 times as 1.36 mg/L, if an incorrect F (0.98) is selected.

4. (a) The one-compartment IV bolus model can be used to estimate the concentration, because VA is rapidly (with very high k_a) and completely absorbed.

For the one-compartment IV bolus model,

$C_{ss,max} = C_0/(1 - e^{-k \cdot \tau})$
$C_{ss,min} = C_{ss,max} \; e^{-k \cdot \tau}$
$= C_0 \; e^{-k\tau}/(1 - e^{-k \cdot \tau})$
$= [(D/V)e^{-k\tau}]/(1 - e^{-k \cdot \tau})$
$D = 250 \text{ mg} \quad \tau = 12 \text{ h}$
$V = (0.14 \text{ L/kg})(25 \text{ kg}) = 3.5 \text{ L}$
$k = Cl/V$

What is the Cl for AH?

$Cl = (13 \text{ mL/kg/h})(25 \text{ kg})$
$= 325 \text{ mL/h} = 0.325 \text{ L/h}$

$k = Cl/V = (0.325 \text{ L/h})/3.5 \text{ L}$
$= 0.093 \text{ h}^{-1}$
$C_{ss,min} = [(D/V) \; e^{-k \cdot \tau}]/(1 - e^{-k \cdot \tau})$
$= [(250 \text{ mg})/(3.5 \text{ L})][e^{-(0.093)(12)}]/$
$[1 - e^{-(0.093)(12)}]$
$= (71.43 \text{ mg/L})(0.328)/(0.672)$
$= 34.8 \text{ mg/L} \sim 35 \text{ mg/L}$

(b) The $C_{ss,min}$ is *below* the therapeutic range of 50–100 mg/L. The current regimen is required to be modified.
Discussion: If Cl of 8 mg/kg/h for adults is misused,

$Cl = (8 \text{ mL/kg/h})(25 \text{ kg})$
$= 200 \text{ mL/h} = \mathbf{0.20 \text{ L/h}}$
$k = Cl/V = (\mathbf{0.20 \text{ L/h}})/3.5 \text{ L}$
$= \mathbf{0.057 \text{ h}^{-1}}$
$C_{ss,min} = [(D/V) \; e^{-k \cdot \tau}]/(1 - e^{-k \cdot \tau})$
$= [(250 \text{ mg})/(3.5 \text{ L})][e^{-(\mathbf{0.057})(12)}]/$
$[1 - e^{-(\mathbf{0.057})(12)}]$
$= (71.43 \text{ mg/L})(\mathbf{0.505})/(\mathbf{0.495})$
$= 72.8 \text{ mg/L} \sim \mathbf{73 \text{ mg/L}}$
    (overestimated for ~ 2 times)

The comment on the regimen will then be mistakenly made as adequate, because the overestimated trough concentration of 73 mg/L is within the therapeutic range of 50–100 mg/L!

$$\frac{\tau_1}{\tau_2} = \frac{(t_{1/2})_1}{(t_{1/2})_2}$$

$$t_{1/2} = 0.5 \text{ h} \qquad\qquad (23.1.3)$$

$$\tau_2 = \frac{4 \times 3.2}{0.5} = 25.6 \text{ h}$$

Therefore, this infant may be given the following dose:

Dose = 4 mg/kg [11 lb/(2.2 lb/kg)]
$= 20 \text{ mg every 24 h}$

Alternatively, 10 mg every 12 hours would achieve the same $C_{ss,ave}$.

REFERENCES

Allegaert K, Rayyan M, Vanhaesebrouck S, et al: Developmental pharmacokinetics in neonates. *Expert Rev Clin Pharmacol* **1**:415, 2008.

Avery MD, First LR: *Pediatric Medicine*, 2nd ed. Baltimore: Williams & Wilkins, 1994.

Barrett JS, Alberighi ODC, Laer S, et al: Physiologically based pharmacokinetic (PBPK) modeling in children. *Clin Pharmacol Ther* **92**:40, 2012.

Bartelink IH, Rademaker CM, Schobben AF, et al: Guidelines on paediatric dosing on the basis of developmental physiology and pharmacokinetic considerations. *Clin Pharmacokinet* **45**:1077, 2006.

Bellibas SE, Siddique Z, Dorr A, et al: Pharmacokinetics of enfuvirtide in pediatric human immunodeficiency virus 1-infected patients receiving combination therapy. *Pediatr Infec Dis J* **23**:1137, 2004.

Benavides S, Huynh D, Morgan J, et al: Approach to the pediatric prescription in a community pharmacy. *J Pediatr Pharmacol Ther* **16**:298, 2011.

Besunder JB, Reed MD, Blumer JL: Principles of drug disposition in neonate: a critical evaluation of the pharmacokinetic-pharmacodynamic interface. Part I & II, *Clin Pharmacokinet* **14**:189, 261, 1988.

Brion LP, Fleischman AR, Schwartz GJ: Gentamicin interval in new born infants as determined by renal function and postconceptional age. *Pediatr Nephrol* **5**:675, 1991.

Burtin P, Jacqz-Aigrain E, Girard P, et al: Population pharmacokinetics of midazolam in neonates. *Clin Pharmacol Ther* **56**:615, 1994.

Chiba K, Ishizaki T, Miura H, et al: Michelis-Menten pharmacokinetics of diphenylhydantoin and application in pediatric age patient. *J Pediatr* **96**:479, 1980.

Edginton AN: Knowledge-driven approaches for guidance of first-in-children dosing. *Padiatr Anesth* **21**:206, 2011.

Ellis JC, L'homme RF, Ewings FM, et al: Nevirapine concentrations in HIV-infected children treated with divided fixed-dose combination antiretroviral tablets in Malawi and Zambia. *Antivir Ther* **12**:253, 2007.

FDA: The Modernization Act 505 (A), Qualifying for Pediatric Exclusivity, http://www.fda.gov/downloads/Drugs/Guidance-ComplianceRegulatoryInformation/Guidances/ucm078751.pdf, 1997.

FDA: Best Pharmaceuticals for Children Act of 2002, http://www.fda.gov/RegulatoryInformation/Legislation/FederalFoodDrugandCosmeticActFDCAct/SignificantAmendmentstotheFDCAct/ucm148011.htm, 2002.

FDA: Pediatric Research Equity Act of 2003, http://www.fda.gov/downloads/Drugs/DevelopmentApprovalProcess/DevelopmentResources/UCM077853.pdf, 2003.

FDA: Guidance for Industry and FDA Staff: Premarket Assessment of Pediatric Medical Devices, March 24, 2014.

FDA Guidance to Industry: Exposure-response Relationships—Study Design, Data Analysis and Regulatory Applications, FDA, 2003.

Gal P, Toback J, Erkan NV, et al: The influence of asphyxia on phenobarbital dosing requirements in neonates. *Dev Pharmacol Ther* **7**:145, 1984.

Heubi JE, Balistreri WF, Suchy FJ: Bile salt metabolism in the first year of life. *J Lab Clin Med* **100**:127, 1982.

Himebauch A, Zuppa A: Methods for pharmacokinetic analysis in young children. *Expert Opin Drug Metab Toxicol* **10**:497, 2014.

Hines R, McCarver G: The ontogeny of human drug-metabolizing enzymes: Phase I oxidative enzymes. *J Pharmacol Exp Ther* **300**:355, 2002.

Hirt D, Urien S, Jullien V, et al: Age-related effects on nelfinavir and M8 pharmacokinetics: a population study with 182 children. *Amtimicrob Agents Chemother* **50**:910, 2006.

Holford N: Dosing in Children. *Clin Pharmacol Ther* **87**:367, 2010.

ICH E11 Guideline: Clinical Investigation of Medicinal Products in the Pediatric Population, December 2000.

Kearns GL, Abdel-Rahman SM, Alander SW, et al: Developmental Pharmacology—Drug disposition, action and therapy in infants and children. *N Engl J Med* **349**:1157, 2003.

Kliegman RM, Stanton BF, St Geme III JW, et al: *Nelson Textbook of Pediatrics*, 19th ed. Philadelphia, Elsevier, 2011, Chap 12.

Korinthenberg R, Haug C, Hannak D: The metabolization of carbamazepine to CBZ-10, 11-epoxide in children from newborn age to adolescence. *Neuropediatrics* **25**:214, 1994.

Knibbe C, Krekels HJ, Danhof M: Advances in pediatric pharmacokinetics. *Expert Opin Drug Metab Toxicol* **7**:1, 2011.

Litterst CL, Mimnaugh EG, Reagan RL: Comparison of *in vitro* drug metabolism by lung, liver, and kidney of several common laboratory species. *Drug Metab Dispos* **3**:165, 1975.

Leong R, Vieira ML, Zhao P, et al: Regulatory experience with physiologically based pharmacokinetic modeling for pediatric drug trials. *Clin Pharmacol Ther* **91**:926, 2012.

Leeder JS, Kearns GL, Spielberg SP, et al: Understanding the relative roles of pharmacogenetics and ontogeny in pediatric drug development and regulatory science. *J Clin Pharmacol* **50**:1377, 2010.

MacKichan JJ: Influence of protein binding and use of unbound (free) drug concentration. In Evans WE, Schentag JJ, Jusko WJ (eds). *Applied Pharmacokinetics: Principles of Therapeutic Drug Monitoring*. Vancouver, WA, Applied Therapeutics Inc., 1992, pp 5-1–5-48.

Maples HD, James LP, Stowe CD: Special pharmacokinetic and pharmacodynamics considerations in children. In Burton ME, Shaw LM, Schentag JJ, Evans WE (eds). *Applied Pharmacokinetics and Pharmacodynamics—Principles of Therapeutic Drug Monitoring*. Philadelphia, Lippincott Williams & Wilkins, 2006, p 222.

Miller RP, Roberts RJ, Fischer LJ: Acetaminophen elimination kinetics in neonates, children and adults. *Clin Pharmacol Ther* **19**:284, 1976.

Morselli PL, Principi N, Tognoni G, et al: Diazepam elimination in premature and full-term infants and children. *J Perinat Med* **1**:133, 1973.

Mortimer O, Persson R, Ladona MG, et al: Polymorphic formation of morphine from codeine in poor and extensive metabolizers of dextromethorphan. Relationship to the presence of immunoidentified cytochrome P 450 IIDI. *Clin Pharmacol Ther* **47**:27, 1990.

Mouksassi MS, Marier JF, Cyran J, et al: Clinical trial simulations in pediatric patients using realistic covariates: application to teduglutide, a glucagon-like peptide-2-analog in neonates and infants with short-bowel syndrome. *Clin Pharmacol Ther* **86**:667, 2009.

Morselli PL: Antiepileptic drugs. In Morselli PL (ed). *Drug Disposition During Development*. New York, Spectrum, 1977, p 311.

Murphy JE: Drug dosing in pediatric patients. In *Clinical Pharmacokinetics*, 5th ed. Bethesda, ASHP, 2012, pp 29–35.

Murry DJ, Crom WR, Reddick WE, et al: Liver volume as a determinant of drug clearance in children and adolescents. *Drug Metab Dispos* **23**:1110, 1995.

Neims AH, Warner M, Loughman PM, et al: Developmental aspects of the hepatic cytochrome P450 mono-oxygenase system. *Ann Rev Pharmacol Toxicol* **16**:427, 1976.

Nguyen L, Leger F, Lennon S, et al: Intravenous busulfan in adults prior to hematopoietic stem cell transplantation: A population pharmacokinetic study. *Cancer Chemother Pharmacol* **57**:191, 2006.

O'Connor WJ, Warren GH, Edrada L, et al: Serum concentrations of sodium nafcillin in infants during the perinatal period. *Antimicrob Agent Chemother* **5**:220, 1965.

Panel on Antiretroviral Therapy and Medical Management of HIV-Infected Children. Guidelines for the Use of Antiretroviral Agents in Pediatric HIV Infection. August 16, 2010 pp 1–219. http://aidsinfo.nih.gov/ContentFiles/PediatricGuidlines.pdf.

Payne K, Mattheyse FJ, Liebenberg D, et al: The pharmacokinetics of midazolam in pediatric patients. *Eur J Clin Pharmacol* **37**:267, 1989.

Rowland M, Tozer TN: Age, weight and gender. In *Clinical Pharmacokinetics and Pharmacodynamics—Concepts and Applications*, 4th ed. Philadelphia: Lippincott Williams & Wilkins, 2011, p 373.

Rudolph C, Rudolph A, Lister G, et al: *Rudolph's Pediatrics*, 22nd ed. New York, McGraw-Hill, 2011.

Schwartz GJ, Brion LP, Spitzer A: The use of plasma creatinine concentration for estimating glomerular filtration rate in infants, children and adolescents. *Pediatr Clin North Am* **3**:571, 1987.

Semchok WM, Shevchuk YM, Sankaran K, et al: Prospective randomized controlled evaluation of a gentamicin loading dose in neonates. *Bio Neonate* **67**:13, 1995.

Shevchuk YM, Taylor DM: Aminoglycoside volume of distribution in pediatric patients. *DICP* **24**:273, 1990.

Sliverio J, Poole JW. Serum concentrations of ampicillin in newborn infants after oral administration. *Pediatrics* **51**:578, 1973.

UNAIDS, Global Report, 2013. http://www.unaids.org/en/media/unaids/contentassets/documents/epidemiology/2013/gr2013/unaids_global_report_2013_en.pdf.

van den Anker JN, Shoemaker RC, Hop WE, et al: Ceftazidime pharmacokinetics I preterm infants: effects of renal function and gastational age. *Clin Pharmacol Ther* **58**:650, 1995.

Vassal G, Michel G, Esperou H, et al: Prospective validation of a novel IV busulfan fixed dosing for pediatric patients to improve therapeutic AUC targeting without drug monitoring. *Cancer Chemother Pharmacol* **61**:113, 2008.

Wang C, Allegaert K, Peeters MYM, et al: The allometric exponent for scaling clearance varies with age: A study on seven propofol datasets ranging from preterm neonates to adults. *Br J Clin Pharmacol* **77**:149, 2013.

Dose Adjustment in Renal and Hepatic Disease

Yuen Yi Hon

Chapter Objectives

► List the common causes of chronic kidney disease (CKD) and describe how CKD affects drug elimination.

► Compare the advantages and disadvantages of the use of drugs or endogenous substances as markers for the measurement of renal function.

► Describe the relationships between creatinine clearance, serum creatinine concentration, and glomerular filtration rate.

► Explain and contrast the methods of Cockcroft–Gault and Modification of Diet in Renal Disease (MDRD) for the calculation of creatinine clearance.

► List the causes for fluctuating serum creatinine concentration in the body.

► Calculate the dose for a drug in a patient with renal disease.

► Describe quantitatively using equations how renal or hepatic disease can alter the disposition of a drug.

► Describe hemoperfusion and the limitations for its use.

RENAL IMPAIRMENT

Chronic kidney disease (CKD) is a worldwide public health problem affecting more than 50 million people, and more than 1 million of them are receiving kidney replacement therapy (Levey et al, 2009). The kidney is an important organ in regulating body fluids, electrolyte balance, removal of metabolic waste, and drug excretion from the body. Impairment or degeneration of kidney function affects the pharmacokinetics of drugs. Some of the more common causes of kidney failure include disease, injury, and drug intoxication. Table 24-1 lists some of the conditions that may lead to chronic or acute renal failure. Acute diseases or trauma to the kidney can cause *uremia*, in which glomerular filtration is impaired or reduced, leading to accumulation of excessive fluid and blood nitrogenous products in the body. Uremia generally reduces glomerular filtration and/or active secretion, which leads to a decrease in renal drug excretion resulting in a longer elimination half-life of the administered drug.

In addition to changing renal elimination directly, uremia can affect drug pharmacokinetics in unexpected ways. For example, declining renal function leads to disturbances in electrolyte and fluid balance, resulting in physiologic and metabolic changes that may alter the pharmacokinetics and pharmacodynamics of a drug. Pharmacokinetic processes such as drug distribution (including both the volume of distribution and protein binding) and elimination (including both biotransformation and renal excretion) may also be altered by renal impairment. Both therapeutic and toxic responses may be altered as a result of changes in drug sensitivity at the receptor site. Overall, uremic patients have special dosing considerations to account for such pharmacokinetic and pharmacodynamic alterations.

PHARMACOKINETIC CONSIDERATIONS

Uremic patients may exhibit pharmacokinetic changes in bioavailability, volume of distribution, and clearance. The oral bioavailability of a drug in severe uremia may be decreased

▶ Distinguish between hemodialysis and peritoneal dialysis and calculate dose adjustments of a drug in patients undergoing dialysis.

▶ Describe the principle of the fraction of drug excreted unchanged (f_e) method and how it is applied to adjust doses in renal disease.

▶ Explain the principle involved in the Giusti–Hayton method.

▶ Describe the effects of hepatic disease on the pharmacokinetics of a drug.

▶ List the reasons why dose adjustment in patients with hepatic impairment is more difficult than dose adjustment in patients with renal disease.

▶ Explain how liver function tests relate to drug absorption and disposition.

▶ List the pharmacokinetic properties of a drug for which dose adjustment would not be required in patients with renal or hepatic impairment.

as a result of disease-related changes in gastrointestinal motility and pH that are caused by nausea, vomiting, and diarrhea. Mesenteric blood flow may also be altered. However, the oral bioavailability of a drug such as propranolol (which has a high first-pass effect) may be increased in patients with renal impairment as a result of the decrease in first-pass hepatic metabolism (Bianchetti et al, 1978).

The apparent volume of distribution depends largely on drug–protein binding in plasma or tissues and total body water. Renal impairment may alter the distribution of the drug as a result of changes in fluid balance, drug–protein binding, or other factors that may cause changes in the apparent volume of distribution (see Chapter 11). The plasma protein binding of weak acidic drugs in uremic patients is decreased, whereas the protein binding of weak basic drugs is less affected. A decrease in drug–protein binding results in a larger fraction of free drug and an increase in the volume of distribution. However, the net elimination half-life is generally increased as a result of the dominant effect of reduced glomerular filtration. Protein binding of the drug may be further compromised due to the accumulation of metabolites of the drug and various biochemical metabolites, such as free fatty acids and urea, which may compete for the protein-binding sites for the active drug.

Total body clearance of drugs in uremic patients is also reduced by either a decrease in the glomerular filtration rate (GFR) and possibly active tubular secretion or a reduced hepatic clearance resulting from a decrease in intrinsic hepatic clearance.

In clinical practice, estimation of the appropriate drug dosage regimen in patients with impaired renal function is based on an estimate of the remaining renal function of the patient and a prediction of the total body clearance. A complete pharmacokinetic analysis of the drug in the uremic patient may not be possible. Moreover, the patient's uremic condition may not be stable and may be changing too rapidly for pharmacokinetic analysis. Each of the approaches for the calculation of a dosage regimen has certain assumptions and limitations that must be carefully assessed by the clinician before any approach is taken. Dosing guidelines for individual drugs in patients with renal impairment may be found in various reference books, such as the *Physicians' Desk Reference,* and in the medical literature (Bennett 1988, 1990; St. Peter et al, 1992). Most newly approved drugs now contain dosing instructions for CKD patients.

TABLE 24-1   Common Causes of Kidney Failure

Pyelonephritis	Inflammation and deterioration of the pyelonephrons due to infection, antigens, or other idiopathic causes.
Hypertension	Chronic overloading of the kidney with fluid and electrolytes may lead to kidney insufficiency.
Diabetes mellitus	The disturbance of sugar metabolism and acid-base balance may lead to or predispose a patient to degenerative renal disease.
Nephrotoxic drugs/metals	Certain drugs taken chronically may cause irreversible kidney damage—eg, the aminoglycosides, phenacetin, and heavy metals, such as mercury and lead.
Hypovolemia	Any condition that causes a reduction in renal blood flow will eventually lead to renal ischemia and damage.
Neophroallergens	Certain compounds may produce an immune type of sensitivity reaction with nephritic syndrome—eg, quartan malaria nephrotoxic serum.

GENERAL APPROACHES FOR DOSE ADJUSTMENT IN RENAL DISEASE

Several approaches are available for estimating the appropriate dosage regimen for a patient with renal impairment. Each of these approaches has similar assumptions, as listed in Table 24-2. Most of these methods assume that the required therapeutic plasma drug concentration in uremic patients is similar to that required in patients with normal renal function. Uremic patients are maintained on the same C_{av}^{∞} after multiple oral doses or multiple IV bolus injections.

For IV infusions, the same C_{ss} is maintained. (C_{ss} is the same as C_{av}^{∞} after the plasma drug concentration reaches steady state.)

The design of dosage regimens for uremic patients is based on the pharmacokinetic changes that have occurred as a result of the uremic condition. Generally, drugs in patients with uremia or kidney impairment have prolonged elimination half-lives and a change in the apparent volume of distribution. In less severe uremic conditions, there may be neither edema nor a significant change in the apparent volume of distribution. Consequently, the methods for

TABLE 24-2   Common Assumptions in Dosing Renal-Impaired Patients

Assumption	Comment
Creatinine clearance accurately measures the degree of renal impairment	Creatinine clearance estimates may be biased. Renal impairment should also be verified by physical diagnosis and other clinical tests.
Drug follows dose-independent pharmacokinetics	Pharmacokinetics should not be dose dependent (nonlinear).
Nonrenal drug elimination remains constant	Renal disease may also affect the liver and cause a change in nonrenal drug elimination (drug metabolism).
Drug absorption remains constant	Unchanged drug absorption from gastrointestinal tract.
Drug clearance, Cl_u, declines linearly with creatinine clearance, Cl_{Cr}	Normal drug clearance may include active secretion and passive filtration and may not decline linearly.
Unaltered drug–protein binding	Drug-protein binding may be altered due to accumulation of urea, nitrogenous wastes, and drug metabolites.
Target drug concentration remains constant	Changes in electrolyte composition such as potassium may affect response to the effect of digoxin. Accumulation of active metabolites may cause more intense pharmacodynamic response compared to parent drug alone.

dose adjustment in uremic patients are based on an accurate estimation of the drug clearance in these patients.

Several specific clinical approaches for the calculation of drug clearance based on monitoring kidney function are presented later in this chapter. Two general pharmacokinetic approaches for dose adjustment include methods based on drug clearance and methods based on the elimination half-life.

Dose Adjustment Based on Drug Clearance

Methods based on drug clearance try to maintain the desired C_{av}^{∞} after multiple oral doses or multiple IV bolus injections as total body clearance, Cl_T, changes. The calculation for C_{av}^{∞} is

$$C_{av}^{\infty} = \frac{FD_0}{Cl_T \tau} \qquad (24.1)$$

For patients with uremic condition or renal impairment, total body clearance will change to a new value, Cl_T^u. Therefore, to maintain the same desired C_{av}^{∞}, the dose must be changed to a uremic dose, D_0^u, or the dosage interval must be changed to τ^u, as shown in the following equation:

$$C_{av}^{\infty} = \frac{D_0^N}{Cl_T^N \tau^N} = \frac{D_0^u}{Cl_T^u \tau^u} \qquad (24.2)$$

(normal)   (uremic)

where the superscripts N and u represent normal and uremic conditions, respectively.

Rearranging Equation 24.2 and solving for D_0^u

$$D_0^u = \frac{D_0^N Cl_T^u \tau^u}{Cl_T^N \tau^N} \qquad (24.3)$$

If the dosage interval τ is kept constant, then the uremic dose D_0^u is equal to a fraction ($Cl_T^u Cl_T^N$) of the normal dose, as shown in the equation

$$D_0^u = \frac{D_0^N Cl_T^u}{Cl_T^N} \qquad (24.4)$$

For IV infusions the same desired C_{ss} is maintained both for patients with normal renal function and for patients with renal impairment. Therefore, the rate of infusion, R, must be changed to a new value, R^u, for the uremic patient, as described by the equation

$$C_{ss} = \frac{R}{Cl_T^N} = \frac{R^u}{Cl_T^u} \qquad (24.5)$$

(normal) (uremic)

Dose Adjustment Based on Changes in the Elimination Rate Constant

The overall elimination rate constant for many drugs is reduced in the uremic patient. A dosage regimen may be designed for the uremic patient either by reducing the normal dose of the drug and keeping the frequency of dosing (dosage interval) constant or by decreasing the frequency of dosing (prolonging the dosage interval) and keeping the dose constant. Doses of drugs with a narrow therapeutic range should be reduced—particularly if the drug has accumulated in the patient prior to deterioration of kidney function.

The usual approach to estimating a multiple-dosage regimen in the normal patient is to maintain a desired C_{av}^{∞}, as shown in Equation 24.1. Assuming the V_D is the same in both normal and uremic patients and τ is constant, then the uremic dose D_0^u is a fraction (k^u/k^N) of the normal dose:

$$D_0^u = \frac{D_0^N k^u}{k^N} \qquad (24.6)$$

When the elimination rate constant for a drug in the uremic patient cannot be determined directly, indirect methods are available to calculate the predicted elimination rate constant based on the renal function of the patient. The assumptions on how these dosage regimens are calculated include the following:

1. The renal elimination rate constant (k_R) decreases proportionately as renal function decreases. (Note that k_R is the same as k_e as used in previous chapters.)
2. The nonrenal routes of elimination (primarily, the rate constant for metabolism) remain unchanged.
3. Changes in the renal clearance of the drug are reflected by changes in the creatinine clearance.

The overall elimination rate constant is the sum total of all the routes of elimination in the body, including the renal rate and the nonrenal rate constants:

$$k^u = k_{nr}^u + k_R^u \tag{24.7}$$

where k_{nr} is the nonrenal elimination rate constant and k_R is the renal excretion rate constant.

Renal clearance is the product of the apparent volume of distribution and the rate constant for renal excretion:

$$Cl_R^u = k_R^u V_D^u \tag{24.8}$$

Rearrangement of Equation 24.8 gives

$$k_R^u = Cl_R^u \frac{1}{V_D^u} \tag{24.9}$$

Assuming that the apparent volume of distribution and nonrenal routes of elimination do not change in uremia, then $k_{nr}^u = k_{nr}^N$ and $V_D^u = V_D^N$.

Substitution of Equation 24.9 into Equation 24.7 yields

$$k^u = k_{nr}^N + Cl_R^u \frac{1}{V_D^N} \tag{24.10}$$

From Equation 24.10, a change in the renal clearance Cl_R^u due to renal impairment will be reflected in a change in the overall elimination rate constant k^u. Because changes in the renal drug clearance cannot be assessed directly in the uremic patient, Cl_R^u is usually related to a measurement of kidney function by the GFR, which in turn is estimated by changes in the patient's creatinine clearance.

Frequently Asked Questions

▶ *What are the main causes of uremia?*

▶ *How does renal impairment affect the pharmacokinetics of a drug that is primarily eliminated by hepatic clearance?*

▶ *What are the main factors that influence drug dosing in renal disease?*

▶ *Name and contrast the two methods for adjusting drug dose in renal disease.*

MEASUREMENT OF GLOMERULAR FILTRATION RATE

Several drugs and endogenous substances have been used as markers to measure GFR. These markers are carried to the kidney by the blood via the renal artery and are filtered at the glomerulus. Several criteria are necessary to use a drug as a marker to measure GFR:

1. The drug must be freely filtered at the glomerulus.
2. The drug must neither be reabsorbed nor actively secreted by the renal tubules.
3. The drug should not be metabolized.
4. The drug should not bind significantly to plasma proteins.
5. The drug should neither have an effect on the filtration rate nor alter renal function.
6. The drug should be nontoxic.
7. The drug may be infused in a sufficient dose to permit simple and accurate quantitation in plasma and in urine.

Therefore, the rate at which these drug markers are filtered from the blood into the urine per unit of time reflects the GFR of the kidney. Changes in GFR reflect changes in kidney function that may be diminished in uremic conditions.

Inulin, a fructose polysaccharide, fulfills most of the criteria listed above and is therefore used as a standard reference for the measurement of GFR. In practice, however, the use of inulin involves a time-consuming procedure in which inulin is given by intravenous infusion until a constant steady-state plasma level is obtained. Clearance of inulin may then be measured by the rate of infusion divided by the steady-state plasma inulin concentration. Although this procedure gives an accurate value for GFR, inulin clearance is not used frequently in clinical practice.

The clearance of creatinine is used most extensively as a measurement of GFR. *Creatinine* is an endogenous substance formed from creatine phosphate during muscle metabolism. Creatinine production varies with age, weight, and gender of the individual. In humans, creatinine is filtered mainly at the glomerulus, with no tubular reabsorption. However, a small amount of creatinine may be actively secreted by the renal tubules, and the values of GFR obtained by the creatinine clearance tend to be higher than GFR measured by inulin clearance. Creatinine clearance tends to decrease in the elderly patient. As mentioned in Chapter 22, the physiologic changes due to aging may necessitate special considerations in administering drugs in the elderly.

Measurement of *blood urea nitrogen* (BUN) is a commonly used clinical diagnostic laboratory test for renal disease. Urea is the end product of protein catabolism and is excreted through the kidney. Normal BUN levels range from 10 to 20 mg/dL. Higher BUN levels generally indicate the presence of renal disease. However, other factors, such as excessive protein intake, reduced renal blood flow, hemorrhagic shock, or gastric bleeding, may affect increased BUN levels. The renal clearance of urea is by glomerular filtration and partial reabsorption in the renal tubules. Therefore, the renal clearance of urea is less than creatinine or inulin clearance and does not give a quantitative measure of kidney function.

SERUM CREATININE CONCENTRATION AND CREATININE CLEARANCE

Under normal circumstances, creatinine production is roughly equal to creatinine excretion, so the serum creatinine level remains constant. In a patient with reduced glomerular filtration, serum creatinine will accumulate in accordance with the degree of loss of glomerular filtration in the kidney. The serum creatinine concentration alone is frequently used to determine creatinine clearance, Cl_{cr}. Creatinine clearance from the serum creatinine concentration is a rapid and convenient way to monitor kidney function.

Creatinine clearance may be defined as the volume of plasma cleared of creatinine per unit time. Creatinine clearance can be calculated directly by dividing the rate of urinary excretion of creatinine by the patient's serum creatinine concentration. The approach is similar to that used in the determination of drug clearance. In practice, the serum creatinine concentration is determined at the midpoint of the urinary collection period and the rate of urinary excretion of creatinine is measured for the entire day

(24 hours) to obtain a reliable excretion rate. Creatinine clearance is expressed in mL/min and serum creatinine concentration in mg/dL or mg%. Other Cl_{cr} methods based solely on serum creatinine are generally compared to the creatinine clearance obtained from the 24-hour urinary creatinine excretion.

The following equation is used to calculate creatinine clearance in mL/min when the serum creatinine concentration is known:

$$Cl_{cr} = \frac{\text{rate of urinary excretion of creatinine}}{\text{serum concentration of creatinine}}$$

$$Cl_{cr} = \frac{C_u V \times 100}{C_{cr} \times 1440} \qquad (24.11)$$

where C_{cr} = creatinine concentration (mg/dL) of the serum taken at the 12th hour or at the midpoint of the urine-collection period, V = volume of urine excreted (mL) in 24 hours, C_u = concentration of creatinine in urine (mg/mL), and Cl_{cr} = creatinine clearance in mL/min.

Creatinine is eliminated primarily by glomerular filtration. A small fraction of creatinine also is eliminated by active secretion and some nonrenal elimination. Therefore, Cl_{cr} values obtained from creatinine measurements overestimate the actual GFR.

Creatinine clearance has been normalized both to body surface area, using 1.73 m² as the average, and to body weight for a 70-kg adult male. Creatinine distributes into total body water, and when clearance is normalized to a standard V_D, similar drug half-lives in adults and children correspond to identical clearances.

Creatinine clearance values must be considered carefully in special populations such as elderly, obese, and emaciated patients. In elderly and emaciated patients, muscle mass may have declined, thus lowering the production of creatinine. However, serum creatinine concentration values may appear to be in the normal range because of lower renal creatinine excretion. Thus, the calculation of creatinine clearance from serum creatinine may give an inaccurate estimation of the renal function. For obese patients, generally defined as patients more than 20% over *ideal body weight* (IBW), creatinine clearance should be based on ideal body weight. Estimation of creatinine clearance based on *total body weight* (TBW) would exaggerate the Cl_{cr} values in obese patients. Women with normal kidney function have smaller creatinine clearance values than men, which are approximately 80%–85% of those in men with normal kidney function.

Several empirical equations have been used to estimate lean body weight (LBW) based on the patient's height and actual (total) body weight (see Chapter 22). The following equations have been used to estimate LBW in renally impaired patients:

LBW (males) = 50 kg
 + 2.3 kg for each inch over 5 ft

LBW (females) = 45.5 kg
 + 2.3 kg for each inch over 5 ft

For the purpose of dose adjustment in renal patients, normal creatinine clearance is generally assumed to be between 100 and 125 mL/min per 1.73 m² for a subject of ideal body weight: $Cl_{cr} = 108.8 \pm 13.5$ mL/1.73 m² for an adult female and $Cl_{cr} = 124.5 \pm 9.7$ mL/1.73 m² for an adult male (*Scientific Tables*; Diem and Lentner, 1973). Creatinine clearance is affected by diet and salt intake. As a convenient approximation, the normal clearance has often been assumed by many clinicians to be approximately 100 mL/min.

Frequently Asked Questions
▶ *Why is creatinine clearance difficult to predict?*
▶ *Why is creatinine clearance used in renal disease?*
▶ *What patient-specific factors influence the accuracy of Cl_cr estimates?*
▶ *How is Cl_cr determined?*

Calculation of Creatinine Clearance from Serum Creatinine Concentration

The problems of obtaining a complete 24-hour urine collection from a patient, the time necessary for urine collection, and the analysis time preclude a direct estimation of creatinine clearance. *Serum creatinine concentration*, C_{cr}, is related to creatinine clearance and is measured routinely in the clinical laboratory.

Therefore, creatinine clearance, Cl_{cr}, is most often estimated from the patient's C_{cr}. Several methods are available for the calculation of creatinine clearance from the serum creatinine concentration. The more accurate methods are based on the patient's age, height, weight, and gender. These methods should be used only for patients with intact liver function and no abnormal muscle disease, such as hypertrophy or dystrophy. Moreover, most of the methods assume a stable creatinine clearance. The unit for Cl_{cr} is mL/min.

Adults

The method of Cockcroft and Gault (1976) shown in Equation 24.12 is used to estimate creatinine clearance from serum creatinine concentration. This method considers both the age and the weight of the patient. For males

$$Cl_{cr} = \frac{[140 - \text{age (year)}] \times \text{body weight (kg)}}{72 \times C_{cr}}$$

(24.12)

For females, use 90% of the Cl_{cr} value obtained in males. In some hospitals, 85% is used for female subjects (Stevens et al, 2006).

The nomogram method of Siersback-Nielsen et al (1971) estimates creatinine clearance on the basis of age, weight, and serum creatinine concentration, as shown in Fig. 24-1. Cockcroft and Gault (1976) compared their method with the nomogram method in adult males of various ages. Creatinine clearances estimated by both methods were comparable. Both methods also demonstrated an age-related linear decline in creatinine excretion, which may be due to the decrease in muscle mass with age.

Children

There are a number of methods for calculation of creatinine clearance in children, based on body length and serum creatinine concentration. Equation 24.13 is a method developed by Schwartz et al (1976):

$$Cl_{cr} = \frac{0.55 \text{ body length (cm)}}{C_{cr}}$$

(24.13)

where Cl_{cr} is given in mL/min/1.73 m². The value 0.55 represents a factor used for children aged 1–12 years.

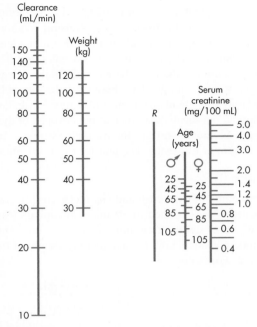

FIGURE 24-1   Nomogram for evaluation of endogenous creatinine clearance. To use the nomogram, connect the patient's weight on the second line from the left with the patient's age on the fourth line with a ruler. Note the point of intersection on R and keep the ruler there. Turn the right part of the ruler to the appropriate serum creatinine value and the left side will indicate the clearance in mL/min. (Reproduced with permission from Kampmann J, et al: Rapid evaluation of creatinine clearance. *Lancet* **1**(7709):1133–1134, 1971.)

Another method of calculating creatinine clearance in children uses the nomogram of Traub and Johnson (1980) as shown in Fig. 24-2. This nomogram is based on observations from 81 children aged 6–12 years and requires the patient's height and serum creatinine concentration.

PRACTICE PROBLEMS

1. What is the creatinine clearance for a 25-year-old male patient with C_{cr} of 1 mg/dL and a body weight of 80 kg?

Solution

Using the nomogram (see Fig. 24-1), join the points at 25 years (male) and 80 kg with a ruler—let the line intersect line R. Connect the intersection point at

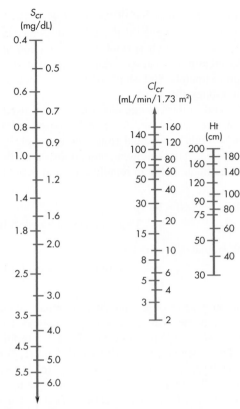

FIGURE 24-2   Nomogram for rapid evaluation of endogenous creatinine clearance (Cl_{cr}) in pediatric patients (aged 6–12 years). To predict Cl_{cr}, connect the child's S_{cr} (serum creatinine) and Ht (height) with a ruler and read the Cl_{cr} where the ruler intersects the center line. (From Traub and Johnson, 1980, with permission.)

line R with the creatinine concentration point of 1 mg/dL, and extend the line to intersect the "clearance line." The extended line will intersect the clearance line at 130 mL/min, giving the creatinine clearance for the patient.

2. What is the creatinine clearance for a 25-year-old male patient with a C_{cr} of 1 mg/dL? The patient is 5 ft, 4 in in height and weighs 103 kg.

Solution

The patient is obese and the Cl_{cr} calculation should be based on ideal body weight.

$$\text{LBW (males)} = 50 \text{ kg} + [2.3 \times 4] = 59.2 \text{ kg}$$

TABLE 24-3 Classification of Renal Function Based on Estimated GFR (eGFR) or Estimated Creatinine Clearance (Cl_{cr})

Stage	Description[b]	eGFR[c] (mL/min/1.73m²)	Cl_{cr}[a,d] (mL/min)
1	Normal GFR	≥90	≥90
2	Mild decrease in GFR	60–89	60–89
3	Moderate decrease in GFR	30–59	30–59
4	Severe decrease in GFR	15–29	15–29
5	End-stage renal disease (ESRD)	<15 Not on dialysis Requiring dialysis	<15 Not on dialysis Requiring dialysis

[a]In some situations, collection of 24-hour urine samples for measurement of creatinine clearance, or measurement of clearance of an exogenous filtration marker, may provide better estimates of GFR than the prediction equations. The situations include determination of GFR for patients in the following scenarios: undergoing kidney replacement therapy; acute renal failure; extremes of age, body size, or muscle mass; conditions of severe malnutrition or obesity; disease of skeletal muscle; or on a vegetarian diet.

[b]Stages of renal impairment are based on K/DOQI Clinical Practice Guidelines for chronic kidney disease (CKD) from the National Kidney Foundation in 2002; GFR: glomerular filtration rate.

[c]eGFR: estimate of GFR based on an MDRD equation.

[d]Cl_{cr}: estimated creatinine clearance based on the Cockcroft-Gault equation.

Using the Cockcroft–Gault method (Equation 24.12), the Cl_{cr} can be calculated.

$$Cl_{cr} = \frac{(140 - 25) \times (59.2 \text{ kg})}{72(1)} = 94.6 \text{ mL/min}$$

The serum creatinine methods for the estimation of the creatinine clearance assume stabilized kidney function and a steady-state serum creatinine concentration. In acute renal failure and in other situations in which kidney function is changing, the serum creatinine may not represent steady-state conditions. If C_{cr} is measured daily and the C_{cr} value is constant, then the serum creatinine concentration is probably at steady state. If the C_{cr} values are changing daily, then kidney function is changing.

Although the Cockcroft–Gault method for estimating Cl_{cr} has some biases, this method has gained general acceptance for the determination of renal impairment (Schneider et al, 2003; Hailmeskel et al, 1999; Spinler et al, 1998). A suggested representation of patients with various degrees of renal impairment based on creatinine clearance is shown in Table 24-3.

The practice problems show that, depending on the formula used, the calculated Cl_{cr} can vary considerably. Consequently, unless a clinically significant change in the creatinine clearance occurs, dosage adjustment may not be needed. According to St. Peter et al (1992),

dose adjustment of many antibiotics is necessary only when the GFR, as measured by Cl_{cr}, is less than 50 mL/min. For aminoglycosides and vancomycin, dose adjustment is individualized according to the wide range of Cl_{cr}. Therefore, dose adjustment for all drugs on the basis of these Cl_{cr} methods alone is not justified.

Estimated Glomerular Filtration Rate (eGFR) Using Modification of Diet in Renal Disease (MDRD) Formula or Using the Chronic Kidney Disease–Epidemiology Collaboration (CKD–EPI) Equations

Various approaches for the estimation of GFR from serum creatinine have been published (Levey et al, 1999, 2009; FDA Guidance for Industry, 2010). The MDRD equation is a simple and effective method and several versions of the MDRD equations have been published. For example,[1]

$$\begin{aligned} \text{eGFR (mL/min/1.73 m}^2) = {}& 175 \times (C_{cr})^{-1.154} \\ & \times (\text{age})^{-0.203} \times (0.742 \text{ if female}) \\ & \times (1.212 \text{ if African American}) \end{aligned}$$

where eGFR is estimated GFR using the MDRD equation.

[1]*FDA Guidance, 2010.*

The MDRD equation does not require weight or height measurements and the results are normalized to 1.73 m² body surface area, which is an accepted average adult surface area.

The Chronic Kidney Disease–Epidemiology Collaboration (CDK-EPI) reviewed various approaches for GFR measurements based on serum creatinine concentration and other factors (Levey et al, 2009). Based on the same four variables as the MDRD equation, the CDK-EPI equation uses a two-slope "spline" to model the relationship between estimated GFR and serum creatinine, and a different relationship for age, sex, and race. In the validation data set, the CKD-EPI equation performed better than the MDRD equation, with less bias (median difference between measured and estimated GFR of 2.5 vs 5.5 mL/min/1.73 m²) especially at higher GFR ($p < .001$ for all subsequent comparisons). The CKD-EPI equation is more accurate than the MDRD equation and could replace it for routine clinical use (Levey et al, 2009). However, no comparison between the CKD-EPI and the Cockcroft–Gault methods has been made, especially in the more important issue of how to relate the calculated GFR to individual drug clearance and, ultimately, an optimized drug dosing regimen in the patients. A limitation of the CKD-EPI method is that the sample contained a limited number of elderly people and racial and ethnic minorities with measured GFR.

Each equation for the calculation of renal function from serum creatinine concentrations gives somewhat different results. The Cockcroft–Gault method for estimating Cl_{cr} has been used most frequently and tends to be the preferred approach at this time. The FDA Guidance for Industry (2010) on impaired renal function includes a classification of renal function based on creatinine clearance (see Table 24-3). Although the two methods, estimated GFR (eGFR) using the MDRD equation and calculated creatinine clearance using the Cockcroft–Gault method, do not give the same values, the classification in Table 24-3 brackets the values for diminishing renal function.

Comparison of Methods for the Measurement of GFR

The estimate of GFR based on serum creatinine concentration is widely used, even though serum creatinine concentrations are known to fluctuate with disease state and patient conditions such as age, gender, and endogenous factors that affect creatinine synthesis and elimination (Table 24-4). These estimation methods are referred to as creatinine-based methods in the clinical literature (Stevens et al, 2006; Levey et al, 2009). Two creatinine-based methods that have been extensively studied and widely applied are the Cockcroft–Gault and the MDRD study equations. The Cockcroft–Gault has a longer history of use but the original equation was based on fewer subjects. The MDRD method is a more recent method based on more subjects with application better defined for certain groups of patients. For example, the relationship of serum creatinine concentration

TABLE 24-4   Factors Affecting Creatinine Generation

Factor	Effect on Serum Creatinine
Aging	Decreased
Female Sex	Decreased
Race or ethnic group	
Black	Increased
Hispanic	Decreased
Asian	Decreased
Body habitus	
Muscular	Increased
Amputation	Decreased
Obesity	No Change
Chronic illness	
Malnutrition, inflammation, deconditioning (eg, cancer, severe cardiovascular disease, hospitalized patients)	Decreased
Neuromuscular diseases	Decreased
Diet	
Vegetarian diet	Decreased
Ingestion of cooked meat	Increased

(From Stevens LA, M.D., Coresh J, Greene T, Levey AS: Assessing Kidney Function—Measured and Estimated Glomerular Filtration Rate, *N Eng J Med* **354**(23):2473–2483, 2006, with permission.)

and GFR may be different between subjects with diabetic nephropathy and those without real renal disease. Some reports indicated that the MDRD method is less biased for obese and diabetic patients, whereas other studies do not find a difference between the two methods.

The Cockcroft–Gault formula was developed initially with the data from 249 men with Cl_{cr} ranging from 30 to 130 mL/min. The equation is described as below.

$$Cl_{cr} = [(140 - \text{age}) \times \text{weight}](72 \times C_{cr})$$
$$\times 0.85 \text{ (for female subjects)} \qquad (24.12)$$

The Cockcroft–Gault formula systematically overestimates GFR because of the tubular secretion of creatinine. In addition, the equation is not adjusted for body surface area, making it difficult to compare creatinine clearance value obtained from this method and that from other methods. Typically, normal values for creatinine clearance are normalized by a body surface area of 1.73 m², which requires a measurement of height of the patients.

The MDRD study equation was developed in 1999 with the use of data from 1628 patients with chronic kidney disease. Its estimated GFR is adjusted for body-surface area. The estimating equation is

$$\text{GFR (mL/min/1.73 m}^2) = 186 \times (C_{cr})^{-1.154}$$
$$\times (\text{age})^{-0.203} \times 0.742 \text{ (if the subject is female)}$$
$$\times 1.212 \text{ (if the subject is black)}$$

This equation was revised in 2005 for use with a standardized serum creatinine assay that yields serum creatinine values that are 5% lower.

$$\text{GFR (mL/min/1.73 m}^2) = 175$$
$$\times (\text{standardized } C_{cr})^{-1.154} \times (\text{age})^{-0.203}$$
$$\times 0.742 \text{ (if the subject is female) or}$$
$$\times 1.212 \text{ (if the subject is black)}$$

In the MDRD study population, 91% of the GFR estimates were within 30% of the measured values, and this approach was more accurate than the use of the Cockcroft–Gault equation. The Cockcroft–Gault equation was reported to be less accurate than the MDRD study equation in older and obese people. Both methods are less accurate in healthy subjects.

While the MDRD method will provide more accurate renal function of the patients, drug clearance is not entirely governed by GFR. Reabsorption and nonrenal elimination are also important for many drugs. Therefore, the MDRD method should be compared with previous methods and see how accurately it adjusts drug doses for different drugs in different uremic patients. For many new drugs, drug dosing information for renal-impaired patients is now available and should be consulted in the package insert. In patients with chronic kidney disease, the following recommendations are good practices that physicians and pharmacists should be aware of (Munar and Singh, 2007):

1. Assess the use of OTC and herbal medicine to ensure proper indication, and avoid medications with toxic metabolites, or use the least nephrotoxic agents.
2. Use alternative medications if potential drug interactions exist.
3. Use caution for drugs with active metabolites that can exaggerate pharmacologic effects in patients with renal impairment.
4. Adjust dosages of drugs cleared renally based on the patient's kidney function (calculated as Cl_{cr} or eGFR); determine initial dosages using published guidelines and adjust based on patient response or monitoring if appropriate.

DOSE ADJUSTMENT FOR UREMIC PATIENTS

Dose adjustment for drugs in uremic or renally impaired patients should be made in accordance with changes in pharmacodynamics and pharmacokinetics of the drug in the individual patient. Whether renal impairment will alter the pharmacokinetics of the drug enough to justify dosage adjustment is an important consideration. For many drugs that are eliminated primarily by metabolism or biliary secretion, uremia may not alter pharmacokinetics sufficiently to warrant dosage adjustment.

Active metabolites of the drug may also be formed and must be considered for additional pharmacologic effects when adjusting dose. For some drugs, the free drug concentrations may need to be considered due to decreased or altered protein binding in uremia. Combination products that contain two or more active drugs in a fixed-dose combination may be differentially affected by decreased renal function and thus, the use of combination drug products in uremic patients should be discouraged.

The following methods may be used to estimate initial and maintenance dose regimens. After initiating the dosage, the clinician should continue to monitor the pharmacodynamics and pharmacokinetics of the drug. He or she should also evaluate the patient's renal function, which may be changing over time.

Basis for Dose Adjustment in Uremia

The loading drug dose is based on the apparent volume of distribution of the patient. It is generally assumed that the apparent volume of distribution is not altered significantly, and therefore, the loading dose of the drug is the same in uremic patients as in subjects with normal renal function.

The maintenance dose is based on clearance of the drug in the patient. In the uremic patient, the rate of renal drug excretion has decreased, leading to a decrease in total body clearance. Most methods for dose adjustment assume nonrenal drug clearance to be unchanged. The fraction of normal renal function remaining in the uremic patient is estimated from Cl_{cr}.

After the remaining total body clearance in the uremic patient is estimated, a dosage regimen may be developed by (1) decreasing the maintenance dose, (2) increasing the dosage interval, or (3) changing both maintenance dose and dosage interval.

Although total body clearance is a more accurate index for drug dosing, the elimination half-life of the drug is more commonly used for dose adjustment because of its convenience. Clearance allows for the prediction of steady-state drug concentrations, while elimination half-life yields information on the time it takes to reach steady-state concentration.

Nomograms

Nomograms are charts available for use in estimating dosage regimens in uremic patients (Bjornsson, 1986; Chennavasin and Craig Brater, 1981; Tozer, 1974). The nomograms may be based on serum creatinine

concentrations, patient data (height, weight, age, gender), and the pharmacokinetics of the drug. As discussed by Chennavasin and Brater (1981), each nomogram has errors in its assumptions and drug database.

Most methods for dose adjustment in renal disease assume that nonrenal elimination of the drug is not affected by renal impairment and that the remaining renal excretion rate constant in the uremic patient is proportional to the product of a constant and the Cl_{cr}:

$$k_u = k_{nr} + \alpha Cl_{cr} \qquad (24.14)$$

where k_{nr} is the nonrenal elimination rate constant and α is a constant.

Equation 24.14 is similar to Equation 24.10, where $\alpha = 1/V_D$, and it can be used for the construction of a nomogram. Figure 24-3 shows a graphical representation of Equation 24.14 for four different drugs, each with a different renal excretion rate constant. The fractions of drug excreted unchanged in the urine (f_e) for drugs A, B, C, and D are 5%, 50%, 75%, and 90%, respectively. A Cl_{cr} of ≥80 mL/min is considered an adequate GFR in subjects with normal renal function. The uremic elimination rate constant (k_u) is the sum of the nonrenal elimination rate constant and the renal elimination rate constant, which is decreased due to renal impairment. If the patient has complete renal shutdown (ie, $Cl_{cr} = 0$ mL/min), then the intercept on the y axis represents the percent of drug elimination due to nonrenal drug elimination routes.

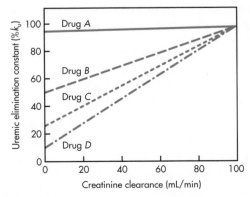

FIGURE 24-3 Relationship between creatinine clearance and the drug elimination rate constant.

Drug D, which is excreted 90% unchanged in the urine, has the steepest slope (equivalent to α in Equation 24.14) and is most affected by small changes in Cl_{cr}. On the other hand, drug A, which is excreted only 5% unchanged in the urine (ie, 95% eliminated by nonrenal routes), is least affected by a decrease in creatinine clearance.

The nomogram method of Welling and Craig (1976) provides an estimate of the ratio of the uremic elimination rate constant (k_u) to the normal elimination rate constant (k_N) on the basis of Cl_{cr} (Fig. 23-4). For this method, Welling and Craig (1976) provided a list of drugs grouped according to the amount of drug excreted unchanged in the urine (Table 24-5). From the k_u/k_N ratio, the uremic dose can be estimated according to Equation 24.15:

$$\text{Uremic dose} = \frac{k_u}{k_N} \times \text{normal dose} \qquad (24.15)$$

When the dosage interval τ is kept constant, the uremic dose is always a smaller fraction of the normal dose. Instead of reducing the dose for a uremic patient, the usual dose is kept constant and the dosage interval τ is prolonged according to the following equation:

$$\text{Dosage interval in uremia, } \tau_u = \frac{k_N}{k_u} \times \tau_N \qquad (24.16)$$

where τ_u is the dosage interval for the dose in uremic patients and τ_N is the dosage interval for the dose in patients with normal renal function.

PRACTICE PROBLEM

Lincomycin is given at 500 mg every 6 hours to a 75-kg healthy patient. What doses would be used (a) in complete renal shutdown ($Cl_{cr} = 0$) and (b) when $Cl_{cr} = 10$ mL/min?

Solution

To use the nomogram method, follow the steps below:

1. Use Table 24-5 to locate the group to which the drug belongs.
2. Find k_u/k_N at the point corresponding to Cl_{cr} of the patient (see Fig. 24-4).

3. Determine k_u for the patient.
4. Make the dose adjustment in accordance with pharmacokinetic principles.
   a. When $Cl_{cr} = 0$,

$$k_u = k_{nr} + k_R$$

In complete renal shutdown ($k_R = 0$), $k_u = k_{nr} = 0.06$ h^{-1} (see Table 24-5, group F).

Alternatively, find k_u/k_N in Fig. 24-4 for group F at $Cl_{cr} = 0$ mL/min:

$$\frac{k_u}{k_N} = 0.425$$

Since $k_N = 0.15$ h^{-1} for group F in Table 24-5, then

$$k_u = 0.425\,(0.15) = 0.0638 \text{ h}^{-1}$$

$$\text{Uremic dose} = 500 \text{ mg} \frac{0.0638}{0.15}$$

$$= 212 \text{ mg every 6 hours}$$

   b. At $Cl_{cr} = 10$ mL/min,

$$\frac{k_u}{k_N} = 0.48$$

$$k_N = 0.15 \text{ h}^{-1}$$

$$k_u = (0.48)(0.15) = 0.072 \text{ h}^{-1}$$

$$\text{Dose} = 500 \text{ mg} \frac{0.072}{0.15} = 240 \text{ mg}$$

Alternatively,

$$\text{Dose} = (0.48)\,(500) = 240 \text{ mg}$$

Fraction of Drug Excreted Unchanged (f_e) Methods

For many drugs, the fraction of drug excreted unchanged (f_e) is available in the literature. Table 24-6 lists various drugs with their f_e values and elimination half-lives. The f_e method for estimating a dosage regimen in the uremic patient is a general method that may be applied to any drug whose f_e is known.

TABLE 24-5   Elimination Rate Constants for Various Drugs[a]

Group	Drug	k_N (h^{-1})	k_{nr} (h^{-1})	k_{nr}/k_N%
A	Minocycline	0.04	0.04	100.0
	Rifampicin	0.25	0.25	100.0
	Lidocaine	0.39	0.36	92.3
	Digitoxin	0.114	0.10	87.7
B	Doxycycline	0.037	0.031	83.8
	Chlortetracycline	0.12	0.095	79.2
C	Clindamycin	0.16	0.12	75.0
	Chloramphenicol	0.26	0.19	73.1
	Propranolol	0.22	0.16	72.8
	Erythromycin	0.39	0.28	71.8
D	Trimethoprim	0.054	0.031	57.4
	Isoniazid (fast)	0.53	0.30	56.6
	Isoniazid (slow)	0.23	0.13	56.5
E	Dicloxacillin	1.20	0.60	50.0
	Sulfadiazine	0.069	0.032	46.4
	Sulfamethoxazole	0.084	0.037	44.0
F	Nafcillin	1.26	0.54	42.8
	Chlorpropamide	0.020	0.008	40.0
	Lincomycin	0.15	0.06	40.0
G	Colistimethate	0.154	0.054	35.1
	Oxacillin	1.73	0.58	33.6
	Digoxin	0.021	0.007	33.3
H	Tetracycline	0.120	0.033	27.5
	Cloxacillin	1.21	0.31	25.6
	Oxytetracycline	0.075	0.014	18.7
I	Amoxicillin	0.70	0.10	14.3
	Methicillin	1.40	0.19	13.6
J	Ticarcillin	0.58	0.066	11.4
	Penicillin G	1.24	0.13	10.5
	Ampicillin	0.53	0.05	9.4
	Carbenicillin	0.55	0.05	9.1

(Continued)

TABLE 24-5   **Elimination Rate Constants for Various Drugs[a] (Continued)**

Group	Drug	k_N (h⁻¹)	k_{nr} (h⁻¹)	$k_{nr}/k_N\%$
K	Cefazolin	0.32	0.02	6.2
	Cephaloridine	0.51	0.03	5.9
	Cephalothin	1.20	0.06	5.0
	Gentamicin	0.30	0.015	5.0
L	Flucytosine	0.18	0.007	3.9
	Kanamycin	0.28	0.01	3.6
	Vancomycin	0.12	0.004	3.3
	Tobramycin	0.32	0.010	3.1
	Cephalexin	1.54	0.032	2.1

[a]k_N is for patients with normal renal function, k_{nr} is for patients with severe renal impairment, and $k_{nr}/k_N\%$ = percent of normal elimination in severe renal impairment.

From Welling and Craig (1976), with permission.

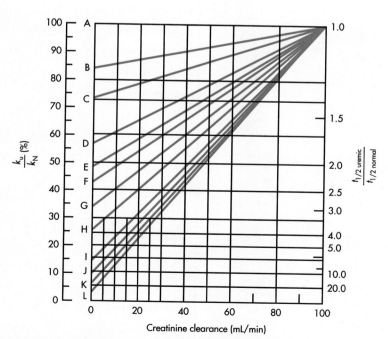

FIGURE 24-4   This nomograph describes the changes in the percentage of normal elimination rate constant (left ordinate) and the consequent geometric increase in elimination half-life (right ordinate) as a function of creatinine clearance. The drugs associated with the individual slopes are given in Table 24-5. (From Welling and Craig, 1976, with permission.)

TABLE 24-6 Fraction of Drug Excreted Unchanged (f_e) and Elimination Half-Life Values

Drug	f_e	$t_{1/2\ normal}$ (h)^a	Drug	f_e	$t_{1/2\ normal}$ (h)^a
Acebutolol	0.44 ± 0.11	2.7 ± 0.4	Cimetidine	0.77 ± 0.06	2.1 ± 1.1
Acetaminophen	0.03 ± 0.01	2.0 ± 0.4	Clindamycin	0.09–0.14	2.7 ± 0.4
Acetohexamide	0.4	1.3	Clofibrate	0.11–0.32	13 ± 3
Active metabolite		16–30	Clonidine	0.62 ± 0.11	8.5 ± 2.0
Allopurinol	0.1	2–8	Colistin	0.9	3
Alprenolol	0.005	3.1 ± 1.2	Cyclophosphamide	0.3	5
Amantadine	0.85	10	Cytarabine	0.1	2
Amikacin	0.98	2.3 ± 0.4	Dapsone	0.1	20
Amiloride	0.5	8 ± 2	Dicloxacillin	0.60 ± 0.07	0.7 ± 0.07
Amoxicillin	0.52 ± 0.15	1.0 ± 0.1	Digitoxin	0.33 ± 0.15	166 ± 65
Amphetamine	0.4–0.45	12	Digoxin	0.72 ± 0.09	42 ± 19
Amphotericin B	0.03	360	Disopyramide	0.55 ± 0.06	7.8 ± 1.6
Ampicillin	0.90 ± 0.08	1.3 ± 0.2	Doxycycline	0.40 ± 0.04	20 ± 4
Atenolol	0.85	6.3 ± 1.8	Erythromycin	0.15	1.1–3.5
Azlocillin	0.6	1.0	Ethambutol	0.79 ± 0.03	3.1 ± 0.4
Bacampicillin	0.88	0.9	Ethosuximide	0.19	33 ± 6
Baclofen	0.75	3–4	Flucytosine	0.63–0.84	5.3 ± 0.7
Bleomycin	0.55	1.5–8.9	Flunitrazepam	0.01	15 ± 5
Bretylium	0.8 ± 0.1	4–17	Furosemide	0.74 ± 0.07	0.85 ± 0.17
Bumetanide	0.33	3.5	Gentamicin	0.98	2–3
Carbenicillin	0.82 ± 0.09	1.1 ± 0.2	Griseofulvin	0	15
Cefalothin	0.52	0.6 ± 0.3	Hydralazine	0.12–0.14	2.2–2.6
Cefamandole	0.96 ± 0.03	0.77	Hydrochloro-thiazide	0.95	2.5 ± 0.2
Cefazolin	0.80 ± 0.13	1.8 ± 0.4	Indomethacin	0.15 ± 0.08	2.6–11.2
Cefoperazone	0.2–0.3	2.0	Isoniazid		
Cefotaxime	0.5–0.6	1–1.5	Rapid acetylators	0.07 ± 0.02	1.1 ± 0.2
Cefoxitin	0.88 ± 0.08	0.7 ± 0.13	Slow acetylators	0.29 ± 0.05	3.0 ± 0.8
Cefuroxime	0.92	1.1	Isosorbide dinitrate	0.05	0.5
Cephalexin	0.96	0.9 ± 0.18	Kanamycin	0.9	2.1 ± 0.2
Chloramphenicol	0.05	2.7 ± 0.8	Lidocaine	0.02 ± 0.01	1.8 ± 0.4
Chlorphentermine	0.2	120	Lincomycin	0.6	5
Chlorpropamide	0.2	36	Lithium	0.95 ± 0.15	22 ± 8
Chlorthalidone	0.65 ± 0.09	44 ± 10			

(Continued)

TABLE 24-6   Fraction of Drug Excreted Unchanged (f_e) and Elimination Half-Life Values (Continued)

Drug	f_e	$t_{1/2\ normal}$ (h)[a]	Drug	f_e	$t_{1/2\ normal}$ (h)[a]
Lorazepam	0.01	14 ± 5	Prazosin	0.01	2.9 ± 0.8
Meperidine	0.04–0.22	3.2 ± 0.8	Primidone	0.42 ± 0.15	8.0 ± 4.8
Methadone	0.2	22	Procainamide	0.67 ± 0.08	2.9 ± 0.6
Methicillin	0.88 ± 0.17	0.85 ± 0.23	Propranolol	0.005	3.9 ± 0.4
Methotrexate	0.94	8.4	Quinidine	0.18 ± 0.05	6.2 ± 1.8
Methyldopa	0.63 ± 0.10	1.8 ± 0.2	Rifampin	0.16 ± 0.04	2.1 ± 0.3
Metronidazole	0.25	8.2	Salicylic acid	0.2	3
Mexiletine	0.1	12	Sisomicin	0.98	2.8
Mezlocillin	0.75	0.8	Sotalol	0.6	6.5–13
Minocycline	0.1 ± 0.02	18 ± 4	Streptomycin	0.96	2.8
Minoxidil	0.1	4	Sulfinpyrazone	0.45	2.3
Moxalactam	0.82–0.96	2.5–3.0	Sulfisoxazole	0.53 ± 0.09	5.9 ± 0.9
Nadolol	0.73 ± 0.04	16 ± 2	Tetracycline	0.48	9.9 ± 1.5
Nafcillin	0.27 ± 0.05	0.9–1.0	Thiamphenicol	0.9	3
Nalidixic acid	0.2	1.0	Thiazinamium	0.41	
Neostigmine	0.67	1.3 ± 0.8	Theophylline	0.08	9 ± 2.1
Netilmicin	0.98	2.2	Ticarcillin	0.86	1.2
Nitrazepam	0.01	29 ± 7	Timolol	0.2	3–5
Nitrofuraniton	0.5	0.3	Tobramycin	0.98	2.2 ± 0.1
Nomifensine	0.15–0.22	3.0 ± 1.0	Tocainide	0.20–0.70 (0.40 mean)	1.6–3
Oxacillin	0.75	0.5	Tolbutamide	0	5.9 ± 1.4
Oxprenolol	0.05	1.5	Triamterene	0.04 ± 0.01	2.8 ± 0.9
Pancuronium	0.5	3.0	Trimethoprim	0.53 ± 0.02	11 ± 1.4
Pentazocine	0.2	2.5	Tubocurarine	0.43 ± 0.08	2 ± 1.1
Phenobarbital	0.2 ± 0.05	86 ± 7	Valproic acid	0.02 ± 0.02	16 ± 3
Pindolol	0.41	3.4 ± 0.2	Vancomycin	0.97	5–6
Pivampicillin	0.9	0.9	Warfarin	0	37 ± 15
Polymyxin B	0.88	4.5			

[a]Half-life is a derived parameter that changes as a function of both clearance and volume of distribution. It is independent of body size, because it is a function of these two parameters (Cl, V_D), each of which is proportional to body size. It is important to consider that half-life is the time to eliminate 50% of the "drug" from the body (plasma), not the time in which 50% of the effect is lost.

Data from Chennavasin P, Brater DC: Nomograms for drug use in renal disease, *Clin Pharmacokinet* **6**(3):193–214, May–June 1981; Dettli L: Drug dosage in renal disease, *Clin Pharmacokinet* **1**(2):126–34, 1976; Gilman AG et al: Pharmacological Basis of Therapeutics, MacMillan, New York, 1980.

The *Giusti–Hayton* (1973) method assumes that the effect of reduced kidney function on the renal portion of the elimination constant can be estimated from the ratio of the uremic creatinine clearance to the normal creatinine clearance.

$$\frac{k_r^u}{k_r^N} = \frac{Cl_{cr}^u}{Cl_{cr}^N} \qquad (24.17)$$

where k_r^u is the uremic renal excretion rate constant and k_r^N is the normal renal excretion rate constant.

$$k_r^u = k_r^N \frac{Cl_{cr}^u}{Cl_{cr}^N} \qquad (24.18)$$

Because the overall uremic elimination rate constant, k_u, is the sum of renal and nonrenal elimination,

$$k_u = k_{nr}^u + k_r^u$$
$$k_u = k_{nr}^u + k_r^N \left(\frac{Cl_{cr}^u}{Cl_{cr}^N}\right) \qquad (24.19)$$

Dividing Equation 24.19 by k_N

$$\frac{k_u}{k_N} = \frac{k_{nr}^u}{k_N} + \frac{k_r^N}{k_N}\left(\frac{Cl_{cr}^u}{Cl_{cr}^N}\right) \qquad (24.20)$$

Let $f_e = k_r^N/k_N$ = fraction of drug excreted unchanged in the urine and $1 - f_e = k_{nr}^u/k_N$ fraction of drug excreted by nonrenal routes. Substitution into Equation 24.20 yields the Giusti–Hayton equation, where G is the Giusti–Hayton factor, which can be calculated from f_e and the ratio of uremic to normal clearance:

$$\frac{k_u}{k_N} = (1 - f_e) + f_e \left(\frac{Cl_{cr}^u}{Cl_{cr}^N}\right)$$

or

$$\frac{k_u}{k_N} = 1 - f_e\left(1 - \frac{Cl_{cr}^u}{Cl_{cr}^N}\right) = G \qquad (24.21)$$

The Giusti–Hayton equation is useful for most drugs for which the fraction of drug excreted by renal routes has been reported in the literature. The ratio k_u/k_N can be calculated from the fraction of drug excreted by the kidney, normal creatinine clearance, and the creatinine clearance in the uremic patient.

PRACTICE PROBLEM

The maintenance dose of gentamicin is 80 mg every 6 hours for a patient with normal renal function. Calculate the maintenance dose for a uremic patient with creatinine clearance of 20 mL/min. Assume a normal creatinine clearance of 100 mL/min.

Solution

From the literature, gentamicin is reported to be 100% excreted by the kidney (ie, $f_e = 1$). Using Equation 24.21,

$$\frac{k_u}{k_N} = 1 - 1\left(1 - \frac{20}{100}\right) = 0.2$$

Because

$$\frac{D_u}{D_N} = \frac{k_u}{k_N} \qquad or \qquad D_u = D_N \times \frac{k_u}{k_N}$$

where D_u = uremic dose and D_N = normal dose,

$$D_u = 80 \text{ mg} \times 0.2 = 16 \text{ mg}$$

The maintenance dose is 16 mg every 6 hours. Alternatively, the dosing interval can be adjusted without changing the dose:

$$\frac{\tau_u}{\tau_N} = \frac{k_N}{k_u} \qquad or \qquad \tau_u = \tau_N \times \frac{k_N}{k_u}$$

$$\tau_u = 6 \text{ h} \times \frac{1}{0.2} = 30 \text{ h}$$

where τ_u and τ_N are dosing intervals for uremic and normal patients, respectively. The patient may be given 80 mg every 30 hours.

Other approaches for using fraction of drug excreted unchanged have been developed by Tozer (1974) and Bjornsson (1986). These methods use f_e for dosing regimen design and the following equation:

$$Q = 1 - f_e(1 - k_f) \qquad (24.22)$$

where Q is the dosage adjustment factor, $k_f = Cl_{cr}^u/Cl_{cr}^N$ and f_e is the fraction of unchanged drug excreted renally. Actually, Q is exactly the same as G in Equation 24.21, as developed by Giusti–Hayton approach in 1973.

The value of Q in Equation 24.22 is multiplied by the normal dose, D_N, to give the uremic dose, D_u:

$$D_u = Q \times D_N \qquad (24.23)$$

PRACTICE PROBLEMS

1. An adult male patient (52 years old, 75 kg) whose serum creatinine is 2.4 mg/dL is to be given gentamicin sulfate for a confirmed Gram-negative infection. The usual dose of gentamicin in adult patients with normal renal function is 1 mg/kg every 8 hours by multiple IV bolus injections. Gentamicin sulfate (Garamycin) is available in 2-mL vials containing 40 mg of gentamicin sulfate per milliliter. Calculate (a) the Cl_{cr} in this patient by the Cockcroft–Gault method and (b) the appropriate dosage regimen of gentamicin sulfate for this patient in mg and mL.

Solution

a. The creatinine clearance is calculated by the Cockcroft–Gault method using Equation 24.12:

$$Cl_{cr} = \frac{(140 - 52)(75)}{72(2.4)} = 38.19 \text{ mL/min}$$

b. The initial dose of gentamicin sulfate in this patient may be estimated using Equation 24.21. Normal creatinine clearance is assumed to equal 100 mL/min. The fraction of dose excreted unchanged in the urine, f_e, = 0.98 for gentamicin sulfate (Table 24-6).

$$\frac{k_u}{k_N} = Q = 1 - 0.98\left(1 - \frac{38.19}{100}\right) = 0.39$$

The usual dose of gentamicin sulfate = 1 mg/kg every 8 hours. Therefore, for a 75-kg adult, the usual dose is 75 mg every 8 hours. The uremic dose may be estimated by:

i. Reducing the maintenance dose and keeping the dosing interval constant:

$$\text{Uremic dose} = \frac{k_u}{k_N} \times \text{normal dose}$$

$$\text{Uremic dose} = 0.39 \times 75 = 29.25 \text{ mg}$$

Give 29.25 mg (about 30 mg) every 8 hours. Because the concentration of gentamicin sulfate solution is 40 mg/mL, 30 mg gentamicin sulfate is equivalent to 0.75 mL.

ii. Increasing the dosing interval and keeping the maintenance dose constant:

$$\text{Dosage interval in uremia, } \tau_u = \frac{k_N}{k_u} \times \tau_N$$

$$\tau_u = 2.564 \times 8 = 20.5 \text{ h (2.564 is the reciprocal of 0.39)}$$

Give 75 mg every 20.5 hours.

iii. Change both the maintenance dose and dosing interval. Using the dosing rate $D_\tau = 29.25 \text{ mg}/8 \text{ h} = 3.66 \text{ mg/h}$, a dose of 23.9 mg every 6 hours or 43.8 mg every 12 hours will produce the same average steady-state plasma drug concentration.

Although each estimated dosage regimen shown above produces the same average steady-state plasma drug concentration, peak drug concentration, and trough drug concentration, the duration of time in which the drug concentration will be above or below the minimum effective plasma drug concentration will be different. The choice of an appropriate dosage regimen requires consideration of these issues: the patient, the safety, and efficacy of the drug.

2. Calculate the dose adjustment needed for uremic patients with (a) 75% of normal kidney function (ie, $Cl_{cr}^u/Cl_{cr}^N = 75\%$); (b) 50% of normal kidney function; and (c) 25% of normal kidney function. Make calculations for (i) a drug that is 50% excreted by the kidney, and (ii) a drug that is 75% excreted by the kidney.

TABLE 24-7   Dosage Adjustment in Uremic Patients

Fraction of Drug Excreted Unchanged (k_r/k_N) or f_e	Percent of Normal Dose			
	50% Normal Cl_{cr}	25% Normal Cl_{cr}	10% Normal Cl_{cr}	0% Normal Cl_{cr}
0.25	87	81	77	75
0.50	75	62	55	50
0.75	62	44	32	25
0.90	55	32	19	10

Solution

The values for percent of normal dose in uremic patients with various renal functions are listed in Table 24-7. The percent of dose adjustment in a given uremic state is obtained using the procedure detailed below. The important facts to remember are (1) although the elimination rate constant is usually composed of two components, only the renal component is reduced in a uremic patient and (2) the kidney function of the uremic patient may be expressed as a percent of uremic Cl_{cr}^u/normal Cl_{cr}^N. The reduction in the renal elimination rate constant can be estimated from the percent of kidney function remaining in the patient. The steps involved in making the calculations are as follows:

   a. Determine f_e or the fraction of drug excreted by the kidney.
   b. Determine k_f by dividing Cl_{cr}^u of the uremic patient by Cl_{cr}^N.
   c. Calculate Q (Equation 24.22).
   d. Multiply Q by the normal dose to give the fraction of normal dose required for a uremic patient.
   3. What is the dose for a drug that is 75% excreted unchanged through the kidney in a uremic patient with a creatinine clearance of 10 mL/min?

Solution

$$f_e = 75\%$$

$$\text{Renal function of uremic patient} = \frac{10}{100}$$

$$= 10\% \text{ normal}$$

Percent of uremic patient's renal elimination constant $= 75\% \times 10\% = 7.5\%$ normal

Percent of uremic patient's overall elimination constant $= 7.5\% + (100\% - 75\%)$
$$= 7.5\% + 25\% = 32.5\%$$

Therefore, the uremic patient's dose should be 32.5% of that of normal patient. Table 24-7 provides some calculated dose adjustments for drugs eliminated to various degrees by renal excretion in different stages of renal failure.

General Clearance Method

The general clearance method is based on the methods discussed above. This method is popular in clinical settings because of its simplicity. The method assumes that creatinine clearance, Cl_{cr}, is a good indicator of renal function and that the renal clearance of a drug, Cl_R, is proportional to Cl_{cr}. Therefore, the renal drug clearance, Cl_R^u, in the uremic patient is

$$Cl_R^u = \frac{Cl_{cr}^u}{Cl_{cr}^N} \times Cl_R \qquad (21.24)$$

$$Cl_u = Cl_{nr} + Cl_R \frac{Cl_{cr}^u}{Cl_{cr}^N} \qquad (24.25)$$

where Cl_u is the total body clearance in the uremic patient.

If the ratio Cl_{cr}^u/Cl_{cr}^N and Cl_R are known, the total body clearance in the uremic patient may be estimated using Equation 24.25. Alternatively, if the normal total body clearance, Cl, and f_e are known,

Equation 24.26 may be obtained by substitution in Equation 24.25:

$$Cl_u = Cl(1 - f_e) + f_e \, Cl \frac{Cl_{cr}^u}{Cl_{cr}^N} \qquad (24.26)$$

Equation 24.26 calculates drug clearance in the uremic patient using the fraction of drug excreted unchanged (f_e), total body clearance of the drug (Cl) in the normal subject, and the ratio of creatinine clearance of the uremic to that of the normal patient.

Dividing Equation 24.26 on both sides by Cl yields the ratio Cl_u/Cl, reflecting the fraction of the uremic/normal drug dose.

$$\frac{Cl_u}{Cl} = (1 - f_e) + f_e \frac{Cl_{cr}^u}{Cl_{cr}^N} \qquad (24.27)$$

PRACTICE PROBLEM

A 34-year-old, 110-lb female patient is to be given tobramycin for sepsis. The usual dose of tobramycin is 150 mg twice a day by intravenous injection. The creatinine clearance in this patient has decreased to a stable level of 50 mL/min. The fraction of tobramycin excreted unchanged is 0.9. Calculate the appropriate dose of tobramycin for this patient.

Solution

$f_e = 0.9$ and apply Equation 24.27:

$$\frac{Cl_u}{Cl} = (1 - f_e) + f_e \frac{Cl_{cr}^u}{Cl_{cr}^N}$$

$$\frac{Cl_u}{Cl} = 1 - 0.9 + 0.9 \left(\frac{50}{100} \right) = 0.55$$

Therefore, the dose for the uremic patient = 150 mg × 0.55 = 82.5 mg (given twice a day).

The Wagner Method

The methods for renal dose adjustment discussed in the previous sections assume that the volume of distribution and the fraction of drug excreted by nonrenal routes are unchanged. These assumptions are convenient and hold true for many drugs. However, in the absence of reliable information assuring the validity of these assumptions, the equations should be demonstrated as statistically reliable in practice. A statistical approach was used by Wagner (1975), who established a linear relationship between creatinine concentration and the first-order elimination rate constant of the drug in patients. The Wagner method is described in greater detail in the third edition of this book.

This method takes advantage of the fact that the elimination rate constant for a patient can be obtained from the creatinine clearance, as follows:

$$k\% = a + b \, Cl_{cr} \qquad (23.28)$$

The values of a and b are determined statistically for each drug from pooled data on uremic patients. The method is simple to use and should provide accurate determination of elimination rate constants for patients when a good linear relationship exists between elimination rate constant and creatinine concentration. The theoretical derivation of this approach is as follows:

$k\%$ = total elimination rate constant
k_{nr} = nonrenal elimination rate constant
k_r = renal excretion rate constant
Cl = total body clearance of drug

$$R = \frac{Cl}{Cl_{cr}} \qquad (24.29)$$

$$Cl = R \, Cl_{cr}$$

Since $k = k_{nr} + k_r$,

$$k = k_{nr} + \frac{R}{V_D} Cl_{cr}$$

$$100k = 100k_{nr} + \frac{100R}{V_D} Cl_{cr} \qquad (24.30)$$

$$k\% = a + b \, Cl_{cr}$$

Equation 24.30 can also be used with drugs that follow the two-compartment model. In such cases, the terminal half-life is used, and the terminal slope of the elimination curve (b) is substituted for the elimination rate constant k. Since the equation assumes a constant nonrenal elimination constant (k_{nr}) and volume of distribution, any change in these two parameters will result in an error in the estimated elimination rate constant.

Frequently Asked Questions

▶ *What are the advantages and disadvantages of using serum creatinine concentrations for the measurement of renal function?*

▶ *What is the most accurate approach for the estimation of glomerular filtration rate?*

▶ *Why does each method based on serum creatinine concentrations for dosage adjustment in renal impairment give somewhat different values?*

▶ *What are the pharmacokinetic considerations in designing a dosing regimen? Why is dosing once a day for aminoglycosides recommended by many clinicians?*

Limitations of Dose Adjustment Methods in Uremic Patients

All of the methods mentioned previously have similar limitations (see Table 24-2). For example, the drug must follow dose-independent kinetics and the volume of distribution of the drug must remain relatively constant in the uremic patient. It is usually assumed that the nonrenal routes of elimination, such as hepatic clearance or k_{nr}, do not change. If there is a change in an active metabolite formation or elimination in uremia, then both parent and active metabolites must be considered when adjusting a dosage regimen for patients with renal disease, because potential side effects may result from an increase in the half-life of the parent drug and/or an accumulation of the active metabolites.

Bodenham et al (1988) have shown that although lorazepam pharmacokinetics were not significantly altered in patients with chronic renal failure, the clearance of lorazepam glucuronide, a major metabolite, was reduced significantly. Therefore, there are potential sedative side effects in the renally impaired patient as a result of the longer metabolite half-life. Bodenham and coworkers (1988) also cited literature references to potentiation of sedative and analgesic drug effects in renal, liver, and other multisystem disease states.

Another assumption in the use of these methods is that pharmacologic response is unchanged in the uremic patient. This assumption may be unrealistic for drugs that act differently in the disease state, and possible changes in pharmacodynamic effects in patients with renal and other diseases must be considered. For example, the pharmacologic response with digoxin is dependent on the potassium level in the body, and potassium level in the uremic patient may be rather different from that of the normal individual. In a patient undergoing dialysis, loss of potassium may increase the potential for toxic effect of the drug digoxin. In addition, neuromuscular-blocking drugs may be potentiated or antagonized by changes in potassium, phosphate, and hydrogen ion concentration brought about by uremic states, and morphine potentiation has been reported in hypocalcemic states.

For many drugs, studies have shown that the incidence of adverse effects is increased in uremic patients. It is often impossible to distinguish whether the increase in adverse effect is due to a pharmacokinetic change or a pharmacodynamic change in the receptor sensitivity to the drug. Serum creatinine concentration may not rise for some time until Cl_{cr} has fallen significantly, thereby adding to the uncertainty of any method that depends on serum Cl_{cr} for dose adjustment. In any event, these observations point out the fact that dose adjustment must be regarded as a preliminary estimation to be followed with further adjustments in accordance with the observed clinical response.

EXTRACORPOREAL REMOVAL OF DRUGS

Patients with *end-stage renal disease* (ESRD) and those who have become intoxicated with a drug as a result of drug overdose require supportive treatment to remove the accumulated drug and its metabolites. Several methods are available for the extracorporeal removal of drugs, including hemoperfusion, hemofiltration, and dialysis. The objective of these methods is to rapidly remove the undesirable drugs and metabolites from the body without disturbing the fluid and electrolyte balance in the patient.

Patients with impaired renal function may be taking other medication concurrently. For these patients, dosage adjustment may be needed to replace drug loss during extracorporeal drug and metabolite removal.

Dialysis

Dialysis is an artificial process in which the accumulation of drugs or waste metabolites is removed by diffusion from the body into the dialysis fluid. Two common dialysis treatments are *peritoneal dialysis* and *hemodialysis*. The principle underlying both processes is that as the uremic blood or fluid is equilibrated with the dialysis fluid across a dialysis membrane, waste metabolites from the patient's blood or fluid diffuse into the dialysis fluid and are removed. The dialysate is balanced with electrolytes and with respect to osmotic pressure. The dialysate contains water, dextrose, electrolytes (potassium, sodium, chloride, bicarbonate, acetate, calcium, etc), and other elements similar to normal body fluids without the toxins.

Peritoneal Dialysis

Peritoneal dialysis uses the peritoneal membrane in the abdomen as the filter. The peritoneum consists of visceral and parietal components. The peritoneum membrane provides a large natural surface area for diffusion of approximately 1–2 m^2 in adults; it is permeable to solutes of molecular weights ≤30,000 Da (*Merck Manual*, 1996–1997). However, only a small portion of the total splanchnic blood flow (70 mL/min out of 1200 mL/min at rest) comes into contact with the peritoneum and gets dialyzed. Placement of a peritoneal catheter is surgically simpler than hemodialysis and does not require vascular surgery and heparinization. The dialysis fluid is pumped into the peritoneal cavity, where waste metabolites in the body fluid are discharged rapidly. The dialysate is drained and fresh dialysate is reinstilled and then drained periodically. Peritoneal dialysis is also more amenable to self-treatment. However, slower drug clearance rates are obtained with peritoneal dialysis compared to hemodialysis, and thus longer dialysis time is required.

Continuous ambulatory peritoneal dialysis (CAPD) is the most common form of peritoneal dialysis. Many diabetic patients become uremic as a result of lack of control of their disease. About 2 L of dialysis fluid is instilled into the peritoneal cavity of the patient through a surgically placed resident catheter. The objective is to remove accumulated urea and other metabolic waste in the body. The catheter is sealed and the patient is able to continue in an ambulatory mode. Every 4–6 hours, the fluid is emptied from the peritoneal cavity and replaced with fresh dialysis fluid. The technique uses about 2 L of dialysis fluid; it does not require a dialysis machine and can be performed at home.

Hemodialysis

Hemodialysis uses a dialysis machine and filters blood through an artificial membrane. Hemodialysis requires access to the blood vessels to allow the blood to flow to the dialysis machine and back to the body. For temporary access, a shunt is created in the arm, with one tube inserted into an artery and another tube inserted into a vein. The tubes are joined above the skin. For permanent access to the blood vessels, an arteriovenous fistula or graft is created by a surgical procedure to allow access to the artery and vein. Patients who are on chronic hemodialysis treatment need to be aware of the need for infection control of the surgical site of the fistula. At the start of the hemodialysis procedure, an arterial needle allows the blood to flow to the dialysis machine, and blood is returned to the patient to the venous side. Heparin is used to prevent blood clotting during the dialysis period.

During hemodialysis, the blood flows through the dialysis machine, where the waste material is removed from the blood by diffusion through an artificial membrane before the blood is returned to the body. Hemodialysis is a much more effective method of drug removal and is preferred in situations when rapid removal of the drug from the body is important, as in overdose or poisoning. In practice, hemodialysis is most often used for patients with end-stage renal failure. Early dialysis is appropriate for patients with acute renal failure in whom resumption of renal function can be expected and in patients who are to be renally transplanted. Other patients may be placed on dialysis according to clinical judgment concerning the patient's quality of life and risk/benefit ratio (Carpenter and Lazarus, 1994).

Dialysis may be required from once every 2 days to 3 times a week, with each treatment period lasting for 2–4 hours. The time required for dialysis depends on the amount of residual renal function in the patient, any complicating illness (eg, diabetes mellitus), the size and weight of the patient, including muscle mass, and the efficiency of the dialysis process. Dosing of drugs in patients receiving hemodialysis is affected greatly by the frequency and type of dialysis machine used and by the physicochemical and pharmacokinetic properties of the drug. Factors that affect drug removal in hemodialysis are listed in Table 24-8. These factors are carefully considered before hemodialysis is used for drug removal.

In hemodialysis, blood is pumped to the dialyzer by a roller pump at a rate of 300–450 mL/min. The drug and metabolites diffuse from the blood through the semipermeable membrane. In addition, hydrostatic pressure also forces the drug molecules into the dialysate by ultrafiltration. The composition of the dialysate is similar to plasma but may be altered according to the needs of the patient. Many dialysis machines use a hollow fiber or capillary dialyzer in which the semipermeable membrane is made into fine capillaries, of which thousands are packed into bundles with blood flowing through the capillaries and the dialysate circulating outside the capillaries. The permeability characteristics of the membrane and the membrane surface area are determinants of drug diffusion and ultrafiltration.

The efficacy of hemodialysis membranes for the removal of vancomycin by hemodialysis has been reviewed by De Hart (1996). Vancomycin is an antibiotic effective against most Gram-positive organisms such as *Staphylococcus aureus,* which may be responsible for vascular access infections in patients undergoing dialysis. In De Hart's study, vancomycin hemodialysis in patients was compared using a cuprophan membrane or a cellulose acetate and polyacrylonitrile membrane. The cellulose acetate and polyacrylonitrile membrane is considered a "high-flux" filter. Serum vancomycin concentrations decreased only 6.3% after dialysis when using the

TABLE 24-8   Factors Affecting Dialyzability of Drugs

Physicochemical and Pharmacokinetic Properties of the Drug	
Water solubility	Insoluble or fat-soluble drugs are not dialyzed—eg, glutethimide, which is very water insoluble.
Protein binding	Tightly bound drugs are not dialyzed because dialysis is a passive process of diffusion—eg, propranolol is 94% bound.
Molecular weight	Only molecules with molecular weights of less than 500 are easily dialyzed—eg, vancomycin is poorly dialyzed and has a molecular weight of 1800.
Drugs with large volumes of distribution	Drugs widely distributed are dialyzed more slowly because the rate-limiting factor is the volume of blood entering the machine—eg, for digoxin, $V_D = 250$–300 L. Drugs concentrated in the tissues are usually difficult to remove by dialysis.
Characteristics of the Dialysis Machine	
Blood flow rate	Higher blood flows give higher clearance rates.
Dialysate	Composition of the dialysate and flow rate.
Dialysis membrane	Permeability characteristics and surface area.
Transmembrane pressure	Ultrafiltration increases with increase in transmembrane pressure.
Duration and frequency of dialysis	

cuprophan membrane, whereas the serum drug concentration decreased 13.6%–19.4% after dialysis with the cellulose acetate and polyacrylonitrile membrane.

In dialysis involving uremic patients receiving drugs for therapy, the rate at which a given drug is removed depends on the flow rate of blood to the dialysis machine and the performance of the dialysis machine. The term *dialysance* is used to describe the process of drug removal from the dialysis machine. Dialysance is a clearance term similar in meaning to renal clearance, and it describes the amount of blood completely cleared of drugs (in mL/min). Dialysance is defined by the equation

$$Cl_D = \frac{Q(C_a - C_v)}{C_a} \qquad (24.31)$$

where C_a = drug concentrations in arterial blood (blood entering kidney machine), C_v = drug concentration in venous blood (blood leaving kidney machine), Q = rate of blood flow to the kidney machine, and Cl_D = dialysance. Dialysance is sometimes referred to as *dialysis clearance*.

PRACTICE PROBLEM

Assume the flow rate of blood to the dialysis machine is 350 mL/min. By chemical analysis, the concentrations of drug entering and leaving the machine are 30 and 12 μg/mL, respectively. What is the dialysis clearance?

Solution

The rate of drug removal is equal to the volume of blood passed through the machine divided by the arterial difference in blood drug concentrations before and after dialysis. Thus,

Rate of drug removal = 350 mL/min
× (30 – 12) μg/mL = 6300 μg/min

Since clearance is equal to the rate of drug removal divided by the arterial concentration of drug,

$$Cl_D = \frac{6300\ \mu\text{g/min}}{30\ \mu\text{g/mL}} = 210\ \text{mL/min}$$

Alternatively, using Equation 24.31,

$$Cl_D = 350\ \text{mL/min} \times \frac{(30 - 12)}{30} = 210\ \text{mL/min}$$

These calculations show that the two terms are the same. In practice, dialysance has to be measured experimentally by determining C_a, C_v, and Q. In dosing of drugs for patients on dialysis, the average plasma drug concentration of a patient is given by

$$C_{av}^{\infty} = \frac{FD_0}{(Cl_T + Cl_D)\,\tau} \qquad (24.32)$$

where F represents fraction of dose absorbed, Cl_T is total body drug clearance of the patient, C_{av}^{∞} is average steady-state plasma drug concentration, and τ is the dosing interval.

In practice, if Cl_D is 30% or more of Cl_T, adjustment is usually made for the amount of drug lost in dialysis.

The elimination half-life, $t_{1/2}$, for the drug in the patient off dialysis is related to the remaining total body clearance, Cl_T, and the volume of distribution, V_D, as shown below.

$$t_{1/2} = \frac{0.693}{Cl_T} V_D \qquad (24.33)$$

Drugs that are easily dialyzed will have a high dialysis clearance, Cl_D, and the elimination half-life, $t_{1/2}$, is shorter in a patient on dialysis.

$$t_{1/2} = \frac{0.693\, V_D}{Cl_T + Cl_D} \qquad (24.34)$$

$$k_{ON} = \frac{Cl_T + Cl_D}{V_D} \qquad (24.35)$$

where k_{ON} is the first-order elimination half-life of the drug in the patient on dialysis.

The *fraction of drug lost* due to elimination and dialysis may be estimated from Equation 24.36.

$$\text{Fraction of drug lost} = 1 - e^{-(Cl_T + Cl_D)t/V_D} \qquad (24.36)$$

Equation 24.36 is based on first-order drug elimination and the substitution of t hours for the dialysis period.

Several hypothetical examples illustrating the use of Equation 24.36 have been developed by Gambertoglio (1984). These are given in Table 24-9.

TABLE 24-9   **Predicted Effects of Hemodialysis on Drug Half-Life and Removal in the Overdose Setting**

Drug	V_D (L)	Cl (mL/min)	Cl_D (mL/min)	$t_{1/2\,off}$ (h)	$t_{1/2\,on}$ (h)	FL[a]
Digoxin[b]	560	150	20	43	38	0.07
Digoxin[c]	300	40	20	86	58	0.05
Ethchlorvynol	300	35	60	99	36	0.07
Phenobarbital	50	5	70	115	8	0.30
Phenytoin	100	5	10	231	77	0.04
Salicylic acid	40	20	100	23	4	0.51

[a]FL = fraction lost during a dialysis period of 4 hours.
[b]Parameters for a patient with normal renal function.
[c]Parameters for a patient with no renal function.
From Gambertoglio (1984), with permission.

Equation 24.36 shows that as V_D increases, the fraction of drug lost decreases. The fraction of drug lost during a 4-hour dialysis period for phenobarbital and salicylic acid was 0.30 and 0.50, respectively, whereas for digoxin and phenytoin, the fraction of drug lost was only 0.07 and 0.04, respectively. Both phenobarbital and salicylic acid are easily dialyzed because of their smaller volumes of distribution, small molecular weights, and aqueous solubility. In contrast, digoxin has a large volume of distribution and phenytoin is highly bound to plasma proteins, making these drugs difficult to dialyze. Thus, dialysis is not very useful for treating digoxin intoxication, but is useful for salicylate overdose.

An example of the effect of hemodialysis on drug elimination is shown in Fig. 24-5. During the interdialysis period, the patient's total body clearance is very low and the drug concentration declines slowly. In this example, the drug has an elimination $t_{1/2}$ of 48 hours during the interdialysis period. When the patient is placed on dialysis, the drug clearance (sum of the total body clearance and the dialysis clearance) removes the drug more rapidly.

CLINICAL EXAMPLES

1. The aminoglycoside antibiotics, such as gentamicin and tobramycin, are eliminated primarily by the renal route. Dosing of these aminoglycosides is adjusted according to the residual renal function in the patient as estimated by creatinine clearance. During hemodialysis or peritoneal dialysis, the elimination half-lives for these antibiotics are significantly decreased. After dialysis, the aminoglycoside concentrations are below the therapeutic range, and the patient needs to be given another dose of the aminoglycoside antibiotic.
2. An adult male (73 years old, 65 kg) with diabetes mellitus is placed on hemodialysis. His residual creatinine clearance is <5 mL/min. The patient is given tobramycin, an aminoglycoside antibiotic, at a dose of 1 mg/kg by IV bolus injection. Tobramycin is 90% excreted unchanged in the urine, is less than 10% bound to plasma proteins, and has an elimination

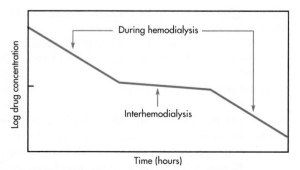

FIGURE 24-5   Effect of dialysis on drug elimination.

half-life of approximately 2.2 hours in patients with normal renal function. In this patient, tobramycin has an elimination $t_{1/2}$ of 50 hours during the interdialysis period and an elimination $t_{1/2}$ of 8 hours during hemodialysis. The apparent volume of distribution for tobramycin is about 0.33 L/kg. For this patient, calculate **(a)** the initial plasma antibiotic concentration after the first dose of tobramycin; **(b)** the plasma drug concentration just before the start of hemodialysis (48 hours after the initial tobramycin dose); **(c)** the plasma drug concentration at the end of 4 hours of hemodialysis; **(d)** the amount of drug lost from the body after dialysis; and **(e)** the tobramycin dose (replenishment dose) needed to be given to the patient after hemodialysis.

Solution

a. Initial plasma antibiotic concentration after the first dose of tobramycin:

$$\text{Patient dose} = \frac{1\ \text{mg}}{\text{kg}} \times 65\ \text{kg} = 65\ \text{mg}$$

$$V_D = \frac{0.33\ \text{L}}{\text{kg}} \times 65\ \text{kg} = 21.45\ \text{L}$$

Plasma drug concentration,

$$C_p^0 = \frac{D_0}{V_D} = \frac{65\ \text{mg}}{21.45\ \text{L}} = 3.03\ \text{mg/L}$$

b. Plasma drug concentration just before the start of hemodialysis (48 hours after the initial tobramycin dose): After 48 hours, the plasma drug concentration declines according to first-order kinetics:

$$C_p = 3.03\ e^{-(0.693/50)\,(48)} = 1.58\ \text{mg/L}$$

c. Plasma drug concentration at the end of a 4-hour hemodialysis:

$$C_p = 1.58\ e^{-(0.693/8)\,(4)} = 0.547\ \text{mg/L}$$

d. Amount of drug lost from the body after dialysis:

Amt of drug lost after dialysis =
Amt of drug in the body before dialysis −
Amt of drug in the body after dialysis

$$\frac{1.58\ \text{mg}}{\text{L}}(21.45\ \text{L}) - \frac{0.547\ \text{mg}}{\text{L}}(21.45\ \text{L})$$

$$= 22.16\ \text{mg}$$

e. Tobramycin dose (replenishment dose) needed to be given to the patient after hemodialysis: The recommended ranges of peak and trough concentrations of tobramycin (Mathews, 1995) are 5–10 mg/L (peak) and 0.5–<2 mg/L (trough). The usual replenishment dose of tobramycin after hemodialysis is 1–1.5 mg/kg.

If a replenishment dose of 65 mg (ie, 1 mg/kg) is given to the patient, then the plasma drug concentration is estimated as

Plasma drug concentration after 65 mg

$$\text{given by IV bolus injection} = \frac{65\ \text{mg}}{21.45\ \text{L}} + 0.547\ \text{mg/L}$$

$$= 3.58\ \text{mg/L}$$

after hemodialysis.

The patient is given 65 mg of tobramycin by IV bolus injection after completion of hemodialysis to produce a tobramycin plasma concentration of 3.58 mg/L.

Hemoperfusion

Hemoperfusion is the process of removing drug by passing the blood from the patient through an adsorbent material and back to the patient. Hemoperfusion is a useful procedure for rapid drug removal in accidental poisoning and drug overdose. Because the drug molecules in the blood are in direct contact with the adsorbent material, any molecule that has great affinity for the adsorbent material will be removed. The two main adsorbents used in hemoperfusion include (1) activated charcoal, which adsorbs both polar and nonpolar drug, and (2) Amberlite resins. Amberlite resins, such as Amberlite XAD-2 and Amberlite XAD-4, are available as insoluble polymeric beads, with each bead containing an agglomerate of cross-linked polystyrene microspheres. The Amberlite resins have a greater affinity for nonpolar organic molecules than activated charcoal.

The important factors for drug removal by hemoperfusion include affinity of the drug for the adsorbent, surface area of the adsorbent, absorptive capacity of the adsorbent, rate of blood flow through the adsorbent, and the equilibration rate of the drug from the peripheral tissue into the blood.

Hemofiltration

An alternative to hemodialysis and hemoperfusion is hemofiltration. *Hemofiltration* is a process by which fluids, electrolytes, and small-molecular-weight substances are removed from the blood by means of low-pressure flow through hollow artificial fibers or flat-plate membranes (Bickley, 1988). Because fluid is also filtered out of the plasma during hemofiltration, replacement fluid is administered to the patient for volume replacement. Hemofiltration is a slow, continuous filtration process that removes non-protein-bound small molecules (<10,000 Da) from the blood by convective mass transport. The clearance of the drug depends on the sieving coefficient and ultrafiltration rate. Hemofiltration provides a creatinine clearance of approximately 10 mL/min (Bickley, 1988) and may have limited use for drugs that are widely distributed in the body, such as aminoglycosides, cephalosporins, and acyclovir. A major problem with this method is the formation of blood clots within the hollow filter fibers.

Continuous Renal Replacement Therapy

Because of the initial loss of fluid that results during hemofiltration, intermittent hemofiltration results in concentration of red blood cells in the resulting reduced plasma volume. Therefore, blood becomes more viscous with a high hematocrit and high colloid osmotic pressure at the distal end of the hemofilter. *Predilution* may be used to circumvent this problem, but this method is rarely used because of cost and inefficiency.

Continuous replacement therapy allows ongoing removal of fluid and toxins by relying on a patient's own blood pressure to pump blood through a filter. The continuous filtration is better tolerated by patients than intermittent therapy and provides optimal control of circulating volumes and ongoing toxin removal. Because continuous replacement

therapies are hemofiltration methods, replacement fluid must be administered to the patient to replace fluid lost to the hemofiltrate, though the volume of fluid removed can be easily controlled compared to intermittent hemofiltration. Heparin infusions are also provided for anticoagulation.

Continuous renal replacement therapy (CRRT) includes *continuous veno-venous hemofiltration* (CVVH) and *continuous arteriovenous hemofiltration* (CAVH). In CAVH, blood passes through a hemofilter that is placed between a cannulated femoral artery and vein. A dialysis filter may be added to CAVH to improve small-molecule clearance. Circulating dialysate on the outside of the filters allows more efficient toxin removal. However, this method is inefficient (10–15 mL filtered per minute) and complex and is not widely used in comparison to CVVH.

CVVH provides a hemofilter that is placed between cannulated femoral, subclavian, or internal jugular veins. Rather than relying on arterial pressure to filter blood, a pump can be used to provide filtration rates greater than 100 mL/min. Like CAVH, a dialysis filter may be added to CVVH to improve clearance of small molecules.

As with other extracorporeal removal systems, hemofiltration methods can alter drug pharmacokinetics. A study by Hansen et al (2001) showed that acute renal failure patients on CVVH demonstrated a 50% decrease in clearance of levofloxacin. However, because of the large volume and moderate renal clearance of fluoroquinolones, levofloxacin does not require dosing adjustment.

Drug Removal during Continuous Renal Replacement Therapy

During CAVH, solutes are removed by convection. The efficiency of the removal of drugs is related to the *sieving coefficient S*, which reflects the solute removal ability during hemofiltration and is equal to the ratio of solute concentration in the ultrafiltrate to the solute concentration in the retentate. When $S = 1$, the solute passes freely through the membrane. When $S = 0$, the solute is retained in the plasma. S is constant and independent of blood flow; therefore,

$$Cl = S \times \text{rate}_{uf} \qquad (24.37)$$

where rate$_{uf}$ is the ultrafiltration rate. The concentration of drug in the ultrafiltrate is also equal to the unbound drug concentration in the plasma. So, the amount of drug removed during CAVH is

$$\text{Amount removed per time unit} = C_p \times \alpha \times \text{rate}_{uf}$$

(24.38)

where α = the unbound fraction.

Frequently Asked Questions

▶ *Which pharmacokinetic properties of a drug would predict a greater or lesser rate of elimination in a patient undergoing dialysis?*

▶ *Drug clearance is often decreased 20%–50% in many patients with congestive heart failure (CHF). Explain how it may affect drug disposition.*

EFFECT OF HEPATIC DISEASE ON PHARMACOKINETICS

Hepatic disease can alter drug pharmacokinetics including absorption and disposition as well as pharmacodynamics including efficacy and safety. Hepatic disease may include common hepatic diseases, such as alcoholic liver disease (cirrhosis) and chronic infections with hepatitis viruses B and C, and less common diseases, such as acute hepatitis D or E, primary biliary cirrhosis, primary sclerosing cholangitis, and α_1-antitrypsin deficiency (FDA Guidance for Industry, 2003). In addition, drug-induced hepatotoxicity is the leading cause of acute liver failure in the United States (Chang and Schiano, 2007).

Drugs are often metabolized by one or more enzymes located in cellular membranes in different parts of the liver. Drugs and metabolites may also be excreted by biliary secretion. Hepatic disease may lead to drug accumulation, failure to form an active or inactive metabolite, increased bioavailability after oral administration, and other effects including possible alteration in drug–protein binding. Liver disease may also alter kidney function, which can lead to accumulation of a drug and its metabolites even when the liver is not primarily responsible for elimination.

The major difficulty in estimating hepatic clearance in patients with hepatic disease is the complexity and stratification of the liver enzyme systems. In contrast, creatinine clearance has been used successfully to measure kidney function and renal clearance of drugs. Clinical laboratory tests measure only a limited number of liver functions. Some clinical laboratory tests, such as the *aspartate aminotransferase* (AST) and *alanine aminotransferases* (ALT), are common serum enzyme tests that detect liver cell damage rather than liver function. Other laboratory tests, such as serum bilirubin, are used to measure biliary obstruction or interference with bile flow. Presently, no single test accurately assesses the total liver function. Usually, a series of clinical laboratory tests are used in clinical practice to detect the presence of liver disease, distinguish among different types of liver disorders, gauge the extent of known liver damage, and follow the response to treatment. A few tests have been used to relate the severity of hepatic impairment to predicted changes in the pharmacokinetic profile of a drug (FDA Guidance for Industry, 2003). Examples of these tests include the ability of the liver to eliminate marker drugs such as antipyrine, indocyanine green, monoethylglycine-xylidide, and galactose. Furthermore, endogenous substrates, such as albumin or bilirubin, or a functional measure, such as prothrombin time, has been used for the evaluation of liver impairment.

Dosage Considerations in Hepatic Disease

Several physiologic and pharmacokinetic factors are relevant in considering dosage of a drug in patients with hepatic disease (Table 24-10). Chronic disease or tissue injury may change the accessibility of some enzymes as a result of redirection or detour of hepatic blood circulation. Liver disease affects the quantitative and qualitative synthesis of albumin, globulins, and other circulating plasma proteins that subsequently affect plasma drug protein binding and distribution (see Chapter 12). As mentioned, most liver function tests indicate only that the liver has been damaged; they do not assess the function of the cytochrome P-450 enzymes or intrinsic clearance by the liver.

TABLE 24-10   Considerations in Dosing Patients with Hepatic Impairment

Item	Comments
Nature and severity of liver disease	Not all liver diseases affect the pharmacokinetics of the drugs to the same extent.
Drug elimination	Drugs eliminated by the liver >20% are less likely to be affected by liver disease. Drugs that are eliminated mainly via renal route will be least affected by liver disease.
Route of drug administration	Oral drug bioavailability may be increased by liver disease due to decreased first-pass effects.
Protein binding	Drug–protein binding may be altered due to alteration in hepatic synthesis of albumin.
Hepatic blood flow	Drugs with flow-dependent hepatic clearance will be more affected by change in hepatic blood flow.
Intrinsic clearance	Metabolism of drugs with high intrinsic clearance may be impaired.
Biliary obstruction	Biliary excretion of some drugs and metabolites, particularly glucuronide metabolites, may be impaired.
Pharmacodynamic changes	Tissue sensitivity to drug may be altered.
Therapeutic range	Drugs with a wide therapeutic range will be less affected by moderate hepatic impairment.

Because there is no readily available measure of hepatic function that can be applied to calculate appropriate doses, enzyme-dependent drugs are usually given to patients with hepatic failure in half-doses, or less. Response or plasma levels then must be monitored. Drugs with flow-dependent clearance are avoided if possible in patients with liver failure. When necessary, doses of these drugs may need to be reduced to as low as one-tenth of the conventional dose for an orally administered agent. Starting therapy with low doses and monitoring response or plasma levels provides the best opportunity for safe and efficacious treatment.

If some of the efflux proteins that normally protect the body against drug accumulation are reduced or not functioning, this could potentially cause hepatic drug injury as drug concentration begins to increase. Compounds that form glucuronide, sulfate, glutathione (GSH), and other substrates that are involved in phase II metabolism (see Chapter 12) may be depleted during hepatic impairment, potentially interrupting the normal path of drug metabolism. Indeed, even albumin or alpha-1-acid glycoprotein (AAG) concentrations can be altered in hepatic impairment and affect drug distribution or drug disposition in many unpredictable ways that can affect drug safety.

Fraction of Drug Metabolized

Drug elimination in the body may be divided into (1) fraction of drug excretion unchanged, f_e, and (2) fraction of drug metabolized. The latter is usually estimated from $1 - f_e$; alternatively, the fraction of drug metabolized may be estimated from the ratio of Cl_h/Cl, where Cl_h is hepatic clearance and Cl is total body clearance. Knowing the fraction of drug eliminated by the liver allows estimation of total body clearance when hepatic clearance is reduced. Drugs with low f_e values (or, conversely, drugs with a higher fraction of metabolized drug) are more affected by a change in liver function due to hepatic disease.

$$Cl_h = Cl(1 - f_e) \qquad (24.39)$$

Equation 24.39 assumes that drug metabolism occurs in the liver and the unchanged drug is excreted in the urine. Assuming that there is no enzyme saturation and a drug exhibits linear kinetics, dosing adjustment may be based on residual hepatic function in patients with hepatic disease as shown in the following example.

PRACTICE PROBLEM

The hepatic clearance of a drug in a patient is reduced by 50% due to chronic viral hepatitis. How is the total body clearance of the drug affected? What should be the new dose of the drug for the patient? Assume that renal drug clearance ($f_e = 0.4$) and plasma drug protein binding are not altered.

Solution

The residual liver function (RL) is estimated by

$$RL = \frac{[Cl_h]_{hepatitis}}{[Cl_h]_{normal}}$$

$$[Cl_h]_{hepatitis} = RL\,[Cl_h]_{normal}$$

Substituting $Cl_{normal}(1 - f_e)$ for $[Cl_h]_{normal}$

$$[Cl_h]_{hepatitis} = RL\,Cl_{normal}(1 - f_e) \qquad (24.40)$$

Assuming no renal clearance deterioration due to hepatitis

$$Cl_{hepatitis} = [Cl_h]_{hepatitis} + [Cl_R]_{normal} \qquad (24.41)$$

Substituting Equation 24.41 with Equation 24.40 and $Cl_{normal}\,f_e$ for $[Cl_R]_{normal}$

$$Cl_{hepatitis} = RL\,Cl_{normal}(1 - f_e) + Cl_{normal}\,f_e \qquad (24.42)$$

$$Cl_{hepatitis} = Cl_{normal}[RL(1 - f_e) + f_e] \qquad (24.43)$$

$$\frac{D_{hepatitis}}{D_{normal}} = \frac{Cl_{hepatitis}}{Cl_{normal}} = \frac{RL(1 - f_e) + f_e}{1} \qquad (24.44)$$

where RL = residual liver function.
$[Cl_h]_{normal}$ = hepatic clearance of drug in normal subject
$[Cl_h]_{hepatitis}$ = hepatic clearance of drug in patient with hepatitis

$[Cl_R]_{normal}$ = renal clearance of drug in normal subject
Cl_{normal} = total clearance of drug in normal subject
$Cl_{hepatitis}$ = total clearance of drug in patient with hepatitis
f_e = fraction of drug excreted unchanged
$1 - f_e$ = fraction of drug metabolized

and $D_{hepatitis}$ and D_{normal} are the doses in a hepatitis patient and in a normal liver function patient, respectively. Substituting in Equation 24.44 with $RL = 0.5$ and $f_e = 0.4$,

$$\frac{D_{hepatitis}}{D_{normal}} = 0.5(1 - 0.4) + 0.4 = 0.3 + 0.4$$

$$= 0.7 \text{ (or } 70\%)$$

The adjusted dose of the drug for the hepatic patient is 70% of that for the normal subject as a result of the 50% decrease in hepatic function in the above case ($f_e = 0.4$).

An example of a correlation established between actual residual liver function (measured by marker) and hepatic clearance was reported for cefoperazone (Hu et al, 1995) and other drugs in patients with cirrhosis. The method should be applied only to drugs that have linear pharmacokinetics or low protein binding, or that are nonrestrictively bound.

Many variables can complicate dose correction when binding profoundly affects distribution, elimination, and penetration of the drug to the active site. For drugs with restrictive binding, the fraction of free drug must be used to correct the change in free drug concentration and the change in free drug clearance. In some cases, the increase in free drug is partly offset by a larger volume of distribution resulting from the decrease in protein binding. Since there are many variables that complicate dose correction for patients with hepatic disease, dose correction is limited to drugs whose hepatic metabolism is approximated by linear pharmacokinetics.

Active Drug and the Metabolite

For many drugs, both the drug and the metabolite contribute to the overall therapeutic response of the drug to the patient. The concentration of both the drug and the metabolite in the body should be known.

When the pharmacokinetic parameters of the metabolite and the drug are similar, the overall activity of the drug can become more or less potent as a result of a change in liver function; that is, (1) when the drug is more potent than the metabolite, the overall pharmacologic activity will increase in the hepatic-impaired patient because the parent drug concentration will be higher; (2) when the drug is less potent than the metabolite, the overall pharmacologic activity in the hepatic patient will decrease because less of the active metabolite is formed.

Changes in pharmacologic activity due to hepatic disease may be much more complex when both the pharmacokinetic parameters and the pharmacodynamics of the drug change as a result of the disease process. In such cases, the overall pharmacodynamic response may be greatly modified, making it necessary to monitor the response change with the aid of a pharmacodynamic model (see Chapter 21).

Hepatic Blood Flow and Intrinsic Clearance

Blood flow changes can occur in patients with chronic liver disease (often due to viral hepatitis or chronic alcohol use). In some patients with severe liver cirrhosis, fibrosis of liver tissue may occur, resulting in intra- or extrahepatic shunt. Hepatic arterial-venous shunts may lead to reduced fraction of drug extracted (see Chapter 12) and an increase in the bioavailability of drug. In other patients, resistance to blood flow may be increased as a result of tissue damage and fibrosis, causing a reduction in intrinsic hepatic clearance.

The following equation may be applied to estimate hepatic clearance of a drug after assessing changes in blood flow and intrinsic clearance (Cl_{int}):

$$Cl_h = \frac{QCl_{int}}{Q + Cl_{int}} \qquad (24.45)$$

Alternatively, when both Q and the extraction ratio, ER, are known in the patient, Cl may also be estimated:

$$Cl = Q\,(ER) \qquad (24.46)$$

Unlike changes in renal disease, in which serum creatinine concentration may be used to monitor changes in renal function such as GFR, the above physiologic model equation may not be adequate for accurate prediction of changes in hepatic clearance. Calculations based on model equations must be corroborated by clinical assessment.

Pathophysiologic Assessment

In practice, patient information about changes in hepatic blood flow may not be available, because special electromagnetic (Nuxmalo et al, 1978) or ultrasound techniques are required to measure blood flow and are not routinely available. The clinician/pharmacist may have to make an empirical estimate of the blood flow change after examining the patient and reviewing the available liver function tests.

Various approaches have been used diagnostically to assess hepatic impairment. The Child–Pugh (or Child–Turcotte–Pugh) score assesses the overall hepatic impairment as mild, moderate, or severe (Figg et al, 1995; Lucey et al, 1997). The score employs five clinical measures of liver disease, including total bilirubin, serum albumin, International Normalized Ratio (INR), ascites, and hepatic encephalopathy (Tables 24-11 and 24-12). Different publications use different measures. Some older references substitute prothrombin time (PT) prolongation for INR. The original classification used nutrition, which

TABLE 24-11   Child-Pugh Classification of Severity of Liver Disease

Parameter	Points Assigned		
	1	2	3
Ascites	Absent	Slight	Moderate
Bilirubin, mg/dL	≤2	2–3	>3
Albumin, g/dL	>3.5	2.8–3.5	<2.8
Prothrombin time			
Seconds over control	1–3	4–6	>6
INR	<1.8	1.8–2.3	>2.3
Encephalopathy	None	Grade 1–2	Grade 3–4

Data from Trey et al (1966).

TABLE 24-12   Severity Classification Schemes for Liver Disease

	Child–Turcotte Classification		
	Grade A	**Grade B**	**Grade C**
Bilirubin (mg/dL)	<2.0	2.0–3.0	>3.0
Albumin (g/dL)	>3.5	3.0–3.5	<3.0
Ascites	None	Easily controlled	Poorly controlled
Neurological disorder	None	Minimal	Advanced
Nutrition	Excellent	Good	Poor

Data from Brouwer et al (1992).

TABLE 24-13   Drugs with Significantly Decreased Metabolism in Chronic Liver Disease

Antipyrine	Caffeine
Cefoperazone	Chlordiazepoxide
Chloramphenicol	Diazepam
Erythromycin	Hexobarbital
Metronidazole	Lidocaine
Meperidine	Metoprolol
Pentazocine	Propranolol
Tocainide	Theophylline
Verapamil	Promazine

Data from Howden et al (1989), Williams (1983), and Hu et al (1995).

was later replaced by PT prolongation. The model for end-stage liver disease, or MELD, is a scoring system for assessing the severity of chronic liver disease based on mortality after liver surgery (Cholongitas et al, 2005; Kamath and Kim, 2007). Unfortunately, neither one of these approaches for assessing hepatic disease and hepatic impairment provides direct predictability or correlation with the pharmacokinetics of a drug.

While chronic hepatic disease is more likely to change the metabolism of a drug (Howden et al, 1989), acute hepatitis due to hepatotoxin or viral inflammation is often associated with marginal or less severe changes in metabolic drug clearance (Farrel et al, 1978). The clinician should make an assessment based on acceptable risk criteria on a case-by-case basis.

In general, basic pharmacokinetics treats the body globally and more readily applies to dosing estimation. However, drug clearance based on individual eliminating organs is more informative and provides more insight into the pharmacokinetic changes in the disease process. A practical method for dosing hepatic-impaired patients is still in the early stages of development. While the hepatic blood flow model (see Chapter 12) is useful for predicting changes in hepatic clearance resulting from alterations in hepatic blood flow, Q_a and Q_v, extrahepatic changes can also influence pharmacokinetics in hepatic-impaired patients. Global changes in

distribution may occur outside the liver. Extrahepatic metabolism and other hemodynamic changes may also occur and can be accounted for more completely by monitoring total body clearance of the drug using basic pharmacokinetics. For example, lack of local change in hepatic drug clearance should not be prematurely interpreted as "no change" in overall drug clearance. Reduced albumin and AAG, for example, may change the volume of distribution of the drug and therefore, alter total body clearance on a global basis.

Chronic liver disease has been shown to decrease the metabolism of many drugs as shown in Table 24-13. However, the amount of decrease in metabolism is difficult to assess.

EXAMPLE ▶ ▶ ▶

After IV bolus administration of 1 g of cefoperazone to normal and chronic hepatitis patients, urinary excretion of cefoperazone was significantly increased in cirrhosis patients, from 23.95% ± 5.06% for normal patients to 51.09% ± 11.50% in cirrhosis patients (Hu et al, 1995). Explain **(a)** why there is a change in the percent of unchanged cefoperazone excreted in the urine of patients with cirrhosis, and **(b)** suggest a quantitative test to monitor the hepatic elimination of cefoperazone (*Hint:* Consult Hu et al, 1994).

Liver Function Tests and Hepatic Metabolic Markers

Drug markers used to measure residual hepatic function may correlate well with hepatic clearance of one drug but correlate poorly with another substrate metabolized by a different enzyme within the same cytochrome P-450 subfamily. Some useful marker compounds are listed below.

1. *Aminotransferase* (normal ALT: male, 10–55 U/L; female, 7–30 U/L; normal AST: male, 10–40 U/L; female, 9–25 U/L): Aminotransferases are enzymes found in many tissues that include serum aspartate aminotransferase (AST, formerly SGOT) and alanine aminotransferase (ALT, formerly SGPT). ALT is liver specific, but AST is found in liver and many other tissues, including cardiac and skeletal muscles. Leakage of aminotransferases into the plasma is used as an indicator for many types of hepatic disease and hepatitis. The AST/ALT ratio is used in differential diagnosis. In acute liver injury, AST/ALT is ≤1, whereas in alcoholic hepatitis the AST/ALT > 2.

2. *Alkaline phosphatase* (normal: male, 45–115 U/L; female, 30–100 U/L): Like aminotransferase, alkaline phosphatase (AP) is normally present in many tissues, and it is also present on the canalicular domain of the hepatocyte plasma membrane. Plasma AP may be elevated in hepatic disease because of increased AP production and released into the serum. In cholestasis, or bile flow obstruction, AP release is facilitated by bile acid solubilization of the membranes. Marked AP elevations may indicate hepatic tumors or biliary obstruction in the liver, or disease in other tissues such as bone, placenta, or intestine.

3. *Bilirubin* (normal total = 0–1.0 mg/dL: direct = 0–0.4 mg/dL): Bilirubin consists of both a water-soluble, conjugated, "direct" fraction and a lipid-soluble, unconjugated, "indirect" fraction. The unconjugated form is bound to albumin and is, therefore, not filtered by the kidney. Since impaired biliary excretion results in increases in conjugated (filtered) bilirubin, hepatobiliary disease can result in increases in urinary bilirubin. Unconjugated hyperbilirubinemia results from either increased bilirubin production or defects in hepatic uptake or conjugation. Conjugated hyperbilirubinemia results from defects in hepatic excretion.

4. *Prothrombin time* (PT; normal, 11.2–13.2 s): With the exception of Factor VIII, all coagulation factors are synthesized by the liver. Therefore, hepatic disease can alter coagulation. Decreases in PT (the rate of conversion of prothrombin to thrombin) are suggestive of acute or chronic liver failure or biliary obstruction. Vitamin K is also important in coagulation, so vitamin K deficiency can also decrease PT.

EXAMPLE ▶ ▶ ▶

Paclitaxel, an anticancer agent for solid tumors and leukemia, has extensive tissue distribution, high plasma protein binding (approximately 90%–95%), and variable systemic clearance. Average paclitaxel clearance ranges from 87 to 503 mL/min/m² (5.2–30.2 L/h/m²), with minimal renal excretion (10%) of the parent drug (Sonnichsen and Relling, 1994). Paclitaxel is extensively metabolized by the liver to three primary metabolites. Cytochrome P-450 enzymes of the CYP3A and CYP2C subfamilies appear to be involved in hepatic metabolism of paclitaxel. What are the precautions in administering paclitaxel to patients with liver disease?

Solution

Although paclitaxel has first-order pharmacokinetics at normal doses, its elimination may be saturable in some patients with genetically reduced intrinsic clearance due to CYP3A or CYP2C. The clinical importance of saturable elimination will be greatest when large dosages are infused over a shorter period of time. In these situations, achievable plasma concentrations are likely to cause saturation of binding. Thus, small changes in dosage or infusion duration may result in disproportionately large alterations in paclitaxel systemic exposure, potentially influencing patient response and toxicity.

Hepatic Impairment and Dose Adjustment

Hepatic impairment may not sufficiently alter the pharmacokinetics of some drugs to require dosage adjustment. Drugs that have the following properties are less likely to need dosage adjustment in patients with hepatic impairment (FDA Guidance for Industry, 2003):

- The drug is excreted entirely via renal routes of elimination with no involvement of the liver.
- The drug is metabolized in the liver to a small extent (<20%), and the therapeutic range of the drug is wide, so that modest impairment of hepatic clearance will not lead to toxicity of the drug directly or by increasing its interaction with other drugs.
- The drug is gaseous or volatile, and the drug and its active metabolites are primarily eliminated via the lungs.

For each drug case, the physician needs to assess the degree of hepatic impairment and consider the known pharmacokinetics and pharmacodynamics of the drug. For example, Mallikaarjun et al (2008) studied the effects of hepatic or renal impairment on the pharmacokinetics of aripiprazole (Abilify), an atypical antipsychotic used to treat schizophrenia. These investigators concluded that there were no meaningful differences in aripiprazole pharmacokinetics between groups of subjects with normal hepatic or renal function and those with either hepatic or renal impairment. Thus, the adjustment of the aripiprazole does not appear to be required in populations with hepatic or renal impairment.

In contrast, Muirhead et al (2002) studied the effects of age and renal and hepatic impairments on the pharmacokinetics, tolerability, and safety of sildenafil (Viagra), a drug used to treat erectile dysfunction. Muirhead et al (2002) observed significant differences in C_{max} and AUC between the young and the elderly subjects for both the parent drug and the metabolite. In addition, the hepatic impairment study demonstrated that pharmacokinetics of sildenafil was altered in subjects with chronic stable cirrhosis, as shown by a 46% reduction in CL/F and a 47% increase in C_{max} compared with subjects with normal hepatic function. Sildenafil pharmacokinetics was affected by age and by renal and hepatic impairments, suggesting that a lower starting dose of 25 mg should be considered for patients with severely compromised renal or hepatic function.

Frequently Asked Questions

▶ *How do changes in drug–protein binding affect dose adjustment in patients with renal and/or hepatic disease?*

▶ *Which pharmacokinetic properties of a drug are more likely to be affected by renal disease or liver hepatotoxicity?*

▶ *Can you quantitatively predict the change in the pharmacokinetics of a drug that normally has high hepatic clearance in a patient with hepatic impairment? Explain.*

CHAPTER SUMMARY

The kidney and liver are important organs involved in regulating body fluids, electrolyte balance, removal of metabolic waste, and drug excretion from the body. Impairment of kidney or liver function affects the pharmacokinetics of drugs as well as safety and efficacy. Renal function may be assessed by several methods. Creatinine clearance calculated by using the serum concentration of endogenous creatinine is used most often to measure glomerular filtration rate. Creatinine clearance values must be considered carefully in special populations such as elderly, obese, and emaciated patients. The Crockcroft–Gault method is frequently used to estimate creatinine clearance from serum creatinine concentration. Dose adjustment in renal disease is based on the fraction of drug that is really excreted and generally assumes that nonrenal drug elimination remains constant. Different approaches for dose adjustment in renal disease give somewhat different values. Patients with ESRD and other patients without kidney function require supportive treatment such as dialysis to remove the accumulated drug and its metabolites. The objective of these dialysis methods is to rapidly remove the undesirable drugs and metabolites from the body without disturbing the fluid and electrolyte balance in the patient. Dosage adjustment may be needed to replace drug loss during extracorporeal drug and metabolite removal. The major difficulty in estimating hepatic clearance in patients with hepatic disease is the complexity and

stratification of the liver enzyme systems. Presently, no single test accurately assesses the total liver function. Various approaches such as the Child–Pugh (or Child–Turcotte–Pugh) score have been used diagnostically to assess hepatic impairment. Hepatic impairment may not sufficiently alter the pharmacokinetics of some drugs to require dosage adjustment. Physicians and/or pharmacists must understand the pharmacokinetic and pharmacodynamic properties of each drug in patients with hepatic and/or renal impairment for proper dose adjustment.

LEARNING QUESTIONS

1. The normal dosing schedule for a patient on tetracycline is 250 mg PO (by mouth) every 6 hours. Suggest a dosage regimen for this patient when laboratory analysis shows that his renal function has deteriorated from a Cl_{cr} of 90 mL/min to a Cl_{cr} of 20 mL/min.

2. A patient receiving antibiotic treatment is on dialysis. The flow rate of serum into the kidney machine is 50 mL/min. Assays show that the concentration of drug entering the machine is 5 μg/mL and the concentration of drug in the serum leaving the machine is 2.4 μg/mL. The drug clearance for this patient is 10 mL/min. To what extent should the dose be increased if the average concentration of the antibiotic is to be maintained?

3. Glomerular filtration rate may be measured by either insulin clearance or creatinine clearance.
   a. Why is creatinine or insulin clearance used to measure GFR?
   b. Which clearance method, insulin or creatinine, gives a more accurate estimate of GFR? Why?

4. A uremic patient has a urine output of 1.8 L/24 h and an average creatinine concentration of 2.2 mg/dL. What is the creatinine clearance? How would you adjust the dose of a drug normally given at 20 mg/kg every 6 hours in this patient (assume the urine creatinine concentration is 0.1 mg/mL and creatinine clearance is 100 mL/min)?

5. A patient on intramuscular lincomycin 600 mg every 12 hours was found to have a creatinine clearance of 5 mL/min. Should the dose be adjusted? If so, (a) adjust the dose by keeping the dosing interval constant; (b) adjust the dosing interval and give the same dose; and (c) adjust both dosing interval and dose. What are the differences in the adjustment methods?

6. Calculate the creatinine clearance for a woman (38 years old, 62 kg) whose serum creatinine is 1.8 mg/dL using the method of Cockcroft–Gault.

7. Would you adjust the dose of cephamandole, an antibiotic that is 98% excreted unchanged in the urine, for the patient in Question 6? If so, why?

8. What assumptions are usually made when adjusting a dosage regimen according to the creatinine clearance in a patient with renal failure?

9. The usual dose of gentamicin in patients with normal renal function is 1 mg/kg every 8 hours by multiple IV bolus injections. Using the nomogram method (see Fig. 24-4), what dose of gentamicin would you recommend for a 55-year-old male patient weighing 72 kg with a creatinine clearance of 20 mL/min?

10. A single intravenous bolus injection (1 g) of an antibiotic was given to a male anephric patient (age 68 years, 75 kg). During the next 48 hours, the elimination half-life of the antibiotic was 16 hours. The patient was then placed on

hemodialysis for 8 hours and the elimination half-life was reduced to 4 hours.

  a. How much drug was eliminated by the end of the dialysis period?

  b. Assuming the apparent volume of distribution of this antibiotic is 0.5 L/kg, what was the plasma drug concentration just before and after dialysis?

11. There are several pharmacokinetic methods for adjustment of a drug dosage regimen for patients with uremic disease based on the serum creatinine concentration in that patient. From your knowledge of clinical pharmacokinetics, discuss the following questions:

  a. What is the basis of these methods for the calculation of drug dosage regimens in uremic patients?

  b. What is the validity of the assumptions upon which these calculations are made?

12. After assessment of the uremic condition of the patient, the drug dosage regimen may be adjusted by one of two methods: **(a)** by keeping the dose constant and prolonging the dosage interval, τ, or **(b)** by decreasing the dose and maintaining the dosage interval constant. Discuss the advantages and disadvantages of adjusting the dosage regimen using either method.

ANSWERS

Frequently Asked Questions

What are the main factors that influence drug dosing in renal disease?

- Renal disease can cause profound changes in the body that must be evaluated by assessing the patient's condition and medical history. Renal dysfunction is often accompanied by reduced protein–drug binding and by reduced glomerular filtration rate in the kidney. Some changes in hepatic clearance may also occur. While there is no accurate method for predicting the resulting *in vivo* changes, a decrease in albumin may increase f_u, or the fraction of free plasma drug concentration in the body. The f_u is estimated from $f_u = 1 - f_b$, where f_b is the fraction of bound plasma drug. For the uremic patient, the fraction of drug bound f_b' is affected by a change in plasma protein: $f_b'/f_b = p'/4.4$, where p is the normal plasma protein concentration (4.4 g/dL assuming albumin is the protein involved) and p' is the uremic plasma protein concentration; f_b' is the fraction of drug bound in the uremic patient. Since f_u' or the fraction of unbound drug is increased in the uremic patient, the free drug concentration may be increased and, sometimes, lead to more frequent side effects. On the other hand, an increase in plasma free drug in the uremic patient is offset somewhat by a corresponding increase in the volume of distribution as plasma protein–drug binding is reduced. Reduction in GFR is more definite; it is invariably accompanied by a reduction in drug clearance and by an increase in the elimination half-life of the drug.

Name and contrast the two methods for adjusting drug dose in renal disease.

- Two approaches to dose adjustment in renal disease are the clearance method and the elimination rate constant method. The methods are based on estimating either the uremic Cl_R or the uremic k_R after the creatinine clearance is obtained in the uremic patient.

What are the pharmacokinetic considerations in designing a dosing regimen? Why is dosing once a day for aminoglycosides recommended by many clinicians?

- Aminoglycosides are given as a larger dose spaced farther apart (once daily). Keeping the same total daily dose of the aminoglycoside improves the response (efficacy) and possibly lessens side effects in many patients. Model simulation shows reduced exposure (AUC) to the effect compartment (toxicity), while the activity is not altered. The higher drug dose produces a higher peak drug concentration. In the case of gentamicin, the marketed drug is chemically composed of three related, but distinctly different, chemical components, which may distribute differently in the body.

How do changes in drug–protein binding affect dose adjustment in patients with renal and/or hepatic disease?

- Hepatic disease may reduce albumin and α_1-acid glycoprotein (AAG) concentrations resulting in decreased drug protein binding. Blood flow to the liver may also be affected. Generally, for a drug with linear binding, f_u may be increased as discussed in FAQ #1. Consult Chapter 10 also for a discussion of restrictive clearance of drugs. Examples of binding to AAG are the protease inhibitors for AIDS.

Drug clearance is often decreased 20%–50% in many patients with congestive heart failure (CHF). Explain how it may affect drug disposition.

- Congestive heart failure (CHF) can reduce renal or hepatic blood flow and decrease hepatic and renal drug clearance. In CHF, less blood flow is available in the splanchnic circulation to the small intestine and may result in less systemic drug bioavailability after oral drug administration. Severe disturbances to blood flow will affect the pharmacokinetics of many drugs. Myocardiac infarction (MI) is a clinical example that often causes drug clearance to be greatly reduced, especially for drugs with large hepatic extraction.

Learning Questions

1. The normal dose of tetracycline is 250 mg PO every 6 hours. The dose of tetracycline for the uremic patient is determined by the k_u/k_N ratio, which is determined by the kidney function, as in Fig. 24-4. From line H in the figure, at Cl_{cr} of 20 mL, $k_u/k_N = 40\%$. In order to maintain the average concentration of tetracycline at the same level as in normal patients, the dose of tetracycline must be reduced.

$$\frac{D_u}{D_N} = \frac{k_u}{k_N} = 40\%$$

$$D_u = (250)(0.40) = 100 \text{ mg}$$

2. The drug in this patient is eliminated by the kidneys and the dialysis machine. Therefore,

$$\text{Total drug clearance} = Cl_T + Cl_D$$

Using Equation 24.31,

$$Cl_D = \frac{Q(C_a - C_v)}{C_a}$$

$$Cl_D = \frac{50(5 - 2.4)}{5} = 26 \text{ mL/min}$$

Total drug clearance = $10 + 26 = 36$ mL/min. Since the drug clearance is increased from 10 to 36 mL/min, the dose should be increased if dialysis is going to continue. Since dose is directly proportional to clearance,

$$\frac{D_u}{D_N} = \frac{36}{10} = 3.6$$

The new dose should be 3.6 times the dose given before dialysis if the same level of antibiotics is to be maintained.

4. The creatinine clearance of a patient is determined experimentally by using Equation 24.11,

$$Cl_{cr} = \frac{C_u V \times 100}{C_{cr} \times 1440}$$

$$Cl_{cr} = \frac{(0.1)(1800)(100)}{(2.2)(1440)} = 5.68 \text{ mL/min}$$

Assuming that the normal Cl_{cr} in this patient is 100 mL/min, the uremic dose should be 5.7% of the normal dose, since kidney function is drastically reduced:

$$(0.057)(20 \text{ mg/kg}) = 1.14 \text{ mg/kg given}$$
$$\text{every 6 hours}$$

5. From Fig. 24-4, line F, at a Cl_{cr} of 5 mL/min,

$$\frac{k_u}{k_N} = 45\%$$

a. The dose given should be as follows:

$$(0.45)(600 \text{ mg}) = 270 \text{ mg every 12 hours}$$

b. Alternatively, the dose of 600 mg should be given every

$$12 \times \frac{100}{45} = 26.7 \text{ h}$$

c. Since it may be desirable to give the drug once every 24 hours, both dose and dosing interval may be adjusted so that the patient will still maintain an average therapeutic blood level of the drug, which can then be given at a convenient time. Using the equation for C_{av}^{∞},

$$C_{av}^{\infty} = \frac{D_0}{kV_D \tau}$$

$$D_0 = 600 \text{ mg}$$

$$\tau = 26.7 \text{ h}$$

$$C_{av}^{\infty} = \frac{600}{kV_D \times 26.7}$$

To maintain C_{av}^{∞} the same, calculate a new dose, D_N, with a new dosing interval, τ_N, of 24 hours.

$$C_{av}^{\infty} = \frac{D_N}{kV_D(24)}$$

Thus,

$$\frac{600}{26.7} = \frac{D_N}{(24)}$$

Therefore,

$$D_N = \frac{24}{26.7} \times 600 = 539 \text{ mg}$$

The drug can also be given at 540 mg daily.

6. For females, use 85% of the Cl_{cr} value obtained in males.

$$Cl_{cr} = \frac{0.85[140 - \text{age(year)}] \text{ body weight (kg)}}{72(Cl_{cr})}$$

$$Cl_{cr} = \frac{0.85[140 - 38]62}{(72)(1.8)} = 41.5 \text{ mL/min}$$

9. Gentamycin is listed in group K (Table 24-5). From the nomogram in Fig. 24-4,

$$Cl_{cr} = 20 \text{ mL/min}$$

$$\frac{k_u}{k_n} = 25\%$$

Uremic dose = 25% of normal dose = (0.25) (1 mg/kg) = 0.25 mg/kg
For a 72-kg patient:

$$\text{Uremic dose} = (0.25)(75) = 18.8 \text{ mg}$$

The patient should receive 18.8 mg every 8 hours by multiple IV bolus injections.

10. a. During the first 48 hours postdose, $t_{1/2} = 16$ h. For IV bolus injection, assuming first-order elimination:

$$D_B = D_0 e^{-kt}$$

$$D_B = 1000 e^{-(0.693/16)\,(48)}$$

$D_B = 125$ mg remaining in body just before dialysis
During dialysis, $t_{1/2} = 4$ h, and
$D_B = 125 e^{-(0.693/4)(8)} = 31.3$ mg after dialysis
Drug eliminated during dialysis = 125 mg − 31.3 mg = 93.7 mg

b. $V_D = (0.5 \text{ L/kg}) (75 \text{kg}) = 37.5 \text{ L}$
Drug concentration just before dialysis:

$$C_p = 125 \text{ mg}/37.5 \text{ L} = 3.33 \text{ mg/L}$$

Drug concentration just after dialysis:

$$C_p = 31.3 \text{ mg}/37.5 \text{ L} = 0.83 \text{ mg/L}$$

REFERENCES

Bennett WM: Guide to drug dosage in renal failure. *Clin Pharmacokinet* **15**:326–354, 1988.

Bennett WM: Guide to drug dosage in renal failure. In Holford N (ed). *Clinical Pharmacokinetics Drug Data Handbook*. New York, Adis, 1990.

Bianchetti G, Graziani G, Brancaccio D, et al: Pharmacokinetics and effects of propranolol in terminal uremic patients and in patients undergoing regular dialysis treatment. *Clin Pharmacokinet* **1**:373–384, 1978.

Bickley SK: Drug dosing during continuous arteriovenous hemofiltration. *Clin Pharm* **7**:198–206, 1988.

Bjornsson TD: Nomogram for drug dosage adjustment in patients with renal failure. *Clin Pharmacokinet* **11**:164–170, 1986.

Bodenham A, Shelly MP, Park GR: The altered pharmacokinetics and pharmacodynamics of drugs commonly used in critically ill patients. *Clin Pharmacokinet* **14**:347–373, 1988.

Brouwer KBR, Dukes GE, Powell JR: Influence of liver function on drug disposition. In Evans WE, Schewtag, J, Jusko, J (eds). *Applied Pharmacokinetics—Principles of Therapeutic Drug Monitoring.* Baltimore, MD, Lippincott Williams & Wilkins, 1992, Chap 6.

Carpenter CB, Lazarus JM: Dialysis and transplantation in the treatment of renal failure. In Isselbacher KJ, et al (eds). *Harrison's Principles of Internal Medicine.* New York, McGraw-Hill, 1994, Chap 238.

Chennavasin P, Craig Brater D: Nomograms for drug use in renal disease. *Clin Pharmacokinet* **6**:193–215, 1981.

Cholongitas E, Papatheodoridis GV, Vangeli M, et al: Systematic review: The model for end-stage liver disease—Should it replace Child-Pugh's classification for assessing prognosis in cirrhosis? *Aliment Pharmacol Ther* **22**(11):1079–1089, 2005.

Cockcroft DW, Gault MH: Prediction of creatinine clearance from serum creatinine. *Nephron* **16**:31–41, 1976.

De Hart RM: Vancomycin removal via newer hemodialysis membranes. *Hosp Pharm* **31**:1467–1477, 1996.

Diem K, Lentner C (eds): *Scientific Tables,* 7th ed. New York, Geigy Pharmaceuticals, 1973.

Farrell GC, Cooksley WG, Hart P, et al: Drug metabolism in liver disease. Identification of patients with impaired hepatic drug metabolism. *Gastroenterology* **75**:580, 1978.

FDA Guidance for Industry: Pharmacokinetics in patients with impaired hepatic function: Study design, data analysis, and impact on dosing and labeling, FDA, Center for Drug Evaluation and Research (CDER), May 2003.

FDA Guidance for Industry: Pharmacokinetics in patients with impaired renal function—Study design, data analysis, and impact on dosing and labeling, Draft Guidance, FDA, Center for Drug Evaluation and Research (CDER), March 2010.

Gambertoglio JG: Effects of renal disease: Altered pharmacokinetics. In Benet LZ, Massoud N, Gambertoglio JG (eds). *Pharmacokinetic Basis of Drug Treatment.* New York, Raven, 1984.

Giusti DL, Hayton WL: Dosage regimen adjustments in renal impairment. *Drug Intell Clin Pharm* **7**:382–387, 1973.

Hailmeskel B, Lakew D, Yohannes L, Wutoh AK, Namanny M: Creatinine clearance estimation in elderly patients using the Cockcroft and Gault equation with ideal, actual, adjusted or no body weight. *Consult Pharm* **14**:72–75, 1999.

Hansen E, Bucher M, Jakob W, Lemberger P: Pharmacokinetics of levofloxacin during continuous veno-venous hemofiltration. *Intensive Care Med* **27**:371–375, 2001.

Howden CW, Birnie GG, Brodie MJ: Drug metabolism in liver disease. *Pharmacol Ther* **40**:439, 1989.

Hu OY, Tang HS, Chang CL: The influence of chronic lobular hepatitis on pharmacokinetics of cefoperazone: A novel galactose single-point method as a measure of residual liver function. *Biopharm Drug Dispos* **15**(7):563–576, 1994.

Hu OY, Tang HS, Chang CL: Novel galactose single point method as a measure of residual liver function: Example of cefoperazone kinetics in patients with liver cirrhosis. *J Clin Pharmacol* **35**(3):250–258, 1995.

Kamath PS, Kim WR: The model for end-stage liver disease (MELD). *Hepatology* **45**(3):797–805, 2007.

Kampmann J, Siersback-Nielsen K, Kristensen M: Rapid evaluation of creatinine clearance. *Acta Med Scand* **196**(6):517–520, 1974.

Levey AS, Bosch JP, Lewis JB, Greene T, Rogers N, Roth D: A more accurate method to estimate glomerular filtration rate from serum creatinine: A new prediction equation, Modification of Diet in Renal Disease Study Group. *Ann Intern Med* **130**(6):461–470, 1999.

Levey AS, Stevens LA, Schmid CH, et al: A new equation to estimate glomerular filtration rate. *Ann Intern Med* **150**(9): 604–612, 2009.

Lucey MR, Brown KA, Everson GT, et al: Minimal criteria for placement of adults on the liver transplant waiting list: A report of a national conference organized by the American Society of Transplant Physicians and the American Association for the Study of Liver Diseases. *Liver Transpl Surg* **3**(6):628–637, 1997.

Mallikaarjun S, Shoaf SE, Boulton DW, Bramer SL: Effects of hepatic or renal impairment on the pharmacokinetics of aripiprazole. *Clin Pharmacokinet* **47**(8):533–542, 2008.

Mathews SJ: Aminoglycosides. In Schumacher GE (ed). *Therapeutic Drug Monitoring.* Norwalk, CT, Appleton & Lange, 1995, Chap 9.

Merck Manual. Merck, Whitehouse Station, NJ, 1996–1997.

Muirhead GJ, Wilner K, Colburn W, Haug-Pihale G, Rouviex B: The effects of age and renal and hepatic impairment on the pharmacokinetics of sildenafil. *Br J Clin Pharmacol* **53**(suppl 1):21S–30S, 2002.

Munar M, Singh H: Drug dosing adjustments in patients with chronic kidney disease. *American Fam Physician* **75**(10): 1489–1496, 2007.

Nuxmalo JL, Teranaka M, Schenk WG, Jr Hepatic blood flow measurement. *Arch Surg* **113**:169, 1978.

Physicians' Desk Reference. Montvale, NJ, Medical Economics (published annually).

Schneider V, Henschel V, Tadjalli-Mehr K, Mansmann U, Haefeli WE: Impact of serum creatinine measurement error on dose adjustment in renal failure. *Clin Pharmacol Ther* **74**:458–467, 2003.

Schwartz GV, Haycock GB, Edelmann CM, Spitzer A: A simple estimate of glomerular filtration rate in children derived from body length and plasma creatinine. *Pediatrics* **58**:259–263, 1976.

Siersback-Nielsen K, Hansen JM, Kampmann J, Kirstensen M: Rapid evaluation of creatinine clearance. *Lancet* **i**:1133–1134, 1971.

Sonnichsen DS, Relling MV: Clinical pharmacokinetics of pacli-taxel. *Clin Pharmacokinet* **27**(4):256–269, 1994.

Spinler SA, Nawarskas JJ, Boyce EG, Connors JE, Charland SL, Goldfarb S: Predictive performance of ten equations for estimat-ing creatinine clearance in cardiac patients. *Ann Pharmacother* **32:**1275–1283, 1998.

St Peter WL, Redic-Kill KA, Halstenson CE: Clinical pharmaco-kinetics of antibiotics in patients with impaired renal function. *Clin Pharmacokinet* **22:**169–210, 1992.

Stevens LA, Coresh J, Greene T, Levey AS: Assessing kidney function: Measured and estimated glomerular filtration rate. *N Eng J Med* **354**(23):2473–2483, 2006.

Tozer TN: Nomogram for modification of dosage regimen in patients with chronic renal function impairment. *J Pharmaco-kinet Biopharm* **2:**13–28, 1974.

Traub SL, Johnson CE: Comparison methods of estimating cre-atinine clearance in children. *Am J Hosp Pharm* **37:**195–201, 1980.

Trey C, Burns DG, Saunders SJ: Treatment of hepatic coma by exchange blood transfusion. *N Engl J Med* **274:**473–448, 1966.

Wagner JG: *Fundamentals of Clinical Pharmacokinetics.* Hamilton, IL, Drug Intelligence, 1975, p 161.

Welling PG, Craig WA: Pharmacokinetics in disease states modi-fying renal function. In Benet LZ (ed). *The Effects of Disease States on Drug Pharmacokinetics.* Washington, DC, American Pharmaceutical Association, 1976.

Williams RL: Drug administration in hepatic disease. *N Engl J Med* **309:**1616, 1983.

BIBLIOGRAPHY

Benet L: *The Effect of Disease States on Drug Pharmacokinet-ics.* Washington, DC, American Pharmaceutical Association, 1976.

Bennett WM, Singer I: Drug prescribing in renal failure: Dosing guidelines for adults—An update. *Am J Kidney Dis* **3:**155–193, 1983.

Bjornsson TD: Use of serum creatinine concentration to determine renal function. *Clin Pharmacokinet* **4:**200–222, 1979.

Bjornsson TD, Cocchetto DM, McGowan FX, et al: Nomogram for estimating creatinine clearance. *Clin Pharmacokinet* **8:**365–399, 1983.

Brater DC: *Drug Use in Renal Disease.* Boston, AIDS Health Science Press, 1983.

Brater DC: Treatment of renal disorders and the influence of renal function on drug disposition. In Melmon KL, Morrelli HF, Hoffman BB, Nierenberg DW (eds). *Clinical Pharmacology— Basis Principlesin Therapeutics,* 3rd ed. New York, McGraw-Hill, 1992, Chap 11.

Brenner BM (ed): *Brenner and Rector's The Kidney,* 8th ed. New York, Elsevier, 2007.

Chang CY, Schiano TD: Drug hepatotoxicity. *Aliment Pharmacol Ther* **25:**1135–1151, 2007.

Chennavasin P, Brater DC: Nomograms for drug use in renal disease. *Clin Pharmacokinet* **6:**193–214, 1981.

Child C, Turcotte J: The liver and portal hypertension. In Child CI (ed). *Surgery and Portal Hypertension.* Philadelphia, WB Saunders, 1964, pp 50–58.

Craig Brater D, Chennavasin P: Effects of renal disease: Pharma-cokinetic considerations. In Benet LZ (eds). *Pharmacokinetic Basis of Drug Treatment.* New York, Raven, 1984.

Cutler RE, Forland SC, St. John PG, et al: Extracorporeal removal of drugs and poisons by hemodialysis and hemoperfusion. *Annu Rev Pharmacol Toxicol* **27:**169–191, 1987.

Dettli L: Elimination kinetics and dosage adjustment of drugs in patients with kidney disease. In Grobecker H, et al (eds). *Progress in Pharmacology,* Vol 1. New York, Gustav Fischer Verlag, 1977.

Fabre J, Balant L: Renal failure, drug pharmacokinetics and drug action. *Clin Pharmacokinet* **1:**99–120, 1976.

Facts and Comparisons: St. Louis, MO, Walter Kluwer Health, (updated monthly), 1992.

FDA Guidance for Industry: Pharmacokinetics in patients with impaired renal function—Study design, data analysis and impact on dosing and labeling, 1998.

Feldman M: Biochemical liver tests. In Feldman M, Friedman LS, Sleisenger MH, et al (eds). *Gastrointestinal and Liver Disease,* 7th ed. New York, Elsevier, 2002, pp 1227–1231.

Figg WD, Dukes GE, Lesesne HR, et al: Comparison of quanti-tative methods to assess hepatic function: Pugh's classifica-tion, indocyanine green, antipyrine, and dextromethorphan. *Pharmacotherapy* **15:**693–700, 1995.

Ford M: *Clinical Toxicology.* Philadelphia, Saunders, 2001, pp 43–48.

Gibaldi M: Drug distribution in renal failure. *Am J Med* **62:** 471–474, 1977.

Gibson TP, Nelson HA: Drug kinetics and artificial kidneys. *Clin Pharmacokinet* **2:**403–426, 1977.

Giusti DL, Hayton WL: Dosage regimen adjustments in renal impairment. *Drug Intell Clin Pharm* **7:**382–387, 1973.

Hallynck TH, Soeph HH, Thomis VA, et al: Should clearance be normalized to body surface or lean body mass? *Br J Clin Pharm* **11:**523–526, 1981.

Jellife RW: Estimation of creatinine clearance when urine cannot be collected. *Lancet* **1:**975–976, 1971.

Jellife RW: Estimation of creatinine clearance in patients with unstable renal function, without a urine specimen. *Am J Nephrol* **22:**320–324, 2002.

Jellife RW, Jellife SM: A computer program for estimation of cre-atinine clearance from unstable serum creatinine concentration. *Math Biosci* **14:**17–24, 1972.

Kampmann JP, Hansen JM: Glomerular filtration rate and creatinine clearance. *Br J Clin Pharmacol* **12:**7–14, 1981.

Lee CC, Marbury TC: Drug therapy in patients undergoing haemo-dialysis. Clinical pharmacokinetic considerations. *Clin Phar-macokinet* **9:**42–66, 1984.

LeSher DA: Considerations in the use of drugs in patients with renal failure. *J Clin Pharmacol* **16:**570, 1976.

Levy G: Pharmacokinetics in renal disease. *Am J Med* **62:** 461–465, 1977.

Lott RS, Hayton WL: Estimation of creatinine clearance from serum creatinine concentration: A review. *Drug Intell Clin Pharm* **12:**140–150, 1978.

Maher JF: Principle of dialysis and dialysis of drugs. *Am J Med* **62:**475–481, 1977.

Paton TW, Cornish WR, Manuel MA, Hardy BG: Drug therapy in patients undergoing peritoneal dialysis. Clinical pharmacokinetic considerations. *Clin Pharmacokinet* **10:**404–426, 1985.

Ratz A, Ewandrowski K: Normal reference laboratory values. *N Engl J Med* **339:**1063–1071, 1998.

Rhodes PJ, Rhodes RS, McClelland GH, et al: Evaluation of eight methods for estimating creatinine clearance in man. *Clin Pharm* **6:**399–406, 1987.

Rosenberg J, Benowitz NL, Pond S: Pharmacokinetics of drug overdosage. *Clin Pharmacokinet* **6:**161–192, 1981.

Schumacher GE: Practical pharmacokinetic techniques for drug consultation and evaluation, II: A perspective on the renal impaired patient. *Am J Hosp Pharm* **30:**824–830, 1973.

Traub SL: Creatinine and creatinine clearance. *Hosp Pharm* **13:**715–722, 1978.

Watanabe AS: Pharmacokinetic aspects of the dialysis of drugs. *Drug Intell Clin Pharm* **11:**407–416, 1977.

Watkins PB, Hamilton TA, Annesley TM, Ellis CN, Kolars JC, Voorhees JJ: The erythromycin breath test as a predictor of cyclosporine blood levels. *Clin Pharmacol Ther* **48:**120–129, 1990.

25

Empirical Models, Mechanistic Models, Statistical Moments, and Noncompartmental Analysis

Corinne Seng Yue and Murray P. Ducharme

Chapter Objectives

▶ Describe the differences between empirical and mechanistic models.

▶ Understand the differences between different types of compartmental analyses.

▶ Describe the physiologic pharmacokinetic model with equations and underlying assumptions.

▶ List the differences in data analysis between the physiologic pharmacokinetic model, the classical compartmental model, and the noncompartmental approaches.

▶ Describe *interspecies scaling* and its application in pharmacokinetics and toxicokinetics.

▶ Describe the statistical moment theory and explain how it provides a unique way to study time-related changes in *macroscopic events*.

▶ Define *mean residence time* (MRT) and how it can be calculated.

The study of pharmacokinetics describes the absorption, distribution, and elimination of a drug and its metabolites in quantitative terms (see Chapter 1). Ideally, a pharmacokinetic model uses the observed time course for drug concentrations in the body and, from these data, obtains various pharmacokinetic parameters to predict drug dosing outcomes, pharmacodynamics, and toxicity.

In developing a model, certain underlying assumptions are made by the pharmacokineticist as to the type of pharmacokinetic model, the order of the rate processes, tissue blood flow, the method for the estimation of the plasma or tissue volume, and other factors. Even with a more general approach such as the non-compartmental method, first-order drug elimination is often assumed in the calculation of AUC_0^∞. In selecting a model for data analysis, the pharmacokineticist may choose more than one method of modeling, depending on many factors, including experimental conditions, study design, and completeness of data. The goodness-of-fit to the model and the desired pharmacokinetic parameters are other considerations. Each estimated pharmacokinetic parameter has an inherent variability because of the variability of the biological system and of the observed data.

In spite of challenges in the construction of these pharmacokinetic models, such models have been extremely useful in describing the time course of drug action, improving drug therapy by enhancing drug efficacy, and minimizing adverse reactions through more accurate dosing regimens. Pharmacokinetic models are used routinely within the development process of new molecules or drug delivery systems.

Models can be broadly categorized as empirical or mechanistic. Empirical models are focused on describing the data with the specification of very few assumptions about the data being analyzed. An example of an empirical model is one that is used for allometric scaling, a type of prediction of PK parameters across diverse species. On the other hand, mechanistic models specify assumptions and attempt to incorporate known factors about the systems surrounding the data into the model, while describing

► Define the mean transit time (MTT) and how it can be used to calculate the mean dissolution time (MDT), or *in vivo* mean dissolution time, for a solid drug product given orally.

► Using MRT, derive equations to estimate other pharmacokinetic parameters such as mean absorption time and total volume of distribution.

the available data (Bonate, 2011). Both physiological modeling and compartmental modeling fall into the latter category. Pharmacokinetic parameters can also be calculated without the specification of compartments in an almost model-independent manner, using noncompartmental analysis derived from statistical moment theory. This chapter will touch upon the aforementioned types of pharmacokinetic models, as well as noncompartmental analysis.

EMPIRICAL MODELS

Allometric Scaling

Various approaches have been used to compare and predict the pharmacokinetics of a drug among different species. *Interspecies scaling* is a method used in toxicokinetics and for the extrapolation of therapeutic drug doses in humans from nonclinical animal drug studies. *Toxicokinetics* is the application of pharmacokinetics to toxicology for interpolation and extrapolation based on anatomic, physiologic, and biochemical similarities (Mordenti and Chappell, 1989; Bonate and Howard, 2000; Mahmood, 2000, 2007; Hu and Hayton, 2001; Evans et al, 2006).

The basic assumption in interspecies scaling is that physiologic variables, such as clearance, heart rate, organ weight, and biochemical processes, are related to the weight or body surface area of the animal species (including humans). It is commonly assumed that all mammals use the same energy source (oxygen) and energy transport systems across animal species (Hu and Hayton, 2001). Interspecies scaling uses a physiologic variable, y, that is graphed against the body weight of the species on log–log axes to transform the data into a linear relationship (Fig. 25-1).

The general allometric equation obtained by this method is

$$y = bW^a \tag{25.1}$$

where y is the pharmacokinetic or physiologic property of interest, b is an allometric coefficient, W is the weight or surface area of the animal species, and a is the allometric exponent. *Allometry* is the study of size.

Both a and b vary with the drug. Examples of various pharmacokinetic or physiologic properties that demonstrate allometric relationships are listed in Table 25-1.

In the example shown in Fig. 25-1, the apparent methotrexate volume of distribution is related to body weight B of five animal species by the equation $V_\beta = 0.859B^{0.918}$.

The allometric method gives an empirical relationship that allows for approximate interspecies scaling based on the size of

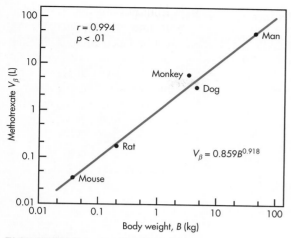

FIGURE 25-1   Interspecies correlation between methotrexate volume of distribution V_β and body weight. Linear regression analysis was performed on logarithmically transformed data. (From Boxenbaum, 1982, with permission.)

relationship between biperiden intrinsic clearance with body weight and MLP:

$$Cl_{int} \times MLP = 1.36 \times 10^7 \times B^{0.892} \qquad (25.2)$$

where MLP is the maximum life-span potential of the species, B is the body weight of the species, and Cl_{int} is the hepatic intrinsic clearance of the free drug.

Although further model improvements are needed before accurate prediction of pharmacokinetic parameters can be made from animal data, some interesting results were obtained by Sawada et al (1985) on nine acid and six basic drugs. When interspecies differences in protein–drug binding are properly considered, the volume of distribution of many drugs may be predicted with 50% deviation from experimental values (Table 25-2).

The application of MLP to pharmacokinetics has been described by Boxenbaum (1982). Initially, hepatic intrinsic clearance was considered to be related to volume or body weight. Indeed, a plot of the log drug clearance versus body weight for various animal species resulted in an approximately linear correlation (ie, a straight line). However, after correcting intrinsic clearance by MLP, an improved log–linear relationship was achieved between free drug Cl_{int} and body weight for many drugs. A possible explanation for this relationship is that the biochemical processes, including Cl_{int}, in each animal species are related to the animal's normal life expectancy (estimated by MLP) through the evolutionary process. Animals with a shorter MLP have higher basal metabolic rates and tend to have higher intrinsic hepatic clearance and thus metabolize drugs faster. Boxenbaum (1982, 1983) postulated a constant "life stuff" in each species, such that the faster the life stuff is consumed, the more quickly the life stuff is used up. In the fourth-dimension scale (after correcting for MLP), all species share the same intrinsic clearance for the free drug.

$$\frac{(MLP)(Cl_{int})}{B} = constant \qquad (25.3)$$

$$Cl_{int} = aB^x \qquad (25.4)$$

the species. Not considered in the method are certain specific interspecies differences such as gender, nutrition, pathophysiology, route of drug administration, and polymorphisms. Some of these more specific cases, such as the pathophysiologic condition of the animal or human, may preclude pharmacokinetic or allometric predictions.

Interspecies scaling has been refined by considering the aging rate and life span of the species. In terms of physiologic time, each species has a characteristic life span, its *maximum life-span potential* (MLP), which is controlled genetically (Boxenbaum, 1982). Because many energy-consuming biochemical processes, including drug metabolism, vary inversely with the aging rate or life span of the animal, this allometric approach has been used for drugs that are eliminated mainly by hepatic intrinsic clearance.

Through the study of various species in handling several drugs that are metabolized predominantly by the liver, some empirical relationships regarding drug clearance of several drugs have been related mathematically in a single equation. For example, the hepatic intrinsic clearance of biperiden in rat, rabbit, and dog was extrapolated to humans (Nakashima et al, 1987). Equation 25.2 describes the

Extensive work with caffeine in five species (mouse, rat, rabbit, monkey, and humans) by Bonati et al (1985)

TABLE 25-1   Examples of Allometric Relationship for Interspecies Parameters

Physiologic or Pharmacokinetic Property	Allometric Exponent[a]	Allometric Coefficient[b]
Basal O_2 consumption (mL/h)	0.734	3.8
Endogenous N output (g/h)	0.72	0.000042
O_2 consumption by liver slices (mL/h)	0.77	3.3
Clearance		
Creatinine (mL/h)	0.69	8.72
Inulin (mL/h)	0.77	5.36
PAH (mL/h)	0.80	22.6
Antipyrine (mL/h)	0.89	8.16
Methotrexate (mL/h)	0.69	10.9
Phenytoin (mL/h)	0.92	47.1
Aztreonam (mL/h)	0.66	4.45
Ara-C and Ara-U (mL/h)	0.79	3.93
Volume of distribution (V_D)		
Methotrexate (L/kg)	0.92	0.859
Cyclophosphamide (L/kg)	0.99	0.883
Antipyrine (L/kg)	0.96	0.756
Aztreonam (L/kg)	0.91	0.234
Kidney weight (g)	0.85	0.0212
Liver weight (g)	0.87	0.082
Heart weight (g)	0.98	0.0066
Stomach and intestines weight (g)	0.94	0.112
Blood weight (g)	0.99	0.055
Tidal volume (mL)	1.01	0.0062
Elimination half-life		
Methotrexate (min)	0.23	54.6
Cyclophosphamide (min)	0.24	36.6
Digoxin (min)	0.23	98.3
Hexobarbital (min)	0.35	80.0
Antipyrine (min)	0.07	74.5
Turnover times		
Serum albumin (1/day)	0.30	5.68
Total body water (1/day)	0.16	6.01
RBC (1/day)	0.10	68.4
Cardiac circulation (min)	0.21	0.44

From Ritschel and Banerjee (1986).

TABLE 25-2 Relationship between Predicted and Observed Values of Various Pharmacokinetic Parameters in Humans for 15 Drugs

Drug	V (L/kg)			Cl_m (mL/min per kg)			$t_{1/2,z}$ (min)		
	Observed	Predicted	Percent[a]	Observed	Predicted	Percent[a]	Observed	Predicted	Percent[a]
Phenytoin	0.640	0.573	10.5	0.574	0.483	15.9	792	822	3.79
Quinidine	3.20	3.69	22.2	2.91	3.25	11.7	470	785	67.0
Hexobarbital	1.27	0.735	42.1	3.57	4.25	19.0	261	120	54.0
Pentobarbital	0.999	1.57	57.2	0.524	0.964	84.0	1340	1126	16.0
Phenylbutazone	0.122[b]	0.0839[c]	31.2	0.0205	0.0162	21.0	4110	3590	12.7
Warfarin	0.108	0.109	0.926	0.0367	0.0165	55.0	2040	4560	124
Tolbutamide	0.112	0.116	3.57	0.180	0.0589	67.3	434	1360	214
Chlorpromazine	11.2[b]	9.05[c]	19.2	4.29	4.63	7.93	1810	1350	25.2
Propranolol	3.62	3.77	4.14	11.2	15.56	38.9	167	135	19.2
Pentazocine	5.56	7.19	29.3	18.3	11.6	36.6	203	408	101
Valproate	0.151	0.482	219	0.110	0.159	44.5	954	2110	121
Diazepam	0.950	1.44	51.6	0.350	2.13	509	1970	469	76.2
Antipyrine	0.869	0.878	1.04	0.662	0.664	3.02	654	917	40.2
Phenobarbital	0.649	0.817	25.9	0.0530	0.0825	55.7	6600	5870	11.0
Amobarbital	1.04	1.21	16.3	0.556	1.01	81.7	1360	827	39.2

[a]Absolute percent of error.

[b]The value of V_{ss}.

[c]Predicted from the value of V_{ss} in the rat.

From Sawada et al (1985).

verified this approach. Caffeine is a drug that is metabolized predominantly by the liver. For caffeine,

$$Q = 0.0554 \times B^{0.894}$$

$$L = 0.0370 \times B^{0.849}$$

where B is body weight, L is liver weight, and Q is the liver blood flow.

Hepatic clearance for the unbound drug did not show a direct correlation among the five species. After intrinsic clearance was corrected for MLP (calculation based on brain weight), an excellent relationship was obtained among the five species (Fig. 25-2).

More recently, the subject of interspecies scaling was investigated using Cl values for 91 substances for several species by Hu and Hayton (2001). These investigators used $Y = a(BW)^b$ in their analysis, similar to Equation 25.1 above but with different symbols: Y = biological variable dependent on the body weight of the species, a = allometric coefficient, b = allometric exponent, and BW = body weight of the species. One issue discussed by Hu and Hayton is the uncertainty in the allometric exponent (b) of

xenobiotic clearance (Cl). Published literature has focused on whether the basal metabolic rate scale is a 2/3 or 3/4 power of the body mass (BW). When the uncertainty in the determination of a b value is relatively large, a fixed-exponent approach might be feasible according to Hu and Hayton. In this regard, 0.75 might be used for substances that are eliminated mainly by metabolism or by metabolism and excretion combined, whereas 0.67 might apply for drugs that are eliminated mainly by renal excretion. The researchers pointed out that genetic (intersubject) difference may be a limitation for using a single universal constant.

Brightman et al (2006) demonstrated the application of a PK-PD model, based on human parameters to estimate plasma pharmacokinetics of xenobiotics in humans. The model was parameterized through an optimization process, using a training set of *in vivo* data taken from the literature. On average, the vertical divergence of the predicted plasma concentrations from the observed data was 0.47 log units, on a semi-log concentration–time plot. They also evaluated the method against other predictive methods that involve scaling from *in vivo* animal data. In terms of predicting human clearance for the test set, the model was found to match or exceed the performance of three published interspecies scaling methods, which tend to give overprediction. The article concludes that the generic physiologically based pharmacokinetic model is a means of integrating readily determined *in vitro* and/or *in silico* data, and useful for predicting human xenobiotic kinetics in drug discovery.

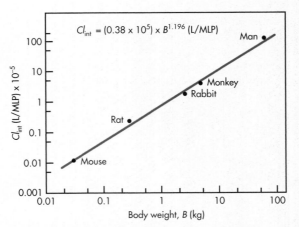

FIGURE 25-2   Caffeine (free drug) Cl_{int} per maximum lifespan potential (MLP) in mammalian species as a function of body weight. MLP values were calculated for monkeys, rabbits, rats, and mice employing the following numeric values: MLP = 10.389 × (brain weight)$^{0.636}$ × (body weight)$^{0.225}$. (Data from Boxenbaum, 1982; Armstrong E: Relative brain size and metabolism in mammals. *Science* **220**(4603):1302–1304, 1983.)

MECHANISTIC MODELS

Compartmental Models

The essence of compartmental analysis is to create a mathematical and statistical model defined by integrated, matrix, and/or partial differential equations (equations that have derivatives with respect to more than one variable) that describe the PK or PD behaviour of a drug. The model is then "fitted" to the data using least squares, Bayesian, and/or maximum likelihood techniques so that mean parameter estimates along with their variability are obtained in an individual or population (most often nowadays)

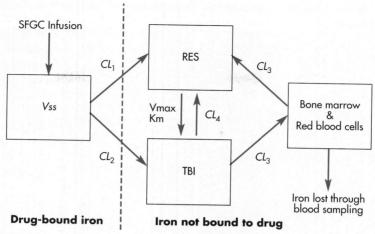

FIGURE 25-3   Final compartmental pharmacokinetic model for sodium ferric gluconate complex. Cl_1: clearance of sodium ferric gluconate complex iron (SFGC-I) to the reticuloendothelial system (RES) compartment; Cl_2: clearance of SFGC-I directly to transferrin; V_{ss}: the apparent steady-state volume of distribution of SFGC-I; Cl_3: clearance of iron entering and exiting the marrow and red blood cell compartment; Cl_4: clearance of TBI to the RES; K_m: iron concentration associated with half of the maximal rate of exchange between the RES and TBI compartments; V_{max}: maximal rate of exchange between the RES and TBI compartments;

along with a residual variability or error component. An illustration of a compartmental model developed to describe the PK of sodium ferric gluconate complex is presented in Fig. 25-3 (Seng Yue, 2013).

Although a compartmental model can never explain the "true" mechanisms underlying PK and/or PD behaviour, important correlations between covariates and parameters may point the way to further studies or provide deeper mechanistic understanding (Sheiner, 1984). Among other advantages of the compartmental method are its use in special populations (such as pediatric or hepatic impairment patients) and its potential partitioning of variability into interindividual, intraindividual, interoccasion, and residual sources (Ette and Williams, 2004).

Various types of compartmental analyses exist, ranging from individual analysis to population PK modeling including the naïve pooled data approach, the standard two-stage approach, and nonlinear mixed-effect modeling that includes among others the iterative two-stage, the first-order conditional estimation (FOCE) and the MLEM (maximum likelihood expectation maximization) approaches (Sheiner, 1984; Rodman et al, 2006; Steimer et al, 1984). In these last approaches, all data are modeled simultaneously while

retaining individual information, in order to obtain estimates of population mean and variance as well as quantify sources of variability (Ette and Williams, 2004; Ludden, 1988). These types of compartmental analyses will be described in this chapter.

At the core of compartmental analyses is nonlinear regression. In contrast with linear regression, where data are being fitted with a straight line defined by a slope and intercept, nonlinear regression depends on equations whose partial derivatives (with respect to each of the parameters) involve other model parameters (Gabrielsson and Weiner, 2006). The equations used to describe the model depicted in Fig. 25-3 are presented in Table 25-3.

Another important difference between the two types of regressions is that linear regressions have analytical solutions, such that the functions can be manipulated to obtain a specific equation for the solution, while only numerical solutions exist for nonlinear regressions. For nonlinear equations, approximate solutions to the equations can only be obtained through iterative processes that are described in further detail below. Various software programs are available to perform such analyses, and many of them are described in more details in Appendix A.

TABLE 25-3   Differential Equations Describing Compartmental Pharmacokinetic Model for Sodium Ferric Gluconate Complex

Compartment	Equation
Serum	$\dfrac{dX(1)}{dt} = R(1) - \dfrac{Cl_1 + Cl_2}{V_{ss}} \cdot X(1)$
Reticuloendothelial system	$\dfrac{dX(2)}{dt} = \dfrac{Cl_1}{V_{ss}} \cdot X(1) + \dfrac{Cl_3}{V\_RBC} \cdot X(4) + \dfrac{Cl_4}{V\_TBI} \cdot X(3) - \dfrac{V_{max}}{Km \cdot V\_RBC + X(2)} \cdot X(2)$
Transferrin bound iron	$\dfrac{dX(3)}{dt} = \dfrac{Cl_2}{V_{ss}} \cdot X(1) + \dfrac{V_{max}}{Km \cdot V\_RBC + X(2)} \cdot X(2) - \dfrac{Cl_4}{V\_TBI} \cdot X(3) - \dfrac{Cl_3}{V\_TBI} \cdot X(3)$
Red blood cells (marrow)	$\dfrac{dX(4)}{dt} = \dfrac{Cl_3}{V\_TBI} \cdot X(3) - \dfrac{Cl_3}{V\_RBC} \cdot X(4) - K0 \cdot R(2)$

Cl_1: Clearance of SFGC-I to the reticuloendothelial system (RES) compartment; Cl_2: Clearance of SFGC-I directly to transferrin; V_{ss}: the apparent steady-state volume of distribution of SFGC-I; V_TBI: volume of distribution associated with TBI; Cl_3: clearance of iron entering and exiting the marrow and red blood cell compartment; V_RBC: marrow and red blood cell compartment; Cl_4: clearance of TBI to the RES; Km: Iron concentration associated with half of the maximal rate of exchange between the RES and TBI compartments; V_{max}: Maximal rate of exchange between the RES and TBI compartments.

Individual Analysis

As its name implies, individual analysis involves the development of a model using data from one source (such as one human or one animal). Because of the error that is always inherent in data, whether it be related to the collection procedures themselves or to analytical assays, a model can never perfectly predict the observed data. The relationship between observed and predicted concentration values must therefore account for this error, as defined in Equation 25.5. In this equation, X_i represents a vector of known values (such as dose and sampling times), C_i represents the vector of observed concentrations, ε_i represents the measurement errors, ϕ_j represents the vector of model parameters (in other words the pharmacokinetic parameters), and f_i is the function that relates C_i to ϕ_j and X_i. The subscript i represents the total number of observations or values.

$$C_i = f_i(\phi_j, X_i) + \varepsilon_i \qquad (25.5)$$

The aim of PK compartmental analysis is to develop a model that is associated with predicted concentration values (or whatever observation is being studied) that are as close as possible to the observed values. In other words, the goal is to minimize the differences between the predicted and observed values (represented by ε_i in Equation 25.5), and generally the least-squares and maximum likelihood approaches are used to quantify these differences (Bonate, 2011).

Various least-squares metrics (often termed "residual sum of squares") can be used to quantify these differences, and they are outlined in Table 25-4 (Gabrielsson and Weiner, 2006; Bonate, 2011).

OLS is inherently biased because it tends to favor model estimates that provide better predictions for larger observations compared to smaller ones. The WLS and ML/ELS approaches are an improvement over the OLS method since they account for the magnitude of observations (and their relative variability) by incorporating a weighting factor into their formulas. The ML/ELS approaches differ from the weighted least-squares approach, because they deal with the probability of observing the actual data given the model and its parameter estimates. In these methods, the function that is being minimized is the log likelihood (LL), or the probability of observing the actual concentration values given a set of model parameter estimates. The function for LL is presented in Equation 25.6. It should be noted that the

TABLE 25-4   Comparison of Least-Squares Methods

Method	Objective Function Formula	Characteristics
Ordinary least squares (OLS)	$O_{OLS} = \sum_{i=1}^{n}(C_i - \hat{C}_i)^2$	No weighting
Weighted least squares (WLS)	$O_{WLS} = \sum_{i=1}^{n}W_i(C_i - \hat{C}_i)^2$	Model and parameters must be defined and stated empirically
Extended least squares (ELS) or Maximum Likelihood (ML)	$O_{ELS} = \sum_{i=1}^{n}[W_i(C_i - \hat{C}_i)^2 + \ln(\text{var}(\hat{C}_i))]$	Models can be defined, but parameters of the models are fitted within the procedure, eg, $W_i = 1/\text{var}(\hat{C}_i)$

$\hat{C}_i$ = predicted ith concentration value, C_i = observed ith concentration value, W_i = weighting factor, n = number of observations, var = variance

only difference between ELS and ML is in the assumptions that are specified about the distribution of the variance parameters. In the ML approach, the distribution is assumed to be normal, while the ELS approach makes no such assumption (Beal and Sheiner, 1989).

$$LL(C \mid \theta) = -\frac{n}{2}\ln(2\pi) - \frac{n}{2}\ln\left[\frac{\sum(C_i - \hat{C}_i)^2}{n}\right] - \frac{n}{2}$$

$$(25.6)$$

Because it is easier to minimize a positive number rather than a negative one, the LL is often multiplied by –2 to obtain a positive number called the "–2 log likelihood" (–2LL).

Population Analysis

Population analysis can be viewed as an extension of individual analyses, since it attempts to develop a model that predicts concentration data associated with different individuals or animals. The general concept is similar to that embraced by individual analysis, except that the model must also take into consideration interindividual variability. The resulting model is therefore able to predict concentration values for each individual within the population, but it also provides an "overall" (mean or population) set of predictions. In other words, the model describes the behavior of the whole population as well as the behavior of each individual within this population. Another distinction is that a population analysis will

always use the same structural model (eg, a two-compartment model) to fit all individuals' data for a specific drug under study, while individual analyses could theoretically use different models to fit data from different subjects (eg, a one-compartment model for some subjects and a two-compartment model for others).

In a population analysis, observed concentrations must be ascribed to specific subjects, as defined in Equation 25.7, which is analogous to Equation 25.5. In this equation, X_{ij} represents a vector of known values (represented by i) for the jth subject, C_{ij} represents the vector of observed concentrations for the jth subject, ε_{ij} represents the measurement errors for the jth subject, ϕ_j represents the vector of model parameters for the jth subject, and f_{ij} is the function that relates C_{ij} to ϕ_j and X_{ij}.

$$C_{ij} = f_{ij}(\phi_j, X_{ij}) + \varepsilon_{ij} \qquad (25.7)$$

Each individual has a distinct set of PK model parameters (ϕ_j) that will provide the best predicted values for that individual's observed data. However, as previously mentioned, there is also a typical profile of "population predictions" that is associated with population PK model parameters (θ) that can be regarded as mean values. The relationship between the mean PK parameters and individual PK parameters is described by Equation 25.8, where g is a known function that relates ϕ_j to θ using the individual's characteristics such as height or weight, denoted by z_j. The last term, η_j, represents random (unexplained or uncontrollable) variability that also causes ϕ_j to deviate from θ.

$$\phi_j = g(\theta, z_j) + \eta_j \qquad (25.8)$$

There are various types of population compartmental analyses, but the most basic type is the "naïve-average data" method, where the average concentration values at given time points are computed from the entire dataset, and then a model is developed using these average values. A similar method is the "naïve pooled data" approach, where data from different individuals are treated as though they were obtained from a single individual, and then analyzed using the individual approach.

The two-stage approach to population compartmental analyses offers some improvement over the previous ones. In essence, data from each subject are first fitted individually (in other words using the individual approach but using the same structural model to fit each individual's data), and in the second step, population parameter estimates are obtained. Different types of two-stage approaches exist, such as the standard two-stage (STS) approach, the global two-stage (GTS) approach, and finally a mixed-effect modeling approach known as the iterative two-stage approach (IT2S or ITS). In the STS approach, the population parameter estimates (for mean and variance) are determined by calculating the mean and variance of the individual PK parameters, while the GTS approach actually estimates expectations for the mean and variance through an iterative process. The ITS method is a nonlinear mixed-effect modeling technique that uses a more refined iterative approach utilizing a mixture of ML and MAP (maximum *a posteriori* probability) techniques. Within each population iteration, prior values are used to estimate individual PK parameters in the first step, while individual values are then used in the second step to recalculate a newer, more probable set of population parameters. Steps one and two are subsequently repeated until there is little to no difference between the new and old prior distributions (eg, until the algorithm "converges").

In contrast with the iterative two-stage approach, other types of nonlinear mixed-effect modeling techniques, such as that of the FOCE method implemented by NONMEM®, proceed by first fitting the data in a reverse manner so they obtain population mean estimates followed in a second step with individual data estimates (therefore called "*post hocs*"). The fixed effects (variables that can be controlled, such as dose or pharmacokinetic parameters) and random effects (uncontrollable factors like interoccasion variability) are fitted simultaneously with respect to population mean and variability estimates as well as the residual variability.

Algorithms for Numerical Problem Solving

Since many combinations of parameter estimates must be evaluated in order to find the parameters that minimize one of the objective functions described previously, many algorithms have been developed to systematically do so. Some algorithms apply linearization techniques to approximate the model using linear equations.

For individual population analyses, Cauchy's method employs a first-order Taylor series expansion, Newton or Newton–Raphson-based methods utilize a second-order Taylor series expansion while the Gauss–Newton method iteratively uses multiple linear regressions via first-order Taylor series expansion. The Levenberg–Marquardt method is another algorithm that includes a modification of the Gauss–Newton method. Finally, in contrast with the algorithms previously described, the Nelder–Mead simplex approach does not involve linearization procedures. This technique involves the examination of the response surface (in order to find the lowest point) using a series of moving and contracting or expanding polyhedra (three-dimensional objects composed of flat polygonal faces joined by vertices). This approach has been implemented in the ADAPT-II to ADAPT 5 software series.

Some of the algorithms used in the context of population compartmental analyses include the first-order (FO) method, first-order conditional estimation (FOCE) approach, the stochastic approximation of EM (SAEM), and the maximum likelihood expectation maximization (MLEM) method, to name a few. In both the FO and FOCE algorithms as implemented within NONMEM, the minimum objective function is sought out by linearization of the model through a series of first-order Taylor series expansions of the error model. The difference between the FO and FOCE algorithms is that in the former, interindividual variability for PK parameters is estimated using estimates of the population mean and variance in a *post hoc* step, while in the latter, interindividual variability is estimated simultaneously with the population mean and variance (Beal and Sheiner, 1998). In other words, within NONMEM the FO algorithm uses a linearization technique that first assumes $\eta = 0$, contrary to the FOCE algorithm which uses the posterior mode of η (that relies on conditional estimates) (Bonate, 2011). A modification of the FOCE algorithm, known as the Laplacian FOCE method, exists also within NONMEM whereby a second-order Taylor series is performed instead of the first-order expansion (Beal and Sheiner, 1998).

The MLEM algorithm is different from the previous methods because it does not rely on any linearization techniques (D'Argenio et al, 2009). This algorithm involves maximizing a likelihood function through an iterative series of two steps that are repeated until convergence. In the first step, termed the expectation step or "E-step," the conditional mean and covariance for each individual's data are computed and the expected likelihood function associated with these parameters is obtained. In the second step, the maximization step or "M-step," the population mean, covariance, and error variance parameters are updated to maximize the likelihood from the previous step (Bonate, 2011; D'Argenio et al, 2009). This algorithm is available within ADAPT 5, as mentioned in Appendix A.

Frequently Asked Questions

▶ *How can we tell if we are using the right model to describe our data?*

▶ *Are certain algorithms better than others?*

▶ *When should individual compartmental analysis be used rather than population analysis?*

Applications of Compartmental Modeling

Compartmental modeling is an extremely versatile tool that allows researchers to do much more than simply estimate pharmacokinetic and/or pharmacodynamic parameters and quantify their variability.

In some cases, it may be of interest to better understand the sources of variability by attributing variability to specific patient characteristics. For example, compartmental models can evaluate whether demographic factors (weight, age, laboratory values, drug polymorphism), drug-related factors (formulation, manufacturer), or other potential variables (disease variables, use of concomitant medication) contribute to interindividual variability in certain parameters. Not only does compartmental modeling allow the identification of important covariates, but it can also quantify their relative importance.

Compartmental models are often used to relate a drug's PK to its response (PD), whether it be efficacy, toxicity, or both. PK-PD modeling can also be used to link preclinical (animal) data to data collected from human subjects by providing a common framework for understanding the data. A well-constructed compartmental model can also be used to answer a wide variety of questions through simulations. Throughout drug development, questions arise at various stages, and compartmental models can be used at all stages to answer these questions. For instance, in Phase 1, questions regarding optimal dosing for Phase 2 can be answered using PK/PD modeling. Among other uses, compartmental modeling can be used to support proof-of-concept claims, select optimal dosing regimens, optimize dosing schedule, and refine study designs (FDA guidance; Chien et al, 2005).

An example of how PK/PD modeling was helpful in making key decisions surrounding the development of a drug is described by Neiforth and colleagues. Interferons are used to treat various viral infections and malignancies. Despite their therapeutic benefits, their short half-life requires frequent administration (three times per week) and they can be highly antigenic. PEGylation of interferons is thought to increase the circulating half-life as well as decrease immunogenicity. In this example a PK/PD model was constructed to relate the exposure to PEG-modified interferon alfa-2a to its effect on the induction of the production of MX protein (Neiforth et al, 1996). Because of their many effects MX proteins were considered to be a useful PD probe. The goal of model development was to provide information to improve dosing strategies as well as guide the drug development of future modified molecules.

The PK/PD model was based on data from a randomized single ascending dose study that included 45 healthy adult male subjects receiving 1 of 4 subcutaneous doses of PEG-modified interferon alfa-2a or interferon alfa-2a. The PK of the interferon products, described by a one-compartment model with first-order absorption and elimination, was related to the PD through an indirect model. The drug stimulated the production of MX protein (stimulation of kin) via an E_{max} function.

The simulations obtained from the PK/PD modeling exercise indicated that, although the addition of a PEG moiety to interferon alfa-2a did indeed prolong the half-life of the drug, the PD properties associated with the PEG-modified interferon alfa-2a would still necessitate a twice-weekly dosing regimen in order to attain a comparable response to the unmodified product. This was a far cry from the anticipated once-weekly dosing for the PEG-modified product and these predictions were confirmed by two Phase II trials.

In conclusion, PK/PD modeling demonstrated that the PEG-modified interferon alfa-2a provided little therapeutic benefit over its unmodified counterpart, which proved to be consistent with Phase II findings. These findings contributed to the decision to discontinue the development of this product for this indication.

Modeling and simulations are not only being used and further developed by the pharmaceutical industry or academia but, from a regulatory perspective, have also been used to enhance decision making and contribute to product labeling (pertaining to dosage and administration, safety, or clinical pharmacology) (Bhattaram et al, 2007). In some submissions to the FDA, drug companies benefitted from modeling and simulations performed by reviewers, who were able to extract information from the data that had not otherwise been presented (Bhattaram et al, 2005, 2007). Lee et al (2011) found that over an 8 year period (2000 to 2008), modeling and simulations contributed to the approval of 64% of products while it influenced the labeling of 67% of products.

Physiologic Pharmacokinetic Models

The human body is composed of organ systems containing living cells bathed in an extracellular aqueous fluid (see Chapter 11). Both drugs and endogenous substances, such as hormones, nutrients, and oxygen, are transported to the organs by the same network of blood vessels (arteries). The drug concentration within a target organ depends on plasma drug concentration, plasma versus tissue protein binding, the rate of blood flow to an organ, and the rate of drug uptake into the tissue. Physiologically, uptake (accumulation) of drug by organ tissues occurs from the extracellular fluid, which equilibrates rapidly with the capillary blood in the organ. Some drugs cross the plasma membrane into the interior fluid (intracellular water) of the cell (Fig. 25-4).

In addition to drug accumulation, some organs of the body are involved in drug elimination, either by excretion (eg, kidney) or by metabolism (eg, liver). The elimination of drug by an organ may be described by drug clearance in the organ (see Chapters 7 and 12). The liver is an example of an organ with drug metabolism and drug uptake (accumulation). Physiologically based pharmacokinetic (PBPK) modeling aims to consider as much as possible all processes of drug uptake, distribution, and elimination.

In physiological PK models, drugs are carried by blood flow from the administration (input) site to various body organs, where the drug rapidly equilibrates with the interstitial water in the organ. Physiological pharmacokinetic models are mathematical models describing drug movement and disposition in the body based on organ blood flow and the organ spaces penetrated by the drug. In its simplest form, a physiologic pharmacokinetic model considers the drug to be blood flow limited. Drugs are carried to organs by arterial blood and leave organs by venous blood (Fig. 25-5).

In such a model, transmembrane movement of drug is rapid, and the capillary membrane does not offer any resistance to drug permeation. Uptake of

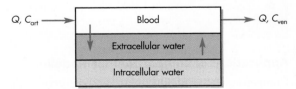

FIGURE 25-4   In describing drug transfer, the physiologic pharmacokinetic model divides a body organ into three parts: capillary vessels, extracellular space, and intracellular space.

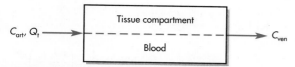

FIGURE 25-5   Noneliminating tissue organ. The extracellular water is merged with the plasma water in the blood.

drug into the tissues is rapid, and a constant ratio of drug concentrations between the organ and the venous blood is quickly established. This ratio is the tissue/blood partition coefficient:

$$P_{\text{tissue}} = \frac{C_{\text{tissue}}}{C_{\text{blood}}} \qquad (25.9)$$

where P is the partition coefficient.

The magnitude of the partition coefficient can vary depending on the drug and on the type of tissue. Adipose tissue, for example, has a high partition for lipophilic drugs. The rate of drug carried to a tissue organ and tissue drug uptake depend on the rate of blood flow to the organ and the tissue/blood partition coefficient, respectively.

The rate of blood flow to the tissue is expressed as Q_t (mL/min), and the rate of change in the drug concentration with respect to time within a given tissue organ is expressed as

$$\frac{d(V_{\text{tissue}}C_{\text{tissue}})}{dt} = Q_t(C_{\text{in}} - C_{\text{out}}) \qquad (25.10)$$

$$\frac{d(V_{\text{tissue}}C_{\text{tissue}})}{dt} = Q_t(C_{\text{art}} - C_{\text{ven}}) \qquad (25.11)$$

where C_{art} is the arterial blood drug concentration and C_{ven} is the venous blood drug concentration. Q_t is blood flow and represents the volume of blood flowing through a typical tissue organ per unit of time.

If drug uptake occurs in the tissue, the incoming concentration, C_{art}, is higher than the outgoing venous concentration, C_{ven}. The rate of change in the tissue drug concentration is equal to the rate of blood flow multiplied by the difference between the blood drug concentrations entering and leaving the tissue organ. In the *blood flow–limited model*, drug concentration in the blood leaving the tissue and the drug concentration within the tissue are in equilibrium, and C_{ven} may be estimated from the tissue/blood partition coefficient in

Equation 25.9. Substituting in Equation 25.11 with $C_{\text{ven}} = C_{\text{tissue}}/P_{\text{tissue}}$ yields

$$\frac{d(V_{\text{tissue}}C_{\text{tissue}})}{dt} = Q_t\left(C_{\text{art}} - \frac{C_{\text{tissue}}}{P_{\text{tissue}}}\right) \qquad (25.12)$$

Equation 25.12 describes drug distribution in a noneliminating organ or tissue group. For example, drug distribution to muscle, adipose tissue, and skin can be represented in a similar manner by Equations 25.13, 25.14, and 25.15, respectively, as shown below. For tissue organs in which drug is eliminated (Fig. 25-6), parameters representing drug elimination from the liver (k_{LIV}) and kidney (k_{KID}) are added to account for drug removal through metabolism or excretion. Equations 25.16 and 25.17 are derived similarly to those for the noneliminating organs above.

Removal of drug from any organ is described by drug clearance (Cl) from that organ. The rate of drug elimination is the product of the drug concentration in the organ and the organ clearance.

$$\text{Rate of drug elimination} = \frac{V_{\text{tissue}}dC_{\text{tissue}}}{dt}$$

$$= C_{\text{tissue}} \times Cl_{\text{tissue}}$$

The rate of drug elimination may be described for each organ or tissue (Fig. 25-7).

$$\text{Muscle:}\ \frac{d(V_{\text{MUS}}C_{\text{MUS}})}{dt} = Q_{\text{MUS}}\left(C_{\text{MUS}} - \frac{C_{\text{MUS}}}{P_{\text{MUS}}}\right)$$

$$(25.13)$$

$$\text{Adipose tissue:}\ \frac{d(V_{\text{FAT}}C_{\text{FAT}})}{dt} = Q_{\text{FAT}}\left(C_{\text{FAT}} - \frac{C_{\text{FAT}}}{P_{\text{FAT}}}\right)$$

$$(25.14)$$

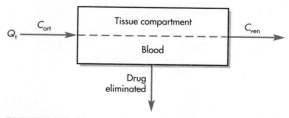

FIGURE 25-6   A typical eliminating tissue organ.

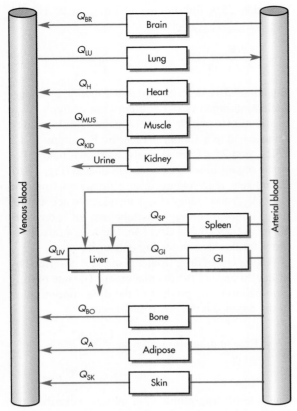

FIGURE 25-7 Example of blood flow to organs in a physiologic pharmacokinetic model.

Skin: $\dfrac{d(V_{SKIN}C_{SKIN})}{dt} = Q_{SKIN}\left(C_{SKIN} - \dfrac{C_{SKIN}}{P_{SKIN}}\right)$

$$(25.15)$$

Liver: $\dfrac{d(V_{LIV}C_{LIV})}{dt} = C_{LIV}(Q_{LIV} - Q_{GI} - Q_{SP})$

$$+ Q_{GI}\left(\dfrac{C_{GI}}{P_{GI}}\right) + Q_{SP}\left(\dfrac{C_{SP}}{P_{SP}}\right) - Q_{LIV}\left(\dfrac{C_{LIV}}{P_{LIV}}\right)$$

$$- C_{LIV}\left(\dfrac{Cl_{int}}{P_{LIV}}\right)$$

$$(25.16)$$

Kidney: $\dfrac{d(V_{KID}C_{KID})}{dt}$

$$= Q_{KID}\left(C_{KID} - \dfrac{C_{KID}}{P_{KID}}\right) - C_{KID}\left(\dfrac{Cl_{KID}}{P_{KID}}\right)$$

$$(25.17)$$

Lung: $\dfrac{d(V_{LU}C_{LU})}{dt} = Q_{LU}\left(\dfrac{C_{LU}}{P_{LU}}\right)$ (25.18)

where LIV = liver, SP = spleen, GI = gastrointestinal tract, KID = kidney, LU = lung, FAT = adipose, SKIN = skin, and MUS = muscle.

The mass balance for the rate of change in drug concentration in the blood pool is

$$\frac{d(V_bC_b)}{dt} = Q_{MUS}\left(\frac{C_{MUS}}{P_{MUS}}\right) + Q_{LIV}\left(\frac{C_{LIV}}{P_{LIV}}\right) + Q_{KID}\left(\frac{C_{KID}}{P_{KID}}\right)$$

$$\qquad\qquad\text{(muscle)}\qquad\quad\text{(liver)}\qquad\quad\text{(kidney)}$$

$$+ Q_{SKIN}\left(\frac{C_{SKIN}}{P_{SKIN}}\right) + Q_{FAT}\left(\frac{C_{FAT}}{P_{FAT}}\right) + Q_{LU}\left(\frac{C_{LU}}{P_{LU}}\right) - Q_bC_b$$

$$\quad\text{(skin)}\qquad\qquad\text{(adipose)}\qquad\quad\text{(lung)}\qquad\text{(blood)}$$

$$(25.19)$$

Lung perfusion is unique because the pulmonary artery returns venous blood flow to the lung, where carbon dioxide is exchanged for oxygen and the blood becomes oxygenated. The blood from the lungs flows back to the heart (into the left atrium) through the pulmonary vein, and the quantity of blood that perfuses the pulmonary system ultimately passes through the remainder of the body. In describing drug clearance through the lung, perfusion from the heart (right ventricle) to the lung is considered venous blood (Fig. 25-7). Therefore, the terms in Equation 25.19 describing lung perfusion are reversed compared to those for the perfusion of other tissues. With some drugs, the lung is a clearing organ besides serving as a merging pool for venous blood. In those cases, a lung clearance term could be included in the general model.

After intravenous drug administration, drug uptake in the lungs may be very significant if the drug has high affinity for lung tissue. If actual drug clearance is at a much higher rate than the drug clearance accounted for by renal and hepatic clearance, then lung clearance of the drug should be suspected, and a lung clearance term should be included in the equation in addition to lung tissue distribution.

The system of differential equations used to describe the blood flow–limited model is usually solved through computer programs, in an analogous manner to what is used with compartmental modeling. Because of the large number of parameters involved in the mass balance, and because "true" solutions to a set of differential equations may not solely exist, more than one set of parameters often fit the experimental data. This is common with human data, in which many of the organ tissue data items are not available. The lack of sufficient tissue data sometimes leads to unconstrained models. As additional data become available, new or refined models are adopted. For example, methotrexate was initially described by a flow-limited model, but later work described the model as a *diffusion-limited model*.

Because invasive methods are available for animals, tissue/blood ratios or partition coefficients can be determined accurately by direct measurement. Using experimental pharmacokinetic data from animals, physiologic pharmacokinetic models may yield more reliable predictions.

Physiologic Pharmacokinetic Model with Binding

The physiologic pharmacokinetic model described above assumed flow-limited drug distribution without drug binding to either plasma or tissues. In reality, many drugs are bound to a variable extent in either plasma or tissues. With most physiologic models, drug binding is assumed to be linear (not saturable or concentration dependent). Moreover, bound and free drug in both tissue and plasma are in equilibrium. Further, the free drug in the plasma and in the tissue equilibrates rapidly. Therefore, the free drug concentration in the tissue and the free drug concentration in the emerging blood are equal:

$$[C_b]_f = [C_t]_f \qquad (25.20)$$

$$[C_b]_f = f_b[C_b] \qquad (25.21)$$

$$[C_t]_f = f_t[C_t] \qquad (25.22)$$

where f_b is the blood free drug fraction, f_t is the tissue free drug fraction, C_t is the total drug concentration in tissue, and C_b is the total drug concentration in blood.

Therefore, the partition ratio, P_t, of the tissue drug concentration to that of the plasma drug concentration is

$$\frac{f_b}{f_t} = \frac{[C_t]}{[C_b]} = P_t \qquad (25.23)$$

By assuming linear drug binding and rapid drug equilibration, the free drug fraction in tissue and blood may be incorporated into the partition ratio and the differential equations. These equations are similar to those above except that free drug concentrations are substituted for C_b. Drug clearance in the liver is assumed to occur only with the free drug. The inherent capacity for drug metabolism (and elimination) is described by the term Cl_{int} (see Chapter 12). General mass balance of various tissues is described by Equation 25.24:

$$\frac{d(V_{tissue}C_{tissue})}{dt} = Q_t(C_{art} - C_{ven})$$

$$\frac{d(V_{tissue}C_{tissue})}{dt} = Q_t\left(C_{art} - \frac{C_t}{P_t}\right) \qquad (25.24)$$

or

$$\frac{d(V_{tissue}C_{tissue})}{dt} = Q_t\left(C_{art} - \frac{C_t f_t}{f_b}\right)$$

For liver metabolism,

$$\frac{d(V_{LIV}C_{LIV})}{dt} = C_b(Q_{LIV} - Q_{GI} - Q_{SP}) - Q_{LIV}\left(\frac{C_{LIV}}{P_{LIV}}\right)$$

(hepatic drug elimination)

$$+ Q_{GI}\left(\frac{C_{GI}}{P_{GI}}\right) + Q_{SP}\left(\frac{C_{SP}}{P_{SP}}\right) \qquad (25.25)$$

The mass balance for the drug in the blood pool is

$$\frac{d(V_b C_b)}{dt} = Q_{MUS} C_{MUS} + Q_{LIV}\left(\frac{C_{LIV}}{P_{LIV}}\right)$$

(muscle)   (liver)

$$+ Q_{KID}\left(\frac{C_{KID}}{P_{KID}}\right) + Q_{SKIN}\left(\frac{C_{SKIN}}{P_{SKIN}}\right) \quad (25.26)$$

(kidney)   (skin)

$$+ Q_{FAT}\left(\frac{C_{FAT}}{P_{FAT}}\right) + Q_{LU}\left(\frac{C_{LU}}{P_{LU}}\right) - Q_b C_b$$

(adipose)   (lung)   (blood)

The influence of binding on drug distribution is an important factor in interspecies differences in pharmacokinetics. In some instances, animal data may predict drug distribution in humans by taking into account the differences in drug binding. For the most part, extrapolations from animals to humans or between species are rough estimates only, and there are many instances in which species differences are not entirely attributable to drug binding and metabolism.

Blood Flow–Limited Versus Diffusion-Limited Model

Most physiologic pharmacokinetic models assume rapid drug distribution between tissue and venous blood. Rapid drug equilibrium assumes that drug diffusion is extremely fast and that the cell membrane offers no barrier to drug permeation. If no drug binding is involved, the tissue drug concentration is the same as that of the venous blood leaving the tissue. This assumption greatly simplifies the mathematics involved. Table 25-5 lists some of the drugs that have been described by a flow-limited model. This model is also referred to as the *perfusion model*. A more complex type of physiologic pharmacokinetic model is called the *diffusion-limited model* or the *membrane-limited model*. In the diffusion-limited model, the cell membrane acts as a barrier for the drug, which gradually permeates by diffusion. Because blood flow is very rapid and drug permeation is slow, a drug concentration gradient is established between the tissue and the venous blood (Lutz and Dedrick, 1985). The rate-limiting step of drug diffusion into the tissue depends on the permeation across the cell membrane rather than blood flow. Because of the time lag in equilibration between blood and tissue, the pharmacokinetic equation for the diffusion-limited model is very complicated.

Physiologic Pharmacokinetic Model Incorporating Hepatic Transporter-Mediated Clearance

It is now well recognized that drug transporters play important roles in the processes of absorption, distribution, and excretion and should be accounted for in PBPK models. Predicting human drug disposition, especially when involving hepatic transport, is difficult during drug development. However, drug transport may be a critical process in overall drug disposition in

TABLE 25-5   Drugs Described by Physiologic Pharmacokinetic Model

Drug	Category	Comment	Reference
Thiopental	Anesthetic	Blood, flow limited	Chen and Andrade (1976)
BSP	Diagnostic	Plasma, flow limited	Luecke and Thomason (1980)
Nicotine	Stimulant	Blood, flow limited	Gabrielsson and Bondesson (1987)
Lidocaine	Antiarrhythmic	Blood, flow limited	Benowitz et al (1974)
Methotrexate	Antineoplastic	Plasma, flow limited	Bischoff et al (1970)
Biperiden	Anticholinergic	Blood, flow limited	Nakashima and Benet (1988)
Cisplatin	Antineoplastic	Plasma, multiple metabolite, binding	King et al (1986)

the body such that without a realistic description of transport processes in the body, model accuracy may be deficient. Watanabe et al (2009) describe a model with hepatobiliary excretion mediated by transporters, organic anion-transporting polypeptide (OATP) 1B1 and multidrug resistance–associated protein (MRP) 2, for the HMG-CoA reductase inhibitor drug, pravastatin. While the classical blood flow–based physiologic pharmacokinetic models developed 40 years ago using systems of differential equations are still useful in describing the mass balance and transfer of drug within major organs, the models are inadequate in light of new discoveries in molecular biology and pharmacogenomics. Drug disposition and drug targeting are better understood based upon using influx/efflux and binding

mechanisms in microstructures such as interior cellular structures, membrane transporters, surface receptors, genomes, and enzymes. The liver is a complex organ intimately connected to drug transport and bile movement. Compartment concepts are needed to track the mass of drug transfer in and out of those fine structures as shown by the example in Fig. 25-8. Human liver microsomes are used to help predict the metabolic clearance of drugs in the body.

The PBPK model with pravastatin (Watanabe et al, 2009) is used to evaluate the concentration–time profiles for drugs in the plasma and peripheral organs in humans using physiological parameters, subcellular fractions (cells lysed and contents fractionated based on density), and drug-related parameters

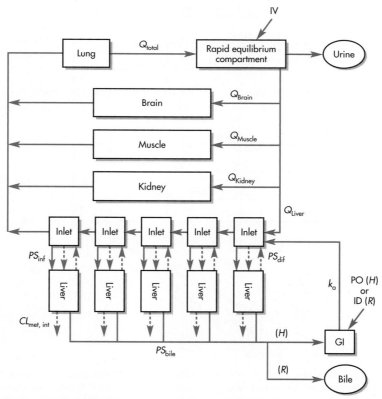

FIGURE 25-8 Schematic diagram of the PBPK model predicting the concentration–time profiles of pravastatin. The liver compartment was divided into five compartments to mimic the dispersion model. Indicated are blood flow (Q), the active hepatic uptake clearance (PS_{inf}), the passive diffusion clearance (PS_{dif}), the biliary clearance (PS_{bile}), and the metabolic clearance ($Cl_{met, int}$), human (H), and rat (R). The enterohepatic circulation was incorporated in the case of humans. (From Watanabe et al, 2009, with permission.)

(unbound fraction and metabolic and membrane transport clearances extrapolated from *in vitro* experiments). The principle of the prediction was as follows. First, subcellular fractions were obtained by comparing *in vitro* and *in vivo* parameters in rats. Then, the *in vitro* human parameters were extrapolated *in vivo* using the subcellular fractions obtained in rats. Pravastatin was selected as the model compound because many studies have investigated the mechanisms involved in the drug disposition in rodents, and clinical data after intravenous and oral administration are available.

When multiple drug metabolites are involved, the physiologic model of the cascade events can be quite complicated and an abbreviated approach may

be used. St-Pierre et al (1988) developed a simple one-compartment open model, based on the liver as the only organ of drug disappearance and metabolite formation. The model was used to illustrate the metabolism of a drug to its primary, secondary, and tertiary metabolites. The model encompassed the cascading effects of sequential metabolism (Fig. 25-9).

The concentration–time profiles of the drug and metabolites were examined for both oral and intravenous drug administration. Formation of the primary metabolite from drug in the gut lumen, with or without further absorption, and metabolite formation arising from first-pass metabolism of the drug and the primary metabolite during oral absorption were

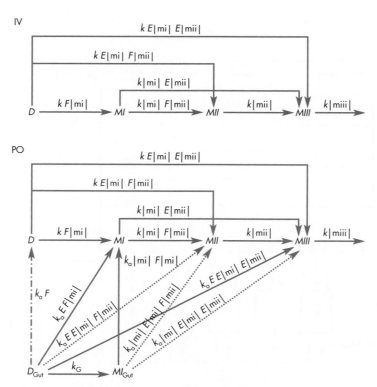

FIGURE 25-9   A schematic representation of the one-compartment open model for drug (*D*) and its primary (*MI*), secondary (*MII*), and tertiary (*MIII*) metabolites after intravenous (IV) and (po) drug dosing (scheme II) The effective rate constants contributing to the appearance of the metabolites in the systemic circulation are presented. The solid lines denote sources pertaining to drug or metabolite species in the circulation; the uneven dashed lines represent sources arising from absorption of drug or the primary metabolite from the gut lumen; and the stippled lines denote sources arising from first-pass metabolism of the drug or primary metabolite. See the glossary for definition of the terms. (From St-Pierre et al, 1988, with permission.)

considered. Mass balance equations, incorporating modifications of the various absorption and conversion rate constants, were integrated to provide the explicit solutions.

Application and Limitations of Physiologic Pharmacokinetic Models

The physiologic pharmacokinetic model is related to drug concentration and tissue distribution using physiologic and anatomic information. For example, the effect of a change in blood flow on the drug concentration in a given tissue may be estimated once the model is characterized. Similarly, the effect of a change in mass size of different tissue organs on the redistribution of drug may also be evaluated using the system of physiologic model differential equations generated. When several species are involved, the physiologic model may predict the pharmacokinetics of a drug in humans when only animal data are available. Changes in drug–protein binding, tissue organ drug partition ratios, and intrinsic hepatic clearance may be inserted into the physiologic pharmacokinetic model.

Most pharmacokinetic studies are modeled based on blood samples drawn from various venous sites after either IV or oral dosing. Physiologists have long recognized the unique difference between arterial and venous blood. For example, arterial tension (pressure) of oxygen drives the distribution of oxygen to vital organs. Chiou (1989) and Mather (2001) have discussed the pharmacokinetic issues

when differences in drug concentrations in arterial and venous are considered (see Chapter 11). The implication of venous versus arterial sampling is hard to estimate and may be more drug dependent. Most pharmacokinetic models are based on sampling of venous data. In theory, mixing occurs quickly when venous blood returns to the heart and becomes reoxygenated again in the lung. Chiou (1989) has estimated that for drugs that are highly extracted, the discrepancies may be substantial between actual concentration and concentration estimated from well-stirred pharmacokinetic models.

NONCOMPARTMENTAL ANALYSIS

Noncompartmental analyses provide an alternative method for describing drug pharmacokinetics without having to assign a particular compartmental model to the drug. Although this method is often considered to be *model independent*, there are still a few assumptions and key considerations that must not be overlooked. This approach is, therefore, better referred to as "noncompartmental" as it does assume a "model" in that, among other things that will be reviewed below, the PK needs to be linear and the terminal phase must be log-linear.

The first assumption is that the drug in question displays linear pharmacokinetics (DiStefano and Landaw, 1984; Gibaldi and Perrier, 2007). In other words, exposure increases in proportion with increasing dose and PK parameters are stable through time. A second important assumption is that the drug is eliminated from the body strictly from the pool in which it is being measured, the plasma, for example (Benet and Ronfeld, 1969; DiStefano and Landaw, 1984). Finally, this approach assumes that all sources of the drug are direct and unique to the measured pool (DiStefano and Landaw, 1984). If these assumptions hold true, noncompartmental analyses can be conducted if sufficient concentration–time data are available (eg, if there are rich data). In most circumstances "rich data" are considered to be a minimum of 12 different concentration time points (eg, includes the predose concentration) associated with a single-dose administration. Any less data may provide inaccurate estimations of pharmacokinetic parameters using the noncompartmental approach.

Statistical Moment Theory

Noncompartmental analyses are based on statistical moment theory, which provides a unique way to study time-related changes in *macroscopic events*. A macroscopic event is considered the overall event brought about by the constitutive elements involved. For example, in chemical processing, a dose of tracer molecules may be injected into a reactor tank to track the transit time (residence time) of materials that stay in the tank. The constitutive elements in this example are the tracer molecules, and the macroscopic events are the residence times shared by groups of tracer molecules. Each tracer molecule is well mixed and distributes noninteractively and randomly in the tank. In the case of all the molecules ($\int_0^{D_0} d\mathrm{De} = D_0$) that exit from the tank, the rate of exit of tracer molecules ($-d\mathrm{De}/dt$) divided by D_0 yields the probability of a molecule having a given residence time t. A mathematical formula describing the probability of a tracer molecule exited at any time is a probability density function. *Mean residence time* (MRT) is the expected value or mean of the distribution.

MRT provides a fundamentally different approach than classical pharmacokinetic models, which involve the concept of dose, half-life, clearance, volume, and concentration. The classical approach does not account for the observation that molecules in a cluster move individually through space and are more appropriately tracked as statistical distribution based on residence-time considerations. Consistent with the concept of mass and the dynamic movement of molecules within a region or "space," MRT is an alternative concept to describe how drug molecules move in and out of a system. The concept is well established in chemical kinetics, where the relationships between MRT and rate constants for different systems are known.

A probability density function $f(t)$ multiplied by t^m and integrated over time yields the moment curve

(Equation 25.27). The moment curve shows the characteristics of the distribution.

$$\mu_m \text{ or } m\text{th moment} = \int_0^{\infty} t^m f(t)\, dt \qquad (25.27)$$

where $f(t)$ is the probability density function, t is time, and m is the mth moment.

For example, when $m = 0$, substituting for $m = 0$ yields Equation 25.28, called the *zero moment*, μ_0:

$$\mu_0 = \int_0^{\infty} f(t)\, dt \qquad (25.28)$$

If the distribution is a true probability function, the area under the zero moment curve is 1. When $f(t)$ represents drug concentration that is a function of time, the zero moment is referred to as area under the curve (AUC). The AUC can be obtained through integration of $f(t)$ or using the trapezoidal method, as described in Chapter 2.

Substituting into Equation 25.27 with $m = 1$, Equation 25.29 gives the first moment μ_1:

$$\mu_1 = \int_0^{\infty} t^1 f(t)\, dt \qquad (25.29)$$

The area under the curve $f(t)$ times t is called the AUMC, or the *area under the first moment curve*. The *first moment*, μ_1, defines the *mean* of the distribution.

Similarly, when $m = 2$, Equation 25.27 becomes the *second moment*, μ_2:

$$\mu_2 = \int_0^{\infty} t^2 f(t)\, dt \qquad (25.30)$$

where μ_2 defines the variance of the distribution. Higher moments, such as μ_3 or μ_4, represent skewness and kurtosis of the distribution. Equation 25.27 is therefore useful in characterizing families of moment curves of a distribution.

The principal use of the moment curve is the calculation of the MRT of a drug in the body. The elements of the distribution curve describe the distribution of drug molecules after administration and the residence time of the drug molecules in the body.

Mean Residence Time

According to statistical moment theory, MRT is the expected value or mean of the distribution of a probability density function. However, MRT can also be viewed from the perspective of the disposition of drug molecules. After an intravenous bolus drug dose (D_0), the drug molecules distribute throughout the body. These molecules stay (reside) in the body for various time periods. Some drug molecules leave the body almost immediately after entering, whereas other drug molecules leave the body at a much later time period. The term MRT describes the average time that drug molecules stay in the body or in a kinetic space.

The equation to calculate the MRT following intravenous bolus or constant infusion administrations is described in Equation 25.31:

$$\text{MRT} = \frac{\text{AUMC}_0^\infty}{\text{AUC}_0^\infty} - \frac{\text{Duration}}{2} \qquad (25.31)$$

where AUMC_0^t is the area under the (first) moment-versus-time curve from $t = 0$ to infinity, AUC_0^∞ (or zero moment curve) is the area under the concentration-versus-time curve from $t = 0$ to infinity, and Duration is the duration of the drug infusion.

The AUMC can be extrapolated to infinity from AUMC_0^t using the following equation and assuming a log-linear terminal phase:

$$\text{AUMC}_0^\infty = \text{AUMC}_0^t + \frac{(C_t \times t)}{\lambda_z} + \frac{C_t}{\lambda_z^2} \qquad (25.32)$$

One major limitation of the AUMC_0^∞ calculation is that it can only be calculated after a single-dose administration, and not at steady-state conditions like the AUC_0^∞. This is because the superposition principle of the AUC (eg, that the AUC_0^∞ after a single dose is exactly equal to the $\text{AUC}_0^t(\text{ss})$ for a drug product exhibiting linear pharmacokinetics, see Chapter 7 for additional details) does not apply to the AUMC calculation. So the AUMC cannot be calculated easily at steady state over a dosing interval like the AUC. In practical terms, it means that the AUMC, and therefore the MRT, can only be calculated readily with the noncompartmental approach after a drug is administered as a single dose.

EXAMPLE ▶ ▶ ▶

An antibiotic was given to two subjects by an IV bolus dose of 1000 mg. Let's assume that the drug's pharmacokinetics is well described by a one-compartment model. The drug has a volume of distribution of 10 L and follows a one-compartment model with an elimination constant (λ_z) of (1) 0.1 h^{-1} and (2) 0.2 h^{-1} in the two subjects. Let's assume that the concentration at time zero was 100 mg/L in each subject. Determine the Cl and the MRT for each subject based on the concentrations listed in Table 25-6 using the noncompartmental approach.

Solution

Noncompartmental Approach

1. From Table 25-6, multiply each time point with the corresponding plasma C_p to obtain points for the moment curve. Use the linear trapezoidal rule and sum the area to obtain the area under the concentration–time curve (AUC_0^t) and the area under the moment curve (AUMC_0^t) for each subject, as demonstrated in Table 25-7.

The AUC_0^t (area from time zero to 30 hours) for subject 1 is 961.6 mg·h/L while it is 509.2 mg·h/L for subject 2. We can then calculate the AUC_0^∞:

$$\text{AUC}_0^\infty = \text{AUC}_0^t + C_t/\lambda_z$$

so $\text{AUC}_0^\infty = 961.605 + 4.979/0.1 = 1011.395$ mg·h/L (subject 1)
$\text{AUC}_0^\infty = 509.243 + 0.248/0.2 = 510.483$ mg·h/L (subject 2)

The Cl is therefore: $Cl = \text{Dose}/\text{AUC}_0^\infty$.

So $Cl = 1000/1011.395 = 0.99$ L/h (subject 1)
$Cl = 1000/510.483 = 1.96$ L/h (subject 2)

We now calculate the AUMC_0^t using Equation 25.32:

$\text{AUMC}_0^t = 1383.135 + 149.37/0.1 + 4.979/0.1^2 = 9963.4$ (subject 1)
$\text{AUMC}_0^t = 525.308 + 7.44/0.2 + 0.248/0.2^2 = 2526.9$ (subject 2)

And, finally the MRT:

$$\text{MRT} = \text{AUMC}_0^\infty/\text{AUC}_0^\infty - (\text{Duration infusion}/2)$$

So MRT = 9963.4/1011.395 = 9.85 h (subject 1)
MRT = 2526.9/510.483 = 4.95 h (subject 2)

TABLE 25-6   Simulated Plasma Data after an IV Bolus Dose, Illustrating Calculation of MRT

Time (h)	C_p (mg/L)	
	Subject 1	Subject 2
0	100	100
1	90.484	81.873
2	81.873	67.032
3	74.082	54.881
4	67.032	44.933
6	54.881	30.119
8	44.933	20.19
12	30.119	9.072
16	20.19	4.076
24	9.072	0.823
30	4.979	0.248

Mean Transit Time (MTT), Mean Absorption Time (MAT), and Mean Dissolution Time (MDT)

After IV administration, the rate of systemic drug absorption is zero, because the drug is placed directly into the bloodstream. The MRT calculated for a drug after IV administration basically reflects the elimination processes in the body, and therefore the MRT that molecules stay in the systemic circulation. When drugs are administered extravascularly, such as after oral administration, the ratio of AUMC to AUC does reflect not only the residence time of molecule once they are in the systemic circulation (MRT) but also the duration of time during which they are absorbed. The AUMC/AUC ratio therefore changes depending on how the drug is administered; hence many refer to this ratio as MRT_{PO} when the drug is orally administered, MRT_{inh} when the drug is administered via inhalation, MRT_{IM} when the drug is administered intramuscularly, and so on. This method of reporting the MRT does suggest that the duration of time that molecules stay in the systemic circulation changes with the method of administration, which is incorrect if the drug displays linear pharmacokinetic properties. In addition, it creates confusion when other parameters need to be calculated, such as the V_{ss}, as we will see later. So although it is not incorrect to label the ratio of AUMC/AUC by calling it an MRT with specification of the administration route, it is recommended to avoid confusion by referring to this ratio as mean transit time (MTT):

$$MTT = AUMC_0^\infty / AUC_0^\infty \text{ after extravascular administration} \qquad (25.33)$$

and as we have seen earlier,

$$MRT = AUMC_0^\infty / AUC_0^\infty - \text{ (duration infusion/2)} \\ \text{after IV administration}$$

such that

$$MTT = MAT + MRT \qquad (25.34)$$

where MAT is the mean absorption time, or the average time it takes for drug molecules to be absorbed into the systemic circulation.

With this nomenclature, the MRT is always obtained after IV administration, and the MTT always represents the total transit time, which is the sum of the MAT and the MRT. With this nomenclature, the route of administration will dictate what the MAT will be and will therefore influence the MTT, but the MRT will stay constant regardless of the route of administration.

So after oral administration $MTT_{PO} = MAT_{PO} + MRT$, after IM administration $MTT_{IM} = MAT_{IM} + MRT$, and so on.

In some cases, IV data are not available and an MTT for a solution may be calculated. The *mean dissolution time* (MDT), or *in vivo* mean dissolution time, for an *immediate-release* (IR) solid drug product would be:

$$MDT_{PO(IR)} = MTT_{PO(IR)} - MTT_{PO(solution)} \qquad (25.35)$$

MDT reflects the time for the drug to dissolve *in vivo*. Equation 25.35 calculates the *in vivo* dissolution time for an immediate-release solid drug product (tablet, capsule) given orally. MDT has been evaluated for a number of drug products. MDT is

TABLE 25-7   **Example of Calculation of MRT**

Time (h)	Subject 1				Subject 2			
	C_p (mg/L)	AUC (mg/L*h)	C_p x t (mg/L*h)	AUMC (mg/L*h^2)	C_p (mg/L)	AUC (mg/L*h)	C_p x t (mg/L*h)	AUMC (mg/L*h^2)
0	100		0		100		0	
1	90.484	95.242	90.484	45.242	81.873	90.9365	81.873	40.9365
2	81.873	86.1785	163.746	127.115	67.032	74.4525	134.064	107.9685
3	74.082	77.9775	222.246	192.996	54.881	60.9565	164.643	149.3535
4	67.032	70.557	268.128	245.187	44.933	49.907	179.732	172.1875
6	54.881	121.913	329.286	597.414	30.119	75.052	180.714	360.446
8	44.933	99.814	359.464	688.75	20.19	50.309	161.52	342.234
12	30.119	150.104	361.428	1441.784	9.072	58.524	108.864	540.768
16	20.19	100.618	323.04	1368.936	4.076	26.296	65.216	348.16
24	9.072	117.048	217.728	2163.072	0.823	19.596	19.752	339.872
30	4.979	42.153	149.37	1101.294	0.248	3.213	7.44	81.576
Sum		961.605		7971.79		509.2425		2483.502

most readily estimated for immediate-release-type products, because the absorption process (or MAT) may be influenced by certain types of modified-release drug products.

EXAMPLE ▶ ▶ ▶

Data for ibuprofen (Gillespie et al, 1982) are shown in Tables 25-8 and 25-9. Serum concentrations for ibuprofen after administration of a capsule and a solution are tabulated as a function of time in Tables 25-8 and 25-9, respectively.

As listed in Table 25-10, the MTT for the solution was 2.65 hours and for the product was 4.04 hours. Therefore, MDT for the product is 4.04 – 2.65 = 1.39 hours.

Other Pharmacokinetic Parameters Calculated by the Noncompartmental Analysis

The reader is referred to Chapter 7, where it is specified in detail how to estimate drug clearance (Cl) using the noncompartmental approach. Using the AUC value (zero moment curve) obtained with the trapezoidal method, total clearance (Cl/F) can be determined as follows:

$$Cl/F = \frac{\text{Dose}}{\text{AUC}_0^\infty}$$

In addition, bioavailability (F) can also be determined using concentration data obtained following intravenous (IV) and oral administration of a

TABLE 25-8   **Serum Concentrations for Capsule Ibuprofen**

Time (h)	C_p	$C_p t$	$t C_p \Delta t$
0	0	0	
0.167	0.06	0.01002	0.000836
0.333	3.59	1.195	0.1000
0.50	7.79	3.895	0.425
1	13.3	13.300	4.298
1.5	14.5	21.750	8.762
2	16.9	33.80	13.887
3	16.6	49.80	41.80
4	11.9	47.60	48.70
6	6.31	37.86	85.46
8	3.54	28.32	66.18
10	1.36	13.60	41.92
12	0.63	7.56	21.16
			Total AUMC = 332.695

$k = 0.347$ h^{-1}, $AUC_0^\infty = 89.1$

AUMC of tail piece (extrapolation to ∞) $= \dfrac{C_p \cdot t}{k} + \dfrac{C_p}{k^2} = \dfrac{0.63 \cdot 12}{0.347} + \dfrac{0.63}{0.347^2} = 27.02$

$AUMC_0^\infty = 332.695 + 27.02 = 359.715$

$MTT_{capsule} = \dfrac{359.715}{89.1} = 4.04$ h

Data adapted from Gillespie et al (1982).

TABLE 25-9 Serum Concentrations for Solution Ibuprofen

Time (h)	C_p	$C_p t$	$t C_p \Delta t$
0	0	0	
0.167	17.8	2.973	0.248
0.333	29.0	9.657	1.048
0.5	29.7	14.85	2.046
1	25.7	25.7	10.14
1.5	19.7	29.55	13.81
2	17.0	34.0	15.88
3	11.0	33.0	33.50
4	7.1	28.4	30.70
6	3.82	22.92	51.33
8	1.44	11.52	34.45
10	0.57	5.70	17.22
12	0.38	4.56	10.26
			Total AUMC = 220.64

$k = 0.455$ h^{-1}, $AUC_0^\infty = 87.7$

AUMC of tail piece (extrapolation to ∞) $= \dfrac{C_p \cdot t}{k} + \dfrac{C_p}{k^2} = \dfrac{0.38 \cdot 12}{0.455} + \dfrac{0.38}{0.455^2} = 11.86$

$AUMC_0^\infty = 220.64 + 11.86 = 232.478$

$MTT_{solution}\ \dfrac{232.478}{87.7} = 2.65$ h

Data adapted from Gillespie et al (1982).

drug (Gibaldi and Perrier, 2007).

$$F = \frac{\text{Dose}_{IV} \cdot \text{AUC}_{oral}}{\text{Dose}_{oral} \cdot \text{AUC}_{IV}} \qquad (25.36)$$

TABLE 25-10 Parameters for Capsule and Solution Ibuprofen

Parameter	Units	Capsule	Solution
AUC_0^∞	(μg/mL)h	89.1	87.7
$AUMC_0^\infty$	(μg/mL)h^2	359.7	232.5
k_a	h^{-1}	0.46	4.90
K	h^{-1}	0.347	0.455
MTT	Hours	4.04	2.65

Parameters were calculated from data of Gillespie et al (1982).

MRT is useful in calculating other pharmacokinetic parameters, particularly the total volume of distribution (V_{ss}).

$$V_{ss} = Cl \times \text{MRT} \qquad (25.37)$$

We have previously seen that the AUMC cannot be readily calculated, unless it is after a single-dose administration. In addition, the MRT can only be calculated after IV administration, as otherwise the MTT is calculated (when an extravascular administration is used) and this parameter includes the MAT in addition to the MRT. So what it means is that the total volume of distribution (V_{ss}) can, therefore, only be readily calculated after a single-dose IV administration. This is a major limitation of the noncompartmental approach, compared to the compartmental approach when the total volume of distribution can always be calculated, but obviously only if a valid compartmental model is used.

COMPARISON OF DIFFERENT APPROACHES

Physiological Versus Compartmental Approach

Both physiological and compartmental models aim to incorporate as much information as possible about the system (biological or other) that encompasses the data being modeled. Both approaches rely on differential equations or partial differential equations to ensure that laws of mass balance are respected.

While physiological models take into consideration biological processes at very specific molecular levels, compartmental models may lump various organs or tissues into groups. For example, a one-compartment model "groups" together all components of the human body such that they are represented by a single box. Thus, compartmental models can be viewed as more simplistic in comparison with their physiologic counterparts.

The major advantage of compartmental models is that the time course of drug in the body may be monitored quantitatively with a limited amount of data. Generally, only plasma drug concentrations and limited urinary drug excretion data are available. Compartmental models have been applied successfully for the prediction of drug pharmacokinetics and the development of dosage regimens. Moreover, compartmental models are very useful in relating plasma drug levels to pharmacodynamic and toxic effects in the body.

The simplicity and flexibility of the compartmental model is the principal reason for its wide application. In many cases, the compartmental model may be used to extract some information about the underlying physiologic mechanism through model testing of the data. Thus, compartmental analysis may lead to a more accurate description of the underlying physiological processes and the kinetics involved. In this regard, compartmental models are sometimes misunderstood, overstretched, and even abused. For example, the tissue drug levels predicted by a compartmental model represent only a composite pool for drug equilibration between all tissue and the circulatory system (plasma compartment). However, extrapolation to a specific tissue drug concentration is inaccurate and analogous to making predictions without experimental data. Although specific tissue drug concentration data are missing, many investigators may make general predictions about average tissue drug levels.

The compartmental model is particularly useful for comparing the pharmacokinetics of related therapeutic agents. In the clinical pharmacokinetic literature, drug data comparisons are based on compartmental models. Though alternative pharmacokinetic models have been available for approximately 20 years, the simplicity of the compartmental model allows easy tabulation of parameters such as V_{ss}, the distribution $t_{1/2}$, and the terminal $t_{1/2}$. The PBPK approach is used much less frequently, even though a substantial body of data has been generated using these types of models.

Because the PBPK model is more detailed, accounting for processes of drug distribution, drug binding, metabolism, and drug flow to the body organs, disease-related changes in physiologic processes are more readily related to changes in the pharmacokinetics of the drug. Furthermore, organ mass, volumes, and blood perfusion rates are often scalable, based on size, among different individuals, and even among different species. This allows a perturbation in one parameter and the prediction of the effect of changing physiology on drug distribution and elimination. The physiological pharmacokinetic model can also be modified to include a specific feature of a drug. For example, for an antitumor agent that penetrates into the cell, both the drug level in the interstitial water and the intracellular water may be considered in the model. Blood flow and tumor size may even be included in the model to study any change in the drug uptake at that site.

The physiological pharmacokinetic model can calculate the amount of drug in the blood and in any tissues for any time period if the initial amount of drug in the blood is known and the dose is given by IV bolus. In contrast, the tissue compartment in the compartmental model is not related to any actual anatomic tissue groups. The tissue compartment is needed when the plasma drug concentration data are fitted to a multicompartment model. In theory, when tissue drug concentration data are available, the multiple-compartment models may be used to fit both tissue and plasma drug data together, including the drug concentration in a specific tissue.

While both types of analyses can be challenging, there are also difficulties specific to each method. In PBPK modeling, obtaining the necessary rates and constants to describe molecular processes is not always obvious or easy. Those who perform compartmental modeling must deal with the challenges of noisy data, or data whose behavior is not easily described by simple models, making the determination of the "best model" more difficult and time consuming.

The compartmental approach is all about "identifiability," which means that a process should not be fitted if it cannot be "identified" or supported by the data, while in the PBPK approach most of the parameters are not identifiable and will be "fixed." For example, a compartmental model will not predict what an oral bioavailability parameter may be if concentration data are only available following IV administration. Predicting an oral bioavailability parameter would then be "unidentifiable." This is in direct contrast to the PBPK modeling approach in which a bioavailability parameter may still be in the model, even though there is no data to support it.

A common descriptor of the compartmental versus the physiological approach is to describe the former as a "top-down" approach, while the later is a "bottom-up" approach. A "top-down" approach means that the compartmental model is created from the data, and the model will therefore need to be identifiable from these data, and ideally will be shown to be perfectly capable of explaining these data. A "bottom-up" approach means that the PBPK model may be created before actual data are obtained, in order to predict what concentration time profiles may look like. It is with this simple comparison, "top-down" versus "bottom-up," that it is easier to reconcile both methods and see when it may be useful to use one more than the other. When a lot of data are available, compartmental modeling may be prioritized. In contrast, when no data are available yet for a drug product, then PBPK may be extremely useful to potentially predict what may happen. For scenarios that are somewhere between these two extreme situations (no data or a lot of data), then both models may coexist and be useful. It is important to note as well that a mixture of the two approaches can be used. For example, compartmental modeling can use "physiological" parameters to predict or explain CYP enzyme activity when drug–drug interaction data are being modeled (Pasternyk et al, 2000).

Noncompartmental Versus Compartmental Approach

Noncompartmental and compartmental analyses are both excellent methods that can be used to characterize the PK and/or PD of a drug, when used in their appropriate context. The disadvantages of each method highlight the advantages of the other method, but when utilized correctly, each approach has its own merits. Table 25-11 summarizes the key advantages and disadvantages of each approach (Ette and Williams, 2004; Tett et al, 1998).

For additional information, the reader is also referred to a section in Chapter 7 that describes the

TABLE 25-11   **Advantages and Disadvantages of Noncompartmental Versus Compartmental Population Analyses**

	Advantages	Disadvantages
Noncompartmental Analysis	– Easy and quick to perform – No special software is needed – Robust and easily reproducible	– Requires rich sampling – Makes assumptions regarding linearity
Compartmental Population Analysis	– Can be performed with rich or sparse data – Can be performed using data from heterogeneous sources or special populations – Can deal with both linearity and nonlinearity	– Requires experienced analyst – Time-consuming and labour intensive – Software is not user-friendly

relationships between clearance, volume of distribution, and rate constants between the noncompartmental and compartmental approaches.

SELECTION OF PHARMACOKINETIC MODELS

Many factors should be considered when using mathematical models to study rate processes (eg, pharmacokinetics of a drug). Ultimately, the type of model that is used will depend on the questions that need to be answered, as well as the nature of the data available. Indeed, adequate experimental design and the availability of valid data are important considerations in model selection and testing. For example, the experimental design should determine whether a drug is being eliminated by saturable (dose-dependent) or simple linear kinetics. A plot of metabolic rate versus drug concentration can be used to determine dose dependence, as in Fig. 25-10.

Metabolic rate can be measured at various drug concentrations using an *in vitro* system (see Chapter 12). In Fig. 25-10, curve *B,* saturation occurs at higher drug concentration.

For illustration, consider the drug concentration–time profile for a drug given by IV bolus. The combined metabolic and distribution processes may result in profiles like those in Fig. 25-11.

Curve *A* represents a slow initial decline due to saturation and a faster terminal decline as drug concentration decreases. Curve *C* represents a dominating distributive phase masking the effect of

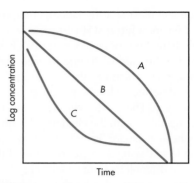

FIGURE 25-11   Plasma drug concentration profiles due to distribution and metabolic process. (See text for description of *A, B,* and *C.*)

nonlinear metabolism. Finally, a combination of *A* and *C* may approximate a rough overall linear decline (curve *B*). Notice that the drug concentration–time profile is shared by many different processes and that the goodness-of-fit is not an adequate criterion for adopting a model. For example, concluding linear metabolism based only on curve *B* would be incorrect. Contrary to common belief, complex models tend to mask opposing variables that must be isolated and tested through better experimental designs. In this case, a constant infusion until steady-state experiment would yield information on saturation without the influence of initial drug distribution.

The use of pharmacokinetic models has been critically reviewed by Rescigno and Beck (1987) and by Riggs (1963). These authors emphasize the difference between model building and simulation. A model is a secondary system designed to test the primary system (real and unknown). The assumptions in a model must be realistic and consistent with physical observations. On the other hand, a simulation may emulate the phenomenon without resembling the true physical process. A simulation without identifiable support of the physical system does little to aid understanding of the basic mechanism. The computation has only hypothetical meaning.

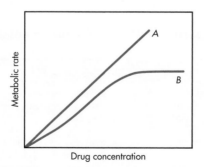

FIGURE 25-10   Metabolic rate versus drug concentration. Drug *A* follows first-order pharmacokinetics, whereas drug *B* follows nonlinear pharmacokinetics and saturation occurs at higher drug concentrations.

Frequently Asked Questions

▶ *Why is statistical moment used in pharmacokinetics?*

▶ *Why is MRT used in pharmacokinetics? How is MRT related to the total volume of distribution (V_{ss})?*

CHAPTER SUMMARY

Various types of models can be used to describe PK data. These include empirical, data-driven models such as allometric scaling. The latter is used to predict pharmacokinetic parameter values for humans based on animal data. Another model category is the mechanistic one, in which models aim to include as much information as possible about the system that surrounds the data being studied. Physiologically based PK models are mechanistic models that use a system of differential equations to describe drug transfer and accumulation in various tissues or organs in the body. Published data in the physiology literature regarding size (mass) of organs and blood flow to each organ and body mass are used. Compartmental models are also mechanistic models that use a system of differential equations to describe drug disposition. In contrast with PBPK models, molecular processes are not specifically modeled; thus a compartment does not usually represent one specific actual organ or tissue. Because they do not include physiological data (organ size, blood flow, etc), compartmental models can be applied to sparse data obtained from individual subjects or groups of subjects. Model-dependent pharmacokinetic parameters can thus be determined with different approaches. Pharmacokinetic parameters can also be determined using noncompartmental analyses based on statistical moment theory. MRT (mean residence time) is a statistical approach that treats drug molecules as individual units that move through organ and body spaces according to kinetic principles, and allows independent development of many equations that are familiar to classical kineticists. MRT allows the determination of the time for mean residence of the molecules (eg, dose administered) in the body according to the route of administration. The variance of the residence time can also be determined using statistical moment theory based on probability density function. The MRT approach allows another way of computing the volume of distribution of a drug through the derived equations. While the noncompartmental approach does not make any assumptions regarding a compartmental model, this approach is not without its own assumptions (linear PK, elimination, and sampling from the same compartment).

LEARNING QUESTIONS

1. After an intravenous bolus dose (500 mg) of an antibiotic, plasma–time concentration data were collected and the area under the curve was computed to be 25 mg/L·h. The area under the first moment-versus-time curve was found to be 100 mg/L·h^2.
   a. What is the mean residence time of this drug?
   b. What is the clearance of this drug?
   c. What is the total volume of distribution of this drug?

2. If the data in Question 1 are fit to a one-compartment model with an elimination k that is found to be 0.25 h^{-1}, MRT may be calculated compartmentally simply as $1/k$. What different assumptions are used in here versus Question 1?

3. What are the principal considerations in inter-species scaling?

4. What are the key considerations in fitting plasma drug data to a pharmacokinetic model?

5. What assumptions must hold true in order to conduct noncompartmental analyses?

ANSWERS

Frequently Asked Questions

How can we tell if we are using the right model to describe our data?

- In reality, there is no "right model" because different combinations of pharmacokinetic parameter estimates can often describe the same set of data using a given model. There can be a model that is superior to another according to predefined criteria, but it is not necessarily the "right" model. The most appropriate model also depends on the objectives of the modeling exercise, as well as the nature of the data that were collected.

Are certain algorithms better than others?

- Each algorithm has its strengths and weaknesses, and depending on the nature of the data being fitted, some algorithms may present certain advantages over others. For example, some of the algorithms that employ linearization may converge more quickly than those that perform no linearization; therefore, results could possibly be obtained more quickly.

When should individual compartmental analysis be used rather than population analysis?

- Besides being used when data are only available from one subject, individual compartmental analysis can be used to perform naïve pooled data analysis with data from a larger population. For example, data from a group of subjects can be pooled together such that a mean concentration–time profile is created from this group. The mean profile can then be fitted using a compartmental PK model, and the results can be used as initial estimates to perform population PK analyses if desired.

Why are differential equations used to describe physiologic models?

- Differential equations are used to describe the rate of drug transfer between different tissues and the blood. Differential equations have the advantage of being very adaptable to computer simulation without a lot of mathematical manipulations.

Why do we assume that drug concentrations in venous and arterial blood are the same in pharmacokinetics?

- After an IV bolus drug injection, a drug is diluted rapidly in the venous pool. The venous blood is oxygenated in the lung and becomes arterial blood. The arterial blood containing the diluted drug then perfuses all the body organs through the systemic circulation. Some drug diffuses into the tissue and others are eliminated. In cycling through the body, the blood leaving a tissue (venous) generally has a lower drug concentration than the perfusing blood (arterial). In practice, only venous blood is sampled and assayed. Drug concentration in the venous blood rapidly equilibrates with the tissue and will become arterial blood in the next perfusion cycle (seconds later) through the body. In pharmacokinetics, the drug concentration is assumed to decline smoothly and continuously. The difference in drug concentration between arterial and venous blood reflects drug uptake by the tissue, and this difference may have important consequences in drug therapy, such as tumor treatment.

Why should transporters be considered in physiological models?

- Drug transporters play important roles in the processes of absorption, distribution, and excretion, and if they are not considered in physiological models, the models may not be as accurate as they should be.

Why is statistical moment used in pharmacokinetics?

- Statistical moment is adaptable to mean residence time calculation and is widely used in pharmacokinetics because of its simplicity and robustness.

Why is MRT used in pharmacokinetics?

- Mean residence time (MRT) represents the average staying time of the drug in a body organ or compartment as the molecules diffuse in and out. MRT is an alternative concept used to describe how long a drug stays in the body. The main advantage of MRT is that it is based on probability and is consistent with how drug molecules behave in the physical world. Concentration in a heterogeneous region of the body may be hard to pinpoint.

How is MRT related to the total volume of distribution (V_{ss})?

- The V_{ss} can be determined from MRT according to the following equation: $V_{ss} = Cl \times MRT$, using data obtained following single-dose, intravenous drug administration.

Learning Questions

1. **a.** MRT = AUMC/AUC = 100/25 = 4 hours
   b. Cl = Dose/AUC = 500/25 = 20 L/h
   c. $V_{ss} = Cl \times MRT = 20 \times 4 = 80$ L

2. MRT = 1/0.25 = 4 hours. In this case, the one-compartment model must be assumed.

3. The principal considerations are size, drug-protein binding, and maximum life span potential of the species.

4. The objectives of the modeling must always be kept in mind, and the simplest model that best explains the data should always be retained.

5. Linear kinetics are assumed, and it is also assumed that drug loss (elimination) only occurs from the compartment from which samples are being collected.

REFERENCES

Beal SL, Sheiner LB: Part I, Users basic guide. In *NONMEM Users Guide*. San Francisco, CA, 1989.

Beal SL, Sheiner LB: Part VII, Conditional Estimation Methods. In *NONMEM Users Guide*. San Francisco, CA, 1988.

Benet LZ, Ronfeld RA: Volume terms in pharmacokinetics. *J Pharm Sci* **58**(5):639–641, 1969.

Benowitz N, Forsyth RP, Melmon KL, Rowland M: Lidocaine disposition kinetics in monkey and man, 1. Prediction by a perfusion model. *Clin Pharmacol Ther* **16**:87–98, 1974.

Bhattaram VA, Booth BP, Ramchandani RP, et al: Impact of pharmacometrics on drug approval and labeling decisions: A survey of 42 new drug applications. *AAPS J* **7**(3):E503–E512, 2005.

Bhattaram VA, Bonapace C, Chilukuri DM, et al: Impact of pharmacometric reviews on new drug approval and labeling decisions—A survey of 31 new drug applications submitted between 2005 and 2006. *Clin Pharmacol Ther* **81**(2):213–221, 2007.

Bischoff KB, Dedrick RL, Zaharko DS: Preliminary model for methotrexate pharmacokinetics. *J Pharm Sci* **59**:149–154, 1970.

Bonate PL: *Pharmacokinetic-Pharmacodynamic Modeling and Simulation.* 2nd ed. New York, NY: Springer; 2011.

Bonate PL, Howard D: Prospective allometric scaling: Does the emperor have clothes? *J Clin Pharmacol* **40**:665–670, 2000.

Bonati M, Latini R, Tognoni G, et al: Interspecies comparison of in vivo caffeine pharmacokinetics in man, monkey, rabbit, rat, and mouse. *Drug Metab Rev* **15**:1355–1383, 1985.

Boxenbaum H: Interspecies scaling, allometry, physiological time, and the ground plan of pharmacokinetics. *J Pharmacokinet Biopharm* **10**:201–227, 1982.

Boxenbaum H: Evolution biology, animal behavior, fourth-dimensional space, and the raison d'etre of drug metabolism and pharmacokinetics. *Drug Metab Rev* **14**:1057–1097, 1983.

Brightman FA, Leahy DE, Searle GE, Thomas S: Application of a generic physiologically based pharmacokinetic model to the estimation of xenobiotic levels in human plasm. *Drug Metab Rev* **34**:94–101, 2006.

Chen CN, Andrade JD: Pharmacokinetic model for simultaneous determination of drug levels in organs and tissues. *J Pharm Sci* **65**:717–724, 1976.

Chien JY, Friedrich S, Heathman MA, de Alwis DP, Sinha V: Pharmacokinetics/Pharmacodynamics and the stages of drug development: Role of modeling and simulation. *AAPS J* **7**(3): E544–E559, 2005.

Chiou WL: The phenomenon and rationale of marked dependence of drug concentration on blood sampling site: Implication in pharmacokinetics, pharmacodynamics, toxicology and therapeutics. Part I, *Clin Pharmacokinet* **17**(3):175–199, 1989; Part II, *Clin Pharmacokinet* **17**(3):275–290, 1989.

D'Argenio DZ, Schumitzky A, Wang X: *ADAPT 5 User's Guide: Pharmacokinetic/Pharmacodynamic Systems Analysis Software.* Los Angeles, CA: Biomedical Simulations Resource; 2009.

DiStefano JI, Landaw E. Multiexponential, multicompartmental, and noncompartmental modeling. I. Methodological limitations and physiological interpretations. *Am J Physiol* **264**:R651–R664, 1984.

Evans CA, Jolivette LJ, Nagilla R, et al: Extrapolation of preclinical pharmacokinetics and molecular feature analysis of "discovery-like" molecules to predict human pharmacokinetics. *Drug Metab Disp* **34**(7):1255–1265, 2006.

Ette EI, Williams PJ: Population pharmacokinetics I: background, concepts, and models. *Ann Pharmacother* **38**(10):1702–1706, 2004.

Gabrielsson J, Bondesson U: Constant-rate infusion of nicotine and cotinine, I. A physiological pharmacokinetic analysis of the cotinine disposition, and effects on clearance and distribution in the rat. *J Pharmacokinet Biopharm* **15**:583–599, 1987.

Gabrielsson J, Weiner D: Parameter Estimation. *Pharmacokinetic & Pharmacodynamic Data Analysis: Concepts and Applications.* 4th ed. Swedish Pharmaceutical Press, Stockholm, SW, 2006.

Gibaldi M, Perrier D: Noncompartmental analysis based on statistical moment theory. In Gibaldi M, Perrier M (eds).

Pharmacokinetics, 2nd ed. Informa Healthcare, New York, NY, 2007, pp 409–417.

Gillespie WR, Disanto AR, Monovich RE, Albert DS: Relative bioavailability of commercially available ibuprofen oral dosage forms in humans. *J Pharm Sci* **71:**1034–1038, 1982.

Hu Teh-Min, Hayton WL: Allometric scaling of xenobiotic clearance: Uncertainty versus universality. *AAPS PharmSci* **3**(4):30–34, article 29, 2001 (www.pharmsci.org).

King FG, Dedrick RL, Farris FF: Physiological pharmacokinetic modeling of *cis*-dichlorodiammineplatinum(II) (DDP) in several species. *J Pharmacokinet Biopharm* **14:**131–157, 1986.

Lee JY, Garnett CE, Gobburu JV, et al: Impact of pharmacometric analyses on new drug approval and labelling decisions: A review of 198 submissions between 2000 and 2008. *Clin Pharmacokinet* **50**(10):627–635, 2011.

Ludden TM: Population pharmacokinetics. *J Clin Pharmacol* **28**(12):1059–1063, 1988.

Luecke RH, Thomason LE: Physiological flow model for drug elimination interactions in the rat. *Comput Prog Biomed* **11:** 88–89, 1980.

Lutz RJ, Dedrick RL: Physiological pharmacokinetics: Relevance to human risk assessment. In Li AP (ed). *New Approaches in Toxicity Testing and Their Application in Human Risk Assessment.* New York, Raven, 1985, pp 129–149.

Mahmood I: Application of allometric principles for the prediction of pharmacokinetics in human and veterinary drug development. *Adv Drug Deliv Rev* **59**(11):1177–92, 2007.

Mahmood I: Critique of prospective allometric scaling: Does the emperor have clothes? *J Clin Pharmacol* **40:**671–674, 2000.

Mather LE: Anatomical-physiological approaches in pharmacokinetics and pharmacodynamics. *Clin Pharmacokinet* **40**(10): 707–722, 2001.

Mordenti J, Chappell W: The use of interspecies scaling in toxicology. In Yacobi A, Skelly JP, Batra VK (eds). *Toxicokinetic and Drug Development.* New York, Pergamon, 1989.

Nakashima E, Benet LZ: General treatment of mean residence time, clearance, and volume parameters in linear mammillary models with elimination from any compartment. *J Pharmacokinet Biopharm* **16:**475–492, 1988.

Nakashima E, Yokogawa K, Ichimura F, et al: A physiologically based pharmacokinetic model for biperiden in animals and its extrapolation to humans. *Chem Pharm Bull* **35:**718–725, 1987.

Nieforth KA, Nadeau R, Patel IH, et al: Use of an indirect pharmacodynamic stimulation model of MX protein induction to compare in vivo activity of interferon alfa-2a and a polyethylene glycol-modified derivative in healthy subjects. *Clin Pharmacol Ther* **59:**636–646, 1996.

Pasternyk Di Marco M, Wainer IW, Granvil CL, Batist G, Ducharme MP. New insights into the pharmacokinetics and metabolism of (R,S)-Ifosfamide in cancer patients using a population pharmacokinetic-metabolism model. *Pharm Res* **17**(6):645–652, 2000.

Rescigno A, Beck JS: Perspective in pharmacokinetics and the use and abuses of models. *J Pharmacokinet Biopharm* **15:** 327–344, 1987.

Riggs DS: *A Mathematical Approach to Physiological Problems.* Baltimore, Williams & Wilkins, 1963.

Ritschel WA, Banerjee PS: Physiological pharmacokinetic models: Principles, applications, limitations and outlook. *Meth Find Exp Clin Pharmacol* **8:**603–614, 1986.

Rodman JH, D'Argenio DZ, Peck CC: Analysis of pharmacokinetic data for individualizing drug dosage regimens. In Burton ME, Shaw LM, Schentag JJ, Evans WE (eds). *Applied Pharmacokinetics & Pharmacodynamics: Principles of Therapeutic Drug Monitoring.* 4th ed. Baltimore, MD: Lippincott Williams & Wilkins, 2006.

Sawada Y, Hanano M, Sugiyama Y, Iga T: Prediction of the disposition of nine weakly acidic and six weakly basic drugs in humans from pharmacokinetic parameters in rats. *J Pharmacokinet Biopharm* **13:**477–492, 1985.

Seng Yue C, Gallicano K, Labbé L, Ducharme MP: Novel population pharmacokinetic method compared to the standard noncompartmental approach to assess bioequivalence of iron gluconate formulations. *J Pharm Pharm Sci* **16**(3):424–440, 2013.

Sheiner LB: The population approach to pharmacokinetic data analysis: Rationale and standard data analysis methods. *Drug Metab Rev* **15**(1–2):153–171, 1984.

Steimer JL, Mallet A, Golmard JL, Boisvieux JF: Alternative approaches to estimation of population pharmacokinetic parameters: comparison with the nonlinear mixed-effect model. *Drug Metab Rev* **15**(1–2):265–92, 1984.

St-Pierre MV, Xu Xin, Pang KS: Primary, secondary, and tertiary metabolite kinetics. *Pharmacokinet Biopharm* **16**(5):493–527, 1988.

Tett SE, Holford NHG, McLachlan AJ. Population pharmacokinetics and pharmacodynamics: An underutilized resource. *Drug Info J* **32:**693–710, 1998.

Watanabe T, Kusuhara H, Maeda K, Shitara Y, Sugiyama Y: Physiologically based pharmacokinetic modeling to predict transporter-mediated clearance and distribution of pravastatin in humans. *J Pharmacol Exper Therap* **328**(2):652–662, 2009.

BIBLIOGRAPHY

Banakar UV, Block LH: Beyond bioavailability testing. *Pharm Technol* **7:**107–117, 1983.

Benet LZ, Galeazzi RL: Noncompartmental determination of the steady-state volume of distribution. *J Pharm Sci* **68:** 1071–1073, 1979.

Benet LZ: Mean residence time in the body versus mean residence time in the central compartment. *J Pharmacokinet Biopharm* **13:**555–558, 1985.

Bischoff KB, Dedrick RL, Zaharko DS, Longstreth JA: Methotrexate pharmacokinetics. *J Pharm Sci* **60:**1128–1133, 1971.

Boxenbaum H, D'Souza RW: Interspecies pharmacokinetics scaling, biological design and neoteny. In Testa B, D'Souza WD (eds). *Advances in Drug Research*, vol 19. New York, Academic, 1990, pp 139–196.

Chanter DO: The determination of mean residence time using statistical moments: Is it correct? *J Pharmacokinet Biopharm* **13:**93–100, 1985.

Coburn WA, Sheiner LB: Perspective in pharmacokinetics: Pharmacokinetic/pharmacodynamic model: What is it! *J Pharmacokinet Biopharm* **15:**545–555, 1987.

Himmelstein KJ, Lutz RJ: A review of the applications of physiologically based pharmacokinetic modeling. *J Pharmacokinet Biopharm* **7:**127–145, 1979.

Kasuya Y, Hirayama H, Kubota N, Pang KS: Interpretation and estimation of mean residence time with statistical moment theory. *Biopharm Drug Disp* **8:**223–234, 1987.

Sawada Y, Hanano M, Sugiyama Y, Iga T: Prediction of the disposition of nine weakly acidic and six weakly basic drugs in humans from pharmacokinetic parameters in rats. *J Pharmacokinet Biopharm* **13:**477–492, 1985.

Smallwood RH, Mihaly GW, Smallwood RA, Morgan DJ: Effect of a protein binding change on unbound and total plasma concentrations for drugs of intermediate hepatic extraction. *J Pharmacokinet Biopharm* **16**(5):529–542, 1988.

Veng-Pedersen P, Gillespie W: The mean residence time of drugs in the systemic circulation. *J Pharm Sci* **74:**791–792, 1985.

Wagner JG: Do you need a pharmacokinetic model, and, if so, which one? *J Pharmacokinet Biopharm* **3:**457–478, 1975.

Wagner JG: Dosage intervals based on mean residence times. *J Pharm Sci* **76:**35–38, 1987.

Wagner JG: Types of mean residence times. *Biopharm Drug Disp* **9:**41–57, 1988.

West GB: The origin of universal scaling laws in biology. *Physica A* **263:**104–113, 1999.

Appendix A: Applications of Software Packages in Pharmacokinetics

Philippe Colucci and Murray P. Ducharme

The term "pharmacokinetics" (PK) is relatively young and was first introduced in 1953 (Wagner 1981). Although some of the concepts associated with pharmacokinetics are much older (eg, Michaelis–Menten equation in 1913, Hill equation in 1908), the study of pharmacokinetics and pharmacodynamics (PD) has only been popularized over the last 60 years. Since the early conceptions of compartmental PK analysis in the 1960s and noncompartmental analysis in the 1970s, the studies of PK and/or PD in drug development have advanced rapidly. These advancements are strongly correlated with the explosion of computers, especially personal computers (PCs). Computer speed and storage capacity have doubled approximately every 2 years over the last 40 years (Keyes 2006). Therefore, mathematical computation time has dramatically shortened over the same period of time.

The increased speed of computers as well as their storage capacity has led to the development of numerous computer software programs that now allow for the rapid solution of complicated pharmacokinetic equations and rapid modeling of pharmacokinetic processes. At its core, a software program is a set of instructions written in a computer language. The computer's operating system must support the computer language of the software in order for this software to function properly. Accordingly, some software may only work in a Windows-based operating system (OS) while others may have been designed to work in Windows, Apple OS, or Linux. It is important to know the software requirements in order to properly choose the software that is most appropriate for the computer that will run the software packages.

These software programs simplify tedious calculations and allow more time for the development of new approaches to data analysis and pharmacokinetic modeling. In addition, computer software is also used for the development of experimental study designs, statistical data treatment, data manipulation, graphical representation of data, pharmacokinetic model simulation, and projection or prediction of drug action.

The improvements in computing have allowed for the estimation of pharmacokinetic (PK) and pharmacodynamic (PD) parameters from increasingly complex PK/PD models. Complex PK/PD and PBPK models are being elaborated today, where they would have been impossible to apply 30 years ago due to the slow computation time (months) in order to obtain parameters. Consequently, these improvements in conjunction with improvements in the analytical analysis of systemic drug concentrations and the capturing of pharmacodynamic parameters have led to a much better understanding of the pharmacokinetics and pharmacodynamics of drugs during drug development. Furthermore, the increased speed of the computer's processors has allowed many more scientists the freedom to simultaneously analyze concentration data (PK) as well as response data (PD) on their personal computers, as most PCs are fast enough to run PK software packages compared to 30 years ago when these PK software packages were often installed on dedicated PK computers or mainframes.

COMPARTMENTAL AND NONCOMPARTMENTAL ANALYSES

In order for the user to decide which PK software package to use, it is important for the user to understand which type of analysis is required. Not all computer programs satisfy all of the user's full requirements. Therefore, the choice of a software package will depend on the objective of the analysis and the PK methodology required.

There are three main PK and PK/PD analysis methodologies. These are the noncompartmental, the individual compartmental, and the population compartmental approaches.

As the name implies, the noncompartmental approach does not need the specification of the number of compartments or exponentials that characterize the shape of the concentration-versus-time curve. This method is described in Chapters 7 and 25. This methodology became popular in the early 1980s and is based on the theory of statistical moments, which is a mathematical concept explaining the distribution of data (Gibaldi et al, 2007; Riegelman et al, 1980; Yamaoka et al, 1978). This methodology requires many concentration samples over a period of time per patient in order to correctly estimate the PK parameters (Gabrielsson et al, 2012). The method utilizes simple analyses that require very little computer power if any. In most cases, a simple spreadsheet such as EXCEL® can be used to calculate all of the required PK parameters associated with this analysis. Nevertheless many scientists will still use a dedicated software program to perform this type of analysis. One reason is that the management of the input data as well as the output tables and profiles is simplified, especially if numerous subjects/patients are analyzed. Another reason can be that some parameters are more tedious to calculate, such as calculating the concentration at time 0 for a bolus administration or determining the optimal elimination rate constant (K_{el}) for all subjects. Furthermore, the use of programs can allow the user to perform curve stripping in a simple manner. An example of a popular program to perform noncompartmental analysis is Certara Phoenix WinNonlin®.

The *compartmental approach* can be considered the classical PK approach, although it started in time more as an individual graphical stripping technique than a true compartmental method due to the absence of computing power and the availability of semilog graph paper. The compartmental approach is still the gold standard since it can be used for any types of drugs, whether they exhibit linear or nonlinear characteristics.

It can be used after single dose or steady-state conditions, and can explain and characterize all different routes of administration. Compartmental analyses try to explain observed concentrations, whether they are PK or PD in nature, or whether they are supporting the data as in the case of clinical covariates. Compartmental analyses use compartment models that have both a mathematical and a statistical basis, and for this the use of specialized PK software packages is mandatory.

There are two main methodological approaches to compartmental analyses, individual or population based. With individual PK analysis, a model is written to explain the observed concentrations in an individual. The model minimizes the error between the predicted and observed concentrations to provide PK parameters that best explain the observed data of the individual. As we have seen in Chapter 25, pharmacokinetic models often use nonlinear equations that often have no definite numerical solutions. Models are therefore often written mathematically with differential equations, and these have to be solved by the software algorithms. With individual compartmental analysis, the data from one individual is analyzed without any influence from the data collected from other individuals who may be in the same study. Multiple functions/algorithms have been proposed to best minimize the error between the observed and predicted concentrations or the "least squares." Most softwares give the user the opportunity to utilize ordinary least squares, weighted least squares, maximum likelihood, and/or Bayesian methods. The Bayesian method requires prior information on the parameters being predicted or fitted. As the model does not attempt to determine the population PK parameters but just the individual's PK parameters, this type of analysis is relatively quick to perform, although much longer than the noncompartmental analysis.

An example of a Microsoft Excel worksheet to generate time–concentration data after n doses of a drug given orally according to a one-compartment model is given in Fig. A-1. The parameter inputs are in column B, time is in column D, and concentration is in column E.

The *population compartmental approach* involves the "simultaneous" analysis of data from all individuals.

	A	B	C	D	E	F
1	D	100000		0	0.00	
2	KA	2		0.1	1.78	
3	K	0.4		0.2	3.16	
4	V	10000		0.3	4.23	
5	TAU	4		0.4	5.04	
6	F	1		0.5	5.64	
7	N	1		0.6	6.07	
8	EXP(-KA*TAU)	0.000335463		0.7	6.36	
9	EXP(-K*TAU)	0.201896518		0.8	6.55	
10	FKAD	200000		0.9	6.65	
11	V(K-KA)	−16000		1	6.69	
12	AA	1		1.1	6.67	
13	BB	1		1.2	6.60	
14				1.3	6.5	
15	FD/VK	25	AUC	1.4	6.38	
16				1.5	6.24	
17	FD/V...	8.86435343	Cmax-ss	1.6	6.08	
18				1.7	5.92	
19				1.8	5.74	
20	TMAX	1.0058987	tmax-1	1.9	5.57	
21				2	5.39	
22				2.1	5.21	
23	TMAX-SS	0.86516026	tmax-ss	2.2	5.03	
24				2.3	4.86	
25				2.4	4.68	
26				2.5	4.51	
27				2.6	4.35	
28				2.7	4.19	
29				2.8	4.03	
30				2.9	3.88	
31				3	3.73	
32				3.1	3.59	
33				3.2	3.45	
34				3.3	3.32	
35				3.4	3.19	
36				3.5	3.07	
37				3.6	2.95	
38				3.7	2.84	
39				3.8	2.73	
40				3.9	2.62	
41			tmin	4	2.52	Cmin
42	PARAMETER	PARAM. Value	PARAM-TERM	TIME (hrs)	CONC (mcg/mL)	

FIGURE A-1   Example of a Microsoft Excel spreadsheet used to calculate time–concentration data according to an oral one-compartment model after *n* doses.

This analysis has been shown to be vastly superior to the individual compartmental analysis in terms of robustness and is therefore the preferred approach when performing compartmental analyses nowadays, now that computing power is no more a limiting factor. Contrary to individual compartmental analyses where PK parameters are estimated for each individual, population compartmental analyses estimate the typical average PK parameters for the population, along with their interindividual variability, as well as the overall residual variability, which includes the intraindividual variability. It is these population parameter estimates (PK parameters and variability parameters) that allow inferences to be made for other populations, as well as provide the possibility to perform simulations of expected concentration–time profiles under different conditions (eg, different dosing regimens, different subpopulations such as renally impaired patients). Numerous algorithms have been proposed to perform population compartmental analysis. These include parametric and nonparametric approaches.

Numerous methods and software packages exist to perform population PK analyses. Scientists should possess the skills and experience to perform compartmental analyses, as it is easy to make an error and there are many steps involved in performing this type of analysis. Many have proposed this to be an "art," not just a "science," as intuition, experience, and collaborative brainstorming sessions are all an essential part of a successful analysis.

The reader is referred to Chapters 7 and 25 for additional details regarding noncompartmental and compartmental approaches. For more in-depth explanations and techniques regarding population compartmental analyses and the "art" of modeling, the fabulous book by Bonate is essential reading (Bonate, 2011).

SOFTWARE USES

Computer programs allow the user to perform one or more of the following analyses:

1. Fitting drug concentration–time data to a series of built-in pharmacokinetic models provided by the software, and choosing the one that best describes the data statistically: Typically, a least-squares program is employed, in which the sum of squared differences between observed data points and theoretic prediction is minimized. Usually, a mathematical procedure is used iteratively (repetitively) to achieve a minimum in the sum of squares (convergence). Some data may allow easier convergence with one procedure rather than another. The mathematical method employed should be reviewed before use.

2. Fitting data into a pharmacokinetic or pharmacodynamic model defined by the user: This method is by far the most useful, because any list of prepared models is often limited. This is where much progress has been made over the last 20 years. The increased speed and storage with computers including PCs have allowed new algorithms and new software packages to be developed or updated that provide the user with more than the one or two alternative softwares/algorithms that were previously the only available. The flexibility of user-defined models allows continuous refinement of models as new experimental information becomes available. This is synonymous with the "Learn and Confirm" approach established by Sheiner (1997). Some software merely provides a utility program for fitting the data to a series of polynomials. This utility program provides a simple, quantitative way of relating the variables, but offers little insight into the underlying pharmacokinetic processes.

3. Simulation: Some software programs generate data based on a model with parameter input by the user. When the parameters are varied, new data are generated based on the model chosen. The user is able to observe how the simulated model data matches the experimental observed data. Another purpose for simulations is to allow the user to answer hypothetical questions. Using simulations, numerous different clinical trials can be simulated to determine the impact of modifying certain clinical characteristics. For example, simulations could determine the predicted concentration profiles in renally impaired patients versus normal subjects.

This could be done for hundreds of different scenarios, whereas it would be impossible in reality to dose all these studies to obtain such information.

4. Experimental design: To estimate the parameters of any model, the experimental design of the study must have points appropriately spaced to allow curve description and modeling. Although statisticians stress the need for proper experimental design, little information is generally available for experimental design in pharmacokinetics when a study is performed for the first time. For the first pharmacokinetic study, an empirical or a statistical experiment design is necessarily based on assumptions that may later prove to be wrong. However, for subsequent studies, certain software packages allow the user to optimize the sampling scheme for upcoming studies to maximize the utility of the data collected.

5. Clinical pharmacokinetic applications: Some software programs are available for the clinical monitoring of narrow-therapeutic-index drugs (ie, critical-dose drugs) such as the aminoglycosides, other antibiotics, theophylline, phenytoin, cyclosporine, tacrolimus, lithium, or others. These programs may include calculations for creatinine clearance using the Cockcroft–Gault method or other equations (see Chapter 21), dosage estimation, pharmacokinetic parameter estimation for the individual patient, and pharmacokinetic simulations.

6. Computer programs for teaching: Software applications for teaching have been reviewed by Charles and Duffull (2001).

SOFTWARE PACKAGES

No PK software package is perfect and each software package will have advantages and disadvantages that can favor the use of different packages at different times or for specific situations. Thus, before deciding on a software, it is imperative to understand the objectives of the PK analyses, the available data, and past experiences of users with certain software packages.

Some software packages are free while others are commercially available at a cost. The quality of the software does not necessarily correlate with its price tag, though, and it is important to research the program's specifications to ensure it will fit the needs of the scientist. Some programs may be free but they may require additional programs in order to work or compile PK and PD models (eg, Fortran compilers), or to perform even basic graphical relationships or summary analyses.

It is also important to note that all software packages should be validated for proper installation in order to ensure the accuracy of the results. Software used for data analyses that depend on statistical and pharmacokinetic calculations should be validated with respect to the accuracy, quality, integrity, and security of the data. One approach for determining the accuracy of the data analysis is to compare the results obtained from two different software packages using the same set of data (Heatherington et al, 1998). Because software packages may have different functionalities, different results (eg, pharmacokinetic parameter estimates) may be obtained. Some PK software packages provide built-in template studies (and results) that can be compared with results from the same model obtained by the user to ensure the accuracy of the installation.

Table A-1 and the following text list some of the popular PK softwares available. Listing of a software package within this text does not mean that it has been endorsed by the authors. The descriptions may not represent the latest versions as features are often added or improved. The user should contact the program vendors directly for more information. The software packages are listed in alphabetical order without regard to personal preferences or ranking.

ADAPT 5

Since 1985, ADAPT-II followed by ADAPT 5 has been developed and supported by the Biomedical Simulations Resource (BMSR) in the Department of Biomedical Engineering at the University of Southern California, under support from the National Institute for Biomedical Imaging and Bioengineering

TABLE A-1 List of Popular PK Software Packages

Software	Version Reviewed	Analysis Type	Operating System	Approximate Price*	URL
ADAPT 5®	5.0.048	Individual compartmental; population compartmental; optimal sampling scheme	Windows	Free (requires Fortran)	http://bmsr.usc.edu/software/adapt/
Bear (to be used with R)	2.6.3	Noncompartmental	Windows	Free	http://pkpd.kmu.edu.tw/bear/
Berkeley Madonna®	8.3.18	Population compartmental	Windows; Apple	$	http://www.berkeleymadonna.com/
GastroPlus® SimCYP®	8.5	Simulation package	Windows	$$$$$$	http://www.simulations-plus.com/Products.aspx?pID=11
Kinetica®	5	Noncompartmental; individual compartmental; population compartmental	Windows	$$$	http://www.adeptscience.co.uk/products/lab/kinetica
Monolix®	4.3.1	Population compartmental	Windows; Linux	$$	http://www.lixoft.eu/
NLINMIX (used with SAS)	NA	Population compartmental	SAS Macro	Free (requires SAS)	http://support.sas.com/kb/25/032.html#pur
NONMEM®	7.3.0	Individual compartmental, population compartmental	Windows; Linux; Apple Solaris	$$$$	http://www.iconplc.com/technology/products/nonmem/
Phoenix NLME®	1.2	Population PK/PD	Windows	(Start-up $$$$) then $$$$ yearly	http://www.certara.com/products/pkpd/phx-nlme
Phoenix WinNonlin®	6.3	Noncompartmental; individual compartmental	Windows	(Start-up $$$$) then $$$ yearly	http://www.certara.com/products/pkpd/phx-wnl
Pmetrics® (to be used with R)	1.2	Individual compartmental; population compartmental	Windows; Apple	Free	http://www.lapk.org/pmetrics.php
PK-Sim®	5.2.1	Individual compartmental; population compartmental	Windows	$$$$$	http://www.systems-biology.com/products/pk-sim.html
PK Solution®	2	Noncompartmental	Windows; Linux; Apple	$	http://www.summitpk.com/pksolutions/pksolutions.htm
Scientist/PK Analyst®	3.0	Curve stripping	Windows	$	http://www.micromath.com/

* $ ≤1000$; $$ >1000$ and ≤2.5k; $$$ >2.5k and ≤5k; $$$$ >5k and ≤10k; $$$$$ >10k and ≤20k; $$$$$$ >20k.

and the National Center for Research Resources of the National Institutes of Health (NIH). With support from the NIH, ADAPT 5 is a software package that has been tested, upgraded, and well published over the last 30 years. ADAPT 5 is a free computational modeling platform (requires user to have a valid Fortran 95 compiler) developed for pharmacokinetic and pharmacodynamic applications. It is intended for basic and advanced clinical research and is designed to facilitate the discovery, exploration, and application of the underlying pharmacokinetic and pharmacodynamic properties of drugs. ADAPT 5 has been developed under the direction of David Z. D'Argenio in collaboration with Alan Schumitzky and Xiaoning Wang (D'Argenio et al, 2009). It allows the user to choose from numerous algorithms both for individual and for population compartmental analyses such as weighted least squares, maximum likelihood (ML), generalized least squares (GLS), maximum *a posteriori* Bayesian estimation (MAP), maximum likelihood estimation via the EM algorithm with sampling (MLEM), iterative two-stage (ITS), standard two-stage (STS), and naive-pooled data (NPD) modeling, each with WLS, ML, and MAP estimators. Other features include a simulation module (SIM) that includes capabilities for single and multisubject Monte Carlo simulations and an optimal sample schedule design module (SAMPLE) that provides the ability to calculate D- and C-optimal samples. The SAMPLE module allows the user to determine the minimum number of sparse samples that should be taken in a future study as well as the optimal timing of these samples.

Bear

This software is an example of a software package written to work with R (see description of the R software). It stands for BE/BA for R. It is a free package created by Hsin-ya Lee and Yung-jin Lee. It is designed to analyze average bioequivalence (ABE) data from a study using noncompartmental PK analysis (NCA) with an analysis of variance (crossover, replicated crossover, parallel designs for single- or multiple-dose studies). Typical noncompartmental PK parameters for a bioequivalence study can be estimated with the calculation of 90% confidence intervals for the ratio of the test to reference products for common pivotal BE parameters such as AUC_{0-t}, AUC_{0-inf}, and C_{max}. One limitation of this software is that data must be obtained according to a typical study design established by Bear, and entered in a very specific manner; otherwise, the software cannot perform the necessary calculations.

Berkeley Madonna

Berkeley Madonna is a commercially available general purpose differential equation solver for constructing mathematical models developed on the Berkeley campus under the sponsorship of the NSF (National Science Foundation) and the NIH. It has a relatively user-friendly graphical interface that allows the user to modify the model by modifying a diagram. The software's powerful algorithms allow for quick convergence and it has been used extensively in the development of multicompartment models such as physiologically based pharmacokinetic models (PBPK) (Amrite et al, 2008). It also allows for easy simulations of profiles at steady state and can determine the impact when the value for one parameter is modified. Although this software package has been widely used in other fields, in pharmacometrics it is mostly used to find preliminary results (priors), which are then used in another software package.

GastroPlus, SimCYP

GastroPlus and SimCYP are mechanistically based simulation software programs that can predict the rate and extent of drug exposure for drugs administered via intravenous, oral, ocular, intranasal, and pulmonary routes in human and preclinical species. The underlying model within these softwares is the Advanced Compartmental Absorption and Transit (ACAT) model. Features include a variety of dosage forms: intravenous (bolus or infusion), immediate release (tablet, capsule, suspension, solution, lingual spray, and sublingual tablet) and controlled release (gastric retention, dispersed release, integral tablet, enteric-coated tablet and capsule, and buccal patch), and *in vitro–in vivo* correlation for immediate- or controlled-release formulations. It allows the user to perform *in vitro–in vivo* extrapolation (IVIVE).

These software packages have gained in popularity with scientists who develop new drugs, who use them to predict the expected PK parameter values in humans.

Kinetica

Kinetica, from Thermo Scientific, allows users to perform a range of analyses, from noncompartmental analysis to population pharmacokinetic–pharmacodynamic analyses. This software also has built-in templates for use with noncompartmental and PK and PD compartmental analyses. Kinetica has a graphical interface that facilitates data analysis, reporting, and file storage. For its population compartmental analysis, Kinetica incorporates the EM algorithm that was originally in P-Pharm. Kinetica has a visual model designer that allows the user to create a model without having to write their own code; a model that is created graphically is converted by the software into the basic code that represents the visual model. Although a variety of analyses can be performed with this software, it is not very user friendly.

Monolix

Monolix (MOdèles Non LInéaires à effets miXtes) is a software package that was developed based on research in statistics and modeling, led by INRIA (Institut National de la Recherche en Informatique et Automatique). Monolix is free of charge for academics, students, and regulatory agencies, but charges a yearly license fee for commercial uses. Like ADAPTs, Monolix has been supported by an agency helping with its development, testing, and use. Although it has not existed for as long as ADAPT, publications with Monolix are becoming more prevalent. This software allows users to apply nonlinear mixed-effect models for advanced population analysis, PK/PD, and preclinical and clinical trial modeling and simulation. Monolix is based on the Matlab scientific environment; however, a stand-alone version is available, and therefore, Matlab does not need to be purchased. This package has numerous built-in and compiled PK and PD models. The primary algorithm utilized by this software is the Stochastic Approximation of EM (SAEM) algorithm coupled with Monte Carlo and Markov Chains (MCMC) for maximum likelihood estimation.

Nlinmix (SAS)

SAS is an all-purpose data analysis system with a flexible application-development language. Over 5000 SAS products are reported to be available including various "PROC" (subroutines) available for statistical as well as general linear and nonlinear regression models. One such subroutine is the NLINMIX macro to fit nonlinear mixed models. It uses PROC NLIN and PROC MIXED and can only be used with SAS version 8 or higher. This subroutine uses a Taylor series expansion point to determine the fixed and random parameters specified in the model. When set to zero, this analysis is similar, but not identical, to Sheiner and Beal's first-order method (Beal and Sheiner, 1982) in NONMEM. The analysis can also be estimated by expanding the nonlinear function about random effects parameters set equal to their current empirical best linear unbiased predictor (EBLUP), which is Lindstrom and Bates' approximate second-order method (Lindstrom et al, 1990). Although the subroutine is freely accessible, the user requires SAS, which is not free. This limits its popular usage and most modeling scientists turn to other software programs.

Nonmem

NONMEM (Nonlinear Mixed Effects Model), developed originally by S. L. Beal and L. B. Sheiner and the NONMEM Project Group at the University of California, is a program used for estimating parameters in population PK/PD. It was one of the first PK/PD modeling software and is considered by many scientists as the gold standard for population compartmental PK and PK/PD analyses. The program first appeared in 1979 and numerous papers featuring NONMEM have been published since then. NONMEM versions up through VI are the property of the Regents of the University of California, but ICON Development Solutions has exclusive rights to license their use. NONMEM 7 up to the current version 7.3 have been updated by ICON (Beal et al, 1989–2009). In addition to its basic applications in population PK and/or PD analysis, NONMEM is useful for evaluating relationships between pharmacokinetic parameters and demographic data (often referred as covariates) such as age, weight, and disease state.

Different algorithms are available in NONMEM to perform population compartmental analyses. With version 7, ITS, and Monte Carlo expectation-maximization and Markov Chain Monte Carlo Bayesian methods have been added to the classical likelihood methods available in previous versions. These included first-order (FO) estimation method, first-order conditional estimation (FOCE), and Laplace conditional estimation algorithms. NONMEM can be used to simulate data as well as fit data.

NONMEM requires Fortran; however, NONMEM works also with free Fortran programs that can easily be downloaded over the Internet.

Phoenix WinNonlin and NLME

These software packages are available from Certara. Phoenix WinNonlin provides a relatively easy-to-use interface for data management, plotting, noncompartmental analysis including bioequivalence testing, as well as individual compartmental PK/PD analysis. It can handle large numbers of subjects or profiles. WinNonlin's input and output data may be managed via Excel (Microsoft)-compatible spreadsheet files. WinNonlin is a powerful least-squares program for parameter estimation. Both a user-defined model and a library of over 20 compartmental models are available to be used for analysis. The program accepts both differential and regular (analytical) equations. Users may select the Hartley-modified or Levenberg-type Gauss–Newton algorithm or the (Nelder and Mead) simplex algorithm for minimizing the sum of squared residuals. Compartmental models, curve fitting, and simulations are specially designed for pharmacokinetics.

Phoenix NLME replaced WinNonMix and is a software package for population PK and PK/PD analyses. Phoenix NLME includes a wide set of optimization engines for nonlinear mixed-effects modeling, including a new EM (expectation maximization) method (QRPEM). Other algorithms include FO, extended least-squares FOCEI, Lindstron–Bates FOCE, naive-pooled, ITS, and nonparametric algorithm. The FO and FOCE algorithms are different from those associated with NONMEM and can provide different results. Scientists can construct their models by selecting through a wide library of models, or by coding them graphically and/or manually. This software is also relatively user-friendly compared to some other programs available. Although the software contains some interesting features, its cost is prohibitive, which is why many scientists continue to rely on software packages such as NONMEM and ADAPT 5, which arguably continue to be academic and industry standards.

Pmetrics

Pmetrics is a free software package developed by the Laboratory of Applied Pharmacokinetics at the University of Southern California to be used within R. Contrary to most other compartmental PK software packages discussed in this chapter, this program provides a nonparametric approach to determine PK and PD parameters. The available algorithms include the ITS Bayesian parametric population PK modeling (IT2B), nonparametric adaptive grid (NPAG), and a semi-parametric Monte Carlo simulator. IT2B is generally used to obtain initial parameter range estimates to be used with NPAG and assumes a normal or transformed to normal distribution of the PK parameters. NPAG creates a nonparametric population model consisting of discrete support points, each with a set of estimates for all parameters in the model plus an associated probability (weight) of that set of estimates. Pmetrics was previously known as USC Pack from Roger Jelliffe and has been around for decades.

PK-Sim

PK-Sim is a comprehensive software tool for PBPK modeling. It allows access to relevant anatomical and physiological parameters for humans and the most common laboratory animals (mouse, rat, minipig, dog, and monkey) that are contained in an integrated database. Further, it provides access to different PBPK calculation methods to allow model building and parameterization. PK-Sim uses both relevant generic passive processes automatically provided (eg, distribution through the blood flow) and specific active processes (eg, metabolization by a certain enzyme) that are specified by the user. PK-Sim is designed for use by nonmodeling experts and only allows minor structural model modifications to be made. However, more experienced modellers can use MoBi, which allows the user full access to all model details including the option for extensive model modifications.

PK Solutions

PK Solutions is an automated Excel-based program that provides noncompartmental single- and multiple-dose pharmacokinetic data analysis of concentration-time data following intravenous or extravascular routes of administration. The program provides comprehensive tables of the most widely used and published pharmacokinetic parameters (up to 75 parameters can be obtained) and graphs. Multiple dose and steady-state parameters are automatically projected from single-dose results using exponential terms (no modeling or differential equations are involved). This allows easy determination of steady-state profiles when certain dosing parameters are changed such as changing the dosing interval.

R

R (http://www.r-project.org/) is a language and environment within which statistical computing and graphics are implemented. R is available as free software under the terms of the Free Software Foundation's GNU General Public License in source code form. It compiles and runs on a wide variety of platforms such as UNIX, Linux, Windows, and Apple OS. R is not a PK software *per se* but provides a wide variety of statistical (linear and nonlinear modeling, classical statistical tests, time-series analysis, classification, clustering, etc) and graphical techniques for data handling and model analysis. It originated in Bell Laboratories and is now maintained as a nonprofit software by a private foundation. It is highly applicable to PK applications. The commercially available S language is often the vehicle of choice for research in statistical methodology, and R provides an open source route to participation in that activity.

Scientist/PKAnalyst

Scientist is specifically designed to fit model equations to experimental data. Scientist is a general mathematical modeling application that can perform nonlinear least-squares minimization and simulation. Scientist can fit almost any mathematical model from the simplest linear functions to complex systems of differential equations, nonlinear algebraic equations, or models expressed as Laplace transforms. A statistics menu is available for AUC, C_{max}, t_{max}, and mean residence time parameter calculations. However, the program does not handle differential equations or user-defined models. Plot outputs are available, as are pharmacokinetic curve stripping, and least-squares parameter optimization.

PKAnalyst for Windows is designed to simulate and perform parameter estimation for pharmacokinetic models. Built-in models can calculate micro rate constants for compartmental models, analyze saturable (Michaelis–Menten) kinetics, handle bolus and zero-/first-order input for finite and infinite time periods, and produce concentration/effect Sigmoid-E_{max} diagrams, including parameter estimation and statistical data analysis.

The last version was released in 2005. Therefore, no changes have been made or supported since then. Other software packages exist that are more recent and more flexible.

SPECIALIZED THERAPEUTIC DRUG MONITORING SOFTWARE

Therapeutic drug monitoring (TDM) is the practice of taking some blood concentrations from an individual in order to optimize the dosing for that individual to ensure that the concentrations of a narrow therapeutic drug remain within a safe and efficacious range. Only limited, sparse samples (one or two) are taken at strategic times. With these limited samples and the patient's characteristics, a Bayesian analysis is performed to predict the expected concentration profile. Many software packages are available with built-in models for the most common narrow therapeutic drugs that are clinically administered. A thorough review of these available software packages is provided by Fuchs et al (2013).

EXAMPLE 1 ▶▶▶

From a series of time–concentration data (Fig. A-2, columns A and B), determine the elimination rate constant using the regression feature of MS Excel.

Solution

a. Type in the time and concentration data shown in columns A and B (see Fig. A-2).

b. Convert in column C all concentration data to ln concentration. Data point #1 may be omitted because ln of zero cannot be determined.

c. From the main menu, select Insert:

Select function

SLOPE

Y data range (select last 4 value)

X data range (select last 4 value)

The slope, given in Fig. A-2, is −0.1. In this case, the ln concentration is plotted versus time, and the slope is simply the elimination rate constant.

Note: To check this result, students may be interested in simulating the data with dose = 10,000 $\mu g/kg$, $V_D = 1000$ mL/kg, $k_a = 0.8$ h^{-1}, and $k = 0.1$ h^{-1}.

EXAMPLE 2 ▶▶▶

Generate some data for a two-compartment model using two differential equations. Initial conditions are dose = 1, $V = 1$, $k_{12} = 0.2$, $k_{21} = 1$, and $k = 3$.

Solution

The data may be generated with ADAPT 5 (Fig. A-3).

EXAMPLE 3 ▶▶▶

After a drug is administered orally, plasma drug concentration–time data may be fitted to a one- or two-compartment model, to estimate the absorption rate constant, elimination rate constant, and volume of distribution. Based on the results of these models, it is possible to determine which model best explains the results using the minimum objective function (MOF). Results from NONMEM (one-, two-compartment models) are shown in Fig A-4A and A-4B. In this case, the plasma concentrations were better fitted using a two-compartment model than a one-compartment model. The MOF was significantly lower with the two-compartment model versus a one-compartment model.

	A	**B**	**C**		
1	Time (hrs)	Conc	Ln (Conc)		
2	0	0			
3	2	7049.53	8.86		
4	4	7194.95	8.88		
5	6	6178.08	8.73		
6	8	5116.2	8.54		
7	10	4200.5	8.34		
8	12	3441.45	8.14	Slope	−0.1
9	14	2818.09	7.94		
10	16	2307.36	7.74		

FIGURE A-2 Example of a Microsoft Excel spreadsheet used to calculate time–concentration data according to an oral one-compartment model after *n* doses.

```
     ADAPT 5       SIM -- MODEL SIMULATION
 Enter file name for storing session run (*.run): Run1.run
       ----- MODEL INPUT INFORMATION -----
 Data file name (*.dat): C:\pt1.csv

    ** This is a population data file:  C:\pt1.csv
       Will analyze 1st subject

 The number of model inputs:      0
 The number of bolus inputs:     1
 Enter the compartment number for each bolus input (e.g. 1,3,...):   1
 The number of input event times:      1

    Input Event Information
           Time    Value for all Inputs
 Event     Units,      B(1)
   1.      0.000         1.000

       ----- MODEL OUTPUT INFORMATION -----
 The number of model output equations:    2
 The number of observations:    15

       ----- SIMULATION SELECTION -----
 The following simulation options are available:
    1. Individual simulation
    2. Individual simulation with output error
    3. Population simulation
    4. Population simulation with output error
 Enter option number:  1

       ----- ENTER PARAMETER INFORMATION -----
 Parameter file name: C:\Priors1.prm
 Enter values for indicated parameters:
  Parameter        Old Value    New Value (<Enter> if no change)
   k               3.000
   k12             .2000
   k21             1.000
   Vc              1.000
   Vp              1.000

 Enter Initial Conditions:
  Parameter        Old Value    New Value (<Enter> if no change)
   IC(   1)        0.000
   IC(   2)        0.000

       ----- RESULTS -----
       --- A. Parameter Summary ---
 Individual simulation

 Parameter         Value
  k                3.000
  k12              0.2000
  k21              1.000
  Vc               1.000
  Vp               1.000
  IC(   1)         0.000
  IC(   2)         0.000
```

FIGURE A-3   A sample of the ADAPT 5 application program used to solve the two-differential equation for a two-compartment model after IV bolus dose. (The first 15 data points are shown. Time is in hours.)

```
        --- B. Simulation Summary ---

Model: 2-cpt model; example 2
Individual simulation
   Obs.Num.     Time            Y(1), ... ,Y(   2)
        1        0.000          0.000       0.000
        2        0.1700E-01     0.9471      0.3281E-02
        3        0.3300E-01     0.8999      0.6160E-02
        4        0.5000E-01     0.8524      0.9008E-02
        5        0.6700E-01     0.8074      0.1165E-01
        6        0.8300E-01     0.7673      0.1397E-01
        7        0.1000         0.7269      0.1625E-01
        8        0.1170         0.6887      0.1836E-01
        9        0.1330         0.6547      0.2020E-01
       10        0.1500         0.6203      0.2201E-01
       11        0.1670         0.5879      0.2367E-01
       12        1.000          0.5076E-01  0.3067E-01
       13        2.000          0.7278E-02  0.1346E-01
       14        3.000          0.2433E-02  0.5446E-02
       15        4.000          0.9586E-03  0.2188E-02
```

FIGURE A-3   (*Continued*)

```
$PROBLEM Run1; Book Chapter 1CPT Oral plasma
$INPUT ID, TIME, RATE, DOSE=AMT, DV, EVID, MDV
$DATA NM1.CSV
$SUBROUTINES ADVAN2 TRANS2
$PK

    ALAG1 = THETA(1)*EXP(ETA(1))
    KA    = THETA(2)*EXP(ETA(2))
    CL    = THETA(3)*EXP(ETA(3))
    V     = THETA(4)*EXP(ETA(4))

    SC = V

        K10 = CL/V
        HALF=LOG(2)/K10

$THETA
     (0      0.3    ) ;  ALAG
     (0      10     ) ;  KA
     (0      1      ) ;  CL
     (0      4      ) ;  VC

$OMEGA 0.05         ;  ALAG
       0.05         ;  KA
       0.05         ;  CL
       0.05         ;  VC

$ERROR
      IPRED = F
      IF(F.GT.0)THEN
        W = F
```

FIGURE A-4A   Sample output from NONMEM showing oral data fitted to (ADVAN 2, TRANS2) a one-compartment model with first-order absorption and first-order elimination.

```
      ELSE
        W = 1
      END IF
      IRES = DV - IPRED
      IWRES = IRES/W

      Y = F + F*EPS(1) + EPS(2)

$SIGMA 0.05 0.05

$ESTIMATION METHOD=1 NOABORT SIGDIGITS=3 MAXEVAL=9999 PRINT=0 POSTHOC

NM-TRAN MESSAGES

WARNINGS AND ERRORS (IF ANY) FOR PROBLEM    1

(WARNING  2) NM-TRAN INFERS THAT THE DATA ARE POPULATION.
CREATING MUMODEL ROUTINE...


 PROBLEM NO.:           1
 Run1; Book Chapter 1CPT Oral plasma
0DATA CHECKOUT RUN:               NO
 DATA SET LOCATED ON UNIT NO.:     2
 THIS UNIT TO BE REWOUND:         NO
 NO. OF DATA RECS IN DATA SET:      378
 NO. OF DATA ITEMS IN DATA SET:   7
 ID DATA ITEM IS DATA ITEM NO.:   1
 DEP VARIABLE IS DATA ITEM NO.:   5
 MDV DATA ITEM IS DATA ITEM NO.:  7
0INDICES PASSED TO SUBROUTINE PRED:
   6   2   4   3   0   0   0   0   0   0   0
0LABELS FOR DATA ITEMS:
 ID TIME RATE DOSE DV EVID MDV
0FORMAT FOR DATA:
 (7E7.0)


 TOT. NO. OF OBS RECS:        340
 TOT. NO. OF INDIVIDUALS:       18
0LENGTH OF THETA:    4
0DEFAULT THETA BOUNDARY TEST OMITTED:    NO
0OMEGA HAS SIMPLE DIAGONAL FORM WITH DIMENSION:    4
0DEFAULT OMEGA BOUNDARY TEST OMITTED:    NO
0SIGMA HAS SIMPLE DIAGONAL FORM WITH DIMENSION:    2
0DEFAULT SIGMA BOUNDARY TEST OMITTED:    NO
0INITIAL ESTIMATE OF THETA:
 LOWER BOUND      INITIAL EST      UPPER BOUND
  0.0000E+00      0.3000E+00      0.1000E+07
  0.0000E+00      0.1000E+02      0.1000E+07
  0.0000E+00      0.1000E+01      0.1000E+07
  0.0000E+00      0.4000E+01      0.1000E+07
0INITIAL ESTIMATE OF OMEGA:
 0.5000E-01
 0.0000E+00     0.5000E-01
 0.0000E+00     0.0000E+00     0.5000E-01
 0.0000E+00     0.0000E+00     0.0000E+00     0.5000E-01
```

FIGURE A-4A   (*Continued*)

```
0INITIAL ESTIMATE OF SIGMA:
 0.5000E-01
 0.0000E+00    0.5000E-01
0ESTIMATION STEP OMITTED:            NO
 CONDITIONAL ESTIMATES USED:         YES
 CENTERED ETA:                       NO
 EPS-ETA INTERACTION:                NO
 LAPLACIAN OBJ. FUNC.:               NO
 NO. OF FUNCT. EVALS. ALLOWED:       9999
 NO. OF SIG. FIGURES REQUIRED:       3
 INTERMEDIATE PRINTOUT:              NO
 ESTIMATE OUTPUT TO MSF:             NO
 ABORT WITH PRED EXIT CODE 1:        NO
 IND. OBJ. FUNC. VALUES SORTED:      NO


 THE FOLLOWING LABELS ARE EQUIVALENT
 PRED=NPRED
 RES=NRES
 WRES=NWRES
1DOUBLE PRECISION PREDPP VERSION 7.2.0


 ONE COMPARTMENT MODEL WITH FIRST-ORDER ABSORPTION (ADVAN2)
0MAXIMUM NO. OF BASIC PK PARAMETERS:    3
0BASIC PK PARAMETERS (AFTER TRANSLATION):
 ELIMINATION RATE (K) IS BASIC PK PARAMETER NO.:   1
 ABSORPTION RATE (KA) IS BASIC PK PARAMETER NO.:   3


 TRANSLATOR WILL CONVERT PARAMETERS
 CLEARANCE (CL) AND VOLUME (V) TO K (TRANS2)
0COMPARTMENT ATTRIBUTES
 COMPT. NO.    FUNCTION    INITIAL    ON/OFF     DOSE      DEFAULT    DEFAULT
                           STATUS     ALLOWED    ALLOWED   FOR DOSE   FOR OBS.
    1          DEPOT       OFF        YES        YES       YES        NO
    2          CENTRAL     ON         NO         YES       NO         YES
    3          OUTPUT      OFF        YES        NO        NO         NO
1
 ADDITIONAL PK PARAMETERS - ASSIGNMENT OF ROWS IN GG
 COMPT. NO.                           INDICES
              SCALE      BIOAVAIL.    ZERO-ORDER   ZERO-ORDER   ABSORB
                         FRACTION     RATE         DURATION     LAG
    1          *          *           *            *            4
    2          5          *           *            *            *
    3          *          -           -            -            -
              - PARAMETER IS NOT ALLOWED FOR THIS MODEL
              * PARAMETER IS NOT SUPPLIED BY PK SUBROUTINE;
                WILL DEFAULT TO ONE IF APPLICABLE
0DATA ITEM INDICES USED BY PRED ARE:
 EVENT ID DATA ITEM IS DATA ITEM NO.:         6
 TIME DATA ITEM IS DATA ITEM NO.:             2
 DOSE AMOUNT DATA ITEM IS DATA ITEM NO.:      4
 DOSE RATE DATA ITEM IS DATA ITEM NO.:        3


0PK SUBROUTINE CALLED WITH EVERY EVENT RECORD.
 PK SUBROUTINE NOT CALLED AT NONEVENT (ADDITIONAL OR LAGGED) DOSE TIMES.
0ERROR SUBROUTINE CALLED WITH EVERY EVENT RECORD.
1
```

FIGURE A-4A   (Continued)

```
 #TBLN:        1
 #METH: First Order Conditional Estimation


 #TERM:
0MINIMIZATION SUCCESSFUL
 NO. OF FUNCTION EVALUATIONS USED:        359
 NO. OF SIG. DIGITS IN FINAL EST.:   3.4
0PARAMETER ESTIMATE IS NEAR ITS BOUNDARY
 THIS MUST BE ADDRESSED BEFORE THE COVARIANCE STEP CAN BE IMPLEMENTED

 ETABAR IS THE ARITHMETIC MEAN OF THE ETA-ESTIMATES,
 AND THE P-VALUE IS GIVEN FOR THE NULL HYPOTHESIS THAT THE TRUE MEAN IS 0.

 ETABAR:          -2.4682E-06  1.3091E-06 -9.0175E-03  1.6093E-03
 SE:               9.5606E-06  5.0353E-06  3.3000E-02  1.8596E-02

 P VAL.:           7.9628E-01  7.9487E-01  7.8465E-01  9.3104E-01

 ETAshrink(%):     9.8133E+01  9.9017E+01 -2.1777E-01  7.8698E+00
 EPSshrink(%):     5.9519E+00  4.7599E+00

 #TERE:
 Elapsed estimation time in seconds:     1.68
1
 ****************************************************************************************************
 ****************
  ********************
  ********************
   ********************                       FIRST ORDER CONDITIONAL ESTIMATION
  ********************
 #OBJT:**************                       MINIMUM VALUE OF OBJECTIVE FUNCTION
 ********************
  ********************
  ********************
  ****************************************************************************************************
 ****************


 #OBJV:******************************************       1497.827       ****************************
 ********************
1
 ****************************************************************************************************
 ****************
  ********************
  ********************
   ********************                       FIRST ORDER CONDITIONAL ESTIMATION
  ********************
  ********************                         FINAL PARAMETER ESTIMATE
 ********************
  ********************
 ********************
  ****************************************************************************************************
 ****************
```

FIGURE A-4A   (*Continued*)

```
THETA - VECTOR OF FIXED EFFECTS PARAMETERS    *********

          TH 1       TH 2       TH 3       TH 4

          3.36E-01  5.56E+00   1.28E+00   4.30E+00



OMEGA - COV MATRIX FOR RANDOM EFFECTS - ETAS  ********

            ETA1       ETA2       ETA3       ETA4

 ETA1
+        5.00E-06

 ETA2
+        0.00E+00   5.00E-06

 ETA3
+        0.00E+00   0.00E+00   2.07E-02

 ETA4
+        0.00E+00   0.00E+00   0.00E+00   7.76E-03



SIGMA - COV MATRIX FOR RANDOM EFFECTS - EPSILONS  ****

            EPS1       EPS2

 EPS1
+        1.13E-02

 EPS2
+        0.00E+00   1.80E+00

1


OMEGA - CORR MATRIX FOR RANDOM EFFECTS - ETAS  *******

            ETA1       ETA2       ETA3       ETA4

 ETA1
+        2.24E-03

 ETA2
+        0.00E+00   2.24E-03

 ETA3
+        0.00E+00   0.00E+00   1.44E-01
```

FIGURE A-4A   (*Continued*)

```
  ETA4
+         0.00E+00  0.00E+00  0.00E+00  8.81E-02



  SIGMA - CORR MATRIX FOR RANDOM EFFECTS - EPSILONS  ***


             EPS1        EPS2

  EPS1
+         1.06E-01


  EPS2
+         0.00E+00  1.34E+00
```

FIGURE A-4A   (*Continued*)

```
$PROBLEM Run1; Book Chapter 2CPT Oral plasma
$INPUT ID, TIME, RATE, DOSE=AMT, DV, EVID, MDV
$DATA NM1.CSV
$SUBROUTINES ADVAN4 TRANS4
$PK

    ALAG1 = THETA(1)*EXP(ETA(1))
    KA    = THETA(2)*EXP(ETA(2))
    CL    = THETA(3)*EXP(ETA(3))
    V2    = THETA(4)*EXP(ETA(4))
    Q     = THETA(5)*EXP(ETA(5))
    V3    = THETA(6)*EXP(ETA(6))

    SC = V2


      K12 = Q/V2
      K21 = Q/V3
      K10 = CL/V2

      C1 = K12 + K21 + K10
      C2 = K21*K10

      Lambda = 0.5*(C1 - SQRT(C1*C1 - 4*C2))

      HALF=LOG(2)/Lambda

$THETA
     (0        0.3    ) ;   ALAG
     (0        10     ) ;   KA
     (0        1      ) ;   CL
     (0        4      ) ;   VC
     (0        0.2    ) ;   CLD
     (0        5      ) ;   VP
```

FIGURE A-4B   Sample output from NONMEM showing oral data fitted to (ADVAN 4, TRANS4), a two-compartment model with first-order absorption and first-order elimination.

```
$OMEGA 0.05         ;  ALAG
       0.05         ;  KA
       0.05         ;  CL
       0.05         ;  VC
       0.05         ;  CLD
       0.05         ;  VP


$ERROR
     IPRED = F
     IF(F.GT.0)THEN
       W = F
     ELSE
       W = 1
     END IF
     IRES = DV - IPRED
     IWRES = IRES/W


     Y = F + F*EPS(1) + EPS(2)


$SIGMA 0.05 0.05

$ESTIMATION METHOD=1 NOABORT SIGDIGITS=3 MAXEVAL=9999 PRINT=0 POSTHOC

NM-TRAN MESSAGES

 WARNINGS AND ERRORS (IF ANY) FOR PROBLEM      1

 (WARNING  2) NM-TRAN INFERS THAT THE DATA ARE POPULATION.
 CREATING MUMODEL ROUTINE...


 PROBLEM NO.:           1
 Run1; Book Chapter 2CPT Oral plasma
0DATA CHECKOUT RUN:              NO
 DATA SET LOCATED ON UNIT NO.:    2
 THIS UNIT TO BE REWOUND:        NO
 NO. OF DATA RECS IN DATA SET:      378
 NO. OF DATA ITEMS IN DATA SET:   7
 ID DATA ITEM IS DATA ITEM NO.:   1
 DEP VARIABLE IS DATA ITEM NO.:   5
 MDV DATA ITEM IS DATA ITEM NO.:  7
0INDICES PASSED TO SUBROUTINE PRED:
   6    2    4    3    0    0    0    0    0    0
0LABELS FOR DATA ITEMS:
 ID TIME RATE DOSE DV EVID MDV
0FORMAT FOR DATA:
 (7E7.0)

 TOT. NO. OF OBS RECS:        340
 TOT. NO. OF INDIVIDUALS:       18
0LENGTH OF THETA:   6
0DEFAULT THETA BOUNDARY TEST OMITTED:    NO
0OMEGA HAS SIMPLE DIAGONAL FORM WITH DIMENSION:    6
0DEFAULT OMEGA BOUNDARY TEST OMITTED:    NO
0SIGMA HAS SIMPLE DIAGONAL FORM WITH DIMENSION:    2
```

FIGURE A-4B (*Continued*)

```
0DEFAULT SIGMA BOUNDARY TEST OMITTED:     NO
0INITIAL ESTIMATE OF THETA:
  LOWER BOUND      INITIAL EST     UPPER BOUND
  0.0000E+00       0.3000E+00      0.1000E+07
  0.0000E+00       0.1000E+02      0.1000E+07
  0.0000E+00       0.1000E+01      0.1000E+07
  0.0000E+00       0.4000E+01      0.1000E+07
  0.0000E+00       0.2000E+00      0.1000E+07
  0.0000E+00       0.5000E+01      0.1000E+07
0INITIAL ESTIMATE OF OMEGA:
 0.5000E-01
 0.0000E+00    0.5000E-01
 0.0000E+00    0.0000E+00    0.5000E-01
 0.0000E+00    0.0000E+00    0.0000E+00    0.5000E-01
 0.0000E+00    0.0000E+00    0.0000E+00    0.0000E+00    0.5000E-01
 0.0000E+00    0.0000E+00    0.0000E+00    0.0000E+00    0.0000E+00    0.5000E-01
0INITIAL ESTIMATE OF SIGMA:
 0.5000E-01
 0.0000E+00    0.5000E-01
0ESTIMATION STEP OMITTED:            NO
 CONDITIONAL ESTIMATES USED:         YES
 CENTERED ETA:                       NO
 EPS-ETA INTERACTION:                NO
 LAPLACIAN OBJ. FUNC.:               NO
 NO. OF FUNCT. EVALS. ALLOWED:       9999
 NO. OF SIG. FIGURES REQUIRED:       3
 INTERMEDIATE PRINTOUT:              NO
 ESTIMATE OUTPUT TO MSF:             NO
 ABORT WITH PRED EXIT CODE 1:        NO
 IND. OBJ. FUNC. VALUES SORTED:      NO


 THE FOLLOWING LABELS ARE EQUIVALENT
 PRED=NPRED
 RES=NRES
 WRES=NWRES
1DOUBLE PRECISION PREDPP VERSION 7.2.0


 TWO COMPARTMENT MODEL WITH FIRST-ORDER ABSORPTION (ADVAN4)
0MAXIMUM NO. OF BASIC PK PARAMETERS:    5
0BASIC PK PARAMETERS (AFTER TRANSLATION):
 BASIC PK PARAMETER NO.   1: ELIMINATION RATE (K)
 BASIC PK PARAMETER NO.   2: CENTRAL-TO-PERIPH. RATE (K23)
 BASIC PK PARAMETER NO.   3: PERIPH.-TO-CENTRAL RATE (K32)
 BASIC PK PARAMETER NO.   5: ABSORPTION RATE (KA)
 TRANSLATOR WILL CONVERT PARAMETERS
 CL, V2, Q, V3 TO K, K23, K32 (TRANS4)
0COMPARTMENT ATTRIBUTES
 COMPT. NO.    FUNCTION    INITIAL    ON/OFF      DOSE      DEFAULT    DEFAULT
                           STATUS     ALLOWED     ALLOWED   FOR DOSE   FOR OBS.
      1        DEPOT       OFF        YES         YES       YES        NO
      2        CENTRAL     ON         NO          YES       NO         YES
      3        PERIPH.     ON         NO          YES       NO         NO
      4        OUTPUT      OFF        YES         NO        NO         NO
1
```

FIGURE A-4B   (*Continued*)

```
ADDITIONAL PK PARAMETERS - ASSIGNMENT OF ROWS IN GG
COMPT. NO.                         INDICES
          SCALE        BIOAVAIL.   ZERO-ORDER  ZERO-ORDER  ABSORB
                       FRACTION    RATE        DURATION    LAG
     1       *            *           *           *          6
     2       7            *           *           *          *
     3       *            *           *           *          *
     4       *            -           -           -          -
             - PARAMETER IS NOT ALLOWED FOR THIS MODEL
             * PARAMETER IS NOT SUPPLIED BY PK SUBROUTINE;
               WILL DEFAULT TO ONE IF APPLICABLE
0DATA ITEM INDICES USED BY PRED ARE:
 EVENT ID DATA ITEM IS DATA ITEM NO.:      6
 TIME DATA ITEM IS DATA ITEM NO.:          2
 DOSE AMOUNT DATA ITEM IS DATA ITEM NO.:   4
 DOSE RATE DATA ITEM IS DATA ITEM NO.:     3

0PK SUBROUTINE CALLED WITH EVERY EVENT RECORD.
 PK SUBROUTINE NOT CALLED AT NONEVENT (ADDITIONAL OR LAGGED) DOSE TIMES.
0ERROR SUBROUTINE CALLED WITH EVERY EVENT RECORD.
1


 #TBLN:      1
 #METH: First Order Conditional Estimation


 #TERM:
0MINIMIZATION SUCCESSFUL
 NO. OF FUNCTION EVALUATIONS USED:      462
 NO. OF SIG. DIGITS IN FINAL EST.:  3.2
0PARAMETER ESTIMATE IS NEAR ITS BOUNDARY
 THIS MUST BE ADDRESSED BEFORE THE COVARIANCE STEP CAN BE IMPLEMENTED

 ETABAR IS THE ARITHMETIC MEAN OF THE ETA-ESTIMATES,
 AND THE P-VALUE IS GIVEN FOR THE NULL HYPOTHESIS THAT THE TRUE MEAN IS 0.

 ETABAR:       -1.8435E-06  1.5359E-06 -1.9829E-02  2.6382E-03  1.0060E-06 -6.2575E-07
 SE:            8.2275E-06  6.3126E-06  3.7159E-02  1.8238E-02  7.1168E-06  2.5343E-06

 P VAL.:        8.2271E-01  8.0777E-01  5.9361E-01  8.8498E-01  8.8758E-01  8.0497E-01

 ETAshrink(%):  9.8394E+01  9.8768E+01 -4.3824E-01  7.8343E+00  9.8611E+01  9.9505E+01
 EPSshrink(%):  1.6718E+01  4.8067E+00

 #TERE:
 Elapsed estimation time in seconds:    3.38
1


 ****************************************************************************************
 ****************
  *******************
 *******************
  *******************            FIRST ORDER CONDITIONAL ESTIMATION
 *******************
```

FIGURE A-4B   (*Continued*)

```
 #OBJT:*************                    MINIMUM VALUE OF OBJECTIVE FUNCTION
********************
 ********************
********************
 *********************************************************************************************
***************

 #OBJV:**********************************   1260.882   ****************************
********************
1
 *********************************************************************************************
***************
 ********************
********************
 ********************                   FIRST ORDER CONDITIONAL ESTIMATION
********************
 ********************                   FINAL PARAMETER ESTIMATE
********************
 ********************
********************
 *********************************************************************************************
***************


 THETA - VECTOR OF FIXED EFFECTS PARAMETERS   *********


         TH 1       TH 2       TH 3       TH 4       TH 5       TH 6

         3.00E-01   4.25E+00   1.17E+00   4.06E+00   1.60E-01   4.61E+00

 OMEGA - COV MATRIX FOR RANDOM EFFECTS - ETAS   ********


           ETA1       ETA2       ETA3       ETA4       ETA5       ETA6

 ETA1
 +        5.00E-06

 ETA2
 +        0.00E+00   5.00E-06

 ETA3
 +        0.00E+00   0.00E+00   2.61E-02

 ETA4
 +        0.00E+00   0.00E+00   0.00E+00   7.46E-03

 ETA5
 +        0.00E+00   0.00E+00   0.00E+00   0.00E+00   5.00E-06

 ETA6
 +        0.00E+00   0.00E+00   0.00E+00   0.00E+00   0.00E+00   5.00E-06
```

FIGURE A-4B   (*Continued*)

```
SIGMA - COV MATRIX FOR RANDOM EFFECTS - EPSILONS   ****


            EPS1        EPS2

 EPS1
 +        1.06E-02

 EPS2
 +        0.00E+00   2.50E-01

 1


 OMEGA - CORR MATRIX FOR RANDOM EFFECTS - ETAS   *******


            ETA1        ETA2        ETA3        ETA4        ETA5        ETA6

 ETA1
 +        2.24E-03

 ETA2
 +        0.00E+00   2.24E-03

 ETA3
 +        0.00E+00   0.00E+00   1.62E-01

 ETA4
 +        0.00E+00   0.00E+00   0.00E+00   8.64E-02

 ETA5
 +        0.00E+00   0.00E+00   0.00E+00   0.00E+00   2.24E-03

 ETA6
 +        0.00E+00   0.00E+00   0.00E+00   0.00E+00   0.00E+00   2.24E-03


 SIGMA - CORR MATRIX FOR RANDOM EFFECTS - EPSILONS   ***


            EPS1        EPS2

 EPS1
 +        1.03E-01

 EPS2
 +        0.00E+00   5.00E-01
```

FIGURE A-4B   (*Continued*)

REFERENCES

Amrite AC, Edelhauser HF, Kompella UB: Modeling of corneal and retinal pharmacokinetics after periocular drug administration. *Invest Ophthalmol Vis Sci* **49**(1):320–332, Jan 2008.

Beal S, Sheiner LB, Boeckmann A, Bauer RJ: *NONMEM User's Guides. (1989–2009)*. Ellicott City, MD, Icon Development Solutions, 2009.

Beal SL, Sheiner LB: Estimating population kinetics. *Crit Rev Biomed Eng* **8**(3):195–222, 1982.

Bonate PL: *Pharmacokinetic-Pharmacodynamic Modeling and Simulation*, 2nd ed. New York, USA, Springer, 2011.

Charles BG, Duffull SB: Pharmacokinetic software for the health sciences: choosing the right package for teaching purposes. *ClinPharmacokinet* **40**(6):395–403, 2001.

D'Argenio DZ, Schumitzky A, Wang X: *ADAPT 5 User's Guide: Pharmacokinetic/Pharmacodynamic Systems Analysis Software*. Los Angeles, Biomedical Simulations Resource, 2009.

Fuchs A, Csajka C, Thoma Y, Buclin T, Widmer N: Benchmarking therapeutic drug monitoring software: A review of available computer tools. *Clin Pharmacokinet* **52**(1):9–22, Jan 2013.

Gabrielsson J, Weiner D: Non-compartmental analysis. *Methods Mol Biol* **929**:377–389, 2012.

Gibaldi M, Perrier D: *Pharmacokinetics*. Second edition revised and expanded. New York, Informa Healthcare, 2007.

Heatherington AC, Vicini P, Golde H: A pharmacokinetic/pharmacodynamic comparison of SAAM II and PC/WIN Nonlin Modeling software. *J Pharm Sci* **87**:1255–1263, 1998.

Keyes, Robert W: The Impact of Moore's Law. Solid State Circuits Newsletter, Sep 2006. Retrieved April 21, 2014.

Lindstrom ML, Bates DM: Nonlinear mixed effects models for repeated measures data. *Biometrics* **46**(3):673–687, Sep 1990.

Riegelman S, Collier P: The application of statistical moment theory to the evaluation of in vivo dissolution time and absorption time. *J Pharmacokinet Biopharm* **8**(5):509–534, Oct 1980.

Sheiner LB: Learning versus confirming in clinical drug development. *Clin Pharmacol Ther* **61**(3):275–291, Mar 1997.

Wagner JG: History of pharmacokinetics. *Pharmacol Ther* **12**(3):537–562, 1981.

Yamaoka K, Nakagawa T, Uno T: Statistical moments in pharmacokinetics. *J Pharmacokinet Biopharm* **6**(6):547–558, Dec 1978.

BIBLIOGRAPHY

Bourne DWA: Mathematical modeling of pharmaceutical data. In Swarbrick J, Boylan JC (eds). *Encyclopedia of Pharmaceutical Technology*, Vol 9. New York, Marcel Dekker, 1994.

Cutler DJ. Theory of the mean absorption time, an adjunct to conventional bioavailability studies. *J Pharm Pharmacol* **30**(8):476–478, 1978.

Ette EI, PJ Williams: *Pharmacometrics the Science of Quantitative Pharmacology*, 1st ed. New Jersey, NJ, John Wiley & Sons Inc., 2007.

Gabrielsson J, Weiner D: *Pharmacokinetics and Pharmacodynamic Data Analysis: Concepts and Applications*, 2nd ed. Stockholm, Swedish Pharmaceutical Press, 1998.

Gex-Fabry M, Balant LP: Consideration on data analysis using computer methods and currently available software for personal computers. In Welling PG, Balant LP (eds). *Handbook of Experimental Pharmacology, Vol 110, Pharmacokinetics of Drugs*. Berlin, Springer-Verlag, 1994.

Karol M, Gillespie WR, Veng-Pederson P: *AAPS Short Course: Convolution, Deconvolution and Linear Systems*. Washington, DC, AAPS, 1991.

Maronda R (ed): Clinical applications of pharmacokinetics and control theory: Planning, monitoring, and adjusting dosage regiments of aminoglycosides, lidocaine, digoxitin, and digoxin. In Jelliffe RW (ed). *Selected Topics in Clinical Pharmacology*. New York, Springer-Verlag, 1986, chap 3.

Rowland M, Tozer TN: *Clinical Pharmacokinetics Concepts and Applications*, 3rd ed. Philadelphia, Lippincott Williams & Wilkins, 1995.

Schumitzky A: Nonparametric EM algorithms for estimating prior distributions. *Appl Math Comput* **45**:143–157, 1991.

Tanswell P, Koup J: TopFit: a PC-based pharmacokinetic/pharmacodynamic data data analysis program. *Int J Clin Pharmacol Ther Toxicol* **31**(10): 514–420, 1993.

Appendix B: Glossary[1]

A, B, C	Preexponential constants for three-compartment model equation	ANDA	Abbreviated New Drug Application; *see also* NDA
a, b, c	Exponents for three-compartment model equation	ANOVA	Analysis of variance
α	Probability of making a type 1 error	API	Active pharmaceutical ingredient
β	Probability of making a type 2 error	AR	Absolute risk
α, β, γ	Exponents for three-compartment model equation (equivalent to a, b, c above)	ARI	Absolute risk increase
		AUC	Area under the plasma level–time curve
$\lambda_1, \lambda_2, \lambda_3$	Exponents for three-compartment-type exponential equation (equivalent to a, b, c above; more terms may be added and indexed numerically with λ subscripts for multiexponential models)	$[AUC]_0^\infty$	Area under the plasma level–time curve extrapolated to infinite time
		$[AUC]_0^t$	Area under the plasma level–time curve from $t = 0$ to last measurable plasma drug concentration at time t
		AUMC	Area under the (first) moment–time curve
Delta (Δ)	Delta is sometimes referred to as the "effect size" and is a measure of the degree of difference between tested population samples	BA	Bioavailability
		BCS	Biopharmaceutics Classification System
μ_0	The null hypothesis value for the mean	BDDCS	Drug disposition classification system
		BE	Bioequivalence
μ_a	μ_a is the alternative hypothesis value expected for the mean	BioRAM	Biopharmaceutics Risk Assessment Roadmap
χ^2	Chi-square test	BLA	Biologic license application
A or Ab	Amount of drug in the body of time t; *see also* D_B	BM	Biomarker
		BMI	Body mass index
Ab^∞	Total amount of drug in the body	BRCP	Breast cancer-resistance protein (an ABC transporter)
ABC	ABC transport protein		
ABW	Average body weight	BUN	Blood urea nitrogen
AE	Adverse event	C	Concentration (mass/volume)
ANCOVA	Analyses of covariance	C_a	Drug concentration in arterial plasma

---

[1]The FDA maintains a list of acronyms and abbreviations at www.accessdata.fda.gov/scripts/cder/acronyms/index.cfm.

C_{av}^{∞}	Average steady-state plasma drug concentration	Cl_{int}	Intrinsic clearance
C_c or C_p	Concentration of drug in the central compartment or in plasma	Cl'_{int}	Intrinsic clearance (unbound or free drug)
C_{cr}	Serum creatinine concentration, usually expressed as mg%	Cl_{nr}	Nonrenal clearance
CE	Clinical endpoint	Cl_R	Renal clearance
C_{eff}	Minimum effective drug concentration	Cl_R^u	Renal clearance of uremic patient
C_{GI}	Concentration of drug in gastrointestinal tract	Cl_T	Total body clearance
		COX-1	Cyclo-oxygenase-1
CI	Confidence interval	CQA	Critical quality attribute
C_m	Metabolite plasma concentration	CMC	Chemistry, manufacturing, and control
C_{max}	Maximum concentration of drug	CRF	Case report form
C_{max}^{∞}	Maximum steady-state drug concentration; *see also* C_{ssmax}	CRFA	Cumulative relative fraction absorbed
C_{min}	Minimum concentration of drug	C_v	Drug concentration in venous plasma
C_{max}^{∞}	Minimum steady-state drug concentration; *see also* C_{ssmin}	%CV	Percent coefficient of variation
C_p	Concentration of drug in plasma	CYP	Cytochrome P-450
C_p^0	Concentration of drug in plasma at zero time ($t = 0$) (equivalent to C_0)	D	Amount of drug (mass, eg, mg)
		D_A	Amount of drug absorbed
C_p^{∞}	Steady-state plasma drug concentration (equivalent to C_{ss})	D_B	Amount of drug in body
		D_E	Drug eliminated
C_{p_n}	Last measured plasma drug concentration	D_{GI}	Amount of drug in gastrointestinal tract
		D_L	Loading (initial) dose
C_{ss}	Concentration of drug at steady state	D_m	Maintenance dose
		DNA	Deoxyribonucleic acid
C_{ssav}	Average concentration at steady state	D_N	Normal dose
C_{ssmax}	Maximum concentration at steady state	D_P	Drug in central compartment
		D_t	Amount of drug in tissue
C_{ssmin}	Minimum concentration at steady state	D_u	Amount of drug in urine
		D_0	Dose of drug
C_t	Concentration of drug in tissue	D^0	Amount of drug at zero time ($t = 0$)
cGMP	Current Good Manufacturing Practices	E	Extraction (extraction ratio)
CKD	Chronic kidney disease	E	Pharmacologic effect
CL	Total body clearance; *see also* Cl_T	E	Intercept on y axis of graph relating pharmacologic response to log drug concentration
Cl_{Cr}	Creatinine clearance		
Cl_D	Dialysis clearance	eGFR	Estimate of GFR based on an MDRD equation
Cl_h	Hepatic clearance		

E_{max}	Maximum pharmacologic effect	k_{el}	Excretion rate constant (first order)
E_0	Pharmacologic effect at zero drug concentration	k_{e0}	Transfer rate constant out of the effect compartment
EC_{50}	Drug concentration that produces 50% maximum pharmacologic effect	k_I	Inhibition constant: $= k_{-I}/k_{I+}$
		K_M	Michaelis–Menten constant
ELS	Extended least square	k_m	Metabolism rate constant (first order)
EMA	European Medicines Agency (http://www.ema.europa.eu/ema/)	k_N	Normal elimination rate constant (first order)
ER	Extraction ratio (constant equivalent to E_h)	k_{nr}^N	Nonrenal elimination constant of normal patient
F	Fraction of dose absorbed (bioavailability factor)	k_{nr}^U	Renal elimination constant of uremic patient
f	Fraction of dose remaining in the body	k_u	Uremic elimination rate constant (first order)
f_e	Fraction of drug excreted unchanged in urine	k_{on}	First-order association rate constant
f_u	Unbound fraction of drug	k_{off}	First-order dissociation constant
FDA	US Food and Drug Administration	k_0	Zero-order absorption rate constant
$f(t)$	Function representing drug elimination over time (time is the independent variable)	k_{le}	Transfer rate constant from the central to the effect compartment
$f'(t)$	Derivative of $f(t)$	k_{21}	Transfer rate constant (from the tissue to the central compartment); first-order transfer rate constant from compartment 2 to compartment 1
GFR	Glomerular filtration rate		
GI	Gastrointestinal tract		
GMP	Good Manufacturing Practice	LBW	Lean body weight
H_o	The null hypothesis	m	Slope (also slope of E vs log C)
H_1	The alternative hypothesis	M_u	Amount of metabolite excreted in urine
$[I]$	$[I]$ is the inhibitor concentration in an enzymatic reaction	mAbs	Monoclonal antibodies
IBW	Ideal body weight	MAT	Mean absorption time
ICH	International Conference on Harmonisation (http://ich.org/)	MDR1	p-Glycoprotein, ABCB1
		MDRD	MDRD equation used to estimate GFR
IVIVC	*In vitro–in vivo* correlation	MDT	Mean dissolution time
K	Overall drug elimination rate constant ($k = k_e + k_m$); first-order rate constant, similar to k_{el}	MEC	Minimum effective concentration
		miRNA	MicroRNA
		MLP	Maximum life-span potential
K_a	Association binding constant	MRP	Multidrug resistance-associated proteins
k_a	First-order absorption rate constant		
K_d	Dissociation binding constant	MRT	Mean residence time
k_e	Excretion rate constant (first order)	MRT_c	Mean residence time from the central compartment

MRT_p	Mean residence time from the peripheral compartment	R_{max}	Maximum pharmacologic response
MRT_t	Mean residence time from the tissue compartment (same as MRT_p)	RLD	Reference-listed drug
		RNA	Ribonucleic acid
MTC	Minimum toxic concentration	RNAi	RNA interference
μ_0	Area under the zero moment curve (same as AUC)	RRR/RRI	Relative risk reductions/increases
		SD	Standard deviation
μ_1	Area under the first moment curve (same as AUMC)	SEM	Standard error of the mean
		SM	Starting material
NDA	New Drug Application	siRNA	Small inhibitory RNA
NNH	Numbers-needed-to-harm	SNP	Single-nucleotide polymorphism
NONMEN	Nonlinear mixed-effect model	t	Time (hours or minutes); denotes tissue when used as a subscript
NTI	Narrow therapeutic index; *see also* critical dose drug	TE	Therapeutic equivalent
OTC	Over-the-counter drugs	t_{eff}	Duration of pharmacologic response to drug
OATP	Organic anion transporting polypeptide	t_{inf}	Infusion period
OAT	Organic anion transporter	t_{lag}	Lag time
P	Amount of protein	t_{max}	Time of occurrence for maximum (peak) drug concentration
PAT	Process analytical technology	t_0	Initial or zero time
PA	Pharmaceutical alternative	$t_{1/2}$	Half-life
PE	Pharmaceutical equivalent	T	Time interval between doses
PD	Pharmacodynamics	USP	*United States Pharmacopeia*
PEG	Polyethylene glycol	V	Volume (L or mL)
P-gp	p-Glycoprotein, MDR1, ABCB1	V	Velocity
PGt	Pharmacogenetics	V_{app}	Apparent volume of distribution (binding)
PK	Pharmacokinetics	V_C	Volume of central compartment
PPI	Patient package insert		
Q	Blood flow	V_D	Volume of distribution
QA	Quality assurance	V_e	Volume of the effect compartment
QbD	Quality by design	V_i	V_i and V are the reaction velocity with and without inhibitor, respectively
QC	Quality control		
QTPP	Quality target product profile	V_{max}	Maximum metabolic rate
R	Infusion rate; ratio of C_{max} after n dose to C_{max} after one dose (see Chapter 9) (accumulation ratio); pharmacologic response (see Chapter 19)	V_p	Volume of plasma (central compartment)
		V_t	Volume of tissue compartment
		$(V_D)_{exp}$	Extrapolated volume of distribution
r	Ratio of mole of drug bound to total moles of protein	$(V_D)_{SS}$ or V_{DSS}	Steady-state volume of distribution

Index

Page numbers followed by *f* indicate figures; page numbers followed by *t* indicate tables.